The SAGE Handbook of

Drug and Alcohol Studies

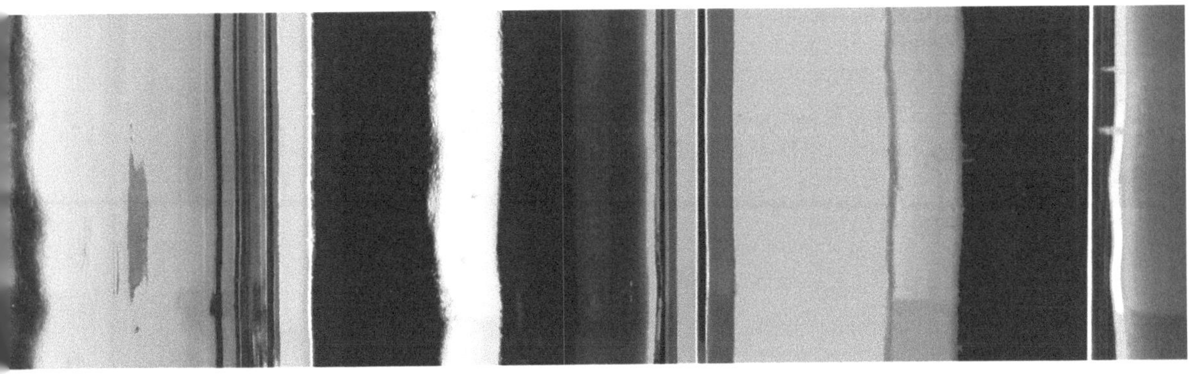

Editorial board

The SAGE Handbook of

Drug and Alcohol Studies

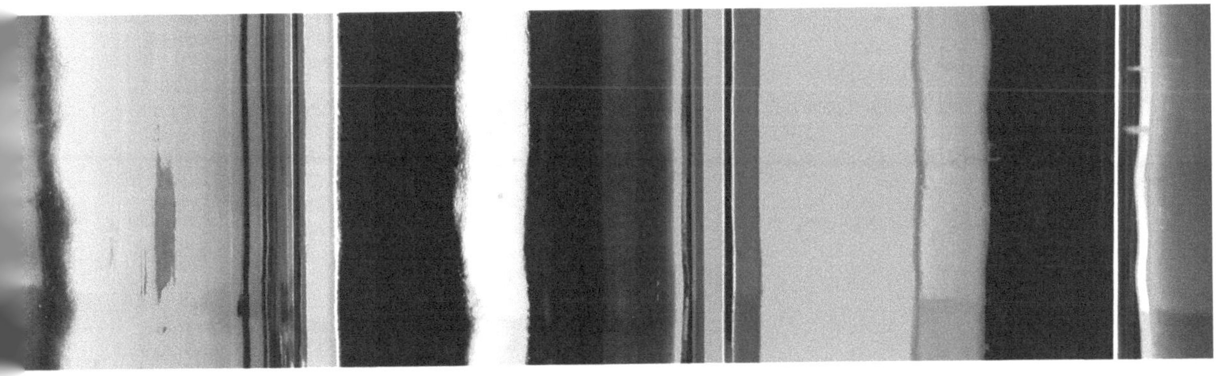

Edited by

Torsten Kolind, Geoffrey Hunt and Betsy Thom

SAGE reference

Los Angeles | London | New Delhi | Singapore | Washington DC | Melbourne

SAGE

Los Angeles | London | New Delhi
Singapore | Washington DC | Melbourne

SAGE Publications Ltd
1 Oliver's Yard
55 City Road
London EC1Y 1SP

SAGE Publications Inc.
2455 Teller Road
Thousand Oaks, California 91320

SAGE Publications India Pvt Ltd
B 1/I 1 Mohan Cooperative Industrial Area
Mathura Road
New Delhi 110 044

SAGE Publications Asia-Pacific Pte Ltd
3 Church Street
#10-04 Samsung Hub
Singapore 049483

Editor: Alex Clabburn
Editorial Assistant: Matthew Oldfield
Production Editor: Sushant Nailwal
Copyeditor: Sunrise Setting Ltd.
Proofreader: Richard Davis
Indexer: Cathryn Pritchard
Marketing manager: Tamara Navaratnam
Cover design: Wendy Scott
Typeset by Cenveo Publisher Services
Printed and bound by CPI Group (UK) Ltd, Croydon, CR0 4YY

At SAGE we take sustainability seriously. Most of our products are printed in the UK using FSC papers and boards. When we print overseas we ensure sustainable papers are used as measured by the PREPS grading system. We undertake an annual audit to monitor our sustainability.

Library of Congress Control Number: 2016933541

British Library Cataloguing in Publication data

A catalogue record for this book is available from the British Library

ISBN 978-1-4462-9866-4

Contents

List of Figures and Tables

FIGURES

TABLES

Notes on the Editors and Contributors

THE EDITORS

Torsten Kolind is Associate Professor at the Centre for Alcohol and Drug Research, Aarhus University. He has a PhD in anthropology and has published widely on drug policy, drug use and drug treatment in prisons. He has taken part in and been principal investigator on several international research projects on drug and alcohol issues including focusses on prisons, youth, ethnicity and drug treatment. He is one of the Editors in Chief of the journal, *Drugs: Education, Prevention and Policy*. He is co-study director of the European Master in Drug and Alcohol Studies.

Betsy Thom is Professor of Health Policy and Head of the Drug and Alcohol Research Centre at Middlesex University, London. She is a social scientist and has focussed her work on alcohol and drug research, with a particular interest in policy and the policy process. She collaborates in a number of European research projects and acted as a consultant on evaluations of the EU Alcohol Strategy. She has published widely on a range of alcohol and drug issues and was Editor-In-Chief of *Drugs: Education, Prevention and Policy* for 20 years.

Geoffrey Hunt is a social and Cultural Anthropologist, who has had over 30 years' experience in planning, conducting and managing research in the field of drugs, alcohol and youth studies. Currently, Dr Hunt is Professor at the Centre for Alcohol and Drugs Research at Aarhus University, Denmark and Senior Research Scientist at the Institute for Scientific Analysis, in San Francisco. Dr Hunt is currently the Principal Investigator (PI) on NIH and NSF funded projects on gender and intoxication and also PI on a Danish Research Council project on the same topic. Dr Hunt has published widely in the field of substance use studies in many of the leading sociology, anthropology and criminology journals in the United States and the UK. His book publications include *Youth Drugs and Nightlife* (Routledge, 2010) and *Drugs and Culture* (Ashgate, 2011).

THE CONTRIBUTORS

Carmen Aceijas graduated in Psychology in 1997, completed her PhD in Psychology with specialty in Health Psychology and Research Methods in 2005 and is a fellow of the Royal Society of Public Health. She started her career in Public Health in the Andalusian School of

Public Health (Spain) until she moved to UK where she worked as full time researcher for Imperial College and the London School of Hygiene and Tropical Medicine until she became a Senior Lecturer and moved to Middlesex University as Senior Lecturer in Applied Public Health and programme leader for the MSc Applied Public Health. She has worked on numerous research studies on different aspects of addiction and has extensively published the findings from those studies in scientific journals. Her previous book, *Assessing Evidence to improve Population Health and Wellbeing* (2011), rapidly became a widely used resource for those at the beginning of their public health career.

Elias Allara, Department of Translational Medicine, Università del Piemonte Orientale, Novara, Italy. Elias Allara is a medical doctor and specialist in public health medicine. He has worked with Professor Fabrizio Faggiano at the Università del Piemonte Orientale, Italy, on several national and international projects regarding prevention of risky behaviours such as substance misuse. Elias Allara is lead author of a large randomized controlled trial aiming to assess the effectiveness of a behaviour prevention intervention tackling four risky behaviours including alcohol misuse. He is co-author of a Cochrane systematic review on the effectiveness of mass-media campaigns for the prevention of illicit drug use and lead author of a related paper.

Tamar Antin is a Research Scientist at the Institute for Scientific Analysis and the Prevention Research Center. She is also the Director of the Center for Critical Public Health. She holds a doctoral degree in public health from the University of California, Berkeley and a Master's degree in applied anthropology from the University of Maryland, College Park. Her research focuses on the lived experience of stigma. In particular, she and her research team are currently investigating to what extent tobacco-related stigma interacts with other stigmatizing social identity statuses to intensify oppression, particularly for Black young adults and sexual and gender minorities.

Rebecca Askew is Lecturer in Criminology at Manchester Metropolitan University, UK. Her academic background spans sociology and criminology, with a broad research interest in illicit substance use. Rebecca is particularly interested in incorporating drug users' experiences and perspectives into policy and research. Her PhD thesis explored how otherwise conforming adults negotiate the criminality and deviance associated with their recreational drug use. Other projects have included novel psychoactive substance use in the UK and evaluations of drug treatment programmes.

Angus Bancroft is a Lecturer in Sociology at the University of Edinburgh. He has written on darknet cryptomarkets, intoxication and society, women's alcohol use and pleasure and the impact of parental drug and alcohol problems on children.

Franca Beccaria, PhD, is a Sociologist, partner in Eclectica, a research institute in Torino (Italy), contract professor for the European Masters on Drug and Alcohol Studies (EMDAS) programme at the Università del Piemonte Orientale in Novara and at the Università di Torino. Her main research interests are drinking cultures, drinking styles, young people and alcohol and drug consumption, health promotion and sociology of health. She has published numerous articles in national and international journals, and has authored, co-authored or edited several books about lifestyle and risky behaviours. The most recent book edited, *Alcohol and Generations. Changes in Style and Changing Styles in Italy and Finland* (Carocci, 2010).

Alcol e giovani. Riflettere prima dell'uso (Alcohol and Youth. Think Before Using) was published in 2013 by Giunti Editore.

Anders Bergmark is Professor at Stockholm University where he has directed the Addiction Research Group for 25 years. His main research areas are substance misuse, interventions against misuse (treatment, prevention), theoretical models regarding misuse aetiology and dynamics, conceptual analysis of key concepts in the addiction field, political doctrines with implications for addiction treatment (alcohol and drug policy, evidence-based practice). During the last 15 years, he has been engaged in both national and international discussions concerning the political and practical problems that have surrounded the attempts to develop an evidence-based practice for substance misuse problems

Bagga Bjerge, PhD, is an Associate Professor at Centre for Alcohol and Drug Research, Business and Social Sciences, Aarhus University. She is trained within anthropology and sociology. She has been involved in a variety of research project, for example, in-depth ethnographic field work amongst methadone users, multi-sited qualitative studies of bureaucratic processes regarding in treatment organizations and case studies of stakeholders in the addiction fields in different European countries.

Jeanett Bjønness is Assistant Professor at Centre for Alcohol and Drug Research, Aarhus University. She holds a PhD degree in anthropology from the Department of Anthropology and Ethnography, Aarhus University. Her research has focused on prostitution, social work, social policy, victimization, agency, gender, drugs, class and the relation between marginalized women and the social system. Presently her research explores non-medical use of prescription drugs in the Danish educational system in relation to wellbeing and risk. Furthermore, she is interested in the methodological and ethical dilemmas inherent in researching politicized and morally loaded fields as prostitution, drug- and medicine use, and more generally, the area of social marginalization.

Caral Brown, PhD, is an early career Research Fellow at Oxford Brookes University. Her background is in Sociology and she has been involved in a range of research projects, all with a focus on addiction and substance use. These include exploring the opinions and experiences of substance users who live in homeless hostels, evaluating a school based drug education programme, exploring the use of online recovery in homeless hostels, and researching social networks and social capital among hostel residents.

Rebecca Brown recently completed her PhD in Gender and Cultural Studies at The University of Sydney. Her thesis, *A Girls' Night Out; Gender, Subjectivity, Pleasure*, explores young British and Australian women's relationship to alcohol. Her broader research interests include women's relationship to femininity, class and post-feminism.

Henry H. Brownstein is the Associate Dean for Research and Professor in the Wilder School of Government and Public Affairs at Virginia Commonwealth University. Previous positions include Senior Vice President and Director of the NORC Division on Substance Abuse, Mental Health and Criminal Justice Studies, Director of the Drugs and Crime Research Division and Executive Director of the Arrestee Drug Abuse Monitoring (ADAM) programme at the National Institute of Justice (NIJ), and Principal Investigator at Narcotic and Drug Research, Inc. (NDRI). For the past 30 years, he has been studying illicit drugs and drug markets, violence and violent crime and qualitative research methods. He earned his PhD in sociology at Temple University in 1977.

Shane Butler is Associate Professor at the School of Social Work and Social Policy, Trinity College Dublin, where his main teaching and research activities are focused on mental health and addictions. Prior to working in TCD, he worked as a mental health social worker with the Eastern Health Board. He is the author of *Alcohol, Drugs and Health Promotion in Modern Ireland* (Institute of Public Administration, 2002) and *Benign Anarchy: Alcoholics Anonymous in Ireland* (Irish Academic Press, 2010). He is a Fellow of Trinity College Dublin.

Glenda Daniels, founder of the Oxford User Team, UK. The Oxford User Team is a service user group that promotes social inclusion, provide opportunities for people who are overcoming drug and alcohol issues and advocate for local drug/service users to gain evidence based, humane drug and alcohol treatment.

Cameron Duff is Vice Chancellor's Senior Research Fellow in the School of Management at RMIT University in Melbourne, Australia. Duff's research investigates complex health and social problems in urban settings, drawing from a range of contemporary social theorists including Gilles Deleuze, Bruno Latour and Michel Foucault. His recent work explores the relationship between health, place and social context with a focus on substance use, mental illness and housing insecurity in youth populations. Duff has developed these interests in empirical studies in Canada and Australia employing qualitative and ethnographic designs. Duff's first book, *Assemblages of Health*, was recently published by Springer.

Karen Duke, PhD, is Associate Professor at Middlesex University, UK. She is a criminologist and policy analyst specialising in research on the development of drugs and alcohol policy and the interfaces with the criminal justice system. She has published articles, chapters and official reports in this area. She is one of the Editors in Chief of the journal, *Drugs: Education, Prevention and Policy* and the author of the book, *Drugs, Prisons and Policy-making* (Palgrave MacMillan). She has over 20 years of experience conducting research and evaluations. She has conducted drugs related research and consultancy for the Home Office, Department of Health, the former Central Drugs Co-ordination Unit (Cabinet Office) and the Royal Society for the Arts. She is currently researching stakeholders in the addiction fields within the EU ALICE RAP research programme (FP7 funded).

Elizabeth Ettorre is an internationally known Feminist Sociologist and has written in the areas of substance misuse, genetics, reproduction and autoethnography. She is Emerita Professor of Sociology, University of Liverpool, Honorary Professor, Aarhuus University, Denmark. Besides publishing in a number of international peer reviewed journals, she has written 10 books and her most recent scholarly work includes *Gendering Addiction: The Politics of Drug Treatment in a Neurochemical World* (with Nancy Campbell) and *Health, Culture & Society* (forthcoming).

Fabrizio Faggiano is Associate Professor of Public Health and Evidence based medicine at the Università del Piemonte Orientale (Novara, Italy). His main research field is the evaluation of prevention interventions, especially in the field of substance abuse, and in the last few years, he has developed research aimed at ensuring effectiveness to public health interventions. Since 1998, he has been a member of the Board of the Cochrane Drugs and Alcohol Review group and carried out several systematic reviews on prevention and treatment of drug abuse. From 2008, he is the Director of the European Masters in Drugs and Alcohol Studies (EMDAS), carried out with the University of Aarhus (Denmark).

Marica Ferri is currently Head of the Sector: Best Practice, knowledge exchange and economic issues at the European Monitoring Centre for Drugs and Drug Addiction (EMCDDA) and is responsible for the Scientific Program of the European Drugs Summer School. Since 1994, she has been working as a researcher and methodologist in the field of drug addiction and other medical disciplines. She coordinated the Cochrane Drugs and Alcohol group for five years (1999–2004) and following this, she acted as a methodologist in the development of several guidelines at national and regional level. She is author of several systematic reviews and meta-analysis and is interested in implementation strategies.

Vibeke Asmussen Frank, PhD, Anthropologist, is the director of Centre for Alcohol and Drug Research, Aarhus University, Denmark and Professor in Social Science Alcohol and Drug Research. Her research is mainly based on qualitative research. She has been involved in the management and conduction of a wide range of national and international research projects. Current projects focus on young people, alcohol, gender and intoxication and non-medical use of prescription drugs. She has written extensively within the field of social science alcohol and drug research, including editing several books. Her articles have appeared in scholarly books and journals, for example, *Addiction*, *Social Science and Medicine* and *International Journal of Drug Policy*.

Mark Hailwood is an Associate Research Fellow at the University of Exeter. His research focuses on the history of the alehouse in England, 1550 to 1700, in particular on government attempts to regulate the institution and on the cultural values associated with drinking by its patrons. These are the subjects of his book *Alehouses and Good Fellowship in Early Modern England*. He has also published on the relationship between alehouses and political culture in early modern England, popular understandings of the effects of alcohol in the seventeenth century, and the relationship between drinking and both occupational and class based identities. He is also a co-convenor of an interdisciplinary alcohol research network: the Drinking Studies Network.

Jennifer Harris, BA Hons, MSc, PsychD, is a Clinical Psychologist in addictions in South London and Maudsley NHS Foundation Trust. She is also a fully trained EMDR therapist with a particular interest in trauma and as well as Yoga Therapy and Mindfulness. Before training as a psychologist she completed her MSc in Health Psychology and worked at the National Addiction Centre on studies investigating alcohol outcomes, the acceptability of Twelve Step meetings and attitudes towards cigarette smoking among drug and alcohol users. She is co-editor of *Principles and Practice of Groupwork in Addictions* (2011) London: Routledge.

Clare Herrick is a Reader in Human Geography in the Department of Geography, King's College London. Her research follows two strands: (i) the intersections between risk behaviours such as eating, drinking and exercise and urban governance in cities and its relationship to (ii) critical global health studies. She has conducted extensive fieldwork in a number of cities – Austin, Texas, London, Addis Ababa, Cape Town and Gaborone – in research funded by the British Academy, ESRC-DFID and the Wellcome Trust. She is the author of the 2011 monograph *Governing Consumption: Sensible Citizens, behaviour and the City* (Policy Press).

Morten Hesse is Associate Professor at the Centre for Alcohol and Drug Research, School of Business and Social Sciences, Aarhus University. His research focuses on substance use disorder, psychopathology and treatment services. He has published extensively on the treatment of patients with substance use disorders, comorbid personality disorders, schizophrenia, mood and anxiety disorders. In addition, he has published a number of papers on attention-deficit/ hyperactivity disorder, biomarkers of alcohol problems, as well as a number of systematic reviews on treatment for patients with substance use disorders. He is the section editor for *Substance-related disorders, addiction and impulse control* in *BMC Psychiatry* and is on the editorial board of *Addictive Behaviors*.

Robert Hill, PhD, PsychD, is a Consultant Clinical Psychologist in addictions at the South London and Maudsley NHS Foundation Trust. He has a particular interest in philosophy and holds an MA in Modern European Philosophy. He has previously worked as a Senior Lecturer and Research Fellow. His most recent publications are Hill, R.G and Harris, J. (2011) (eds) *Principles and Practice of Groupwork in Addictions*. London: Routledge and Mitcheson, L., Maslin,J., Meynon, T., Morrisson, T., Hill, R. and Wanigaratne, S. (2010). *Applied Cognitive and Behavioural Approaches to the Treatment of Addiction: A practical treatment guide*. London: Wiley-Blackwell.

Sarah Holloway is Professor of Human Geography at Loughborough University, UK. She is a social and cultural geographer, with twin interests in 'Geographies of Children, Youth and Families' and 'Geographies of Social Difference', key themes that have shaped her engagement with alcohol research. She is an Academician of the Social Sciences, a previous Philip Leverhulme Prize winner and a British Academy Mid-Career Fellow and a recipient of funding from RCUK, major charities and government sources.

Esben Houborg, PhD, is an Associate Professor at Centre for Alcohol and Drug Research, Business and Social Sciences, Aarhus University. He is trained in public administration and sociology. His main areas of research are drug policy in a historical and contemporary perspective, criminological research particularly concerning law enforcement, the relationship between science and politics in policy making and policy implementation and urban sociology in relation to drugs.

Lena Hübner is Senior Lecturer at Stockholm University and has been a member of the Addiction Research Group since the beginning of the 2000s. Her main areas are substance misuse, especially interventions against misuse within the Swedish compulsory care system, and public opinion on alcohol and drugs and the Swedish policies concerning alcohol and drugs. Recently, her research interests have been directed towards the Swedish social services' agencies handling of substance misusers, in light of recurrent demands to develop evidence-based practice.

Caitlin Hughes, PhD, is a Criminologist and Senior Research Fellow at the National Drug and Alcohol Research Centre. She works as part of the multi-disciplinary Drug Policy Modelling Program (DPMP) which seeks to improve Australian drug policy by identifying what works, translating research evidence and engaging directly with policy makers. Dr Hughes' prime focus is improving understanding of the effects of different legislative regimes and law enforcement approaches and the role of law enforcement relative to other aspects of drug policy. Dr Hughes' research is undertaken in collaboration with Australian policy makers, including Health and Police Departments.

Phillip Hull worked as a Research Officer with DPMP (2013 to 2104) on the Review of Drug and Alcohol Prevention and Treatment Services. He has 14 years of experience in the alcohol and drug and tobacco control sectors as a counsellor, project officer, trainer and manager. He is a former clinical manager of NSW Alcohol and Drug Information Service (ADIS) and NSW Quitline.

Mark Jayne is Professor of Human Geography at the Cardiff University, UK. He is a social and cultural geographer whose research interests include consumption, the urban order, city cultures and cultural economy. Mark has published around 75 journal articles, book chapters and official reports and has undertaken empirical research in the UK, Ireland, Slovakia, the Netherlands, New Zealand, Australia, USA and China. Mark is author of *Cities and Consumption* (Routledge, 2005), co-author of *Alcohol, Drinking, Drunkenness: (Dis)Orderly Spaces* (Ashgate, 2011) and *Childhood, Family, Alcohol* (Ashgate, 2016). Mark is also co-editor of *City of Quarters: Urban Villages in the Contemporary City* (Ashgate, 2004), *Small Cities: Urban Experience Beyond the Metropolis* (Routledge, 2006), *Urban Theory Beyond the West: A World of Cities* (Routledge, 2012) and *Urban Theory: New Critical Perspectives* (Routledge, 2016).

Helen Keane is an Associate Professor in the School of Sociology at the Australian National University in Canberra, Australia. Her research focuses on drug and alcohol use, including pharmaceutical, recreational and illicit drugs (and the relationships between these categories and forms of use). She has a particular interest in concepts of addiction. She is the co-author of *Habits: Remaking Addiction* (Palgrave Macmillan, 2014) with Suzanne Fraser and David Moore. This book examines addiction in an era of neuroscience and expanding pathologies of compulsive consumption and builds on her 2002 work *What's Wrong with Addiction?* (New York University Press, 2002).

Harald Klingemann, who lives in Warsaw, studied at Cologne University (Germany), where he received the degree of Doctor of Economics and Social Science. He has taught at the University of Bonn, where he was a Senior Researcher in criminology, and has been Research Director at the Swiss Institute for the Prevention of Alcohol and Drug Problems and the Swiss consortium for alcohol treatment research. At present, he is a research professor at Bern University of the Arts in communication design. His main research interests include the Sociology of Time, the cross cultural analysis of treatment systems and the natural history of addiction careers, for which he received an honorary doctorate from Stockholm University in 2003. Together with G. Hunt and J.-P. Takala he coordinated, from 1990 to 1998, the International Studies in the Development of Alcohol and Drug Treatment Systems (ISDATS and ISDRUTS).

Karen Joe Laidler is a Professor of Sociology and Director of the Centre for Criminology at the University of Hong Kong. Her current research focuses on drugs, sex work, youth gangs and women's imprisonment. As a native San Franciscan, she has been involved in criminological research since the 1980s, working with several non-profit organizations and government agencies in Northern California. She moved to Hong Kong in the 1990s and has witnessed the development of the city's drug market over the past two decades. Her recent projects include a study on social supply and drug use, and parallel trading between Hong Kong and mainland China and its implications for identity politics.

Philip Lalander has written books and scientific articles about phenomenon such as youth culture, ethnicity, alcohol, heroin, gambling, criminality and exercise of power and processes of stigmatization in relation to people who are seen as strange and inferior in society. Through ethnographic studies, including participant observation and interviews, he develops an understanding for the life of other people and how they navigate in everyday life. He is the author of *Hooked on Heroin: Drugs and Drifters in a Globalized World* (Oxford/New York: Berg Publishers, 2003) and *Respekt: Gatukultur, ny etnicitet och droger* (*Respect: Street Culture, New Ethnicity and Illicit Drugs*. Stockholm: Liber). The last years he has directed extra focus in understanding the consequences of segregation and social injustice and to study how hidden dimensions of power can be understood, discussed and be made visible. He is the head of research at the Department of Social Work, Malmö University, Malmö, Sweden.

Lisa Maher is a Program Head at the Kirby Institute for Infection and Immunity, Professor in the Faculty of Medicine at UNSW Australia and an Australian National Health and Medical Research Council (NHMRC) Senior Research Fellow. She leads an internationally recognized programme of research focusing on innovative approaches to the prevention of infectious disease in vulnerable populations. Her research is based on effective and sustained engagement with people who use drugs, female sex workers, men who have sex with men, marginalized youth and Indigenous people, in North America, South East Asia, Australia and the Pacific. In 2015, she was awarded the Order of Australia for significant services to medicine in the field of epidemiology.

Paula Mayock is Assistant Professor at the School of Social Work and Social Policy, Trinity College Dublin, where she is Course Director of the Masters in Applied Social Research. Her research focuses primarily on the lives and experiences of marginalized youth, covering areas such as homelessness, drug use and drug problems. Paula is a NIDA (National Institute on Drug Abuse) INVEST Post-Doctoral Fellow (2006 to 2007) and an IRC (Irish Research Council) Research Fellow (2009 to 2010). She is the founder and Co-Director of the Women's Homelessness in Europe Network (WHEN), which aims to foster international collaborative research on gender dimensions of homelessness. Paula is the author of numerous articles, chapters and research reports and is Assistant Editor to the international journal, *Addiction.*

Susanne MacGregor is Honorary Professor of Social Policy at the London School of Hygiene and Tropical Medicine, University of London, attached to the Centre for History in Public Health. She is also Professor Emerita at Middlesex University London, attached to the Drug and Alcohol Research Centre. From 2000 to 2009, she was Programme Coordinator for the UK Department of Health *Drug Misuse Research Initiative*, which involved 24 projects focusing on issues such as treatment, comorbidity, service organization and parental substance use. She edited a book based on some of this work *Responding to Drug Misuse: Research and Policy Priorities in Health and Social Care* (Routledge, 2010). She was an Associate Editor of the *International Journal of Drug Policy* to July 2015 and serves on the international advisory board of *Drugs: Education, Prevention and Policy.* She is a Fellow of the Academy of Social Sciences and a member of an ACMD Working Group on Older Drug Users.

Fiona Measham was appointed Professor of Criminology at Durham University in 2013. Fiona has conducted research for over two decades exploring changing trends in legal and illegal drugs, the night time economy and the socio-cultural context to consumption; new psychoactive substances and broader policy implications. Fiona was appointed to the Advisory Council on the Misuse of Drugs in 2009: currently, she is Chair of the ACMD Polysubstance Use Working Group and Mephedrone review sub-group and sits on the new psychoactive substances standing committee and NPS Watch List sub-group. Fiona was appointed to the Home Office Ministerial Expert Panel on New Psychoactive Substances in 2014 and Public Health England's Drug Treatment Expert Reference Group in 2015.

Richard Midford is Professor of Health in Education, in a joint appointment between Charles Darwin University and the Menzies School of Health Research. Richard also holds an adjunct appointment at the National Drug Research Institute (NDRI). His academic research focuses on social and emotional wellbeing, on how alcohol and other drug harm prevention programmes can be developed in partnership with local communities, prevention of alcohol and other drug harm in workplace settings and in the development of health programmes in schools. He has worked as a consultant to a number of industry groups, government departments and international organizations, including WHO, and he has sat on numerous boards and committees. He has published over 100 journal articles, monographs, books and book chapters on his work. The Drug Education in Victorian Schools (DEVS) intervention research project, of which he was the grant holder, received the 2012 Australian National Drug and Alcohol Award for excellence in prevention and community education.

Jacek Moskalewicz, PhD, works as a Head of the Department of Studies on Alcoholism and Drug Dependence at the Institute of Psychiatry and Neurology in Warsaw, Poland. Sociologist, for over 30 years involved in alcohol and drug research as well as in psychiatric studies, including epidemiology, policy-oriented studies, action research and social history. Member of the World Health Organization experts' advisory panel on drug dependence and alcohol problems. Consultant or technical adviser to international organizations including WHO, EMCDDA and UNODC. Deputy-chairman of the Science Group of the Alcohol and Health Forum at the European Commission (2008-2015). Recipient of Jellinek Memorial Award (2001) and Chevalier Cross of Polonia Restituta (2004). Editor-in-Chief of a quarterly journal *Alkoholizm i Narkomania/Alcoholism and Drug Addiction*, member of advisory boards of *Addiction, European Addiction Research, Journal of Substance Use, Drugs: Education, Prevention and Policy*.

Anna Nelson began her career in the alcohol and other drug sector in New Zealand in 1996 when she worked as a dual diagnosis social worker with the Salvation Army Bridge Programme. In 2000, she graduated as a Master of Social Work with Honours from Massey University in New Zealand having completed a thesis on effective interventions with substance using adolescents in Aotearoa New Zealand. Since this time, she has worked in a variety of addiction settings including in outpatient and residential settings and in prisons, as well as in education throughout New Zealand and in London. She is currently the Programme Manager at Matua Raḵi New Zealand's National Addiction Workforce Development Centre, supporting workforce development initiatives that build capability and capacity for the specialist addiction sector and other health and social care organizations. Her other publications include the book *Social Work with Substance Users* (2012).

Russell Newcombe has been a Researcher, Lecturer, Trainer and Consultant on drug use and drug services for 32 years. In 2010, he received the National Rolleston Award from Harm Reduction International for outstanding contributions to reducing drug-related harm. Since 2010, Russell has been running 3D Research, based in Liverpool, and specializing in research on new drugs (NPS) and harm reduction. His books include *The Reduction of Drug-Related Harm* (co-editor 1992) and '*Tripology*' (2004).

James Nicholls is Director of research and Policy Development at Alcohol Research UK and Honorary Senior Lecture in the Centre for History in Public Health at the London School of Hygiene and Tropical Medicine.

Anette Søgaard Nielsen, PhD, is Associate Professor at the Unit of Clinical Alcohol Research, Clinical Institute, Faculty of Health, University of Southern Denmark. Professionally, she has concentrated on the implementation of evidence based treatment methods (in particular motivational interviewing) and continuous quality assurance in operating alcohol treatment organizations. Her research interests include the matching hypothesis in treatment planning, patient perceptions and how to prevent premature drop out of treatment. She is currently the director of the RESCueH studies, which is a series of five randomized controlled trials in the field of clinical alcohol research.

Isidore Silas Obot is a Professor in the Department of Psychology, University of Uyo, Nigeria. Prior to this he was Professor of Public Health and Chair, Department of Behavioral Sciences, Morgan State School of Public Health in Baltimore, MD, USA. He also worked as a Scientist in the Department of Mental Health and Substance Abuse, World Health Organization, Geneva and at the Johns Hopkins University Bloomberg School of Public Health. Obot is the author of many papers on drug and alcohol epidemiology and policy, Editor-in-Chief of the *African Journal of Drug and Alcohol Studies* and Director of the non-profit Centre for Research and Information on Substance Abuse (CRISA) devoted to research on drugs in Africa. Obot consults for many organizations on drug-related issues in Africa and serves as a member of several committees and commissions on drugs and health. He received a PhD in psychology from Howard University, Washington, DC and a Master of Public Health (MPH) degree from the Harvard School of Public Health.

J. Bryan Page, PhD, is Professor in the Department of Anthropology at the University of Miami, with secondary appointments in the Department of Psychiatry and Behavioral Sciences and the Department of Sociology. He has engaged in anthropological study of street-based drug use in many different settings during the last four decades. His studies have ranged from examination of long-term marijuana use to poly-drug use among Native Americans (Seminole Tribe) Cuban Americans and African Americans, as well as Spanish heroin users. These studies involved productive collaborations with diverse disciplines, including molecular biology, virology, immunology, ophthalmology, internal medicine, psychology and psychiatry. Each of his studies begins by establishing a perspective on the use of drugs in the natural habitat of the user. From this level of understanding, he builds layers of perspectives and parameters to derive conclusions beyond the reach of a single discipline.

Franco Prina, Sociologist, PhD in Sociology of Law. Full Professor of Sociology of Law and Sociology of Deviance in the Department of Cultures, Politics and Society, Università di Torino. His main research interests are: theories of sociology of deviance, penal and social control policies, juvenile delinquency and functions of juvenile prisons, prostitution and connection with trafficking in human beings, young people and alcohol, legislation and social policies on drugs and alcohol. He has published numerous articles in national and international journals. His books include: *Il bere giovane. Saggi su giovani e alcol* (1997);

Devianza e politiche di controllo (2003); *I cambiamenti nei consumi di bevande alcoliche in Italia* (2006), *Youth and Alcohol: Consumption, Abuse and Policies.* (2010), *Consumo di droghe e sanzioni amministrative* (2011).

Kane Race is Associate Professor of Gender and Cultural Studies at the University of Sydney. His work has explored embodied engagements with medicine across various different contexts and cultures of consumption: HIV/AIDS, sexual practice, drug use (both licit and illicit), and more recently, markets in bottled water. He is the author of *Pleasure Consuming Medicine: The Queer Politics of Drugs* (Duke University Press, 2009) and (with Gay Hawkins and Emily Potter), *Plastic Water: The Social and Material Life of Bottled Water* (MIT Press, 2015). He is currently investigating the emergence of new sexual and drug practices among gay men in the digital context.

Alison Ritter, BA (Hons), MA (Clin Psych), PhD, is the Professor Director of the Drug Policy Modelling Program (DPMP) at the National Drug and Alcohol Research Centre (NDARC) at the University of New South Wales. She is an NHMRC Senior Research Fellow leading a multi-disciplinary programme of research on drug policy. She is the immediate past President of the International Society for the Study of Drug Policy, Vice-President of the Alcohol and Drug Council of Australia and an Editor for a number of journals, including *Drug and Alcohol Review* and the *International Journal of Drug Policy*. Professor Ritter has an extensive research grant track record and has published widely in the field.

Bill Sanders, PhD, is Professor of Criminal Justice at California State University, Los Angeles. He is a sociologist who has conducted qualitative research on high-risk behaviours among at risk youth in London, New York and Los Angeles. Dr Sanders has published about substance use, violence, crime and unsafe sexual behaviours, including HIV/HCV risk among young offenders, gang members, injection drug users and homeless youth. He has also published on drug selling, club drug use, prescription drug misuse, gang intervention and diversion, qualitative research methods and on the intersections of criminal justice and public health. His latest book, *Gangs: An Introduction* (2016), is published by Oxford University Press.

Anthony Shakeshaft is Professor and Deputy Director at the National Drug and Alcohol Research Centre (NDARC), based at the University of NSW (UNSW Australia). He was appointed to the Council of Australia's National Health and Medical Research Council (NHMRC) for the 2012 to 2015 triennium, which is Australia's leading expert body for administering health and medical research grants, developing health advice for consumers, professionals and government and providing guidelines for health care and research ethics. He has held conjoint appointments and visiting research fellow positions at universities in Australia, the UK, Canada, Italy and The Netherlands. His research has been widely published (more than 140 publications) and he is regularly sought to present his work internationally and nationally. His principal research interest is the development and evaluation of interventions that are embedded into the routine delivery of health and other services. He is interested in increasing the capacity of communities and services to conduct high-quality evaluations of their own strategies and in developing more effective models of integrating research into practice. His research has examined the cost-effectiveness of interventions implemented in a range of services (e.g. primary care, community counselling, emergency departments, hospitals, Indigenous Medical Services, non-government organizations), across defined populations (mainstream, Indigenous and disadvantaged communities) and targeting multiple harms (alcohol, illicit drug use, psychological stress, resilience, unnecessary blood transfusions). Most recently, he led the largest whole-of-community cluster randomized controlled trial ever undertaken internationally, the Alcohol Action in Rural Communities (AARC) trial.

Merrill Singer, PhD, a Medical and Cultural Anthropologist, is a professor in the departments of Anthropology and Community Medicine and a Senior Research Scientist at the Center for Health, Intervention and Prevention at the University of Connecticut. Additionally, he is affiliated with the Center for Interdisciplinary Research on AIDS at Yale University. The central issue in his work is the social origins of health inequality. Over his career, his research and writing have addressed HIV/AIDS in highly vulnerable and disadvantaged populations, illicit drug use and drinking behaviour, community and structural violence and the political ecology of health including the impacts of climate change. His current drug-related research focuses on assessment of harm reduction with injection drug users in Kabul, Afghanistan. Dr Singer has published over 265 articles and book chapters and has authored or edited 29 books. He is a recipient of the Rudolph Virchow Professional Prize, the George Foster Memorial Award for Practicing Anthropology, the AIDS and Anthropology Paper Prize, the Prize for Distinguished Achievement in the Critical Study of North America, the Solon T. Kimball Award for Public and Applied Anthropology from the American Anthropological Association and the AIDS and Anthropology Research Group's Distinguished Service Award.

Jessica Storbjörk, Associate Professor and Senior Lecturer at the Centre for Social Research on Alcohol and Drugs (SoRAD), Stockholm University, received her degree of Doctor of Sociology in 2008. She has held research positions at SoRAD and taught at Stockholm University since 2000. She is the coordinator of a Swedish national research network (Alcohol and Drug Research within Social Sciences), arranging annual conferences. Her research has focused on substance users in treatment, often from a client perspective, and includes: barriers and paths to treatment; living situation and social marginalization; treatment experiences and satisfaction; coercion and social control; service user involvement; and treatment outcomes and mortality. Recent interests include cross cultural comparisons of treatment systems, organizational changes and New Public Management in health, welfare and addiction treatment systems.

Heino Stöver is Professor of Social Scientific Addiction Research at the University of Applied Sciences in Frankfurt/ Germany, Faculty of Health and Social Work and director of the 'Institute of Addiction Research of the University of Applied Sciences in Frankfurt am Main'. His main fields of expertise are health promotion for vulnerable and marginalized groups, drug services, prisons and related health issues (especially HIV/AIDS, hepatitis C, drug dependence and gender issues). His has worked as a consultant for the European Commission, United Nations Office on Drugs and Crime (UNODC), WHO, European Monitoring Centre for Drugs and Drug Addiction (EMCDDA), International Committee of the Red Cross (ICRC) and Open Society Institute (OSI) in various contexts. He has published several articles in peer reviewed international journals and books on preventing and treating infectious diseases adequately (HIV/AIDS, hepatitis, STIs and TB), opioid substitution programmes (including the provision of heroin) in the community and in prisons and general health care issues in prisons. He is co-founder of the *International Journal of Prisoner Health.*

Thomas Thurnell-Read is Lecturer in Cultural Sociology at Loughborough University, UK. His work explores identity and, in particular, masculinity in relation to leisure and consumption practices. His research interests include the sociology of the body and the sociological study of alcohol and drinking cultures. He is a Convenor of the British Sociological Association Alcohol Study group and is editor of *Drinking Dilemmas: Space, Culture and Identity*, published by Routledge in 2015.

Birgitte Thylstrup is Associate Professor at the Centre for Alcohol and Drug Research, School of Business and Social Sciences, Aarhus University. Her main research interests are treatment research, the evaluation of treatment services and their development, user perspectives and treatment satisfaction, psychopathology and mental illness, criminal lifestyle and behaviour. Currently, she is engaged in a randomized effect study on outpatient treatment for substance users with comorbid antisocial behaviour. She is on the editorial board for *Substance-related disorders, addiction and impulse control* in *BMC Psychiatry*.

Gill Valentine is Professor of Human Geography and Pro-Vice Chancellor for Social Sciences at the University of Sheffield, UK. Gill has secured over £4m of research funding, published 15 books, nearly 200 journal articles and book chapters, 10 official reports and supervised over 20 PhD students. Gill was Co-founder and co-editor of *Social and Cultural Geography*, as well as Co-editor of *Gender, Place and Culture*.

Łukasz Wieczorek, PhD, is an Assistant Professor at the Institute of Psychiatry and Neurology, Warsaw, Poland. He is interested in alcohol and drug research, especially alcohol policy studies, epidemiology of addiction, stigmatization of alcohol and drug dependents and alcohol and drug treatment systems. Recently engaged in a study on availability of treatment for people with gambling disorder. He is a member of the Polish Society on Addiction Research.

Lisa Williams is Lecturer in Criminology at the Centre for Criminology and Criminal Justice, School of Law, University of Manchester, UK. For over a decade she has undertaken research on both recreational and dependent forms of drug taking. Her recent research has focussed upon recreational drug journeys during the life course, exploring onset, stability, change and desistance. In particular, she is interested in how and why recreational drug use persists into adulthood. Methodologically, her research employs a longitudinal mixed methods approach.

PART I

Central Social Science Theories in Drug and Alcohol Studies

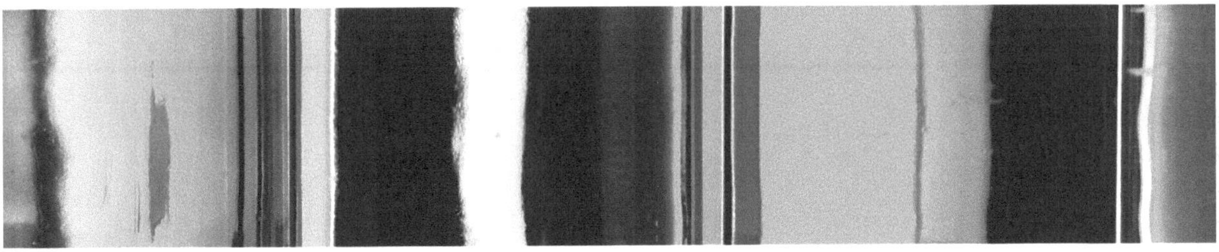

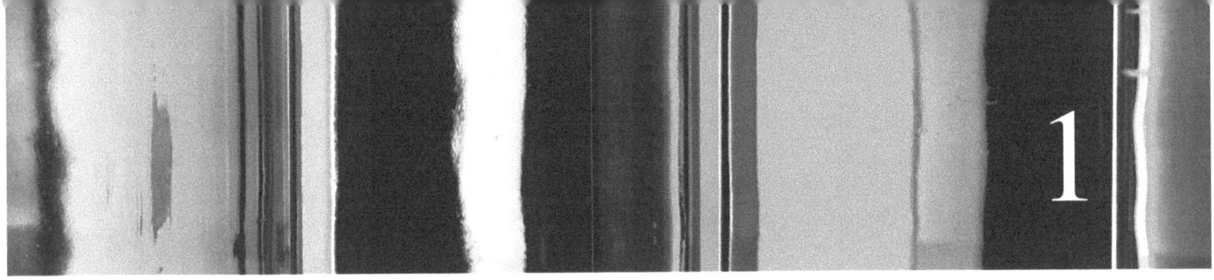

1

Central Social Science Theories in Drug and Alcohol Studies Introduction

Torsten Kolind, Betsy Thom and Geoffrey Hunt

THE GROWING IMPORTANCE OF DRUG AND ALCOHOL RESEARCH FOR POLICY AND INTERVENTION

Our general aim in producing this Handbook has been to map drug and alcohol research disciplines and to illustrate the contribution of different disciplines to the study of substance use. To our knowledge no such map currently exists. This *map* includes historical perspectives, and contemporary theoretical paradigms, it provides a state-of-the-art current debates and controversies, as well as sketching out emerging themes and new developments in the field.

In the last two to three decades, the interest in drug and alcohol issues has increased markedly in many societies. This is due both to an increase in worldwide use of substances and an increased political focus on both illegal and legal drug use. This societal interest is also reflected in academia, in social and health policy developments at national and international levels, and in the growth and diversification of professional services. Research on prevention, treatment, harm reduction, policy and recreational consumption has been conducted from a range of different disciplinary perspectives, e.g. sociology, political science, history, biology, psychology, psychiatry, pharmacology, cultural studies, gender studies, geography, anthropology and economics. Consequently, the field by its very nature is inter-disciplinary and this characteristic is reflected in the Handbook. As a result, the Handbook is divided in two volumes reflecting both a social science and a biological approach. While for many researchers, students and professionals both areas are important, the division into two sections allows a more meaningful way of compiling the contents in order to address the core interests of different groups of readers.

During the last 15 years or so, drug and alcohol studies has become a more established academic field of research involving researchers from different countries across the globe. Currently, drug and alcohol research centres and specialist units exist in a wide range of countries, either as departments in universities or as independent (public or private) research institutions. As a consequence, programmes and courses in drug and alcohol studies are offered at a number of academic levels, including foundation programmes, undergraduate and postgraduate degrees, as well as specific training for professionals in the field and also bespoke courses for students from a range of other academic disciplines. The exponential growth in specialist alcohol and drug peer reviewed journals is a further testament to the growing importance of this area of research. In addition, drug and alcohol research is also being funded by both national and international funding agencies including for example, the Medical Research Council (MRC) and the Economic and Social research Council (ESRC) in the UK, National Institute on Drug Abuse (NIDA) and National Institute on Alcoholism and Alcohol Abuse (NIAAA) in the US, the National Health and Medical Research Council (NHMRC) and the Australian Research Council (ARC) in Australia, and the European Union. Consequently, the title 'Handbook of drug and alcohol studies' has been deliberately chosen as a way of reflecting this growing importance.

It has been our aim, that the Handbook reflects the state-of-the-art analytical and theoretical advances in the drug and alcohol research fields. As stated above, these advances stem from a range of different disciplines and research traditions. However, many issues and even key concepts are still contested, debated and discussed and therefore, the Handbook also covers such discussions and controversies. In this way, while we have not aspired to settle discussions about controversial issues by offering final authoritative arguments and summaries, we do hope that the Handbook will be an inspiration for readers to continue their engagement in reflecting on and debating contemporary and controversial areas of drug and alcohol issues. For instance, there is a growing discussion in the field about the concept of addiction, a concept which has now spread to other areas of research far beyond the confines of substance use. Also, we have witnessed recently an increased interest in issues of pleasure as essential components in drug and alcohol research, a situation rarely seen before. Other examples of the flux within the drug and alcohol research field include a growing interest in the use of new psychoactive substances, non-medical use of prescription medicine, and alcohol use among the elderly. In the Handbook we have found it useful to recognize such developments and to offer critical discussion of concepts and changes in empirical focus. Moreover, the drug and alcohol research field also involves a broad, debated and continuously changing terminology. Terms like use, misuse, substance use disorder or recreational use are used by researchers and policy makers alike to serve different purposes. Such multifaceted, unsettled and debated use of terminology is also reflected in the Handbook chapters in which one will find different definitions and perspectives, reflecting the diversity of the field.

Increasingly, the issue of 'evidence' underlies much of the debates, the fluctuating use of different concepts and terminologies and the proliferation of variable perspectives on drug and alcohol policy and practice. The demand for policy and practice to be 'evidence based' or at least 'evidence informed' has become a core element and even mantra of the research-policy-practice nexus. The chapters in the Handbook invite reflection on the nature of evidence, the types of evidence produced from research studies and the use – or lack of use – of research findings in policy and practice. Chapters draw extensively on a wide range of empirical studies that employ both quantitative and qualitative methods – experimental trials of different sorts, documentary analyses, focus group discussions, interviews and observational approaches, to name a few. But they also provide a critical approach to this evidence, illustrating the often different and conflictual nature of evidence; the ways in which evidence develops and changes over time; the importance of considering the sources of evidence; the different types of evidence available to policy makers and practitioners and the ways in which evidence is produced and used in the alcohol and drugs field. These themes run throughout the chapters and offer the reader a window of opportunity to look more carefully and critically at the findings and insights derived from academic research.

Finally, although we intend the Handbook to provide an overview of a very disparate research field, we also believe that by demonstrating the role of the diverse disciplinary theories and methodological approaches in providing research based 'evidence' and insights, the Handbook also shows how the drug and alcohol research field thrives in its interdisciplinary approach and how it can contribute usefully to policy and practice.

It is our intention that the Handbook can provide academics, postgraduate and undergraduate students and drug and alcohol professionals with a high quality interdisciplinary reference book that covers contemporary key issues and central controversies in the drug and alcohol research fields. Moreover, currently, an increasing number of universities are offering programmes and courses in drug and alcohol studies, schools' curricula cover alcohol and drug issues, and healthcare providers seek to equip those working in a variety of disciplines (such as, accident and emergency, mental health, social work/welfare, forensic services and the judiciary) with the skills to manage drug and alcohol use. Hopefully, the Handbook will be a resource for the growing academic drug and alcohol research community, especially at a time when the issues are gaining prominence in both policy and practice domains.

The Handbook contributors to this volume represent a wide range of expertise in the various disciplines in the social sciences. These authors have, we believe, been able to offer critical and up-to-date articles on contemporary issues and debates within drug and alcohol research. However, even though we have aimed at a geographically dispersed group of authors (Africa, Asia, Australia, Europe and US), we must also recognize that most authors are from the Global North or Anglophone countries. This may reflect our inability to engage a more geographically dispersed group of contributors. More likely, it also reflects the fact that most current written social science drug and alcohol research comes from a relatively small group of (affluent) countries and is published in English language journals. When reading the Handbook therefore, one should recognize and reflect on possible bias in the content and analyses in order to judge the potential global relevance of the different discussions in the chapters. In other words, maybe even the perspectives and assumptions which informed the development, content and approach of the Handbook are biased toward what was seen to be relevant within a Western context at the time this Handbook was assembled. In two chapters of the Handbook (chapter 31 and 32) such issues are addressed. Here the authors reflect on whether a Western discussion and issues of concern in the drug and alcohol field can be exported to non-western countries. We acknowledge that there are other biases and gaps in the Handbook coverage. The enormous range of issues in this field meant that choices had to be made about what to include and exclude. In particular, a decision was made not to focus on research into smoking. At the time when we were planning the Handbook there were few controversial issues or new debates in this field, although subsequently the widespread availability and growth in the use of e-cigarettes has brought renewed vigour into discussions and research around smoking. At the same time, many of the debatable and critical issues covered in the chapters could also be used to reflect on current policy and intervention in smoking behaviours (or other areas of addiction)

OUTLINE OF THE HANDBOOK

This volume includes 39 chapters, divided between three parts. Part I focuses on theoretical and historical issues, whereas Parts II and III have been chosen to reflect key substantive areas in drug and alcohol research, with particular emphasis on emerging issues. Part II is divided into four subsections, which cover the central 'pillars' within the area: *regulation, prevention, treatment* and *consumption*, focusing on the most important research areas as well as on new developments. Part III covers central controversies in policy as well as within drug and alcohol research. Some chapters deal with classic controversies, while others look towards emerging and future debates.

Part I

Part I introduces the field, first, by outlining the interdisciplinary nature of the drug and alcohol research field. Second, it provides an historical view of the production, consumption and distribution of substances in human societies focusing on the last two centuries. Third, it introduces the theoretical resources available for addressing current research areas in drug and alcohol studies. Together Part I provides an overview on how research and social science paradigms have developed in the field of drug and alcohol studies. While specific theoretical "ancestors" do not exist, it is nevertheless the case that the ancestors have been "borrowed" from other disciplines including sociology, psychology, anthropology, history and criminology, and most recently cultural and geographical studies. It should be noted, that while the Handbook does not include a specific theoretical chapter on economics, nevertheless a discussion of economic aspects of the drug and alcohol research are addressed directly in two of the chapters in Part III, focusing respectively on the legal (chapter 38) and illegal (chapter 37) drug and alcohol economy. Also, the Handbook does not have a theoretical perspective from the field of Epidemiology. The reason is that while critical reflections exist in Epidemiology itself, we found it difficult to uncover a similar critical reflection on public health and epidemiology from within the field of drug and alcohol research. Epidemiological thinking and research is however represented in chapter 12 on *National preventive approaches* and in chapter 36 on *Public Health approaches to psychoactive substance use – a critique*. Such 'omissions' however, also reflect the interdisciplinary status of (social science) drug and alcohol research. In fact, we argue that it can be difficult to determine exactly where the field begins and ends, and which disciplines and approaches should be included and which left out. In the Handbook the chapters in Part I represent our view as editors on those disciplines we believe have contributed most significantly to the theoretical development of drug and alcohol research. Part I also lays the basis for the rest of the Handbook by providing the historical and theoretical framework within which the *Pillars* and *Controversies* can be understood.

Part II

This section focuses on what we see as the four central pillars in drug and alcohol research: *regulation, prevention, treatment* and *consumption*. These pillars thematically encompass much of the pertinent social science research on drug and alcohol issues, in spite of the possible overlaps that exist between the categories. In Part II we have deliberately included articles examining the four central pillars from different levels of analyses. These analyses include: i) an examination of the role of global alcohol and drug policy in regulating policy internationally and nationally – raising questions of the extent to which international policy does in fact impact on national policy and action;

ii) an exploration of national policy and its links with strategic action at community level, which illustrate the potential and the constraints arising from growing trends towards devolved policy making and local governance of alcohol and drug service provision; iii) a consideration of changing perspectives regarding what is considered appropriate policy and practice responses – reflected in the chapter on harm reduction and recovery; iv) a discussion of organizational and practice based aspects of treatment, including issues around workforce development, a neglected area of research which, nevertheless, has become increasingly relevant as the drug and alcohol field in many countries experiences rapid structural, ideological and political change; and, finally, v) an interest in identities, context and discourses related to consumption. The different theoretical perspectives, which are presented in Part I are illustrated here as they link with the four pillars.

Part III

The final section has a focus on key debates and controversies that have existed in the drug and alcohol research fields, both historically and in the contemporary period. The controversies included here are not necessarily comprehensive as the field is fast moving, with new issues constantly emerging as knowledge, novel substances or political and policy contexts change and demand fresh thinking and new research. Some chapters present classic controversies, for instance, on the definition and understanding of 'addiction', on the (de)criminalization of drug use, and on the links between individual characteristics such as gender, ethnicity and socio-economic status, substance use and the effects of use. These issues have been the focus of research and debate for the past two centuries and continue to spark lively exchanges and a stream of publications. Other chapters reflect controversies which have arisen in the past, died away and been re-awakened. For instance, the more recent shift to a broader population based view of consumption and harm from legal substances and the implications for policy and practice, is addressed in chapter 36 on public health approaches to substance use. Although, in some national contexts, there have been earlier population-wide measures aimed at regulating substance use, notably alcohol, we are again witnessing a rise in debates around the merits of adopting interventions, which target individuals compared to interventions aiming to influence the behaviour of populations as a whole. The role played by different stakeholders and interest groups in the alcohol and drugs field runs through the chapters with chapters 37 and 38 taking up current controversies on legal and illegal economies and drawing attention to the part played by major economic players as well as by less visible players in influencing the direction of policy. Emerging and possible future debates also find a place in this section in chapters which, for example, consider drug and alcohol consumption and responses to problematic use among prisoners, sex workers and among homeless populations, and development of interest in the ontological contingency of drugs and the discussion of possible policy implication hereof. Discussions merge and complement each other across chapters and may prove difficult to disentangle. However, while each chapter stands on its own, together the chapters provide a critical portrayal of the extent to which the drug and alcohol research fields are lively, politically value-laden, and highly contested.

CREATING THE HANDBOOK

We started work on this Handbook in 2011, submitting a proposal for the structure and chapter outline to Sage. Based on the valuable comments received from a comprehensive review panel and from our editorial board members, we revised our outline; adding new chapters, modifying some and merging others. We then began the process of identifying potential authors and experts in order to represent the complexity and diversity of the field. We wanted to include authors from different parts of the globe, from different social science backgrounds, and at different stages of their careers. Completion of this task was lengthy and elaborate and we faced many challenges in recruiting the writers we wanted. As is increasingly the case, many of our colleagues felt that they were currently over-worked and when asked to contribute to the Handbook some declined because they did not wish to take on yet another commitment. Nevertheless, we were fortunate in achieving most of the objectives we had set ourselves and in gaining collaboration from an excellent range of experts in the field. Having chosen the authors, we encouraged them to amend, augment or, indeed, change, our initial summary outline of the chapter that we wished them to write, and add their own interpretations, views and ideas about the topic. Consequently, each of the chapters can be seen as a highly individual and original expert contribution. All chapter submissions were then anonymously reviewed by at least one external reviewer and by two people from the Editorial Board. Revised chapters were then re-reviewed and further revised until we considered them to be of a publishable standard. In sum, the Handbook can be seen as a collaborative project characterised by lively debates and discussions between us as editors, the individual authors, the editorial board, reviewers, and the publisher. Hopefully readers of the Handbook will also add their own layer of interpretation to the perspectives, insights and conclusions offered in the chapters, ensuring that the drug and alcohol research fields will continue to be debated, developed and never completely finalised.

2

Historical Perspectives

Mark Hailwood

INTRODUCTION

There is now a considerable literature on the history of alcohol and drugs. The past two decades have seen an ever-increasing interest in these subjects on the part of historians, in large part due to insights from other fields in the social sciences being adopted by historians and applied to their own field. Historians were once happy to cursorily conclude that levels of alcohol and drug consumption in the past were straightforward responses to economic hardship and social dislocation. They have now learned from an engagement with anthropology and sociology that the rituals, symbols and debates that surrounded the use of alcohol and drugs in past societies can offer a guide to the underlying social, cultural and political structures of those societies, and not just to their breakdown. The consumption of what historians have come to refer to as 'intoxicants' or 'psychoactive substances' is now seen as central to forms of social exchange and cultural expression across the social scale. As Thomas Brennan put it, in calling for a cultural history of alcohol in France, historians now believe 'we can learn a great deal about society through the prism of a wine glass' (Brennan, 1989: 85).

This chapter will provide an introduction to this body of historical work on alcohol and drugs. The first part of the chapter will offer a literature review. It will sketch out the changing approaches, priorities and definitions that historians have adopted when researching alcohol and drug issues, and outline the broad range of topics relating to alcohol and drug consumption that historians now deal with, highlighting important works in these areas and possible future directions in the field. The second part of the chapter will be more historical in focus. It will provide a broad overview of the history of alcohol and drugs, and then discuss three case studies of key moments in that history:

- The first nationwide attempt to regulate alcohol consumption: the campaign against alehouses in seventeenth-century England.

- The first major 'epidemic' of intoxicant use: the eighteenth-century 'gin craze'.
- The trade wars and domestic tensions associated with the mass consumption of opium in nineteenth-century England and China.

In addition to providing historical background on a range of contemporary alcohol and drug issues, these case studies will demonstrate a number of ways in which the findings of historians working in the field of alcohol and drug research might usefully inform the approaches taken in other social sciences and even in the biological sciences and in policy debates.

The perspective offered here is that of a historian whose own specialism lies in the social and cultural history of England in the early modern period, c.1500 to 1700, and more with the history of alcohol than of drugs, and that undoubtedly shapes the contours of what follows. There is some justification for such a historian to write a survey of recent developments in the field, as historians of early modern England – and Europe – have been at the forefront of the growth of historical research on alcohol and drugs (Kümin and Tlusty, 2002; Brennan, 2011; Withington, 2011). I have endeavoured to include references to important works on other historical periods and geographical areas where appropriate and to reflect broader trends within the historical profession, although inevitably, many of the examples and works cited are weighted towards my own field of expertise.

HISTORICAL APPROACHES TO ALCOHOL AND DRUGS

The emergence of a cultural history of alcohol and drugs

The major shift that has occurred in the way historians approach alcohol and drugs in recent decades has seen them focus less on them as 'problems' and more on the social and cultural significance of their use and its contexts. This change can be seen especially clearly in work on the history of alcohol. An earlier generation of historians, such as Keith Thomas and Fernand Braudel, sought to explain rising levels of concern about drinking in sixteenth and seventeenth century Europe – expressed in the newly emerging print literature and in legislation – as responses to real rises in alcohol consumption. These were in turn understood as a consequence of growing social tensions and poverty in a period of rapid population growth and socio-economic pressures, as the poor in society took to drink to 'blot out some of the horror in their lives' (Thomas, 1971: 19; Braudel, 1981: 236–7). This 'drink-as-despair' model has since given way, having been challenged by the work of historians such as Thomas Brennan, who explored the drinking of the lower-classes in eighteenth-century Paris, and B. Ann Tlusty, focusing on the tavern culture of the German city of Augsburg in the sixteenth and seventeenth centuries (Brennan, 1988; Tlusty, 2001). Both emphasised that their subjects did not drink primarily in pursuit of narcotic oblivion, but rather to participate in the rituals of sociability that accompanied alcohol consumption. Sharing drinks, buying rounds and drinking toasts were all important gestures that served to express and reinforce important bonds between drinkers and helped to foster collective identities amongst them. Drunken oblivion may have sometimes been the outcome of these drinking bouts, but it was not their principal intention (Tlusty, 2001: 6).

This change of perspective owes much to the influence of other social science disciplines on historians. Brennan, the pioneer of this new approach, was heavily influenced by Natalie Zemon Davis, who pioneered the application of anthropological insights to historical research (Davis, 1975). Historians were particularly receptive to the findings of anthropologists – especially those published in Douglas (1987) – who emphasised that 'while alcohol clearly has a physiological impact on the body, there is extensive cultural variation in drinking rituals and drunken comportment, suggesting that drunken behaviour is learned behaviour, and a form of calculated social interaction rather than merely an alcohol-induced physical condition' (Shepard, 2005: 120). Certain strands of sociological research on intoxication had long been making a related argument: that the way people experienced the effects of drugs and behaved when consuming them were to some extent determined by the meanings associated with them by their consumers – in other words, by culture (Lindesmith, 1938; Becker, 1953, 1967; Weinberg, 1997, 2002; Herring et al., 2013: 11). Such sociological works appear in the footnotes of historians rather less than Mary Douglas does, but they nonetheless fed into a broader shift of thinking across the social sciences that had come to influence the approaches of historians. Coming to understand that people drink not simply to induce a physiological state, and that intoxicated behaviour is not simply biologically determined, historians have started to examine the precise form that drinking rituals took in past societies as a way of uncovering some of the broader social and cultural values that informed drinking behaviour.

Terminology

This emphasis on the consumption of alcohol and drugs as forms of 'ritual' that can be decoded to lay bare the underlying mentality of consumers and their culture has also influenced the way historians now prefer to label the objects of their research. The use of the term 'drugs' has come to be seen as unhelpful. It carries negative connotations in present day debates and it is closely associated with the perspective that their consumption is inherently problematic. Not only are historians trying to get beyond this paradigm, they have also come to argue that the idea that certain drugs are illicit is largely a development of the nineteenth and twentieth centuries and not one widely recognised by many of their historical subjects (Courtwright, 2001; Berridge, 2013a). Instead, historians have tended to prefer the term 'intoxicants', or in David Courtwright's case 'psychoactive substances'. These have the advantage of being more ideologically neutral, but they are also more inclusive: they allow historians to draw comparisons between substances that have come to be labelled as 'drugs' – such as opium, cannabis and cocaine – and other licit psychoactive substances – such as alcohol, tea, coffee and tobacco. Whilst we now tend to divide such substances into neat categories – drugs, medicine, food and alcohol, as well as licit and illicit – these classifications were much more blurred, and flexible, in the past. Substances from across the range of 'intoxicants' or 'psychoactives' often have important historical resemblances as trade commodities, subjects of licensing or taxation, fashionable symbols of social status or subjects of debates over their medicinal or harmful qualities. As such, historians prefer to treat them as a whole, rather than structuring their focus around more restricted and ideological modern categories such as 'drugs' (Schivelbusch, 1992; Courtwright, 2001: 2; Goodman et al., 2007: 1–10; Withington and McShane, 2014: 12–15).

AREAS OF RESEARCH

Regulation

This inclusive approach is also reflected in the wide range of topics in the history of intoxicants that have opened up as active areas of research. Some of these are best described as having received a new lease of life rather than being entirely new concerns. The growth of historical interest in alcohol and drugs has, for instance, reignited interest in the history of attempts to regulate and police them. Subjects such as the temperance movement of the nineteenth century and prohibition in the USA in the 1920s have long interested historians, and in the 1980s, historians of sixteenth-and seventeenth-century England examined the campaign to restrict the proliferation of alehouses in that society as part of a pre-occupation with the concepts of social control and class conflict (Harrison, 1971; Clark, 1978; Cashman, 1981; Wrightson, 1981). More recently, historians have been revisiting the issue of the regulation of alcohol and emphasising a more nuanced interpretation of the range of factors that influence decisions about when and how to restrict consumption. Regulatory impulses are not now generally seen as straightforward responses to real rises in levels of consumption, or as part of a clear-sighted 'top down' strategy to oppress the lower orders, but as more complex processes. Work on early modern England has sought to demonstrate that authorities and elites did not always understand intoxicants simply as a problem: they were often motivated by conflicting concerns about the disorderly behaviour of their social inferiors and the opportunities to benefit or profit from the trade in intoxicants (Warner, 2002; Brown, 2013; Withington, 2013b; Hailwood, 2014). Historians charting developments into the nineteenth and twentieth centuries have shown that ideas about the role of the state; the power of vested and especially economic interests; forms of activism; local and national tensions; varying professional interests; international interests and relations; and changing or enduring cultural values and paradigms have all impacted on the variety of responses to the regulation of alcohol and drugs (Nicholls, 2009; Berridge, 2013a: 5; Yeomans, 2014). There is now a sophisticated literature on how and why our present day regulatory frameworks have developed over time, often in response to historical circumstances that have now changed.

Commerce

The economic history of intoxicants is another subject that has become the focus of renewed interest. An established tradition of work on the brewing industry in particular has now been supplemented by a plethora of works treating a range of psychoactive substances as important commodities in the emergence of global markets (Mathias, 1959; Bennett, 1996; Unger, 2004). This is in part a consequence of the rise of two other especially vibrant fields of historical study: the history of consumerism and global history. Much of this work focuses on the centrality of must-have 'colonial groceries' such as tobacco, coffee and tea in establishing closer trading links – often bolstered by imperialism and slavery – between the New World and the Old (Shammas, 1990; Goodman, 1993; Walvin, 1997; Cowan, 2005; Smith, 2007; De Vries, 2008). Others highlight the fact that long-established Old World intoxicants such as wine also became increasingly integrated into these developing markets, or focus on the later development of global markets in cannabis, opium and coca (Courtwright, 2001; Mills, 2007; Hancock, 2009). As a consequence, 'psychoactive commerce' is now seen as central to the development of the global economy and the trade in intoxicants as very much in 'the vanguard of capitalism' (Courtwright, 2001: 3; Withington, 2014: 23). There is also a literature focused on how states have seized the opportunity to bolster their own revenues through the taxation of the lucrative trade in intoxicants, creating a tension between their role as policemen of consumption on one hand and that of beneficiaries of vibrant markets in alcohol and drugs on the other (Brewer, 1989; Courtwright, 2001; Price, 2007). The importance of such taxation can be seen in the fact that by the second half of the eighteenth century, two-thirds of the revenue of the British state derived from the taxation of intoxicants, and tensions over the attempt to collect tea taxes in Boston played their part in triggering Americans to rebel against British rule (Withington, 2014: 27). The monopolies over psychoactive commerce of powerful corporate interests such as the East India Company, virtually a state in its own right, have also received attention as crucial factors in the origins of global empire (Stern, 2011). Intoxicants are now situated by historians at the centre of various processes of modernisation: the emergence of capitalism, imperialism and globalisation.

Identity formation

This resurgence of interest in the political and economic histories of intoxicants has occurred alongside the substantial growth of research into the social and cultural histories of psychoactive substances. Such histories have often emphasised the centrality of alcohol and drug consumption to the expression of various forms of social identity, especially those centred on class, gender and race. In terms of class, there has been important work revising the way historians have traditionally understood the relationship between alcohol and the working class. Moving away from a 'drink-as-despair' model, studies of lower class drinkers in early modern England and eighteenth-century France have demonstrated that these groups often drank alcohol as an expression of their industriousness – as a form of conspicuous consumption – or with co-workers to express a positive occupational identity (Brennan, 1988; Hailwood, 2011). Alcohol consumption has come to be seen as a vehicle for expressing an affirming sense of lower-class identity, rather than an indicator of desperation and misery on the part of these groups. Another interesting development in the literature on class has challenged the tradition of seeing alcohol consumption in the past as a story of lower class excess and upper class disapproval, arguing that drinking has historically been as much a part of elite culture and identity (O'Callaghan, 2007; Withington, 2011, 2014: 23–4). Civic elites in early modern Germany, Italy and England consumed considerable quantities of beer and wine in city taverns, engaging in rituals of sociability that were crucial to forging bonds among this segment of the ruling classes (Tlusty, 2001; Barzman, 2009; Withington, 2013b). Alcohol consumption has also been seen as playing its part in the literary culture of elites, and Renaissance writers in particular often drew on classical traditions of the symposia to extol the virtues of wine as an adjunct to creativity (Withington, 2014: 25). If the colonial groceries tea and coffee have conventionally been seen by historians as the drugs of the elites, this recent body of work has reminded us that high levels of alcohol consumption were also driven by the upper, and not just the working, classes.

Gender

Gendered patterns of alcohol and drug consumption have also attracted the attention of historians. There has been particular focus on the contexts in which women could be found drinking in past societies and an examination of the attitudes that prevailed towards female drinkers. Much of this work has emphasised a drinking 'double standard', whereby female drinking has tended to be viewed by societies as more problematic than male drinking, and routinely linked with sexual promiscuity (Martin, 2001). Others have cautioned that whilst historical discourses about female drinking have often been overwhelming negative, this did not prevent many women from frequenting alehouses or taverns in practice, and there were many contexts in which they could do so without necessarily compromising their reputation (Capp, 2007; Kümin, 2007: 70–4). Mixed-gender alehouse sociability has emerged as an area that would repay further investigation, and may cast light on mixed gender forms of social interaction more generally (Hailwood, 2014). Masculinity has served as a useful concept for analysing all-male forms of sociability. Rituals of heavy drinking have been reconfigured as deliberate acts of bravado and courage, holding a particular appeal for young men determined to find ways to express their masculine prowess in an era when mainstream ideals of masculinity were generally associated only with middle-aged married men (Roberts, 2004; Shepard, 2005). These bachelor drinking cultures were often markedly misogynistic, placing a high status on boasts of sexual prowess and conquest. They could turn alehouses into dangerous and hostile environments for female patrons and especially those working in the drinks trade, who were regularly victims of sexual assault (Hitchcock, 1999). Behaviours and attitudes associated with alcohol consumption have come to be seen as important avenues of research for those interested in gender roles and relations in past societies. Work in this area has generally emphasised the ambiguities of their operation, rather than simply reinforcing a view of pre-industrial society as harshly patriarchal.

Race and ethnicity

Race and ethnicity have received less attention from historians of drinking in early modern Europe than have class and gender, but there have been important considerations of these issues focused on their operation within the context of Spanish and North America (Lender and Martin, 1982: 21–9; Toner, 2012; Earle, 2014). This work has paralleled the efforts of work on early modern Europe in challenging the notion that alcohol consumption is a symptom of cultural breakdown. The post-conquest drinking of Amerindians, for instance, had often been seen by historians as evidence of cultural trauma induced by the destructive forces of colonialism (Mancall, 1995: 7–8). This view has now been challenged by historians – influenced by anthropological and ethnographic studies of indigenous drinking cultures – who have argued that the patterns of heavy drinking among indigenous people observed by colonials often reflected pre-conquest rituals. These were imbued with religious significance and operated in accordance with a different interpretation of moderation to that held by European colonists, one based more on the context within which drinking took place than the level of intoxication achieved. It has been argued therefore that what looked to colonists like drunken stupor was rather a form of communal drinking that served as an act of cultural affirmation, not a marker of 'cultural devastation' (Taylor, 1979; Earle, 2014: 92). Indigenous drinking cultures, like those of the European lower classes, are being rehabilitated as socially and culturally significant.

Political drinking

Political significance is also being increasingly attributed to historical drinking cultures. Lower class drinking and the development of subversive political views have long been associated in the minds of both ruling elites and historians (Clark, 1978; Hailwood, 2010). Yet there is now a growing recognition that the consumption of intoxicants, and especially the public spaces that facilitate the same, provide fertile contexts for the development of political discourse and debate across the social scale. This link is well-established in the case of England's Restoration coffeehouses, but the taverns of revolutionary France and America have also come to be seen as essential breeding grounds of the powerful political ideas that shaped modern nationhood (Thompson, 1998; Cowan, 2005; Brennan, 2006). Drink has not always been on the side of rebels and revolutionaries. Rituals such as health-drinking or toasting have acted as central components of loyalist political cultures. This was particularly notable among the defeated Royalists who remained committed to the English crown after the Civil Wars of the 1640s, and drinking loyal toasts became a widespread national trend after the Restoration of the crown in 1660 (McShane, 2004, 2010, 2014). Drinking was also entwined with political loyalties in eighteenth-century Stockholm, and the particular type of wine consumed by elites in eighteenth-century England could act as an indicator of party political affiliations (Luddington, 2010; Sennefelt, 2014). Political parties, persuasions and movements have often been fuelled by alcohol and its associated rituals and sociability.

Literary approaches

As social and cultural historians have explored the ways in which a variety of drinking rituals were imbued with significance in past societies they have drawn heavily on literary studies. If sociologists and anthropologists have inspired historians to investigate the meanings invested in alcohol and drug use, it has often been literary scholars that they have turned to for help in recovering these meanings. Close attention to a range of literary texts originating in the society under study has been a favoured methodology for recovering the discourses associated with alcohol in a given time and culture. Historians of early modern England in particular have benefited from a parallel upsurge of interest in drinking culture on the part of their literary studies colleagues. The attitudes and drinking habits of early seventeenth-century metropolitan elites; the ambivalent judgements of religious moralists; the perspectives of Renaissance medical and conduct writers; and the discourses on drink and drunkenness circulating in popular print, have all been scrutinised to enhance our understanding of the ways in which early modern men and women thought about alcohol, its effects and how it should be appropriately consumed (Smyth, 2004; O'Callaghan, 2007; Shrank, 2013; Withington, 2013a; Hailwood, 2014; Richards, 2014). Scholars have also explored the meanings associated with drinking and drugs in early modern theatre, and subjected the visual media of the period to analysis, ranging from the Italian classical and Northern European realist traditions of art, to representations of gin drinkers in William Hogarth's famous prints (White, 2003; Pollard, 2005; Glanville and Lee, 2007; Nichols, 2014). The valuable contribution of literary, dramatic and art history approaches extends beyond the early modern European context. Steven Earnshaw has examined literary representations of the pub from Geoffrey Chaucer to Martin Amis – via Shakespeare, of course – and Deborah Toner's pioneering work has combined literary and historical approaches to explore the symbolic importance of alcohol consumption to Mexican national identity in the nineteenth century (Earnshaw, 2000; Toner, 2012). The pursuit of the historical meanings of alcohol consumption – something not necessarily easily retrieved from historical sources such as legal records – has been heavily dependent on the analysis of literary sources and the techniques of literary scholars.

Epistemological shifts

This concern with the way contemporaries in the past thought about alcohol and drugs has led historians to reflect upon the broader epistemological frameworks within which they did so. There has been considerable emphasis on the way in which classical values and ideas about drinking came, via the Renaissance, to play an important part in structuring the way early modern society related to alcohol consumption. A belief in alcohol as an adjunct to creativity, and an obsession with striking a balance between this positive form of intoxication and staying in control of mental and physical faculties, were two particularly prominent features of early modern drinking culture that had their roots in classical thought (Withington, 2013a; Osborne, 2014; Richards, 2014). Other historians have charted the way in which the development of medical thought over time has influenced attitudes towards drinking and drunkenness. Once again, the classical inheritance was important to ideas in the early modern period, which often saw drinking as compatible with good health (Grieco, 2009), but most historians emphasise that the emergence of the notion of medical 'expertise' and more 'scientific' ways of understanding the world eventually came to configure alcohol and drugs as harmful substances that needed stronger policing. Whilst there is disagreement about the precise chronologies of these changes – for instance, over when the notion of addiction as a disease first emerged – it is clear that medico-scientific epistemologies had by the end of the nineteenth century become more significant in shaping understandings of alcohol and drugs than classical and Christian frameworks of thought (Porter 1985; Berridge, 1990, 2013b; Warner, 1994; Ferentzy, 2001; Nicholls, 2008; Clemis, 2013; Withington, 2014: 29–30).

The list of topics now explored by historians through a focus on alcohol and drugs could be expanded yet further: there has been fascinating work on the material culture of alcohol and drug consumption (Glanville and Lee, 2007; McShane, 2014); on the way the spaces and places of consumption have helped to shape its meanings and associations (Nicholls and Owen, 2000; Brown, 2008); and on historical legal understandings of intoxication and drunkenness (Rabin, 2005; Hailwood, 2013). There is, then, a vibrant, diverse and growing body of work on the histories of alcohol and drugs that uses them as a lens through which to explore a wide range of historical issues and processes.

Future directions

What directions might historical approaches to alcohol and drugs take in future? One trend that is already emerging is that historians are keen to adopt what might be termed integrated or holistic approaches to the history of intoxicants. Whilst historians often tend to specialise in a particular subdiscipline within history – political history, economic history or cultural history, for instance – the study of intoxicants, especially when the focus is narrowed to one particular intoxicant, can provide an opportunity to examine the connections between these facets of history. David Hancock's brilliant study of the Madeira wine trade between 1640 and 1815, for instance, combines a detailed reconstruction of the production and distribution of the wine – classic topics of economic history – with analysis of the social and cultural factors that helped to explain and shape its consumption – the territory of social and cultural history (Hancock, 2009). Others have sought to emphasise that the political and cultural histories of consumption cannot be separated, and that for marginal groups, such as women or subordinate classes, the meanings they invested in drinking or drug-taking often took shape within a context of prohibition or at least severe disapproval that strongly influenced their own drinking culture (Hailwood, 2014). These more holistic approaches are likely to necessitate collaboration between historians trained in different sub-disciplinary traditions, which may also make large-scale collaborative projects the standard model for future research (See, for example: http://www.intoxicantsproject.org/). Historians, who have long tended to operate as individual researchers, may finally be coming to adopt the research-team approach found across many other disciplines in the social and physical sciences.

Another sense in which the field of alcohol and drug history is likely to become further integrated is in relation to its geographical coverage. Much of the literature at present focuses on Western Europe and North America, albeit whilst seeking to emphasise that the histories of alcohol and drugs are in very important ways global, or at least transnational, stories (other works on North America not mentioned above include: Rorabaugh, 1979; Salinger, 2002; Burns, 2004; Meacham, 2009). The most recent collection of essays in the field reflects a growing concern to develop conversations between historians working on the history of intoxicants in a range of different geographical contexts: the Islamic Middle East, South and West Africa and Japan all feature (Withington and McShane, 2014), and a recent book by Gina Hames attempts the first comprehensive global history of alcohol (Hames, 2012). There is also literature available on the history of alcohol in China (Huang, 2000); the significance of the trade and consumption of rum in the Caribbean (Smith, 2005); and a sizeable literature on the history of alcohol in Russia (Segal, 1986; White, 1996; Herlihy, 2002; Phillips, 2002; Transchel, 2006; Schrad, 2014). There is, therefore, considerable scope for an increasingly comparative approach to the history of alcohol and drugs to develop in the future. The field at present is also characterised by a much higher concentration of work on alcohol, tea, coffee and tobacco than on other drugs, and this may be something else that future study will seek to address.

Future research is also likely to maintain and develop the interdisciplinary interactions that have been at the heart of the recent growth of historical studies of alcohol and drugs. Interdisciplinary research networks such as the Drinking Studies Network (go.warwick.ac.uk/wdsn) provide an important context for these exchanges, and recent collaborative publications have even sought to expand the conversation beyond historians, sociologists, literary scholars and anthropologists to also include lawyers and to start a dialogue between the social sciences and the biological sciences (Herring et al., 2013). The study of intoxicants provides an opportunity for a uniquely broad interdisciplinary conversation and it is one that historians are keen to learn from and contribute to. To do the latter effectively, however, historians need to work harder to integrate their work into a coherent overall narrative of the history of alcohol and drugs that is comprehensible to non-historians. The following section turns to this issue.

THE HISTORY OF ALCOHOL AND DRUGS

Historians tend to specialise in their work, whether that be within a particular sub-discipline, or by focusing on a specific country or time period. As a consequence, the vast array of literature on the history of alcohol and drugs outlined above is largely comprised of relatively narrowly focused studies of particular intoxicants in given places and historical periods. Whilst the findings of these studies, taken together, may be of considerable interest to those researching alcohol and drugs outside of the discipline of history, many of these individual studies may appear too narrow in focus to merit the attention of a busy non-specialist. If greater interdisciplinary dialogue in the field of alcohol and drug research is to be encouraged, historians will need to produce more works of synthesis that draw together the findings of specialist studies into a coherent overview.

This type of endeavour is one that historians in general have become more and more reluctant to undertake, as the discipline becomes more specialised, more heavily populated and more epistemologically averse to constructing over-arching and inevitably simplified grand narratives that are often then co-opted for political or ideological purposes. The preference of most historians is to emphasise complexity, ambiguity and the particularities of given events or processes in various geographical or temporal contexts (Withington, 2014: 20). These are important principles, but they do risk making research in the discipline increasingly esoteric. The challenge that many historians are currently wrestling with, therefore, is how to provide more general accounts of historical change that are comprehensible to non-specialists whilst still doing justice to the complexities of historical processes.

There have been important works in the history of alcohol and drugs that have attempted to strike this balance. The most ambitious and stimulating general history has been provided by David Courtwright, who ranges across the last 500 years, from caffeine to heroin, combining detailed case studies with some bold overarching conclusions (Courtwright, 2001). Wolfgang Schivelbusch's *Tastes of Paradise* is another, offering a wide-ranging social history of spices, stimulants and intoxicants from the middle ages to the nineteenth century (Schivelbusch, 1992). Both make interesting introductions to the more general history of alcohol and drugs, though neither has gone unchallenged in their conclusions by more specialist historians of some of the territory they traverse (Withington, 2014: 23) Nonetheless, when taken together with the findings of more focused research, it is possible to identify some broad contours of a general history of alcohol and drugs – albeit a relatively Western-centric one – that can serve as a useful overview for non-specialists.

Historical levels of consumption

We might reasonably look to start by reconstructing how levels of alcohol and drug consumption have changed over time, but this is no easy task. The available historical evidence makes only crude estimates possible, especially as we look further back in time, but there are some patterns we can usefully identify if we narrow the focus to alcohol and England. The earliest work on consumption levels relates to the period after the Black Death of 1348, and suggests that the period 1350 to 1500 saw a significant rise in alcohol consumption as the lower orders began to drink ale instead of water as their everyday staple drink (Galloway, 1998; on late medieval and early modern levels of consumption see also Martin, 2009: Chapter 3). The period from 1500 to 1700 was marked by beer coming to replace ale as the drink of choice (the former was hopped, the latter was not), as well as high levels of wine and tobacco consumption, with the early 1700s witnessing rising levels of spirit drinking, as well as the emergence of tea and coffee drinking. If the period from 1350 to 1750 had witnessed fairly high levels of alcohol consumption, the two centuries from 1750 to 1950 saw a relative decline: tea came to replace beer as the everyday staple and the emergence of opium in this period may also have had an effect. From the 1960s, levels of alcohol consumption have again been rising (Spring and Buss, 1977; Burnett, 1999; Withington and McShane, 2009).

Pre-classical and classical

Establishing changing patterns of consumption with any precision may be difficult, but historians have not been put off from identifying distinct phases and periods in the history of alcohol and drugs. Such a story can begin as far back as 3000 BCE, by which time the production, trade, consumption and regulation of both wine and beer were already central features of the pre-classical civilisations of Egypt and Mesopotamia: societies that had taverns, that taxed alcohol and that used it in recreational and religious rituals as well as for medicinal purposes. Wine, in particular, continued to be central to the culture and economy of Greek and Roman civilisations (800 BCE to 500 AD), most famously perhaps in the form of the symposia (Osborne, 2014), and the expansion of the Roman Empire helped to spread classical drinking culture across Europe (Hames, 2012: Chapters 1 and 2).

Middle Ages

The period from 500 AD to 1000 AD is not as well documented, but there is evidence that ale production was widespread, if small-scale, especially in England and northern Europe. Due to the spread of Christianity throughout western Europe in these years the monasteries, in particular, came to play an important role in alcohol production (Unger, 2004: Chapter 2) From the High Middle

Ages, c.1000 to 1300, population expansion in Europe drove increased demand for wine, and taverns became an increasingly prominent feature of society (Hames, 2012: Chapter 3; Skoda, 2013). The period from 1300 to 1500, and especially the years after the Black Death, saw important developments in the commercialisation of brewing, and alongside a rise in real wages this meant ale and beer consumption enjoyed a notable rise amongst the lower orders (Bennett, 1996; Galloway, 1998; Unger, 2004), whilst wine continued to be an important part of renaissance elite culture (Barzman, 2009; Grieco, 2009). Throughout the Middle Ages, then, alcohol in particular continued to play an important role in European society as an everyday staple, a trade commodity and as a marker of social status.

The early modern period

If traditional alcoholic drinks such as beer and wine had long been established at the centre of European societies, the years from 1500 to 1700 – the early modern period – was notable for the introduction of a number of new intoxicants, as the emergence of Spanish, Portuguese, Dutch and English colonies contributed to a considerable expansion of oceangoing commerce. This brought new commodities on to the market. First tobacco, then coffee and tea, took their place alongside alcoholic drinks, with each following a pattern of first being considered attractive for their putative medicinal qualities, then becoming important and fashionable symbols of elite social status, before in the eighteenth century coming to enjoy mass consumption and widespread popularity in western Europe. They made the transition from exotic and novel imports to everyday and essential items of consumption. The sixteenth, seventeenth and eighteenth centuries had witnessed a 'psychoactive revolution' and the emergence of 'psychoactive commerce' (Courtwright, 2001).

Whilst undoubtedly tied to processes of colonial and overseas expansion, this story is often seen as intimately connected to another major historical development of the early modern period: the supposed occurrence of a 'civilising process' among European elites (Elias, 2000). Put simply, the twin influences of the Renaissance and the Protestant Reformation are thought to have encouraged early modern elites, and indeed, an emerging bourgeoisie, to turn away from the violent, drunken excesses characteristic of medieval society and to instead adopt soberer, controlled and 'civil' forms of behaviour. Thus, the popularity of caffeinated drinks has been explained by historians as a consequence of the desire of early modern elites for a psychoactive that served as a stimulating yet more sober alternative to traditional alcoholic drinks (Schivelbusch, 1992: Chapter 2; Goodman, 2007; Smith, 2007). Of course, such a narrative does not account for the dramatic rise of spirit consumption in the eighteenth century, in which the strongest form of intoxicant then known in Europe also enjoyed unprecedented popularity (Warner, 2002). There has been a tendency to see this as a parting of the ways between elite and popular cultures, as the elites turned to milder caffeine-based stimulants and the working classes began to drink more heavily in response to the pressures of an increasingly commercialised, capitalist, industrial and urban world (Schivelbusch, 1992: Chapter 5). Yet we have seen already that elites did not stop drinking in this period, and that trade in wine, for instance, was an important strand of the market in psychoactives (Hancock, 2009; Luddington, 2010; Withington, 2011). It is also the case that the 'gin craze' in London – which occurred between 1720 and 1750 – predated the serious onset of industrialisation in England, and brandy and gin were both already popular recreational drinks in Germany in the sixteenth and seventeenth centuries (Tlusty, 1998). Whilst the eighteenth century undoubtedly witnessed important developments in the history of intoxicants, the precise causes and explanations for this remain the subject of much debate.

Nineteenth and twentieth centuries

The nineteenth century was also a period of significant new developments. Not the least of which was the fact that opium, coca products and cannabis all came to enjoy much wider global circulation, and their consumption became a more pronounced feature of nineteenth-century European life (Courtwright, 2001: Chapter 2). This did not, at first, create a particular backlash of regulatory efforts, and a laissez-faire climate seems to have operated in relation to the trade and consumption of both alcohol and drugs for much of the century, despite the emergence of temperance movements at this time (Harrison, 1971; Blocker et al., 2003; Berridge, 2013a: 7). By its end, however, there was a growing counterrevolution to what Courtwright has labelled the 'psychoactive revolution' of the early modern period. Its causes were numerous and are debated, but historians have suggested that industrialisation played a role. It both contributed to new technologies that facilitated the production of larger quantities of stronger drugs and heightened the levels of concern that employers had over the impact of such intoxicants on the productivity of their workers (Courtwright, 2001: 173–9). The growth of medical and scientific paradigms also contributed to a greater emphasis on the harmful effects of alcohol and drugs. In the early part of the twentieth century these concerns began to translate into a climate of stricter control and regulation, and the classification of some drugs – especially opium, cannabis and cocaine – as illicit, whilst also seeing a tightening of controls on some licit intoxicants such as alcohol (although some areas, such as the United States, Russia and India, also saw attempts at the prohibition of alcohol: Courtwright, 2001: Chapters 9 and 10; Hames, 2012: Chapters 5 and 6). The modern categories of illicit 'drugs' on one hand, and of licit alcohol, tobacco and caffeine on the other, began to crystallise.

This overview is, of course, one of very broad brush strokes, but it serves to highlight what have emerged as several of the key contours of a general history of alcohol and drugs: a very long history of wine and ale playing a key role in Western societies, stretching from the pre-classical era through the Middle Ages; a period of commercial expansion in the period 1500 to 1800, especially in relation to spirits, caffeine and tobacco; a period of further expansion in the trade and consumption of intoxicants in the nineteenth-century to include opium, cannabis and cocaine; and then a shift around the turn of the twentieth century to greater restriction and prohibition of at least some of these substances. Within this, historians have also tended to see governments and ruling classes as broadly supportive of many of these developments: they were keen to see vibrant markets in intoxicants that bolstered state revenues through the period 1500 to 1900, but then shifted their position to one of greater control and prohibition. All of these conclusions may be challenged by future research, and are certainly nuanced by more focused existing work, but they stand as broadly accepted generalisations. However, to be able to draw out useful conclusions about the histories of alcohol and drugs it is necessary to move beyond the level of the overview and to consider some of the key moments in these histories in greater detail. What follows, then, is a series of case studies of such moments as they relate to England, my area of expertise, and comments on what their study can contribute to broader debates and approaches within the field of alcohol and drug research beyond the discipline of history.

THE CAMPAIGN AGAINST THE ALEHOUSE IN SEVENTEENTH-CENTURY ENGLAND

News headlines about Britain's supposed 'binge-drinking' problem are now rife, but such concerns are not novel to the twenty-first century. In fact, very similar complaints were voiced as long as 400 years ago, when it was thought that young men wasted 'their time in idleness and their money in excessive drinking' (Hailwood, 2014: 7). Concerns about alehouses and drunkenness in England date back even further (McIntosh, 1998), but they reached unprecedented levels in the early seventeenth century, when the sermons of clergymen, printed treatises and even petitions sent to the authorities from local communities, all echoed the sentiment that England had developed a drink problem (Shrank, 2013; Withington, 2013a; Hailwood, 2014). Whether it did or not is a moot point. We do not have reliable figures for this period, but estimates suggest that alcohol consumption may have been lower than in the medieval period, even though the number of alehouses was increasing (Clark, 1983: 39–63; Martin, 2009: 61–79). Again, we can see from history that scares about alcohol or drugs consumption do not necessarily always tie in with actual rising levels. Why was there such concern then? Poverty was rising in this period, causing anxiety and fears about social breakdown and disorder which heightened concern about drinking. The Reformation is also important. England's conversion from Catholicism to Protestantism in the sixteenth century gave impetus to attempts to reform society as a whole and create a more 'godly' nation: drunkenness became a target for those who wanted to bring about a moral reformation of peoples' behaviour (Wrightson, 1981).

This clamour of complaint led to the first nationwide attempt on the part of the government to limit levels of alcohol consumption. There had been legislation passed as far back as the 1300s that had given magistrates the power to shut down unruly or disorderly alehouses in their locale, and from 1552, all alehouses had to obtain a license to sell ale. But it was in the early years of the seventeenth century that the English government went beyond providing the powers to close down the most disreputable drinking dens and embarked on the first nationwide attempt to try and limit how much people were drinking in all alehouses. Drunkenness was made a criminal offence: you were only permitted to drink for an hour in an alehouse unless you were travelling and lodging there overnight and a closing time of 9pm was introduced (Nicholls, 2009; 13–16; Hailwood, 2014: 23–9). These attempts to control alcohol consumption were not particularly effective. They were very difficult to enforce in a period when the state had only a limited bureaucracy and no police force (Hailwood, 2014: Chapter 2). Yet it is worth emphasising that these features of 'modern' states were not a prerequisite for attempts to limit alcohol or drugs consumption. Moreover, the alehouse 'epidemic' was not a response to the pressures of urbanisation or industrialisation: there was as much concern with the institution in rural as urban areas. Alcohol and drug scares are not an exclusive feature of urban modernity.

Another interesting comparison between the regulation of alehouses in early modern England and modern regulatory efforts relates to the use of pricing policy as a means of controlling consumption. It is a major plank of government strategies today and it was also central to policy in the early modern period. Since the 1300s, there had been laws in place about the price of ale and beer, but these actually stipulated a *maximum* price, and were intended to keep the cost of drink low. Why? Ale and beer were not just recreational in this period, they were also a crucial part of peoples' diets. They were a valuable source of nutrients and calories, and for men, women and children they were a daily staple of their diet, although the beer that was drunk regularly was a weaker version of that drunken recreationally (Muldrew, 2011: 65–83). Regulations were in place to keep the price down because it was essential that the poor could afford their daily beer. Therefore, the early modern government had to balance ensuring that people had access to beer as food, whilst trying to stop people drinking recreationally and to excess. Our neat modern categories that separate off food, recreational drugs and medicine are just that, modern categories: in the early modern period – and indeed in some contemporary cultures – such categories were blurred.

THE GIN CRAZE, 1720 TO 1750

Whilst the campaign against the alehouse may have been the first concerted nation-wide attempt to regulate alcohol and drug consumption, the first major 'craze' or 'epidemic' of consumption is generally regarded to be the explosion of gin consumption in eighteenth-century London. As such, the craze has been the subject of a number of studies within the field of alcohol and drugs research (Clark, 1988; Dillon, 2002; Warner, 2002; White, 2003; Nicholls, 2009: Chapter 3). The years from 1720 to 1750 saw an even greater level of social comment and concern about alcohol consumption than in the early years of the seventeenth century, directed against the distilled spirit gin. Gin, and other spirits, especially brandy, had been consumed long before this time, but prior to the 1700s they were generally consumed for their perceived medicinal qualities, not as a recreational drink. Again, we can see the blurred boundaries between our modern categories, here between alcohol and medicine. This changed in the eighteenth century, partly due to tax policies introduced by the new King, William III, in the 1690s, to encourage a domestic gin production industry in England to compete with the lucrative brandy market operated by the nation's great geo-political rival at that time, France (Warner, 2002: Chapter 1). It is a reminder that government interventions in the alcohol and drugs markets are not always attempts to restrict consumption. In this instance, they made gin cheap to produce and buy.

Combined with an easing of the socio-economic pressures of the century 1550 to 1650, which led to improved rates of real wages and an increase in disposable income, levels of consumption subsequently and dramatically rose, as much as eightfold between 1700 and the peak of the craze in the 1740s (Spring and Buss, 1977; Nicholls, 2009: 36–7). There was a real change in the levels of consumption here and there were also genuine social consequences. Part of the problem was that gin was a substance of unprecedented potency, ten times stronger than the ale people were used to drinking. Given that ale had traditionally been consumed in sessions of heavy drinking by the working classes this proved particularly dangerous. Indeed, this is often identified as a key feature of major drug scares or epidemics, the emergence of a new more potent substance that is incompatible with old rituals of consumption and this is arguably the first time this had happened in European society. Again, there was a raft of legislation in response to the craze, and although this was initially hit and miss, it does appear to have been more effective than that aimed at alehouses (Nicholls, 2009: Chapter 3).

A key feature of the gin craze that alerts us to another important conclusion of historical research in this field is the way in which 'drug scares' can often be manipulated for political ends, and the way in which 'alcohol or drugs can easily become exaggerated symbols in what are in fact cultural or political skirmishes' (Warner, 2002: 218). There was, for sure, a real rise in gin consumption that had very real consequences that needed to be addressed, but the way ruling elites responded to that situation was deeply politicised and ideological. Take, for instance, William Hogarth's famous print Gin Lane, issued in 1751, depicting the deleterious effects of the spirit's consumption on London society. Jessica Warner sees this as an effective piece of propaganda that, when taken alongside its partner print Beer St – a contrasting celebration of the wholesome effects of beer consumption – sends a clear message: it is gin that causes poverty, rather than the other way round. Take away gin for more wholesome beer and poverty recedes. It is a convenient message for eighteenth-century elites, as it takes away the imperative to deal with poverty. The substance and its feckless users are to blame: responsibility is configured as that of the individual, not of society or social problems. Moreover, the print, like much of the concern over gin consumption in the period, points the finger firmly at women's consumption of gin as the heart of the problem. Marginal political groups are burdened with the responsibility for the crisis, which shifts that away from governing elites. Warner draws parallels here between the discourses surrounding the gin craze and those surrounding the 'crack epidemic' in the US in the 1980s, which sought to demonise users and play down social factors (Warner, 2002: Chapter 9). So, history here can remind us of the need to be sensitive to the manipulation of discourses surrounding the causes and effects of alcohol and drugs consumption, even in cases where there clearly is a dramatic rise in levels of use.

OPIUM: EVERYDAY CONSUMPTION AND TRADE WARS

Opium was the first psychoactive to be widely consumed in England that would today be labelled a 'drug' (Berridge, 1999). Much like spirits, it had a long history of medicinal use that predated its more widespread and more recreational consumption, but by the nineteenth century it had for many become a drug of everyday use. The working classes of Manchester, the cotton-manufacturing heart of the industrial revolution, were notorious for opium-eating – it was at this time taken in pills bought legally from the pharmacist – but so too were the working class inhabitants of East Anglia's rural Fens: again, the rise of the drug was not an exclusively urban phenomenon (Schivelbusch, 1992: 206–15; Berridge, 2013a: 14–29). To some extent, it inherited a mantle that had earlier been associated with alcohol – as an anaesthetic for the downtrodden lower classes. But if its use was at least part medicinal, intended to blunt the aches and pains of working life, it no doubt shaded into the recreational too. It certainly did so in elite culture, and opium played an important role, as wine had done in the seventeenth century, in elite forms of cultural expression. The literary and artistic avant-garde of the first half of the nineteenth century consumed opium excessively. Coleridge, Shelley, Byron and Keats, for instance, all saw it as an adjunct to creativity and it is a role reflected in Thomas De Quincey's famous *Confessions of an Opium Eater*, published in 1821 (Schivelbusch, 1992: 206–15). These features of opium consumption in nineteenth-century England serve as a useful example of why historians are reluctant to draw too clear a distinction between the histories of alcohol and drugs: there are many similarities in the way societies relate to them. Perhaps most strikingly in this case is the fact that opium, now considered an illicit and highly problematic drug, was consumed across the social scale on a routine basis in nineteenth-century England, and enjoyed something similar to the widely accepted place of alcohol in society.

Long before its consumption started to be significant in England, opium had played an important part in England's colonial and economic history. In the eighteenth century, demand for another intoxicant, tea, had taken off in England, and as such the country was importing significant amounts from China. This created a balance of payment problem, as there was little that the Chinese wanted in return except for silver. However, when the British East India Company gained control of India in the 1750s, the English opted to exploit India's opium harvest and illegally import this into China to help cover the costs of their tea purchases. Opium smoking was already established in China, but had been made illegal there in 1729. Demand for illicit opium was still strong though, and the English sought to exploit this. As they flooded China with supply, consumption increased 70-fold between 1767 and 1850 (Schivelbusch, 1992: 218–9). In the 1830s, the Chinese Emperor declared an early 'war on drugs' in an attempt to restrict this illegal market. The British responded by declaring war on China and thousands were killed in clashes that ultimately resulted in Chinese markets being forced open to the opium trade (Schivelbusch, 1992: 215–23; Courtwright, 2001: 31–6). Here, then, we can see another aspect of contemporary drugs and alcohol issues that have a long history: the geo-politics of the drugs trade also has its origins back in the early modern period (see also Hsu, 2014).

The mass consumption of opium in China would, in turn, have an impact on English society. The social problems and concerns caused by its use in China, which had parallels with those of the gin craze, began to feed into attitudes to the drug in the West. The diaspora of Chinese workers that headed to the United States and to London's East End in the nineteenth century also changed the image of the drug: now it was associated with a minority group, contemporaries' fears about its effects grew stronger (Berridge, 2013: Chapter 5). As influential authors, such as Charles Dickens, began to take up this mantle, opium became increasingly associated with the type of seedy East End 'opium dens' portrayed in his final novel, *Edwin Drood* (Berridge, 2013: 78–81). Combined with the development of medical and scientific concerns about addiction, the tide was turning, and in the early part of the twentieth century, some of the first international agreements on drugs were reached to strictly control its use (Berridge, 2013a: Chapter 7). As shifts in cultural discourses, epistemological frameworks, global labour migration and international relations all intertwined, opium was one of the first psychoactives to make the historic transition from toleration to prohibition.

CONCLUSION

This chapter has sought to demonstrate that there is now a considerable and constantly expanding field of research into the histories of alcohol and drugs. This covers a wide range of political, economic, social and cultural history approaches, and in the best cases, looks to integrate them. The field is in important ways an interdisciplinary one, albeit more in the sense that historians have found it fruitful to engage with other disciplinary perspectives on alcohol and drugs rather than having had any major impact on the way other disciplines conduct their research. In part, this is because historians are often reluctant to direct their work at non-specialists and they are certainly uncomfortable engaging explicitly with contemporary policy debates or issues. This is, however, changing, and recent collections of essays in particular have begun to engage in such conversations (Herring et al., 2013). What this chapter has aimed to do is highlight some of the important findings of historical research that may be of value to those researching alcohol and drugs in any discipline. In particular, history encourages us to challenge the categories, and indeed the attitudes, that prevail in discussions of drugs and alcohol in our own society, highlighting the ways in which they are determined by a complex range of factors and historical developments. They are not fixed, or natural, and can change, for better or worse.

REFERENCES

Barzman, KE (2009) '"Wine should taste like wine"': drinking at court in early modern Italy', *Mediaevalia*, 30(1): 137–61.
Becker, H (1953) 'Becoming a marijuana user', *American Journal of Sociology*, 59: 235–42.
Becker, H (1967) 'History, culture, and subjective experience: an exploration of the social bases of drug-induced experiences', *Journal of Health and Social Behaviour*, 8: 162–76.

Bennett, J (1996) *Ale, Beer and Brewsters in England: Women's Work in a Changing World, 1300–1600*. Oxford: Oxford University Press.

Berridge, V (1990) 'Dependence: historical concepts and constructs', In G Edwards and M Lader (eds), *The Nature of Drug Dependence*. Oxford: Oxford University Press, pp. 1–18.

Berridge, V (1999) *Opium and the People: Opiate Use and Drug Control Policy in Nineteenth and Early Twentieth Century England*, revised edn, original 1981. London: Free Association.

Berridge, V (2013a) *Demons: Our Changing Attitudes to Alcohol, Tobacco and Drugs*. Oxford: Oxford University Press.

Berridge, V (2013b) 'Intoxicants: the formation of health expertise in the twentieth century', In J Herring, C Regan, D Weinberg and P Withington (eds), *Intoxicants and Society: Problematic Pleasures of Drugs and Alcohol*. Basingstoke: Palgrave Macmillan, pp. 69–83.

Blocker, J, Fahey, D and Tyrrell, I (eds) (2003) *Alcohol and Temperance in Modern History: An International Encyclopedia*, 2 Vols. Santa Barbara and Oxford: ABC-CLIO.

Braudel, F (1981) *Civilization and Capitalism, 15th–18th Century*. Vol. I, *The Structure of Everyday Life: The Limits of the Possible*. Translated by S Reynolds. London: Collins.

Brennan, T (1988) *Public Drinking and Popular Culture in Eighteenth-Century Paris*. Princeton: Princeton University Press.

Brennan, T (1989) 'Towards the cultural history of alcohol in France', *Journal of Social History*, 23(1): 71–92.

Brennan, T (2006) 'Taverns and the public sphere in the French Revolution', In M Holt (ed.), *Alcohol: A Social and Cultural History*. Oxford: Berg, pp. 107–20.

Brennan, T (ed.) (2011) *Public Drinking in the Early Modern World. Voices from the Tavern*, 4 Vols. London: Pickering & Chatto.

Brewer, J (1989) *The Sinews of Power: War, Money and the English State, 1688–1783*. London: Routledge.

Brown, J (2008) *The Landscape of Drink: Inns, Taverns and Alehouses in Early Modern Southampton*. PhD diss. Coventry: University of Warwick.

Brown, J (2013) 'Alehouse licensing and state formation in early modern England', In J Herring, C Regan, D Weinberg and P Withington (eds), *Intoxicants and Society: Problematic Pleasures of Drugs and Alcohol*. Basingstoke: Palgrave Macmillan, pp. 110–32.

Burnett, J (1999) *Liquid Pleasure: A Social History of Drinks in Modern Britain*. London: Routledge.

Burns, E (2004) *The Spirits of America: A Social History of Alcohol*. Philadelphia: Temple University Press.

Capp, B (2007) 'Gender and the culture of the alehouse in late Stuart England', In A Korhonen and K Lowe (eds), *The Trouble with Ribs: Women, Men and Gender in Early Modern Europe*, Vol. 2. Helsinki: COLLeGIUM: Studies across Disciplines in the Humanities and Social Sciences, pp. 103–27.

Cashman, S (1981) *Prohibition: The Lie of the Land*. London: Macmillan.

Clark, P (1978) 'The alehouse and the alternative society', In D Pennington and K Thomas (eds), *Puritans and Revolutionaries: Essays in Seventeenth-Century History Presented to Christopher Hill*. Oxford: Clarendon Press, pp. 47–72.

Clark, P (1983) *The English Alehouse: A Social History 1200–1830*. London: Longman.

Clark, P (1988) 'The "Mother Gin" controversy in the early eighteenth century', *Transactions of the Royal Historical Society*, 5th series 38: 63–84.

Clemis, D (2013) 'Medical Expertise and the Understanding of Intoxication in Britain, 1660 to 1830', In J Herring, C Regan, D Weinberg and P Withington (eds), *Intoxicants and Society: Problematic Pleasures of Drugs and Alcohol*. Basingstoke: Palgrave Macmillan, pp. 33–51.

Courtwright, D (2001) *Forces of Habit: Drugs and the Making of the Modern World*. Cambridge and London: Harvard University Press.

Cowan, B (2005) *The Social Life of Coffee: The Emergence of the British Coffeehouse*. London: Yale University Press.

Davis, NZ (1975) *Society and Culture in Early Modern France*. Stanford: Stanford University Press.

De Vries, J (2008) *The Industrious Revolution: Consumer Behaviour and the Household*

Economy, 1650 to the Present. Cambridge: Cambridge University Press.
Dillon, P (2002) *The Much-Lamented Death of Madam Geneva: The Eighteenth-Century Gin Craze*. London: Review.
Douglas, M (ed.) (1987) *Constructive Drinking: Perspectives on Drink from Anthropology.* Cambridge: Cambridge University Press.
Earle, R (2014) 'Indians and Drunkenness in Spanish America', In P Withington and A McShane (eds), *Past and Present*, Supplement 9: *Cultures of Intoxication*. Oxford: Oxford University Press, pp. 81–99.
Earnshaw, S (2000) *The Pub in Literature*. Manchester: Manchester University Press.
Elias, N (2000) *The Civilizing Process*. Translated by E Jephcott, original published 1939. Oxford: Blackwell Publishers.
Ferentzy, P (2001) 'From sin to disease: differences and similarities between past and current conceptions on "chronic drunkenness"', *Contemporary Drug Problems*, 28: 362–90.
Galloway, J (1998) 'Driven by drink? Ale consumption and the agrarian economy of the London region c. 1300–1400', In M Carlin and J Rosenthal (eds), *Food and Eating in Medieval Europe*. London: Hambledon Press, pp. 87–100.
Glanville, P and Lee, S (2007) *The Art of Drinking*. London: V&A Publications.
Goodman, J (1993) *Tobacco in History: The Cultures of Dependence*. London: Routledge.
Goodman, J (2007) 'Excitantia: or, how Enlightenment Europe took to soft drugs', In J Goodman, PE Lovejoy and A Sherratt (eds), *Consuming Habits: Global and Historical Perspectives on How Cultures Define Drugs*, 2nd edn. London: Routledge, pp. 121–41.
Goodman, J, Lovejoy, PE, Sherratt, A (eds) (2007) *Consuming Habits: Global and Historical Perspectives on How Cultures Define Drugs*, 2nd edn. London: Routledge.
Grieco, A (2009) 'Medieval and Renaissance wines: taste, dietary theory, and how to choose the "right" wine (14th–16th centuries)', *Mediaevalia*, 30(1): 15–42.
Hailwood, M (2010) 'Alehouses, popular politics and plebeian agency in early modern England', In F Williamson, F (ed.), *Locating Agency: Space, Power and Popular Politics*. Newcastle: Cambridge Scholars Publishing, pp. 51–76.
Hailwood, M (2011) 'Sociability, work and labouring identity in seventeenth-century England', *Cultural and Social History,* 8(1): 9–29.
Hailwood, M (2013) '"It puts good reason into brains": popular understandings of the effects of alcohol in seventeenth-century England', *Brewery History*, 150: 39–53.
Hailwood, M (2014) *Alehouses and Good Fellowship in Early Modern England*, Woodbridge: Boydell and Brewer.
Hames, G (2012) *Alcohol in World History*. London: Routledge.
Hancock, D (2009) *Oceans of Wine: Madeira and the Emergence of American Trade and Taste*. New Haven and London: Yale University Press.
Harrison, B (1971) *Drink and the Victorians: The Temperance Question in England, 1815–1872*. London: Faber and Faber.
Herlihy, P (2002) *The Alcoholic Empire: Vodka and Politics in Late Imperial Russia*. Oxford: Oxford University Press.
Herring, J, Regan, C, Weinberg, D, and Withington, P (eds) (2013) *Intoxicants and Society: Problematic Pleasures of Drugs and Alcohol*. Basingstoke: Palgrave Macmillan.
Hitchcock, T (1999) 'Sociability and misogyny in the life of John Cannon, 1684–1743', In T Hitchcock and M Cohen (eds), *English Masculinities, 1660–1800*. London: Longman, pp. 25–43.
Hsu, HB (2014) 'The taste of opium: science, monopoly, and the Japanese colonization in Taiwan, 1895-1945', In P Withington and A McShane (eds), *Past and Present*, Supplement 9: *Cultures of Intoxication*. Oxford: Oxford University Press, pp. 227–46.
Huang, HT (2000) *Science and Civilisation in China, Volume 6. Biology and Biological Technology, Part 5. Fermentations and Food Science*. Cambridge: Cambridge University Press, Chapter 3.
Kümin, B (2007) *Drinking Matters: Public Houses and Social Exchange in Early Modern Central Europe*. Basingstoke: Palgrave Macmillan.
Kümin, B and Tlusty, BA (eds) (2002) *The World of the Tavern: Public Houses in Early Modern Europe*. Aldershot: Ashgate.
Lender, ME and Martin, JK (eds) (1982) *Drinking in America: A History*. New York: Free Press.

Lindesmith, A (1938) 'A sociological theory of drug addiction', *American Journal of Sociology*, 43: 593–609.

Luddington, C (2010) *The Politics of Wine in Britain: A New Cultural History*. Basingstoke: Palgrave Macmillan.

Mancall, P (1995) *Deadly Medicine: Indians and Alcohol in Early America*. Ithaca and London: Cornell University Press.

Martin, AL (2001) *Alcohol, Sex, and Gender in Late Medieval and Early Modern Europe*. Basingstoke: Palgrave Macmillan.

Martin, AL (2009) *Alcohol, Violence and Disorder in Traditional Europe*. Kirksville: Truman State University Press.

Mathias, P (1959) *The Brewing Industry in England, 1700–1830*, Cambridge: Cambridge University Press.

McIntosh, MK (1998) *Controlling Misbehavior in England, 1370–1600*. Cambridge: Cambridge University Press.

McShane Jones, A (2004) 'Roaring Royalists and ranting brewers: the politicisation of drink and drunkenness in political broadside ballads from 1640 to 1689', In A Smyth (ed.), *A Pleasing Sinne: Drink and Conviviality in Seventeenth-century England*. Cambridge: Cambridge University Press, pp. 69–87.

McShane, A (2010) 'The extraordinary case of the flesh eating and blood drinking cavaliers', In A McShane and G Walker (eds), *The Extraordinary and the Everyday in Early Modern England*. Basingstoke: Palgrave Macmillan, pp. 192–210.

McShane, A (2014) 'Material culture and "political drinking" in seventeenth-century England', In P Withington and A McShane (eds), *Past and Present*, Supplement 9: *Cultures of Intoxication*. Oxford: Oxford University Press, pp. 247–76.

Meacham, SH (2009) *Every Home a Distillery: Alcohol, Gender and Technology in the Colonial Chesapeake*. Baltimore: Johns Hopkins University Press.

Mills, JH (2007) 'Globalizing *ganja*: the British Empire and international cannabis traffic c.1834 to c.1939', In J Goodman, PE Lovejoy and A Sherratt (eds), *Consuming Habits: Global and Historical Perspectives on How Cultures Define Drugs*, 2nd edn. London: Routledge, pp. 178–93.

Muldrew, C (2011) *Food, Energy and the Creation of Industriousness: Work and Material Culture in Agrarian England, 1550–1780*. Cambridge: Cambridge University Press.

Nicholls, J (2008) '*Vinum Britannicum*: the "drink question" in early modern England', *The Social History of Alcohol and Drugs*, 22(2): 6–25.

Nicholls, J (2009) *The Politics of Alcohol: A History of the Drink Question in England*. Manchester: Manchester University Press.

Nicholls, J and Owen, SJ (2000) *A Babel of Bottles: Drink, Drinkers and Drinking Places in Literature*. Sheffield: Sheffield Academic Press.

Nichols, T (2014) 'Double vision: the ambivalent imagery of drunkenness in early modern Europe', In P Withington and A McShane (eds), *Past and Present*, Supplement 9: *Cultures of Intoxication*. Oxford: Oxford University Press, pp. 146–67.

O'Callaghan, M (2007) *The English Wits: Literature and Sociability in Early Modern England*. Cambridge: Cambridge University Press.

Osborne, R (2014) 'Intoxication and sociality: the symposium in the ancient Greek world', In P Withington and A McShane (eds), *Past and Present*, Supplement 9: *Cultures of Intoxication*. Oxford: Oxford University Press, pp. 34–60.

Phillips, LL (2002) *Bolsheviks and the Bottle: Drink and Worker Culture in St. Petersburg, 1900–1929*. DeKalb: Northern Illinois University Press.

Pollard, T (2005) *Drugs and Theatre in Early Modern England*. Oxford: Oxford University Press.

Porter, R (1985) 'The drinking man's disease: the pre-history of alcoholism in Georgian Britain', *British Journal of Addiction*, 80: 385–96.

Price, JM (2007) 'Tobacco use and tobacco taxation: a battle of interests in early modern Europe', In J Goodman, PE Lovejoy and A Sherratt (eds), *Consuming Habits: Global and Historical Perspectives on How Cultures Define Drugs*, 2nd edn. London: Routledge, pp. 158–77.

Rabin, D (2005) 'Drunkenness and responsibility for crime in the eighteenth century', *Journal of British Studies*, 44: 457–77.

Richards, J (2014) 'Health, intoxication and civil conversation in Renaissance England', In P Withington and A McShane (eds), *Past and Present*, Supplement 9: *Cultures of Intoxication*. Oxford: Oxford University Press, pp. 168–86.

Roberts, B (2004) 'Drinking like a man: the paradox of excessive drinking for seventeenth-century Dutch youths', *Journal of Family History*, 29(3): 237–52.

Rorabaugh, WJ (1979) *The Alcoholic Republic: An American Tradition*. New York: Oxford University Press.

Salinger, SV (2002) *Taverns and Drinking in Early America*. Baltimore: Johns Hopkins University Press.

Schivelbusch, W (1992) *Tastes of Paradise: A Social History of Spices, Stimulants and Intoxicants*. Translated by D Jacobson. New York: Pantheon.

Schrad, ML (2014) *Vodka Politics: Alcohol, Autocracy, and the Secret History of the Russian State*. New York: Oxford University Press.

Segal, BM (1986) *Russian Drinking: Use and Abuse of Alcohol in Pre-Revolutionary Russia*. New Brunswick: Publications Division, Rutgers Center of Alcohol Studies.

Sennefelt, K (2014) 'Wine, corruption and the politics of intoxication in eighteenth-century Stockholm', In P Withington and A McShane (eds), *Past and Present*, Supplement 9: *Cultures of Intoxication*. Oxford: Oxford University Press, pp. 277–95.

Shammas, C (1990) *The Pre-Industrial Consumer in England and America*. Oxford: Clarendon Press.

Shepard, A (2005) '"Swil-bols and tos-pots": drink culture and male bonding in England, c.1560-1640', In L Gowing, M Hunter and M Rubin (eds), *Love, Friendship and Faith in Europe, 1300–1800*. Basingstoke: Palgrave Macmillan, pp. 110–30.

Shrank, C (2013) 'Beastly metamorphoses: losing control in early modern literary culture', In J Herring, C Regan, D Weinberg and P Withington (eds), *Intoxicants and Society: Problematic Pleasures of Drugs and Alcohol*. Basingstoke: Palgrave Macmillan, pp. 193–209.

Skoda, H (2013) *Medieval Violence: Physical Brutality in Northern France, 1270–1330*. Oxford: Oxford University Press.

Smith, FH (2005) *Caribbean Rum: A Social and Economic History*. Gainesville: University Press of Florida.

Smith, WD (2007) 'From coffeehouse to parlour: the consumption of coffee, tea and sugar in north-western Europe in the seventeenth and eighteenth centuries', In J Goodman, PE Lovejoy and A Sherratt (eds), *Consuming Habits: Global and Historical Perspectives on How Cultures Define Drugs*, 2nd edn. London: Routledge, pp. 142–57.

Smyth, A (ed.) (2004) *A Pleasing Sinne: Drink and Conviviality in Seventeenth-Century England*. Cambridge: Cambridge University Press.

Spring, JA and Buss, DH (1977) 'Three centuries of alcohol in the British diet', *Nature*, 270: 567–72.

Stern, PJ (2011) *The Company-State: Corporate Sovereignty and the Early Modern Foundation of the British Empire in India*. Oxford: Oxford University Press.

Taylor, WB (1979) *Drinking, Homicide and Rebellion in Colonial Mexican Villages*. Stanford: Stanford University Press.

Thomas, K (1971) *Religion and the Decline of Magic: Studies in Popular Beliefs in Sixteenth- and Seventeenth-Century England*. London: Weidenfeld and Nicolson.

Thompson, P (1998) *Rum Punch and Revolution: Taverngoing and Public Life in Eighteenth-Century Philadelphia*. Philadelphia: University of Pennsylvania Press.

Tlusty, BA (1998) 'Water of life, water of death: the controversy over brandy and gin in early modern Augsburg', *Central European History*, 31: 1–30.

Tlusty, BA (2001) *Bacchus and Civic Order: The Culture of Drink in Early Modern Germany*. Charlottesville and London: University Press of Virginia.

Toner, DF (2012) 'Drinking to fraternity: alcohol, masculinity, and national identity in the novels of Manuel Payno and Heriberto Frías', *Bulletin of Hispanic Studies*, 89(4): 397–412.

Transchel, K (2006) *Under the Influence: Working-Class Drinking, Temperance, and Cultural Revolution in Russia, 1895–1932*. Pittsburgh: University of Pittsburgh Press.

Unger, R (2004) *Beer in the Middle Ages and the Renaissance*. Philadelphia: University of Pennsylvania Press.

Walvin, J (1997) *Fruits of Empire: Exotic Produce and British Taste, 1660–1800*. Basingstoke: Macmillan Press.

Warner, J (1994) '"Resolv'd to drink no more": addiction as a preindustrial concept', *Journal of Studies on Alcohol*, 55: 85–91.

Warner, J (2002) *Craze: Gin and Debauchery in an Age of Reason*. New York: Four Walls Eight Windows.

Weinberg, D (1997) 'Lindesmith on addiction: a critical history of a classic theory', *Sociological Theory*, 15(2): 150–61.

Weinberg, D (2002) 'On the embodiment of addiction', *Body and Society*, 8(4): 1–19.

White, J (2003) 'The slow, but sure poyson: the representation of gin and its drinkers in England, 1736–51', *Journal of British Studies*, 42(1): 35–64.

White, S (1996) *Russia Goes Dry: Gorbachev, Alcohol, and the Policy Process*. Cambridge: Cambridge University Press.

Withington, P (2011) 'Intoxicants and Society in Early Modern England', *The Historical Journal*, 54(3): 631–57.

Withington, P (2013a) 'Renaissance drinking cultures and popular print', In J Herring, C Regan, D Weinberg and P Withington (eds), *Intoxicants and Society: Problematic Pleasures of Drugs and Alcohol*. Basingstoke: Palgrave Macmillan, pp. 135–52.

Withington, P (2013b) 'Intoxicants and the early modern city', In S Hindle, A Shepard, and J Walter (eds), *Remaking English Society*. Woodbridge: Boydell and Brewer, pp. 135–63.

Withington, P (2014) 'Cultures of intoxication', In P Withington and A McShane (eds), *Past and Present*, Supplement 9: *Cultures of Intoxication*. Oxford: Oxford University Press, pp. 9–33.

Withington, P and McShane, A (2009) *Fluctuations in English Drinking Habits: An Historical Overview*. London: Parliamentary Health Committee Memorandum, AL57.

Withington, P and McShane, A (eds) (2014) *Past and Present*, Supplement 9: *Cultures of Intoxication*. Oxford: Oxford University Press.

Wrightson, K (1981) 'Alehouses, order and reformation in Rural England, 1590–1660', In E Yeo and S Yeo (eds), *Popular Culture and Class Conflict 1590–1914: Explorations in the History of Labour and Leisure*. Brighton: Harvester, pp. 1–27.

Yeomans, H (2014) *Alcohol and Moral Regulation: Public Attitudes, Spirited Measures and Victorian Hangovers*. Bristol: Policy Press.

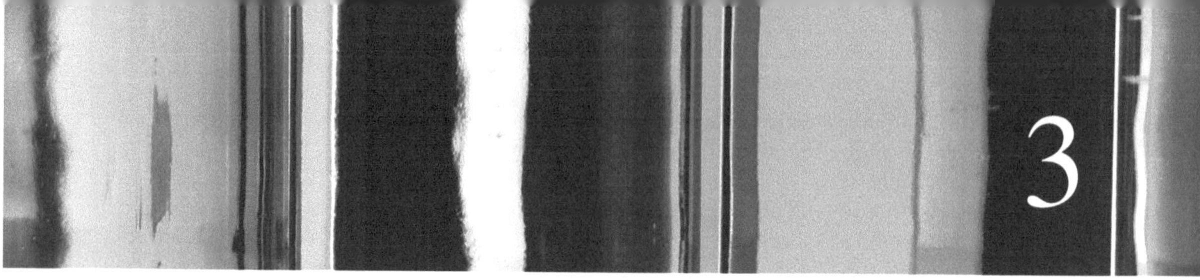

Sociological Perspectives

Franca Beccaria and Franco Prina

INTRODUCTION

Studying drugs and alcohol from a sociological perspective means looking at the relationship between individuals, groups of individuals and psychoactive substances in the context of the social, economic and cultural conditions that inform this relationship. The sociology of drugs and alcohol is closely related to other disciplinary approaches: epidemiology (measurement of drug and alcohol related behaviour), psychology (attention to individually ascribed meanings associated with drug and alcohol practices), anthropology (the socio-contextual meanings of psychoactive substances and the 'functions' that they can fulfil) and criminology (crimes related to the consumption, production and distribution of illegal substances and the role of control institutions). However, in this chapter we will attempt to illustrate the sociological approach in the fields of alcohol and drug research even where it overlaps with other disciplines.

There are many sociological theories on the relationship between individuals, social groups and psychoactive substances in different social and cultural contexts. Sociological theories have been useful in attempting to explain the distinction between use, abuse and addiction, the multiple functions ascribed to psychoactive substances, socially acceptable and socially condemned drug and alcohol consumption and the question of legality.

Across most societies and at most times, a key distinction is the difference between legal and illegal substances. On the one hand, the legal nature of alcohol consumption in most societies and cultures made it possible to focus on different uses, different levels of problems and on the function of alcohol in society, including positive functions as well as negative effects. This way of thinking about the substance is reflected in lay and professional and policy discourse and has a bearing on the use and development of sociological research and theories. On the other hand, the study of illegal substances has been more focussed on the deviant aspects related to consumption and on addictions as social problems.

More recently, however, other perspectives on the use of illegal substances, similar to those on alcohol, have broadened the theoretical frameworks used to understand use and problem use and to analyse consumption and behaviour. The tendency to 'normalize' some forms of consumption, the discovery of a 'regulated' area of consumption and addiction, the emergence of a discussion about the possibility of challenging a prohibitionist approach (in particular, but not only, regarding cannabis) – these ideas have shifted thinking about illicit drug use away from a largely deviance framework towards a more mainstream 'consumptionist' viewpoint which, as well as employing a broader range of sociological theories to explain illicit drug use and drug-related problems, has also helped to generate theory. Thus, within the broad range of sociological theories used in the substance use/misuse field, we can distinguish a focus on studying social problems on the one hand, and on the other, an emphasis on gaining insight into the pleasures, functions and meanings related to drug and alcohol use. Consequently, many different branches of sociology have dealt with drug and alcohol issues: for example, the sociology of deviance, sociology of youth, sociology of lifestyles, sociology of health and medicine, sociology of law and political sociology.

In this chapter, we will discuss some of the central theories that have been applied in the drug and alcohol field. We will group them into three categories: social structural theories, social process theories and social reaction theories. Within these theoretical categories, drug and alcohol use has often been viewed as a form of social pathology – linking substance use closely to the field of deviance, as noted earlier. But the three groups of sociological theories also offer alternative views that challenge the social pathology analysis: for example, focusing on the social construction of phenomena draws attention to a problem definition – how a legal drug such as opium comes to be defined as an illegal substance. With the intention of providing some critique of the social pathology approach, we include theoretical approaches that, especially in recent times, have put individual choice and decision making at the centre of attention, that refer to concepts of rationality, normalization and the search for risk and pleasure and that denote the relationship with psychoactive substances in its various forms, more broadly than in problematic terms.

Finally, in thinking about how sociological theories have explained substance use, problem use and addiction, it is worth keeping in mind some of the issues that arise in developing theory in this subject area. The development of theory in any field is a product of the insights gained from empirical research. Theory is dependent, at least partly, on the strength of the methods and the quality of the research. For example, a sociologist needs to consider the following: the nature of the samples (their representativeness, size, cost, respondent availability, etc.); how questions are formulated; the setting and type of interaction between researcher and those who are the object of study; and the reliability of responses received. Considerations such as these are not unique to the drug and alcohol research field and other chapters in this *Handbook* will address such issues in more detail. However, as in many areas of deviance research, studies on drug and alcohol issues face methodological problems in that individuals tend to conceal behaviour that could be judged negatively for fear of social and institutional responses. In brief, social acceptance or non-acceptance of behaviours and relationships or of individual characteristics and attributes (e.g. being disabled, being an 'addict') may well influence the research that tests theory, amends theory and generates new theory. Thus, the drug and alcohol sociologist is called upon to be especially critical when examining the empirical basis of the theories used to frame our understanding of substance use and misuse or when using data to critique existing theory and devise new knowledge.

SOCIAL STRUCTURAL THEORIES

Social structural theories focus on the role of social structure, including socio-economic background and environmental context, in explaining in particular the problematic use of drugs and alcohol. We examine the Chicago School of sociology and strain theories as examples of how theoretical perspectives consider psychoactive substance abuse respectively as a social problem and as deviant adaptation.

The Chicago School

The social pathological approach to alcohol and drugs can be traced back to the 'Chicago School', which consisted of a group of sociologists in the Sociology Department of the University of Chicago. The work of the Chicago School was primarily conducted in the 1920s and 1930s, a period in which American society, and especially Chicago, was growing rapidly (Bulmer, 1984). As a result, they were particularly interested in studying the community, that is, the city, its districts, specific ethnic groups and ghettos, as these developed and changed during this period of rapid transformation. In general, the Chicago School, inspired initially by Durkheim's (1897) thinking on anomy and social disorganisation, concluded that the uneven distribution of deviance and criminality (including alcohol misuse and a few cases of drug consumption) in the town should not be explained by individuals' characteristics, but should be examined in terms of different degrees of social disorganization (Downes and Rock, 2003).

In investigating the city of Chicago, they found the degree of social disorganization to be particularly high in the so-called 'transitional zone', with its higher proportion of immigrants who had just arrived in the city (Park et al., 1925). In the same way, and according to the view that has been summarized as the ecological paradigm of the Chicago School, crime rates were seen as primarily linked to neighbourhood environmental characteristics. In summary, extreme poverty, transient residents and deteriorated housing were all seen as factors that contributed to the weakening of social bonds, thereby making social control less effective. Social problems and deviance, it was argued, occurred when social bonds are weak or lacking, whereas in well-organized communities, social control can be strong and individuals will have fewer opportunities to violate social norms and values (Anderson, 1923; Thrasher, 1927; Burgess and Bogue, 1964). In line with this, Dai (1935) discovered, in the first ecological study on opium addicts in Chicago – which, actually, was virtually ignored in the main accounts of the Chicago School – a higher rate of addicts in the downtown area decreasing in accordance with the distance from it. The ecological distribution of drug addicts was, in this way, seen as similar to the distribution of other social problems.

The classic study of Thomas and Znaniecki (1918), in which they meticulously analysed the changes that occurred in the Polish community after immigration to the US, can be seen as an early example of the Chicago School approach, focusing on social structures (families, neighbourhoods and communities) in order to explain change and social disorganization. In this work, the authors also addressed the problem of alcoholism. In a peasant community, they argued, social control was effective in sanctioning alcohol abuse, so that it was more difficult for a member to drink to the point of ruining himself and his family. In American society, however, the immigrant's economic uncertainty and the lack of social ties could make him more likely to seek refuge in alcoholic beverages. According to Thomas and Znaniecki, alcoholism, therefore, like many other social phenomena, is strongly related to processes of social disorganization, that is, the reduction of the influence of social norms shared by the group on the single individual. Moreover, such weakening of group control and solidarity is not attributed to the individual or the group, but to more general structural factors and changes.

Another early contribution to the sociology of alcohol use within the Chicago School tradition is the study of Park et al. (1925), written during Prohibition, in which they analyse individual alcohol misuse in the light of structural factors such as commercialized vice and liquor traffic and the effects of governmental control policies.

The early work of the Chicago School and their focus on the role of social disorganization, urban poverty and social inequity in the onset and development of so-called antisocial or delinquent behaviour (Burgess, 1925; Park, 1926) is still influential in present day sociological studies of drug and alcohol-related problems, in research seeking to identify the contributions of neighbourhood disadvantage, urban poverty, gangs and the drug street market to understanding of the onset of drug use and the development of drug and alcohol consumption careers (see for instance: Geis and Ross, 1998; Brody et al., 2001; Bennett and Holloway, 2004; Brenner et al., 2011; Taniguchi et al., 2011; Taniguchi and Salvatore, 2012; Parks, 2014). However other contemporary studies, also influenced by the structural approach of the Chicago School, have called the role of disadvantaged neighbourhoods into question by arguing that even though drug problems are more visible in these areas, drug use is equally distributed across different communities (Saxe et al., 2001).

Strain theory

One of the most important contributions to social structural theories was made by the sociologist, Robert K. Merton, who worked on understanding the relation between social and cultural structures and individual deviant behaviour. According to his functionalist perspective, society can be seen as a normative system exercising pressure on its members to act in conformity with social expectations and members who are adequately socialized into prevailing norms and values comply with the rules. In such a balanced society, deviant people are those who transgress social and cultural norms (Merton, 1938).

To understand deviance, Merton identifies two important elements that produce different levels of strain in a society: cultural goals that people are expected to reach and legitimate means for reaching them. The different distribution of means in a society and the emphasis attributed to goals instead of legitimate means for reaching them can produce a strain between means and goals; consequently, some people may decide to use illegal means to obtain legitimate goals. It should be noted that Merton's theory was developed in an American society where the emphasis on attaining goals – mainly personal success – was stronger than that on complying with institutional means (Downes and Rock, 2003: 104–41). Merton developed a typology of five ways people adapt to dominant societal values, known as Merton's paradigm of deviant behaviour: conformity, innovation, ritualism, retreatism and rebellion. Conformity is attaining cultural goals by socially accepted means, while innovation is achieving those goals in illegitimate or deviant ways. Ritualism is accepting the means even if the goals are rejected. Ritualists are unlike retreaters, who, after having assimilated both cultural goals and socially accepted means, find themselves in a situation where they are unable to reach goals by legitimate means, and – as they feel they cannot use illegitimate means to solve their frustration – they refuse both. Rebellion entails rejecting goals and means and substituting them with new goals and means that will be accepted.

According to Merton, alcoholics and especially drug addicts can be seen as retreatist, as they have abandoned both dominant goals and conventional life styles for behaviours that often break the law. Such persons have retreated from pursuing the goals proposed by society; antisocial individuals who solve the conflict between goals and means by escaping with the help of alcohol or drugs. In this view, drug use is a consequence of social marginalization. By contrast, one could argue that the 1960s drug counterculture revolving around cannabis and hallucinogens could be classified as rebellion, as both mainstream societal goals and means were rejected and new one were proposed by these countercultures (Young 1971).

Likewise, in recent years, the innovation adaptation could help explain both illegal and legal recreational drug consumption among upper social classes as well as drug use aimed at performance enhancement (Moisan et al., 1999; Berridge, 2013). That is, these socially integrated drug consumers have accepted social goals, such as better performance at work, in arts or sports, but they set aside norms that prohibit drug use in order to reach these goals.

While the notion of 'subculture' was not new during the 1950s and 60s, building on Merton's strain theory, Cohen (1955) and Cloward and Ohlin (1960) developed the concept of subculture more fully. They interpreted deviant adaptation not only as individual choice and adaption but as related to common values held within social groups whose members are subject to similar conditions and strains. In his study, *Delinquent Boys*, Cohen (1955) showed that beliefs are more stable if they can be compared and shared with significant others. When boys or girls are exposed to illegal drugs for the first time, their decision whether to try them out will depend on their peer group's opinion of drug consumption, as well as on the judgements expressed by parents, the school and mass media. But, according to Cohen, peer judgement will probably outweigh the other influences, and the individual is more likely to be involved in drug behaviour if such significant others characterize drug use in positive terms.

Cloward and Ohlin (1960) depicted three types of delinquent subcultures in American society: criminal, conflict and retreatist. The consolidation of deviant behaviour depends on the pressure exerted by subcultures with norms and values that oppose the dominant culture and which make available both legitimate or illegitimate opportunities. The authors suggested that, beyond the initiation and early experimentation stages of drug use, illegal drug consumers are retreatists suffering from a 'double failure', as they have failed in achieving economic success by both legitimate and illegitimate means.

Although strain theories dominated drug use research during the 1960s, they were soon called into question and lost importance (Aseltine, 2000). While recognizing the work of Robert Merton as seminal in the development of sociological theory, Fazey (1973) stated that the application of his theories to specific patterns of behaviour – such as drug addiction – 'does not seem to have attracted the attention of many of those engaged in empirical research'. One possible explanation for the neglect of Merton's theory in drug addiction research is that, even if for some addicts, addiction is an expression of retreat from social pressure towards socially shared goals that are not possible to achieve, 'the pressures towards addiction seemed, for most, to have roots in other areas and addiction was for them a successful problem solving activity' (Fazey, 1973: 431). In other words, drug use was a successful way of coping with problems such as poverty, violence, homelessness, unemployment, etc.

Among several revisions of classic strain theory, Agnew's *general strain theory of delinquency and drug use* focuses on negative life events and negative relationships in order to explain drug use. Agnew argues that 'strain theory has typically focused on relationships in which others prevent the individual from achieving positively valued goals' (Agnew, 1992: 48–9). According to this author, the contribution of strain theory to understanding drug use should be to focus on negative relationships and their role in pressuring adolescents into deviant behaviours, adding that strain may result not only from the failure to achieve positively valued goals but also from the inability to escape from painful situations as a result of unpleasant circumstances, for example, the loss of a boyfriend/girlfriend, moving to a new school district or adverse conditions at work. In this way, Agnew's revitalization of strain theory consists of adding a social-psychological level to Merton's preoccupation with social and cultural structures.

In fact, according to Kandel (1980), Merton's adaptation concepts developed to describe features of social structures – where the incongruities between goals and means are seen as a pressure for illegitimate behaviours – used by the classic sociological theories of drug behaviour – opened the way to social-psychological frameworks (Jessor and Jessor, 1977) as the adaptation concepts 'have been translated into individual characteristics, such as perceived approval-disapproval for specific behaviors' (Kandel, 1980: 250). Consequently, the great success of social-psychological orientations in the field of drug research has neglected the role of larger social-structural factors.

SOCIAL PROCESS THEORIES

Social process theories explaining why people engage in deviant behaviours focus on how values, expectations, beliefs, relationships and norms influence individuals' attitudes towards breaking or respecting the law.

In assigning primary importance to structural strain, strain theory distinguishes itself from social process theories, which explain deviant behaviour as learned behaviour not necessarily linked to disorganization, exclusion and marginalization (Sutherland, 1934).

The explanatory power of strain theory is limited by the fact that homogeneous normative systems do not exist in contemporary complex societies, as social norms vary from one society to another and also within subsectors of society. Consequently, behaviour defined as deviant on the basis of a certain normative system will be seen as non-deviant on the basis of another. In taking this view, social process theories – the most important of which is social learning theory – focus on the roles of subcultures in the deviance process.

Sutherland and Cressey (1974) contributed to social learning theory by challenging the causal link between poverty and deviance. They showed that all segments of society have some values and norms that conflict with dominant views and which are learned through group interactions and learning processes. Likewise, Sutherland (1949) rejected the understanding of deviance as reflecting social and personal conditions such as poverty, mental illness, and family disorganization. As illegal drug use is not only found in the lower social classes or among sick people, this means that in order to understand such behaviour, the focus has to be on the process whereby the deviant behaviour is learned. It should be noted, that already in 1934, Edwin Sutherland's *differential association theory* suggested that to understand deviant behaviours, it is necessary to look at the interaction among individuals, as it is through this that people learn values, attitudes and techniques for deviant behaviour. Deviant behaviour, therefore (and one could include illegal drug use), is learned by direct or indirect association with those who are already involved in criminal acts.

Social learning theory has played a significant role in the sociology of drug and alcohol use. It has, for instance, been shown that differential association (direct and indirect interaction with others), differential reinforcement (instrumental learning through rewards and punishments), definitions (attitudes) and imitation (observational learning) play significant roles in explaining legal and illegal substance use among adolescents and offenders (Akers et al., 1979; Akers and Lee, 1996; Yun and Kim, 2015). As argued by Akers:

> Whether individuals will abstain from or take drugs (and whether they will continue and desist) depends on the past, present and anticipated future rewards and punishments perceived to be attached to abstinence and use (differential reinforcement). The person learns attitudes, orientations, or evaluative knowledge which are favourable or unfavourable to using drugs (definitions). These are themselves verbal and cognitive behaviour which can be directly reinforced and can also act as cue stimuli for drug use. The more individuals define the behaviour as good or at least as justified or excusable rather than holding to general beliefs or specific attitudes counter to a drug, the more likely they are to use it. (Akers, 1992: 12)

Reinforcements however, do not only come from peers, but also in interaction with the drug per se. If initial effects of drugs are perceived as pleasant, they can provide a positive reinforcement to continue, if they are unpleasant they can provide strong motives to discontinue use. As an example of how social learning and the drug intersect, it is interesting to look at Becker's (1953, 1963) theory of how one has to engage in a learning process in order to become familiar with the effects of different drugs. According to Becker, such learning can be seen as a process: learning the techniques of using the drug (inhaling deeply and holding in the smoke), learning to recognize the effects and connect them with drug use (the drug-using subculture provides information to normalize the experiences) and learning to enjoy the sensations perceived. This learning (including learning to get high) is, therefore, to be seen as a socialization process conducted by more experienced users who behave as mentors. Moreover, such a mentor not only teaches new members techniques and how to recognize positive effects, but also transmits motives, *techniques of neutralization* (Sykes and Matza, 1957) – that make it possible to ignore the inner call to respect norms – and justifications, as well as rules of behaviour to reduce the risk of being discovered.

Although Becker's social-process-based theory has survived the test of time, Hallstone (2002) suggests that changes in the marijuana scene necessitate a revision of this theory. Hallstone tested Becker's theory of the three-step social process to becoming a marijuana smoker by replicating a similar study in a more recent period. His research suggests that most smokers become intoxicated the first time they smoke marijuana and many no longer have to learn that they are intoxicated through social interaction with other users. Most immediately find the experience enjoyable, as 'the process of learning to define the effects of marijuana as pleasurable now happens at a much faster rate' (Hallstone, 2002: 840).

Drug learning processes have also been found among users of other illegal drugs, generally considered much more addictive than marijuana (Harding, 1988). To reduce risks and optimize the pleasure, heroin consumers, for instance, have to learn how to cook heroin, to prepare their veins and to insert the needle correctly without damage (Faupel, 1991). Therefore, according to Zinberg (1984: 17), 'although the opportunities for learning how to control illicit drug consumption are extremely limited, rituals and social sanctions that promote control do exist within subcultures of drug users'.

In contemporary society, the opportunities for learning how to control alcohol consumption are much more widespread than for illicit drugs (Akers et al., 1989; see also Chapter 26 in this Handbook). Social learning theory postulates that adolescent alcohol use is a learned behaviour acquired through social interactions and social reinforcement that could encourage pro-social or anti-social definitions of drinking, depending on the drinking culture involved, for instance, whether it is Mediterranean or Nordic (Ennett et al., 2008, Østergaard, 2009; Beccaria, 2010;

Rolando et al., 2012). Finally, social learning theory is also confirmed in the explanation of nonmedical prescription drug use among adolescents (Ford, 2008).

SOCIAL REACTION THEORIES

With social reaction theories, the interpretative paradigm for explaining drug and alcohol use shifts radically. The core question is no longer why people use drugs, but why and how society reacts to drug use, how this reaction can be a form of social control and which consequences this reaction has on individuals. Both labelling theory and conflict theory (in critical criminology contributions of the 1970s and 1980s) will be considered here as examples of social reaction theories and their role in explaining the social construction of drug and alcohol phenomena will be discussed.

While acknowledging that conflict theory deals with structural issues, the choice to consider conflict theory among social reaction theories is due to the fact that it calls into question the 'naturalness' of what is considered deviant and especially emphasizes the role of laws (as defined by dominant groups) to determine acceptable or deviant behaviours, that have 'real' consequences on individuals.

Labelling theory

Without denying that drug use is a concrete social phenomenon that can be observed and measured, labelling theory focuses its interest on the socially produced definition of deviance. Labelling theory thus deals with the process whereby some drug users are labelled as deviant, rather than on definitions of use, misuse and addiction. Basically, labelling theorists posit that there is no absolute definition of deviance. Deviance is relative, as it acquires meaning within a society's normative system that changes with time and setting.

For instance, according to Becker (1963), who can be characterized as both a social learning and labelling theorist, the act of injecting heroin into a vein is not inherently deviant. A nurse who provides a prescribed opioid intravenously to a patient is following the rules, but when such provision occurs in a way not defined as proper it becomes deviant. Another typical example concerns the distinction between legal drugs (e.g. alcohol) and illegal drugs (e.g. marijuana). Marijuana consumption is not defined as deviant because it has been found to be more dangerous than alcohol, but because it has been defined as illegal by law, with *moral entrepreneurs* playing a significant role in attaching this label (Becker, 1963; see also Christie and Bruun, 1985). Indeed, the scientific findings on the potential harms of individual drugs often do not parallel general societal ideas of their risks or how they are regulated by law (Nutt et al., 2007).

In the labelling perspective, deviance is seen as a *social and political construction*, and as a consequence, the deviant is defined as a person to whom the label of deviance has been successfully applied: a behaviour is deviant when it has been labelled as deviant (Becker, 1963). Furthermore, when people are labelled as such by society, they are likely to accept this label as a part of themselves, assuming a deviant identity. At times, this deviant identity may even assume the role of a *Master status* – the primary signifier of a person's identity ((Becker, 1963). According to this perspective, then, assuming the identity of an alcohol or drug addict is the result of a process of social interaction, as an individual's self-definition is influenced by the perception that others have of him.

Lemert (1951) contributed to labelling theory by distinguishing between two stages of deviance: primary deviance and secondary deviance. Primary deviance implies that an individual commits deviant acts, even accidentally, but does not become labelled as deviant. As long as the individual is perceived to behave according to socially acceptable roles, he does not assume a new 'deviant' identity, as he/she does not symbolically reorganize the self and his/her social roles. Secondary deviance is the consequence of societal disapproval and labelling of individuals who have broken the social norm. When the labelling process takes place and one accepts a deviant identity as 'a junkie' or 'a doper', for instance, it is likely that a deviant career will then be followed. In such deviant careers, both the individually labelled person and his or her social relations will participate in the often laborious work of managing (or at times resisting) such a 'spoiled identity' (Goffman 1974).

Most people who use legal and illegal drugs have an ordinary life, as shown by national and international surveys, and they are mostly able to hide their 'bad' habits in the majority of settings (Harding, 1988; Scarscelli, 2006). Frequently, the transition from primary to secondary deviance occurs when this habit becomes public for some reason, or becomes visible in new settings, so that other people begin to observe the person as 'a drug user' and his identity acquires a master status: from worker or student to addict or alcoholic. The subject then may gradually acquire a deviant identity, and consequently, compromises his quality of life and opportunities. The deviance process can, in this way, be seen as a self-fulfilling prophecy.

According to Robin Room (2005: 143), alcohol and drug use are 'heavily moralized territories', and this moralization often produces stigma and marginalization with important adverse consequences. A process of stigmatization may accompany the deviant label and in the case of illegal drug consumption, often entails substantial consequences as, in most countries, it can incur an institutional/formal reaction that often results in the person being sent to prison or to other institutions. Accordingly, the label assumes greater significance because of its consequences compared to the consequences that might follow from informal reaction (Goffman, 1961). Looking at alcoholism and drug addiction, in a WHO study in 14 countries, both conditions were ranked near the top in terms of social disapproval among a list of 18 conditions: above being 'dirty and unkempt' and 'having a criminal record for burglary' (Room et al., 2001: 276). Of course, there is no necessary relation between substance use and stigma or marginalization. Indeed, as will be seen below, if we look at drinking in contemporary society, we will note that it is mostly associated with positive values and even high-prestige activities, and drugs such as cannabis, and to an extent amphetamine and cocaine, have, at least in some milieus, been 'normalized' (Parker et al., 1998).

Finally, an important role in the stigma process is played by social institutions and professions that tend to participate in creating or strengthening particular governing images or rubrics of 'a problem' (Room et al., 2015). Some authors have termed such creation of troubled identities as 'institutional selves' (Gubrium and Holstein, 2001). However, having recognized the role and the magnitude of the labelling process, it remains to be explored 'how much of the stigmatization of those with a particular problem is affected by changing its rubric, or even its social handling procedures' (Room, 2005: 146).

Labelling theory has been applied largely to drug studies. According to Room (1983: 66): 'alcoholism pretty much drops out of the labelling literature after its appearance as a chapter in what is often regarded as a foundation document of the labelling literature, Lemert's *Social Pathology* (1951) – except for the special arena of Skid Row'. In fact, Becker in his seminal book on *Social Problems* (1966) mentioned alcohol use and alcohol problems only in the introduction. An exception to this can be found in the work of Roman and Trice (1968), who used labelling theory to support the disease concept of alcoholism, seeing alcoholism as a consequence of the social fact of the application of the diagnosis more than of the drinker's inner predisposition (Room, 1983). Here, the labelling function is performed by the medical authorities that attribute the 'sick role' to the alcoholic or deviant drinker.

Inspired by the labelling perspective, Roizen's criticism (1977a, 1977b) of the dominant concept of alcoholism as a disease (see Pattison et al., 1977) took into consideration the role played by the alcoholism movement in convincing the alcoholic that he is different.

Once labelled as a sick person in an AA group or in a clinic, the alcoholic begins an educational process that leads to the adoption of the 'alcoholic' identity:

> The treatment attempts to educate him to the acceptance of the belief that he is different, and that this difference is not a piecemeal or transitory thing. In short, alcoholism treatment, as it is seen in the classical model, is largely a didactic and persuasional effort that attempts to treat an alcoholic by getting him to accept a particular theory of alcoholism, and his acceptance of that theory is itself the essence of alcoholism treatment. (Roizen, 1977a: 172)

Conflict theory

The critical macro-societal approaches that go by the name of conflict theory argue that, given a low level of consent around norms and values in society, the law is a means of enforcing the dominant social class interests and that social institutions are entrenched structures of power that affect the entire society (see for instance Box 1992).

This theory focuses more on drug and alcohol abuse among marginal social groups than on, for instance, patterns of drinking and marijuana smoking among socially integrated young people. In a conflict theoretical approach, drug problems are perceived as a consequence of the political marginalization of entire communities, as problems linked to alcohol and drug abuse are much more widespread and serious in neighbourhoods with little opportunities, high unemployment and low educational level (Lo, 2003; McCrystal et al., 2007; Karjalainen et al., 2011; Bakhromov and Levy, 2013). Conflict theories stress the role of structural factors, considering drug and alcohol abuse as a problem of structural inequality (Currie, 1993, 1997). In a study of such 'political economy of drug problems', Bourgios (2003) has, for instance, showed that crack use and selling among marginalized Porto Ricans in East Harlem strongly relates to the disappearance of unskilled work in that area. The illegal drug economy then becomes the only possible (illegal) means to acquire legitimate goals (a prestigious masculine identity) for the new generation of Porto Ricans. Very similar arguments are also used about the black community in New York (Dunlap, 1995). From the perspective of conflict theories, laws regulating drug and alcohol use are seen as an instrument of power; an expression of the interests of dominant groups used to maintain the existing social and symbolic order. So that the link with the social process theories consists in placing it in a macro framework (the power, the economy, etc.), the insights of labelling and its reflection on building regulatory systems are an expression of dominant interests. Even if American and British radical schools of the 1970s dealt more with criminal behaviours than with deviance, they put together macro (structural) and micro (relations, reactions, treatment of deviants) variables. This power relationship is illustrated in a seminal study by Gusfield (1981).

Gusfield (1981) shows how the way in which the scientific – media – policy 'system' responds to drink-driving – by exclusively blaming guilty individuals (*the Killer-Drunk*) – is a key factor in the construction of the problem. And, importantly, such a construction is consistent with the defence of dominant economic interests and with the aim of maintaining traditional moral order in society. The drink-driving issue and its social construction is revealed in almost dramaturgical terms: each time alcohol is identified in an accident, its presence is translated in terms of causality, obscuring any other cause '*as if* it were the only, or the major, cause in drinking-driver accidents' (Gusfield, 1981: 72). In summary, the scene is a drama, there is a culprit, there is a solution at hand, the conviction of the offender. The exclusive focus on individual responsibility obscures other relevant factors, some of which are supported by substantial, powerful interests.

Looking at the history of the regulation of psychoactive substances, it emerges that some substances have been prohibited or strictly regulated because they were associated with the 'dangerous social classes' (Snowdon, 2011). In eighteenth century England, for example, gin and whisky were regulated differently, with much higher taxes applied to gin. The official reason for this different policy was that gin was more dangerous than whisky, but the real reason was that gin was mainly consumed by the working class (see Chapter 2 this Handbook). Alcohol laws were in this way used by the dominant class to control marginalized or potentially dangerous social groups. In addition, the treatment of alcohol problems has been theorized as a form of social control, as has been shown by the prevalence of indigent clients in treatment agencies that emphasize custody rather than real cure and offer only short-term services (drop-in centres), while some treatment programmes – especially in the US – accept mainly clients who can pay (Weisner, 1983). This is in line with a general tendency towards the medicalization of deviance represented by a general shift in the twentieth century from crime to illness models of deviance (Conrad and Schneider, 1980). According to Conrad (1992: 209) 'medicalization describes a process by which non-medical problems become defined and treated as medical problems, usually in terms of illnesses or disorders'. Recent studies of the relation between law, drugs and power similarly show that lower social class drug users and marginalized ethnic drug users have a significantly higher probability of being targeted and sentenced for drug law violations than members of high social classes (Gordon, 1994; Acevedo, 2007; Monaghan, 2014; see also Chapter 24 this Handbook).

CONTEMPORARY SOCIOLOGICAL APPROACHES

After having explored the more classical sociological theories that have provided important keys to interpret alcohol and drug use, misuse and addiction, in this section, we will examine more contemporary sociological approaches that refer to concepts such as rational choice, pleasure, normalization and risk.

In contrast to the theories outlined so far, the framework is no longer the sociology of deviance, but the broader agency of individuals, the meanings attributed to the opportunities and choices, the cultures that permeate social action (including the pleasure and risk culture).

Already in the 1940s, Selden Bacon, a young assistant professor at the *Center of Alcohol Studies* at Yale University directed by E.M. Jellinek, urged sociologists to move their focus on alcohol studies from the biomedical approach – mainly concentrating on pathological alcohol consumption and on alcoholism as a clinical entity – to the social meaning of individual actions (Bacon, 1943). According to Bacon, drinking should be studied as part of social life in line with other social behaviours such as religion, family and politics. Moreover, alcohol studies should employ the same theoretical and methodological approaches as used in the study of other social aspects and avoid focusing only on deviant and pathological behaviour (Levine, 1991).

> The sociologist is interested in the customs of drinking, the relationship between these customs and other customs, the way in which drinking habits are learned, the social controls of this sort of behaviour, and those institutions of society through which such control issues. The sociologist wishes to know the social categories in which much or little or no drinking occurs, he seeks correlations of amount and type of drinking with occupational,

> marital, nationality, religious, and other statuses. More importantly, he poses the broad questions: What are the societal functions served by the drinking of alcoholic beverages? What are the social rubs concerned with drinking? What are the pressures for and against this practice? (Bacon, 1943: 407)

According to Levine (1991), however, Bacon's appeal remained largely unheeded within the sociology of alcohol as the main interest for a long time remained on the problematic aspects of drinking and alcohol problems as testified by social-problems textbooks. As Room (1983: 50) noted: 'particularly those written by sociologists with no research experience in alcohol studies, would reveal a presentation of alcohol problems in terms of an orthodox alcoholism disease concept'.

Nevertheless, from the 1960s to the 1980s, sociologists working in the alcohol field gradually managed to distance themselves from the dominant disease paradigm (Room, 1983). Such scholars recognized that sociology's contribution to alcohol studies would be more significant if the object of the study moved beyond drinking problems to include a focus also on different drinking and non-drinking contexts, social factors that promote or discourage alcohol consumption, the role played by the alcohol industry and other stakeholders and the processes related to developing different forms of laws and regulations.

Different kinds of drinking patterns and the socially integrated consumption of legal and illegal drugs have also received more attention in sociological studies, with a growing focus on recreational use and pleasure and consumption in leisure contexts. This means to privilege the relationship between individuals and drugs in a context of normality, taking into consideration consumers who are not necessarily marginalized. The same consideration is valid when we observe the use of psychoactive substances with the aim of self-medication to face performance anxieties and social expectations.

The explanation of these behaviours has tended to be cast in a theoretical framework that favours individual choice and rationality, although aspects of culture, emotions and norms are also often included in such studies. In this regard, Elster's contribution (1999) appears important: it highlights how in drug and alcohol consumption behaviour and in the establishment of conditions of addiction a complex mixture of neurobiology, culture and choice, including the rational one, play an important role. That is, rational choice is also driven by emotions, circumstances and beliefs around the meaning of a particular behaviour.

Elster belongs to what has been termed analytical sociology (such as Coleman, 1990; Goldthorpe, 2000; Barbera, 2004; Hedstrom, 2005) analysing the 'social mechanisms' that constitute the central element of the connection between the influence of macro and micro variables on the behaviour of individuals. On the micro level, it is possible to identify the factors (e.g. personal relationships, life context, personal incomes, etc.) that make individuals develop certain strategies of action, elaborate preferences or make specific choices. While on the macro level, social and cultural structures define the boundaries and opportunities for such individual decisions making (for example, the nature of the markets – legal or illegal – on which the availability of substances depends). In contemporary society, such dominant cultural structures relate especially to individualism, the search for pleasure, consumerism, the need for group acceptance and the culture of efficiency (Bauman 1998, 2007), elements that among other consequences induce for instance the need for self-medication or lack of compliance with social and legal norms. Moreover, such cultural structures also take part in normalising the use of psychoactive substances – particularly alcohol, cannabis, cocaine and designer drugs –by a large portion of the population and not just in marginal and/or deviant subcultures (Parker et al., 1998, 2002; Parker, 2005; Manning, 2013).

Alongside these contributions, since the end of the 1980s, theories of risk and risk-taking have acquired growing importance and influenced the study of drugs and alcohol. According to Beck (1992), whereas modernity relied on rationality and science, in contemporary 'risk society', science is no longer able to provide answers and solutions to the new risks that are emerging. Uncertainty and insecurity are the main features of our world, so that individuals and societies are more and more concerned about preventing or removing risks. Beck acknowledges that risk is not equally distributed in society, as poor social classes show greater exposure to risky situations, nevertheless, he posits that risks have become individualized making it the subject's own responsibility to make the right choices, and thereby, avoiding risk.

Theories on reflexive individualism and the globalization and individualization of risk (Giddens, 1991; Beck, 1992; Bauman, 1998) have been applied in the sociology of drugs and alcohol to explain how young people weigh pleasure and risk before deciding to take drugs or to drink heavily (Beccaria and Sande, 2003). It has, for instance, been argued that, when young people use psychoactive substances, this is linked to a process of rational choice, that is, young drug and alcohol users are depicted as reflexive agents who integrate drug and alcohol use in their planning of their biography in a world of globalized risks. Or to put it in another way, living in a post-modern risk society requires young people to make rational choices about self-identity and drug consumption, weighing up costs and benefits (Plant and Plant, 1992; Szmigin et al., 2008).

In line with this, France's work (2000) on young people's risk-taking identifies three areas of interest for research: the importance of lay beliefs, the importance of social interaction and power relations and the habituation of risk and risk-taking. As in other areas of risky behaviour, lay beliefs about drugs are actively constructed to make sense of contradictory experiences. First, research shows that young people often react to the bombardment of messages on drug and danger by relying more on experiential sources (Shiner and Newburn, 1997). Second, risk has to be considered as a negotiated process that is a product of social interactions, as shown by risk management among illicit drug injectors (Power et al., 1996). In this study, even if almost all drug injectors (97 per cent) were very aware of the risks of sharing needles and said that they took measures to reduce risk, a number of them stated that one effective strategy for reducing risk is to share needles only with sexual partners. In a more activist approach, the concept of the 'risk environment' has been suggested as a way to analytically overcome the limits of individualism by focussing on how drug related risk is produced institutionally, politically and economically and that changes in these spheres are necessary in order to reduced individual risk (Rhodes, 2002). Third, the habituation of risk-taking affects the process of decision-making. When certain behaviour has become normalized, it is perceived as being at limited risk rather than high risk. In this perspective, 'risk-taking is more a result of how young people interact and negotiate with their social worlds, putting culture and context at the centre of these processes' (France, 2000: 327). Clearly, sociology can play an important role in understanding risk-taking by considering it as a result of an interaction and negotiation process, influenced by broader forces such as gender, power and social exclusion. In this connection, a further area that needs more empirical investigation and theoretical framing is the link between risk and pleasure (Hunt, 2008; Bancroft, 2009). In this direction, a range of studies have emerged such as Duff (2008) and Goulding et al. (2009).

Beck's and Giddens' perspectives on risk have been broadly criticized as having assumed an over-rationalistic and individualist model of human action. Such criticisms are well illustrated by Hilary Pilkington (2007), who posits that research on alcohol and drug use among young people clearly struggles with finding a balance between social structure, context and agency. Young people's response to risk 'is contradictory and complex as they seek to control risk whilst simultaneously professing the importance of selective voluntary risk-taking' (Pilkinton, 2007: 379).

Investigating Russian young people's narratives, Pilkington extended the reflexive self to recognize not only the cognitive mode of reflexivity but also the hermeneutic and aesthetic dimensions of reflexivity. From her field research, it emerges that even if young people may narrate their risk experiences and decisions in making their alcohol and drug choices as individual, they 'draw heavily on narratives of risk and security that are developed collectively within their friendship groups' (Pilkington, 2007: 388). Decisions to consume or not consume are motivated by the group atmosphere and informed by situated non-expert experiences and knowledge. Recognizing that young people's primary point of reference in making decisions on alcohol and drug consumption is other young people, casts doubt on theories of individual rational choice.

This complexity has also been well described by an ethnographic study on drug use in an inner-city Dublin locality with a high concentration of drug problems. In her analysis, Mayock (2005: 351) shows the complexity of the risk practices and the failure of the rational choice approach to capture the 'context-dependent nature of risk decisions and the complex social negotiations and constraints that characterize much drug-taking'. Young people construct an alternative discourse on risk based on daily life and practices, which is frequently in contrast with the official messages on drugs, as their views and beliefs are rarely based on expert warnings about the dangers of psychoactive substances.

Postmodern risk society tends to develop a tension between science, represented by 'experts' in risk assessments and 'lay knowledge', represented by those who have direct experience. This struggle between different types of knowledge expresses its influence on alcohol and drug policies (Duff, 2003).

CONCLUSIONS

As we wrote in the introduction, attempting to adequately cover in one chapter the theories that provide explanations and interpretations of the relationship between individuals, social groups and psychoactive substances (legal and illegal) in the context of the social, economic and cultural conditions that characterize this relationship is not an easy task. There are many ways in which this relationship is structured – from considering substance use as part of everyday normality to extreme marginalisation of some practices. There are many environmental, cultural and social contexts that open opportunities for substance use and that have significance and meaning for people; in addition, there are political and legal contexts that regulate access and opportunities for consumption.

Over time, understanding the link between individuals, social groups and psychoactive substances has benefitted from sociological analyses coming from a number of different perspectives: for example, from a social problem perspective for which solutions should be offered; as harmful behaviour that helps to explain other forms of deviance, for instance, crime; as an example of non-compliant behaviour learned individually or in groups, in the context of subcultures or as part of broader social relationships; as a reaction to stigmatizing definitions within a 'social construction' perspective that relates problem construction to power interests; and finally, within a 'normalization' framework, as consumption that is part of everyday life and is capable of enhancing the positive functions of substances (as well as incurring negative effects).

Contemporary drug and alcohol sociology seems to have abandoned the quest for one-dimensional theoretical explanations, acknowledging that interpreting empirical reality cannot ignore the plurality of situations, conditions, opportunities, representing the structural, cultural and legal frameworks within which individuals move. At the same time, it is not possible to avoid consideration of the choices that individuals make, even in defined contexts, relating to expectations, desires, needs, beliefs, values and rationally pursued goals.

The contribution of recent approaches, discussed above, that aim to theorize the relationship between the macro and micro dimensions, can be useful as they introduce a perspective that continues to value the differences that characterize the real world, differences in the context of structural conditions, in everyday practices and in the different meanings given to these practices by individuals and groups. The advantage of these theories is even more pronounced in societies characterized by 'normative pluralism' that can affect individuals' choices in very different ways.

Moreover, sociology has a significant contribution to make in considering the uses of different psychoactive substances across the ages and the various forms of regulation and control in force at different times and in different cultures. Sociology can enhance our understanding not only in the analysis of current reality, but also in assessing how behaviours (and related issues) change or could change in relation to structural, cultural and legal changes in control policies.

REFERENCES

Acevedo, B. (2007). Creating the cannabis user: a post-structuralist analysis of the re-classification of cannabis in the United Kingdom (2004–2005). *International Journal of Drug Policy*, 18(3): 177–86.

Agnew, R. (1992). Foundation for a general strain theory of crime and delinquency. *Criminology*, 30(1): 47–88.

Akers, R.L. (1992). *Drugs, Alcohol and Society*. Belmont: Wadsworth.

Akers, R.L. and Lee, G. (1996). A longitudinal test of social learning theory: adolescent smoking. *Journal of Drug Issues,* 26: 317–43.

Akers, R.L., Krohn, M.D., Lanza-Kaduce, L. and Radosevich, M. (1979). Social learning and deviant behavior: a specific test of a general theory. *American Sociological Review*, 44: 636–55.

Akers, R.L., La Greca, A.J., Cochran, J. and Sellers, C. (1989). Social learning theory and alcohol behavior among the elderly. *The Sociological Quarterly*, 30(4): 625–38.

Anderson, N. (1923). *The Hobo: The Sociology of Homeless Men*. Chicago: University of Chicago Press.

Aseltine Jr, R.H., Gore, S. and Gordon, J. (2000). Life stress, anger and anxiety, and delinquency: an empirical test of general strain theory. *Journal of Health and Social Behavior*, 41(3): 256–75.

Bacon, S.D. (1943). Sociology and the problems of alcohol: foundations for a sociologic study of drinking behavior. Introduction by E.M. Jellinek. *Quarterly Journal of Studies on Alcohol,* 4: 402–45.

Bakhromov, M. and Levy, J. A. (2013). Double jeopardy through social marginalization: HIV risk among Tajik Male labor migrants in Moscow. *Drug and Alcohol Dependence,* 132: S53–5.

Bancroft, A. (2009). *Drugs, Intoxication and Society*. Cambridge: Polity Press.

Barbera F. (2004). *Meccanismi Sociali. Elementi di Sociologia Analitica*, Bologna: Il Mulino.

Bauman, Z. (1998). *Globalization: The Human Consequences*. New York: Columbia University Press.

Bauman, Z. (2007). *Consuming Life*. Cambridge: Polity.

Beccaria, F. (2010). Drinking styles of the young generations: twenty years' qualitative research. *Salute e Societa,* IX(3): 58–78.

Beccaria, F. and Sande, A. (2003). Drinking games and rite of life projects a social comparison of the meaning and functions of young people's use of alcohol during the rite of passage to adulthood in Italy and Norway. *Young*, 11(2): 99–119.

Beck, U. (1992). *Risk Society. Towards a New Modernity*. London: Sage.

Becker, H.S. (1953). Becoming a Marijuana User. *American Journal of Sociology*, 59: 235–42.

Becker, H.S. (1963). *Outsiders: Studies on the Sociology of Deviance*. New York: The Free Press.

Becker, H. S. (Ed.). (1966). *Social Problems: a Modern Approach*. New York: J. Wiley and Sons.

Bennett, T. and Holloway, K. (2004). Gang membership, drugs and crime in the UK. *British Journal of Criminology*, 44(3): 305–23.

Berridge, V. (2013). *Demons: Our Changing Attitudes Towards Alcohol, Tobacco and Drugs*. Oxford: Oxford University Press.

Brenner, A.B., Bauermeister, J.A. and Zimmerman, M.A. (2011). Neighborhood variation in adolescent alcohol use: examination of socioecological and social disorganization theories. *Journal of Studies on Alcohol and Drugs*, 72(4): 651–9.

Bourgios, P. (2003). *In Search of Respect*. Cambridge: Cambridge University Press.

Box, S. (1992). *Power, Crime, and Mystification*. London: Routledge.

Brody, G.H., Conger, R., Gibbons, F.X., Ge, X., McBride Murry, V., Gerrard, M. and Simons, R.L. (2001). The influence of neighborhood disadvantage, collective socialization, and parenting on African American children's affiliation with deviant peers. *Child Development*, 72(4): 1231–46.

Bulmer, M. (1984). *The Chicago School of Sociology: Institutionalization, Diversity, and the Rise of Sociological Research*. Chicago: University of Chicago Press.

Burgess, E.W. (1925). The growth of the city. In R.E. Park, E.W. Burgess and R.D. McKenzie (eds), *The City*. Chicago: University of Chicago Press, pp. 47–62.

Burgess, E.W. and Bogue, D.J. (1964). *Contributions to Urban Sociology*. Chicago: University of Chicago Press.

Christie, N. and Bruun, K. (1985). *Den Gode Fiende*. Oslo: Universitetsforlaget.

Cloward, R. and Ohlin, L. (1960). *Delinquency and Opportunity*. New York: Free Press.

Cohen, A.K. (1955). *Delinquent Boys*. Glencoe: Free Press.

Coleman, J.S. (1990). *Foundations of Social Theory*. Cambridge: The Belknap Press of the Harvard University Press.

Conrad, P. (1992). Medicalization and social control. *Annual review of Sociology*, 18: 209–32.

Conrad, P. and Schneider, J.W. (1980). *Deviance and Medicalization: From Badness to Sickness*. St. Louis: The CV Mosby Company.

Currie E. (1993). *Reckoning: Drugs, the Cities, and the American Future*. New York: Hill & Wang.

Currie, E. (1997). Market, Crime and community toward a mid-range theory of post-industrial violence. *Theoretical Criminology*, 1(2): 147–72.

Dai, B. (1935). *Opium Addiction in Chicago*. Montclair: Patterson Smith.

Downes, D. and Rock, P. (2003). *Understanding Deviance*. Oxford: Oxford University Press.

Duff, C. (2003). The importance of culture and context: rethinking risk and risk management in young drug using populations. *Health, Risk and Society*, 5(3): 285–99.

Duff, C. (2008). The pleasure in context. *International Journal of Drug Policy*, 19(5): 384–92.

Dunlap E. (1995). Inner-city crisis and drug dealing: portrait of a New York drug dealer and his household. In S. MacGregor and A. Lipow (eds), *The Other City: People and Politics in New York and London*. Atlantic Highlands: Humanities Press, pp. 114–31.

Durkheim, E. (1897). *Le Suicide: Étude de Sociologie*. Paris: Alcan.

Elster J. (1999). *Strong Feelings: Emotion, Addiction and Human Behavior*. Cambridge: MIT Press.

Ennett, S.T., Foshee, V.A., Bauman, K.E., Hussong, A., Cai, L., Reyes, H.L.M., Faris R., Hipp J. and Durant, R. (2008). The social ecology of adolescent alcohol misuse. *Child Development*, 79(6), 1777–91.

Faupel, C.E. (1991). *Shooting Dope: Career Patterns of Hard Core Heroin Users*. Gainesville: University Florida Press.

Fazey, C. (1973). Merton, retreatism and drug addiction: the testing of a theory. *The Sociological Review*, 21(3): 417–36.

Ford, J.A. (2008). Social learning theory and nonmedical prescription drug use among adolescents. *Sociological Spectrum*, 28(3): 299–316.

France A. (2000). Towards a sociological understanding of youth and their risk-taking. *Journal of Youth Studies*, 3(3): 317–31.

Geis, K.J. and Ross C.E. (1998). A new look at urban alienation: the effect of neighborhood disorder on perceived powerlessness. *Social Psychology Quarterly*, 61(3): 232–46.

Giddens, A. (1991). *Modernity and Self-Identity*. Cambridge: Polity.

Goffman, E. (1961). *Asylums*. Garden City: Doubleday.

Goffman, E. (1974). *Stigma. Notes of the Management of Spoiled Identity*. Harmondsworth: Penguin Books.

Goldthorpe J.H. (2000). *On Sociology*. Oxford: Oxford University Press.

Gordon, D.R. (1994). *The Return of the Dangerous Classes: Drug Prohibition and Policy Politics*. New York: W.W. Norton.

Goulding, C., Shankar, A., Elliott, R. and Canniford, R. (2009). The marketplace management of illicit pleasure. *Journal of Consumer Research*, 35(5): 759–71.

Gubrium, J.F. and Holstein, J.A. (eds) (2001). *Institutional Selves: Troubled Identities in a Postmodern World*. Oxford: Oxford University Press.

Gusfield, J. (1981). *The Culture of Public Problems. Drinking-Driving and the Symbolic Order*. Chicago: The University of Chicago Press.

Hallstone, M. (2002). Updating Howard Becker's theory of using marijuana for pleasure. *Contemporary Drug Problems*, 29(4): 821–45.

Harding, G. (1988). Patterns of heroin use: what do we know? *British Journal of Addiction*, 83(11): 1247–54.

Hedstrom P. (2005). *Dissecting the Social. On the Principles of Analitical Sociology*. Cambridge: Cambridge University Press.

Hunt, G. (2008). 'The great unmentionable': exploring the pleasures and benefits of ecstasy from the perspectives of drug users. *Drugs: Education, Prevention and Policy*, 15: 329–49.

Jessor, R. and Jessor, S.L. (1977). *Problem Behavior and Psychosocial Development: A Longitudinal Study of Youth*. New York: Academic Press.

Kandel, D.B. (1980). Drug and drinking behavior among youth. *Annual Review of Sociology*, 6: 235–85.

Karjalainen, K., Lintonen, T., Impinen, A., Lillsunde, P., Mäkelä, P., Rahkonen, O., Haukka J. and Ostamo, A. (2011). Socio-economic determinants of drugged driving – a register-based study. *Addiction*, 106(8): 1448–59.

Lemert, E.M. (1951). *Social Pathology*. New York: McGraw-Hill Book Co.

Levine, H.G. (1991). The promise and problems of alcohol sociology. In P.M. Roman (ed.), *Alcohol: The Development of Sociological Perspectives on Use and Abuse*. New Brunswick: Rutgers Center of Alcohol Studies, pp. 87–112.

Lo, C.C. (2003). An application of social conflict theory to arrestees' use of cocaine and opiates. *Journal of Drug Issues*, 33(1): 237–66.

Manning, P. (2013). *Drugs and Popular Culture in the Age of New Media*. New York: Routledge.

Mayock, P. (2005). 'Scripting' risk: young people and the construction of drug journeys. *Drugs: Education, Prevention and Policy*, 12(5): 349–68.

McCrystal, P., Percy, A. and Higgins, K. (2007). Exclusion and marginalisation in adolescence: the experience of school exclusion on drug use and antisocial behaviour. *Journal of Youth Studies*, 10(1): 35–54.

Merton, R.K. (1938). Social structure and anomie. *American Sociological Review*, 3: 672–82.

Moisan, J., Bourbonnais, R., Brisson, C., Gaudet, M., Vezina, M., Vinet, A. and Regoire, J.P. (1999). Job strain and psychotropic drug use among white-collar workers. *Work and Stress*, 13(4): 289–98.

Monaghan, M. (2014). Drug policy governance in the UK: lessons from changes to and debates concerning the classification of cannabis under the 1971 Misuse of Drugs Act. *International Journal of Drug Policy*, 8(2): 171–91.

Nutt, D., King, L.A., Saulsbury, W. and Blakemore, C. (2007). Development of a rational scale to assess the harm of drugs of potential misuse. *Lancet*, 369(9566): 1047–53.

Østergaard, J. (2009). Learning to become an alcohol user: adolescents taking risks and parents living with uncertainty. *Addiction Research and Theory*, 17: 30–53.

Park, R.E. (1926). The urban community as a special pattern and moral order. In E.W. Burgess (ed.), *The Urban Community*. Chicago: University of Chicago Press, pp. 3–18.

Park, R., Burgess, E. and McKenzie, R.D. (1925). *The City: Suggestions for the Study of Human Nature in the Urban Environment*. Chicago: University of Chicago Press.

Parker, H. (2005). Normalization as a barometer: recreational drug use and the consumption of leisure by younger Britons. *Addiction Research and Theory*, 13(3): 205–15.

Parker H.J., Aldridge, J. and Measham, F. (1998). *Illegal Leisure: The Normalization of Adolescent Recreational Drug Use*. London: Routledge.

Parker, H., Williams, L. and Aldridge, J. (2002). The normalization of 'sensible' recreational drug use: further evidence from the North West England Longitudinal Study. *Sociology*, 36(4): 941–64.

Parks, M.J. (2014). Urban poverty traps: neighbourhoods and violent victimisation and offending in Nairobi, Kenya. *Urban Studies*, 51(9): 1812–32.

Pattison, E.M., Sobell, M.B. and Sobell, L.C. (1977). *Emerging Concepts of Alcohol Dependence*. New York: Springer Publishing Company.

Pilkington, H. (2007). In good company: risk, security and choice in young people's drug decisions. *The Sociological Review*, 55(2): 373–92.

Plant, M. and Plant M. (1992). *Risk-Takers: Alcohol, Drugs, Sex and Youth*. London: Routledge.

Power R., Jones S., Kearns G. and Ward J. (1996). An ethnography of risk management amongst illicit drug injectors and its implications for the development of community-based interventions. *Sociology of Health and Illness*, 18(1): 86–106.

Rhodes, T. (2002). The 'risk environment': a framework for understanding and reducing drug-related harm. *International journal of drug policy*, 13(2): 85–94.

Roizen, R. (1977a). Comment on the 'Rand Report'. *Journal of Studies on Alcohol*, 38: 170–8.

Roizen, R. (1977b). *Alcoholism Treatment's Goals and Outcome Measures: Conceptual, Pragmatic, and Structural Sources of Controversy in the Outcome Debate*. Berkeley: University of California.

Rolando, S., Beccaria, F., Tigerstedt, C. and Törrönen, J. (2012). First drink: what does it mean? The alcohol socialization process in different drinking cultures. *Drugs: Education, Prevention and Policy*, 19(3): 201–12.

Roman, P.M. and Trice, H.M. (1968). The sick role, labelling theory, and the deviant drinker. *International Journal of Social Psychiatry*, 14(4): 245–51.

Room, R. (1983). Sociological aspects of the disease concept of alcoholism. In R. Smart (ed.), *Research Advances in Alcohol and Drug Problems*. New York and London: Plenum Press, pp. 47–91.

Room, R. (2005). Stigma, social inequality and alcohol and drug use. *Drug and Alcohol Review*, 24(2): 143–55.

Room, R, Hellman, M. and Stenius, K. (2015). Addiction: the dance between concepts and terms. *International Journal on Alcohol and Drug Research*, 4(1): 27–35.

Room, R., Rehm, J., Trotter, R.T., Paglia A. and Üstün, T.B. (2001). Cross-cultural views on stigma, valuation, parity and societal attitudes towards disability. In T.B. Üstün, S. Chatterji, J.E. Bickenbach, J.R. Trotter, R. Room, J. Rehm and S. Saxena (eds), *Disability and Culture: Universalism and Diversity*. Seattle: Hogrefe & Huber, pp. 247–91.

Saxe, L., Kadushin, C., Beveridge, A., Livert, D., Tighe, E., Rindskopf, D., Ford, J. and Brodsky, A. (2001). The visibility of illicit drugs: implications for community-based drug control strategies. *American Journal of Public Health*, 91: 1987–94.

Scarscelli, D. (2006). Drug addiction between deviance and normality: a study of spontaneous and assisted remission. *Contemporary Drug Problems*, 33(2): 237–74.

Shiner, M. and Newburn, T. (1997). Definitely, maybe not? The normalisation of recreational drug use amongst young people. *Sociology*, 31(3): 511–30.

Snowdon, C. (2011). *The Art of Suppression*. Ripon: Little Dice.

Sutherland, E.H. (1934). *Principles of Criminology*. Chicago, Philadelphia, New York: Lippincott Company.

Sutherland, E.H. (1949). *White Collar Crime*. New York: Holt, Rinehart & Winston.

Sutherland, E.H. and Cressey, D.R. (1974). *Criminology*. Philadelphia: Lippincott.

Sykes, G.M. and Matza, D. (1957). Techniques of neutralization: a theory of delinquency. *American Sociological Review*, 22(6): 664–70.

Szmigin, I., Griffin, C., Mistral, W., Bengry-Howell, A., Weale, L. and Hackley, C. (2008). Re-framing 'binge drinking' as calculated hedonism: empirical evidence from the UK. *International Journal of Drug Policy*, 19(5): 359–66.

Taniguchi, T.A. and Salvatore, C. (2012). Exploring the relationship between drug and alcohol treatment facilities and violent and property crime: a socioeconomic contingent relationship. *Security Journal*, 25(2): 95–115.

Taniguchi, T.A, Ratcliffe, J.H. and Taylor, R.B (2011). Gang set space, drug markets, and crime around drug corners in Camden. *Journal of Research in Crime and Delinquency*, 48(3): 327–63.

Thomas, W.I. and Znaniecki, F. (1918). *The Polish Peasant in Europe and America*. Boston: Richard G. Badger.

Thrasher, F. (1927). *The Gang. A Study of 1313 Gangs in Chicago*. Chicago: University of Chicago Press.

Weisner, C. M. (1983). The alcohol treatment system and social control: a study in institutional change. *Journal of Drug Issues*, 13(1): 117–33.

Young, J. (1971). *The Drugtakers. The Social Meaning of Drug Use*. London: Paladin.

Yun, M. and Kim, E. (2015). Illicit drug use among South Korean offenders: assessing the generality of social learning theory. *International Journal of Offender Therapy and Comparative Criminology*, 59(11): 1166–87.

Zinberg, N.E. (1984). *Drug, Set and Setting. The Basis for Controlled Intoxicant Use*. New Haven: Yale University Press.

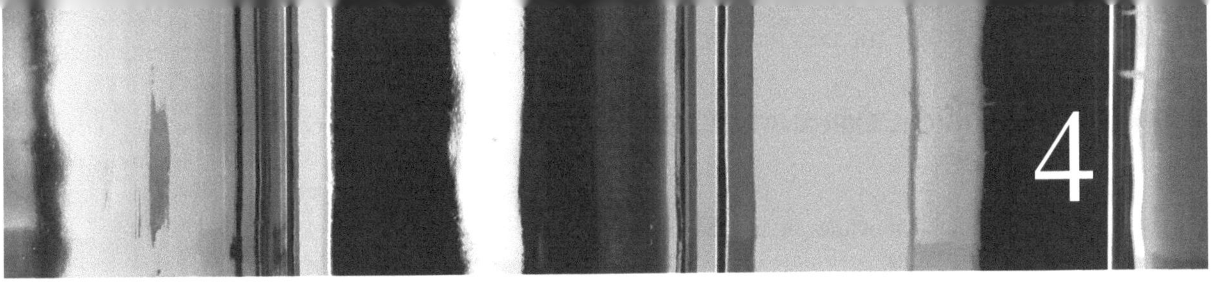

4

Psychological Explanations of Addiction

Robert Hill and Jennifer Harris

INTRODUCTION

Terms such as 'addiction', 'dependence' and 'excessive appetites' are used to describe an individual's overwhelming, intense desire to engage in a particular behaviour, despite the negative consequences of doing so. Addiction is typically thought of as relating to psychoactive substances but encompasses other behaviours that can become compulsive such as eating, gambling, sexual activity, exercising and shopping. While these behaviours are thought to share similar psychological processes, psychoactive substances exert an additional unique neurobiological impact on the brain, psyche and body. With repeated use, the body and mind can adapt to the substance so that, if prevented from taking the substance, they can enter a withdrawal state. This triggers the urge to use in order to gain relief and regain equilibrium. Tolerance develops so that the individual experiences the need for increasingly frequent doses of the substance to maintain biological, neurological and psychological homeostasis. Alongside the typical cycle of craving, substance-seeking and use, relief and withdrawal, there is a concomitant narrowing of interests, social contact and lifestyle in order to focus on the substance. It may seem perplexing that the behaviour continues despite the dwindling positive effects of substance use over time, together with the considerable negative impact on physical and mental health, social, financial and legal aspects of life. Moreover, substance dependence has historically been viewed in terms of a chronic relapsing condition with periods of remission and relapse. The two major psychiatric diagnostic systems, the World Health Organisation's International Classification of Mental and Behavioural Disorders (ICD-10; WHO, 1992) and the American Diagnostic and Statistical Manual of Mental Disorders, Version 5 (DSM-5; APA, 2014), clearly describe the above physiological, behavioural, cognitive and social features of excessive and dependent substance use.

PSYCHOLOGICAL EXPLANATIONS OF ADDICTION

It is intriguing that while all psychoactive substances have the potential for addiction and a not insignificant number of people use such drugs at some point in their lives, only a minority develop dependence.

Psychological formulations of addiction typically view the behaviour as serving some function for the individual, for instance, a desire for social belonging, euphoria or relief from negative emotions. Behaviourist theories focus on external contingencies driving forward addiction, whereas others focus more on individual vulnerabilities such as mental health, inadequate coping skills or cognitive deficits; still others, such as psychodynamic theories, focus more on universal but distorted unconscious developmental patterns. Inconsistencies between goals, thoughts, feelings and behaviours, also raises intriguing questions about the interplay of conscious, controlled responses, sometimes referred to as 'explicit social cognition', and non-volitional drives that are unconscious, automatic responses or so called 'implicit social cognition'.

Our current understanding of addiction tends to adopt elements from a number of theories and in this chapter we focus on: (i) psychodynamic thinking; (ii) behavioural theory; (iii) social learning theory; (iv) cognitive theory; (v) dual process perspectives; (vi) the role of personality and mental health; and (vii) neurobiological and neuropsychological markers. We then introduce addiction-specific models that integrate psychological thinking into an overall framework centred around: (i) motivation; (ii) excessive appetites; and (iii) relapse prevention.

Psychodynamic theories of addiction

Psychodynamic theories provided one of the earliest ways of thinking about addiction. Different schools of psychoanalytic thinking have different theories as to how the personality is shaped, psychopathology develops and change takes place. However, they all share a common belief that our current feelings, thoughts and experiences are affected by our early life experiences and that some of our mental activity is unconscious. Addiction is thought to relate to early experiences of deprivation or over-indulgence, which results in unmet attachment needs, disturbances in the sense of self and difficulties with drive and affect, self-care, dependency and need satisfaction.

Drive/structural models

Freud writing at the turn of the twentieth century viewed the mind as being structured into three entities: the id, ego and superego (Freud, 1984). He saw addiction as being driven from unconscious conflicts between the super-ego and unacceptable id drives. Addiction was thought to result from a fixation at the oral stage of psychosexual development, where early needs for nurturing were frustrated or over-indulged, making the individual vulnerable to excessive nurturance seeking behaviour, including comfort through substances. Defence mechanisms help to maintain the addiction through protecting the individual from full realisation of its harmful effects. Defence mechanisms that are characteristics of addiction include denial, paranoid projection, isolation of affect, rationalisation and intellectualisation. Freudian theory suggests that recovery from addiction might involve making the unconscious conscious and resolving unconscious conflict, and strengthening the ego so that it might better mediate between the id's drive for instant gratification and the high standards set by the super-ego's ideals.

Ego psychology

Ego psychology (Hartmann, 1964) derives from Freudian psychology and focuses on enhancing and maintaining ego function in accordance with the demands of reality. It suggests that early deprivation or over-indulgence can result in varying degrees of ego impairment. This can result in disturbances in the sense of self, difficulties with drive and affect, self-care, dependency and need satisfaction. Substances can come to be used to compensate for these developmental ego defects. The specific effects of different substances can facilitate or impede the attempts of the ego to balance the needs of the internal emotional environment with the demands of external social and physical environment (Khantzian and Treece, 1977).

Object relations

Object relations theorists such as Melanie Klein, Donald Fairbairn and Donald Winnicott link current addiction to the oral stage of development where the infant processes how much they can trust the world to love and care for them (Gomez, 1997). Addiction can be said to reflect early oral modes of relating whereby an individual's basic needs for love and care during infancy have not been met by caretakers and substances later take 'the place of a human relationship' so that the substance is treated 'as the answer to all personal needs without the requirement for reciprocity' (Gomez, 1997: 181).

Attachment theory

John Bowlby (1980) added a relational perspective to object relations, emphasising the impact of real-life events and care-giving over internal psychic or fantasy experiences on psychological development. Attachment theory suggests that all humans have a biological need for attachment, to feel safe and secure (Holmes, 1993) and for mutual affect regulation (Flores, 2004). Bowlby proposed that infants developmental representations of their sense of self and others based on repeated interactions with others. These guide the individual in their later relationships and also influence their ability to regulate affect.

Early caregiving that is sensitive, attuned and responsive encourages infants to develop a secure attachment. Securely attached infants feel confident that they will receive protection and support when alarmed, thereby feeling free to explore and attach to others in a manner that is helpful to meeting their emotional needs. Early caregiving that is inconsistent, disrupted, neglectful or even abusive is likely to interfere with healthy attachment and can result in insecure or disorganised attachment styles. Individuals with an insecure attachment style are more likely to have difficulty forming relationships, may view the world as dangerous, may be more prone to anxiety and less able to tolerate distress and self-soothe, particularly in the absence of supportive relationships. This increases the chances that they might self-medicate their emotional pain through substance use. From this perspective, therapy might offer a safe base to explore the self and develop a secure attachment thus modifying their internal working model and gaining optimal balance between intimacy and autonomy.

Philip Flores has contributed greatly to the concept of addiction as an attachment disorder (2004, 2011). He cites Maclean and Panseep's theory that addiction might replace the endogenous opiates and neuropeptides (dopamine and oxytocin) normally provided by adult attachment so that attachment and addiction might share common neuro-pathways and neurobiology (Flores, 2011). Flores (2004) acknowledged that whilst impaired attachment may cause, or indeed result, from addiction, recovery requires the capacity for healthy interpersonal affect regulation and secure attachment. Flores (2004) emphasises the importance of detaching oneself from the addiction and attaching oneself to treatment, informing approaches such as attachment-oriented therapy (Weegman, 2011).

Self-psychology

Heinz Kohut's (1977) self-psychology places great emphasis on the individual's sense of self and attributed much psychopathology, including addiction, to lack of a cohesive sense of self resulting from early failings in empathic nurturing and unmet early needs. Addiction is viewed as an attempt to repair developmental deficits in the self, where the substance becomes a substitute self-object that meets subconscious developmental needs and is a defence against fragmentation of the self and psychic annihilation (Hoyt, 2011). Recovery comes through developing a cohesive self, internalising qualities previously not internalised from early self-objects and developing healthy intimacy (Hoyt, 2011).

Jungian theory

Carl Jung (1976) felt that substance use changes both the individual's mood and their inner world by merging their fragmented inner world and allowing the experience of (illusory) wholeness. Individuals find that this feeling of wholeness dissolves on sobering up, driving them to repeat their substance use. The AA Historical Materials (http://hindsfoot.org/archive3.html) record how Carl Jung advised Rowland Hazard III, who was influential in the formation of Alcoholics Anonymous (AA), to immerse himself in a spiritual life as another way of achieving completeness in order to overcome alcoholism. Rowland achieved sobriety through the then Oxford Group whose approaches were taken up by Bill Wilson and Dr Bob, co-founders of AA (Schoen, 2009). Flanagan (2013) in discussing AA suggests that it works, not because it is right or correct on many of its core principles, for example, that alcoholism is a disease that necessarily involves loss of control, but rather that it works because it is a repository of collective wisdom about self-control and recovery.

Behavioural theories of addiction

Whilst psychodynamic theories focused on the internal world, behavioural theories adopted the opposite approach. As humans, when we engage in behaviours that are rewarding we tend to try and repeat them. We gain pleasure from natural rewards such as water, food, sex and nurturing and the feelings of pleasure derived from such activities provide positive reinforcement; therefore, the behaviour is repeated. We also gain reward from psychoactive substances such as opiates, cocaine and alcohol. While different substances may have different, specific, psychoactive effects, they appear to activate the same dopamine reward pathway in the brain. This is discussed further within the 'Neurobiological and Neuropsychological' section.

Classical conditioning

Pavlov (1927) in his work on classical conditioning found that an unconditioned stimulus can, if accompanied by a neutral stimulus, result in the development of a conditioned response. With enough repeated exposures, the neutral stimulus becomes a conditioned stimulus provoking a conditioned response. In addiction, this means that when a specific stimulus (neutral stimulus) is repeatedly paired with the effects of substance use (unconditioned stimulus and unconditioned response), the previously neutral stimulus develops the power to trigger the drug effects or craving (i.e. conditioned response). In this way, drug-seeking or craving can be triggered by stimuli that have been paired to substance use (such as a place, person, smell) or by acute stressors/state of stress. Whilst extinction of a paired stimulus and response is extremely difficult, the link between cue and response can be weakened by a number of factors, for instance, (i) cue exposure where the cue (and urge) is not followed by drug-use; (ii) by increasing the range of coping responses to craving; or (iii) aversion therapy where the unwanted behaviour is paired with an unwanted response, for example, taking Disulfiram (Antabuse) so that alcohol ingestion is followed by vomiting.

Operant conditioning

Skinner's (1938) research on operant conditioning is useful in understanding how the consequences of behaviour influence the continuation of that behaviour. Substance use can be both positively and negatively reinforcing. A behaviour that brings pleasure or enjoyment is positively rewarding and increases the likelihood that it will be repeated, thereby reinforcing the behaviour. For example, if drinking alcohol results in a positive effect, such as increased sociability, then sociability is the positive consequence that will reinforce the act of drinking alcohol. Behaviour that brings escape or avoidance from a negative consequence is also rewarding and likely to be repeated. For instance, if drinking alcohol provides relief from anxiety, then the alcohol will be acting as a negative reinforcer. As the addiction continues, the substance misuse may be more negatively reinforced than positively reinforced, although as Orford (2001: 209) points out, there has been a 'move away from a deficit-reduction, escape-avoidance, negative reinforcement model of addiction towards one based upon the pleasure seeking, approach, positive reinforcement of appetitive objects and activities'. Where a behaviour results in negative consequences or a penalty, it is said to be punished and is thought to reduce the probability of repeating the behaviour. Punishment early on in substance use may alter the behaviour; however, it may have less power as the addiction becomes more established.

The timing of the reinforcement can be important in shaping the likelihood of the behaviour continuing. Immediate consequences are more powerfully reinforcing than delayed consequences. As substance use brings an immediate neurobiological reward, it can begin to replace other healthier but slower-acting sources of reward/relief, a concept explored in hyperbolic discounting (Ainslie, 2013). Operant conditioning also highlights how it is harder to extinguish behaviours that are reinforced intermittently than those with predictable consequences, as demonstrated in problematic gambling (Dickerson and O'Connor, 2006). This theory helps to explain how individuals continue to seek out the effects of substances despite overall delayed negative consequences, but is not explicit as to why some people develop a problem. Clinically, recovery may be supported through increasing the immediate salient rewards for healthy choices and/or the development of behaviours incompatible with substance use. These principles have been applied with good effect in approaches such as contingency management (CM), to encourage treatment attendance and adherence. Positive behaviours, such as group attendance, adherence to methadone scripts, drug-free urines and health screening, are systematically reinforced, rewarded with vouchers, weekend methadone scripts, prizes or special privileges. The UK Department of Health recommend CM within their National Institute of Health and Care Excellence (NICE) guidelines as an evidence-based, best practice for addictions (NICE, 2007, CG51).

Hyperbolic discounting

Hyperbolic discounting is a term used to describe a time delay method of judging which alternate activities are worth pursuing and relates to addiction through judgements about present and future behaviours. This theory proposes that immediate, small short-term rewards ('small-soon') are preferred over larger, longer term rewards ('large-later') and that individuals show greater impulsivity, less waiting and lower self-control in the face of immediately accessible rewards, even if waiting longer would bring larger rewards (Ainslie, 2013). Whilst individuals vary in their tendency towards such discounting behaviour, those with addiction difficulties show a stronger tendency towards this than those who are not addicted. Ida (2014), for example, found that smokers placed greater value on the immediate relief gained from smoking than on longer-term health benefits of not smoking. This has important implications for judgements made in the face of high-risk situations, craving states, emotional dysregulation and ambivalence and it is similar to the problem of immediate gratification discussed in the relapse prevention literature (Marlatt and Gordon, 1985).

Social learning theory of addiction

Social learning theory or as it later became known 'social-cognitive theory' elaborates on behavioural ideas to include cognitive processes. Bandura (1977) in his idea of 'reciprocal determinism' suggested that not only does the environment influence the individual but that the individual also influences the environment such that there is 'a continuous interaction between cognitive, behavioural, and environmental determinants' (Bandura, 1977: 7). He proposed that while we do learn by direct experience, we also learn indirectly by observing others around us ('observational learning'; 'social modelling'). Through watching, making sense of and encoding ('symbolising'), how, for example, a parent uses alcohol to relax or socialise, we develop our own substance-related 'outcome expectancies' (Brown et al., 1987). Such expectancies can consciously or unconsciously mediate our own behaviour towards initiating and continuing substance use (Brown, 1993). We are more likely to imitate models of the same sex and those of higher status and we are also motivated to model behaviour we have previously been rewarded for, have observed being rewarded ('vicarious learning') or imagine will bring rewards ('incentives'). We are motivated not to copy behaviour where we have previously been punished for this, observe/recall others being punished or are threatened with punishment. There is some evidence to support this from research investigating the intergenerational transmission of addiction. Children of parents with an addiction do show an increased risk for later developing their own addiction, as well as other mental health and interpersonal difficulties. However, parental addiction in itself is not a sufficient risk factor and it interacts with numerous other risk factors such as stressors, poverty, unemployment, neglect, trauma, disrupted education and protective factors within the child, parent and community relationships (Evans et al., 2014). Social learning theory also gives powerful support to the importance of being around others who are also in recovery, for instance, in various Fellowship groups. Bandura's ideas around 'self-regulation' and 'self-efficacy' also lend themselves to understanding addiction and they are important components of the relapse prevention model.

Cognitive theory of addiction

Cognitive theory as applied to addiction focuses on how addictive beliefs shape addiction and can be targeted to promote recovery. As many high-risk situations are internal or inevitable, cognitive therapy helpfully focuses on individuals modifying their belief systems rather than simply relying on avoiding or coping with high-risk situations. The cognitive perspective focuses on how the individual's interpretation of situations influences their subsequent feelings and behaviours and that these interpretations are shaped from core beliefs developed during early life. Core beliefs broadly fall into two themes, 'I am unlovable' and 'I am helpless' (Beck et al., 1993). The cognitive theory of addiction proposes that individuals also develop addictive beliefs alongside their beliefs about the self; these may reflect social learning processes (e.g. seeing family members cope by drinking alcohol), fit with core beliefs about the self (e.g. 'I am powerless') and become activated in response to life stressors, particular contexts or emotions.

The cognitive theory of addiction suggests that beliefs are activated in a particular sequence starting with *anticipatory beliefs* about the expected effects from using drug/alcohol such as 'drinking will help me to relax'. As the individual begins to rely on substances to cope with distress, they will also develop *relief-oriented beliefs* that have a more imperative quality (e.g. 'I need a drink to cope'). These sets of beliefs, which are sometimes referred to under the term 'positive outcome expectancies', trigger cravings and they are likely to be acted upon if they remain unchallenged. Furthermore, inhibitions about using/drinking are overcome by *permission-giving beliefs* that justify drinking/using or minimise harm ('I've worked hard this week and deserve a line of coke'; 'just one drink won't matter'), thereby allowing the individual to act on plans to seek out and use/drink. Beliefs also shape an individual's reaction to physiological sensations associated with anxiety and craving (Beck et al., 1993). Orford (2001: 221) notes that whilst 'cognitive processes may operate outside or on the borders of consciousness' it is 'self-talk, self-statements and the use of self-instruction' that may both contribute to the development of, and the solution to, excessive behaviours.

Dual process perspectives of addiction

Dual system models focus on understanding addiction from the perspective of the joint operation of a controlled, reflective response system and an automatic, impulsive response system (Norman and Shallice, 1986). More recent work on non-reflective approaches to addiction includes the idea of implicit cognition, which is seen as a default in human decision and as 'automatic, implicit and associative' (Stacy and Wiers, 2010: 17). Implicit cognition suggests that 'influential cognitions are the ones that are spontaneously activated during critical decision points' (Stacy and Wiers, 2010: 1). It is thought that such activations occur due to associations in memory but remain below conscious awareness. This unconscious or automatic processing does not refer to the stimuli or content (i.e. the drug or drug-related cues), but refers to the process of activation itself, so that there is conscious awareness of the stimuli but unconscious awareness of the effects of the stimuli (Stacy and Wiers, 2010: 2). Such activations can be viewed in terms of a default mechanism that can only be overridden with sustained practice and where there are efficient executive and working memory process at work, although, as Borland (2014) notes below, such executive processes may not be sufficient in order to sustain the maintenance of changed behaviour.

Borland's context, executive and operational systems model (2014)

Borland's model (2014) focuses on 'hard to maintain' behaviour changes such as changing/eliminating negative behaviour and achieving/sustaining positive behaviour change. Borland acknowledges that what is needed for initial behaviour change is not the same as that needed to maintain such behaviour change. This model assumes that all behaviour change occurs within the matrix of the particular individual and their external environment and that these interact with two internal processes, the operational system (OS) and executive system (ES). The OS controls the means by which we act on the world on a moment by moment basis; it operates automatically and it is focused on action. The ES is essentially linguistic and logical, and it is involved in self-regulation and determining preferential future courses of action. It is the ES's function to monitor the OS, particularly in novel and/or complex situations, and where necessary, override the OS's automatic response. While addiction and dependence can be thought of as becoming part of the OS, the ES is necessary to initiate changes in substance use, for example, overcome automatic responses such as craving states. However, in order for behaviour change to be sustained, the OS needs to take over the function of the ES, so that the newly changed behaviour operates on a more automatic basis.

Reflective-impulsive model (Strack and Deutsch, 2004)

Strack and Deutsch's (2004) reflective-impulsive model (RIM) views addiction as the outcome of two classes of process, one that is relatively automatic, appetitive and impulsive (the 'impulsive system', IS) and a second class that is relatively controlled, effortful and reflective (the 'reflective system', RS). Both processes can occur consciously and unconsciously. The 'impulsive system' processes information rapidly, drawing on its long-term memory storage of associative networks to influence cognitive and behaviour schemata/sets. Associations do not have time-codes so that there is no differentiation between past, present and future. When representations (sensory, affective, behaviour information) repeatedly co-occur, they form associative clusters. Associations activate behavioural schemata and repetition develops the connections between antecedents (e.g. setting, cues, context, mood), behaviour (e.g. drink alcohol) and consequences (e.g. relief). Chronic substance use leads to changes in associative structure and therefore influences future processing of behaviour. The IS is thought to be involved in addiction phenomena such as conditioned withdrawal and tolerance, drug habits and incentive sensitisation. As the short-term memory of the 'reflective system' has no longer-term memory to draw from, it must process stimuli each time they are encountered and activate behaviour through deliberate, effortful decision-making. The RS can use information stored in the IS to form judgements and decisions. Within addiction, the RS is thought to be involved in rational choice and outcome expectancies. A state of deprivation (e.g. withdrawal, craving) will rapidly make the representation of immediate drug-effects accessible in the IS and activate thoughts/behaviours that lead to consumption (Deutsch and Strack, 2005). Appetite can be triggered by outside awareness and then receive little control by the conscious processes, helping to explain the seemingly irrational behaviour observed within addiction. During the acute effects of a substance, automatic appetitive processes (IS) become stronger and executive functions (RS) become weaker. The imbalance between increased impulsive appetite, reduced motivation to regulate and weakened executive control increases with repeated use, an effect that seems most pronounced in individuals with weak pre-morbid executive functioning.

According to the dual process model, neuro-adaptation results in sensitisation of the impulsive system to substance-related cues, these cues automatically and preferentially capture attention and result in an automatic approach action. There is also a concurrent down-regulation or interference of the controlled reflective system that might reflect on the cost-benefit of doing this and inhibit the approach action. Hence, longer term substance use results in impaired executive functions (inhibition) that regulate the impulsive system and simultaneously sensitise the impulsive system. These ideas have led to the development of tests to assess attentional bias and memory associations and interventions such as attentional retraining and techniques to help recovery oriented action plans become more automatic.

The above explanations tend to start with an assumption of homogeneity or population normality in that they do not distinguish between individuals and treat everyone as essentially the same. This is clearly far from the case clinically and the next section highlights disorders, whether developmental or acquired, which may either be the determining factor in addiction or at least as a cofounding variable in relation to the above models.

Neurobiological and neuropsychological theories of addiction

It is obviously a matter of some debate whether neurobiological and neuropsychological models of addiction fit into a psychological framework or a strict biological one. Both look to locate the source of addiction within the biology or neuropsychology of an individual. The evidence for over-activation of the brain's reward pathways is accumulating and it is the mesolimbic dopamine pathway that seems to be mainly responsible for the rewarding use of both alcohol and drugs irrespective of the amount of effort associated with their use. This reward circuit is designed for survival, to grab our attention and drive us towards activities that ensure pleasure and survival. Within addiction, these same processes of motivation and compulsion are hijacked and taken over. While each substance has its own distinct neurobiological effect, all drugs directly or indirectly activate the reward circuit to bring feelings of pleasure. Repeated use leads to neuro-adaptation and behaviour moves from being voluntary and mediated by the frontal lobe/executive functioning to being more habitual and automatic and focused on processes in the midbrain.

As part of striving for homeostasis and the process of neuro-adaptation, neurons respond to the increased levels of dopamine activated by chronic drug use by down regulating their receptors. Not only does the reward system become dependent on ingesting drugs to feel normal, it also needs increasing doses to achieve normality and normal rewards lose their salience. Dysphoria replaces euphoria and negative reinforcement takes over from positive reinforcement. Thombs (2006) suggests that preserved memories for such rewards and/or diminishing ability to create natural highs may be the explanation for the focus on drugs and alcohol as the primary source of gratification. As well as neuro-adaptation, substance use causes cell death.

Neuropsychological approaches to addiction tend to focus on those deficits that make self-regulation of behaviour and emotions more difficult and thereby contribute to the development and maintenance of addictive behaviours. Executive functioning (EF) is particularly important in this respect due to its role as a mediator of self-regulation. Neuro-anatomically, EF is often used to refer to the frontal lobes or pre- frontal cortex due to its role in planning, rule-switching, inhibition, working memory and, more generally, self-regulation (Barkley, 2012). EF also supports other neuropsychological processes such as intellectual functioning, working and prospective memory (Griffiths et al., 2012). Given the importance for recovery of forming and sustaining goals and plans, maintaining motivation and altering plans and goals in response to new information, any deficit in EF and memory will, it could be argued, have a huge effect on the ability to pursue substance regulation and treatment goals. Indeed, damage to any of the components of the memory system as well as frontal executive type difficulties have both been shown to be associated with poorer outcomes amongst those with substance use (Manning et al., 2008, Griffiths et al., 2012).

Around half of all clients entering treatment for alcohol dependence have some cognitive impairment (Wang et al., 1993; Morgenstern and Bates, 1999). This may be due to impact of high levels of alcohol on the body and brain and thiamine deficiency, as in Wernicke's disease (Kopelman, 1995), as well as the increased risk of head injury and accident (Knight and Longmore, 1993; Walker et al., 2001). There is some debate as to whether EF deficits persist after detoxification in all clients (Noel et al., 2001) or just in those with Korsakoff's syndrome (Van der Plas et al., 2009: 715).

Despite a renewed interest in neuropsychological deficits and functioning, treatment approaches in addiction have tended to adopt either a knowledge deficit model or, more recently, a psychological/emotional regulation deficit model in which the role of psychological factors in the initiation and maintenance of addictive behaviours is given more prominence than cognitive deficits. The result is that deficits associated with mild-moderate neuropsychological impairments in alcohol dependence are rarely incorporated into current treatment modalities. Where such deficits are not recognised an over emphasis on rationality can take place, whereas a focus on those factors such as reduced attention, poor memory and poor self-regulatory control may actually, be more beneficial for longer-term behavioural change.

The role of personality and mental health in addiction

The prevalence of dual diagnosis, whereby an individual experiences an addiction together with a mental health disorder, personality disorder and/or cognitive impairment is extremely high. Difficulties with substance use are high in those with a primary mental health problem and levels, particularly of anxiety and depression, are elevated within populations of substance users. Weaver et al. (2003) found that 44 per cent of a sample of clients presenting at mental health services had also used drug/alcohol at a problematic level in the last year. Similarly, they found that 75 per cent of clients attending drug services and 80 per cent of those attending alcohol services had mental health difficulties. It is well established that mental health and substance misuse problems can precipitate and perpetuate each other (Tiet and Mausbach, 2007) and that dual diagnosis adds complexity to the individual's needs and if left unaddressed can contribute to difficulty engaging in, and adhering with, treatment (Department of Health, 2007).

There are a number of mechanisms that explain the high comorbidity between substance misuse and mental health. Zimberg (1999) identifies three different types of dual diagnosis. He identifies Type 1 as a primary mental health problem where substances are used as a means of self-medication for that disorder (Zimberg, 1999), that is, an adaptive attempt to heal, self-repair and self-care (Khantzian et al., 1990). For example, an individual with post-traumatic stress disorder (PTSD) may use alcohol to dampen the experiences of hyperarousal. Khantzian is credited with coining the term '*self-medication*' hypothesis and also proposed a specific psychopharmacological match between the individual's psychological needs and their drug of choice. He proposed that heroin may be preferred to manage uncontrollable rage and aggression; alcohol to allow the ordinarily cut-off individual to connect with others to experience comfort, closeness and manage aggression; and cocaine to counter depression, hypomania and hyperactivity. While it is useful to consider the substance's psychological function for the individual, specific predictions about drugs of choice have not been supported by psychometric studies of clinical samples (Greene et al., 1993; Schinka et al., 1994). Where there is a primary mental health problem, associated distress and negative feelings are likely to surface during or after detoxification and become significant predictors of craving and relapse. Clients with an untreated diagnosed anxiety disorder are shown to be significantly more likely to meet criteria for drinking relapse in the months after entering alcohol treatment (Kushner et al., 2005) and depression is a significant predictor of craving among alcohol dependent clients (Yoon et al., 2006). This highlights the importance of screening for mental health and offering interventions that target both the mental health and substance misuse.

Zimberg (1999) defines a Type 2 problem as a primary substance misuse problem with substance-induced mental health problems. This might be thought of as a '*toxicity*' hypothesis; the substance may directly or indirectly contribute to the development of mental health difficulties, cognitive impairment, and sometimes, perceived personality disorder. Individuals can experience acute psychological symptoms such as paranoia, delusions, hallucinations, anxiety, suicidal thoughts during intoxication or withdrawal. Alcohol use is likely to be a causative factor in anxiety disorder development (Allan, 1995) and dependent drinkers have a higher prevalence of head injury than the non-dependent population, placing them at greater risk of acquired cognitive deficits. Increasing evidence shows that smoking skunk increases the risk of developing psychosis (Di Forti et al., 2009). The psychosocial consequences of addiction, such as isolation, poverty, stigma, loss and narrowing of interests, are also likely to indirectly contribute to poor mental health. Individuals who engage in risky behaviours, or who are intoxicated, may place themselves at a greater risk of trauma and subsequent PTSD, or substance misuse itself, via neurobiological processes, unhelpful coping or avoidance of processing, may increase the likelihood of a PSTD reaction after a trauma (Ouimette and Read, 2014).

Zimberg (1999) classifies a Type 3 problem as a co-existing mental health problem and/or personality disorder together with substance misuse. Such comorbidity might reflect shared predisposing factors that may underlie both the mental health and addiction presentations. Evans et al. (2014) offer a useful description of possible shared predisposing factors, including those relating to demographics, family (modelling of substance use, mental health, disrupted attachments), social factors and environment (earlier trauma, poverty, isolation), genetics (foetal alcohol syndrome, assortative mating), neurobiology and personality characteristics (e.g. unstable personality disorder, anti-social personality disorder).

Controversy continues over whether there is evidence to support the idea of personality traits that predispose an individual to addiction, namely an 'addictive personality'. However, Lang (1983) has identified some personality characteristics that seem typical of those who develop addiction, namely difficulty tolerating stress, impulsivity, nonconformity, sense of social alienation, little value on socially valued achievements and tolerance for deviance.

SPECIFIC/INTEGRATIVE MODELS OF ADDICTION

Despite there being a number of different theories as to why individuals develop problems with substances, no one theory is sufficient for explaining the complexity of addiction. In this next section, we examine some thinking around motivation, excessive appetites and relapse prevention.

Approaches to understanding motivation

Addiction might be understood as a motivation problem (Miller, 1998). Motivation can be thought of as steering us, providing energy and direction for our behaviour. We have instinctive drives towards food, water and sexual activity for survival but also motives for social contact and curiosity (Mitcheson and Grellier, 2011). Motivation is also thought of as part of the drive-reduction theory or as a mechanism to maintain homeostasis. Motivation may be 'extrinsic' in that it is driven by gaining rewards and/or avoiding punishments or it may be 'intrinsic' in that it exists within the individual for its own sake.

Incentive salience theory (Robinson and Berridge, 1993)

Motivation biases our attention and cognitive processing towards goal-related stimuli (such as addiction-stimuli) and subsequent achievement of our goals is positively or negatively reinforced. Substance use produces a dopaminergic response that becomes sensitised with each use ('incentive salience'). Conditioning also causes stimuli/cues to elicit conditioned dopaminergic responses (Franken, 2003). Substance use and related stimuli are therefore automatically processed and as they are perceived as salient and preferential, they acquire strong motivational properties and become an important goal that triggers craving and activation of approach behaviours. Through classical conditioning, cues acquire incentive-motivational properties and grab attention (Robinson and Berridge, 2008). Addiction is likely when this occurs together with reduced executive control over impulses (Stacy and Wiers, 2010).

Motivational interviewing (Miller and Rollnick, 2013)

Motivational interviewing (MI) is a counselling style that addresses what Miller and Rollnick (2013) view as core to addiction and recovery, namely ambivalence and motivation. They view ambivalence, the being 'in two minds' or 'feeling strongly towards two incompatible choices' as normal and expected within the process of addiction and recovery. From this viewpoint, motivation is a state that fluctuates in response to shifting personal, cognitive, behavioural and environmental determinants (Bandura, 1986) and requires harnessing before other techniques such as relapse prevention (RP) can be successful. Miller and Rollnick (2013) coined the phrase 'ready, willing and able'. Discrepancy between present reality and future values is registered by the self-regulation system and creates a state of discomfort, 'ambivalence' or 'cognitive dissonance' as Festinger (1957) described it. This may well result in the individual seeing the importance of change ('willing') and searching for options for positive change. However, the individual needs to feel confident of succeeding in their plans ('able'), if not, they may well rationalise their thinking ('my drinking isn't such a problem') to be in line with the problem behaviour (carry on drinking). Actions are only likely to be taken when the individual also feels that these are important now ('ready'). MI offers some extremely useful therapist skills that help build therapeutic relationships, explore and resolve ambivalence and enhance intrinsic motivation for change.

The transtheoretical model of change (Prochaska and DiClemente, 1986)

The transtheoretical model of change (Prochaska and DiClemente, 1986) suggests that the process of change involves moving through five stages: *pre-contemplation, contemplation, preparation, action, maintenance* (and *relapse*). This model is best understood as a motivational model and is useful for helping us to understand where an individual may be in their addiction and their readiness for change, thereby allowing interventions to be more effectively targeted. It does not offer an understanding of how an addiction may have developed or be maintained. An individual who is in *pre-contemplation* may not be aware that they have a problem with addiction or may have no intention to change. While others may see there is a problem, the individual may become defensive when pressure is placed on them to change. In *contemplation*, the individual may begin to show some distress about the addiction and begin to consider the pros and cons of making a change. Those in *preparation* are more clearly ready to change their attitudes and behaviour and with appropriate support can move into the *action* stage, which is marked by taking steps to change and learning skills to make these changes. During the *maintenance* stage the individual is focused on sustaining and strengthening their recovery. Individuals can exit the cycle at any time and return to an earlier stage. *Relapse* prevention is most appropriate during the *action* and *maintenance* stages together with Twelve-Step approaches and structured treatments.

The PRIME theory of motivation (West, 2006)

Robert West (2006) has pieced together the wealth of knowledge about motivation in order to formulate an integrated model, called the PRIME theory of motivation. PRIME is an acronym for 'plans', 'responses', 'impulses/inhibitory forces', 'motives' and 'evaluations'. West (2006) proposes that this theory has significant implications for the formulation of addiction's interventions.

PRIME theory proposes that the motivational system operates at different levels of complexity from simple reflex responses to motives and evaluations. *Motives* allow us to consider the possible outcomes of our behaviour and manifest themselves in our conscious awareness as feelings such as 'want', 'desire' or 'need'. Past experience will influence the generation of these motives. When motives are in competition, avoidance behaviours may be used. *Evaluations* involve the world being represented in terms of 'beliefs', which through their influence on motives, can indirectly affect our behaviour. Competing evaluations result in dissonance: an uncomfortable state that motivates us to suppress, change or add new beliefs to try and resolve the dissonance. *Plans* are formulated when we cannot act upon an evaluation immediately. Of particular importance are plans for lifestyle change (e.g. giving up drugs/alcohol). Such plans are internally dictated, lack discrete action sequences, can exist even when we are not acting in accordance with those plans and are long-term requiring a sustained level of commitment and motivation.

While this theory lacks the ability to make explicit predictions and recommendations, West (2006) does highlight some resulting principles of key relevance for addiction and relapse prevention. He suggests that any of these motivational levels can malfunction and an effective intervention needs to address the whole motivational system. However, many interventions, for example, motivational interviewing, assume 'rationality' as integral to their execution and target higher levels of the motivational system, such as *Evaluations*, whilst arguably neglecting lower level processes, such as emotional forces, drives, habits and impulse control. West (2006) recommends that the full range of abnormalities needs to be identified, including dysfunctional beliefs, feelings, impulses, sense of identity, propensity to self-control and habit. This requires that different treatment elements should be combined or when limited by resources, the PRIME theory can help determine which element of the motivational system is best to target in which cases.

West (2006) therefore views current approaches to relapse prevention as unlikely to provide clear benefits. He proposes that for effective relapse prevention to happen, a radical change in identity is necessary, the individual's social and physical environment requires remodelling as far as possible and long-term medication is important to dampen drives and enhance impulse control. He proposes that in extreme cases, abnormalities and imbalances can be reduced but no 'cure' is possible and recovery is best viewed as long-term management.

Excessive appetites (Orford, 2001)

Jim Orford provides a neat attempt to explain why some people develop excessive appetites and describes his model as a Social-Behavioural-Cognitive-Moral model. In his book, *Excessive Appetites*, Orford (2001) has written two chapters that are particularly important for considering 'how appetites that mostly give pleasure, delight, joy or harmless entertainment can sometimes become so excessive that they threaten to spoil our lives' (Orford, 2001: 201). 'Overcoming Restraint', looks at those factors that differentiate one person's ability to regulate their use of substances from another who cannot. 'The Development of Strong Attachment', focuses on the development of what he terms 'highly troublesome and noticeable excess'.

Orford examines the so called 'conformity curve', or skewed distribution of problematic substance use, and identifies two factors that predispose an individual to excess, namely unconventionality and non-conformity. In essence, it appears that the majority of the population will restrict their behaviour on the basis of social conformity or other similar deterring forces, such as the presence of other incompatible rewarding behaviours that results in an inter-play of inclining and restraining forces, as highlighted earlier through social learning theory. Orford then proposes a number of factors that tip the balance into noticeable excess, beginning with social change or transition that is a deeper immersion into the world of substance use and a subsequent reduction in non-using social activities. This factor ties in with ICD-10 criteria for dependence, namely the 'progressive neglect of alternative pleasures or interests because of psychoactive substance use, increased amount of time necessary to obtain or take the substance or to recover from its effects'. Orford also notes a reduction in discrimination, so that restrictions and judgements about when, where and in what circumstances it is appropriate to use become less frequent, contributing to a sort of normalisation process to the changed behaviour state. Finally, Orford, cites how appetite or substance specific attention and memory schemata contribute to excessive use.

Models of relapse prevention

Model of relapse prevention (Marlatt and Gordon, 1985)

Traditional models of addiction tended to view substance use in dichotomous terms with relapse as an end point or treatment failure, attributable to endogenous factors such as cravings and withdrawals, symptoms of an underlying disease state or lack of willpower or motivation. Marlatt and Gordon's (1985) model introduced an important conceptual shift in viewing relapse not as a spontaneous event but rather the last step in a series of events. Their model emphasised the role of contextual factors in triggering relapse and viewed relapse/recovery as a fluctuating process. Lapses were viewed as temporary setbacks ('a fork in the road') that offered opportunities for therapeutic intervention and learning. Within this model, return to full blown use also allowed the possibility of re-instating positive changes and recovery. Hence, it offered a flexible more optimistic view of behaviour change/lapse/relapse (Hendershot et al., 2011). It also offered a framework to intervene in this process to prevent and manage relapse. Indeed, alongside motivational interviewing (Miller and Rollnick, 2002) and Prochaska and DiClemente's transtheoretical model, relapse prevention has had the greatest influence in the addictions field over the last 20 years (Mitcheson et al., 2010).

Marlatt and Gordon (1985) combined cognitive, behavioural and Bandura's social learning thinking about addiction to offer a conceptual model of relapse and a set of cognitive and behavioural strategies to prevent or limit relapse episodes. It focuses on how an individual might effectively cope with encountering a high-risk situation (HRS), that is, any situation or mood state that threatens an individual's resolve to maintain change. A positive coping response is likely to lead to increased self-efficacy and reduced likelihood of relapse. However, failure to cope with a HRS is likely to result in lowered self-efficacy and positive expectancies from using/drinking, and therefore, lead into an initial slip or lapse. The model suggested that whether or not the slip leads into a relapse may depend on subsequent cognitive processes such as dissonance, rule violation effect and positive outcome expectancies.

A second part of Marlatt and Gordon's model addresses the longer-term maintenance of change through highlighting the covert factors that can contribute to later relapse. They highlight the risk of lifestyle imbalance where inadequate coping skills for everyday life can result in the accumulation of stressors and individuals starting to feel 'hard done by' and desiring indulgence. The probability of lapse is further increased by urges and cravings combined with positive outcome expectancies from using and supported by cognitive processes such as seeking immediate gratification, denial, justification and seemingly irrelevant decisions where one sets oneself up for a lapse by a series of decisions over time. Therefore, RP strategies aimed to teach individuals to anticipate, recognise and cope with the possibility of relapse using specific techniques such as identifying and coping with high-risk situations, enhancing self-efficacy, lapse management, cognitive restructuring, balanced lifestyle, stimulus control, urge management, and individualised relapse road maps.

The dynamic model of relapse (Witkiewitz and Marlatt, 2004)

While the original relapse model offered a useful framework and set of techniques, it was criticised for being rather a static, linear, two-dimensional model that did not adequately account for negative emotional states, craving and withdrawal, motivation, cultural differences and social support. Clients, clinicians and researchers observed how a seemingly insignificant shift in one factor can kindle a downward spiral in other factors that result in relapse. Witkiewitz and Marlatt (2004) looked to explain the observed fluctuations in abstinence and relapse, and found this to fit well with catastrophe theory, the study of sudden discontinuous changes in behaviour resulting from slight continuous changes in system parameters (Witkiewitz and Marlatt, 2007). They therefore developed their thinking to account for these criticisms and new research findings to put forward their dynamic model of relapse (Witkiewitz and Marlatt, 2004).

This model does not abandon the original structure but rather adds more dimensions. This is a complex model that incorporates the multidimensional, dynamic, unpredictable nature of lapse/relapse. It presents relapse as a complex system of multiple elements that interact dynamically within a high-risk situation to maintain the status quo or tip the balance towards changes in substance use. Tonic processes are conceptualised as those factors that confer chronic vulnerability to relapse/substance use such as background factors (family history, social support, degree of dependence, comorbid psychiatric conditions, cognitive impairment) ('distal relapse risks'). Phasic processes are conceptualised to reflect characteristics and responses to the immediate HRS ('proximal relapse risks') and include cognitive processes, physical withdrawal, craving, coping behaviours, affective state and shift in social support. Cognitive processes and physical withdrawal are said to span both chronic vulnerability and phasic responses. The relationship between distal and proximal factors is contextual. The phasic response represents the 'turning point' in this dynamic model that can lead to sudden changes in substance use.

The dynamic model of relapse awaits scientific investigation and clinical application and some authors, such as Hunter-Reel et al. (2009), consider the dynamic model continues to downplay the importance of interpersonal factors as these are represented as distal factors. One study, the COMBINE measures (Anton et al., 2006), used a multi-method approach to evaluate latent class models of 1383 participants over 68 weeks post alcohol treatment. They found support for components of the dynamic model and the relationships between static and dynamic factors during and post treatment. Their conclusions highlighted the importance of targeting craving, negative affect and stress during treatment, particularly among individuals with dual diagnosis and targeting craving and negative affect post treatment. Small changes in mood resulted in large changes to drinking behaviours. Relapse road maps and warnings to clients about the HRS of negative emotions.

Mindfulness-based relapse prevention (Witkiewitz et al., 2005)

While relapse prevention remains a proficient tool for recovery, it could be argued that it emphasises the deliberate, conscious, controlled processes of behaviour and may overlook the automatic, habitual processes of addiction, processes that are highlighted in dual process models. The incorporation of mindfulness training or so called third wave CBT approaches with RP techniques into a comprehensive treatment programme called mindfulness-based relapse prevention (MBRP; Witkiewitz et al., 2005) has attempted to counter habitual processes. MBRP has been shown to result in improved abstinence rates, reduced drug and alcohol use (Kadden, 2001), reduced relapse rates (Carroll, 1996; Irving et al., 1999; Bowen et al., 2009) and to be effective for individuals with dual diagnosis (Witkiewitz and Bowen, 2010). Practicing mindfulness allows individuals to develop awareness, acceptance and tolerance of thoughts, feelings and sensations that may arise as internal triggers to substance use, and encourages using this awareness to activate explicit skills and strategies early on in the high-risk situation. Marlatt and Ostafin (2005) usefully explain how mindfulness targets some of the automatic processes of addiction, for example, countering attentional bias by enhancing attention and countering avoidance by nurturing acceptance. They note how the accepting attitude of mindfulness towards present moment experience, 'having a different agenda' as they put it, without seeking to change or avoid it, can lead to a reduction in use. Recent work has also begun to look towards how best to combine Alcoholics Anonymous, CBT and Buddhist Mindfulness (Dermatis and Egelko, 2014).

CONCLUSION

This chapter has been primarily about psychological models and theories of addiction. As will hopefully have become apparent there is a great deal of crossover between seemingly different theories. Thus, whilst psychodynamic models and implicit cognition may be quite different, both highlight the importance of sub-threshold awareness within addiction. This idea may also, to some extent, relate to the impact of neuropsychological deficits. Consequently, one might conclude that our current state of knowledge regarding the psychology of addiction would best acknowledge processes occurring both at the conscious level, such as self-efficacy and contingency management, as well as those occurring unconsciously and more implicitly. This has implications for treatment approaches and highlights the important role that lifestyle balance, recovery and mindfulness-based approaches can have. This chapter does not, however, discuss some of the other significant factors that influence addiction, such as social, economic and cultural determinants, systems theory or rational choice theory. It is important to note their potential causal influence when considering addiction-and acknowledge that psychological understanding always operates in a particular context, and that certainly, as far as prevention and treatment outcomes go, it is both the external as well as the internal world of clients that matters.

REFERENCES

Ainslie, G. (2013). Money as MacGuffin: A factor in gambling and other process addictions. In: *Addiction and Self-Control. Perspectives from Philosophy, Psychology and Neuroscience*, N. Levy (ed.). Oxford. Oxford University Press, pp. 16–37.

Allan, C.A. (1995). Alcohol problems and anxiety disorders–a critical review. *Alcohol and Alcoholism*, 30(2): 145–51.

Anton, R.F., O'Malley, S.S., Ciraulo, D., Cisler, R.A., Couper, D., Donovan, D.M., Gastfriend, D.R., Hosking, J.D., Johnson, B.A., LoCastro, J.S., Longabaugh, R., Mason, B.J., Mattson, M.E., Miller, W.R., Pettinati, H.M., Randall, C.L., Swift, R., Weiss, R.D., Williams, L.D. and Zweben, A. (2006). Combined pharmacotherapies and behavioral interventions for alcohol dependence. The COMBINE study: a randomized controlled trial. *JAMA*, 295(17): 2003–17.

APA. (2014). *Diagnostic and Statistical Manual of Mental Disorders, Fifth Edition (DSM-5)*.

Arlington, VA: American Psychiatric Publishing.

Bandura, A. (1977). Self-efficacy: toward a unifying theory of behavioral change. *Psychological Review,* 84(2): 191–215.

Bandura, A. (1986). *Social Foundations of Thought and Action: A social Cognitive Theory.* Englewood Cliffs, NJ: Prentice-Hall.

Barkley, R.A. (2012). *Executive Functions: What They Are, How They Work and Why They Evolved.* London: The Guilford Press.

Beck, A.T., Wright, F.D., Newman, C.F. and Liese, B.S. (1993). *Cognitive Therapy of Substance Abuse.* London: The Guildford Press.

Borland, R. (2014) *Understanding Hard to Maintain Behaviour Change: A Dual Process Approach.* Chichester: Wiley.

Bowlby, J. (1980). *Attachment and Loss Vol III. Loss.* New York: Basic Books.

Bowen, S., Chawla, N., Collins, S.E., Witkiewitz, K., Hsu, S., Grow, J., Clifasefi, S., Garner, M., Douglass, A., Larimer, M.E. and Marlatt, A. (2009). Mindfulness-based relapse prevention for substance use disorders: a pilot efficacy trial. *Substance Abuse,* 30(4): 295–305.

Brown, S.A. (1993). Drug effect expectancies and addictive behavior change. *Experimental and Clinical Psychopharmacology,* 1: 55–67.

Brown, S.A., Christiansen, B.A. and Goldman, M.S. (1987). The Alcohol Expectancy Questionnaire: an instrument for the assessment of adolescent and adult alcohol expectancies. *Journal of Studies on Alcohol,* 48: 483–91.

Carroll, K.M. (1996). Relapse prevention as a psychosocial treatment: A review of controlled clinical trials. *Experimental and Clinical Psychopharmacology,* 4: 46–54.

Department of Health (England) and the Devolved Administrations (2007). Drug misuse and dependence: UK guidelines on clinical management. London: Department of Health (England), the Scottish Government, Welsh Assembly Government and Northern Ireland Executive.

Dermatis, H. and Egelko, S. (2014). Buddhist mindfulness as an influence in recent empirical CBT approaches to addiction: convergence with the Alcoholics Anonymous model. *Alcoholism Treatment Quarterly,* 32: 194–213.

Dickerson, M. and O'Connor, J. (2006). *Gambling as an Addictive Behaviour: Impaired Control, Harm Minimisation, Treatment and Prevention.* Cambridge: Cambridge University Press.

Di Forti, M., Morgan, C., Dazzan, P., Pariante, C., Mondelli, V., Marques, T.R., Handley, R., Luzi, S., Russo, M., Paparelli, A., Butt, A., Stilo, S.A., Wiffen, B., Powell, J. and Murray, R.M. (2009). High-potency cannabis and the risk of psychosis. *British Journal of Psychiatry,* 195(6): 488–91.

Deutsch, R. and Strack, F. (2005). Reflective and impulsive determinants of addictive behaviour. In: R. Wiers and A. Stacy (eds). *Handbook of Implicit Cognition and Addiction.* Thousand Oaks, CA. Sage Publications, pp. 45–57.

Evans, A.C., Lamb, R. and White, W.L. (2014). Promoting Intergenerational Resilience and Recovery: Policy, Clinical, and Recovery Support Strategies to Alter the Intergenerational Transmission of Alcohol, Drug, and Related Problems. Philadelphia: Department of Behavioral Health and Intellectual Disability Services. Posted at www.williamwhitepapers.com

Festinger, L. (1957). *A Theory of Cognitive Dissonance.* Stanford, CA: Stanford University Press.

Flanagan, O. (2013). Phenomenal authority: the epistemic authority of Alcoholics Anonymous. In: N. Levy (ed.). *Addiction and Self-Control.* Oxford: Oxford University Press, pp. 67–93.

Flores, P.J. (2004). Addiction as an attachment disorder. New York, NY: Rowman & Littlefield.

Flores, P.J. (2011). Addiction as an Attachment Disorder. http://www.santecenter.com/wp-content/uploads/2013/05/files_Flores_Addiction_as_an_Attachment_Disorder-Part_1.pdf

Franken., I.H. (2003). Drug craving and addiction: integrating psychological and neuropsychopharmacological approaches. *Progress in Neuropsychopharmacology & Biological Psychiatry,* 27: 563–79.

Freud, S. (1984). *On Metapsychology: The Theory of Psychoanalysis.* Harmondsworth: Penguin.

Gomez, L. (1997). *An Introduction to Object Relations.* London: Free Association Books.

Greene, R.L., Adyanthaya, A.E., Morse, R.M. and Davis, L.J. Jr (1993). Personality variables in cocaine- and marijuana-dependent patients. *Journal of Personality Assessment,* 61(2): 224–30.

Griffiths, A., Hill, R.G., Morgan, C., Rendell, P.G., Karimi, K., Wanigaratne, S. and Curran, V. (2012). Prospective memory and future event simulation in individuals with alcohol dependence. *Addiction*, 107(10): 1809–16.

Hartmann, H. (1964). *Essays on Ego Psychology*. London: The Hogarth Press.

Hendershot, C.S., Witkiewitz, K.A., George, W.H. and Marlatt, G.A (2011). Relapse prevention for addictive behaviors. *Substance Abuse Treatment Prevention Policy,* 6: 17.

Holmes, J. (1993). *John Bowlby & Attachment Theory*. London: Routledge.

Hoyt, T.J. (2011). An overview of Heinz Kohut's self psychology and object relations theory. http://www.practicalphilosophy.net.

Hunter-Reel, D., McCrady, B. S. and Hildebrandt, T. (2009). Emphasizing interpersonal factors: An interpersonal extension of an intra-individual model of relapse. *Addiction*, 104(8): 1281–90.

Ida, T. (2014). A quasi-hyperbolic discounting approach to smoking behaviour. *Health Economics Review*, 4:5.

Irving, J.E., Bowers, C.A., Dunn, M.E. and Wang, M.C. (1999). Efficacy of relapse prevention: a meta-analytic review. *Journal of Consulting & Clinical Psychology*, 67(4): 563–70.

Jung, C.G. (1976). *Letters Volume 2*. London: Routledge and Kegan Paul.

Kadden R.M. (2001). *Cognitive-Behaviour Therapy for Substance Dependence: Coping Skills Training*. Storrs, CT: University of Connecticut.

Khantzian EJ, Treece CJ. Psychodynamics of drug dependence: an overview. NIDA Res Monogr. 1977 May; (12): 11-25. PMID: 97532. https://archives.drugabuse.gov/pdf/monographs/12.pdf

Khantzian, E.J., Halliday, K.S. and McAuliffe, W.E. (1990). *Addiction and the Vulnerable Self*. New York, NY: Guildford Press.

Knight, R.G. and Longmore, B.E. (1993). *Clinical Neuropsychology of Alcoholism*. Hove: Lawrence Erlbaum Associates.

Kohut, H. (1977). *The Restoration of the Self*. New York, NY: International Universities Press.

Kopelman, M.D. (1995). The Korsakoff syndrome. *British Journal of Psychiatry*, 166: 67–85.

Kushner, M.G., Abrams, K., Thuras, P., Hanson, K. L., Brekke, M. and Sletten, S. (2005). Follow-up study of anxiety disorder and alcohol dependence in comorbid alcoholism treatment patients. *Alcoholism: Clinical and Experimental Research*, 29(8): 1432–43.

Lang, A. R. (1983). Addictive personality: a viable construct? In: P.K. Levison, D.R. Gerstein and D.R. Maloff (eds). *Commonalities in Substance Abuse and Habitual Behavior.* New York, NY: Lexington Books, pp. 157–236.

Manning, V., Wanigaratne, S., Best, D., Hill, R., Reed, L.J, Strang, J. and Gossop, M. (2008). Changes in neuropsychological functioning during alcohol detoxification. *European Addiction Research*, 484: 1–8.

Marlatt, G.A. and Gordon, J.R. (1985). *Relapse Prevention: Maintenance Strategies in the Treatment of Addictive Behavior*. New York, NY: Guilford Press.

Marlatt, A.G. and Ostafin, B.D. (2005). Being mindful of automaticity in addiction: a clinical perspective. In: R. Wiers and A. Stacy (eds). *Handbook of Implicit Cognition and Addiction*. Thousand Oaks, CA. Sage Publications, pp. 489–93.

Miller, W. (1998). Towards a motivational definition and understanding of addiction. *Motivational Interviewing Newsletter for Trainers*, 5(3): 2–6.

Miller, W., and Rollnick, S. (2002). Motivational Interviewing: Preparing People for Change. 2nd edition. NY: Guilford Press

Miller, W. and Rollnick, S. (2013). *Motivational Interviewing: Preparing People for Change*. 3rd edn. New York, NY: Guilford Press.

Mitcheson, L., Maslin, J., Meynon, T., Morrison, T., Hill, R. and Wanigaratne, S. (2010). *Applied Cognitive and Behavioural Approaches to the Treatment of Addiction: A practical Treatment Guide*. Chichester: Wiley-Blackwell.

Mitcheson, L. and Grellier, B. (2011). Motivation and change: the role of motivational interviewing in substance use groups. In: R. Hill and J. Harris (eds). *Principles and Practice of Group Work in Addictions*. London: Routledge, pp. 17–29.

Morgenstern, J. and Bates, M. E. (1999). Effects of executive function impairment on change processes and substance use outcomes in 12-step treatment. *Journal of Studies on Alcohol and Drugs*, 60(6):846–55.

NICE. (2007). Drug Misuse: Psychosocial Interventions (NICE Clinical Guideline 51). http://www.nice.org.uk/CG51.

Noel, X., Van der Linden, M., Schmidt, N., Sferrazza, R., Hanak, C., Le Bon. O., De Mol, J., Kornreich, C., Pelc, I. and Verbanck, P. (2001). Supervisory attentional system in nonamnesic alcoholic men. *Archives of General Psychiatry,* 58: 1152–8.

Norman, W. and Shallice, T. (1986). Attention to action. In: R.J. Davidson, G.E. Schwartz and D. Shapiro (eds). *Consciousness and Self-regulation: Advances in Research and Theory,* vol. 4. New York, NY: Plenum, pp. 1–18.

Orford, J. (2001). *Excessive Appetites: A Psychological View of Addictions.* Chichester: John Wiley & Sons Ltd.

Ouimette, P. and Read, J.P. (eds). (2014). *Trauma and Substance Abuse: Causes, Consequences and Treatment of Comorbid Disorders.* 2nd Edn. Washington, DC: American Psychological Association.

Pavlov, I. P. (1927). *Conditional Reflexes*. New York, NY: Dover.

Prochaska, J.O. and DiClemente, C.C. (1986). Toward a comprehensive model of change. In: W. R. Miller and N. Heather (eds.) *Treating Addictive Behaviors: Processes of Change*. New York, NY: Plenum Press, pp. 3–27.

Robinson, T.E. and Berridge, K.C. (1993). The neural basis of drug craving: an incentive-sensitization theory of addiction. *Brain Research Review,* 18: 247–91.

Robinson, T.E. and Berridge, K.C. (2008). The incentive sensitization theory of addiction: some current issues. *Philosophical Transactions of the Royal Society B.,* 363: 3137–46.

Schinka, J. A., Curtiss, G. and Mulloy, J.M. (1994). Personality variables and self-medication in substance abuse. *Journal of Personality Assessment,* 63(3): 413–22.

Schoen, D.E. (2009). *The War of the Gods in Addiction: C.G. Jung, Alcoholics Anonymous and Archetypal Evil*. New Orleans, LA: Spring Journal Books.

Skinner, B.F. (1938). *The Behavior of Organisms: An Experimental Analysis*. New York, NY: Appleton-Century.

Stacy, A.W. and Wiers, R.W.H.J. (2010). Implicit cognition and addiction: a tool for explaining paradoxical behaviour. *Annual Review Clinical Psychology*, 6: 551–75.

Strack, F. and Deutsch, R. (2004). Reflective and impulsive determinants of social behaviour. *Personality and Social Psychology Review,* 8(3): 220–47.

Thombs. D.L. (2006). *Introduction to Addictive Behaviours.* New York, NY: Guilford Press.

Tiet, Q.Q & Mausbach, B. (2007) Treatments for patients with dual diagnosis: a review. *Alcoholism: Clinical and Experimental Research*, 31(4): 513–536.

Van der Plas, Ellen, A.A., Crone, E.A., van den Wildenberg, W.P.M., Tranel, D. and Bechara, A (2009). Executive control deficits in substance-dependent individuals: a comparison of alcohol, cocaine and methamphetamine and of men and women. *Journal of Clinical and Experimental Neuropsychology,* 31(6): 706–19.

Walker, R., Staton, M. and Leukefeld, C.G. (2001). History of head injury among substance users: preliminary findings. *Substance Use and Misuse,* 36(6&7): 757–70.

Wang, G.J., Volkow, N.D., Roque, C.T., Cestaro, V.L, Hitzemann, R.J., Cantos, E.L., Levy, A.V. and Dhawan, A.P. (1993). Functional importance of ventricular enlargement and cortical atrophy in healthy subjects and alcoholics as assessed with PET, MR imaging and neuropsychological testing. *Radiology*, 186: 59–65.

Weaver, T., Madden, P., Charles, V., Stimson, G., Rention, A., Tryer, P., Barnes, T., Bench, C., Middleton, H., Wright, N., Paterson, S., Shanahan, W., Seivewright, N. and Ford, C. (2003). Comorbidity of substance misuse and mental illness in community mental health and substance misuse services. *The British Journal of Psychiatry,* 183: 304–13.

Weegman, M. (2011). Psychodynamics in groups or psychodynamic groups? In: R. Hill and J. Harris (eds). *Principles and Practice of Group Work in Addictions*. London: Routledge, pp. 224–40.

World Health Organization. (1992). The ICD-10 classification of mental and behavioural disorders: Clinical descriptions and diagnostic guidelines. Geneva: World Health Organization.

West, R. (2006). *Theory of Addiction*. Chichester: Wiley-Blackwell.

Witkiewitz, K. and Marlatt, M. (2004). Relapse prevention for alcohol and drug problems: that was Zen, this is Tao. *American Psychologist,* 59(4): 224–35.

Witkiewitz, K., Marlatt, G.A. and Walker, D. (2005). Mindfulness-based relapse prevention for alcohol and substance use disorders. *Journal of Cognitive Psychotherapy,* 19(3): 211–28.

Witkiewitz, K. and Marlatt, A. (2007). Modelling the complexity of post-treatment drinking: it's a rocky road to relapse. *Clinical Psychology Review*, 27(6): 724–38.

Witkiewitz, K. and Bowen, S. (2010). Depression, craving, and substance use following a randomized trial of mindfulness-based relapse prevention. *Journal of Consulting & Clinical Psychology*, 78(3): 362–74.

Yoon, G., Kim, S.W., Thuras, P., Grant, J.E. and Westermayer, J. (2006). Alcohol craving in outpatients with alcohol dependence-rate and clinical correlates. *Journal of Studies on Alcohol*, 67(5): 770–7.

Zimberg, S. (1999). A dual diagnosis typology to improve diagnosis and treatment of dual disorder patients. *Journal of Psychoactive Drugs,* 31(1): 47–51.

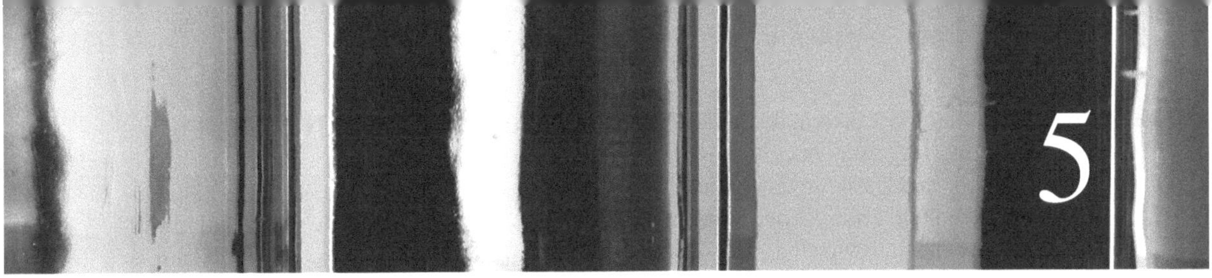

Anthropological Study of Drug Use: Methodological and Theoretical Considerations

John Bryan Page and Merrill Singer

INTRODUCTION

Among disciplinary platforms for studying drug use, anthropology occupies an advantageous position. We provide evidence supporting this notion. Examples from our own and our anthropological colleagues' research experiences provide the bulk of that evidence. Our presentation of these experiences includes settings and circumstances of research that occurred in many different cities and several different countries. In keeping with the overall theme of a handbook, we emphasize how to go about this kind of research, avoiding dangerous situations and maximizing the value of the information obtained. We begin by placing the relationship between ethnography and the study of drug use in historic context.

Although the full story of drug ethnography probably began with Herodotus (Page and Singer 2010: 25–49), from our prospective as researchers who have been involved in this work for many decades, the key juncture in the history of drug ethnography occurred in the latter part of the last century. The largest source of funding for research on drug use in the world, the National Institute on Drug Abuse (NIDA), came to the realization that in order to learn fully about patterns of illegal drug use and related health risks, the agency needed ethnographic studies of the behaviors, conceptions, and social worlds of drug users. One project officer at NIDA, Eleanor Carroll, was an especially effective advocate for ethnographic approaches to drug studies. She recognized that no amount of short-answer interviewing of at-large populations would give the agency what it needed to know about the nature and forms of illegal drug consumption. As a result, she vigorously advocated for ethnographic studies, such as those conducted by Agar (1973), Partridge (1974), Rubin and Comitas (1975), and Carter (1980). With the exception of Agar's (1973) initial investigation of heroin users in a treatment facility, all of these studies included individual ethnographers or teams of field workers whose task was to make initial contact with active drug users in culturally unfamiliar territory and learn directly about their use of drugs through observation, casual conversation, formal interviewing, and related strategies.

Certainly, the anthropological canon is replete with accounts of how ethnographic researchers went about introducing themselves to the people in the communities they had chosen to study. Each of the cultural contexts in which Western social/behavioral scientists attempted to study the behavior of culturally distinct people presented barriers and difficulties ranging from needing to understand the nuances of a totally unfamiliar language to arranging for edible food and adequate shelter. Most anthropological ethnographers of the early twentieth century, however, sought, in the cultural setting chosen for study, to understand how the patterns of ordinary life fit together. Mead's study of becoming an adult in Samoa (1928) provided an example of this kind of ethnography in which she related the process of re-defining children as adults to division of labor, gender roles, religion, and family structure, among many other aspects of Samoan life. Similarly, Evans-Pritchard's study of Nuer life (1940) encompassed subsistence, gender roles, marriage, puberty, and conflict resolution. In the late 1960s, ethnographers of drug use in urban settings in developed countries attempted to learn about patterns of behavior that were covert to varying degrees and defined by the larger society as deviant and threatening. This chapter first addresses the place of theory in the endeavor of studying drug use ethnographically. In keeping with the purpose of the chapter to provide the information expected from a handbook, it focuses on key aspects of the most difficult part of initiating drug ethnography – making contact with active drug users in their natural habitats. Subsequently, it defines some principles of ethnographic practice for the study of drug use and discusses variants of that practice.

ETHNOGRAPHY AND THEORY

Investigations involving social and behavioral science often begin with the identification and appraisal of pre-existing theories about the phenomena to be studied. For example, sociological and social work studies of gang behavior among North American youth have invoked various theories through which the investigators seek to explain how and why young people come to participate in gangs. Among the theories used to explain participation in youth gangs are stress or strain theory, in which the conditions of poverty and deprivation lead to the formation of youth gangs (cf. Cloward and Ohlin 1960; Cohen 1955), differential association or subcultural theory, where youth in specific neighborhood environments associated themselves with delinquent peers (cf. Johnson 1979; Miller 1958; Sutherland 1966; Voss 1963), or social control theory, which posited a lack or weakening of institutions of social control, allowing youth to overstep the boundaries of acceptable behavior (cf. Elliot et al. 1979; Hirschi 1969; Nye 1958) (see also chapter 3 on Sociological approaches in this Handbook). These and other theories have provided preliminary justification for pursuing specific lines of inquiry into the nature and process of delinquent youth gangs (Page 1997). They have also served would-be sociological investigators of illegal drug use. Inspection of the content of the publications cited above reveals that the theoretical approaches they describe include considerable overlap. In conditions of neighborhood stress, the formation of subcultural complexes would seem inevitable, as would the breakdown of institutional supervision of youth.

In contrast to the theory-driven research initiatives in sociology, anthropological sorties into the worlds of illegal drug use often have tended not to set out with a theoretical explanatory model at their core (cf. Page and Trotter 1999). Rather, they began as theory building exercises, intended to develop some hypotheses about drug using practices and their origins. For example, the studies of cannabis use in Jamaica (Rubin and Comitas 1975) and Costa Rica (Carter 1980) did not begin with a priori theoretically formulated hypotheses about the etiology and impact of that drug plant among marijuana users. Because they were both multidisciplinary in nature, these studies had formulated theories in some disciplinary aspects, such as ophthalmology and psychology, about the health impact of cannabis use, based on the literature to date. For example, much of the literature suggested that intraocular pressure might be affected by regular cannabis use; therefore, the Costa Rican study conducted examinations of eyeball tonometry in pursuit of this theorized effect, related conceptually to cannabis' vasodilation. Effects on short-term and long-term memory, both in terms of storage processes and retrieval processes, led the investigators in the Costa Rica study to test these particular aspects of memory in its study group. The anthropologists on these research teams, however, did not know enough about the patterns of cannabis use or the circumstances in which it was consumed to posit any hypotheses about the impact of cannabis use on long-term users. Rather, they were assigned first with the task of finding users and determining the extent of their experience and then characterizing patterns of use through participant observation and informal interviewing. The field anthropologists operated only under one quasi-theoretical assumption: that users of marijuana participated by necessity in some kind of subcultural context that enabled them to continue to use, despite the drug's illegality and disapproval. Therefore, the field team worked under the assumption that by making the acquaintance of one marijuana user, one could tap into a network of users. This assumption was borne out by the final form of the Costa Rican cannabis study (cf. True et al. 1980).

One theoretical approach that received attention in the studies of drug users before 1980 (Agar 1973; Spradley 1970) involved ethnoscience as defined by Goodenough (1956). Using an analogy with field studies of linguistics, Goodenough suggested methods to determine the meaning of cultural components in order to provide a cognitive map of cultural systems. This theoretical stance posited the existence in all cultural systems of a system of related meanings among cultural components, along the lines of phonemes in language. Spradley (1970) applied this approach to his study of street alcoholics in Seattle, and Agar (1973) did something similar in his study of heroin addicts at the Lexington treatment facility. In *Ripping and Running* (1973), Agar attempted to delineate the structure of heroin users' activities aimed at obtaining their drug of choice through a standard anthropological procedure of convening a group of informants, engaging in free listing and pile sorting activities, and developing a conceptualization of the essential behavioral domains of hustling, copping, and getting off. This work is the first example that involved the development of an ethnographic perspective on drug use based on work conducted in an institutional setting rather than an uncontrolled 'natural habitat', that is, the street. None of the aforementioned domains had previously been characterized in the literature on heroin use, and so Agar's ethnographic study essentially used a quasi-linguistic theory/method (componential analysis) to build a mid-level theory about the need of heroin users to be constantly on the move.

Variants of this approach appeared in numerous other ethnographies of drug use during the twentieth century, including Koester (1994), Carlson (1996), Carlson and Siegal (1988), and Sterk (1999) among many others. In developing their understanding of drug use, anthropologists have embraced several different explanatory frameworks. The core component of the anthropological approach to human interaction with psychotropic drugs is known as the 'cultural model' (Page and Singer 2010: 5–7). This model stresses that human interaction with drugs is determined to a large degree by cultural expectations and understanding (sometimes called 'local knowledge') about the expectable effects of a particular drug on the human mind/body. These cultural constructs are products of the social history of a sociocultural group, their contact with neighboring peoples, and the configuration of opportunities and challenges encountered in their social and physical environment. The cultural model has informed a large body of anthropological literature on drug use, addiction, and the behavioral strategies of drug addicts. An especially useful aspect of this work has been its revealing accounts of previously less studied subgroups, such as female drug addicts (cf. Page and Singer 2010; 149–162). The cultural model also has guided anthropological research on the lifestyles or distinctive subcultural traditions shared among groups of drug users. The primary aim of the subculture approach is the development of a holistic description of the people for whom drug use has become a central organizing mechanism in their lives. This approach counters simplistic stereotypes and narrow pathological portrayals of drug users. Further, it has provided the framework for studies of: (i) the survival strategies used to sustain a drug-focused lifestyle in light of drug laws and law enforcement (Agar 1973); (ii) the components and organization of the underground drug economy (Johnson 1985); (iii) processes and routines of socialization into drug use social networks and the street drug use subculture (Becker 1953; Johnson et al. 1998); (iv) the social settings and key locations, such as places to 'cop' (acquire) drugs and shooting galleries, that comprise drug users' social environments (Agar 1973; Page et al. 1990a); (v) the cultural frameworks used by drug users to classify various social statuses within the subculture (Page et al. 1990b); (vi) risk behaviors and risk environments (Koester 1994; Page and Salazar 1999); (vii) the street jargon that developed to communicate issues of concern to drug users as well as a sense of in-group membership (Page 1977); (viii) the daily routines and experiences of active drug users (Ripoll et al. 2003); and (ix) drug users' interactions with social welfare institutions (Bourgois 2000).

An alternative theoretical model in the anthropology of drug studies is the political economic approach (Singer 2001). Its development reflected a recognition that whatever its strengths, the cultural model fails to consider the importance in drug use of macrolevel structures (e.g. significant economic inequalities, institutions of social control), social processes and dominant institutions (such as the activities of corporations, the effects of the dominant media portrayal of drug users, and systems of discrimination), and relations of power (e.g. social classes, unequal relations among nations). Within the domain of drug use, the political economic model has emphasized three issues: the social production of suffering, the use of drugs to self-medicate the emotional injuries of injustice and mistreatment, and the political economy of legal and illegal drug markets. For example, Philippe Bourgois' *In Search of Respect* presents an examination of socioeconomic marginalization in an urban setting (East Harlem) under the influence of theories about political economy and power forwarded by Foucault (2003, 2011) and Bourdieu (1991). Once in the field, Bourgois soon concluded that the salient feature of marginalization in his chosen neighborhood was the management of the crack cocaine market. Therefore, he aimed his focus at that complex of behavior. Because it had not received much anthropological attention by that time, Bourgois also began his study as a theory building process. This process is typical of most ethnographic studies of drug use and it is accurate to characterize the studies cited here as attempts to build theories of street based drug use.

PRINCIPLES OF GETTING STARTED IN DRUG ETHNOGRAPHY

In keeping with the handbook theme of this chapter, we have identified several principles that have emerged from our experience in initiating ethnographic drug studies. The set of principles is intended to provide guidance for the field worker who may be attempting this kind of ethnography for the first time:

1) Time spent in the setting of interest is never wasted

A well-trained, culturally sensitized observer needs time to become familiar with the specific cultural context in which prospective key informants and other study participants conduct the behaviors of interest. Every hour spent in the chosen locale contributes to the array of cultural features that the field researcher will be able to apply to interactions with local people and eventually, to establishing trusting human relationships with the people of most interest in that locale. This principle is equally true for the post-contact stage of the research as for the pre-contact phase. In the latter, the field researcher is accruing cultural understanding that enables him/her to push beyond the initial contact and broaden his/her relations and store of cultural knowledge. Pre-contact presence in the locale also gives prospective study participants time to size up the researcher. In the post-contact phase of ethnographic research, the participant observer continues learning about the cultural context of interest, especially how the behaviors of interest relate to specific aspects of that socio-spatial context. Family relations, labor and economic activity, ritual and religion, and health practices gradually become available to the observer, and these opportunities for enriching the field researcher's cultural understanding merit the same attention (i.e. being recorded in field notes) given to pre-contact observations. The field researcher should uphold this principle throughout the duration of the field research project.

2) Be cautious about approaching people you think are drug users

There have been occasions when new-to-the-scene ethnographers have observed behaviors that reveal the faces of some of the local drug users. In some contexts, such as the open-air drug dealing sites where dozens of people would gather in groups that Singer commonly observed in Washington, D.C., or the corner drug selling units he routinely observed in Hartford, CT, it was possible to spot specific individuals who could be approached when they were encountered alone elsewhere in the community (Weeks et al. 2001). In some cases, this approach can lead to shunning, threats, or actual risk to the drug researcher. Frustration in not being able to gain permitted access to local drug scenes has prompted some researchers to pursue contact with drug users aggressively, but we recommend patience and allowing the users who are curious about the researcher's presence to bring about voluntary contact.

3) Engage in casual conversation

As you visit targeted neighborhoods, engage people on the street who you do not necessarily think are involved in the local drug scene (although at the outset, you can never assume that you know who is) in casual conversation, such as local merchants, health and social service workers, and civil employees, always being sure to present your purpose for being there accurately.

Word gets around, especially about people from the outside who are new to a local setting. Ethnographers generally stand out, and their presence generates curiosity. Being friendly and self-revealing in casual conversations with people around the neighborhood is part of the process of breaking through the understandable protective barriers that drug users and others maintain. The first people to come forward in contexts where drug use is reportedly taking place, however, often are not the most knowledgeable individuals in local drug using social networks. These individuals may be marginal to the locale under study but hope that through their contact with the field worker they will gain some regard among the non-marginal participants in that locale's drug using scene. Others may be sent by a curious (and knowledgeable) observer who wishes to determine whether or not it is risky to make contact him/herself. The observer sends the latter people forward because they are not particularly knowledgeable, and therefore, are unlikely to divulge valid information, if the interloper, in fact, is a police officer. These first contact individuals should be treated just as the field worker would handle an important, knowledgeable participant, politely and with interest in what they have to say. With skilled interviewing, they could offer up the name of the person who sent them, and that is the person the field researcher really wants in the study.

4) Networks

Informal social relations among users of illegal drugs can be assumed to exist in the locales targeted for ethnographic study. Shared experience in common places for using drugs and participation in systems for distributing drugs (e.g. shooting galleries, or get-off houses, opium dens, street corners, alleys, parked cars) depend heavily on the networks that exist among the individuals involved in these activities. While Page (True et al. 1980) was gaining familiarity with the neighborhood, the network of marijuana users was transmitting information about him to their fellows, being warned to proceed with caution, and being counseled to give the process time. Once he established contact and the beginnings of trust, the network opened up to him through initial introductions to additional participants. The methodological implications of network tracing in drug ethnography will receive attention elsewhere in this chapter. For purposes of identifying a principle for drug ethnography, it suffices to say that drug ethnographers must, at all times, be aware that networks are present and active in all cultural contexts involving illegal drug use. It may not be possible to characterize fully these social structures in the course of a single ethnographic study, but it is essential to pay attention to network relations among the people under investigation.

5) Finding common ground

The anthropological canon is full of features that succeeded in helping to attract the attention of community members in all kinds of research settings. In Singer's case (2003), initial experience with drug research was preceded by local community activism rooted in a health-oriented community-based organization. Public involvement in such activities gave him a degree of initial credibility and suggested he was probably not a police agent and may even be of some benefit to drug users. Conversation about such work, and why he was involved in it, was subsequently initiated by participants in his various drug use studies. Agar (1973), by contrast, simply played basketball with the inmates at the Lexington Narcotics Treatment facility, establishing initial rapport through sport. Far less elaborate ethnographic gambits involved simply bringing extra cigarettes to observation spots to share with the people encountered there.

6) Be constantly open to contacts from unexpected quarters

The field team in the Costa Rican marijuana project fully expected the bars located in neighborhoods identified with marijuana use to be major sources of contact. They were not. Page, for example, spent many hours engaging clientele of the corner bars in Barrio Cuba, a neighborhood known for housing marijuana smokers, but that time yielded no productive contacts. Rather, encounters with individuals who, unbeknownst to the field workers, were observing them for weeks before the encounters seemed to be the rule. In another project in Miami (Page 1990), Page opened a conversation with a local young man who had been hanging out in the shopping center across the street from Page's office. He had been aware of Page's presence for weeks, but at this particular moment, he chose to engage in conversation about his extensive drug use experience.

7) Accept that some participants in the drug scene will never agree to talk to you

In every locale that has a reputation for drug use and trafficking, there will always be individuals who refuse to speak to the field researcher, regardless of the researcher's skill in engagement and positive reputation in the rest of the drug users' networks. To know who these people are is in fact a form of ethnographic information. Each locale studied by Page had at least one person who took that stance. In Little Havana, a man named Ruben, known to all of Page's other contacts, never agreed to talk to him, even informally. Often times, however, it is likely that a field researcher will never learn much about such individuals or their specific reasons for enhanced wariness. No doubt, drug users who have only lower level involvement in the local drug trade are easier to access than those further up the illicit drug chain. Singer has encountered drug users who were quite open about their activities from the beginning simply because they were well known to the local police, who harassed them often, and felt they had little left to hide.

PARTICIPANT OBSERVATION

The researcher's senses and the information they record about the surrounding environment are the baseline for the inclusion of various other approaches to collecting data. Also, the field researcher is not just present in a cultural context of interest, but seeks to become engaged with people in their routine activities as a better means of learning just what they do, their understandings of why they do it, and how they feel about things in their cultural world. We use the term participant observation in research on illicit drug use, even though it implies that the field researcher will engage in the illegal behaviors involved. This implication requires examination of the precise meaning of participant observation in this kind of research. According to Patricia and Peter Adler (1991), the role of the participant must be meaningful to the inhabitants (whom they call 'members') of the social context chosen for observation:

> When researchers take membership roles they are recognized and treated by others as members. They become privy to members' innermost thoughts, activities and emotions. This is particularly important in settings characterized by secrecy and/or exclusiveness (which, to some degree, most settings are). (Adler and Adler 1991: 22)

Participation, then, primarily involves the defining and enacting of a role for the participant observer in the social context being studied. In the setting described here, the Adlers' participation did not involve any illegal or risky activity, but it did involve accessing exclusive information, which they needed as researchers to keep confidential. Participant observation among drug users need not include the entire repertoire of behaviors involved in drug use and/or trafficking, but it often will involve developing a holistic perspective on the lives of the participants. Some drug ethnographers maintain that participant observation should not include any form of drug use or any other illegal activity (Rubin and Comitas 1975). Others would permit limited involvement, such as smoking marijuana or giving automobile rides to people who may be in possession of illegal drugs. It is possible to conduct field research on drugs under either of these conditions, although the approach involving no drug use or illegal activity is somewhat more difficult to pursue in some contexts than field efforts characterized by a more involved approach.

In other contexts, the opposite is true. As the director of a team study of drug use and HIV risk, Singer was told by several drug users that one of the researchers he had hired was seen buying drugs from the same dealers they frequented. This left them distrustful of this individual because they had come to view researchers as people they could count on never to expose them to the police. A researcher who was involved in drug use, however, could potentially be pressured by the police into identifying or entrapping other drug users and drug sellers. Some behaviors among drug users, such as self-injection of drugs, are laden with risk, and therefore, they are to be avoided by ethnographers. Other behaviors, such as carrying drug material or paraphernalia as a favor for study participants, place the field worker in jeopardy of arrest and incarceration.

It is possible for field workers to protect themselves from risk of incarceration by arranging for immunity from police harassment with the local law enforcement authorities. This strategy itself carries potential risks, including the possibility that identification of field workers can make them targets of police who do not intend to comply with the prior arrangement. Police can observe the activities of field workers to identify new potential arrestees who use drugs or otherwise participate in the activities of drug consumption and traffic. Also, police who have become corrupt can come to perceive anthropological ethnographers as threats to their sources of income. This kind of perception can become extremely dangerous to the field workers. In Miami, there have been instances in which drug traffickers who were in business with police officers were murdered to keep them quiet, as in the River Cops case of 1985 (Kissell 2000). The mere discovery of police complicity with drug trafficking is therefore extremely dangerous, and a prior arrangement with police may be riskier than not entering an immunity agreement (Page 2006). Our approach to mitigating that kind of risk has involved avoiding any indication of interest in the process of trafficking drugs. Suspicions tend to arise when field researchers ask pointed questions about sources or origins of drugs. Our field teams are specifically instructed to avoid all inquiries about trafficking at any level. In over 40 years of research on patterns of illegal drug use, Page has never experienced any untoward incidents involving suspicious traffickers in illegal drugs.

We have, in some of our various studies made prior arrangements with the police, and in others not done so. Even without any arrangements, we have informed local police who we are and why we are out and about in places where illicit behaviors are known to occur. In one study in which Singer and his colleagues were collecting discarded syringes from abandoned buildings, alleys, and other sites for laboratory testing, we were warned by the police that we would be arrested if caught in the possession of these items without a doctor's prescription, although no arrests ever occurred (Singer et al. 2005). In neighborhoods where there is high activity related to drug trafficking, contact with police is almost inevitable, but strategies developed over years of experience with these kinds of studies have helped to minimize difficulties. This has been possible by being mindful of three key field strategies:

1 When going to a place where drug activity is prevalent that you have not previously visited, take a cultural guide with you. A cultural guide is someone who knows the lay of the land, has experience in avoiding police and other trouble,

and who has broad network contacts in the site to be visited. They may be active or former drug users or community outreach workers. We have, in some cases, employed cultural guides full-time, and in others, engaged them for brief periods. Their presence is helpful in avoiding or disarming potentially dangerous situations.

2 Adopt and enforce a project-wide policy of field researchers never giving any police officer encountered in the field the least excuse for detaining or arresting them. Before entering into field situations, each field researcher must receive training in how to address police officers in field encounters. Short of providing information about study participants' activities or whereabouts, the field worker must be unfailingly polite, regardless of the behavior of the officers, never resisting the officers' actions, nor exhibiting the least disagreement with, or disdain for, the officers in the encounter.
3 Establish and enforce a set of rules of the road for field research on drug use (Singer et al. 1999). This is a list of locally informed behaviors that should be adhered to or avoided to minimize problems, reduce risk, and avoid ethical dilemmas for field researchers. For example, on the street, field workers may be approached to buy items at what appear to be significantly reduced rates. Because these items may be stolen, purchasing them should be avoided even if interest in buying them is motivated by a desire to develop relations with the item's seller, who may be a drug user seeking to raise funds to purchase drugs.

Because researchers on our respective field teams usually have been accompanied by cultural guides, negative encounters with the police have been infrequent. Also, field workers in our grant-funded projects, even in situations of high stress, always identified themselves and the studies for which they worked, giving the officers the telephone numbers of the respective principal investigators.

Our experience and that of our colleagues tells us that useful research on drug use must include some form of participant observation (Page and Singer 2010). Not only can it be carried out ethically and safely, avoiding harm to participants and field researchers, but its scientific payoffs have been essential to advancing our understanding of drug using behavior. Agar's (1973) ethnoscientific characterization of copping behavior among heroin users provided key insights into the daily pursuits of this little understood population. Page's observations in Miami get-off houses (Page et al. 1990a, 1990b) re-defined the risk of HIV infection incurred in those settings. Dunlap conducted extensive participant observation of households in which three generations of a family participated in the crack cocaine epidemic of the 1990s (Dunlap et al. 1994, 2001; Dunlap and Johnson 1996). Koester's (1994) participant observation uncovered the reasons for IDUs choosing not to carry their own personal syringes, and led to health-related recommended changes in police handling of minor offenses. Singer's study of drug user narratives suggested key lessons for improved program outreach and treatment of drug users (Singer et al. 2001). Findings from these and similar field-based investigations have important implications for drug abuse prevention and treatment, law enforcement, violence prevention, HIV and other disease prevention, and policy formation.

Field notes

The methodological literature has range of opinions on how to take anthropological field notes (Pelto and Pelto 1978; Schensul and LeCompte 2013). When it comes to doing drug research, however, we would like to highlight the following:

1 Drug use is an especially apt topic for anthropological study because it impinges on so many different aspects of the human condition. Drug use affects family relations, economics, spirituality and religion, sexual behavior, labor patterns, food and nutrition, social control and hierarchy, policy and polity, art and value formation, and health-related behavior, to name a few. In the contemporary world, in light of the War on Drugs, drug use affects global relations among nations and can be an issue of social conflict.

2 The primary goal of the field observer in studying drug use is to have their field notes, and the observations on which they are based, reflect the behaviors of primary interest and other relevant aspects of the human condition as thoroughly as possible. Events or settings recorded early in field work that seem quite tangential to the issue of drug use may later prove to be of considerable importance. For instance, Singer's field team who studied drug user narratives did not begin with this focus or with a specific idea about these components of cultural production. Singer and his colleagues simply wrote down in their notes stories drug users told them about things that had happened in their lives. One day at a project meeting, one member of the team mentioned that a drug user had used the term 'war stories', by which he meant somewhat stylized accounts (with a beginning, middle, and ending) that seemed intended to convey a lesson or make a point. A review of field notes led to the discovery of many such narratives of various sorts, each type with their own cultural message about the trials and tribulations, hopes and surprising experiences that shaped the world of drug users in a social context that condemned and punished them and their behavior. This discovery prompted the researchers to collect more war stories and to analyze them as encapsulated sources of information on drug user experience, emotion, and perspective.

3 In describing a person, field notes should record his/her height, body build, eye and hair color, and observable age category (Schensul and LeCompte 2013). They should not, however, infer age, socioeconomic status, sexual preference, or use of drugs. Taking field notes is a process in which not all questions are answered after a first, second, or third visit to a site of interest. Rather, the process of field observation is a strategy for getting increasingly closer to the information desired and the understanding of that information. It is, in short, a process of discovery, not a quick assessment. Thus, the field researcher does not have to find out on the first try whether or not the people in the observational session are drug users, or whether or not traffickers operate in the area, although in many contexts evidence of these may be abundant. As the notes accumulate, the field researcher should gradually obtain not only the needed information about the behaviors of interest, but a rounded, anthropological view of the cultural and built physical context in which they occur.

Interviewing

Besides observational studies, elicitation of cultural content, interpretations of actions, and conceptualizations of social and economic process occurs in at least three different ways in the course of ethnographic research on drug use: (i) informal interviews guided by a general set of research questions; (ii) structured, short answer interviews with an established list of questions; and (iii) in-depth interviews. The narratives that follow delineate the place of each kind of interview in ethnographic research on drug use.

Informal interviews

During participant observation, the field researcher will frequently have opportunities to engage in conversation with the actors in a site of observation. These opportunities may occur early in the first observational phase of a given study, involving people with whom the researcher has not yet established a relationship. Informal interviews can be valuable to the understanding of local context and actors' attitudes about their, or others', behavior, but they can only be documented in field notes. The reason for this principle of documenting informal interviews is that at this point in the research, the field observer has not yet obtained expressed consent for recording conversations, and obtaining that consent can interfere with the spontaneity of the observational moment. The canons of ethical research require informed consent, especially if the investigator is collecting voice recording and/or linking the content of the conversation to a specific individual. In the circumstances of early observation and informal interview, it is preferable to ask the question, listen to the answer, and incorporate the gist of the conversation into field notes for that observational session without recording personal identifiers of the interviewee.

Certain occasions for informal interviewing can yield telling results. For example, Page had occasion, early in a study of HIV risk among IDUs, to observe a person who, during a previous interview, claimed only to use new needle/syringes. Page had just seen him remove one from a coffee can, and asked, 'Didn't you tell me you only used new needles?' He replied, 'It *was* new'. This encounter afforded the opportunity to probe on what 'new' meant in the context of a 'get-off' house. At later junctures in the same study, at a time when some actors in an observational site have fully consented to participate in the study, audio recording may be appropriate in informal interviews. The principal caveat in those circumstances involves avoiding calling too much attention to the conversation in a street setting.

Because these interviews occur spontaneously while the actors are doing what they normally do, it is possible to gain insight into how they perceive what they are doing and what it means to them, or what ethnographers call the 'emic' point of view (Eiserman et al. 2003; Goodenough 1956). The observer's questions can be framed about events that just happened and involve asking what the actors think of that occurrence. This spontaneous quality can be very useful in exploring such issues as self-perception of deviance, feelings about stigma, solidarity with fellow users, and avoidance of police contact.

Short answer interviews

This variety of interview should not occur until the investigator or investigative team has conducted enough background participant observation and informal interviews to have a grasp of the forms in which the drug users of interest consume their drugs of choice or at least drugs of current availability. The questionnaires in this variety of interviewing have to contain the words and depict the behaviors that characterize the specific variants of drug use being investigated. The specific purpose of short answer interviews is to obtain a sense of the distribution of the variants of drug use in the population under study. The questionnaire format allows the investigators to find out as efficiently as possible how widespread the drug using patterns they have described are. Rather, they reflect the relative distribution of the drug use forms defined by participant observation among the specific respondents to the survey. Often, with large numbers of respondents, the administration of the questionnaire may identify additional variants not picked up in the ethnographic work.

At no time should such a convenience sample of drug users ever be considered generalizable to the whole population of drug users, even the drug users in the locale of the study. The main reason for avoidance of over-interpreting these results is because the behavior being studied is illegal and possibly stigmatized, we have no way of defining the universe of drug users, even in the locale being studied. Rather, generalizable results should be based upon a sample of respondents produced through a rigorous sampling procedure in which the universe of drug users is defined and each person in that universe has an equal chance of being in the sample. The impossibility of obtaining a rigorously framed probability sample of illegal drug users exists because we cannot define the universe of illegal drug users. Nevertheless, responses to a survey instrument can be useful in suggesting how widespread certain risky behaviors might be and which ones to concentrate on first. If the questions included in the short answer interview include the terminology and meanings discovered during observation and in-depth interviews, the response process will be smooth. Questions that do not use familiar terms for drugs and paraphernalia (for example, in Miami, 'gimmick' is universal for 'needle/syringe', but it is not be necessarily used or understood in other parts of the country) confuse and frustrate the respondents.

In-depth interviews

Interviews in which the interviewer tries to deepen his/her understanding of the relationship between the respondent and the behaviors of interest require a markedly different approach from those used in informal interviewing and short answer interviewing. In-depth interviewing has as its primary objective the uncovering of fundamental values, motivations, social contexts, behaviors, social relations, and meanings that underlie the behaviors of interest. This kind of probing encourages the respondent to begin a discursive narrative in which the structure is a direct product of the respondent's own perception of the topic. The task of the interviewer is to ask open-ended questions that cannot be answered with a simple yes or no answer and to listen attentively, encouraging the respondent to continue, and occasionally asking a probing follow-up question in pursuit of something mentioned in the midst of the flowing narrative. That something may simply require definition or clarification, but sometimes it opens a whole new line of inquiry. The interviewer should have an interview guide that serves as a list of topics to be covered in the respondent's narrative. Without interrupting the flow of the narrative, the items on the guide can be checked off as they are covered by the ongoing speech of the respondent. Sometimes, however, it is easy to think a question has been fully answered only to realize later that it has not, and thus, the interviewer should be cautious in checking off a topic area.

When an interviewee mentions something unexpected, however, the interviewer has to be alert to pursue this emergent information enthusiastically. It may take the form of a different way to inject drugs, as in the case of using lemon juice to dissolve heroin (see Page and Salazar 1999), or an approach to carrying or not carrying disposable needle/syringe sets (see Koester 1994) to avoid police arrest and warrant checks. It may also involve the use of a drug not previously known to researchers (e.g. Singer et al. 2000). Each of these emergent revelations resulted in new perspectives on the behavior of drug users with regard to risk. Because not all in-depth interviewees are spellbinding narrators, the vigil for emergent information is especially demanding for the interviewer, who must remain alert for important facts in the midst of halting, ungrammatical, self-aggrandizing, or sorrow-filled and self-deprecating narratives. Towards this end, it may be helpful to the interviewer to think of these interviews as a kind of proxy space exploration in which the interviewee is an 'alien' who has been to places the interviewer has never been, and neither have most potential readers. As the lone 'explorer' on this particular expedition, it is up to the interviewer to make the most of the opportunity, with great attention to detail, especially with reference to emergent information.

In-depth interviews can also be conducted in 'focus groups'. Agar and MacDonald (1995) provided an anthropological model for group interviews among drug users which, although not ideal, made this process more anthropological than other focus group techniques. The principal utility of the anthropological focus group is to derive a sense of cultural consensus on a set of topics as discussed in a group of active drug users. Individual interviews can be laden with small conceits, self-deceptions, and artifacts of self-presentation that face no disagreement in the setting where only the interviewer and interviewee are present. When other actors in the same sociocultural setting are present, the prospect of contradiction and disagreement can reduce sometimes outrageous assertions that can occur in one-on-one interviews. Furthermore, statements about major aspects of a given context (e.g. police presence, drug availability, attitude of dealers about clientele) made and agreed upon in a group setting tend to be more valid and reliable than statements made in individual interviews.

A skillful group interviewer can elicit large volumes of information in a relatively short time, and this fact has tempted some researchers to try to replace labor intensive ethnography with focus groups. A series of focus groups does not constitute ethnography, however, for the following reasons:

1 Preliminary ethnographic study is necessary to learn what the significant behaviors are and how to talk about them.
2 In the absence of some participant observation and on-site informal interviewing, focus group declarations may have little relation to actual behavior.
3 The relationships among participants prior to coming to the focus will be unknown, making the interpersonal dynamics in the focus group difficult to understand.
4 If not preceded by ethnographic field research, the interviewer will have no field hypotheses to check with the group.

In all of the varieties of interviews mentioned above, the process of gathering information involves an ongoing and highly personal contact between interviewer and interviewee in which rapport and trust make the difference between guarded, laconic responses and open, self-disclosing ones. In order to attain rapport and trust, the interviewer must exhibit genuine interest in the topic at hand and assure the interviewee that none of the interview content will be identified with the interviewee by name or other identifier in any public medium. This kind of relationship is not easy to establish and maintain for the duration of an ethnographic study. It demands that the field researcher have special skills in managing and maintaining social relationships, even with people to whom he/she is not attracted personally. It also involves the need for the researcher to be responsive to questions raised by the interviewee, including those about the researcher's motives.

CONCLUSION

While there are complications and challenges in drug ethnography, there are also rewards, as when findings are used productively to address the real issues drug users face, such as avoiding diseases, struggling with police harassment, or lacking access to appropriately designed treatment systems. The methods we have described here have repeatedly proven useful in these problems because findings obtained through methods that include ethnography and quantitative analysis have a very firm footing in the life experiences of drug users. Singer and his colleagues, for example, have repeatedly put their study findings to use in implementing programs to prevent HIV infection (Singer et al. 2001, 2003, 2005). Similarly, Page and colleagues (Page and Llanusa-Cestero 2006; Page et al. 2006) have used ethnographic research findings in combination with other methods to prevent HIV infection among drug users. Ethnographic perspective on health risks and other aspects of drug users' lifestyles has been the key to identifying and addressing key factors in the risks taken by people when they use drugs. By applying a fresh pair of eyes to specific sets of drug using behaviors, whether the drugs in question are legal or illegal, ethnographic research on drug use enhances the specificity and validity of findings on the impact of drug use on the lives of the users.

REFERENCES

Adler, Patricia A. and Adler, Peter (1991) *Backboards and Blackboards: College Athletes and Role Engulfment*. New York: Columbia University Press.

Agar, Michael (1973) *Ripping and Running: A Formal Ethnography of Urban Heroin Addicts*. New York: Academic Press.

Agar, Michael and MacDonald, James (1995) Focus groups and ethnography. *Human Organization* 54: 78–86.

Becker, Howard S. (1953) Becoming a marijuana user. *American Journal of Sociology* 59: 235–42.

Bourdieu, Pierre (1991) *Métier de Sociologue*. Chicago: University of Chicago Press.

Bourgois, Phillippe (2000) Disciplining addictions: the bio-politics of methadone and heroin in the United States. *Culture, Medicine, and Psychiatry* 24(2): 165–95.

Bourgois, Phillippe (2003) *In Search of Respect: Selling Crack in El Barrio*. 2nd edn. Cambridge: Cambridge University Press.

Carlson, Robert G. (1996) The political economy of AIDS among drug users in the United States: Beyond blaming the victim or powerful others. *American Anthropologist* 98(2): 266–78.

Carlson, Robert G. and Siegal, Harvey A. (1988) The crack life: an ethnographic overview of crack use and sexual behavior among African Americans in a Midwest metropolitan city. *Journal of Psychoactive Drugs* 23(1): 11–20.

Carter, William E. (ed). (1980) *Cannabis in Costa Rica*. Philadelphia: ISHI Press.

Cloward, Richard A and Ohlin, Lloyd E. (1960) *Delinquency and Opportunity: A Theory of Delinquent Gangs*. New York: Free Press.

Cohen, Albert K. (1955) *Delinquent Boys: The Culture of the Gang*. New York: Free Press.

Dunlap, Eloise, Golub, Andrew, Johnson, Bruce D. and Wesley, Damaris (2001) Intergenerational transmission of conduct norms for drugs, sexual exploitation, and violence: a case study. *British Journal of Criminology* 42(1): 1–20.

Dunlap, Eloise and Johnson, Bruce D. (1996) Family and human resources in the development of a female crack-seller career: case study of a hidden population. *Journal of Drug Issues* 26(1): 175–98.

Dunlap, Eloise, Johnson, Bruce D. and Manwar, Ali (1994). A successful female crack dealer: case-study of a deviant career. *Deviant Behavior* 15(1): 1–25.

Elliot, Delbert S., Ageton, Suzanne S. and Canter, Rachelle J. (1979) An integrated theoretical perspective on juvenile delinquency. *Journal on Research in Crime and Delinquency* 16 (1): 3–27.

Eiserman, Julie, Singer, Merrill, Schensul, Jean and Broomhall, Lorie (2003) Methodological Challenges in Club Drug Research. *Practicing Anthropology* 25(3): 19–22.

Evans-Pritchard, Edward Evan (1940) *The Nuer, A Description of the Modes of Livelihood and Political Institutions of a Nilotic People*. Oxford: The Clarendon Press.

Foucault, Michel (2003) *Il Faut Defendre la Societé*. New York: Picador.

Foucault, Michel (2011) *Courage de la Verité*. New York: Palgrave Macmillan.

Goodenough, Ward H. (1956) Componential analysis and the study of meaning. *Language* 32: 195–216.

Hirschi, Travis (1969) *Causes of Delinquency*. Berkeley: University of California Press.

Johnson, Bruce (1985) *Taking Care of Business: The Economics of Crime by Heroin Abusers*. Lexington: Lexington Books.

Johnson, Bruce D., Dunlap, Eloise E. and Maher, Lisa (1998) Nurturing for careers in drug use and crime: Conduct norms for children and juveniles in crack-using households. *Substance Use and Misuse* 33(7): 1511–46.

Johnson, Robert E. (1979) *Juvenile Delinquency and its Origins*. Cambridge: Cambridge University Press.

Kissell, Ted B. (2000) River of sleaze: a top Miami-Dade schools cop is the focus of a probe that recalls the area's biggest police scandal. *New Times*. http://www.miaminewtimes.com/2000-04-06/news/river-of-sleaze; Accessed May 26, 2014.

Koester, Stephen K. (1994) Copping, Running, and paraphernalia laws: contextual variables and needle risk behavior among injection drug users. *Human Organization* 53(3): 287–95.

Mead, Margaret (1928) *Coming of Age in Samoa: A Psychological Study in Primitive Youth for Western Civilization*. New York: W. Morrow.

Miller, Walter B. (1958) Lower class culture as a generating milieu of gang delinquency. *Journal of Social Issues* 14: 5–19.

Nye, Francis, Ivan (1958) *Family Relationships and Delinquent Behavior*. New York: Wiley.

Page, J. Bryan (1977) The study of San José, Costa Rica Street Culture: codes and communication in lower class society. In Brian M. DuToit (ed.), *Drugs, Rituals, and Altered States of Consciousness*. Rotterdam: Balkema, pp. 207–14.

Page, J. Bryan (1990) Streetside drug use among Cuban drug users in Miami, Florida. In R. Glick and J. Moore (eds), *Drug Use in Hispanic Communities*, New Brunswick: Rutgers Press, pp. 169–91.

Page, J. Bryan (1997) Vulcans and Jutes: Cuban fraternities and their disappearance. *Free Inquiry in Creative Sociology* 25(1): 65–74.

Page, J. Bryan (2006) International research and local authorities: interplay between research and police agendas in the field of drug abuse and AIDS. *Journal of Urban Health* (special issue) iv: 16–23.

Page, J. Bryan and Salazar, Jose (1999) Lemon juice as a solvent for heroin in Valencia, Spain (letter) *Substance Use and Misuse* 34(8): 1193–7.

Page, J. Bryan and Trotter, II, Robert T. (1999) To theorize or not to theorize. In Patricia Marshall and Merrill Singer (eds), *Anthropological Contributions to the Study of Drug Use*. Washington, D.C.: U.S. Government Printing Office, National Institute on Drug Abuse.

Page, J. Bryan and Llanusa-Cestero, Renée (2006) Changes in the get-off: social process and intervention in risk locales. *Substance Use and Misuse* 41(6–7): 1017–28.

Page, J. Bryan and Singer, Merrill (2010) *Comprehending Drug Use: Ethnographic Research at the Social Margins*. New Brunswick: Rutgers University Press.

Page, J. Bryan, Chitwood, Dale D., Smith, Prince C., Kane Normie and McBride, Duane C. (1990a). Intravenous drug abuse and HIV infection in Miami. *Medical Anthropology Quarterly* 4(1): 56–71.

Page, J. Bryan, Smith, Prince C. and Kane, Normie (1990b) Shooting galleries, their proprietors, and implications for prevention of AIDS. *Journal of Drug Issues* 5(1/2): 69–85.

Page, J. Bryan, Shapshak, Paul, Duran, Elena M., Even, Gerardo, Moleon-Borodowski, Ines and Llanusa-Cestero, Renée (2006) Detection of HIV-1 in injection paraphernalia: risk in an era of heightened awareness. *AIDS Patient Care* 20 (8): 576–85.

Partridge, William L. (1974) Exchange relationships in a community on the north coast of Colombia with special reference to Cannabis. *Ph.D. dissertation*. Gainesville: University of Florida.

Pelto, Pertti J. and Pelto, Gretel (1978) *Anthropological Research: The Structure of Inquiry*, 2nd edn. New York: Cambridge University Press.

Ripoll, Carmen A., Page, J. Bryan and Salazar, José M. (2003) Drug use in sex workers on the streets of Valencia. *Ethnicity in Drug Abuse* 1(4): 1–27.

Rubin, Vera and Comitas, Lambros (1975) *Ganja in Jamaica*. The Hague: Mouton.

Schensul, Jean J. and LeCompte, Margaret D. (2013) *Essential Ethnographic Methods: A Mixed Methods Approach*. New York: Altamira Press.

Singer, Merrill (2001) Toward a bio-cultural and political economic integration of alcohol, tobacco and drug studies. *Social Science and Medicine* 53(2): 199–213.

Singer, Merrill (2003) The Hispanic Health Council: an experiment in applied anthropology. *Practicing Anthropology* 25(3): 2–7.

Singer, Merrill, Marshall, Patricia, Trotter, Robert, Schensul, Jean, Weeks, Margaret, Simmons, Janie and Radda, Kim (1999) Ethics, ethnography, drug use and AIDS: dilemmas and standards in federally funded research. In Patricia Marshall, Merrill Singer and Michael Clatts (eds), *Cultural, Observational, and Epidemiological Approaches in the Prevention of Drug Abuse and HIV/AIDS*. Bethesda: National Institute on Drug Abuse, pp. 198–222.

Singer, Merrill, Juvalis, Joy Ann and Weeks, Margaret (2000) High on illy: studying an emergent drug problem in Hartford, CT. *Medical Anthropology* 18: 365–88.

Singer, Merrill, Scott, Glen, Wilson, Scott, Easton Delia and Weeks, Margaret (2001) 'War Stories': AIDS prevention and the street narratives of drug users. *Qualitative Health Research* 11(5): 589–611.

Singer, Merrill, Stopka, Thomas, Shaw, Susan, Santilices, Claudia, Buchanan, David, Teng, Wei, Khoosnood, Kaveh and Heimer, Robert (2005) Lessons from the field: from research to application in the fight against AIDS among injection drug users in three New England Cities. *Human Organization* 64(2): 179–91.

Spradley, James P. (1970) *You Owe Yourself a Drunk: An Ethnography of Urban Nomads*. Boston: Little, Brown.

Sterk, Claire (1999) *Fast Lives: Women Who Use Crack Cocaine*. Philadelphia: Temple University Press.

Sutherland, Edwin Hardin (1966) *Criminology*. Philadelphia: Lippincott.

True, William Ray, Hovey, Mary Ann, Page, J. Bryan and Doughty, Paul (1980) Marijuana user lifestyles. In William E. Carter (ed.), *Cannabis in Costa Rica*. Philadelphia: ISHI Press, pp. 98–115.

Voss, Harlan L. (1963) Ethnic differentials in delinquency in Honolulu. *Journal of Criminal Law and Criminology* 54: 322–7.

Weeks, Margaret, Clair, Scott, Singer, Merrill, Radda, Kim, Schensul, Jean, Wilson, Scott, Martinez, Maria, Scott, Glenn and Knight, Glenn. (2001) High risk drug use sites, meaning and practice. *Journal of Drug Issues* 31(1): 781–808.

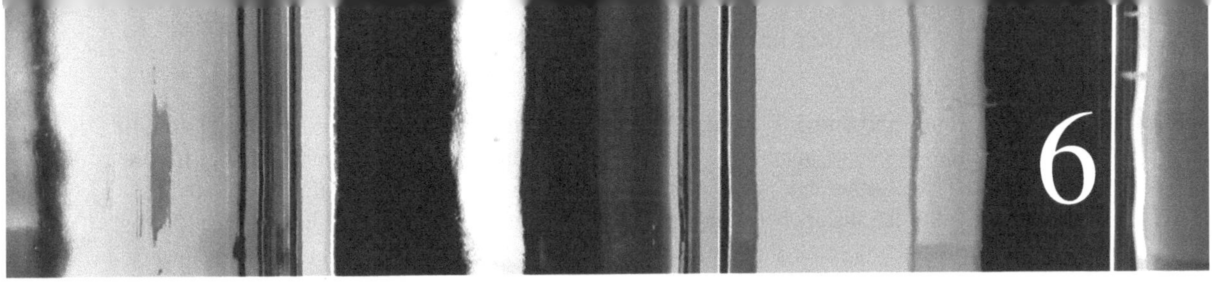

Criminological Perspectives

Karen Joe Laidler

INTRODUCTION

Criminology lies at a somewhat peculiar juncture in the study of drugs and alcohol. This is largely because the discipline, while commonly understood as a field in its own right, is in fact an eclectic mix of – naming only a few of the dominant ones – history, psychology, sociology, politics, public health, medicine, and law. These disciplines, with their own assumptions, paradigms, and policy concerns, have, to some extent, converged, blending to create a criminological lens on drugs and alcohol. This chapter traces the development of three key themes and debates in drug and alcohol studies in criminology.

One of the key themes in drug studies across disciplines is consumption. As social historians have underscored, consumption of pleasurable substances has at various social political points in time, become the subject of moral contestation and legal controls. It is therefore not surprising that criminologists too, with their interests in criminalization, have debated over the causes and consequences of alcohol and drug use. A spectrum of other explanatory frameworks has emerged, reflecting the disciplinary concerns from within and outside criminology, and range from psychological traits of individuals at one end to collective attributes of social groups at the other end. At issue with all of these explanations is the balance between the individual, free will, and the collective, or agency and social structure.

The connection between drugs and crime has been a second dominant theme, emerging as a key research agenda in the 1930s through the 1970s as crime rates rose, as did the use of narcotics, most notably, heroin. Here too, we see a focus on understanding the relationship between alcohol and violence. In the 1980s, the emergence of a distinct crack cocaine scene and the impending war on drugs had a significant impact for criminology. It was at this time, that criminology stepped up its efforts to establish the precise links between drugs and crime, and moving beyond the more specialized focus on narcotics. Policy calls resulted in American criminology focusing on the relationship between drugs and crime, and later became the subject of much interest in other locales including the UK and Australia. Popular characterizations portrayed drug users, especially those using crack cocaine, as being 'driven' to commit crime and violent acts because of their consuming addiction. Goldstein's 1985 tripartite model of the drugs crime link became a focal point in the ongoing debates on the relationship between drugs, crime, and violence.

A focus on this tripartite relationship was also linked to a focus on particular social groups, including youth gangs, who were popularly assumed, at least in the 1980s and early 1990s, to control much of the crack cocaine markets in the US. Drug markets have become another, third, key theme emerging from the expansion and proliferation of local to national and global drug use.

The chapter concludes with a look at recent criminological directions in understanding drug use and markets, with a particular focus on the role of social relationships in the contemporary drug market. As will become evident throughout the chapter, criminological research on drugs and crime has largely been shaped by scholars working in the North American, the UK, and Australian context and traditions. While the North/South debate in criminology is beyond the scope of this chapter, there are a few points to bear in mind (see Aas, 2012; Carrington et al., 2016). First, it is only in recent years that voices from the periphery have emerged in criminology, including in the area of drugs and crime. Historically, there has been a tendency to adopt the Northern paradigm, applying and testing concepts and theories in 'other' cultures (Karstedt, 2001; Carrington et al., 2016). Second, the lack of voices from the South on drugs and crime, in many sites in the periphery, is related to their geopolitical positioning where drugs may be linked to political movements, and, in turn, raise different sorts of questions than the Northern focus on etiology and domestic trade. It may also be related to cultural values and colonial politics. As Lee and Joe Laidler (2013) have described, the historical dominance of administrative criminology in Asia has shaped the kind of questions that have and could be asked, but this is changing with the theoretical challenges of global criminology.

THE CRIMINOLOGICAL LENSES ON CONSUMPTION

As this handbook attests to, the study of drugs and alcohol has emerged as an area of inquiry with distinct disciplinary and interdisciplinary frameworks. One key question running through these frameworks is that of causation or etiology. Why do individuals or groups of individuals use drugs? Despite over a century of research and debate among psychologists, psychiatrists, public health experts, sociologists, criminologists, legal scholars, and economists, it seems we are no closer to a definitive answer. This is due in part to differences in disciplinary assumptions about human nature and social structure, but also to moral and political agendas.

Criminology's presence in these debates emerged slowly, in part because of its comparatively more recent origins, and its early interdisciplinary connections with anthropology, sociology, and psychology. Many of the ideas and groundwork for contemporary criminological studies originated in sociological and psychological studies, some of which were responding to biomedical approaches, during the first half of the 1900s.

Early etiological work in the nineteenth century emerged in the biomedical field, with physicians, psychiatrists, biologists, social reformists, and others focusing on alcohol, narcotics (or opiates), and addiction. Several explanatory models about alcohol, drugs and addiction emerged in the 1800s and early 1900s (see Nicholls, 2009; Room,

1984; Barrows and Room, 1991; Berridge, 1999). Historians observed that many medical professionals described habitual and chronic alcohol use as a disease of the will in the nineteenth century; this view gained momentum, resulting with the American Medical Association formally endorsing the disease model in the 1950s. Treatment under this model largely focused on identification and admission of the disease and a commitment to abstinence. The disease of the will, however, has never been precisely defined, and has remained a highly contested idea. A second explanation is that of the temperance model with social reformists advocating the view that alcohol was a dangerous and detrimental substance to the individual and society at large, therefore requiring abstinence. This argument was the basis for the prohibition movement in the late 1800s. A third explanation – the criminological model – described in further detail below, also emerged in the work of Lombroso and others, who suggested that alcohol and drug use was connected to inherent individual deficits.

In addition, observers have noted that the sustained and greater preoccupation with alcohol rather than opiate addiction until the 1950s was due in part to the alcoholic's potential for volatile behavior as compared with the narcotic addict's sedated state (Parker and Rebhun, 1995; Courtwright, 1997; Chen, 2014). As Courtwright (1997) points out, many addicts at the time were typically white women, whose opiate addiction resulted from chronic use for self or physician prescribed pain relief. These women, unlike the dominant male alcoholic addict, were unlikely to pose a criminal or health threat. While some physicians viewed alcohol and narcotic addiction as neuropsychiatric disorders or hereditary defects, others agreed with psychologists believing addicts suffered from psychological defects or poor socialization (Chen 2014). The view of narcotic addicts as unrestrained pleasure seeking psychopaths gained prominence through the work of Kolb (1925), and helped shift the focus in the US., from the declining numbers of medical opiate addicts to the increasingly visible heroin street addicts (Courtwright 1997). Bean (2014) observed that narcotics use emerged as a visible social problem in the 1960s with its association to a bohemian lifestyle and it was cast as an individual pathology. Few in the medical field acknowledged the significance of social structure and environment nor that use did not necessarily equate with addiction, but these issues were central to the growing counterview among Chicago sociologists. As Franca and Franco, this volume, details the contributions of the Chicago school, here I reference Lindesmith's shift to study the social processes of addiction, as this has served as an important marker for sociological criminology.

Lindesmith (1938) challenged Kolb's addiction model of psychopathology on the grounds that it was unable to explain cases in which, despite repeated administration of opiates, some individuals became 'incurable addicts' while others did not. A theory of addiction, he argued, must be able to explain this differential. A social process orientation does this by taking into account individual differences and the definitional process of group interaction.

Addiction is established in the first instance in a process involving: 1) the interpretation of the withdrawal symptoms as being caused by the absence of opiates, followed by; 2) the use of the drug for the consciously understood purpose of alleviating these symptoms or of keeping them suppressed.

> As a result of this process there is established in the addict the typical desire for the drug, a constant sense of dependence upon it, and the other attendant features of addiction. The attitudes, which arise in this experience, persist when the drug has been removed and predispose toward relapse. When the point is reached at which withdrawal symptoms intrude themselves upon the attention of the individual and compel him to go on using the drug, he also has forced upon him the unwelcome definition of himself as a 'dope fiend'. He realizes then what the craving for drugs means, and applying to his own conduct the symbols,

> which the group applies to it, he is compelled to readjust his conception of himself to the implications of this collective viewpoint. (Lindesmith, 1938: 606)

Lindesmith's focus on the sociological nature of drug addiction provided the groundwork for a critical questioning of causation and an in-depth examination of the processes and micro-interactions involved not just in addiction but across the spectrum of use. As Waldorf (1973) notes, in the first half of the twentieth century in the US, the FBI's political propaganda about the evils of drugs, especially heroin and marijuana, created the stereotype that addiction followed from one's first use, and blinded scientists from making distinctions between experimentation and addiction. Instead, scientists were preoccupied in the quest for the single cause or grand theory of narcotic addiction. Waldorf's study (1973) was one of the few at the time to examine the initial use of heroin, and the importance of the cultural and social setting in defining and facilitating use. He found that the stereotype of immediate addiction did not match with respondents reports about their first use. Initial use was motivated by a range of reasons, including stress relief, curiosity, and peer sociability. In the UK, Young (1971) similarly found that the drug taker's experience was connected not only to the drug's pharmacological effects, but also intimately related to the cultural context of use (a setting where the meaning of use is understood by others). Like other legal and illegal drugs, first use occurred in a distinct social cultural milieu in interaction with others (Waldorf, 1973). This focus on the social processes of drug use provided an alternative paradigm to the disease and temperance models, and in doing so, opened the path to examine questions about why some experiment and others go on to develop dependence to different types of drugs emerging in the drug market. Psychiatrist, Norman Zinberg, developed this framework further with drug, set and setting, which demonstrated that the drug experience varied, and did not necessarily result in dependence as the effects of particular drugs were dependent on the interaction of individual expectations, his/her mindset, and the cultural milieu (Zinberg, 1984). Subsequent efforts have focused on the distinctions in types of consumers – experimenters, social recreational users, regular users, and dysfunctional or problematic users – as well as the types of drugs – stimulants, depressants, and hallucinogens (Orcutt and Rudy, 2003; Inciardi and McElrath, 2010).

The idea of pleasure as a causal explanation for drug use seems obvious, as most accounts of intoxication indicate that the feelings derived from using (a range of drugs) are associated with unique sensory experiences. The essence of pleasure opens up newfound feelings of freedom, liberation, empathy, euphoria, excitement, or calmness, depending on the type of substance. The use of substances to alter consciousness, has featured as a 'universal human theme' from the early Bronze Age's affinity with alcohol to the Neolithic period's cultural use of cannabis and the classical epoch's rituals with opium to today's youthful fascination with dance drugs like ecstasy. Although historical accounts document these sensory pleasures, there has been much silence on this in scholarly and policy arenas (Joe Laidler et al., 2014).

Notable exceptions to this silence occurred first with Becker's (1953) treatise on social learning and the process of becoming a marijuana user. Following the lead of Lindesmith, Becker countered the dominant view that use was equivalent to addiction. Instead, an individual could, through interaction with others, learn to smoke marijuana, what to expect from the drug and take pleasure in the experience. His objective was to demonstrate that '*the use of marijuana for pleasure*' was a 'non-compulsive and casual behavior', indicative of recreational use (as distinct from addiction) (Becker's emphasis, 1953: 235).

The idea of pleasure and altered states was pursued in earnest in the 1960s when many of the Harvard school and others pursued the study of the ways in which drugs, such as

LSD and MDMA, could be incorporated into therapy (Leary, 2008). For Leary, the ability to 'turn on, tune in, and drop out' with psychedelics held the promise of not just pleasure but spiritual awakening (Joe Laidler et al., 2014: 63). Weil (1972) similarly argued that the desire for altered states was not morally wrong but a natural impulse. It alleviated pain and stress, facilitated spirituality and self-awareness in relation to others and the world around him/her through 'deep thinking'. Although the psychedelic project was fraught with political and moral tension, it led to new alternative ways of understanding the spiritual dimensions of drug use. With the rise of ecstasy use in the dance drug scene, observers have pointed to the spirituality of the drug in the context of raves (Hutson, 2000; St John, 2004; Partridge, 2005; Joe Laidler and Hunt 2013). Alongside the increasing interest in the link between spirituality and drugs, there has been a renewed focus on pleasure, particularly in theorizing intoxication, risks and governance (Chatterton and Hollands, 2003; O'Malley and Valverde, 2004; Hunt and Evans, 2008; Hunt et al., 2009; Zajdow, 2010).

At the same time, on another front, we are reminded that the current American 'brain disease' paradigm in the form of addiction neuroscience bears a striking resemblance to the early twentieth century (Courtwright, 2010; Vrecko, 2010; Hammer et al., 2013). The current 'brain disease' paradigm is couched in politically neutral and rational terminology in an attempt to facilitate treatment, although many within the science and social sciences communities contest the disease paradigm in treating drug dependence. The consequence, however, has been to advance the neurobiological addiction approach, and an alliance between a select group of policymakers and scientists in the War on Drugs, and to further the link between drugs and crime (Vrecko, 2010).

It seems, from this review of some of the shifts and turns in the etiological question from different disciplines (of which criminology's presence has been largely influenced by sociology and psychology) that the very idea of causation is a highly contested one, shaped by 'policy funders' with particular political agendas (Allen, 2007). The research project – questions, designs, objectives, findings – are framed within the context of political priorities (Hunt and Barker, 2001). Reflecting on the polemics of drug addiction, over half a century ago (but certainly relevant today), Schur (1963: 211)[1], aptly raises the question, 'is addiction a crime or is it a disease?'

THE PURSUIT AND PARADOX OF A DRUGS CRIME CONNECTION

For criminologists, one of the most vexing research questions centers on the relationship between alcohol, drugs and crime, originating well over a century ago (Ball et al., 1981; Inciardi, 1981; Nurco et al., 1991). Early work on alcohol assumed a deterministic and moral stance. In the latter part of the nineteenth century, while chemists, biologists, pathologists and others identified the 'true nature' of alcohol and its attendant social evils (Howard, 1918), the pioneer of criminology, Lombroso (1895), followed the natural science model, and subscribed to a hereditary explanation for the alcoholic criminal. For Lombroso, alcoholism and drugs were inextricably linked to crime and mental illness. Despite its hereditary link, Lombroso believed that a stay in prison could 'cure' the alcoholic's insanity and affliction to crime because the isolation would help to rid the body and soul of the poisons of alcohol.

> It is well known that drunkenness causes crime… All stimulants have the capacity to drive us to crime, suicide, or insanity, phenomena that are inextricably intertwined. Alcohol and drugs irritate the nervous centers…From the perspective of criminal anthropology; I have no doubt that the criminal alcoholic is a special variant of the epileptic even though he often lacks physical degenerative anomalies. However, there is one important difference between

the two groups: if alcoholics give up drinking entirely, they have a greater possibility of cure than epileptics. (Lombroso, 1895: 280)

The inborn nature of alcoholic criminals (Lombroso 1899), however, was supplanted not long after, and even Lombroso recognized, that the social environment played a critical role in predicting who was among the criminal classes. Howard (1918), reflecting on sociological and criminological studies at the time, argued that alcoholic criminals were 'creatures of their environment'. Citing prison studies, he noted that a substantial proportion of convicts had committed their crimes because of intemperance. Among the convict population, however, there were distinctions. The 'notoriously' hardest drinking groups, including the Scots, Irish, Scandinavians, and the English, were greater in numbers in prison for their drinking and serious crimes. Germans, by contrast, were fewer in numbers, due likely, he argues, to their 'superior social environment', which discourages excessive drinking (Howard, 1918).

Although this view placed more emphasis on environmental influences, its stance was similar with its assumption that stricter regulatory controls over alcohol would protect particular groups from the temptations and evils associated with alcohol. Howard advocated the following:

Under the shield of heredity the social conscience may no longer shift its burden to the shoulders of the Almighty. If directly or indirectly criminality is mainly the fruit of bad social conditions, the remedy is in society's own hands; for intellectual man, unlike the lower animal, is able to transform his environment. Sometimes the task is titanic. To master the crime-producing environment which consists in alcohol and the organized alcohol traffic may cost more courage, wisdom, and toil than it cost to abolish human slavery, than it may cost to destroy the 'great white plague' or the 'great black plague'; but it can be done and it will be done when its nature is clearly understood by the majority. (Howard, 1918: 63–4)

This environmental view was aligned with the push for stricter controls with narcotics. By 1914, the Harrison Act, in the US, had criminalized the unauthorized sale, possession, or purchase of narcotics, and it was followed by a number of acts further criminalizing the importation of narcotics. Not surprisingly, with this criminalization came the redefinition of practices as well as the increase in cost and scarcity of narcotics. In the 1920s, the public call for the complete criminalization of drugs was clear and based on the rationale that there was a natural and inevitable link between drug addiction and crime. The visibility of the 'new' street addict demanded new legal controls. As Greenberg and Adler (1974) document, it was at this time that the 'dope fiend' – driven to crime by his need for the drug to alleviate the pains of withdrawal – entered the public imagination.

Sara Graham-Mulhall, then president of the Narcotic Control League, in outlining the 'Ten Basic Facts about Drug Addiction and Preventable Crime', spoke authoritatively about this link, despite little evidence.

No one knows scientifically the relation between drug addiction and crime and no one is trying to find out on a scale large enough to justify current belittling conclusions (Fact 3) [but] the addict is an incurable criminal so long as he is an uncured addict (Fact 4). Every addict, no matter how cultivated, is under our laws a potential criminal, because violation of law bulks small compared with the pain of going without the drug (Fact 5)... The ten basic facts... point the way to preventing all crime of and from addiction by making addiction impossible. Safety lies in annihilating drugs for addiction, not in the philosophical distinctions as to *whether the egg preceded or followed the chicken*. (Graham-Mulhall, 1926: 163–5; my emphasis)

This testament notably came at the heels of the World Opium Conference of 1924, where, as Graham-Mulhall pointed out, 'when Britain taunted us with holding the Christian World's record of opium consumption' (1926: 163). Despite increasing pressure on Britain, prohibitive controls on opium would have dire effects on its colonial enterprises. In Hong Kong, the colonial government conceded with slight revisions to regulations and controls, but it would not stop one of its major sources of revenue. Opium revenue accounted for nearly one-half of the colonial government's revenues at its height in 1918 (Joe Laidler et al., 2000). The colonial administration relied for a large proportion of its revenue from opium sales until the start of the Second World War (Joe Laidler et al., 2000). Despite ever increasing restrictions and eventual criminalization in many locales, the same question continued to plague the drug field, followed with years of research and debate.

In the 1920s, research suggested that drug use, specifically of opiates, occurred prior to engagement with crime, yet there were other studies suggesting the onset of drug use prior to criminal involvement. From the start, the temporal sequence between crime and drugs was identified as the primary issue. From the 1920s through the 1940s, US studies generally showed more support for the view that narcotics addicts, who increasingly were from the lower socioeconomic class, did not have money to buy drugs, and had little choice but to commit crime to support his/her addiction. Still, there were studies indicating that the addict had to be immersed in a criminal lifestyle in order to obtain his/her knowledge and networks for using (Greenberg and Adler, 1974). From the 1950s to the 1970s, the number of studies in the US and elsewhere appeared to be increasing, perhaps related to the growing visibility of street addicts and resulting public policy concerns.

While there appeared to be growing support for the view that the criminal lifestyle preceded narcotics addiction, Greenberg and Adler (1974) argued that these studies had a number of methodological problems including issues related to representativeness and control groups. While there was evidence to support the alternative view, several observers offered explanations as to why narcotics addicts prior to the 1950s were less likely to have a criminal history and those from the 1950s onwards were criminally active. Finestone, for example, explained the increase in narcotics addiction and crime among young people as due to relative deprivation and criminal subculture they find themselves in. This is, he argues, part of the 'street corner society' (Finestone 1957: 73). Others explained the shift as the result of changes in federal laws, including a mandatory two-year minimum sentences (The Boggs Act 1951), which resulted in market changes, with addicts needing more money to pay for higher prices, despite a decline in quality (Musto, 1973; Abrams et al., 1968; cited by Greenberg and Adler, 1974: 234).

The debate continued into the 1980s, and Ball et al. (1981) underscore the importance of the micro and macro situational factors that need to be considered in the drug crime nexus. As they point out:

> This difference in the sequence of events between the early and later studies suggests that there is no invariant relationship between heroin addiction and crime. Instead, it seems that the relationship is contingent upon the particular historical period and population of heroin addicts selected. Thus, if heroin is being introduced into a noncriminal or low criminal population (e.g. medical professionals or middle class adults) it would be highly unlikely to find criminality preceding heroin use. Conversely, higher levels of preexisting criminality among heroin addicts would be expected within a population with a high endemic crime rate (e.g. youthful lower class males in metropolitan slums...It seems reasonable to conclude, therefore that the issue of the sequence of unique events (first heroin use or a first act of delinquency) may be less significant than determining the continuing influences that sustain criminality and opiate addition over a period years or decades. (Ball et al., 1981: 40)

Despite decades of research, criminologists were still no closer to a definitive answer to, what Graham-Mulhall (1926), and later Inciardi (1981), referred to, as the 'chicken and egg' question. That is, does drug consumption lead an individual to commit crime to support his addiction? Or does involvement in a criminal lifestyle include or lead one to drug use? What is the temporal sequence of drugs and crime? In addition to this question of temporal sequence, the type of criminal behavior of drug users was also an aspect of the drug crime debate from the 1920s to the 1970s. Not surprisingly, studies generally indicated that drug users' crimes were largely for monetary gain and violence was not necessarily involved (Greenberg and Adler, 1974)

From the 1980s onwards, criminologists' interest in the crime nexus shifted, with increased attention on drug use and types of crime. Why at this particular point in time? How was it distinct from the earlier period? At this time, the US witnessed the rise of crack cocaine use in many inner cities, including Los Angeles, New York City, and Chicago, with devastating effects on individuals, their families, and communities. Policymakers and the police were particularly concerned with the rise in drug related violence. Goldstein's tripartite model identified three frameworks for understanding the link between drug use and crime, including the economic compulsive model (income generating), the psychopharmacological motive (impaired cognition), and the systemic frame (instrumentally associated with drug dealing). This model led to attempts to replicate, modify, and debate the connections (Entorf and Winker, 2008; Bennett and Holloway, 2009).

The popular image of those involved in the crack cocaine market was of violence prone, gun-toting youth gang members in deathly competition with each other. In a number of cities across the US, researchers found a great deal of variation in the link between gangs, drugs, and violence. Some observers found gangs organized in a corporate style, acting in accordance with rational and instrumental codes in California and Detroit (Skolnick et al., 1989; Taylor 1989). Others documented more opportunistic and less organized approaches among some gangs in New York and Chicago (Williams, 1989; Padilla, 1992). Other studies suggested that gang members were dealing drugs as individuals, without a formal or hierarchal structure. Waldorf et al. (1993) argued that San Francisco and much of California's drug market was organized around many small entrepreneurs moving drugs across the Mexican border working against any formal organization (Joe Laidler and Hunt, 2012).

Although there was great variation in whether gangs acted as collectives or its members were individual entrepreneurs, research did support the view that gangs were involved in drug distribution, with some participation in trafficking, but predominantly involvement at the street level. Importantly, studies also suggested that many gang members did use and sell drugs, but certainly not all (Howell and Decker, 1999). The emergence of the crack cocaine scene and gang involvement was linked to the devastating economic restructuring in many of American's inner cities (Hagedorn, 1988). But what of violence and gangs? The public imagination, and no less the 'criminologists' gang' (Katz and Jackson-Jacobs, 2004) portray gang members as heavily involved in violence, often related to territorial protection of their drug and turf. Research appears to show, however, that there is great variability in whether, and how, gang violence is related to drug dealing and it is dependent on other factors such as space and drug types. Levitt and Venkatesh (2000) found gangs are likely to discourage violence, as this may bring unwanted police and community attention, and at the same time, keep potential customers away for fear of their safety. In our own work (Joe Laidler and Hunt 2012), gang violence related to drug dealing was generally avoided as it was bad for business. Instead, gang violence was likely to be due to individual masculinity contests of honor in the context of everyday life. Taniguichi et al. (2011) found drug gangs were engaged in violence in open-air drug distribution spaces, and resorted to higher levels of violence and property offenses where other groups competed in the same space. In the UK, researchers began to study the gang, drug and crime connection much later as that country witnessed the rise of a 'gang phenomenon' (Bennett and Holloway, 2004).

UK observers have also pointed to the distinctions between occasional recreational users (who perceive 'hard' drugs such as heroin as unacceptable), serious recreational users (who are respectable but start using 'hard drugs' as an alternative to chill out), and problematic users (who are regularly using 'hard drugs') (Parker et al., 1998, 2002; Allen 2007). Those with problematic use are believed to be concentrated in marginalized communities where the supply and accessibility of heroin is greater, and therefore, for policymakers, of greater political concern because of a perceived association between 'hard' drug use and acquisitive crime (Allen 2007). Simpson (2003) further demonstrates that by going beyond the recreational/problematic dichotomy, and including the 'persistent drug user', we can observe the ways in which shifts in drug use and type operate in relation to engagement with crime.

FROM LOCAL TO GLOBAL DRUG MARKETS

International work on drug markets has detailed the structure, organization, and layers of drug distribution for different drugs, particularly heroin, cocaine, and cannabis. There is general agreement on several points: (i) there is no clear unified definition of the market; (ii) two general structures exist with one of a hierarchical nature connected to criminal syndicates and the other fluid networks of entrepreneurs; and (iii) distribution chains are loosely understood at the international trafficking level, the middle market, and the retail level (McSweeney et al., 2010).

One reason for the lack of consensus on the definition of the market lies in the different frameworks used. As Dwyer and Moore (2010) observe, particularly in the Australian context, economists define the market in relation to supply and demand, and drawing from surveillance data, provide detailed knowledge about trends (price, purity, and availability). Criminologists define the market in relation to the illegal practices of different parties – (users, deals, wholesalers, and producers) and the impact of enforcement on these practices, often drawing from enforcement and professional sources as well as self-reports of those involved in distribution. Although both approaches operate from different definitions, they share common theoretical and methodological assumptions, which hamper our understanding of drug distribution, including the reification of the market as an object. In other words, 'the market is seen to exist prior to the social relations and processes by which it is constituted…[yet] markets are socially produced… constituted by networks of social relations and transactions' (Dwyer and Moore, 2010: 88). Moreover, the standpoint of 'market as object' assumes a deterministic view of those involved in transactions (buyers and sellers) that act in accordance to calculated rational self-pursuit, and as such, are likely to be deterred if the costs outweigh the benefits. However, these assumptions fail to explain how buyers and sellers accommodate and adapt to market changes (Dwyer and Moore, 2010). Sociological and anthropological work on drug markets, drawing from qualitative methods, have made these social processes central to their investigations (Adler 1985; Murphy et al., 1990; Morgan and Joe Laidler 1995; Bourgois 1996; Hamid et al., 1997; Jacobs 1998; Maher et al., 1998; Curtis and Wendel 2000; Sandberg and Pedersen 2008). Ruggiero and South (1997) observed that drug markets are indeed affected by changes in economic structures. Yet the history of drug markets in the US and the UK suggests that they can be likened to a city bazaar – a hub of licit and illicit activity with a range of individuals performing and moving between legal and illegal work. Despite the appearance of a fluid market, it is subject to a number of 'conditions', including the constant threat of police intervention, and consequently, a division of labor emerges, introducing barricades from within. Others have also has found that markets are fluid, flexible, and involve networks of relationships built on trust, reciprocity, and differential opportunities. Møller and Sandberg (2015) found that fronting, though disliked for its risks, is important in building trust, and credit is inextricably linked to social and economic relationships. Denton and O'Malley (1999) similarly underscore the importance of trust for women drug dealers.

What becomes clear from drug market research is that social relations, between the consumer and the supplier, are crucial to the market exchange. While drugs are indeed a commodity, its use is part of a social activity – embedded with meaning and entailing social processes and relations. This process starts from the point of planning the event with others and determining how to obtain the drugs for the event with consideration of the supplier's reputation, quality, quantity, price, purchase location, risks of victimization and detection, safety, and expected reciprocity of others from past events. Moore and Miles (2004) make a similar point, noting that club drug use involves rituals and processes as users organize the night, purchase the drug, and plan pre, during, and after activities (see also Chapter 37, this volume)

Among researchers documenting the emergent youth drug culture (where consumption has been the primary focus), there has been a small but growing number who have picked up on this exact point: that social relations are key to understanding drug transactions in this emergent youth context. Parker (2000) was among the first to observe that most young British recreational drug users get their drugs free or share in the purchasing from relatives, friends, and acquaintances. As he observes, most users are also suppliers for their peer networks, deriving little financial gain from being the supplier (just enough to cover costs or get own supply free). Thus the process of obtaining drugs involves 'complex social arrangements' (Parker 2000: 75) whereby peer networks 'sort' out and share with each other, based on reciprocity and trust. As such, they do not identify themselves as 'real drug dealers', but instead, attempt to keep a distance from 'real dealers'. This is evident from Parker's description of the 'rules of engagement with the drugs market: Never make a transaction (money for drugs) yourself. Always rely on a partner, friend or "friend of a friend" of a drugs dealer. Ideally "club" your financial contribution with others' (Parker 2000: 76).

As Coomber and Turnbull (2007) and South (2004) observe, this transactional arena is a distinctly social one within the UK drug marketplace and it has become relatively normalized among recreational users. Other countries, such as the US and Australia, report similar social arrangements (Hamilton 2005; Schensul et al., 2005; Jacinto et al., 2008). Thus, despite the local culture of drug markets, there are emergent commonalities internationally. The boundaries between young recreational users and sellers are blurring and raise theoretical questions about the changing nature of young people's social consumption and identity processes. Research thus far suggests that 'social supply' enhances social interaction among peers, and is embedded in a culture governed by rules, rituals, and norms of reciprocity, sharing, trust, and gifting. Exchange through sharing and gifting serve to solidify relationships as well as set boundaries for inclusiveness and distinction (Hamilton 2005; Coomber and Turnbull 2007; Jacinto et al., 2008).

Such socially oriented transactions are distinct from conventional drug dealing arrangements in open street-level sales and closed systems, which typically operate within a hierarchal and controlled structure (May et al., 2000). They are also distinct from the 'semi-open' system that has emerged in the nightclub scene where dealers sell to unknown buyers providing the latter 'looks the part', typically in private or semipublic locales (e.g. clubs) (May et al., 2000; May and Hough 2004; Ward 2010). Semi-public systems, such as nightclub floor dealing, are typically operated through bouncers and doormen (Hobbs et al., 2003; Sanders 2006; Pearson 2007).

This complex and fluid arena for drug transactions challenges conventional notions about public definitions and legal penalties associated with drug selling and trafficking, as young people who are embedded in networks of users and suppliers perceive themselves as distinct from 'real drug dealers'. Moreover, 'sharing' and 'gifts' in the context of social relationships are an important aspect of culture and daily life, and in the context of youth drug use, present challenges for demand reduction – with its emphasis on abstinence and recovery (Hamilton 2005).

CONCLUSION

In this chapter, I have attempted to review the history and role of criminology in understanding alcohol and drug use, its connections to crime and participation in the drug market. Criminologists' focus on consumption, at least in its early years, occurred in the context of the disease model advocated by the biomedical field. Given the dominance of the disease model, it should not be so surprising then that early criminological studies, as evidenced in Lombroso's work, followed a similar paradigm – one that focused on individual deficits and pathologies. A counter framework to the individual pathologies emerged in the 1930s, gathering momentum over the next three decades. This alternative view, advocated by sociologists and psychiatrists, underscored the range, variability and distinctions among drug users, and therefore, the need to bring the social processes and the cultural milieu of drug taking to the foreground. This analytical shift has also broadened the lens to challenge assumptions about individual pathologies and environmental stressors, and examine pleasure and spirituality as fundamental to the drug taking experience.

Although Lombroso's work set the stage, suggesting that alcohol and drug use was inextricably linked to crime, this view was relatively short-lived as an environmental view provided a more expansive explanation for, what was perceived to be, an addict population concentrated within particular groups and communities. The environmental view provided the 'evidence' for criminalization. For criminologists, the drug crime nexus became a major area of debate with the challenges of determining temporal order (i.e. the chicken and egg phenomenon), and subsequently, disentangling the role of gangs and violence in the nexus. Despite the advances in understanding causes of drug taking and the drug-crime connection, these links are still far from being definitively established. But perhaps this should not be so surprising given the ways in which criminological research questions on alcohol, drugs, and crime are framed by assumptions about human agency and social structure, and relatedly, within particular political and moral paradigms (Allen, 2007; Hunt and Barker, 2001). Although these connections are likely to continue to be the subject of debate and controversy, criminological and sociological discussions have facilitated a broader and more nuanced lens for looking at the range of alcohol and drug consumers in modern society, the ways they obtain their supplies, and importantly, that users – experimenters, occasional, regular, or chronic – do not necessarily engage in crime.

Although criminologists have not developed a consensus on a definition of the market, perhaps partly due to its cultural and geopolitical variability, research, especially in the US, UK, and Australia has focused on unpacking the organization and layers of the market. Recent research has underscored the importance of understanding the marketplace less as an 'object' and more as a fluid and flexible scene, with some suggesting it be understood as a city 'bazaar' with mobile actors and barricades. With the diversification of the drug scene and its connection to youth leisure, questions have also emerged over how young people obtain, share, and use drugs. Social supply – a cultural feature of drug taking with norms of trust and reciprocity – raise further questions about assumptions in existing drug laws.

There are areas beyond the scope of this discussion including the work of positive criminology with their interest in the role of the criminal justice system in the recovery process, cultural criminology with their focus on popular portrayals of drug use, and crime and evaluations of drug courts.

While one could argue that much progress has been made in criminology in these three areas, one of the key challenges ahead is to move beyond a domestic framework. As I noted earlier, much of the criminological work on drugs and crime has been from the US, the UK, and Australia. Yet global criminology reminds us that the histories, culture, and geopolitics of the peripheries are essential to understanding the core.

NOTE

1 Schur's study on narcotic addiction compared the British medical approach to that of America's punitive criminal laws.

REFERENCES

Aas, K. (2012) 'The earth is one but the world is not': criminological theory and its geopolitical divisions. *Theoretical Criminology,* 16(1): 5–20.

Abrams, A., Gagnon, J.H. and Levin, J.J. (1968) Psychosocial aspects of addiction. *American Journal of Public Health*, 58(11): 2142–55.

Adler, P. (1985) *Wheeling and Dealing: An Ethnography of an Upper-Level Drug Dealing and Smuggling Community.* New York: Columbia University Press.

Allen, C. (2007) *Crime, Drugs and Social Theory: A Phenomenological Approach*. Surrey: Ashgate.

Ball, J., Rosen, L., Flueck, J. and Nurco, D. (1981) The criminality of heroin addicts: when addicted and when off opiates. In J. Inciardi (ed.), *The Drugs Crime Connection*. Beverley Hills: Sage, pp. 39–66.

Barrows, S. and Room, R. (1991) *Drinking: Behavior and Belief in Modern History*. Berkeley: UC Press.

Bean, P. (2014) Drugs and Crime. 4th edition. Abington, Oxon: Routledge.

Becker, H. (1953) Becoming a marijuana user. *The American Journal of Sociology*, 59(3): 235–42.

Bennett, T. and Holloway, K. (2004) Gang membership, drugs and crime in the UK. *British Journal of Criminology*, 44: 305–23.

Bennett, T. and Holloway, K. (2009) The causal connection between drug misuse and crime. *British Journal of Criminology*, 49(4): 513–31

Berridge, V. (1999). *Opium and the People: Opiate Use and Drug Control Policy in Nineteenth and Early Twentieth Century England*. London: Free Association Books.

Bourgois, P. (1996) *In Search of Respect*. Cambridge: Cambridge University Press.

Carrington, K., Hogg, R. and Sozzo, M. (2016) Southern criminology. *British Journal of Criminology*, 56(1): 1–20.

Chatterton, P. and Hollands, R. (2003) *Urban Nightscapes: Youth Cultures, Pleasure Spaces and Corporate Power*. New York: Routledge.

Chen, J.S. (2014) Revisiting early sociological studies on addiction: interactions with collectives. *History of the Human Sciences*, 27(5): 111–25.

Coomber, R. and Turnbull, P. (2007) Arenas of drug transaction: adolescent cannabis transactions in England - 'social supply'. *Journal of Drug Issue*, 37(4): 845–66.

Courtwright, D. (1997) Morality, religion and drug use. In A. Brandt and P. Rozin, P (eds), *Morality and Health*. New York: Routledge, pp. 231–50.

Courtwright, D. (2010) The NIDA brain disease paradigm: history, resistance and spinoffs. *BioSocieties*. 5(1): 137–47.

Curtis, R. and Wendel, T. (2000) Toward the development of a typology of illegal drug markets. In M. Natarajan and M. Hough (eds), *Illegal Drug Markets: From Research to Policy.* Monsey: Criminal Justice Press, pp. 121–52.

Denton, B. and O'Malley, P. (1999) Gender, trust and business: women drug dealers in the illicit economy. *British Journal of Criminology*, 39(4): 513–30.

Dwyer, R. and Moore, D. (2010) Understanding illicit drug markets in Australia. *British Journal of Criminology*, 50: 82–101.

Entorf, H. and Winker, P. (2008) Investigating the drugs crime channel in economics of crime models: empirical evidence from panel data of the German States. *International Review of Law and Economics*, 28: 8–22.

Finestone, H. (1957) Narcotics and criminality. *Law and Contemporary Problems*, 22(1): 69–85.

Graham-Mulhall, S. (1926) Drug addiction and crime. *Annals of the American Academy of Political and Social Science*, 125: 162–5.

Greenberg, S. and Adler, F. (1974) Crime and addiction: an empirical analysis of the literature, 1920–1973. *Contemporary Drug Problems*, 3: 221–70.

Hagedorn, J. (1988) *People and Folks: Gangs, Crime and the Underclass in a Rustbelt City*. Chicago: Lakeview Press.

Hamid, A., Curtis, R., McCoy, K., McGuire, J., Conde, A., Bushell, W., Lindenmayer, R., Brimberg, K., Maia, S., AbdurRashid, S. and Settembrino, J. (1997). The heroin epidemic in New York City: current status and prognoses. *Journal of Psychoactive Drugs*, 29(4): 375–91.

Hamilton, J. (2005) Receiving marijuana and cocaine as gifts and through sharing. *Substance Use and Misuse*, 40: 361-368.

Hammer, R., Dingel, M., Ostergren, J., Partridge, B., McCormick, J. and Koenig, B.A. (2013) Addiction: current criticism of the brain disease paradigm. *AJOB Neuroscience*, 4(3): 27–32.

Hobbs, D., Hadfield, P., Lister, S. and Winslow, S. (2003) *Bouncers: Violence and Governance in the Night-time Economy*. Oxford: Oxford University Press.

Howard, G.E. (1918) Alcohol and crime: a study in social causation. *American Journal of Sociology*, 24(1): 61–80.

Howell, J. and Decker, S. (1999) The youth gangs, drugs and violence connection. *Juvenile Justice Bulletin*. Washington, D.C.: Office of Juvenile Justice and Delinquency Prevention. United States Department of Justice.

Hunt, G. and Barker, J. (2001) Socio-cultural anthropology and alcohol and drug research: towards a unified theory. *Social Science and Medicine*, 53: 165–88.

Hunt, G. and Evans, K. (2008) 'The great unmentionable': exploring the pleasures and benefits of ecstasy from the perspectives of drug users. *Drugs*, 15(4): 329–49.

Hunt, G.P., Bailey, N., Evans, K. and Moloney, M. (2009) Combining different substances in the dance scene: enhancing pleasure, managing risk and timing effects. *Journal of Drug Issues*, 39(3): 495–522.

Hutson, S. (2000) The rave: spiritual healing in modern Western subcultures. *Anthropological Quarterly*, 73(1): 35–49.

Inciardi, J. (1981) *The Drugs Crime Connection*. Beverley Hills: Sage.

Inciardi, J. and McElrath, K. (eds) (2010) *The American Drug Scene: An Anthology*. Los Angeles: Roxbury.

Jacinto, C., Duterte, M., Sales, P. and Murphy, S. (2008) 'I'm not a real dealer': the identity process of ecstasy sellers. *The Journal of Drug Issues*, 38(2): 419–44.

Jacobs, B. (1998) *Dealing Crack: The Social World of Street Corner Selling*. Boston: Northeastern University Press.

Joe Laidler, K. and Hunt, G. (2012) Moving beyond the gang drug violence connection. *Drugs: Education, Prevention and Policy*, 19(6): 442–52.

Joe Laidler, K. and Hunt, G. (2013) Unlocking the spiritual with club drugs: a case study of two youth cultures. *Substance Use and Misuse*, 48(12): 1099–108.

Joe Laidler, K., Hodson, D. and Traver, H. (2000) *The Hong Kong Drug Market. Report for UNICRI on The UNDCP Global Study in Illicit Drug Markets*. Hong Kong: Centre for Criminology, University of Hong Kong.

Joe Laidler, K., Hunt, G. and Moloney, M. (2014) 'Tuned out or tuned in': spirituality and youth drug use in global times. *Past and Present*, 222(Suppl. 9): 61–80.

Karstedt, S. (2001) Comparing cultures, comparing crime: challenges, prospects and problems for a global criminology. *Crime, Law and Social Change*, 36: 285–308.

Katz, J. and Jackson-Jacobs, C. (2004) The criminologists' gang. In C. Summer (ed.),

Companion to Criminology. Oxford: Blackwell, pp. 91–124.

Kolb, L. (1925) Pleasure and deterioration from narcotic addiction. *Mental Hygiene*, 9: 699–724.

Leary, T. (2008) *Leary on Drugs: Writings and lectures from Timothy Leary (1970–1996)*. San Francisco: Re/Search Publications.

Lee, M. and Joe Laidler, K. (2013) Doing criminology from the periphery: crime and punishment in Asia. *Theoretical Criminology*, 17(2): 141–57.

Levitt, S. and Venkatash, S. (2000) An economic analysis of a drug selling gang's finances. *The Quarterly Journal of Economics*, 115: 755–89.

Lindesmith, A. (1938) A sociological theory of drug addiction. *American Journal of Sociology*, 43(4): 593–613.

Lombroso, C. (1895) *Criminal Man*. Translated by Gibson, M. and Rafter, N. (2006) Durham: Duke University.

Lombroso, C. (1899) *Crime: Its Causes and Remedies*. New York: Little, Brown and Co.

Maher, L., Dixon, D., Lynskey, M. and Hall, W. (1998) Running the risks: heroin, health and harm in South West Sydney. *NDARC Monograph 38*. Sydney: NARC, University of South Wales.

May, T., Harocopos, A., Turnbull, P. and Hough, M. (2000) Serving up: the impact of low level police enforcement on drug markets. *Police Research Series*, Paper 133. London: Home Office.

May, T. and Hough, M. (2004) Drug markets and distribution systems. *Addiction, Theory and Research*, 12(6): 549–63.

McSweeney, T., Turnbull, P.J. and May, T. (2010) Drug supply and possession. In F. Brookman, M. Maguire, H. Pierpoint and T. Bennett (eds), *Handbook On Crime*. Abingdon: Routledge, pp. 598-625.

Møller, K. and Sandberg, S. (2015) Credit and trust: management of network ties in illicit drug distribution. *Journal of Research in Crime and Delinquency*, 52(5): 691–716.

Moore, K. and Miles, S. (2004) Young people, dance and the sub-cultural consumption of drugs. *Addiction, Theory and Research*, 12(6): 507–23.

Morgan, P. and Joe Laidler, K. (1995) Citizens and outlaws: the private lives and public lifestyles of women in the illicit drug economy. *Journal of Drug Issues*, 26: 125–42.

Murphy, S., Waldorf, D. and Reinarman, C. (1990). Drifting into dealing: becoming a cocaine seller. *Qualitative Sociology*, 13(4): 321–43.

Nicholls, J. (2009). *The Politics of Alcohol: A History of the Drink Question in England*. Oxford: Oxford University Press.

Musto, D. (1973) *The American Disease*. New Haven: Yale University Press.

Nurco, D.N., Kinlok, T.W. and Hanlon, T.E. (1991) The drugs crime connection. In J. Inciardi (ed.), *Handbook of Drug Control in the United States*. Westport: Greenwood, pp. 71–90.

O'Malley, P. and Valverde, M. (2004) Pleasure, freedom and drugs: the uses of 'pleasure' in liberal governance of drug and alcohol consumption. *Sociology*, 38: 25–42.

Orcutt, J. and Rudy, D. (eds) (2003) *Drugs, Alcohol and Social Problems*. Oxford: Roman and Littlefield.

Padilla, F. (1992) *The Gang as an American Enterprise: Puerto Rican Youth and the American Dream*. New Brunswick: Rutgers University Press.

Parker, H. (2000) How young Britons obtain their drugs: drugs transactions at the point of consumption. *Crime Prevention Studies*, 11: 59–81.

Parker, H., Aldridge, J. and Measham, F. (1998) *Illegal Leisure: The Normalization of Recreational Drug Use*. London: Routledge.

Parker, H., Williams, L. and Aldridge, J. (2002) The normalization of 'sensible' recreational drug use. *Sociology*, 36(4): 941–64.

Parker, R.N. and Rebhun, L.A. (1995). *Alcohol and Homicide: A Deadly Combination of Two American Traditions*. Albany: SUNY Press.

Partridge, C. (2005) *The Re-enchantment of the West: Alternative Spiritualities, Sacralization, Popular Culture and Occulture*. New York: T&T Clark Publishers.

Pearson, G. (2007) Drug markets and dealing: from street dealer to Mr. Big. In M. Simpson, T. Shildrick and R. MacDonald (eds), *Drugs: Supply, Consumption and Control*. London: Palgrave, pp. 76–91.

Room, R. (1984) Alcohol control and public health. *Annual Review of Public Health*, 5: 293–317.

Ruggiero, V. and South, N. (1997) The late modern city as a bazaar: drug markets, illegal enterprise and the 'barricades'. *British Journal of Sociology*, 48(1): 54–70.

Sandberg, S. and Pedersen, W. (2008) A magnet for curious adolescents: the perceived dangers of an open drug scene. *International Journal of Drug Policy*, 19(6): 459–66.

Sanders, B. (2006) *Drugs, Clubs and Young People*. Surrey: Ashgate.

Schensul, J., Diamond, S., Disch, W., Bermudez, R. and Eiserman, J. (2005) The diffusion of ecstasy through urban youth networks. *Journal of Ethnicity in Substance Abuse*, 4(2): 39–71.

Schur, E. (1963) *Narcotic Addiction in Britain and America*. London: Tavistock.

Simpson, M. (2003) The relationship between drug use and crime: a puzzle inside an enigma. *International Journal of Drug Policy*, 14: 307–19.

Skolnick, J. Correl, T, Navarro, E. and Rabb, R. (1989) *The Social Structure of Street Drug Dealing*. Sacramento: Office of the State Attorney General, State of California.

South, N. (2004) Managing work, hedonism and 'the borderline' between the legal and illegal markets: two case studies of recreational heavy drug users. *Addiction, Theory and Research*, 12(6): 525–38.

St John, G. (2004) The difference engine: liberation and the rave imaginary. In G. St John (ed.), *Rave Culture and Religion*. London: Routledge.

Taniguichi, T., Ratcliffe, J. and Taylor, R. (2011) Gang set space, drug markets and crime around drug corners in Camden. *Journal of Research in Crime and Delinquency*, 48(3): 327–63.

Taylor, C. (1989) *Dangerous Society*. East Lansing: Michigan State University Press.

Vrecko, S. (2010) Birth of a brain disease: science, the state and addition neuropolitics. *History of the Human Sciences*, 23(4): 52–67.

Waldorf, D. (1973) *Careers in Dope*. Englewood Cliffs: Prentice Hall.

Waldorf, D., Hunt, G., Joe, K. and Murphy, S. (1993) *Final Report of the Crack Sales, Gangs and Violence Study to the National Institute on Drug Abuse*. San Francisco: Institute for Scientific Analysis.

Ward, J. (2010) *Flashback: Drugs and Dealing in the Golden Age of the London Rave Scene*. Devon: Willan.

Weil, A. (1972) *The Natural Mind: An Investigation of Drugs and the Higher Consciousness*. New York: Houghton Mifflin Harcourt.

Williams, T. (1989) *The Cocaine Kids*. Reading: Addison-Wesley.

Young, J. (1971) *Drug Takers: The Social Meaning of Drug Use*. London: Judson, McGibbon and Kee.

Zajdow, G. (2010) It blasted me into space: intoxication and an ethics of pleasure. *Health Sociology Review*, 19(2): 218–29.

Zinberg, A. (1984) *Drug, Set and Setting: The Basis for Controlled Intoxicant Use*. New Haven: Yale University.

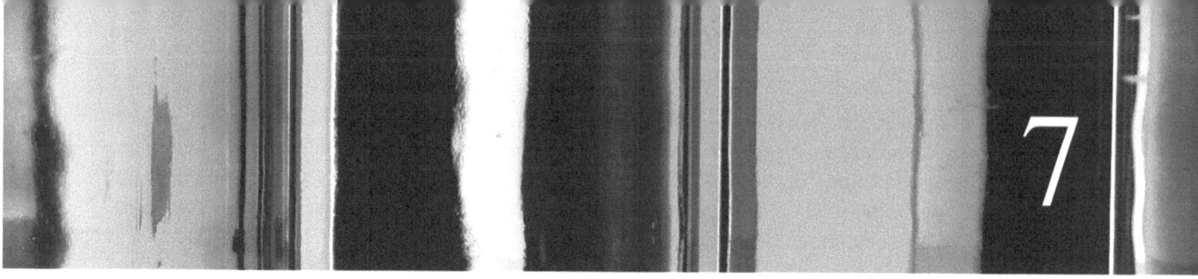

7

Cultural Studies Approaches to Drugs and Alcohol

Kane Race and Rebecca Brown

INTRODUCTION

As an interdisciplinary space that draws quite liberally on the methods of established disciplines – philosophy, sociology, semiotics, anthropology, history, education and literary criticism among them – the heterogeneity of what takes place under the sign of cultural studies can make it difficult to pin down as a coherent field. Emerging in the 1970s as part of a critical project that sought to investigate the political implications and opportunities of the social upheavals and transformations of post-war Britain, the field has expanded internationally to become a major source of theoretical and critical innovation at the forefront of the new humanities, even while its institutional status and academic legitimacy can often seem precarious in some locations. Graeme Turner positions cultural studies 'as an enabler of the development or renovation of other disciplines' (Turner, 2012: 26), serving as a kind of 'academic *lingua franca* for the new humanities' (2012: 12). Conceived as an attractor for yet-to-be-devised cross-fertilisations of theory, method and approach, cultural studies has certainly functioned as an experimental horizon, enabling innovation and movement to take place in other disciplines – and this would be no less true of drug and alcohol studies. Indeed, we suspect that many drug and alcohol researchers (those working in qualitative traditions in particular) would affiliate themselves or significant aspects of their scholarly formation with work from cultural studies, at least in part. This complicates the problem of what to include in any discussion of 'Cultural Studies Approaches', making it all the more prone to those crimes of omission borne of inadvertent oversight, personal investments, the impossibility of reading everything and constraints of word count.

To deal with this problem, we have chosen to focus our attention on developments in the field as it has been instituted in field-defining journals, anthologies and books classified as cultural studies. We consider how these developments have conditioned approaches to drugs and alcohol, rather than attempting to conduct any exhaustive survey of all the work within drug and alcohol studies that might recognise itself under the sign of cultural studies. But what immediately stands out when adopting this approach is the relative absence of drug use as an explicit point of focus or source of more than cursory attention in this literature. We searched the indexes of more than ten collections and anthologies devoted to the institutionalisation of cultural studies, and found fewer references to drugs, alcohol and intoxication than you can count on one hand. This is surprising when one considers that youth subcultures, popular culture, and the identities, meanings and pleasures of consumption have featured as constitutive themes and analytic objects for the field of cultural studies. All the more so, given the conspicuousness of drugs and alcohol as elements of popular culture – a trend that has become only more pronounced over the period in which cultural studies has grown and consolidated itself as a scholarly field. For their part, drug and alcohol researchers have invoked cultural studies as a potential corrective to the predominance of scientific and pathologising accounts that tend to provide a narrow picture of drug use in terms of its health risks or prevalence (Hunt et al., 2009). We agree that cultural studies has had considerable impact and continues to have a great deal to contribute to the analysis of meanings, pleasures and social contexts of drug and alcohol practices, their discursive classification and the regulatory effects of these processes. Indeed, there is a burgeoning literature within alcohol studies that owes a great deal to cultural studies, with its focus on how drinking cultures generate social and identity work related to modes of consumption.[1] But this work tends to take place in other disciplines such as critical health psychology, critical public health, sociology and criminology, which have a more established relation to health policy and a more consistent tradition of empirical qualitative research undertaken for policy purposes. We discuss the relationship between the policy field and cultural studies in the concluding section of this chapter. More generally, the relative absence of drugs and alcohol as explicit points of focus within mainstream cultural studies remains something of a mystery that opens up questions about the historical trajectories of the field, its critical and conceptual investments and how the latter have shaped its analytic objects.

There are three references to drug use in *Resistance Through Rituals* (Hall and Jefferson, 1993 [1975]), the collection of Birmingham studies of youth subcultures that is widely regarded as one of the foundational texts for cultural studies as a field. The first occurs in Dick Hebdige's analysis of Mod subculture, in which the use of amphetamines by Mods is depicted as a way of magnifying their activities and maintaining an 'imaginary relationship [...] to their real conditions of existence' (Hebdige, 1993: 71). The second appears in Paul Willis' study of the Hippie subculture and consists of an extended discussion of the cultural meaning of drug use within this context (Willis, 1993: 88). In the third, Geoffrey Pearson and John Twohig take issue with the emphasis they find in this literature on how drug experiences are socially constructed and culturally learned, which, in their view, unfairly subordinates the physiological or pharmacological properties of drugs to socio-cultural factors (Pearson and Twohig, 1993: 100). Quarrelling with proponents of this approach and the sociology of deviance and symbolic interactionism they cite as precedents [Howard Becker's *The Outsiders* (1963) and Jock Young's *The Drugtakers* (1972) in particular], the authors propose the need for a more 'materialist' focus on what they call 'technologies of ingestion' (1993: 103).

We begin with these drug references in one of the seminal texts of cultural studies because they are the first – and until recently remained among the most detailed – discussions of drug use to appear within the field. After the publication of this volume, the topic of drug use largely drops out of mainstream cultural studies, only to re-emerge with the rise of ecstasy use, rave culture, club cultures and the 'dance generation' of the 1990s. Even in this context, drugs tend to appear as a subsidiary or minor feature of larger cultural forms, discussion of which is typically consigned to the margins of most analyses. What are the reasons for the partial constitution of drugs as an object of cultural studies? How can we explain their elusive, fragmentary and unfinished figuration within this literature?

The treatment of drug use in *Resistance Through Rituals* offers clues towards this question, so we begin this chapter with a consideration of this text. Alongside the insight this process provides into some of the main tenets of cultural studies, we argue that a consideration of the trickiness of drugs as a cultural object allows them to emerge as an object with uniquely generative potential for the field of cultural studies, despite (indeed perhaps because of) their elusive and recalcitrant character. Drugs function in these early studies as a kind of irritant that spurs articulation of some of the key tensions and problems confronted by the field. These include questions regarding the meaning of consumption, and in particular, how to conceive relations between agency and passivity; the cultural and the material, subjects and objects; and the work of semiosis and conceptions of the political. Drugs even come to figure prominently in some of the positions that scholars adopt in response to these problems, which serve to distinguish cultural studies as a critical project and scholarly field. In the second part of the chapter, we suggest that a consideration of drugs opens up new avenues of empirical and conceptual experimentation within cultural studies that may generate new modes of encounter between science and aesthetics – those conventionally distinct faculties that have structured the divisions of modern thought in major ways. We consider the usefulness of newly influential concepts and approaches from affect theory and science and technology studies for these purposes, before concluding with some remarks about the political ambitions of cultural studies.

RESISTING CULTURAL DOPES

Dick Hebdige's study of Mod subculture serves as a useful starting point, because it illustrates several of the tensions mentioned above (Hebdige 1993). The Mods' use of amphetamines is conceived by Hebdige as a means of bridging the gap between the carefully controlled stylisation of their self-presentation and leisure time and the somewhat harsher 'real conditions of existence' they experienced, which stemmed mainly from employment in semi-skilled office work, manual labour or menial jobs in the service industry. Hebdige sensitises the reader to the symbolism of 'speed' and movement within this subculture, in which values of sharpness, opportunism, arrogance and hyperactivity reigned supreme. But amphetamine is also associated with a sense of hopelessness in Hebdige's analysis, evoking images of physical deterioration, stunted development and going nowhere rapidly. In this regard, Hebdige's analysis reveals its commitments to class analysis, and in particular, the relation between social structure and cultural practices. Like other studies in *Resistance Through Rituals*, Hebdige is informed by Gramsci's theory of hegemony and Althusser's work on the 'relative autonomy' of the interconnected domains, 'society' and 'culture' (Hall and Jefferson, 1993: ix). Early practitioners of cultural studies developed a keen interest in any signs that the lives of the groups they studied were not completely determined by economic and structural forces. The symbolic practices of youth subcultures thus emerge as an opportunity to theorise the complex relations between cultural processes and social structure. The 'cultural' and the symbolic are positioned as spaces of resistance to the formal determinations of the social structure, even while socio-economic forces are largely seen to make up these youth's 'real conditions of existence'. Hence the title of this early collection of cultural studies, which finds some evidence of class resistance in the symbolic practices of youth subcultures: '*Resistance Through Rituals*'.

If, for Hebdige, amphetamine is expressive of the material depletion and enervation of the Mods' social situation, drugs are also bound up in a countervailing dynamic in his analysis. Drugs feature as one of a number of consumer objects whose meaning is actively transformed through their subcultural use and active appropriation. Just as the Mods appropriated the scooter, 'a formerly ultra-respectable means of transport' and converted it into 'a weapon and symbol of social solidarity', drugs and their meanings are depicted as subject to similar cultural transformations through their subcultural use and enunciation (Hebdige, 1993: 76). 'Thus pills, medically diagnosed for the treatment of neuroses, were appropriated and used as an end-in-themselves' (1993: 76). Their meaning and purpose changes in the very act of consumption. For Hebdige, the 'semantic rearrangement of components of the objective world' was 'repeated at every level of the mod experience' and supplies crucial evidence that 'the mod was never a passive consumer' (1993: 76).

This move – from a model of passive consumption to an insistence on the *activity* of the consumer – becomes practically foundational for early cultural studies, which take up the general interest in how subordinate groups borrow objects from the world of consumer commodities and transform their meaning by working them into new stylistic ensembles. This generates considerable interest in the analysis of situated meanings, symbolic creativity, the play of semiosis and signification-in-context – foci that quickly become mainstays of the field. Meaning is not fixed once and for all in consumer objects: rather, it depends on the way these objects are taken up and used, the cultural practices in which they are embedded. Consumers are not dupes who passively soak up the messages of the culture industries: they are actively involved in practices of symbolic re-signification from which new identities and forms of group belonging emerged (for a fuller discussion see Race, 2009: 71–9). This focus on the contextual production and negotiation of meanings certainly contributes a great deal to qualitative and cultural studies of drug and alcohol use, which set out to explore the negotiation of meaning in different contexts of use. And yet in a curious way, the figure of drug use comes to function as a sort of limit point to the active character of consumption, as is evident in some of the field's most axiomatic and politically invested passages:

> Now, if the forms and relationships on which participation in this commercially provided 'culture' depend are purely manipulative and debased, then the people who consume and enjoy them must either themselves be debased by these activities or else living in a permanent state of 'false consciousness'. They must be 'cultural dopes' who can't tell that what they are being fed is an updated form of the opium of the people [...] I don't know that [this] is a view that can survive very long as an adequate account of cultural relationships [...] Ultimately, the notion of the people as a purely *passive* outline force is a deeply unsocialist perspective. (Hall, 1981: 232).

THE 'CULTURAL MEANING' OF DRUG USE

If drugs figure somewhat ambiguously in the field's initial attempts to address the political valences of consumer culture, they are also subject to a full-blown skirmish in *Resistance Through Rituals* (Hall and Jefferson 1993). Paul Willis' chapter on the drug practices of Hippies places great emphasis on how drug experiences are culturally defined, socially constructed and learnt, aligning itself with interactionist and ethnographic traditions in the sociology of deviance found, for example, in Howard Becker's marijuana essays in *The Outsiders* (1963) and Jock Young's argument in *The Drugtakers* (1972). By contrast, in their short chapter 'Ethnography through the looking glass', Geoffrey Pearson and John Twohig criticise this sociological approach to drug experience and its apparent neglect of the physiological properties of drugs. They even relay a joke made provocatively by one of their participants, that 'if Becker's subjects needed to learn to spot the effects, then they had been given a "bum deal"' (Pearson and Twohig, 1993: 103). It is difficult to ascertain the impact of this academic stoush on subsequent cultural studies: certainly, Pearson and Twohig's essay is not widely cited. And yet the conspicuous absence of drug use as an analytic focus within cultural studies over the next two decades suggests it may have had a dissuasive influence on the exploration of drug use as a topic. Much hinges in this early debate on whether drugs are properly associated with physiology or culture. Indeed, the exchange can be read as an early attempt to work out the scope and limits of cultural analysis, and in particular, the relation between 'the cultural' and 'the material', and for this reason it is worth revisiting and closer inspection.

In 'The cultural meaning of drug use', Paul Willis charts a complicated course through the physiological and symbolic aspects of drug use and their significance for his participants, who are drawn from the Hippie subculture of a large industrial city. According to his informants, it was 'possible to take acid and not "trip", and possible to "trip" without taking acid' (Willis, 1993: 89): only when the drug was used to counter the values of 'straight' society was it functioning as a subcultural element. Willis argues on this basis that drugs did not 'intrinsically contain' the values of Hippie subculture, but could be 'thought of as cultural placebos – keys to experience, rather than experience itself' (1993: 91) – mere tools that could be used to achieve an existential state. Significantly, for Willis, this existential state may be achieved in 'non-physical ways' – an interpretation that minimises the significance of the physiological attributes of drugs on user experience (1993: 89). So, while Willis acknowledges that acid and hash have 'marked chemical effects', he argues these could 'equally well be interpreted in a thousand different *cultural* forms', thus maintaining a distinction between drugs' 'intrinsic properties' and 'cultural meanings' (1993: 91). Willis even distinguishes between different types of drugs – LSD, hash, heroin and barbiturates – in terms of the degree of connection between 'the cultural meaning ascribed to the drug and the drug's 'objective' pharmacological effects' (1993: 99). Significantly, a decisive link is only claimed in the case of heroin.

While Willis works hard to carve out a space for the cultural analysis of drug use, drugs also serve in his analysis as a source of insight into how individuals are 'determined by the structures around [them]' within the subculture he investigates (1993: 90). For the Hippies, the experience of LSD 'symbolised a fundamental ontological change from the sense of feeling oneself as an autonomous determining agent, to feeling oneself, in part, as a determined variable in the world' – a feeling that is not confined to drug experience but extends to 'the economy, politics, society, industry, pollution, the police, upbringing', etc. (1993: 90). This feeling induces an inclination to live for the 'now' and 'feel the moment'; a 'yielding to experience' that is said to break down conventional notions of 'industrial and job-oriented time' and the forms of personal responsibility associated with them (1993:92). In this sense, drugs are implicated in a cultural or symbolic movement to 'drop out' of material modes of production, in a reading that is remarkably reflective of some of the questions and anxieties that inform distinctions between the 'cultural' and the 'social' at this critical juncture – specifically, those concerning agency versus structure. Indeed, the feeling of being determined by external structures that is attributed to drugs within the Hippie subculture is remarkably reminiscent of some of the key sociological debates and concerns of the period.

Pearson and Twohig's critique of sociological and cultural analyses of drug use displays some suspicion of disciplinary tendencies to reinstate the need for their own existence in drug analyses (1993: 100). These authors take aim at the imputed overreach of social constructionist theories in ethnographic studies of drug experience and their supposed propagation of sociological dogma. They criticise Howard Becker's (1963) emphasis on how cultural definitions and expectations shape drug experiences, claiming it disregards the physiological attributes of drugs (including their toxicity). They propose an alternative emphasis on 'technologies of ingestion' – a term that seems to refer to practical strategies and material contexts of consumption [they differentiate 'heavy technology' from a 'party technology' (1993: 103), but these stand as their sole examples]. 'How the drug is ingested' is said to inform the production of different effects – and much more so than cultural expectations, as proposed by Becker. Their argument appears to target the emphasis on the symbolic and representational aspects of cultural processes and in this sense hinges on quite a limited conception of 'the cultural', as we discuss in a later section.

To be fair, Willis does pay some attention to the ritualistic aspects of drug ingestion, in which subcultural participants are depicted as 'preparing themselves quite meticulously for the experience' (Willis, 1993: 97). His chapter includes quite a generous discussion of different drug-taking techniques, including limited discussion of harm reduction techniques specific to this subculture, such as 'skin popping' heroin, crushing up barbiturates and LSD dosing rituals that determine the intensity of the physiological experience that becomes 'open to specific cultural interpretation' (1993: 90). That is to say, Willis does not exactly ignore 'technologies of ingestion', though neither do they form an explicitly named thematic of his discussion.

We will return to this materialist emphasis on technologies of ingestion and the question of how to theorise drug effects in the final section. This will enable us to elaborate some of the theoretical trajectories of cultural studies and track some of critical shifts and conceptual repertoires it has engaged with. For now, we turn to a consideration of how drugs have been approached in later studies on dance and rave culture and the critical trends shaping their characterisation in this literature. Until this point, the association of drug use with images of passive consumption and material determination appears to have made it an uninviting ground on which to stake affirmative visions of political relevance for the field of cultural studies.

JUST DANCE: CULTURAL POLITICS AND (A)POLITICAL CULTURES

From its original concern with class analysis, to its nascent consideration of the politics of race, gender, sexuality, cultural identity and everyday life over the 1980s and 1990s, cultural studies has always borne the mark of the theories it has used to conceive 'the political'. So far, we have noted the Gramscian and Althusserian inheritance of early subcultural studies and the attention this directed towards the symbolism of resistance. In the following section, we suggest that this critical emphasis has tended to hamstring detailed analyses of drug use, even rendering the latter a paradigmatic instance of de-politicisation in some cultural studies. But in the context of the 'dance generation' and the popularisation of ecstasy, alternative readings have become possible, thanks to an emerging feminist and Foucauldian emphasis on the embodied dimensions of power, subjection and subjectification. The cultural studies literature on dance and rave culture is large, and so we have chosen to proceed by picking out only a few examples that we see as illustrative of broader trends and approaches within this literature.

A good example of the drugs-as-depoliticisation tendency is the analysis of rave culture that appears in *The Clubcultures Reader* (Redhead, 1997). This collection emanates from the Manchester Institute for Popular Culture and sets out to continue the ethnographic tradition of Birmingham cultural studies in the very different political climate of the 1990s. In his chapter, 'Rave culture: living dream or living death', Simon Reynolds is concerned with the dissipation of rave's utopian promise and what he sees as the diminishing political potential of this collective moment (Reynolds, 1997). While rave starts off as a promising expression of collectivity and is credited minimally with shifting gender relations among working-class youth, Reynolds disputes the idea that 'something radical is at stake in this music' (1997: 103). Here, ecstasy becomes a particularly evocative signifier of the political failure of rave, or at least the critic's disappointment with the political development of this culture. 'My sense is that the intransitive, go-nowhere aspects of rave culture are almost chemically programmed into MDMA itself' he writes. 'Among all its other effects, E incites a sort of free-floating fervour, a will-to-belief [...] radiant with MEANING. But at the end of even the most tearing night out, there can be a disenchanting sense of futility: all that energy and idealism mobilized to no end' (1997: 105–6). Rave is characterised as the ultimate postmodern experience, with 'no goal beyond its own propagation' (1997: 104) that finally 'boils down to little more than music and drugs' (1997: 110). So disillusioned is Reynolds with the political potential of rave that he is led to pose what he regards as 'the real question': 'whether any form of drug use is an adequate basis for a culture?' (1997: 109).

Here we can see how Reynolds' (actually quite poetic) engagement with ecstasy is informed and constrained by his critical investments. The suggestion seems to be that only those cultures that bear out predetermined political impacts are worthy of study – or even worthy of designation as a 'culture'. Because questions of political value function as a motivation for analysis here, exploration of drug use is subordinated to their terms. This has the effect of circumscribing the sort of attention brought to bear on drugs, reducing them to a grotesque figure of political disenchantment.

Angela McRobbie's discussion of rave culture bears comparison here, because of its concern to extend subcultural analysis while taking it 'in a slightly different direction' (McRobbie, 1993: 406). In this article, McRobbie attempts to expand the conception of the political to include not only gender but also the cultural activities of middle class youth in post-Thatcher Britain. She wants to move considerations of the political beyond a symbolism of resistance grounded in questions of class authenticity and towards the forms of cultural production where new modes of femininity were being elaborated, among other 'youth culture' or 'subcultural' values. Rather than selling out, she reads youth participation in music, fashion and magazine production as empowering activities, involving choices about 'how to live' that diverge from mainstream values (1993: 407). For McRobbie, the activities of young people engaging in the post-Thatcher 'frenzy of cultural production' involve staking out an investment in society and making a statement; an 'absolute engagement with the social' as she puts it. 'It is in this sense they are political' (1993: 407).

McRobbie devotes considerable space to a discussion of rave culture in this article, though women are not as visible as cultural producers within this culture. Like Reynolds, McRobbie draws attention to the shifting gender relations that are apparent here, which include a friendlier, more malleable embodiment of masculinity associated with ecstasy use, whereby young men 'enter into a different relationship to their own bodies, more tactile, more sensuous, less focussed round sexual gratification' (1993: 419). For women, self-abandon is balanced by 'caution and the exercise of control in sex' (1993: 421), something that is effected (in part) by adopting the vestiges of a childlike and pre-Oedipal version of bodily pleasure (the use of dummies, ice lollies, whistles, smiley faces, etc.). In the context of AIDS, raves allow for a form of physical abandon that is not premised on narratives of sex and romance but locates its 'orgiastic frenzy' in the intensities of friendship (1993:421).

When it comes to its political implications, McRobbie argues that rave culture manifests a series of social tensions and might be characterised not only in terms of pleasure and excitement but also 'a text of avoidance' (1993: 422). 'It is as though young ravers cannot bear the burden of the responsibilities they are expected to carry', she ventures (1993: 422). At a time when youth confront multiple dangers and social demands, 'rave turns away from this heavy load and dips headlong into a culture of avoidance and almost pure abandonment' (1993: 422). McRobbie questions the extent to which 'a subcultural aesthetics which asks of its fans that they "shut up and dance" produces in the haze of pleasure and enjoyment a cultural politics of any sort?' (1993: 422). If this question echoes some of the terms and commitments of Reynolds' (1997) analysis, McRobbie is more circumspect about the possibility of characterising the politics of youth at all, recalling that youth is not a 'stable undifferentiated category' with a 'unity of focus and direction' but is 'cut across by gender, ethnic, class and other differences' (1993: 422). Considering this heterogeneity, she proposes a focus on new and emergent 'structures of feeling' within specific youth populations (young women for instance), arguing that this may constitute a meaningful component of critical analyses of cultural transformation (1993: 422).

Such an emphasis is developed and extended in Maria Pini's work on women's experience of the early British rave scene (Pini, 1997). Challenging the focus on men and masculinity in work on youth subcultures, especially as it emerges in the literature on the symbolism of resistance, she describes how early rave spaces provided an opportunity for women to experience themselves outside the prescribed structures of normative femininity. Pini argues that for many women 'rave represents an undoing of the traditional cultural associations between dancing, drugged, "dressed-up" women and sexual invitation, and as such opens up a new space for the exploration of new forms of identity and pleasure' (1997: 154). Significant here is the kind of 'self' or 'subjectivity' that rave produces, which on Pini's analysis provides an opportunity to experience oneself differently. This attention to subjectivity connects Pini's analysis with McRobbie's interest in 'structures of feeling' and their capacity to articulate new 'modes of femininity' (McRobbie, 1993: 422).

'Obviously central to the production of "excitement" was the heavy use of "Ecstasy", and the bodily "rushes" associated with it' Pini states (1997: 157). All of the participants in her study had used ecstasy at raves and felt it was necessary to have taken the drug at least once to fully appreciate the pleasures of raving. While for Pini, the cultural atmosphere of excitement and friendliness at raves is connected to ecstasy and its effects, she argues that the drug is only one part of the ensemble of rave experience, and that a significant component involves the activation of subjectivities. 'The holistic self of rave becomes the primary target to be "worked", "pleasured", "drugged", "taken higher" and, in Foucauldian terms, otherwise "produced". Having stamina, the "right attitude", and being "positive" are similarly sought after states and the techniques through which a particular mind/body/spirit/technology assemblage is produced' (1997: 165). This arguably de-centres physiological accounts of drug effects, or at least contextualises them as contingent on a range of other conditions. Meanwhile, the emphasis on self-technologies here reveals the influence of Foucault's work, and in particular, the political significance accorded to experiments with subjectivity. Here, work on the self and 'an ethics of pleasure' play a noteworthy part in counteracting the effects and pressures of disciplinary norms, and drug use may form part of this collective/subjective working on 'bodies and pleasures' (Foucault, 1978, 1985). A number of other cultural scholars pursue a similar emphasis (see Martin, 1999; Race, 2008; and Malins, 2004, for a comparable Deleuzean approach to drug-using assemblages). If the body is conceived as a central locus of disciplinary power, it also becomes significant as a site in or through which new self-relations and relations to power are experimented.

Scholars such as Malbon (1999) and Jackson (2004) similarly explore the experiential dimensions of clubbing in a way that takes account of the sensual and visceral effects of ecstasy and its implication in the production of states of feeling.[2] Drawing on sociological theories of habitus, for example, Jackson explores how club drug experiences change the way people 'negotiate their passage through the social realm' including its ideological dimensions (Jackson 2004: 5). 'Through clubbing, people create and socialise through novel bodies that underpin new social practices, which eventually become embodied and taken up beyond club space' (2004: 2). These transformations are said to include 'the way people engage with each other socially [...] people's knowledge of how their world can feel and the limits of their own pleasure in that world; their capacity to know and perceive their own lives from alternative emotional perspectives' (2004: 55). On this basis, Jackson argues that the club experiences he studied were neither 'resistance nor capitulation, but an ongoing process of socially creative experimentation, which created alternate modes of socio-sensual knowledge that impacted on people's lives to varying degrees' (2004: 174). Here, experiments in subjectivity are treated as politically significant projects. Such an approach is not confined to analyses of ecstasy culture. For example, Rebecca Brown (2014) conducted a comparable analysis of young women's drinking practices on 'girls' nights out' to reveal how normative ideals of hyper-femininity are not only performed, but also undercut, enjoyed, exhausted, subverted and poked fun at in these excursions. Taken together, these studies model cultural approaches that prioritise contextually specific analysis of the meanings, pleasures and embodied experiences of drug and alcohol use, generating an impressive array of analytic approaches and resources for these purposes.

DECONSTRUCTION AND GENEALOGY

A significant strand of cultural studies work in this area focuses less on experiences of drug and alcohol use than their discursive categorisation. Drawing on deconstructive techniques and Foucauldian genealogies of the emergence of modern terms, these studies set out to question the stability and self-evidence of the categories used to understand and regulate drug and alcohol experience such as addiction. In her influential essay 'Epidemics of the Will', Eve Sedgwick draws from Foucault's account of the invention of the homosexual (1978) explicitly to generate critical interest in the 'the taxonomic reframing of the drug user as an addict' and its connection to new forms of medical-juridical power that idealise 'healthy free will' (Sedgwick, 1993: 131). In *What's Wrong with Addiction*? Helen Keane develops and extends this line of inquiry to develop a critical analysis of 'the production of addiction as a disorder [and] the range of pathological subjects and disordered bodies that are thereby constituted as objects of medical and therapeutic knowledge' (Keane, 2002: 5). Informed by similar theoretical commitments,

Kane Race explores how the distinction between legal and illegal drugs is used to identify figures of 'excessive consumption' in consumer society and subject them to forms of policing that carve out a normalised sphere of compliance and 'proper consumption' (Race, 2009: 60). These studies exert critical pressure on the categories used to demarcate 'normal' from 'abnormal' identities, highlighting their participation in disciplinary regimes that have major impacts on the lives of those subjected to them. They seek to generate possibilities for drug and alcohol use to be conceived in alternative terms, less encumbered by normalizing imperatives.

With their genealogical focus on the instability and historicity of social, medical and legal categories, these studies mobilise Foucauldian arguments about the involvement of expert discourses in the exercise of power. Deconstructive techniques are commonly used to critical effect here: For example, Keane proceeds by exposing inconsistencies in, and contradictory connections between, the dichotomies that produce addiction as the binary opposite of a realm of experience designated as 'healthy' and 'normal' (Keane, 2002). One of the values of this approach is the critical reflection it provokes on the application of categories normally understood as natural or self-evident to drug and alcohol practices. Foucault's work is an obvious source of influence and analytic energy here, but it bears noting that the effects of labelling and the social construction of deviance were already concerns of the early sociology of deviance that cultural studies cites as a precedent, including the studies of drug use by Howard Becker (1963) and Jock Young (1972) mentioned earlier, as well as Erving Goffman's well-known and influential work on stigma (Goffman, 1968). Indeed, it might be argued that one of the principal impacts of Foucault's work has been to extend the analysis of discursive categories to include consideration of the socio-material technologies and political assemblages through which they become embodied. In the next section we consider how this interest is taken up in the 'material turn' and the turn towards affect.

AFFECTS, ASSEMBLAGES AND EVENT-NETWORKS

From the early 2000s, a number of works of cultural theory aimed to move beyond the prevailing focus on representation and signification found in most cultural studies (Massumi, 2002; Sedgwick, 2003; Thrift, 2007). An interest in affect, emotion and broader questions of materiality began to emerge, stemming from developments in queer theory (Probyn, 2005; Sedgwick, 2003), corporeal feminism (Grosz, 1994; Wilson, 2004), Deleuzean studies (Massumi, 2002), as well as engagements with intersecting disciplines such as human geography (Thrift, 2007; Whatmore, 2002). As part of this turn, many scholars' interests shifted from questions of identity and representation to becoming, effectivity, processes of materialisation. While the theoretical resources cultural scholars drew on to theorise affect and materiality were disparate and occasionally incommensurable (ranging from biological psychiatry to Deleuzean philosophy, for example) their attention to bodily dynamics, often conceived as part of hybrid assemblages composed of human and non-human elements, has served as a source of inspiration and conceptual/methodological innovation for a range of recent drug and alcohol studies (e.g. Duff, 2014; Malins, 2004; McLeod, 2014; Vitellone, 2010).

Another recent source of influence is the constructivist approach to nature and materiality developed by proponents of actor-network theory within science and technology studies (Latour, 2005a). Perhaps first introduced to health researchers through the work of feminist science scholar Donna Haraway (1991) and medical anthropologist Annemarie Mol (2003), this body of work has a great deal to offer drug research by virtue of the path it charts beyond disciplinary distinctions between nature and culture, between whose cracks the topic of drugs often falls. Here we examine some work from this tradition that analyses cultural processes – in particular, the cultural attachments, activities and passions of 'amateurs' (Gomart and Hennion, 1999). This provides a useful point of contrast with earlier cultural studies that take meanings and representations as the parametric scope of their analysis. In 'A sociology of attachment: music amateurs, drug users', Emilie Gomart and Antoine Hennion (1999) develop an analysis of 'event-networks' – those hybrid arrangements and practical set-ups that enable people to 'enter into a world of strong sensations; of accepting that "external" forces take possession of the self; of being "under the influence" of something else; of bracketing away one's own control and will in order to be expelled or rendered "beside oneself"' (1999: 221). On their analysis, music amateurs and drug users 'establish conditions' in order to be moved or seized by their passions (1999: 227). The authors concentrate on the 'mechanisms through which this kind of "active passion" is performed or "made to happen" ("faire faire")' (1999: 221) – a process they understand with reference to the Foucauldian concept of the *dispositif*. On their argument, amateurs actively experiment with the socio-material arrangements that enable them to feel the effects they seek. It is users – rather than the sociologists – who attribute agency and the determining sources of pleasure here, 'and are more innovative about it' (1999: 235).

Gomart and Hennion's approach is instructive for the course it weaves between some classic sociological dualisms – determinism/agency, nature/culture, active/passive among them. They achieve this through a pragmatist focus on practical encounters and their generative affects and the mediating impact of objects in their practical arrangement.

> Taste is neither the affirmation of a free subject nor the action of determinism. Instead, it is a concrete activity whose modes, dispositifs and practices can be described. A rock concert, or a sculpture exhibit, does not bring together already existing objects, subjects and social groupings – rather, this is a conjunctural event in which the relevant objects, subjects and social groupings are co-produced. (Gomart and Hennion, 1999: 228).

Here, the properties of drugs or music are not intrinsic, but neither are they socially constructed or completely arbitrary. Rather, they are what emerge from a field of differences in local and practical encounters between users, objects and intermediating environments: 'The drug or the music is "potentialized" as the user acquires the skills to condition the arrival of pleasure' (1999: 243). The subject is not fixed here but rather grasped in terms of how they are moved by the encounter. Meanwhile, the 'event-network' enables the analyst to dispense with problematic notions of sovereign agency or complete abandon, each of which are typically attributed to drug and alcohol use at different moments in the history of their analysis. For Gomart and Hennion, like other actor-network theorists, agency is distributed among human and nonhuman actors, a position which enables an appreciation of the socio-material arrangements that enable the subject's movements 'between activity and passivity' (1999: 243).

There is much to be said for this approach and the attention it levies towards the contingencies of drug experience. It adopts a materialist focus on what Pearson and Twohig once called 'technologies of ingestion' (Pearson and Twohig, 1993), but it does so without resorting to biological determinism, nor does it negate the mediating potential of cultural meanings and definitions. By expanding the range of mediating variables to include nonhuman objects as well as cultural forces, it enables a more thoroughgoing and far-reaching constructivist approach. What is also worth noticing about this expanded attention to the mediating capacity of techniques, object and procedures is the new domains it opens up for cultural analysis and intervention. The practices of science can now be viewed as cultural practices, including the specific arrangements of devices and procedures that characterises any given experiment or analysis. Indeed, opening up nature and science to constructivist analysis may be regarded as one of the key achievements of actor-network theory (Haraway, 1991; Latour, 2005a; Mol, 2003: 19–22). Not only are laboratories assembled, they can always be assembled differently. Their facts, while material, are contingent.

The significance of this approach for drug and alcohol studies should be clear. It opens up the field of scientific and medical practice for critical engagement. Indeed, one of the problems that has beset scholars concerned with affect and the material turn has been what status to accord the claims of the natural and the biological sciences (Hemmings, 2005; Ley, 2011; Papoulias and Callard, 2010). In this regard, it is useful to return to some of cultural studies' foundational quarrels to see what difference these science and technology studies approaches make for cultural analyses of drug use. In seeking to temper the reach of cultural analysis, Pearson and Twohig cede a great deal of ground, not simply to the physiological effects of drugs, but to the disciplines that purport to be able to determine these definitively (Pearson and Twohig 1993). These authors criticise Becker (1963) for his social constructionist suggestion that drug users 'learn to perceive the effects' (Pearson and Twohig, 1993: 101). But if we put the propositions of actor-network theory to work, we can begin to appreciate how scientists, as much as drug users, must 'learn to perceive the effects' of drugs – by means of an 'artificially created set-up' – of the clinical trial or experiment in their case (Latour, 2005b: 209). Actor-network theory provides tools for investigating the socio-material arrangements that selectively potentialise the properties of drugs and establish the terms through which they may be registered. This in turn provides a more robust basis for querying the classificatory and regulatory practices surrounding drugs, including the licit/illicit distinction, expanding our capacity to imagine how they might be practiced otherwise. As Race has written, 'a drug is not a thing – or not only. Its safety and specific effects vary according to complex assemblages of composition, interaction, timing, conduct [etc.]' (Race 2009: 54). This conduct includes the medical, legal, social and policy practices that differentially enact drugs and alcohol – their harms, pleasures, benefits and broader impacts – as each of these are presently materializing (see Fraser and Moore, 2011; Fraser et al., 2014). Whether one is concerned with the legal apparatuses of drug prohibition, or the design and conduct of randomised control trials – each of which can be regarded as major institutions centrally involved in the identification, classification, intervention into and generation of drug effects – attention to the hybrid assemblages that mediate these engagements opens up new avenues for critically addressing drug and alcohol events and practices (Race, 2011b, 2012).

CONCLUSION

In tracing some of the key historical and theoretical trajectories of cultural studies, this chapter has attempted to give insight into the multiple affordances and analytical tools the field offers for the investigation of drugs and alcohol. From its origins in class politics, subcultural analysis and the symbolic dimensions of resistance, to its expanding interest in the dynamics and politics of embodiment, we have seen how the political aspirations of this interdisciplinary field have shaped its approach to these topics. In addition, we have seen how these approaches have themselves transformed in the context of changing conceptions of the political, not to mention social, cultural and material processes. Of course, this account does not pretend to be exhaustive; we have had to leave out a great deal of potentially relevant work.

The connections between drug and alcohol practices and media practices, especially in the context of changes wrought by digital media, is a topic that deserves a whole chapter, given its relation not only to questions of representation but other topics that are highly relevant, such as moral panics, the construction of drug markets, new consumption and procurement practices and user quality control assurance.[3] By way of conclusion, we would like to comment on another feature of cultural studies we have not yet mentioned – one that creates vexing difficulties for cultural studies practitioners working in the field, but which may also form a powerful basis for interventions into drug and alcohol policy as it is constituted in the context of drug prohibition, not to mention the intensifying problematisation of youth drinking practices.

As John Frow and Meaghan Morris have argued, the scholarly project of cultural studies is always at some level marked by 'a discourse of social involvement' (Frow and Morris, 1993: xviii). Such scholarship tends to be critically and politically motivated, and for this reason, it is often 'openly incomplete, and it is partisan in its insistence on the political dimensions of knowledge' (1993: xviii). This openness resounds with feminist and post-structuralist critiques of objectivity (e.g. Haraway, 1991) and may be regarded as a refreshingly honest and explicit attempt to put these commitments into practice. Perhaps more than any other field of scholarship, cultural studies is marked by its appreciation of the insights that can come from 'acknowledging partiality and admitting one's attraction to the culture under investigation' – and indeed, one's involvement in it, where relevant (Gregg, 2006: 142). This orientation has also had a range of additional benefits, most notably a refusal to exoticise the cultural forms it investigates. This is particularly welcome given how prone drug cultures can be to the sort of exoticisation that can attend the use of ethnographic methods.

Despite these advantages, the inclination to situate one's analytic perspective can also create problems for the status of the claims its practitioners make and in particular the value these claims are accorded in the field of public health policy. In the context of drug and alcohol research especially, being explicit about one's immersion in the culture under study can create problems. In many public health circles, any admission of drug use or immersion in a culture deemed 'unhealthy' is liable to disqualify claims to authoritative knowledge on these topics and confer upon everyone else 'a power of irrefutable judgment' over the maker of them (Race, 2009: 149). No doubt this is a primary reason behind the 'reluctant reflexivity' that Measham and Moore have discussed as a characteristic feature of club studies (Measham and Moore, 2006). And yet, many of the most valuable insights of these studies have been built on the perspectives afforded by insider knowledge and embodied participation in these cultures, whether explicitly or implicitly acknowledged.

> Without a reflexive consideration of the social, emotional and intellectual location of the researcher and its implications for the research process, club research risks doing an injustice to the millions of people for whom clubs and clubbing have become an integral part of their leisure time and possibly their identity. (Measham and Moore, 2006: 25; see also Gilbert and Pearson, 1999: 18–19)

We agree with this argument. To illustrate the stakes of this conundrum, we would like to invoke a local policy context. The film *Rampant* (2007, dir. Midwinter-Pitt) tells the remarkable story of how three criminalised, highly marginalised populations – 'junkies, pooftahs and whores', as the film dubs them – came to play a key part in the design of governmental policies and programmes in the context of the early AIDS crisis in Australia. What is so remarkable about this story is how the 'sordid' knowledge of these previously abject subjects was transformed through this process into a form of technical know-how with an immediately practical and practicable function for government.

Questions such as how people score, how sex takes place and how drugs are used – the practical meanings and logics of a whole range of illicit activities – become highly relevant for the design of effective public health interventions. The film depicts how members of affected groups came to serve as spokespeople for these worlds in a relatively sudden trajectory from deviant status to that of policy partners and situated experts. Judging by HIV incidence rates in Australia, this formula has been highly effective, at least in terms of policy measures.[4]

We mention this example, not because we wish to idealise this moment as some utopian or un-conflicted policy development, nor do we mean to suggest that cultural studies played an especially important role in this trajectory (it did not). Such policy designs are never simple or straightforwardly positive in their impacts, to be sure, but often conflicted and double-edged.[5] We only wish to suggest that the complexities that inhere in this situation mirror those faced by the field of cultural studies at various points in its development. The creation of new speaking positions, the valorisation and redeployment of degraded forms of knowledge, the whole problem of speaking for others and existential tensions between practical utility and critical dissent have each figured as key problematics for the field at various points in the course of its development.

In practice, the 'self-situating' propensity of cultural studies has been a source of rigorous inquiry and critically informed, inventive responses (Haraway, 1991; Morris 1990, 2006; Probyn, 1993). There is now a robust literature that consists of non-naïve and systematic reflections on how to navigate 'the odd duality that splits the critic into participant and observer, practitioner and reflexive intellectual, on the basis of [their relation] to the institutions of knowledge that make such reflexivity possible' (Frow and Morris, 1993: xvii). This does not by itself address the risks that admissions of drug use, for example, pose to one's professional authority, by virtue of drugs' criminalised status, not to mention their cultural association with cognitive impairment, etc. Indeed, such admissions are risky and likely to place drug and alcohol scholars in particularly precarious positions, professionally speaking. Taking such risks also involves considerable professional bravery, it must be said, and has the potential to impact the affective climate in which policy thinking and practices take place in positive ways.

Therefore, while we want to avoid an overly idealistic celebration of community partnerships in the context of HIV/AIDS, neither do we wish to downplay the historical impact of these new configurations, nor minimise their significance as more democratic approaches to citizenship, social arrangements of knowledge and the governmentality of public health more generally. The inclusion of members of affected communities in the apparatus of government is an ongoing source of critical energy and innovation in these policy fields. Brokering the entry of previously unrecognised subjects into given conventions of practice and knowledge is a no less familiar process to most communities of cultural studies practitioners, to draw a connection here. In Melissa Gregg's assessment:

> One of [cultural studies] key achievements has been to question the conventions of traditional academic discourse, reworking some of its expectations and functions to keep step with contemporary events. In doing so, [it] has widened the participants for scholarly debate, making the academic vocation a more attractive and likely prospect for different kinds of people. (Gregg, 2006: 2).

Largely on the basis of this experience, the field contains a plethora of models for how to frame one's situated experience as a viable position from which to make critical claims and compelling interventions into given regimes of knowledge. Cultural studies might be seen as a pedagogical space that is uniquely well adapted to the sort of situated exchanges and collective encounters that would usefully inform drug and alcohol policy from this vantage point. Indeed, we believe that this space affords distinctive opportunities for sparking reflection on how best to *inhabit* the public roles and identities that drug users – among health consumers more generally – are increasingly invited to occupy. Of course, addressing such propositions is by no means easy, but calls for ongoing conceptual, methodological and practical experimentation. Cultural Studies has long provided a hospitable environment for precisely such experiments, both within the university and at its various community and institutional interfaces.

NOTES

1 See, for example, de Visser et al. (2013); Emslie et al. (2015); Griffin et al. (2009); Hutton et al. (2013); Lindsay (2006); Lyons and Willott (2008); MacLean and Moore (2014); Measham and Brain 2005; Szmigin et al. (2008). There is also a growing body of literature in Emotional Geography that explores alcohol, gender and identity formation. See, for example, Hubbard (2005); Leyshon (2008); Waitt et al. (2011).

2 See Race (2003, 2011a) for a comparable analysis of how ecstasy was productively involved in the generation of a sense of gay community in the context of the AIDS crisis.

3 See, for example, Manning (2014), McRobbie and Thornton (1995) and Reeves and Campbell (1994) on drugs, moral panic and media formations; and Barratt (2012), Brown and Gregg (2012) and Race (2014) on new drug and alcohol consumption practices in the digital context.

4 One per cent of Australian drug users are HIV positive, compared to 20 per cent in the USA; relative to the USA, the general incidence of HIV infection is 10 times less in Australia. There has not been a single recorded instance of transmission from a female sex worker to a man and Australia's death toll from AIDS is below 7000.

5 Conflicted, because the claim to represent any identity necessarily opens a can of worms in which questions of authenticity, representativeness and the terms of inclusion and exclusion invariably squirm. Double-edged; because the rationale that drives such moves towards expanded participation has disciplinary trade-offs insofar as it presumes some shared investment in governmental objectives.

REFERENCES

Barratt, Monica (2012) Silk Road: Ebay for drugs. *Addiction*, 107(3): 683.

Becker, Howard (1963) *Outsiders: Studies in the Sociology of Deviance*. New York: Free Press.

Brown, Rebecca (2014) *A Girls' Night Out: Gender, Subjectivity, Pleasure*. PhD thesis. Sydney: Department of Gender and Cultural Studies, University of Sydney.

Brown, Rebecca and Gregg, Melissa (2012) The pedagogy of regret: Facebook, binge-drinking and young women. *Continuum*, 26(3): 357–69.

de Visser, Richard. O., Wheeler, Zoe, Abraham, Charles and Smith, Jonathan. A. (2013) 'Drinking is our modern way of bonding': young people's beliefs about interventions to encourage moderate drinking. *Psychology and Health*, 28(12): 1460–80.

Duff, Cameron (2014) *Assemblages of Health*. New York: Springer.

Emslie, Carol, Hunt, Kate and Lyons, Antonia (2015) Transformation and time-out: the role of alcohol in identity construction among Scottish women in early midlife. *International Journal of Drug Policy*, 26(5): 437–45.

Foucault, Michel (1978) *The History of Sexuality, Volume 1: An Introduction*. London: Penguin.

Foucault, Michel (1985) *The Use of Pleasure: The History of Sexuality Volume 2*. New York: Vintage.

Fraser, Suzanne and Moore, David (2011) *The Drug Effect: Health, Crime and Society*. Melbourne: Cambridge University Press

Fraser, Suzanne, Moore, David and Keane, Helen (2014) *Habits: Remaking Addiction*. London: Palgrave MacMillan.

Frow, John and Morris, Meaghan (1993) Introduction. In John Frow and Meaghan Morris (eds), *Australian Cultural Studies: A Reader*. Urbana: University of Illinois Press, pp. vii–xxxii.

Gilbert, Jeremy and Pearson, Ewan (1999) *Discographies: Dance, Music, Culture and the Politics of Sound*. London: Routledge.

Goffman, Erving (1968) *Stigma*. London: Penguin.

Gomart, Emilie and Hennion, Antoine (1999) A sociology of attachment: music amateurs, drug users. In Law, J. and Hassard, J. (eds), *Actor Network Theory and After*. London: Blackwell, pp. 220–47.

Gregg, Melissa (2006) *Cultural Studies' Affective Voices*. London: Palgrave MacMillan.

Griffin, Christine, Bengry-Howell, Andrew, Hackley, Chris, Mistral, Willm and Szmigin, Isabelle (2009) 'Every time I do it I absolutely annihilate myself': loss of (self-) consciousness and loss of memory in young people's drinking narratives. *Sociology*, 43(3): 457–67.

Grosz, Elizabeth (1994) *Volatile Bodies: Towards a Corporeal Feminism*. Sydney. Allen and Unwin.

Hall, Stuart (1981) Notes on deconstructing 'the popular'. In Raphael Samuel (ed.), *People's History and Socialist Theory*. London: Routledge and Kegan Paul, pp. 227–39.

Hall, Stuart and Jefferson, Tony (eds) (1993) *Resistance Through Rituals: Youth Subcultures in Post-War Britain*, 2nd edn. London and New York: Routledge.

Haraway, Donna (1991) *Simians, Cyborgs, Women: The Reinvention of Nature*. London: Free Association Books.

Hebdige, Dick (1993) The meaning of Mod. In Stuart Hall and Tony Jefferson (eds), *Resistance Through Rituals: Youth Subcultures in Post-War Britain*, 2nd edn. London and New York: Routledge, pp.71–9.

Hemmings, Claire (2005) Invoking affect: cultural theory and the ontological turn. *Cultural Studies*, 19(5): 548–67.

Hubbard, Phil (2005) The geographies of 'going out'. In Joyce Davidson, Liz Bondi and Mick Smith (eds.), *Emotional Geography*. Aldershot: Ashgate, pp. 117–34.

Hunt, Geoffrey, Moloney, Molly and Evans, Kristin (2009) Epidemiology meets cultural studies: studying and understanding youth cultures, clubs and drugs. *Addiction Research and Theory*, 17(6): 601–21.

Hutton, Fiona, Wright, Sarah and Saunders, Emma (2013) Cultures of intoxication: young women, alcohol and harm reduction. *Contemporary Drug Problems*, 40(Winter): 451–80.

Jackson, P. (2004) *Inside Clubbing: Sensual Experiments in the Art of Being Human*. Oxford and New York: Berg.

Keane, Helen (2002) *What's Wrong with Addiction?* Melbourne: Melbourne University Press.

Latour, Bruno (2005a) *Reassembling the Social*. Oxford: Oxford University Press.

Latour, Bruno (2005b) How to talk about the body: the normative dimension of science studies. *Body and Society*, 10(2–3): 205–29.

Ley, Ruth (2011) The turn to affect: a critique. *Critical Inquiry*, 37(3): 434–72.

Leyshon, Michael (2008) 'We're stuck in the corner': young women, embodiment and drinking in the countryside. *Drugs: Education, Prevention and Policy*, 15(3): 267–89.

Lindsay, Jo (2006) A big night out in Melbourne: drinking as an enactment of class and gender. *Contemporary Drug Problems*, 33: 29–61.

Lyons, Antonia C. and Willott, Sara A. (2008) Alcohol consumption, gender identities and women's changing social positions. *Sex Roles*, 59(9–10): 694–712.

MacLean, Sarah and Moore, David (2014). 'Hyped up': assemblages of alcohol, excitement and violence for outer-suburban young adults in the inner-city at night. *International Journal of Drug Policy*, 25(3): 378–85.

Malbon, Ben (1999) *Clubbing: Dancing, Ecstasy, Vitality*. London: Routledge.

Malins, Peta (2004) Machinic assemblages: Deleuze, Guattari and an ethico-aesthetics of drug use. *Janus Head*, 7(1):84–104.

Manning, Paul (2014) *Drugs and Popular Culture in the Age of New Media*. New York: Routledge.

Massumi, Brian (2002) *Parables of the Virtual: Movement, Affect, Sensation*. Durham: Duke University Press.

Martin, D. (1999) Power play and party politics: the significance of raving. *Journal of Popular Culture*, 32(4): 77–99.

McLeod, Kim (2014) The missing work of collaboration: using assemblages to rethink antidepressant action. *Contemporary Drug Problems*, 41:109–42.

McRobbie, Angela (1993) Shut up and dance: youth culture and changing modes of femininity. *Cultural Studies*, 7(3): 406–26.

McRobbie, Angela, and Sarah L. Thornton (1995) Rethinking 'moral panic' for multi-mediated social worlds. *The British Journal of Sociology*, 46(4): 559–574.

Measham, Fiona and Moore, Karenza (2006) Reluctant reflexivity and the development of club studies. In Bill Sanders (ed.), *Drugs, Clubs and Young People*. Aldershot: Ashgate, pp. 13–25.

Measham, Fiona and Kevin Brain (2005) 'Binge' drinking, British alcohol policy and the new culture of intoxication. *Crime, Media, Culture*, 1(3): 262–83.

Midwinter Pitt, Victoria (2007) *Rampant: How a City Stopped a Plague*. Sydney: Chapman Pictures Pty Ltd.

Mol, Annemarie (2003) *The Body Multiple: Ontology in Medical Practice*. Durham: Duke University Press.

Morris, Meaghan (1990) Banality in cultural studies. In Patricia Mellencamp (ed.), *Logics of Television*. Indianapolis: Indiana University Press, pp.14–43.

Morris, Meaghan (2006) *Identity Anecdotes: Translation and Media Culture*. London: Sage.

Papoulias, Constantina and Callard, Felicity (2010) Biology's gift: interrogating the turn to affect. *Body and Society*, 16(1): 29–56.

Pearson, Geoffrey and Twohig, John (1993) Ethnography through the looking glass. In Stuart Hall and Tony Jefferson (eds), *Resistance Through Rituals: Youth Subcultures in Post-War Britain*, 2nd edn. London and New York: Routledge, pp. 100–5.

Pini, Maria (1997) Women and the early British rave scene. In Angela McRobbie (ed.) *Back to Reality? Social Experience and Cultural Studies*. Manchester and New York: Manchester University Press, pp. 152–69.

Probyn, Elspeth (1993) *Sexing the Self: Gendered Positions in Cultural Studies*. London: Routledge.

Probyn, Elspeth (2005) *Blush: Faces of Shame*. Minneapolis: University of Minnesota Press.

Race, Kane (2003) The death of the dance party. *Australian Humanities Review*, 30.

Race, Kane (2008) The use of pleasure in harm reduction: perspectives from The History of Sexuality. *International Journal of Drug Policy*, 19(5): 417–23.

Race, Kane (2009) *Pleasure Consuming Medicine: The Queer Politics of Drugs*. Durham: Duke University Press.

Race, Kane (2011a) Party animals: the significance of drug practices in the materialization of modern gay identity. In Suzanne Fraser and David Moore (eds), *The Drug Effect: Health, Crime and Society*. Melbourne: Cambridge University Press, pp. 35–56.

Race, Kane (2011b) Drug effects, performativity and the law. *International Journal of Drug Policy*, 22(6): 410–12.

Race, Kane (2012) Framing responsibility: HIV, biomedical prevention and the performativity of the law. *Journal of Bioethical Inquiry*, 9: 327–38.

Race, Kane (2014) Complex events: drug effects and emergent causality. *Contemporary Drug Problems*, 41(3): 301–34.

Redhead, Steve, Wynne, Derek and O'Conner, Justin (eds) (1997) *The Clubcultures Reader*. Oxford: Blackwell.

Reeves, Jimmie L. and Campbell, Richard (1994) *Cracked Coverage: Television News, the Anit-Cocaine Crusade and the Reagan Legacy*. Durham: Duke University Press.

Reynolds, Simon (1997) Rave culture: living dream or living death. In Steve Redhead, Derek Wynne and Justin O'Connor (eds), *The Clubcultures Reader*. Oxford: Blackwell.

Sedgwick, Eve K. (1993) *Tendencies*. Durham: Duke University Press.

Sedgwick, Eve K. (2003) *Touching Feeling: Affect, Pedagogy, Performativity*. Durham: Duke University Press.

Szmigin, Isabelle, Christine Griffin, Willm Mistral, Andrew Bengry-Howell, Louise Weale and Chris Hackley (2008) Re-framing 'binge drinking' as calculated hedonism: empirical evidence from the UK. *International Journal of Drug Policy*, 19(5): 359–66.

Thrift, Nigel (2007) *Non-Representational Theory: Space, Politics, Affect*. London: Routledge.

Turner, Graeme (2012) *What's Become of Cultural Studies?* London: Sage.

Vitellone, Nicole (2010) Just another night in the shooting gallery? The syringe, space and affect. *Environment and Planning D: Society and Space*, 28(5): 867–80.

Waitt, Gordon, Jessop, Loretta and Gorman-Murray, Andrew (2011) 'The guys in there just expect to be laid': embodied and gendered socio-spatial practices of a 'night out' in Wollongong, Australia. *Gender, Place and Culture*, 18(2): 255–75.

Whatmore, Sarah (2002) *Hybrid Geographies: Natures, Cultures, Spaces*. London and Thousand Oaks: Sage.

Willis, Paul E. (1993) The cultural meaning of drug use. In Stuart Hall and Tony Jefferson (eds), *Resistance Through Rituals: Youth Subcultures in Post-War Britain*, 2nd edn. London and New York: Routledge, pp. 88–99.

Wilson, Elizabeth (2004) *Psychosomatic: Feminism and the Neurological Body*. Durham: Duke University Press.

Young, Jock (1972) *The Drugtakers: The Social Meaning of Drug Use*. London: Paladin.

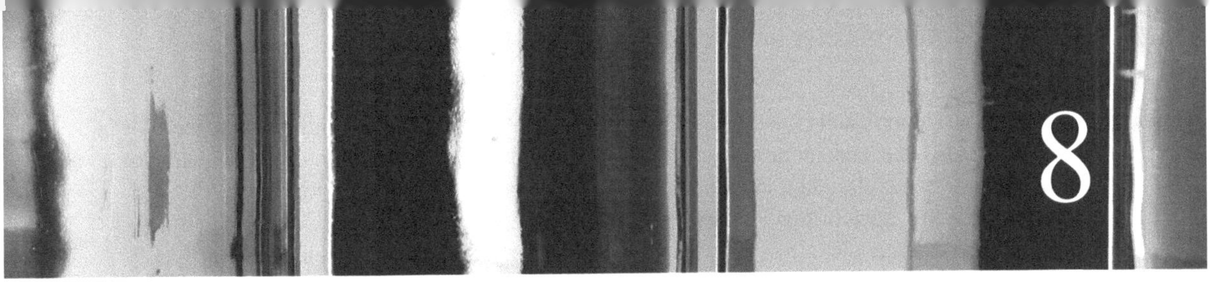

Geographical Perspectives on Drug and Alcohol Studies

Mark Jayne, Gill Valentine and Sarah L. Holloway

INTRODUCTION

This chapter investigates the ways in which spatialities of drugs and alcohol have been considered within and beyond the discipline of geography.[1] The first half of the paper shows how drugs and alcohol research includes significant and sustained consideration of geographical issues. For example, studies undertaken by scholars in a variety of disciplines including medical and health studies, psychology, sociology, politics, criminology, economics and cultural studies have considered issues relating to drugs and alcohol via 'geographical' issues such as spatial scale, national, regional and local identities, distinctions between public and private space, urbanity and rurality, boundaries and transgressions, visibility and invisibility, centrality and marginality and so on. In the second half of the paper, we suggest that while being relatively slow to engage with drug and alcohol research, recent studies have highlighted that geographers have much to offer academic and policy debate.

In reviewing geographical contributions to drug and alcohol studies this paper presents two main arguments. First, we show that a large amount of rich, detailed and relevant geographical work has been undertaken by drug and alcohol researchers relating to a diverse set of topics, social groups and spaces and places. However, although voluminous, research has under-theorized the ways in which space and place are key to understanding practices and processes relating to drugs and alcohol. Drugs and alcohol researchers have tended to consider space and place as a passive backdrop, rather than as an active constituent to the topic being researched (Jayne et al., 2008a; DeVerteuil and Wilton, 2009). Moreover, studies have also overwhelmingly failed to pursue an understanding of connections, mobilities, similarities or differences between case studies (including consideration of policy transfer, legislation, planning, design and policing strategies, everyday drug and alcohol production and consumption cultures and so on) and consideration of space and place has been undertaken via a de facto and/or fragmented agenda that, while being based on particular people or places, does not enable generalizations to be made (Castree, 2005). In these terms, drugs and alcohol studies that have had a geographical focus rarely move beyond specificities and have thus failed to generate a convincing case to assert the importance of geography as a key feature of research agendas.

Second, despite being a fledgling disciplinary research agenda, geographers' consideration of drugs and alcohol has produced critically rich and detailed case study research that has sought to unpack complex spatialities (Wilton and DeVerteuil, 2006; Jayne et al., 2008a, 2008b, 2011; DeVerteuil and Wilton, 2009; McShane and Kneale, 2011; Wilton and Moreno, 2012). As DeVerteuil and Wilton (2009) highlight, geographers have considered a remarkably diverse range of 'intoxicants' including alcohol and drugs via consideration of production and consumption, regulation, treatment and prevention with reference to critical consideration of urban life, families, life-course, gender, ethnicity, masculinity/femininity, work and employment, criminal justice, violence and so on. More recently, geographers have also pointed to an impasse where drugs and alcohol are 'pathologised as a health, social, legislative, crime or policy problem *or* as being embedded in social and cultural relations – with limited dialogue between these approaches' and thus sought to engage with ontologies and epistemologies that have dominated research agendas (Jayne et al., 2008a: 247; Jayne and Valentine 2016).

However, despite this progress, a major failing of geographers' engagement with drugs and alcohol has been an inability to transcend disciplinary boundaries. Concern over the impact of geographical research beyond the discipline has been a long running debate (Harvey, 1974; Peck, 1999; Martin, 2001). In this paper, we signpost the need for geographical research into drugs and alcohol that not only continues to pursue theoretical and empirical advances, but which does a better job of offering policy relevant 'public geographies' that speak to diverse non-academic audiences (Ward, 2005).

DRUG AND ALCOHOL STUDIES AND GEOGRAPHY

A large amount of drug and alcohol research has importantly discussed the ways in which a diverse range of practices and processes unfold in specific spaces and places. For example, if we focus on alcohol, an indicative (and non-exhaustive) list includes research focused on local, regional or national contexts, studies of 'national' drinking cultures (see, for example, Kubicka et al., 1998; Campbell, 2000; McGovern, 2002) or how consumption, identity, lifestyle and forms of sociability unfold in specific regional, rural or urban settings (Bloomfield, 1993; Robbins and Martin, 1993; Plant, 1997; Gough and Edwards, 1998; Harnett et al., 2000; Shaikh and Nax, 2000; Waterson, 2000). A similar review of drugs research also highlights a large amount of research that focuses on different spatial scales, social groups and specific spaces and places.[2]

Nonetheless, despite a voluminous amount of valuable studies, researchers have overwhelmingly considered space and place as a passive backdrop. For example, Thrift (2009) summarized geographers' progressive and critical engagement with space and place as sharing:

> A common ambition: that is to abandon the idea of any pre-existing space in which things are embedded for an idea of space an undergoing continual construction exactly through the agency of things encountering each other in more or less organized circulations. This is a *relational* view of space in which, rather than space being viewed as a container within which the world proceeds,

space is seen as a co-product of those proceedings. (Thrift, 2009: 95)

Thrift (2009) goes on to suggests four foundational elements of geographical thinking; first, a focus on the empirical construction of space and the need to consider 'houses, cars, mobiles, knives and forks, offices, bicycles, computers, clothes and dryers, cinemas, trains, televisions, garden paths – but because these things are usually so mundane we tend to overlook them. So we often forget just what an extraordinary achievement the fabric of our daily lives actually is'. Second, to theorize space as 'a series of carefully worked-up connections through which what we know as the world interacts. These connections consist of pathways which bind often quite unalike things together, usually on a routine, circulating basis' (Thrift, 2009: 95). Third, to understand how space is represented in images, pictures, words and so on. And finally, to unpack 'place' through engagement with 'particular rhythms of being that confirm and naturalize the existence of certain spaces (Thrift, 2009: 95), or, as Massey suggests, to investigate how places are 'constructed out of a particular constellation of social relations, meeting and weaving together at a particular locus' (Massey, 1991: 28).

Such insights highlight that space and place must not be considered as static, bounded territories but as constituted through complex interpenetrations of political, economic, social and cultural processes, flows and power relations, occurring at various scales (e.g. the body, the neighbourhood, the city, region, nation and so) and which gives places their uniqueness (see Massey 1991, 2005; Cresswell 2004). Drugs and alcohol studies, while generally undertaking research in specific space and places or at different spatial scales, tend to undertheorize the kind of above spatialities that constitute the topics at hand. If reflected upon at all, context, location and the relationships between the people and places being studied, tends to be considered as a peripheral issue. This failing is best exemplified by a lack of research that seeks to compare or contrast research in different contexts and at different spatial scales. The impact of this impasse has ensured that overwhelmingly drugs and alcohol research across the social sciences have failed to take geography seriously.

Such criticisms notwithstanding, there are, nonetheless, a number of examples where drugs and alcohol studies have attempted a more geographically nuanced approach. For example, consideration of the trade-offs and conflicts between legal and 'common-sense' definitions of intoxication and policing policy (including sensitivity towards differences in local cultural practices, behaviour, speech and so on), have shown how discourses of pleasure are accounted for in policy making in different locations (Levi and Valverde, 2001; Valverde, 2003; O'Malley and Valverde, 2004). Similarly, consideration of the characterization of the 'lager lout' by the Thatcherite government and studies of young male drinkers in the north east of England and street drinking in Vietnam (see Hunt and Slatterlee, 1986, 1987; Gofton, 1990; Hunt, 1991; Thomas, 2002; Nayak, 2003) have identified how local, regional and national identities are constructed in terms of broader processes.

Other useful research has addressed geographies of production, regulation and policy regimes, despite the spatialities that constitute the topic at hand being undertheorized. For example, national, regional and local policy related studies have focused on the relationship between drinking and gender in nine European countries (Allaman et al., 2000), a study of students' drinking in 18 countries (Smart and Ogbourne, 2000), a survey of the Russian population's drinking habits (Bobak et al., 1999) and various local initiates in Europe (Ramsey, 1990), the UK, the US (Wittman, 1997) and Australia (Lindsay, 2005). Moreover, there is also a growing number of large transnational surveys such as World Health Organization (2000, 2001, 2004), ESPAD

(2004) and ECAS (2002). Research has also considered how increasingly globalized alcohol supply and international supply side initiatives impact on strategies to reduce alcohol related harm and how international trade treaties effect alcohol regulation and policy in local contexts (Alavaikko and Osterberg, 2000). These studies show that while there is an increasingly integrated global system of production and distribution, and also less restriction on cross-border trading of alcohol, the collection of cross-cultural data on alcohol remains patchy. Thus, there is often an underreporting of consumption in many countries. As such, a key concern of the work on production, regulation and policy regimes has been to highlight the conflict between health concerns and economic and social development at national, regional and local contexts, with little implicit attention to the geographies that underpin the case studies at hand (Grieshaber-Otto et al., 2000; Room and Jernigan, 2000).

More recent work by drugs researchers have offered a more sophisticated understanding of spatialities with regards to the role of 'place' based drug resource and policy strategies (Duff, 2010), public/private injection of illegal drugs (Fitzgerald et al., 2004; Rhones, 2007), the role of urban neighbourhoods in terms of substance use and treatment (Mason et al., 2004; Stahler, 2007; Best et al., 2012) and the development of more critical geographical analysis of national drug recovery programmes (Bourgois, 2000). With a focus on the social, cultural and material conditions of drug use in public and domestic spaces such research has relevantly shown how drugs and alcohol related concerns are mobilized in particular places in comparison with others, around specific issues and specific groups of people.

However, despite these interesting studies, theoretical arguments relating to drugs and alcohol generally fail to translate beyond specific people and spaces and places, other than dialectical approaches of alcohol as a social/medical problem or as a social or cultural practice (Jayne et al., 2008b). Moreover, while there have been attempts to conjoin these issues in studies at transnational, national and local levels (for example, Harrison, 1996; Holder, 2000), perspectives have not been developed that translate beyond the empirical evidence relating to particular spatial scales (see Jayne et al., 2008b).

Despite the large amount of valuable research, broader theoretical and empirical weaknesses of drug and alcohol research highlights the important work that human geography has to undertake in order to impact on future research agendas. By addressing the conceptual connections between spaces and places, by tracing general relations, practices and processes in order to identify those that are common (and unique) 'on the ground', and the need to imagine different kinds of practical responses shows that a nuanced geographical approach has much to contribute to debate. Indeed, with a focus on both historical and contemporary spatial practices and processes relating to drugs and alcohol and their unique position in wider constellations of political, economic, social, cultural and spatial relations, geographers' spatial knowledges can be utilized in order to make theoretical, political and policy connections (Massey, 1995).

GEOGRAPHY AND DRUG AND ALCOHOL STUDIES

In comparison with the voluminous canon of research across the medical and social sciences, geography's engagement with academic, popular and policy debate focused on drugs and drink has been limited. Despite this, geographers have nonetheless pursued a wide variety of issues with relation to different spaces and places throughout the world. For example, Purvis (1998), Dion (1959) and Unwin (1991) have looked at the proliferation of working men's clubs in the nineteenth century and historical geographies of the production and consumption of wine and Hall (1992) has considered nostalgic ideas of pub life. Kneale (2001), Beckingham (2008, 2010, 2012) and Howell and Beckingham (2015) focused on historical geographies of moral supervision relating to alcohol consumption and Lagendijk's (2003) study of global wine producing networks showed how local socio-cultural bindings of distinctiveness, identity and cultural values impacted upon the economic logic of globally integrated networks of production and distribution. Field and Beale (2004) investigated the use of GIS in modelling incidences, prevalence and spread of non-legal drug use and Wylie et al. (2007) offered a sophisticated understanding of the spatialities of social networks bound up with injecting drug users and the prevalence of blood borne pathogens.

Over a relatively short period of time it is clear that there has been a bourgeoning interest in drugs and alcohol amongst geographers. Indeed, it is arguably more difficult to identify an area of human geography where drugs and alcohol does *not* have potential resonance for research agendas. However, perhaps the most important research by geographers that engages with drugs and alcohol is that which has sought to make critical contributions to theoretical and empirical debates not only within, but beyond the discipline. For example, an indicative (and non-exhaustive) list of the kinds of topics and issues where geographers have offered critical commentary on drug and alcohol studies includes the nature and form of liberalization policy both in terms of legislative and policy regimes in specific spatial contexts (Shaw, 2010, 2014, 2015), consideration of how national, regional and local drug and drinking cultures are changing and how issues relating to regulation and production and geographies of drug and alcohol consumption play out in the global south have been considered (Herrick, 2012; Herrick and Charman, 2013).

Other theorists have focused on ways in which the proliferation of supermarkets has impacted on domestic drinking patterns and habits (Holloway et al., 2009). Lowe et al. (1993), Jayne et al. (2012a, b), Valentine et al. (2014) and Jayne and Valentine (2016) have investigated family life and transmission of drinking cultures. Indeed, there is clearly a need to build on current research with more sustained investigation of domestic/public drug and alcohol consumption cultures to address the relational geographies of how, why and when people take drugs and drink alcohol at home or in public spaces and commercial venues (see Dovey et al., 2001; Hembree, 2005; Robertson, 2007). Similarly, geographical perspectives on how the life course affects ethnic drug and drinking patterns and intergenerational change in different places at different times is of importance to research agendas across the social sciences (Valentine et al., 2009, 2010a). The geographies of drug taking and alcohol consumption on holiday are also clearly potentially productive future areas of study (Bell, 2008; Jayne et al., 2012a, b).

Similarly, other studies have focused on a number of issues relating to legislation, production, consumption, service provision and health issues by concentrating on social geographies of class, gender, ethnicity, sexuality, age, urbanity/rurality, public/private and so on. Valentine et al. (2007) discussed how drinking alcohol is discursively constructed as a 'problem', and when and for whom, government intervention and the development and enactment of specific tailored policing strategies in the UK are unfolding (also see Valentine et al., 2011; Jayne and Valentine, 2015b). By considering the spatialized ways in which drinking is constructed as a problem (and when it is not) – differently in private and public space, in urban and rural areas and different city spaces and places – research by geographers is highlighting the importance of a more sustained and nuanced consideration of the ways in which alcohol, drinking and drunkenness is problematized (also see Maye et al., 2005; Jayne et al., 2006, 2008b; Jayne and Valentine, 2015a, b; Holloway et al., 2008; Valentine et al., 2007; Valentine et al., 2011).

In a similar vein, Leyshon (2005, 2008), Holloway et al. (2009) and Wilton et al. (2014) have discussed the role of masculinity/femininity in both alcohol consumption and drug treatment. Leyshon (2005), for example, traces the ways in which young men who dominate the backrooms of rural pubs construct and perform hegemonic masculinity. Central to these young men's performance was bodily management in which, for example, they proved they could hold their drink by holding conversations, their bladders and playing pub sports well whilst drinking. This bodily performance, along with phallocentric language and sexist and homophobic discourses mark these as the 'in' young men and relegate other young men and women to marginal areas of the pub or from it completely. Leyshon (2005) himself notes that 'the ritual is interestingly unrebellious'. Unlike the young people in Kraack and Kenway's (2002) study, who upset older residents by holding parties outside as there were no other places for them to go, these young men reproduce hegemonic masculinity with the landlord's consent and the tactic approval of the older men who occupy the front bar.

Heley (2008) and Nayak (2003) also show how middle-aged and young men's drinking landscapes are cross-cut by class and ethnicity. Heley's (2008) study starts to trace the emergence of a new 'squirearchy', as middle-class male incomers to a rural area seek to position themselves in the local class structure, in part through drinking practices that ape those of farmers they regard as the 'old squires' of the village. This is not a smooth process, both because their interpretation of the class structure is not always shared by locals, and because the economics of the drinks industry are changing rural drinking landscapes. At the other end of the class system, Nayak (2003) traces the ways in which working-class white men from the north east of England maintain a Geordie identity in the context of deindustrialisation. Central to this are hedonistic displays of circuit drinking, which Nayak interprets as a contemporary form of promenading, as well as support for the local football team, as the identity which previous generations of men gained through industrial employment has been replaced by 'its re-enactment through an exaggerated display of white industrial masculinity' in the sphere of consumption (Nayak, 2003: 22)

However, while studies undertaken by geographers suggest that the discipline has much to add to theoretical and empirical debates, to a certain degree geography has tended to mirror drugs and alcohol studies by focusing on a diverse range of issues in specific places that while generating rich and detailed findings has been based on a de facto and fragmented research agenda. Such comments notwithstanding, when writing by geographers *is* adding value to knowledge and debates within geography and across the social sciences – as well as to drug and alcohol studies – theoretical and empirically nuanced research has sought to consider the interpenetration of political economic, social, cultural and spatial practices and processes and also challenge ontological and epistemological orthodoxies that have dominated drug and alcohol research.

For example, the most sustained drug and alcohol related issue that geographers have engaged with in the past few years has concerned public space and the night-time economy. For example, on the one hand – and in parallel with alcohol research – Chatterton and Hollands (2003), Bromley et al. (2003) and Thomas and Bromley (2000) have considered the increased corporatization of the night-time economy in the UK (see for example, Hadfield, 2006; Hobbs et al., 2003; Plant and Plant, 2006; Winlow and Hall, 2006; and so on). While adding much to understanding of alcohol and the night-time-economy, this research tends to depict an overly neat picture of city centres populated by young people who are drunken and disorderly. Others writers, such as Latham (2003), Bell (2005), Edensor (2006) and Jayne et al.

(2006, 2008b) have begun to move beyond such generalized depictions arguing that far from being homogenized, drug taking and alcohol consumption is a varied activity constructed through diverse practices and experiences. Mirroring such arguments, geographers focused on drug consumption, regulation and policy in the urban night time economy have also sought to move beyond generalized depictions to understand the complexities and spatialities of everyday experience of a diverse range of drug taking with reference to neo-liberal urban policy and policing agendas (Punch, 2005; Corva, 2008; McCann, 2008, 2011; Draus et al., 2010). McCann (2008), for example, considers drug policy in Vancouver, British Columbia, with regards to the mundane of a 'four-pillar' drug strategy (prevention, treatment, enforcement and harm reduction), which was essentially policy learned from cities outside North America. Drawing on a neo-Foucauldian governmentality approach to emphasize the role of expertise (specialized knowledge held by many actors, not just credentialed professionals) McCann critiques the mobilities of drug policy transfer and the deployment of powerful truths in the development of the policy, and gives everyday examples of how drugs policy is not transferable from one place to another. These examples of work being undertaken into geographies of drugs and alcohol highlight how geographers are offering diverse and critical contributions to academic and policy debate. In the remainder of this section, however, we will focus on one specific burgeoning area of human geography in order to highlight in more detail how geographers are progressing our understanding of drugs and alcohol.

Drawing on similar arguments about the importance of taking geography seriously, studies of our emotional life are an emerging and exciting field of geography and focuses on the interplay between emotions, space and place (McCormack, 2003; Davidson and Bondi, 2004; Thrift, 2004). In this work, emotions are investigated as important aspects of our daily lives; 'embodied and mindful phenomena that partially shape, and are shaped by our interaction with people, places and politics that make up our unique, personal geographies' (Davidson and Bondi, 2004: 373). This includes joy, sadness, confusion, excitement, fear, conviviality, love, hate, arousal, reciprocity and so on. In these terms, drug taking and alcohol, drinking and drunkenness can be seen as part of a process of 'performative experience... which encourages new configuration and twists of ideas and experience' (Thrift, 2004: 57). This argument has allowed geographical approaches to drug and alcohol studies to begin to engage with the ways in which drug and alcohol consumption are bound up with economic and cultural life, supported and nurtured (or not) not only at the level of vernacular everyday life but through political and planning discourses.

Importantly, this literature has been successful in unpacking emotional and embodied geographies in the context of broader political, economic, social, spatial and cultural practices and processes. We suggest that such an approach has a vital role to play in contributing to drug and alcohol studies more broadly. For example, Philo et al. (2002) look at the relationship between alcohol and mental health in rural areas. Their research investigates both the important symbolic contribution of drinking to regional identity, but also how excessive drinking and drunkenness are an accepted and important element of local social relations. Elaborating on this position, Philo et al. show how alcohol is bound up with emotional geographies around a number of issues. These include hospitality, a lack of leisure opportunities, relaxation and a reward, coping strategies and both isolation and belonging. Philo et al. also show the ways in which these geographies are gendered, with men's heavy drinking tending to take place in public whilst women's heavy drinking is more private and solitary and thus a constitutive element of exclusionary social relations.

Similarly, Hubbard (2005) unpacks the experience of 'going out' in the 'evening economy'. Hubbard describes how danger, unpleasantness, frustration, resentment, pleasure, desire, fun, anger, happiness and fear are central to a night out. He shows that the occasion of 'a big night out' is saturated with emotion, and indeed, that these emotions help us to make sense of particular spaces and places and how we manage our emotional selves (also see Latham and McCormack, 2004; Waitt et al., 2011). Moreover, Briggs (2013) also undertook ethnographic research in order to understand how emotions regarding space and place are bound up with the use of crack cocaine. Love et al. (2012) focused on emotions and 'therapeutic landscapes' of drug treatment for women (also see Moreno, 2009)

While there is much work to be done to explore the co-constitutive relations between emotions, space and place and drugs and alcohol, drinking and drunkenness, as yet, drugs and alcohol studies have not caught onto the importance of this field of enquiry in a sustained way (although see Seeman et al. (1988) on drinking and alienation and Fennell et al. (1981) on alcohol and stress). Indicative areas of study could include, for example, the relationships between excitement, anticipation, apprehension, affection and sociability bound up with drug and alcohol consumption, performativity and national, regional and local and identities. Indeed, health geographers have usefully begun to contribute to these debates by discussing self-reporting of drinking and concerns over consumption levels (Twigg and Jones, 2000; Twigg et al., 2002). Drug taking and drinking as a reward, or to relax, as well as hangovers, come-downs regret, sadness and 'boozer's gloom' will also be important topics for study. We suggest that study of such issues will not only play an important part in the bourgeoning geographical literature in terms of emotional and embodied geographies and drugs and alcohol, drinking and drunkenness, but also has much to offer the broader theoretical, empirical and policy debates. Indeed, our own work on 'units' and everyday understandings and experiences of drunkenness (Jayne et al., 2010, 2011a, b) works at the intersection of theoretical debates concerning biopower and governmentality, emotional, embodied and affective geographies and actor network theory in order to consider ontological and epistemological approaches to studying alcohol, drinking and drunkenness. In doing so, we call for dialogue between social, health and medical scientists in order to develop more pertinent ways of understanding and representing the risks and benefits of alcohol consumption (also see Jayne and Valentine 2016).

Throughout this section, we have introduced work by geographers that includes both case study based research and studies that seek to unpack the connections, similarities, differences and mobilities relating to drugs and alcohol at different spatial scales. In light of such progress, that geographers have failed to impact on drugs and alcohol studies agendas is nonetheless disappointing. While this is perhaps unsurprising given the voluminous amount of 'geographical study' being undertaken throughout drug and alcohol research by writers in diverse disciplines that have a longer tradition of working in this field, it is clear that there is a significant challenge for geographers to ensure that our work resonates throughout drug and alcohol studies debates. However, we suggest that it is vital that a central tenant of this challenging project must be that geographers engage in research agendas that are not only of importance to broad academic audiences, but which also impact on policy and popular discourses.

CONCLUSION

We have shown in this chapter that, in the context of the broad variety of different issues, topics and concerns bound up in the drug and alcohol literature, a geographical perspective has much to contribute to theoretical and empirical debate. At present however, drug and alcohol research tends to under-theorize the importance of space and place, and while geographers are contributing research that offers both case study, and more nuanced research that looks at connections, similarities, differences and mobilities between drug and alcohol related issues and different people and places, these studies have failed to have a significant impact beyond the discipline. In these terms, it is clear that geographers must work hard to assert the importance of geography to drug and alcohol research agendas through the usual routes of visibility in interdisciplinary alcohol studies conferences, journals, contributions to edited collections and book series and so on and in policy and consultancy realms, but also by offering theoretically and empirically informed interventions into political and popular debates.

Our own research regarding alcohol, drinking and drunkenness in the UK has been undertaken in partnership with the Joseph Rowntree Foundation, in collaboration with a diverse range of partners including Alcohol Concern and the Drinkaware Trust (see Valentine et al., 2008, 2010b) and, along with other geographers, we contributed to the Royal Geographical Society (with the Institute of British Geographers) *Consumption Controversies: Alcohol Policies in the UK* (2010) highlighting the productive ways that geographers can contribute to policy debate. To this end, we challenge human geographers from all areas of study, and drug and alcohol studies researchers engaging in 'geographical' issues and approaches, to play a major and definitive role in contributing to the development of a more critical and coherent approach to studying geographies of drugs and alcohol. To readers of this book, then, we hope that your theoretical, empirical, policy or professional and practice work focused on drugs and alcohol might in the future include more thought and action on how geography matters.

NOTES

1 This paper draws on, updates and advances previous arguments made in Jayne, M., Valentine, G., and Holloway, S. L. (2008) The place of drink: geographical contributions to alcohol studies. *Drugs: Education, Prevention and Policy*, 15(3): 219–32.

2 Just as with alcohol research, there is a voluminous body of academic research that considers drugs at various spatial scales and with reference to specific spaces and places, social groups and different legal and illegal drugs. As well as such academic work there is a very large number of governmental, policy and think-tank studies focusing on drugs at various spatial scales throughout the world that similarly fail to take geography seriously.

REFERENCES

Alavaikko, M. and Osterberg, E. (2000) 'The influence of economic interests on alcohol control policy: a case study from Finland', *Addiction*, 93(4): S565–79.

Allaman, A., Voller, F., Kubicka, L. and Bloomfield, K. (2000) 'Drinking and the position of women in nine European countries', *Substance Abuse*, 21(4): 231–47.

Beckingham, D. (2008) 'Geographies of drink culture in Liverpool: lessons from the drink capital of nineteenth-century England', *Drugs: Education, Prevention and Policy* 15:3: 305–13.

Beckingham, D. J. (2010) 'An historical geography of liberty: Lancashire and the inebriates act', *Journal of Historical Geography* 36: 388–401.

Beckingham, D. J. (2012) 'Gender space and drunkenness: Liverpool's licensed premises 1860–1914', *Annals of the Association of American Geographers*, 20 (2): 647–66.

Bell, D. (2005) 'Commensality, urbanity, hospitality', In C. Lashley, P. Lynch and A. Morrison (eds.), *Critical Hospitality Studies*. London: Butterworth Heineman, pp. 34–42.

Bell, D. (2008) 'Destination drinking: toward a research agenda on alcotourism', *Drugs: Education, Prevention and Policy*, 15: 291–304.

Best, D., Gow, J., Knox, T., Taylor, A., Groshkova, T. and White, W. (2012) 'Mapping the recovery stories of drinkers and drug users in Glasgow: quality of life and its associations with measures of recovery capital', *Drug and Alcohol Review*, 31: 334–41.

Bloomfield, K. (1993) 'A comparison of alcohol consumption between lesbians and heterosexual women in an urban population', *Drug and Alcohol Dependence*, 33: 257–69.

Bobak, M., Mckee, M., Rose, R. and Marmot, M. (1999) 'Alcohol consumption in a sample of the Russian population', *Addiction*, 94(4): 857–66.

Bourgois, P. (2000) 'Disciplining addictions: the bio-politics of methadone and heroin in the United States', *Medicine and Psychiatry*, 24: 165–95.

Briggs, D. (2013) 'Emotions, ethnography and crack cocaine users', *Emotions, Space and Society*, 7: 1–12.

Bromley, R., Tallon, A. and Thomas, C. (2003) 'Disaggregating the space-time layers of city-centre activities and their uses', *Environment and Planning A*, 35: 1831–51.

Campbell, H. (2000) 'The glass phallus: pub(lic) masculinity and drinking in rural New Zealand', *Rural Sociology*, 65(4): 562–81.

Castree, N. (2005) 'The epistemology of particulars: human geography, case studies and 'context'. *Geoforum*, 36: 541–4.

Chatterton, P. and Hollands, R. (2003) *Urban Nightscapes: Youth Culture, Pleasure Spaces and Corporate Power*. London: Routledge.

Cresswell, T. (2004) *Place: A Short Introduction*. Oxford: Blackwell.

Corva, D. (2008) 'Neoliberal globalisation and the war on drugs: transationalizing liberal governance in the Americas', *Political Geography*, 27: 176–93.

Davidson, J. and Bondi, L. (2004) 'Spatialising affect; affecting space: an introduction', *Gender, Place and Culture*, 11(3): 373–4.

DeVerteuil, G and Wilton, R. (2009) 'The geographies of intoxicants: from production and consumption to regulation, treatment and prevention', *Geography Compass*, 3: 478–94.

Dion, R. (1959) *Hisotrie de la Vigne et du Vin en France des Origines au Xixie Siecle*. Paris: Flammarion.

Dovey, K., Fitzgerald, J. and Choi, Y. (2001) 'Safety becomes danger: dilemmas of drug-use in public space', *Health and Place*, 7: 319–31.

Draus, P., Roddy, J. and Greenwald (2010) "A hell of a life": addiction and marginality in post-industrial Detroit', *Social and Cultural Geography*, 11: 663–80.

Duff, C. (2010) 'Enabling places and enabling resources', *Drug and Alcohol Review*, 29: 337–44.

ECAS (2002) *European Comparative Alcohol Study 1998–2001*. Brussels: European Union.

ESPAD (2004) *European Schools Project on Alcohol and Drugs 1995–2003*. Brussels: European Union.

Edensor, T. (2006) 'Caudan: domesticating the global waterfront', In D. Bell and M. Jayne (eds.), *Small Cities: Urban Experience beyond the Metropolis*. London: Routledge, pp. 205–16.

Fennell, M. L, Rodin, M. B. and Kantor, G. K. (1981) 'Problems in work setting, drinking and reasons for drinking', *Social Forces*, 60(1): 114–32.

Field, K. and Beale, L. (2004) 'Using GIS to model incidence, prevalence and spread of non-legal drug use', *Transactions in GIS*, 8: 423–9.

Fitzgerald, J., Dovey, K. and Dieteze, P. (2004) 'Health outcomes and quasi-supervised settings for street injecting drug use', *International Journal of Drug Policy*, 15: 247–57.

Gofton, L. (1990) 'On the town: drink and the "new" lawlessness' *Youth and Policy*, 29: 33–9.

Gough, B. and Edwards, G. (1998) 'The beer talking: four lads, a carry out and the reproduction of masculinities', *Sociological Review*, 46(3): 409–435.

Grieshaber-Otto, J., Sinclair, S. and Schacter, N. (2000) 'Impacts of international trade, services and investment treaties on alcohol regulation', *Addiction*, 95(4): S491–S504.

Hadfield, P. (2006) *Bar Wars: Contesting the Night in Contemporary British Cities*. Oxford: Oxford University Press.

Hall, T. (1992) *The Postmodern Pub, Hegemonic Narrative, Nostalgia and Collective Identity in the Construction of Postmodern Landscapes: A Problem for Research*. Discussion paper. Birmingham: Department of Geography, University of Birmingham.

Harrison, L. (ed.) (1996) *Alcohol Problems in the Community*. London: Routledge.

Harnett, R., Thom, B., Herring, R. and Kelly, M. (2000), 'Alcohol in transition: towards a model of young men's drinking styles'. *Journal of Youth Studies*, 3(1): 61–77.

Harvey, D. (1974) 'What kind of geography for what kind of public policy?' *Transactions of the Institute of British Geographers*, 63: 18–24.

Heley, J. (2008), 'Rounds, Range Rovers and rurality: the drinking geographies of a new squirarchy', *Drugs: Education, Prevention and Policy* 15(3): 315–21.

Hembree, C. (2005) 'The urban built environment and overdose mortality in New York City neighbourhoods', *Health and Place*, 11: 147–156

Herrick, C. (2012) 'The political ecology of alcohol as disaster in South Africa's Western Cape'. *Geoforum*, 43(6): 1045–56.

Herrick, C. and Charman, C. (2013) 'Shebeens and crime: the multiple criminalities of South African liquor and its regulation', *South African Crime Quarterly*, 45: 25–33.

Holloway, S. L., Jayne, M. and Valentine, G. (2008) '"Sainsbury's is my local": English alcohol policy, domestic drinking practices and the meaning of home', *Transactions of the Institute of British Geographers*, 33: 532–47.

Holloway, S. L., Jayne, M. and Valentine, G. (2009) 'Masculinities, femininities and the geographies of public and private drinking landscapes', *Geoforum*, 40(5): 821–31.

Hobbs, D., Hadfield, P., Lister, S. and Winslow, S. (2003) *Bouncers: Violence and Governance in the Night-time Economy*. Oxford: Oxford University Press.

Holder, H. D. (2000) 'The supply side initiative as an international collaboration to study alcohol supply, drinking and consequences: current knowledge, policy issues and research opportunities', *Addiction*, 95(4): S416–63.

Howell, P. and Beckingham, D. (2015) 'Time geography, gentleman please: chronotypes of publand in Patrick Hamilton's London Trilogy', *Social and Cultural Geography*, 16(8): 931–49.

Hubbard, P. (2005) 'The geographies of "going out": emotion and embodiment in the evening economy', In J. Davidson, L. Bondi and M. Smith (eds.), *Emotional Geographies*. Aldershot: Ashgate, pp. 117–34

Hunt, G. and Satterlee, S. (1986) 'The pub, the village and the people', *Human Organisation*, 54(1): 62–74.

Hunt, G. and Satterlee, S. (1987) 'Darts, drink and the pub: the culture of female drinking', *Sociological Review*, 35: 575–601.

Hunt, G. (1991) 'The middle class revisited: eating and drinking in an English village', *Western Folklore*, 50: 401–20.

Jayne, M. and Valentine, G (2015a) *Childhood, Families, Alcohol*. Aldershot: Ashgate.

Jayne, M. and Valentine, G. (2015b) '"It makes you go crazy": children's knowledge and experience of alcohol consumption', *Journal of Consumer Culture*: doi: 10.1177/1469540515574450.

Jayne, M. and Valentine, G. (2016) 'Alcohol-related violence and disorder: new critical perspectives', *Progress in Human Geography*, 40(1): 67–87.

Jayne, M., Holloway, S. and Valentine, G. (2006) 'Drunk and disorderly: alcohol, urban life and public space' *Progress in Human Geography*, 30(4): 451–88.

Jayne, M., Valentine, G. and Gould, M. (2012a) 'Family life and alcohol consumption: the transmission of "public" and "private" drinking cultures', *Drugs: Education, Prevention and Policy*, 19(3): 192–200.

Jayne, M., Valentine, G. and Holloway, S. L. (2008a) 'Geographies of alcohol, drinking and drunkenness: a review of progress' *Progress in Human Geography*, 32(2): 243–59.

Jayne, M. Valentine, G and Holloway, S. L. (2008b) 'Fluid boundaries—British binge drinking and european civility: alcohol and the production and consumption of public space', *Space and Polity*. 12(1): 81–100.

Jayne, M., Valentine, G. and Holloway, S. L. (2010) 'Emotional, embodied and affective geographies of alcohol, drinking and drunkenness', *Transactions of the Institute of British Geographers,* 35(4): 540–54.

Jayne, M., Valentine, G. and Holloway, S. L. (2011a) *Alcohol, Drinking, Drunkenness: (Dis)Orderly Spaces.* Aldershot: Ashgate.

Jayne, M., Valentine, G. and Holloway, S. L. (2011b) 'What use are units? Critical geographies of alcohol policy', *Antipode,* 44(3): 828–46.

Jayne, M., Gibson, C., Waitt, G. and Valentine, G. (2012) 'Drunken mobilties: backpackers, alcohol, "doing place"', *Tourist Studies*, 12(3): 211–31.

Kneale, J. (2001) 'The place of drink: temperance and the public, 1956–1914', *Social and Cultural Geography*, 2(1): 43–59.

Kraack, A. and Kenway, J. (2002) 'Place, time and stigmatised youthful identities: bad boys in paradise', *Journal of Rural Studies* 18, 145–55.

Kubicka, L., Csemy, L., Duplinsky, J. and Kozeny, J. (1998) 'Czech men's drinking in changing political climates 1983-93: a three-wave longitudinal study', *Addiction*, 93(8): 1219–30.

Lagendijk, A. (2003) 'Global "lifeworlds" versus local "systemworlds": how flying winemakers produce global wines in interconnected locales', *Tijdschift Voor Economische en Sociale Geographie*, 95(5): 511–26.

Latham, A. (2003) 'Urbanity, lifestyle and making sense of the new urban cultural economy: notes from Auckland, New Zealand', *Urban Studies*, 40(9): 1699–724.

Latham, A. and McCormack, D. P. (2004) 'Moving cities: rethinking the materialities of urban geographies', *Progress in Human Geography,* 28(6): 701–24.

Leyshon, M. (2005) 'No place for a girl: rural youth pubs and the performance of masculinity', In J. Little and C. Morris (eds.), *Critical Studies in Rural Gender Issues*. Aldershot: Ashgate, pp. 104–22.

Leyshon, M. (2008) '"We're stuck in the corner": young women, embodiment and drinking in the countryside', *Drugs: Education, Prevention and Policy* 15(3): 267–89.

Levi, R. and Valverde, M. (2001) 'Knowledge on tap: police science and common knowledge in the legal regulation of drunkenness', *Law and Social Inquiry*, 21(3): 819–46.

Lindsay, J. (2005) *Drinking in Melbourne Pubs and Clubs: A Study of Alcohol Consumption Contexts*. Melbourne: Monash University.

Love, M. N, Wilton, R. and DeVerteuil, G. (2012) '"You have to make a new way of life": woman's drug treatment programmes in therapeutic landscapes in Canada', *Gender, Place and Culture,* 19(3): 382–96.

Lowe, G., Foxcroft, D. R. and Sibley, D. (1993) *Adolescent Drinking and Family Life*. London: Harwood Academic Publishers.

Mason, M., Cheung, I. and Walker, L. (2004) 'Substance use, social networks and the geography of urban adolescents', *Substance Use and Misuse*, 39: 1751–77.

Martin, R. (2001), 'Geography and public policy: the case of the missing agenda', *Progress in Human Geography*, 25: 189–210.

Massey, D. (1991) 'A global sense of place', *Marxism Today*, June: 24–9.

Massey, D. (1995) *Spatial Divisions of Labour: Social Structures and the Geography of Production*, 2nd edn. New York: Routledge.

Massey, D. (2005) *For Space*. London: Sage.

Maye, D., libery, B. and Kneafsy, M. (2005) 'Changing places: investigating the cultural terrain of village pubs in south Northamptonshire', *Social and Cultural Geography,* 6(6): 831–47.

McCormack, D. (2003) 'An event of geographical ethics in spaces of affect', *Transactions of the Institute of British Geographers*, 28(4): 488–507.

McCann, E. J. (2008) 'Expertise, truth, and urban policy mobilities: global circuits of knowledge in the development of Vancouver, Canada's 'Four Pillar' drug strategy', *Environment and Planning A,* 40(4): 885–904.

McCann, E. (2011) 'Points of reference: knowledge of elsewhere in the politics of urban drug policy', In E. McCann and K. Ward (eds), *Mobile Urbanism: Cities and Policy-making in the Global Age*. Minneapolis: University of Minnesota Press, pp. 97–122.

McGovern, M. (2002), 'The 'criac' market': Irish theme bars and the commodification of

Irishness in contemporary Britain', *Irish Journal of Sociology,* 11(2): 77–98.

McShane, A. and Kneale, J. (2011) 'Histories and geographies of intoxicants and intoxication: an introduction', *Social History of Alcohol and Drugs*, 25: 6–14.

Moreno, C. (2009) 'Body politics and spaces of addiction in Daren Aronofsky's Requiem for a Dream', *Geojournal*, 74: 219–26.

Nayak, A. (2003) "Last of the 'real Geordies'? White masculinities and the subcultrual response to deindustrialisation', *Environment and planning D: Society and Space*, 21: 7–25.

O'Malley, P. and Valverde, M. (2004) 'Pleasure, freedom and drugs: the use of "pleasure" in liberal governance of drugs and alcohol consumption', *Sociology,* 38(1): 25–42.

Philo, C., Parr, H. and Burns, N. (2002), *Alcohol and Mental Health* (draft), published by the Department of Geography and Topographical Science, University of Glasgow at: http://www.geog.gla.ac.uk/olpapers/cphilo015.pdf.

Plant, M. (1997) *Women and Alcohol: Contemporary and Historical Perspectives*. London: Free Association Books.

Plant, M. and Plant, M. (2006) *Binge Britain: Alcohol and the National Response*. Oxford: Oxford University Press.

Peck, J. (1999) 'Grey geography?', *Transactions of the Institute of British Geographers,* 24: 131–6.

Punch, M. (2005) 'Problem drug use and the political economy of urban restructuring: heroin class and governance in Dublin', *Antipode,* 37: 754–74.

Purvis, M. (1998) 'Popular institutions', In J. Langton and R. J. Morris (eds.), *Atlas of Industrial Britain 1780–1914*. London: Methuen, pp. 34–42.

Ramsey, M. (1990) *Lagerland Lost? An Experiment in Keeping Drinkers off the Streets in Central Coventry and Elsewhere*. Crime prevention Unit: paper 22. London: Home Office.

Rhones, T. (2007) 'Risk, shame and the public injector: a qualitative study of drug injecting in South Wales', *Social Science and Medicine*, 65: 572–85.

Robbins, C. A. and Martin, S. S. (1993) 'Gender, styles of deviance and drinking problems', *Journal of Health and Social Behaviour,* 34(4): 302–21.

Robertson, L. (2007) 'Taming space: drug use, HIV and homemaking in downtown eastside Vancouver', *Gender, Place and Culture*, 14: 527–49.

Room, R. and Jernigan, D. (2000) 'The ambiguous role of alcohol in economic and social development', *Addiction*, 95(4): S523–35.

Royal Geographic Society (with Institute of British Geographers (2010) *Consumption Controversies: Alcohol Policies in the UK*. London: RGS. Available at: http://www.rgs.org/NR/rdonlyres/88DF6837-E68B-4301-9376-B30E0FA72F21/0/RGSPolicyAlcohol5c_AWSingle.pdf.

Seeman, M., Seeman, A. Z. and Burdos, A. (1988) 'Powerlessness, work and community: a longtitudinal study of alienation and alcohol use', *Journal of Health and Social Behaviour*, 29(3): 185–98.

Shaikh, Z. and Nax, F. (2000) *A Cultural Cocktail: Asian Women and Alcohol Misuse*. Warks: Aldgate Press.

Shaw, R. (2010) 'Neoliberal Subjectivities and the Development of the Night-Time Economy in British Cities', *Geography Compass*, 4: 893–903.

Shaw, R. (2014) 'Beyond night-time economy: affective atmospheres of the urban night', *Geoforum*, 51:87–95.

Shaw, R. (2015) '"Alive after five": constructing the neoliberal night in Newcastle-upon-Tyne', *Urban Studies*, 52(3): 456–70.

Smart, R. G. and Ogborne, A. (2000) 'Drinking and heavy drinking by students in 18 countries', *Drug and Alcohol Dependence*, 60: 315–18.

Stahler G. (2007) 'The effect of individual, programme, and neighbourhood watch variables on continuity and treatment among dually diagnosed individuals', *Drug and Alcohol Dependence,* 87: 54–62.

Thomas, C. J. and Bromley, R. D. F. (2000), 'City-centre revitalization: problems of fragmentation and fear in the evening and night-time city', *Urban Studies*, 37(8): 1403–29.

Thomas, M. (2002) 'Out of control: emergent cultural landscapes and political change in urban Vietnam', *Urban Studies*, 39(9): 1611–24.

Thrift, N. (2004) 'Intensities of feeling: towards a spatial politics of affect'. *Geografiska Annaler Series B Human Geography*, 86B(1): 57–78.

Thrift, N. (2009) 'Space: the fundamental stuff of geography', In N. Clifford, S. L. Holloway, S. P. Rice and G. Valentine (eds), *Key Concepts in Human Geography*. Sage: London, pp. 95–107.

Twigg, L. and Jones, K. (2000) 'Predicting small-area health related behaviour: a comparison of smoking and drinking indicators', *Social Science and Medicine*, 80(11): 9–20.

Twigg, L, Moon, G., Duncan, G. and Jones, K. (2002) 'Consumed with worry: 'unsafe' alcohol consumption and self-reported drinking in England', *Health Education Research*, 15(5): 569–80.

Unwin, T. (1991) *Wine and the Vine: An Historical Geography of Viticulture and the Wine Trade*. London: Routledge.

Valentine, G., Jayne, M. and Gould, M. (2011) 'Do as I say, not as I do: the affective space of family life and the transmission of drinking cultures', *Environment and Planning A*, 44(1): 776–92.

Valentine, G., Jayne, M. and Gould, M. (2014) 'The proximity effect: the role of the affective space of family life in shaping children's knowledge about alcohol and its social and health implications', *Childhood: A Journal of Global Child Research*, 21(1): 103–18.

Valentine, G, Jayne M. and Holloway, S. (2009) 'Contemporary cultures of abstinence and the night-time economy: Muslim attitudes towards alcohol and the implications for social cohesion', *Environment and Planning A*, 42(1): 8–22.

Valentine, G, Jayne, M. and Holloway, S. L. (2010a) 'Generational patterns of alcohol consumption: continuity and change', *Health and Place*, 16: 916–25.

Valentine, G., Jayne, M., Gould, M. and Keenan, J. (2010b) *Family Life and Alcohol Consumption: The Transmission of Drinking Cultures*. York: Joseph Rowntree Foundation.

Valentine, G., Holloway, S. L., Jayne, M. and Knell, C. (2008) *Drinking Places: Where People Drink and Why*. York: Joseph Rowntree Foundation.

Valentine, G., Holloway, S. L., Knell, C. and Jayne, M. (2007) 'Drinking places: young people and cultures of alcohol consumption in rural environments', *Journal of Rural Studies*, 24: 28–40.

Valverde, M. (2003) 'Police science, British style: pub licensing and knowledges of urban disorder', *Economy and Society*, 32(2): 234–52.

Waitt, G., Jessop, A. and Gormely-Murray, A. (2011) '"The guys in there just expect to be laid?": embodied and gendered socio-spatial practices of a "night out" in Wollongong, Australia', *Gender, Place and Culture*, 18(2): 255–75.

Ward, K. (2005) 'Geography and public policy: a recent history of "policy relevance"', *Progress in Human Geography*, 29(3): 310–19.

Waterson, J. (2000) *Women and Alcohol in Social Context: Mothers Ruin Revisited*. London: Palgrave.

Wilton R., DeVerteuil, G. and Evans, J. (2014) '"No more macho bullshit" drug treatment, place and the reworking of masculinity', *Transactions of the Institute of British Geographers*, 39(2): 291–303

Wilton, R. and DeVerteuil, G. (2006) 'Spaces of sobriety/sites of power', *Social Science and Medicine*, 63: 649–61.

Wilton, R. and Moreno, C. M. (2012) 'Critical geographies of drugs and alcohol', *Social and Cultural Geography*, 13(2): 99–108.

Winlow, S. and Hall, S. (2006) *Violent Night: Urban Leisure and Contemporary Culture*. Oxford: Berg.

Wittman, F. D. (1997) 'Local control to prevent problems of alcohol availability; experience in Californian communities', In M. Plant, E. Single and T. Stockwell (eds), *Alcohol: Minimizing the Harm*. London: Free Association Books, pp. 43–71.

World Health Organization (2000) *International Guide for Monitoring Alcohol Consumption and Related Alcohol Harm*. Stockholm: World Health Organisation.

World Health Organization (2001) *Alcohol in the European Region – Consumption, Harm and Policies*. Stockholm: World Health Organisation.

World Health Organization (2004) *Global Status Report: Alcohol Policy*. Stockholm: World Health Organisation.

Wylie, J., Shah, L. and Jolly, A. (2007) 'Incorporating geographic settings into a social network analysis of injecting drug users and bloodborne pathogen prevalence', *Health and Place*, 13: 617–28.

PART II

Pillars in Social Science Drug and Alcohol Studies

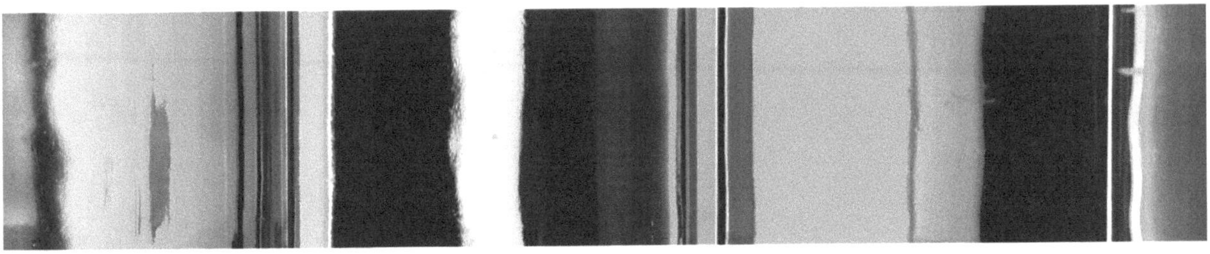

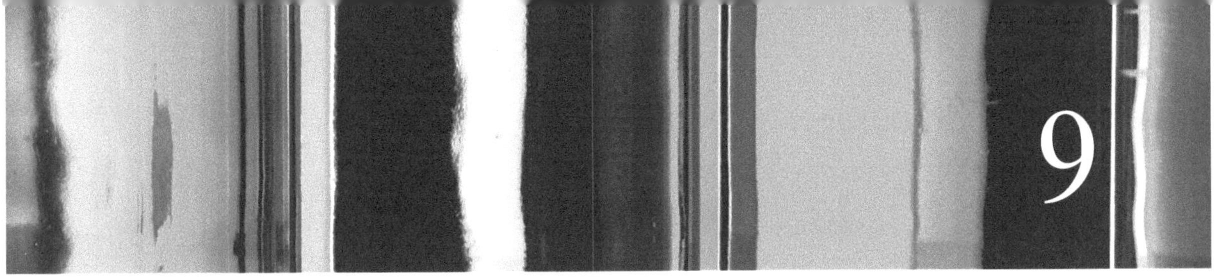

Drug Policy

Alison Ritter, Caitlin Hughes
and Phillip Hull

INTRODUCTION

Illicit drug policy is at a time of flux. The last few years have seen the first legally regulated cannabis markets in the United States (Pardo, 2014; Room, 2014). There has been an increasing concern about the rise of new synthetic drugs – commonly referred to as new psychoactive substances (NPS) – drugs that mimic the effects and/or chemical structure of illicit psychoactive drugs such as cannabis and ecstasy (Griffiths et al., 2013). There is concern that new technologies (such as the internet) are profoundly changing drug markets and the ways in which drugs are purchased and consumed (Barratt and Lenton, 2013). Misuse of legal drugs, especially pharmaceutical opioids, is a rising issue (Executive Office of the President of the United States, 2014b; United Nations Office on Drugs and Crime, 2014). Finally, at the time of writing, UNGASS 2016 (the United Nations General Assembly 2016) is approaching: a meeting involving all UN member states that has been explicitly brought forward following the pleas from the Presidents of Mexico, Colombia and Guatemala that the UN facilitate a real dialogue on alternative approaches to the global drug problem. Given the plea was supported by 95 other member states, this is seen by many as a potential tipping point for reform of the UN Conventions and/or to re-frame drug policy debates (Fordham and Tinasti, 2014).

In this chapter we capitalise on this rich period in drug policy to:

- Trace the historical development of the regulation of drugs
- Analyse the varieties of domestic drug policy today – in terms of (i) national drug strategies (goals, pillars and strategy comprehensiveness); (ii) drug laws; and (iii) security, human rights, welfare and development
- Discuss analytic tools for studying drug policy

We chose nine countries as case examples across these issues: Australia, Colombia, New Zealand, Nigeria, Portugal, Sweden, the USA, the United Kingdom (UK) and Vietnam.

INTERNATIONAL DRUG CONVENTIONS

At its inception the international drug control regime can be traced back to the eighteenth century opium wars and subsequent signing of the 1912 Hague Convention, limiting trade in opium (Babor et al., 2010). However, contemporary international drug control centres around the adoption of three United Nations treaties: the 1961 Single Convention on Narcotic Drugs, as amended by its 1972 protocol; the 1971 Convention on Psychotropic Substances; and the 1988 Convention Against the Illicit Traffic in Narcotic Drugs and Psychotropic Substances. The first convention prohibited the production and use of narcotic drugs – defined as cannabis, opioids and cocaine – except for medical and scientific purposes (United Nations, 1961). The second convention extended this approach to synthetic pharmaceutical drugs, such as amphetamine-type stimulants and benzodiazepines, and the chemical precursors used to manufacture these agents (United Nations, 1971). The 1988 Convention increased controls surrounding drug trafficking and money laundering. It also explicitly required member states to prohibit as criminal offences the production, manufacturing, sale and 'possession or purchase of any narcotic drug or psychoactive substance' for non-medical and non-scientific purposes (United Nations, 1988).

The main aim of the international drug control system was to reduce illicit use and supply. This cemented two pillars or approaches: supply reduction and demand reduction (Babor et al., 2010). The role of harm reduction was largely ignored (Room, 2012).

The treaties are overseen by a number of bodies (Room, 2012). These include the Commission on Narcotics Drugs (CND) – comprising representatives of all member states – which meets every year in Vienna to negotiate, adopt resolutions and approve the budget for the UN system (Commission on Narcotic Drugs, 2014); the United Nations Office on Drugs and Crime (UNODC), which serves as a secretariat to the CND, collates international data on drug use patterns via the World Drug Report (e.g. United Nations Office on Drugs and Crime, 2014) and provides advice on effectiveness of treatment and law enforcement responses; and the International Narcotics Control Board (INCB), which oversees operation of the treaties and operates as the guardian of treaty compliance (e.g. International Narcotics Control Board, 2014a), 'challenging any policy or activity that does not correspond with what it perceives as the original vision of the control system' (Bewley-Taylor and Trace, 2006: 1). A fourth body – the World Health Organization (WHO) – plays a technical role providing medical and scientific advice on which drugs should be included, and in which schedules, and international guidelines and protocols for health responses (World Health Organization, 2012).

Given that the treaties form the basis for domestic drug policy, the member states, NGOs and advocacy bodies have often expressed frustration over the limited 'room to manoeuvre' afforded to member states (Bewley-Taylor and Trace, 2006: 1). This is particularly with regard to the laws that must be applied and the lack of support for measures to ameliorate harms from use (Room and Reuter, 2012). However, over the last decade there have been a number of important shifts, as exemplified by the UNODC, WHO and even the INCB, with a reducing emphasis on 'criminalisation' per se and an embracing of the need for a more public-health-oriented approach to drug policy. An early example was the 1988 UNGASS statement supporting demand reduction (Ghodse, 1999; United Nations General Assembly, 1998). More recently, in 2013, the UNODC Executive Director, Yury Fedotov, issued an important document highlighting UNODC support for depenalisation of illicit drug possession, the rebalancing of efforts – and funding – away from law enforcement and into health, the valuing of harm reduction and evidence-based treatment and for ensuring that drug responses are 'in line with human rights standards' (United Nations Office on Drugs and Crime, 2013). Moreover, in July 2014, the WHO gave express support for the decriminalisation of illicit drug use and access to harm reduction services including needle syringe programmes, opioid substitution treatment and naloxone (for people who use drugs) (World Health Organization, 2014). Finally, in July 2014, INCB President, Lochan Nadioo, noted that drug use is essentially a health problem and that HIV/AIDS prevention programmes and drug treatment are part of a comprehensive approach (International Narcotics Control Board, 2014b). Hence, 50 years after the adoption of the international drug policy regime there are a number of signs of change. That said, drug policy, at least at the highest level, remains highly supply focussed and narrow in its perspective. As will be shown, this differs to how many domestic drug policies are considering issues today.

DESCRIBING DRUG POLICY REGIMES IN THE TWENTY-FIRST CENTURY

There is no agreed or internationally recognised way of describing or categorising national drug policies. Here, we consider multiple aspects or frameworks for understanding drug policy regimes: a nation's overarching drug strategy (including the goals, pillars and strategy comprehensiveness); a nation's drug laws; the social welfare arrangements; security and governance; and development and human rights approaches (see Table 9.1). Any one of these frameworks in isolation will throw light on a nation's drug policies, but a comprehensive approach requires consideration across all aspects. This is shown in the recently published 'Governance of Addictions' (Ysa et al., 2014), an explanatory framework for drug policy that comprises state factors, such as welfare regime and well-being indicators, along with policy factors, which include the structures for addiction policy as well as the

Table 9.1 Frameworks for describing drug policy regimes

Type	*Definition*
Overarching drug strategy (goals, "pillars", and strategy comprehensiveness)	What is the central purpose of the drug strategy? e.g. zero tolerance versus to reducing harms What are the key areas of drug policy response? e.g. prevention, treatment, harm reduction, supply reduction How comprehensive is the approach? e.g. does it include only illicit drugs or both illicit and licit drugs?
Drug laws	What is the criminal status for drug use, and drug supply offences? Eg criminalisation, depenalisation, legalisation How is this applied/implemented? e.g. court precedent, police, prosecutorial and judicial discretion, availability of non-criminal sanctions
Social welfare	What is the level of welfare support provided in a nation? e.g. unemployment benefits What specific social welfare policies are afforded for illicit drug users?
Security and governance	What is the extent of political stability, democracy and good governance? e.g. level of corruption (especially of government, police and courts), transparency and accountability, and implicit acceptance of illicit economic activities, including drug trafficking and other commodities
Development	To what extent is drug policy implemented in a developmental perspective? e.g. what is the economic growth, GDP, and income distribution of the nation and what avenues for income generation exist outside the drug trade?
Human rights	To what extent is drug policy implemented in a human rights framework? e.g. do laws infringe the human rights of people who use drugs including rights to life, to privacy, to health and to avoid discrimination?

types of drug strategies. In this sense, the governance of addiction approach taken by Ysa et al. (2014) conforms to consideration of factors beyond just drug policy itself.

National drug policies have traditionally been compared in terms of their overarching goals and central pillars for action or control. These are important indicators of drug policy as they represent the formal policies, and thus, their implementation (MacCoun and Reuter, 2001, 2002; Ritter and Lancaster, 2013). One common framework is the three pillars: supply reduction, demand reduction and harm reduction. Supply reduction is concerned with controlling and eliminating the production, traffic and distribution of illicit drugs. Demand reduction is focussed on preventing the uptake of drug use, or through providing effective treatments that reduce use in existing consumers. Harm reduction, the third pillar, is concerned less with controlling supply or demand, but reducing the harmful consequences of drug use to users and society (Ritter and Lancaster, 2013). It can be useful to examine the extent to which these pillars form part of a nation's drug policy and the relative balance between the pillars (Ritter, 2010). However, the three pillars approach has been critiqued as insufficient, with five rather than three possible categories: domestic law enforcement, international supply-side reduction, treatment, prevention and harm reduction (Kilmer et al., 2012). Furthermore, the categories can conflate law enforcement with supply reduction (for example, tighter regulation of medicines is not law enforcement) and, as we will see, most national policies have additional or variant categories. Finally, as noted earlier, the three pillars as a foundation for a nation's drug policies appear to contradict the international treaties that focus on supply reduction and demand reduction but exclude harm reduction.

Two other traditional ways of thinking about nations in relation to drug policy are first, the extent to which a country is classified as a producer/manufacturer, consumer or transit country (United Nations Office on Drugs and Crime, 2009: 35). Second, the ways in which drug laws are classified – how a country's laws define and respond to drug use and drug supply and related offences (MacCoun and Reuter, 2001; Rolles, 2009). The distinctions between producer, transit and consumer countries is increasingly unhelpful, as will be seen with reference to the nine countries analysed here. Drug laws have been compared in terms of the extent to which they criminalise drug possession and drug supply, or 'decriminalise' or 'legalise' such activities (MacCoun and Reuter, 2001; Rolles, 2009; Rosmarin, 2013); however, other aspects of drug laws, including penalty regimes, legal quantity thresholds and rights afforded to the accused are also central to a country's response to drug use and drug supply. Drug laws impact on the extent of social, economic and health harms associated with drug use (Babor et al., 2010) and are thus central instruments in drug policy and drug harm. Beyond the laws or statutes themselves, there are other important factors that can affect how laws are enforced and implemented (including sentencing guidelines, court precedent, ministerial/political directives and priorities, police, prosecutorial and judicial discretion, policing practice and other appointed regulations and regulators that operate outside of the criminal justice system). In analysing and comparing drug laws the devil is in the detail – as Pacula and colleagues (Pacula et al., 2015) show – for example, medicinal cannabis laws may appear the same in the statutes (particularly when conceptualised as a binary construct that is either present or absent), but vary greatly in their design and implementation, and hence, impacts.

Social welfare is inextricably linked to drug policy. Stevens has shown that there is a statistically significant negative correlation between the prevalence of injecting drug use and the level of welfare support – based on unemployment benefits, sickness pay and the levels of pensions (Stevens, 2011). Those countries that provide the lowest levels of welfare support tend to have higher rates of injecting drug use. This suggests that welfare policy is a crucial element of an effective approach to reducing problematic drug use and the harms that are associated with it. Furthermore, Stevens (2011) argues that drug policy per se may only have a weak influence on drug use and related harms – policies concerned with inequality, welfare and sentencing law may be much more influential. Hence, drug policy analysis needs to adopt a lens beyond drug strategy and drug laws and consider social welfare policies.

In the last decade it has become clear that issues of development, governance and human rights can have critical impacts on both the likelihood and shape of drug problems and effectiveness of drug policies. For example, there is a complex interrelationship between illicit drug use/drug markets and political, social and economic development of a nation/region, particularly in relation to sites of production and transit. The issue of human rights is also integral to drug policy (Barrett, 2010; Barrett and Nowak, 2010). The Universal Declaration of Human Rights, to which all member states have signed, enshrines the rights to life, to privacy, to avoid cruel, inhumane or degrading treatment or punishment, to be presumed innocent, to proportionate sanction, to avoid arbitrary arrest, to avoid discrimination and to vote (United Nations General Assembly, 1948). Other conventions explicitly include rights to health (e.g. United Nations General Assembly, 1966). Many of these rights are constrained by current international and domestic drug policies and it is increasingly clear that this reduces the effectiveness of drug policy (Barrett, 2010; Barrett and Nowak, 2010). For example, stigma reduces the likelihood of accessing drug treatment services and a criminal record impedes community integration through barriers to employment. The extent and means by which nations identify and ameliorate human rights infringements that are inherent in drug laws, and in approaches to drug treatment, is thus another way of understanding and describing drug policies.

In summary, none of the frameworks, whether overarching drug strategy goals, drug laws, social welfare or security, development and human rights, comes as an uncomplicated way of describing and analysing drug policies. Each of these approaches can make a unique contribution to understanding any one nation's drug policies, but drawing together multiple approaches will afford a more nuanced and full picture, something we demonstrate by application to our nine countries.

THE VARIETY OF DRUG POLICIES: FROM AUSTRALIA TO VIETNAM

We apply these descriptive frameworks (from Table 9.1) to analyse drug policy in nine nations: Australia, Colombia, New Zealand, Nigeria, Portugal, Sweden, the USA, the UK and Vietnam. The prevalence rates of illicit drug use vary considerably between these countries and between drug classes. The countries with the highest rates of annual use (as recorded by the World Drug Report, 2014) are Australia, the USA, New Zealand and the UK, possibly with the inclusion of Nigeria (United Nations Office on Drugs and Crime, 2014). The countries with the lowest prevalence of annual use are Portugal, Sweden, Colombia and Vietnam (United Nations Office on Drugs and Crime, 2014). (The data are provided in Appendix 1 to this chapter.) The rate of blood borne viruses (HIV and HCV) also vary substantially between countries (United Nations Office on Drugs and Crime, 2014) with Vietnam and Portugal having the highest HIV rates and New Zealand, Australia and the UK the lowest amongst the nine countries. Thus, there is not an automatic association between rates of use and rates of harm. Some countries have high consumption rates and high harm (e.g. the USA); others have high consumption but low rates of drug-related harm (e.g. Australia and New Zealand); and still others have low consumption but high rates of drug-related harms (e.g. Vietnam and Sweden).

These nine countries also differ in terms of whether they are regarded as producer/manufacturer, consumer or transit countries. Australia, New Zealand, Sweden, the UK and the USA are each regarded as consumer countries. Colombia and Nigeria are regarded as manufacture or producer countries and Vietnam, Nigeria and Portugal are considered as transit countries. Rates of drug use (United Nations Office on Drugs and Crime, 2014) are generally lower in most producer/transit countries, providing at least some face validity for the distinction between producer and consumer nations. However, like any simplified categorisation system, such distinctions may obscure relevant complexity, and/or the effects of change over time. As the Global Commission on Drugs has pointed out 'the distinction [between producer, consumer and transit countries] is increasingly blurred, as many countries now experience elements of all three' (Global Commission on Drug Policy, 2011: 8). Nigeria, for example, has been discussed as a transit country for heroin and cocaine (passing through to Europe) but Nigeria is also a high consumer nation and producer country, notably for cannabis (indeed rates of cannabis use are similar to the USA, Australia and New Zealand) (Obot, 2004; United Nations Office on Drugs and Crime, 2014; West Africa Commission on Drugs, 2014). Nations such as Australia and the USA, while traditionally high consumer nations, also have increasing levels of domestic production particularly of cannabis and methamphetamine (Central Intelligence Agency, 2014; Ritter et al., 2011). Added to this is the emergence of the global drug trade through the internet which enables drug production and transit in any part of the world (Griffiths et al., 2013). All such factors mean that the traditional distinction between producer and consumer countries affords significantly less explanatory power.

OVERARCHING DRUG STRATEGY (GOALS, PILLARS AND COMPREHENSIVENESS)

National drug policy goals across the nine countries range from a drug free society (Sweden and Vietnam) to reducing harms and negative health, social and economic consequences from drug use (Australia and New Zealand) as summarised in Table 9.2. Core principles also differ. Of note, Portugal has placed a strong emphasis upon humanism and pragmatism; factors that have fostered an emphasis on human rights and drug decriminalisation (see later).

Supply reduction dominates across all countries. For example, Colombian drug policy has had a strong focus on the control of production and trafficking in coca and cocaine, and also heroin (Meija, 2015; Quintero, 2012; Thoumi, 2012). Supply control efforts have focused, under Plan Colombia and the National Consolidation Plan (Integrated Network for Societal Conflict Research, 2012) on herbicidal crop eradication and militarised policing of cocaine and heroin production and trafficking, coupled with alternative development, and more recently, a focus on reducing social marginalisation and increasing democratic security and economic development (see later sections) (Elhawary, 2010; Meija, 2015). Supply reduction across many countries appears to take the lion's share of drug budget expenditure. Notwithstanding the limits to comparability due to data gaps/methodological and conceptual differences (European Monitoring Centre for Drugs and Drug Addiction, 2008), we note that USA, Australia, UK, Colombia and Sweden have published estimates of the split in expenditure between the three pillars. In each case, supply reduction is the largest

Table 9.2 Nine country profile: drug policy objectives, strategic frameworks and pillars

Country	*Overall objective of drug policy*	*National strategic framework and key elements, pillars, components*
Australia	The Australia goal is: "to build safe and healthy communities by minimising alcohol, tobacco and other drug-related health, social and economic harms among individuals, families and communities." (Ministerial Council on Drug Strategy, 2011, p. ii)	National Drug Strategy 2010-2015: a framework for action on alcohol, tobacco and other drugs (Ministerial Council on Drug Strategy, 2011) Elements: Three pillars: Supply reduction; Demand reduction; Harm reduction.
Colombia	As expressed by Acevedo, the Colombian drug goal is: "Eliminating drug trafficking and promoting social and economic development" (Acevedo, Bewley-Taylor, & Youngers, 2008)	Focus on supply reduction (crop eradication and alternative development); democratic security; and economic development. (National Consolidation Plan (2009). National Policy for the Reduction of Psychoactive Substance Consumption and Its Impact (2007) emphasises need for prevention and treatment: reduce incidence, prevalence, and negative effects substance use on the individual, family, community, society (Ministry of Social Protection, 2007)
New Zealand	The New Zealand goal is to: "Prevent and reduce the health, social and economic harms that are linked to tobacco, alcohol, illegal and other drug use." (Ministerial Committee on Drug Policy, 2007, p. 4)	National Drug Policy 2007-2012. Elements: Supply control; Demand reduction; Problem limitation (Ministerial Committee on Drug Policy, 2007)
Nigeria	The vision/mission for Nigeria is: "…cutting off the supply of illicit drugs, reducing the demand for illicit drugs and other substances of abuse, tracing and recovering drug-related proceeds… for the total eradication of illicit trafficking in narcotic drugs and psychotropic substances; suppression of demand for illicit drugs and other substances of abuse; recovery of ill-gotten wealth, acquired from proceeds of illicit drug trade (National Drug Law Enforcement Agency, 2009)	National Drug Control Master Plan 2008-2011 (Inter Ministerial Committee on Drug Control, 2008) (extended to 2013). Elements: Control of illicit drug supply; drug demand reduction; adequacy and effectiveness of legal framework; control of licit drug supply (Inter Ministerial Committee on Drug Control, 2008, p. v)
Portugal	The vision for Portugal is: "To consolidate and build an integrated and effective public policy for addictive behaviours and dependencies based on inter-sectoral coordination, and sustainable improvements in health and social well-being" (Serviço de Intervenção nos Comportamentos Aditivos e nas Dependências, 2013). Eight principles guide the Portugese national plan on drugs: (i) international cooperation; (ii) prevention; (iii) the humanistic principle; (iv) pragmatism; (v) security; (vi) coordination and rationalisation of resources; (vii) subsidiarity; and (viii) participation. (European Monitoring Centre for Drugs and Drug Addiction, 2014)	National Plan for the Reduction of Addictive Behaviours and Dependencies 2013–2020; Strategic Plan 2013-2015 (available in Portuguese only). Elements: Supply reduction: reducing supply of illicit substances; regulation of licit substances; and harmonisation of legal frameworks. Demand reduction: prevention; dissuasion; treatment; harm and risk reduction; and social reintegration (Serviço de Intervenção nos Comportamentos Aditivos e nas Dependências, 2013).

(Continues)

Table 9.2 (Continued)

Country	*Overall objective of drug policy*	*National strategic framework and key elements, pillars, components*
Sweden	The Swedish national drug policy has as its goal: "A society free from illegal drugs and doping, with reduced alcohol-related medical and social harm, and reduced tobacco use." (Ministry of Health and Social Affairs, 2011)	National Action Plan on Drugs (2011–15) (ANDT). A Cohesive Strategy for Alcohol, Narcotic drugs, Doping and Tobacco (ANDT) Policy, covering the period between 2011 and 2015 (Ministry of Health and Social Affairs, 2011, p. 8) Elements: 1. Zero tolerance for illegal drugs and doping 2. Measures to reduce tobacco use, and prevent uptake 3. Prevention harmful consumption of alcohol (Ministry of Health and Social Affairs, 2011)
UK (England and Wales)	The UK Strategy gaols are: "Stopping people taking drugs in the first place and bearing down relentlessly on those involved in the drugs trade" (HM Government, 2010) Two overarching aims: "reduce illicit and other harmful drug use; and increase the numbers recovering from their dependence" (HM Government, 2010)	Drug Strategy 2010 "Reducing demand, restricting supply, building recovery": supporting people to live a drug free life (HM Government, 2010) Elements: Three themes: (i) reducing demand; (ii) restricting supply; and (iii) building recovery in communities
USA	The National Drug Control Strategy (2014) goals are to: 1. Curtail illicit drug consumption in America; 2. Improve the public health and public safety of the American people by reducing the consequences of drug abuse (Executive Office of the President of the United States, 2014b, p. 4).	National Drug Control Strategy 2014 (Executive Office of the President of the United States, 2014b) Elements: 1. Prevention 2. Early intervention 3. Treatment and expanded support for recovery 4. Breaking the cycle of drug use, crime, delinquency and incarceration 5. Disrupt domestic drug trafficking and production 6. Strengthen international partnerships and reduce the availability of foreign-produced drugs in the United States (Executive Office of the President of the United States, 2014b)
Vietnam	As described by Baldwin (2013), the objectives of the Vietnamese drug strategy are "1. To enhance the accountability of individuals, families and the broader society to prevent and eliminate drug use; and 2. to reduce the number of drug users by 30 to 40 percent with 70 percent of communes free of drug use" (Baldwin, 2013). From another source, the objectives of the strategy include: reduction in drug use (number of drug addicts); provision of treatment (to 100%), increase drug seizures; and strict control of legal trading in precursors, drugs and psychotropics. (National Committee on AIDS, No date) https://www.unodc.org/documents/southeastasiaandpacific//2012/05/ats-report-vietnam/Natl_Committee_on_Aids-ATS_prevention.pdf	Strategy on preventing, combating and controlling drug abuse in Vietnam till 2020 (signed 27 June, 2011 Decision No.1001/QD-TTg). "preventing and combating drug abuse must be closely combined with reduction in drug supply and demand as well as harm reduction" (National Committee on AIDS, No date) Elements: Six main tasks: 1. Public awareness 2. Strict control of all drug addicts 3. Regular surveys of plant cultivation 4. Control legal drug-related activities 5. Law enforcement (raids, border control) 6. International commitments (National Committee on AIDS, No date)

share of the drug policy expenditure: USA 59 per cent, federal only (Executive Office of the President of the United States, 2014a); Australia 66 per cent (Ritter et al., 2013); UK 65 per cent (European Monitoring Centre on Drugs and Drug Addiction, 2014, July 3); Sweden 75 per cent (Ramstedt, 2006); and Colombia 98 per cent (Gomez, 2013). The focus on supply reduction is consistent with the primary focus of the international treaties.

However, all countries examined here also have a focus on demand reduction. Notably those countries with a primary focus on supply reduction, such as Colombia and Nigeria, do not exclude demand reduction. In the case of Colombia, recent years have seen efforts to improve treatment and the introduction of nascent harm reduction initiatives. While the explicit drug policy goal in Nigeria is to cut off the supply of illicit drugs (Inter Ministerial Committee on Drug Control, 2008; Klantschnig, 2009), demand reduction is listed in the vision and mission, albeit minimally applied (Obot, 2004).

Unsurprisingly, those countries regarded as consumer countries have a primary focus on demand reduction. For example, in the USA, the 2014 National Drug Control Strategy focusses on prevention, early intervention, treatment and recovery support (not though to the exclusion of criminal justice, law enforcement and international cooperation; Executive Office of the President of the United States, 2014b). The latest USA drug strategy is explicitly linked to health care reform and the newly introduced Affordable Care Act, which now provides for substance use disorder treatment (Kilmer et al., 2012). It also aligns with the somewhat uniquely USA focus on addiction as a brain disease (Courtwright, 2010; Volkow, 2001). Despite the commonly-held view regarding America as championing the 'war on drugs' (Bertram et al., 1996; Caulkins et al., 2005), the current national strategy appears to align more closely with domestic issues, notably access to affordable treatment and the neuroscience agenda.

In the case of the UK, we also see a focus on demand reduction with supply reduction as the second listed goal (HM Government, 2008). The UK also demonstrates another trend in drug policy: a move towards 'recovery' (Duke, 2013). As the 2010 UK strategy explicitly states: 'a fundamental difference between this strategy and those that have gone before is that instead of focussing primarily on reducing the harms caused by drug misuse, our approach will be to…offer support for people choosing recovery' (HM Government, 2010: 2). In this way, demand reduction appears to have evolved from a focus on reducing harms to eliminating use. The USA national strategy also refers to recovery ('celebrate and support recovery from addiction'; page 23).

The USA strategy does not use the term 'harm reduction' (or refer to reducing harms). Likewise, the UK strategy does not use the term 'harm reduction'. Explicit mention of harm reduction within national goals and strategies is limited to Australia (Ministerial Council on Drug Strategy, 2011), New Zealand (Ministerial Committee on Drug Policy, 2007), Vietnam (Reid and Higgs, 2011) and Portugal (Serviço de Intervenção nos Comportamentos Aditivos e nas Dependências, 2013a). Harm reduction remains controversial. For example, in Vietnam, there are continued tensions in establishing harm reduction due to cultural factors, funding and policy goals of eliminating use (Baldwin and Thomson, 2013; Vuong et al., 2012; Windle, 2015). Investment in harm reduction programmes (national and international donor programmes) is substantially short of what is required (Cook et al., 2014).

Lastly, the countries vary in terms of strategy comprehensiveness: the inclusion of both licit and illicit drugs. Many national drug strategies now include alcohol (and sometimes tobacco) as is the case for Australia (Ministerial Council on Drug Strategy, 2011), Portugal (which also includes gambling) (Serviço de Intervenção nos Comportamentos

Aditivos e nas Dependências, 2013a), Sweden (Ministry of Health and Social Affairs, 2011), Nigeria (Inter Ministerial Committee on Drug Control, 2008) and New Zealand (Ministerial Committee on Drug Policy, 2007). In the UK drug strategy, alcohol is included in the scope (HM Government, 2010) but the strategies are focussed almost solely on illicit drugs (e.g. under restricting supply there is no mention of alcohol licensing laws, alcohol pricing or availability measures). Prescription drug abuse is now a prominent concern and it also blurs the boundary between legal and illegal drugs. For example, the USA drug strategy explicitly includes prescription drug abuse (Executive Office of the President of the United States, 2014b) with the drug control strategy referring to four pillars in this area: education, monitoring, disposal and enforcement. In Nigeria, a recent political announcement (July 2014) noted special attention to misuse of pharmaceutical medicines in the new national drug control plan (NAFDAC, 2014).

DRUG LAWS

Drug laws across the globe are set in the context of the three international conventions – which prohibit the use, sale and supply of illicit drugs. The nine case example countries are signatories to all three conventions. Some have made reservations to the treaties but most are minor, such as regarding powers of extradition from a member state (Vietnam – 1971, 1988; USA – 1988; Colombia – 1988; Sweden - 1988). A noted exception was the reservation of Colombia, which declared the requirement of the 1988 Convention to criminalise the cultivation of coca leaf 'discriminatory' and 'restrictive' and argued that this requirement 'must be harmonised with a policy of alternative development, taking into account the rights of indigenous communities involved' (United Nations, 2014). As of July 2014, 184 countries are signatories to the 1961 Convention, as amended, 183 to the 1971 Convention, and 189 to the 1988 Convention: many similarly with minor reservations. For a complete overview see Room (2012).

Here we look at domestic laws, distinguishing between laws on drug use (use, acquisition and possession for personal use) and laws on drug supply (importation, cultivation, manufacture, trafficking) (see Table 9.3). We also consider two aspects of their implementation: first, the likelihood that people who use drugs receive a criminal sanction; and second, the likelihood of traffickers being imprisoned. Despite all being signatories to the Conventions, there is substantial diversity in the drug laws (Table 9.3).

Clarification of terminology is essential in any such exercise. For our purposes, legalisation is defined as the complete removal of sanctions, making a certain behaviour legal and applying no criminal or administrative penalty; decriminalisation is defined as the removal of sanctions under the criminal law, with optional use of administrative sanctions (e.g. provision of civil fines or court-ordered therapeutic responses); and depenalisation is the decision in practice not to criminally penalise offenders, even though criminal sanctions are available, such as non-prosecution or non-arrest. One common depenalisation strategy involves the use of 'diversion' or 'drug courts'. Drug diversion involves the provision of a warning, caution, civil penalty or a referral to drug education and treatment often (but not always) instead of a criminal charge or sanction (Hughes and Ritter, 2008). A final issue of definition is 'de jure' versus 'de facto': that is whether countries change law (de jure) or change practice (de facto).

As outlined in Table 9.3, there have been a number of significant changes in recent years: most notably, the adoption of the first legal and regulated models for cannabis supply and use in Colorado and Washington (Pardo, 2014; Room, 2014) (Alaska, Oregon and Washington D.C. have since legalised use and/or supply, albeit regulatory models

Table 9.3 Nine country profile: statutes and laws on drug use and drug supply

Country	*Statutes/Acts*	*Law regarding drug use*	*Laws regarding drug supply*
Australia	Criminal Code Act 1995 (Cth) Each state/territory has its own drug laws. e.g. New South Wales: Drugs Misuse and Trafficking Act 1985 (NSW). Drugs and Poisons Legislation Amendment (New Psychoactive and Other Substances) Act 2013 (NSW).	Personal use and possession of cannabis decriminalised in some states. Other illicit drugs criminalised. Prison possible (2 years if imported; or < 2 years in most states) but rarely applied. Diversion and drug courts widespread. Hence main response: police diversion or fine. NPS: Criminal penalties apply. Often ineligible for diversion programs.	Illicit drugs: Cultivation of cannabis for personal use decriminalised in some states. Production and trafficking other drugs criminalised. Penalties: <21 yrs prison or life imprisonment. But alternatives to prison common for low level supply offences. NPS: Criminal penalties apply. Max of 2-5 years prison.
Colombia	Law 30 of 1986 (National Narcotics Statute/(Estatuto Nacional de Estupefacientes—ENE). Law 1566 (2012).	Drug use and possession of 'personal doses' was decriminalised in 1994 by the Constitutional Court. It was re-criminalised by the Ubide Government in 2009, but in 2012 the Constitutional Court again ruled it unconstitutional: effectively decriminalising it.	Production, cultivation, export and supply subject to criminal offences. Penalty: 1-3 years (minor); 4-12 years imprisonment (major) and 10 to 100 minimum monthly salary's fine.
New Zealand	Misuse of Drugs Act 1975. Class A drugs: cocaine, heroin, methamphetamine, LSD, magic mushrooms. Class B: ATS, ecstasy, cannabis oil. Class C: cannabis seeds/plants. Psychoactive Substances Act 2013.	Drug use and possession criminalised. Max penalty: 6 mths prison (class A) or 3 mths (class B/C). Long history of diversion. Drug courts since Nov 2012. NPS laws passed to make personal possession of approved NPS legal and possession of unapproved substances - a civil fine (no criminal conviction) of up to NZD 500. However system is not yet operational.	Production and supply criminalised. Max penalty: life imprisonment (class A) or 14 yrs (class B) or 8 yrs (class C). However, moderate rate of use of imprisonment: 36% and 54% imprisoned for dealing and importation respectively in 2013 (NZ Stats, 2014). 2013 act allows legal production and regulated sale of NPS provided trials conducted and classified low risk. As of July 2014 all NPS banned prior to approval.
Nigeria	Tribunal (Miscellaneous Offenses) Decree 1984 National Drug Law Enforcement Agency Act (1989)	Personal use and possession criminalised. Penalty: 15-25 years imprisonment. Forfeiture of assets and passports also possible. Corporal punishment for AOD use under Sharia law in some northern states. Diversion to treatment and social reintegration an option under law but rarely applied.	Import, cultivation and supply criminalised. Max penalty: life imprisonment. Most of those sanctioned are low level. Importation of drugs by Nigerian citizens can lead to 5 years prison: even if already sanctioned by another country.
Portugal	Law 30/2000 Decree Law 15/93 Decree Law 54/2013 (prevention and protection against sale of new psychoactive substances)	Acquisition, possession and use of all illicit substances decriminalised when for personal use. Prison not used. Referral to panels involving social workers, medical professionals who provide administrative sanctions e.g. fines, community service, suspended sentences. But principal goal is to encourage dependent users to enter treatment. Since 2013 use and possession of NPS is also decriminalised.	Illicit drugs: Trafficking and trafficking-consumption prohibited as criminal offences. Penalties: < 3 years prison (trafficking-consumption); 1-5 years (minor trafficking); 4-12 years (major trafficking). NPS: Production and trafficking prohibited as an administrative offence and subject to fines of < 44,890 euro (group). Other sanctions can also be applied e.g. closure of premises and suspension of licenses.

(Continues)

Table 9.3 (Continued)

Country	*Statutes/Acts*	*Law regarding drug use*	*Laws regarding drug supply*
Sweden	Penal Law on Narcotics (1968) Narcotic Drugs Punishment Act (1992) The Act on the Destruction of Certain Substances of Abuse Dangerous to Health (2011)	Personal use and possession criminal offence. Prison possible (up to 6 mths) but conviction and fine is usual. Compulsory drug treatment used (albeit rarely). NPS: Criminal penalties apply once harms have been assessed and drug is scheduled. Otherwise administrative offence: drug may be seized but no criminal penalties apply.	Production and supply criminalised. Max penalty: ≤ 18 yr prison. Low use of prison. Further declined following a 2011 Supreme Court ruling to increase use of alternatives.
UK (England and Wales)	Misuse of Drugs Act 1971. Class A drugs: heroin, cocaine, methamphetamine, LSD. Class B: cannabis, amphetamines, ketamine, synthetic cannabinoids, synthetic cathinones (eg mephedrone). Class C: GHB, khat (since 2014). Temporary class drugs e.g. NBOMe.	Drug use per se not an offence, but possession is. Max penalties vary e.g. 2, 5 or 7 years prison for class C, B and A drugs respectively. Prison in approx. 20% cases. Cannabis: warnings and penalty notices and drug courts used. Courts can mandate treatment. NPS: Criminal penalties apply once harms have been assessed and drug is scheduled. Otherwise drug may be seized but no criminal penalties apply.	Production and supply of illicit drugs criminalised. Max penalty for class A drugs: life imprisonment (class A drug) or 14 yrs (class B or C drug). High rate of imprisonment but new drug sentencing guidelines enacted in 2012 seek to increase proportionality of sanctions: and reduce prison for some groups of offenders e.g. mules. Supply of any NPS is a criminal offence with max penalty of 14 years prison.
USA	The United States Code (USC) Controlled Substances Act Schedule I: heroin, MDMA, LSD, cannabis, BZP, GHB Schedule II: methamphetamine, cocaine. Schedule III: ketamine. Federal Analog Act (1986) Each state has their own drug laws. e.g. Washington: *Washington Initiative 502* (I-502) (legalisation of cannabis) Uniform Controlled Substances Act (RCW 69.50)	Possession and personal use of cannabis is legalised in four states (CO, WA, OR & AK) and Washington D.C. and decriminalised in 20+ states. Possession of other drugs or drug paraphernalia e.g. syringes criminalised. Federal: Max penalty of prison (<3 years) but a conviction for possession can also lead to loss of federal benefits, including school loans, grants, and licenses. State: Penalties vary hugely. For example in Georgia possession of any amount of a heroin, cocaine or ecstasy is a felony punishable with 2-15 yrs prison. But, in most states fines, diversion and drug courts are used instead of prison. NPS: Criminal penalties apply in most jurisdictions.	Cannabis cultivation and supply was legalised in 2012 in Colorado (CO) and Washington State (WA) and in 2014 in OR and AK following public referenda. Cannabis cultivation (but not supply) was also legalised in Washington D.C. in 2014 following public referenda. Restrictions on retail sales apply on price, tax, packaging, products, advertising etc. Retail sales commenced in CO and WA 2014: sales in OR and AK have not yet commenced. Production and trafficking of other drugs criminalised with max penalty of life imprisonment (or death penalty – but not applied). History of mandatory minimums (e.g. the federal penalty for trafficking 1kg heroin carries a minimum of 10 years prison; 20 years if a second offence), quantity thresholds, habitual offender laws, and other sentence enhancements (both federal and state). This has led to very high rates of imprisonment. e.g.in 2013 98% federal drug traffickers received a sentence of imprisonment. Federal sentencing guidelines enacted in 2013 and 2014 reduce sentences for some drug trafficking offenders and encourage alternatives to imprisonment. NPS: Criminal penalties apply: often equivalent to mimicked illicit drug.

Vietnam	Vietnamese Penal Code No. 15/1999/ QH10 The Criminal Code (2009) Law on Drug Prevention and Control 2000 (amended 2008) HIV Law (2006) Decree 135/2004 & Decree 94/2009/ ND-CP (re compulsory drug treatment centres)	Drug use decriminalised in 2009, but it remains an administrative offence and there is high use (60,000+) of compulsory drug treatment with forced labour (2 years). Crack downs on drug users by police common. Requirement for drug users to register with the Government.	Manufacture, cultivation, storage, transport and trafficking is criminalised. Vietnam remains one of the few countries to use the death penalty for drug trafficking, however executions remain a state secret and figures are not publicly released. Other sanctions range from 2-7 years (low level) to life imprisonment (high level). Penalty is determined by factors including type and weight of drug e.g. low level < 5 g heroin or cocaine vs high level ≥ 100g heroin or cocaine, and whether it is a first/repeat offence, whether offender holds positions of power. Penalty for cultivation of crops is lower: max penalty of 3-7 years, with admin sanctions also available. Offenders can also be subject to property confiscation and bans on undertaking particular professions.

Notes:

NPS: New psychoactive substances

This is a summary: hence not all drug laws have been included.

The laws were correct at the time of writing: July 2015.

differ, as does the stage of implementation.) We also note that the New Zealand model for potential legal sale of new psychoactive substances has been tested and approved as safe for human consumption (Wilkins et al., 2013). These changes explicitly embrace variants of a public health approach, to consider how to best minimise unintended harms through, for example, controlling the extent of commercial enterprise allowed, what products to sell, underage sales, whether and how to tax and restrictions on labels, advertising, purity, maximum purchase amounts and places of consumption (Pacula et al., 2014; Pardo, 2014; Room, 2014; Winstock and Ramsey, 2010).

Looking across the nine countries, one can see increasing diversity in the nature of legal change (Table 9.3). For example, while there remain 'de jure' drug law reforms (such as Portugal, Washington and Colorado) the police, prosecutors and courts are playing an increasingly important role in shaping drug laws in practice. This is most evident with regard to Colombia, where it was the Constitutional and Supreme Courts that have decriminalised possession for personal use and where continued efforts to introduce de jure reforms have yet to succeed. While the role of the Courts can, in part, be attributed to the features of the Colombian political system, they have also been commended for ensuring that controversial issues can be addressed in the absence of the requisite political conditions to undertake de jure reform (Cepeda-Espinosa, 2004). Another noted example of the increasing role of other criminal justice actors has been in the United States. While the decision of Colorado and Washington State to legalise and regulate cannabis was noteworthy, it was well acknowledged that to do so went against federal laws and federal powers to prosecute any person who cultivated, sold, possessed or used cannabis (Kilmer et al., 2012). Hence it was highly significant that in August 2013 the US Attorney General issued a directive that federal prosecutors do not pursue prosecutions in any state that has legalised cannabis (unless in exceptional circumstances) (United States Attorney General, 2013).

Across most countries, and those we have examined in detail here, there is now a significant take-up of non-criminal options for people who use drugs (Table 9.3, column 3). For example, seven of our nine countries afford some form of decriminalisation or legalisation and the other two provide diversion to treatment. This means that drug use is increasingly being responded to as a health and social issue: not a criminal issue. This is in line with the calls of organisations, such as the UNODC and WHO, for a more public-health oriented approach to drug use and the evidence on the benefits of their take up (Babor et al., 2010). That said, there can be clear differences in the extent of implementation. The clearest example of this is that while both Portugal and Vietnam have adopted policies of decriminalisation, Portugal employs a policy aimed at humanising and de-stigmatising people who use drugs (Hughes and Stevens, 2010) whereas Vietnam retains compulsory drug treatment and forced labour (Amon et al., 2014; Vuong et al., 2012; Windle, 2015).

Coupled with the growing use of non-criminal sanctions for people who use drugs, many countries are embracing laws to ensure the rights of users to healthcare and harm reduction. Noted examples here are Colombia: Law 1566 of 2012 recognised drug use as a public health issue and created guaranteed rights, for example, voluntary drug treatment (Observatorio de Drogas de Colombia, 2014). This bill has been used to roll out a range of new policy responses including the first drug consumption rooms (in Bogota) and first needle syringe programmes [in Medellin, Bogota, Cali, Cucuta and Armenia (McKenzie, 2014)]. In Vietnam, aided by the 2006 HIV Law, there has been an expansion of harm reduction services (Jardine et al., 2012; Vuong et al., 2012).

There are also more nations seeking to increase the proportionality of drug sanctions and encourage alternatives to imprisonment. For example, in Sweden, a Supreme court ruling in 2011 to reduce sentences for drug offenders led to 200 fewer people imprisoned in the subsequent year (Orange, 2013). In 2012, the UK introduced new sentencing guidelines for drug offences (Sentencing Council, 2012); a move that was specifically designed to reduce disproportionate sanctions, particularly for 'drug mules' (those who carry drugs for mid or high level drug traffickers often under pressure, influence or intimidation) (Sentencing Council, 2011). Finally, in recent years the USA drug policy has explicitly identified the toll from over-imprisonment of drug offenders and sought to 'redress the balance' through reforms to the criminal justice system (Attorney General Eric Holder, 2013; President Obama, 2015; US Department of Justice, 2013; US Sentencing Commission, 2014).

There remain, however, instances of countries that apply highly punitive drug sanctions for drug use, especially Vietnam with the death penalty and Nigeria with a penalty for possession [15 to 25 years in prison that equals or exceeds penalties for supply in many nations (Ashley and Boehlke, 2011; Klantschnig, 2011)]. However, such punitive sanctions are the exception rather than the rule within the nine countries examined here.

Despite the seeming trend towards harmonisation of drug laws, reducing penalties and/or therapeutic responses for use/possession, increasing the proportionality of sanctions for drug supply and increasing legal rights to harm reduction and treatment, there remain important inter-country differences. For example, while, as noted above, there has been an increase in the use of decriminalisation and diversion approaches, these differ in terms of their reach; that is, the proportion of drug offenders they can or will affect. For example, while the USA has received a lot of attention for the rise of drug courts, the USA drug court system can serve a maximum of 110,000 to 130,000 offenders in any one year: 7 per cent of drug-involved offenders (Bhati et al., 2008; Sevigny et al., 2013). In contrast, Australian states often divert between 25 to 55 per cent of use/possess offenders and 16 per cent of drug-involved offenders (Hughes and Ritter, 2008; Hughes et al., 2014). The additional reach is fostered in part by the explicit emphasis on front-end police diversion programmes rather than back-end drug courts (Hughes and Ritter, 2008). However, the broader policy environment also plays a role: namely that drug diversion is congruent with Australian and New Zealand objectives of harm minimisation. In contrast, as shown by Sevigny et al. (2013), drug courts in the USA have been constrained by the predominance of strict sentencing laws such as mandatory minimums, sentencing guidelines and three-strikes laws that limit the pool of eligible offenders.

New psychoactive substances are an interesting case in point regarding newer laws concerned with drugs (see Table 9.3) showing the breadth of possible legal and regulatory responses (see also Measham and Newcombe, this volume). Some countries (e.g. UK, Sweden) use a temporary drug class (with no sanctions) for new and emerging substances, pending assessment of harms and subsequent criminalisation. Others (e.g. Portugal) decriminalise use and possession of all NPS (regardless of whether or not the harms have been assessed), providing all NPS users with 'existing programs and structures of prevention, risk reduction and harm minimisation, social care and treatment' (Serviço de Intervenção nos Comportamentos Aditivos e nas Dependências, 2013b). Still other countries criminalise all NPS, even those that have yet to be invented (USA and Australia). In the reverse direction, the New Zealand approach is a legal regulatory market (Wilkins et al., 2013). Aside from the legal and regulatory differences, there are also differences in the extent to which sanctions for NPS are the same as those for illicit drugs. While many countries treat NPS more leniently (e.g. Sweden), Australia is a noted exception, as while people who use illicit drugs commonly receive diversionary sanctions, NPS are ineligible for diversion programmes. A new national framework released in July 2014 recognised the conflict this creates with Australia's NDS objective of 'harm minimisation' and called on diversion programmes to include NPS users (Intergovernmental Committee on Drugs, 2014).

Finally, one country of note that warrants specific attention is Colombia: both for the rapid pace of legal change and potential for future change. In recent years, Colombia, under the leadership of President Santos, has seen the introduction of significant laws to reframe drugs as a health issue, negotiations with the FARC rebel/guerrilla movement to obtain peace, and an increasing role on the international stage calling for alternatives to the War on Drugs. Also issued were two important (albeit unsuccessful) legal proposals in 2012/2013 in the lead up to the end of Santos first term. The first sought to decriminalise by law (rather than court ruling) possession of all illicit drugs and NPS; the second sought to decriminalise the cultivation of cannabis, coca and opium poppy plants (but not trafficking in these drugs). The first would significantly build upon the Constitutional Court rulings. The second would build upon the original objectives to the 1988 UN Convention on the rights of Colombian farmers. Following the re-election of President Santos in June 2014, it is deemed highly likely that significant drug law reform will be enacted in the years to come.

SECURITY, WELFARE, DEVELOPMENT AND HUMAN RIGHTS

It is impossible to consider drug policy in isolation from the social, political and governance arrangements within any one country. A nation's political stability and strength of governance, its social welfare regime and its compliance with human rights are important contextual factors in understanding the development of and current status of illicit drug policies. Two relationships are of note: (i) the ways in which political instability can shape and influence the extent of drug trafficking (Thoumi, 2012); and (ii) the ways in which social welfare and human rights policies can shape and influence the extent of drug-related harm (Rhodes, 2002).

Political stability, security and governance

There is an important association between political stability and good governance and drugs. The reinforcing cycle of illicit economic activities leading to corruption and political instability, which create fertile grounds for further illicit activities has been well-documented (Aning and Pokoo, 2013; Klein, 2005; Mannava et al., 2010; Schultze-Kraft, 2014; Thoumi, 2012; West Africa Commission on Drugs, 2014). Thoumi noted, in relation to Colombia, that 'drug interests have deeply permeated the political system' (Thoumi, 2012: 999). The illicit drugs issue may be viewed by both the population and some political elites as a useful source of much needed national income (Felbab-Brown and Forest, 2012).

Commentators such as Felbab-Brown and Forest (2012) point out that West African drug policy, including Nigerian policy, cannot be considered in isolation from systemic governance problems. Relevant issues include political instability, violence and corruption, weak institutional structures including in the justice system, politicisation and corruption of law enforcement and the military and the presence of other illicit economies and organised crime, such as the illicit economy in oil in Nigeria. The interrelationship of illicit markets that include human trafficking, terrorism, money laundering, weapons and drugs suggests that drug policies in isolation may be less effective than policies which cover the range of transnational crime. That said, the extent and nature of inter-relationships between illicit drug and other illicit markets requires more theorisation and research (Hughes et al., in press).

Development

The UN Millennium Development Goals (United Nations, 2000) aimed to reduce poverty and improve social development. Both of these are inextricably linked to the drugs issue. Countries with lower levels of development, whether defined in terms of economic growth, income distribution, employment, productivity, social capital, political stability, governance, health and education have higher involvement in the drug trade (Babor et al., 2010; Barrett, 2010; Rhodes et al., 2003). The level of development also affects the likelihood of drug-related problems and harms, such as rates of HIV, with less developed nations often lacking the capacity to provide effective prevention, treatment and/or harm reduction responses (Babor et al., 2010; Mannava et al., 2010). It has been noted, however, that the actors involved in drug policy and those involved in development tend to work in isolation (Mannava et al., 2010). For countries such as Colombia and Nigeria, the drug trade can be seen as 'development' inasmuch as it represents short-term increases in disposable income and GDP (Mannava et al., 2010). However, as noted earlier, there are longer-term negative consequences (corruption, violence, political instability). Specific examples of problems when drugs policy is considered independently from development are the well-documented issues associated with crop substitution (alternative development) (Babor et al., 2010; Lupu, 2004), as shown in Colombia where the switch from growing coca leaf to coffee beans can lead to reduced income as there is not the necessary road and transport infrastructure to compete on the international market for coffee (Veillette and Navarrete-Frías, 2005).

In spite of the clear difficulties in bringing development and drug policy together, it is notable that the national drug strategies of Nigeria and Colombia, both nations with poor governance and security, focus on 'democratic security' and legal frameworks respectively (see Table 9.2). For example, Colombia's National Development Plan 2010–14 explicitly seeks to enhance economic development and regional integration (through social welfare, developing avenues for income generation, short and long-term infrastructure) and also promote social participation and good governance mechanisms to enable ownership of development planning (Observatorio de Drogas de Colombia, 2014). However, this appears to be rare for other countries.

Social welfare policies and drug polices

As noted earlier, drug policy is likely to be shaped and influenced by a country's social welfare approach. The nine nations vary in the extent of decommodification (citizen's social welfare entitlements), and levels of inequality. Research has shown a relationship between these variables and the extent of drug-related harm (Stevens, 2011). We suspect, although it has yet to be studied extensively, that drug policies themselves can be driven by, and inextricably linked to, social welfare policies.

Examination of welfare policies highlights that countries with low decommodification indexes (albeit as at 1980; Scruggs and Allan, 2006), which include Australia, New Zealand and the USA, and the one country with high decommodification, Sweden, may not have such divergent drug policies. In these four countries national drug policy balances supply and demand reduction. Unfortunately, we could not locate research (published in English) examining decommodification in other countries, such as Nigeria, Colombia or Portugal. Given the significant relationships between welfare policies, and drug-related harm, this is an important research topic. The ways in which social welfare policy evolves is also linked to drug policy. One example is the emergence of 'mutual obligation' (as it is referred to in Australia) or conditional benefits (UK) and the impact on drug policies. The growing movement from an approach characterised by a universal right to welfare to an approach characterised by conditional entitlements (Dwyer, 2004) impacts on people who use drugs and on drug policy. Policies concerned with drug testing and drug treatment are thus linked to welfare policies (Monaghan, 2012; Monaghan and Wincup, 2013; Wincup, 2014).

Sweden has long been a prominent proponent of a social net for people who use drugs: indeed, this has been deemed a key contributor to Sweden's low levels of use and drug-related problems (Babor et al., 2010). Since 1999, Portugal has had a similar focus on social issues, including policies of social reintegration, housing support and incentives for employers to hire people who use drugs. The more recent Portuguese 2013–15 drug strategy further identifies the interrelationship between social and economic factors and drug-related harms and how rising unemployment levels and increasing inequity can increase the vulnerability of many people in society to drug dependence, as well as the necessity of good social supports (Serviço de Intervenção nos Comportamentos Aditivos e nas Dependências, 2013a, 2013b).

Poverty reduction is also now explicitly acknowledged in the USA drug strategy (Executive Office of the President of the United States, 2014b). To what extent this impacts on policies on the ground is not yet clear but it would appear to be an important first step. New Zealand is another nation that has specific policies designed to reduce known elevated rates of drug-related harms amongst marginalised groups. Their drug strategy includes an explicit focus to reduce inequalities amongst minorities (Maori and Pacific people) and young people.

Despite these positive examples, discriminatory and inequitable practices exist and they are receiving increasing attention: particularly as they pertain to USA and UK drug laws (Reuter, 2013). For example, in the United States state prison system, black inmates are imprisoned for drug offences at eight times the rate of white inmates (Kilmer et al., 2012). This has led not only to overimprisonment, but also disenfranchisement of large segments of black populations through flow on effects including eviction from public housing, reduced access to social security benefits (e.g. food stamps and student loans), employment restrictions and loss of rights to vote (Caulkins et al., 2005). In the UK, large inequities have been found in the rates of stop and search by police (and subsequent prosecution) (Eastwood et al., 2013). Both nations have introduced a number of drug policy reforms that aim to rectify these inequalities including USA legislative reforms to reduce disparity in the sentencing of crack cocaine and cocaine offenders (US Congress, 2010).

Human rights and drug policies

Human rights are argued to be a foundational principle underpinning drug policy (Barrett, 2010). As of 2010, however, the International Narcotics Control Board and the Commission on Narcotic Drugs had 'yet to affirm the human rights of people who use drugs' (Wolfe and Saucier, 2010: 145). Conversely, UN agencies have been concerned with, and called for, the closure of compulsory detention centres that abuse the rights of people who use drugs (Amon et al., 2014).

It is possible to find examples of human rights conflicts in most countries, including those with explicit 'harm minimisation' policies. For example, the human rights principles of avoiding arbitrary arrest and discrimination can conflict with Australian (Hughes et al., 2015) and USA deemed supply laws, where deemed supply laws mean that people carrying more than a particular quantity of drug can be presumed guilty of an offence of drug trafficking.

At the most extreme of the nine countries examined here are Nigeria and Vietnam. Nigeria retains corporal sanction in northern parts of the country (Iakobishvili, 2011). Vietnam is noted for human rights abuses with respect to drug policy (Baldwin, 2013; Human Rights Watch, 2011; Reid and Higgs, 2011; Vuong et al., 2012). Human rights organisations argue that nations risk being complicit in the human rights abuses: either through engagement in the international drug control system, direct law enforcement assistance or provision of funds to member states that retain the death penalty (Gallahue, 2011; Lines et al., 2010). Human rights organisations have thus argued there exists a 'shared responsibility' to abolish the death penalty for drug offences (Gallahue, 2011: 22). As noted earlier, Portugal is the only nation of our nine to explicitly mention a humanistic and human rights approach in its current drug strategy; something that has meant the rights of people who use drugs to access treatment, harm reduction and social reintegration services remain of central focus (Hughes and Stevens, 2010).

DISCUSSION AND IMPLICATIONS

The evolution of drug policy across the globe is a fascinating and evolving story. This chapter shows that some of the traditional ways of viewing drug policies are increasingly unhelpful and may miss the complexity, similarity and difference that characterises drug policy around the world. For example, the analysis in this chapter suggests that the distinction between producer versus consumer versus transit countries is less relevant; the categorisation of national drug laws into prohibition, decriminalisation, and legalisation is inaccurate and limited; the distinction between legal and illegal drugs is no longer germane; and there are important differences between policy as stated versus policy as implemented. This reinforces the necessity of a comprehensive approach to analysing and discussing drug policy.

Even though all nine countries under examination in this chapter are signatories to the three international conventions, we observe substantial variety in domestic policies. The explicit goals and objectives listed in national drug strategies vary, as does the relative focus on supply reduction compared to demand reduction and harm reduction. A clear trend in drug laws can be observed: a shift away from criminal sanctions and towards health responses and legal regulatory approaches, notwithstanding the preponderance of developed countries in our analysis. What is interesting is that in many cases the policy changes have not necessarily conformed to the drug law reform agenda of legalisation per se.

The varieties of drug laws are as numerous as the number of countries. It is necessary to consider the laws together with their implementation – this includes police and sentencing practices. An example is Australia, where, in spite of maintaining criminal penalties for possession and sometimes use in most states, less than 1 per cent are imprisoned (Australian Bureau of Statistics, 2014a, 2014b). Likewise, a focus solely on the laws can miss the importance of regulation. Regulations, which often sit outside formal laws and statutes, are coming to define a substantial number of approaches to drugs: New Zealand for NPS and the USA for cannabis are cases in point. Implementation may be influenced by international forces (such as international donor programmes in Vietnam) or by other non-drug related practices (such as the example of court rulings in Colombia) or through the difference between state and national policies (as shown in the USA with legalisation of cannabis use) or through a nation's level of development (such as in the case of introducing alternative development measures in Colombia in the absence of adequate transport infrastructure to enable a viable coffee trade). Which factors have the greatest impact on implementation remains unclear. Moreover, in many countries, analysis of the implementation impact of new drug policy directions (such as the UK recovery agenda and USA cannabis legalisation) are yet to occur.

By comparing the international conventions against those of the domestic policies, it is increasingly clear that the international conventions are no longer fit for purpose: they do not address legal drugs, they focus on laws (not implementation), they focus overly on supply reduction and they do not articulate with a social welfare, human rights and development approach. That said, there may also be important lessons from the regulatory experiences of alcohol and tobacco. Given the blurred distinction between legal and illegal drugs, and the explicit inclusion of both in some national policies, it is likely that important lessons for drug policy can be gained from alcohol and tobacco regulation. This is all the more important as further drug law reform and drug law reform discussions are highly likely given the re-election of President Santos in Colombia, further USA states voting on cannabis legalisation in 2016 and the 2016 UNGASS meetings.

Lessons can be learnt from all national approaches. For example, the experience from Colombia shows the importance of a balanced approach – demand as well as supply reduction – in order to be responsive to changing drug problems, in this case, the emergence of heightened consumption. Sweden shows the benefit of a high social welfare net for people who use drugs, but also highlights the potential costs of having minimal harm reduction. There is not an 'ideal' drug policy stance: drug policy evolves as the political, social and economic circumstances change in countries. The analyses also show inherent conflicts within national approaches: for example, in spite of the objective of harm minimisation, Australia has some of the most punitive laws and responses on NPS, and Vietnam retains and uses the death penalty for drug offences but is one of the few countries to explicitly emphasise harm reduction in their drug strategy.

We have shown there is rich opportunity to systematically compare and contrast drug policy between nations. In such an analysis, we have argued for consideration of frameworks or dimensions beyond merely the traditional 'drug policy'. A rich qualitative case study approach across the various frameworks can lay productive groundwork for systematic quantitative comparative policy analysis. In such quantitative analyses, policy impacts and outcomes are compared (examples include Belackova et al., 2015; Hughes and Stevens, 2010; Kelly and Rasul, 2014; McMorris et al., 2011; Simons-Morton et al., 2010; Vuolo, 2013). The use of an Index score, which summarises a nation's drug policy and its implementation is another quantitative approach to comparative analysis. Index scores can compare policy outcomes across time between the same nation, or compare different nations (McFadden, 2006; Ritter, 2009; United Nations Office on Drugs and Crime, 2005), Quantitative approaches can only be deployed where there is available, reliable and comparable quantitative data, across a sufficient number of cases. This is often not the case.

Importantly, much of the comparative analyses conducted to date on drug policies (see above references) do not consider the broader frameworks that we have explored here. There is not an Index that we are aware of that covers all aspects of drug harm as well as social welfare, human rights and other components. Rarely do comparative policy analyses include considerations beyond drug laws and strategies per se (exceptions are Corman et al., 2013; Stevens, 2011). Data are frequently lacking and a key challenge in all such analyses is the importance of good theorising with respect to the relationship between drug policy and the outcomes.

The relationship between drug policy and drug use outcomes assumes causality – that is, drug use rates are determined by the policies under study. This is a significant and problematic assumption. The causal pathways between policy and practice (in this case consumption and harm) are under-studied and under-theorised (Babor et al., 2010; MacCoun and Reuter, 2001). There is an essential dynamic between policy and drug use and harms: that high rates of harms can lead to policy is as reasonable as policy leading to high rates of harm. For example, the policy focus can drive harms, such as a focus on imprisonment resulting in social and economic harms (Milloy et al., 2008). But it is also the case that policy reform often follows rising consumption and harm: for example, the Portuguese decriminalised all illicit drug use in 2001 in large part due to increasing concerns about the rising levels of problematic drug use and harm (Hughes and Stevens, 2010). The dynamic interplay between drug policies and rates of drug use and harms is perhaps best understood as a mutually self-correcting dynamic system, where there is neither a clear leader nor clear follower, rather a confluence of both factors evolving over time.

Aside from comparative analysis of drug policy (whether qualitative or quantitative), there are other analytic tools for studying policy, less concerned with comparisons between nations, and more concerned with understanding the evolution of policies and the various influences on policy. This tradition of policy analysis aims to understand how drug policies came into place and takes into account the multiple influences and dynamics of policy development. These influences include the media, public opinion, political processes, interest groups, researchers, international laws including the UN Conventions and so on (Lancaster et al., 2011; MacGregor, 2013; Monaghan, 2010; Ritter and Bammer, 2010; Ritter and Lancaster, 2013) Studies in this tradition provide detailed analysis of the ways in which actors and institutions dynamically interact such that a particular policy comes to the fore (e.g. Lancaster et al., 2014; Monaghan, 2012).The work of Thom and colleagues (2013) exemplifies this kind of analytic approach. In their study of the development of OST across six European nations, they analyse the differences in stakeholder power and dynamics, administrative and regulatory structures, treatment goals and problematisation and legitimisation. The analysis provides insights into cultural differences, historical trends and factors that influence policy implementation. Finally, social constructivist approaches provide an alternate analytic tool to studying drug policy. In this frame, drug policy is considered as a process of social construction (Lancaster, 2014) constituted and maintained through stabilising practices (Fraser and Moore, 2011; Fraser et al., 2014). Here the policy analysis concerns the ways in which the policy solution comes to represent the problem of drugs (Bacchi, 2009).

It appears we have a potentially rich array of methodologies: qualitative case studies, quantitative comparative analysis and policy development analyses, whether from an historical, public policy or social constructivist epistemology. All of these approaches can include attention to the variety of frameworks (Table 9.1) and to analyses that move beyond traditional and now out-dated dichotomies. As we have shown, a focus solely on drug strategies and drug laws excludes factors that may indeed have a much greater influence on consumption and harm. Political stability, security and good governance have potent influences on drug use and drug-related harm, and hence, drug policies, as shown in the cases of Colombia and Nigeria. The social welfare regime within any one country can also be an important determinant, as seen in Sweden. Likewise, discrimination and equity are centrally linked to drug policy impacts, as shown in the USA and UK policies. Finally, human rights have emerged as a central theme in drug policy considerations, as seen in Vietnam and Portugal. This indicates that a nation's drug problems may be more directly tied to broader economic and social policies than anything specific to do with drug policies. This sets a new research agenda for scholars of drug policy.

ACKNOWLEDGEMENTS

We are very grateful for the assistance we received from Thu Vuong, UNSW, in relation to the details for Vietnam and from the Colombian Ministry of Justice (Andres Lopez) and Prof Daniel Meija, Universidad de los Andes, for details regarding Colombia. Alison Ritter is supported by funding from an NHMRC Senior Research Fellowship (APP1021988). The Drug Policy Modelling Program has received funding from philanthropy (Colonial Foundation Trust) and the National Drug and Alcohol Research Centre receives funding from the Commonwealth Department of Health Australia.

REFERENCES

Acevedo, B., Bewley-Taylor, D. and Youngers, C. (2008). *Ten years of Plan Colombia: An Analytical Assessment*. Oxford: The Beckley Foundation, Drug Policy Programme.

Amon, J. J., Pearshouse, R., Cohen, J. E. and Schleifer, R. (2014). Compulsory drug detention in East and Southeast Asia: evolving government, UN and donor responses. *International Journal of Drug Policy,* 25(1): 13–20.

Aning, K. and Pokoo, J. (2013). *Drug Trafficking and Threats to National and Regional Security in West Africa*. West African Commission on Drugs.

Ashley, L. and Boehlke, K. (2011). Vietnam. In M. A. R. Kleiman and J. E. Hawdon (eds), *Encyclopedia of Drug Policy* (Vol. 2). Los Angeles: Sage, pp. 831–3.

Attorney General Eric Holder. (2013). *Remarks at the Annual Meeting of the American Bar Association's House of Delegates*. Retrieved from http://www.justice.gov/iso/opa/ag/speeches/2013/ag-speech-130812.html.

Australian Bureau of Statistics. (2014a). *4517.0 - Prisoners in Australia, 2013*. Canberra: Australian Bureau of Statistics.

Australian Bureau of Statistics. (2014b). *4519.0 - Recorded Crime - Offenders, 2012–13*. Canberra: Australian Bureau of Statistics.

Babor, T., Caulkins, J., Edwards, G., Fischer, B., Foxcroft, D., Humphreys, K., Obot, I. S., Rehm, J., Reuter, P., Room, R., Rossow, I. and Strang, J. (2010). *Drug Policy and the Public Good*. Oxford: Oxford University Press.

Bacchi, C. (2009). *Analysing Policy: What's The Problem Represented To Be?* Sydney: Pearson Education.

Baldwin, S. (2013). Emerging from a black box: drug policymaking in Vietnam. In F. Rahman and N. Crofts (eds), *Drug Law Reform in East and Southeast Asia*. Lanham: Lexington Books, pp. 211–19.

Baldwin, S. and Thomson, N. (2013). Compulsory 'rehabilitation' in Asia: problems and possible solutions. In F. Rahman and N. Crofts (eds), *Drug Law Reform in East and Southeast Asia*. Lanham: Lexington Books, pp. 139–49.

Barratt, M. J. and Lenton, S. (2013). Drugs and the internet. In A. Ritter, T. King and M. Hamilton (eds), *Drug Use in Australian Society*. South Melbourne: Oxford University Press.

Barrett, D. (2010). Security, development and human rights: legal normative and policy challenges to the international drug control system. *International Journal of Drug Policy,* 21(2): 140–4.

Barrett, D, and Nowak, M. (2010). The United Nations and drug policy: towards a human rights-based approach. In A. Constantinides and N. Zaikos (eds), *The Diversity of International Law: Essays in Honour of Professor Kalliopi K Koufa*. Leiden: Brill/Martinus Nijhoff, pp. 449–77.

Belackova, V., Maalsté, N., Zabransky, T. and Grund, J. P. (2015). 'Should i buy or should i grow?' How drug policy institutions and drug market transaction costs shape the decision to self-supply with cannabis in the Netherlands and the Czech Republic. *International Journal of Drug Policy*, 26(3): 296–310.

Bertram, E., Blachman, M., Sharpe, K. and Andreas, P. (1996). *Drug War Politics: The*

Price of Denial. Berkeley, Los Angeles and London: University of California Press.

Bewley-Taylor, D. and Trace, M. (2006). *The International Narcotics Control Board: Watchdog or Guardian of the UN Drug Control Conventions?* London: The Beckley Foundation.

Bhati, A. S., Roman, J. K. and Chalfin, A. (2008). *To Treat or Not to Treat: Evidence on the Prospects of Expanding Treatment to Drug-Involved Offenders*. Washington, DC: Urban Institute, Justice Policy Centre.

Caulkins, J. P., Reuter, P. H., Iguchi, M. Y. and Chiesa, J. (2005). *How Goes the 'War on Drugs'?* Santa Monica: RAND Drug Policy Research Center.

Central Intelligence Agency. (2014). The World Factbook. Available from https://www.cia.gov/library/publications/the-world-factbook/.

Cepeda-Espinosa, M. J. (2004). Judicial activism in a violent context: the origin, role, and impact of the Colombian Constitutional Court. *Global Studies Law Review*, 3(4): 529–700.

Commission on Narcotic Drugs. (2014). *Report on the Fifty-Seventh Session (13 December 2013 and 13–21 March 2014)*. New York: United Nations, Economic and Social Council.

Cook, C., Bridge, J., McLean, S., Phelan, M. and Barrett, D. (2014). *The Funding Crisis for Harm Reduction: Donor Retreat, Government Neglect and the Way Forward*. London: International Harm Reduction Association.

Corman, H., Dave, D. M., Das, D. and Reichman, N. E. (2013). Effects of welfare reform on illicit drug use of adult women. *Economic Inquiry*, 51(1): 653–74.

Courtwright, D. T. (2010). The NIDA brain disease paradigm: history, resistance and spin-offs. *BioSocieties*, 5(1): 137–47.

Duke, K. (2013). From crime to recovery the reframing of British drugs policy? *Journal of Drug Issues*, 43(1): 39–55.

Dwyer, P. (2004). Creeping conditionality in the UK: from welfare rights to conditional entitlements? *The Canadian Journal of Sociology*, 29(2): 265–87.

Eastwood, N., Shiner, M. and Bear, D. (2013). *The Numbers in Black and White: Ethnic Disparities in the Policing and Prosecution of Drug Offences in England and Wales*. London: Release.

Elhawary, S. (2010). Security for whom? Stabilisation and civilian protection in Colombia. *Disasters*, 34(Suppl 3): S388–405.

European Monitoring Centre for Drugs and Drug Addiction. (2008). *Towards a Better Understanding of Drug-Related Public Expenditure in Europe*. Luxembourg: Office for Official Publications of the European Communities.

European Monitoring Centre for Drugs and Drug Addiction. (2014). *Country Overview: Portugal*. Luxembourg: Office for Official Publications of the European Communities.

European Monitoring Centre on Drugs and Drug Addiction. (2014, July 3). *National Drug-Related Public Expenditure: United Kingdom*. Available from http://www.emcdda.europa.eu/countries/public-expenditure/united-kingdom.

Executive Office of the President of the United States. (2014a). *National Drug Control Budget: FY 2015 Funding Highlights*. Washington, DC: Executive Office of the President of the United States, Office of National Drug Control Policy.

Executive Office of the President of the United States. (2014b). *National Drug Control Strategy 2014*. Washington, DC: Executive Office of the President of the United States, Office of National Drug Control Policy.

Felbab-Brown, V. and Forest, J. J. (2012). Political violence and the illicit economies of West Africa. *Terrorism and Political Violence*, 24(5): 787–806.

Fordham, A. and Tinasti, K. (2014). UNGASS 2016 on drugs, the first challenge for HIV advocates in the post-2015 era. *Journal of the International AIDS Society*, 17: 19274.

Fraser, S. and Moore, D. (2011). Governing through problems: the formulation of policy on amphetamine-type stimulants (ATS) in Australia. *International Journal of Drug Policy*, *22*(6): 498–506.

Fraser, S., Moore, D. and Keane, H. (2014). *Habits: Remaking Addiction*. Hampshire: Palgrave MacMillan.

Gallahue, P. (2011). *The Death Penalty for Drug Offences - Global Overview in 2011: Shared Responsibility and Shared Consequences*. London: International Harm Reduction Association.

Ghodse, H. (1999). Guiding principles of drug demand reduction: an international response. *British Journal of Psychiatry,* 175: 310–12.

Global Commission on Drug Policy. (2011). *[War] On Drugs: Report of the Global Commission on Drug Policy*. Rio de Janeiro: The Global Commission on Drug Policy.

Gomez, A. P. (2013). Out of the eye of the hurricane, but still close. *Adicciones,* 25(2): 106–8.

Griffiths, P., Evans-Brown, M. and Sedefov, R. (2013). Getting up to speed with the public health and regulatory challenges posed by new psychoactive substances in the information age. *Addiction,* 108(10): 1700–3.

HM Government. (2008). *Drugs: Protecting Families and Communities: the 2008 Drug Strategy*. London: HM Government.

HM Government. (2010). *Drug Strategy 2010 - Reducing Demand, Restricting Supply, Building Recovery: Supporting People to Live a Drug Free Life*. London: HM Government.

Hughes, C. and Ritter, A. (2008). *Monograph No. 16: A Summary of Diversion Programs for Drug and Drug-Related Offenders in Australia*. Sydney: National Drug and Alcohol Research Centre.

Hughes, C., Shanahan, M., Ritter, A., McDonald, D. and Gray-Weale, F. (2014). *Monograph No. 25: Evaluation of Australian Capital Territory Drug Diversion Programs*. Sydney: National Drug and Alcohol Research Centre.

Hughes, C., Chalmers, J., Bright, D. and McFadden, M. (in press). *Trafficking in Multiple Commodities: Exposing Australia's Poly-drug and Poly-crime Networks. NDLERF Report*. Canberra: National Drug Law Enforcement Research Fund.

Hughes, C. E. and Stevens, A. (2010). What can we learn from the Portuguese decriminalization of illicit drugs? *British Journal of Criminology,* 50(6), 999–1022.

Hughes, C. E., Cowdery, N. and Ritter, A. (2015). Deemed supply in Australian drug trafficking laws: a justifiable legal provision. *Current Issues in Criminal Justice*, 27(1): 1–20.

Human Rights Watch. (2011). *The Rehab Archipelago: Forced Labor and Other Abuses in Drug Detention Centres in Southern Vietnam*. New York: Human Rights Watch.

Iakobishvili, E. (2011). *Inflicting Harm: Judicial Corporal Punishment for Drug and Alcohol Offences in Selected Countries*. London: Harm Reduction International.

Integrated Network for Societal Conflict Research. (2012). *Colombia*.

Inter Ministerial Committee on Drug Control. (2008). *National Drug Control Master Plan (NDCMP): 2008–2011*. National Drug Law Enforcement Agency.

Intergovernmental Committee on Drugs. (2014). *Intergovernmental Committee on Drugs (IGCD): Framework for a National Response to New Psychoactive Substances*. Retrieved from http://www.nationaldrugstrategy.gov.au/internet/drugstrategy/Publishing.nsf/content/F1C8C74524B4A214CA257D0E0017F4CC/$File/NPS%20Framework.pdf.

International Narcotics Control Board. (2014a). *Report of the International Narcotics Control Board for 2013*. New York: United Nations, International Narcotics Control Board.

International Narcotics Control Board. (2014b). *Statement by Dr Lochan Naidoo, President, International Narcotics Control Board. Economic and Social Council high level panel discussion: 'Sustainable Development and the World Drug Problem: Challenges and Opportunities' 15 July 2014, New York*. Vienna: International Narcotics Control Board.

Jardine, M., Crofts, N., Monaghan, G. and Morrow, M. (2012). Harm reduction and law enforcement in Vietnam: influences on street policing. *Harm Reduction Journal*, 9(1): 27.

Kelly, E. and Rasul, I. (2014). Policing cannabis and drug related hospital admissions: evidence from administrative records. *Journal of Public Economics,* 112: 89–114.

Kilmer, B., Caulkins, J. P., Pacula, R. L. and Reuter, P. H. (2012). *The U.S. Drug Policy Landscape: Insights and Opportunities for Improving the View*. Santa Monica: RAND Drug Policy Research Center.

Klantschnig, G. (2009). The politics of law enforcement in Nigeria: lessons from the war on drugs. *The Journal of Modern African Studies,* 47(4): 529–49.

Klantschnig, G. (2011). Nigeria. In M. A. R. Kleiman and J. E. Hawdon (eds), *Encyclopedia of Drug Policy* (Vol. 2). Los Angeles: Sage, pp. 584–5.

Klein, A. (2005). International pressure, drug control and political culture: a comparison between Jamaica and Nigeria. *African Journal of Drug and Alcohol Studies,* 4(1&2): 54–66.

Lancaster, K. (2014). Social construction and the evidence-based drug policy endeavour *International Journal of Drug Policy*, 25(5): 948–51.

Lancaster, K., Hughes, C., Spicer, B., Matthew-Simmons, F. and Dillon, P. (2011). Illicit drugs and the media: models of media effects for use in drug policy research. *Drug and Alcohol Review,* 30(4): 397–402.

Lancaster, K., Ritter, A. and Colebatch, H. (2014). Problems, policy and politics: making sense of Australia's 'ice epidemic'. *Policy Studies* 35(2): 147–71.

Lines, R., Barrett, D. and Gallahue, P. (2010). *Complicity or Abolition: The Death Penalty and International Support for Drug Enforcement*. London: International Harm Reduction Assocation.

Lupu, N. (2004). Towards a new articulation of alternative development: lessons from coca supply reduction in Bolivia. *Development Policy Review,* 22(4): 405–21.

MacCoun, R. and Reuter, P. (2001). *Drug War Heresies: Learning from Other Vices, Times, and Places*. Cambridge: Cambridge University Press.

MacCoun, R., and Reuter, P. (2002). The varieties of drug control at the dawn of the twenty-first century. *Annals of the American Academy of Political and Social Science,* 582(1): 7–19.

MacGregor, S. (2013). Barriers to the influence of evidence on policy: are politicians the problem? *Drugs: Education, Prevention and Policy,* 20: 225–33.

Mannava, P., Zegenhagen, S. and Crofts, N. (2010). *Dependent on Development: The Interrelationships Between Illicit Drugs and Socioeconomic Development*. Melbourne: The Nossal Institute for Global Health.

McFadden, M. (2006). The Australian Federal Police drug harm index: a new methodology for quantifying success in combating drug use. *Australian Journal of Public Administration,* 65: 68–81.

McKenzie, V. (2014). Colombia kicks off 1st clean needle program for drug addicts. July 4, *Colombia Reports*. Retrieved from http://colombiareports.co/colombia-announces-needle-exchange-program/.

McMorris, B. J., Catalano, R. F., Kim, M. J., Toumbourou, J. W. and Hemphill, S. A. (2011). Influence of family factors and supervised alcohol use on adolescent alcohol use and harms: similarities between youth in different alcohol policy contexts. *Journal of Studies on Alcohol and Drugs,* 72(3): 418–28.

Meija, D. (2015). Plan Colombia: an analysis of effectiveness and costs. In V. Felbab-Brown and H. Trinkunas (eds), *Improving Global Drug Policy: Comparative Perspective and UNGASS 2016*. Washington, DC: Brokkings Institution.

Milloy, M. J., Wood, E., Small, W., Tyndall, M., Lai, C., Montaner, J. and Kerr, T. (2008). Incarceration experiences in a cohort of active injection drug users. *Drug and Alcohol Review,* 27(6): 693–9.

Ministerial Committee on Drug Policy. (2007). *National Drug Policy: 2007–2012*. Wellington: Ministry of Health, New Zealand.

Ministerial Council on Drug Strategy. (2011). *National Drug Strategy: 2010–2015*. Canberra: Ministerial Council on Drug Strategy, Australia.

Ministry of Health and Social Affairs. (2011). *A Cohesive Strategy for Alcohol, Narcotic Drugs, Doping and Tobacco (ANDT) Policy: A Summarised Version of Government Bill 2010/11:47*. Stockholm: Ministry of Health and Social Affairs, Sweden.

Ministry of Social Protection. (2007). *National Policy for the Reduction of the Consumption of Psychoactive Substances and their Impact: Executive Summary*. Bogota: Republic of Colombia.

Monaghan, M. (2010). The complexity of evidence: reflections on research utilisation in a heavily politicised policy area. *Social Policy and Society,* 9(1): 1–12.

Monaghan, M. (2012). The recent evolution of UK drug strategies: from maintenance to behaviour change. *People, Place and Policy Online,* 6(1): 29–40.

Monaghan, M. and Wincup, E. (2013). Work and the journey to recovery: exploring the implications of welfare reform for methadone maintenance clients. *International Journal of Drug Policy,* 24(6): e81–6.

NAFDAC. (2014). NAFDAC partners NDLEA on National Drug Control Masterplan. Available from http://www.nafdac.gov.ng/component/k2/item/245-nafdac-partners-ndlea-on-national-drug-control-masterplan.

National Committee on AIDS, Drugs and Prostitute Control of Vietnam. (No date). *Ceremony for the Public Announcement of the Strategy on Preventing, Combating and Controlling Drug Abuse in Vietnam Till 2020 and Orientation Till 2030.*

National Drug Law Enforcement Agency. (2009). *Our Vision, Our Mission.*

NZ Stats. (2014). Adults convicted in court by sentence type – all offence types. Available from http://nzdotstat.stats.govt.nz/wbos/Index.aspx?DataSetCode=TABLECODE7355#.

Obot, I. S. (2004). Assessing Nigeria's drug control policy, 1994–2000. *International Journal of Drug Policy,* 15(1): 17–26.

Observatorio de Drogas de Colombia. (2014). *El Problema de las Drogas en Colombia 2011–2013 Acciones y Resultados.* Observatorio de Drogas de Colombia.

Orange, R. (2013). Sweden closes four prisons as number of inmates plummets. *The Guardian,* November 12. Retrieved from http://www.theguardian.com/world/2013/nov/11/sweden-closes-prisons-number-inmates-plummets.

Pacula, R. L., Kilmer, B., Wagenaar, A. C., Chaloupka, F. J. and Caulkins, J. P. (2014). Developing public health regulations for marijuana: lessons from alcohol and tobacco. *American Journal of Public Health,* 104(6): 1021–8.

Pacula, R. L., Powell, D., Heaton, P., and Sevigny, E. L. (2015). Assessing the effects of medical marijuana laws on marijuana use: the devil is in the details. *Journal of Policy Analysis and Management,* 34(1): 7–31.

Pardo, B. (2014). Cannabis policy reforms in the Americas: a comparative analysis of Colorado, Washington, and Uruguay. *International Journal of Drug Policy,* 25: 727–35.

President Obama. (2015). *Remarks by the President at the NAACP Conference, Pennsylvania Convention Center, Pennsylvania, 14 July*: https://www.whitehouse.gov/the-press-office/2015/07/14/remarks-president-naacp-conference.

Quintero, J. (2012). *Bogota's Medical Care Centres for Drug Addicts (CAMAD): An Initiative Wedged Between Political Discourse and Technical Action, Series on Legislative Reform of Drug Policies Nr. 22.* Amsterdam: Transnational Institute, Drugs and Democracy Programme.

Ramstedt, M. (2006). What drug policies cost. Estimating drug policy expenditures in Sweden, 2002: work in progress. *Addiction,* 101(3): 330–8.

Reid, G., and Higgs, P. (2011). Vietnam moves forward with harm reduction: an assessment of progress. *Global Public Health,* 6(2): 168–80.

Reuter, P. (2013). Why has US drug policy changed so little over 30 years? *Crime and Justice,* 42: 1–66.

Rhodes, T. (2002). The 'risk environment': a framework for understanding and reducing drug-related harm. *International Journal of Drug Policy,* 13(2): 85–94.

Rhodes, T., Lilly, R., Fernández, C., Giorgino, E., Kemmesis, U. E., Ossebaard, H. C., Lalm, N., Faasen, I. and Spannow, K. E. (2003). Risk factors associated with drug use: the importance of 'risk environment'. *Drugs: Education, Prevention and Policy,* 10(4): 303–29.

Ritter, A. (2009). Methods for comparing drug policies - the utility of composite Drug Harm Indexes. *International Journal of Drug Policy,* 20: 475–9.

Ritter, A. (2010). Conceptualising 'balance' in national drug policy *Drug and Alcohol Review,* 29(4): 349–51.

Ritter, A. and Bammer, G. (2010). Models of policy-making and their relevance for drug research. *Drug and Alcohol Review,* 29(4): 352–7.

Ritter, A. and Lancaster, K. (2013). Policy models and influences on policy processes. In A. Ritter, T. King and M. Hamilton (eds), *Drug Use in Australian Society.* South Melbourne: Oxford University Press, pp. 99–132.

Ritter, A., Lancaster, K., Grech, K. and Reuter, P. (2011). *Monograph No. 21: An assessment of illicit drug policy in Australia (1985–2010): Themes and Trends.* Sydney: National Drug and Alcohol Research Centre.

Ritter, A., McLeod, R. and Shanahan, M. (2013). *Mongraph No. 24: Government Drug Policy Expenditure in Austrralia - 2009/10*. Sydney: National Drug and Alcohol Research Centre.

Rolles, S. (2009). *After the War on Drugs: Blueprint for Regulation*. London: Transform.

Room, R. (2012). *Roadmaps to Reforming the UN Drug Conventions*. Oxford: The Beckley Foundation.

Room, R. (2014). Legalizing a market for cannabis for pleasure: Colorado, Washington, Uruguay and beyond. *Addiction,* 109(3): 345–51.

Room, R. and Reuter, P. (2012). How well do international drug conventions protect public health? *The Lancet,* 279(9810): 84–91.

Rosmarin, A. and Eastwood, N. (2013). *A Quiet Revolution: Drug Decriminalisation Policies in Practice Across the Globe*. London: Release.

Schultze-Kraft, M. (2014). Why a governance perspective could contribute to improving drug policy and engaging the international development community: lessons from Colombia. *International Journal of Drug Policy*, 25: 1038–9.

Scruggs, L. and Allan, J. (2006). Welfare-state decommodification in 18 OECD countries: a replication and revision. *Journal of European Social Policy,* 16(1): 55–72.

Sentencing Council. (2011). *Drug Offences Guideline: Professional Ponsultation*. London: Sentencing Council.

Sentencing Council. (2012). *Drug Offences Definitive Guideline Final*. London: Sentencing Council.

Serviço de Intervenção nos Comportamentos Aditivos e nas Dependências. (2013a). *Plano estratégico 2013–2015*. Lisboa: SICAD.

Serviço de Intervenção nos Comportamentos Aditivos e nas Dependências. (2013b). *Portugal – New Developments, Trends and in-depth information on selected issues – 2013 Draft National Report (2012 data) to the EMCDAA*. Lisbon: EMCDDA.

Sevigny, E. L., Pollack, H. A. and Reuter, P. (2013). Can drug courts help to reduce prison and jail populations? *The Annals of the American Academy of Political and Social Sciences,* 647(1): 190–212.

Simons-Morton, B., Pickett, W., Boyce, W., ter Bogt, T. F. and Vollebergh, W. (2010). Cross-national comparison of adolescent drinking and cannabis use in the United States, Canada, and the Netherlands. *International Journal of Drug Policy,* 21(1): 64–9.

Stevens, A. (2011). *Drugs, Crime and Public Health: The Political Economy of Drug Policy*. Abingdon: Routledge.

Thom, B., Duke, K., Frank, V. A. and Bjerge, B. (2013). Stakeholders in opioid substitution treatment policy: similarities and differences in six European countries. *Substance Use and Misuse,* 48(11): 933–42.

Thoumi, F. E. (2012). Illegal drugs, anti-drug policy failure, and the need for institutional reforms in Colombia. *Substance Use and Misuse,* 47(8-9): 972–1004.

United Nations. (1961). *Single Convention on Narcotic Drugs, as amended by the 1972 protocol*. New York: United Nations.

United Nations. (1971). *Convention on Psychotropic Substances*. New York: United Nations.

United Nations. (1988). *United Nations Convention against the Illicit Traffic in Narcotic Drugs and Psychotropic Substances*. New York: United Nations.

United Nations. (2000). *United Nations Millenium Declaration*: United Nations General Assembly. New York: United Nations.

United Nations. (2014). *Status of treaties: United Nations Convention against Illicit Traffic in Narcotic Drugs and Psychotropic Substances Vienna, 20 December 1988*. New York: United Nations. Available from https://treaties.un.org/Pages/ViewDetails.aspx?src=TREATY&mtdsg_no=VI-19&chapter=6&lang=en#3.

United Nations General Assembly. (1948). *The Universal Declaration of Human Rights G.A. res. 217A (III), U.N. Doc A/810 at 71*. Paris: United Nations.

United Nations General Assembly. (1966). *International Covenant on Economic, Social and Cultural Rights, resolution 2200A (XXI)*. New York: United Nations.

United Nations General Assembly. (1998). *Declaration on the Guiding Principles of Drug Demand Reduction. A/S - 20/11*. Vienna: United Nations.

United Nations Office on Drugs and Crime. (2005). *World Drug Report 2005: Volumes I and II*. Vienna: UNODC.

United Nations Office on Drugs and Crime. (2009). *Political Declaration and Plan of Action on International Cooperation Towards an Inegrated and Balanced Strategy to Counter the World Drug Problem*. New York: United Nations.

United Nations Office on Drugs and Crime. (2013). *Contribution of the Executive Director of the United Nations Office on Drugs and Crime to the high-level review of the implementation of the Political Declaration and Plan of Action on International Cooperation towards an Integrated and Balanced Strategy to Counter the World Drug Problem - UNODC/ED/2014/1*. Vienna: United Nations.

United Nations Office on Drugs and Crime. (2014). *World Drug Report: 2014*. Vienna: United Nations Office on Drugs and Crime.

United States Attorney General. (2013). *Directive of the US Attorney General - Memorandum for all United States Attorneys - Guidance regarding marijuana enforcement*. Washington, DC: United States Department of Justice.

US Congress. (2010). Fair Sentencing Act of 2010 (US). Washington, DC: US Congress.

US Department of Justice. (2013). *Smart of Crime Initiative: Reforming The Criminal Justice System for the 21st Century*. Washington, DC: US Department of Justice.

US Sentencing Commission. (2014). *Media release: US Sentencing Commission Unanimously Votes To Allow Delayed Retroactive Reduction In Drug Trafficking Sentences*. Available from http://www.ussc.gov/sites/default/files/pdf/news/press-releases-and-news-advisories/press-releases/20140718_press_release.pdf.

Veillette, C. and Navarrete-Frías, C. (2005). *Drug Crop Eradication and Alternative Development in the Andes*. Washington, DC: The Library of Congress, Congressional Research Service.

Volkow, N. (2001). *Teacher's Guide: The Essence of Drug Addiction*. Maryland: National Institute of Drug Abuse.

Vuolo, M. (2013). National-level drug policy and young people's illicit drug use: a multilevel analysis of the European Union. *Drug and Alcohol Dependence,* 131(1-3): 149–56.

Vuong, T., Ali, R., Baldwin, S. and Mills, S. (2012). Drug policy in Vietnam: a decade of change? *International Journal of Drug Policy,* 23(4): 319–26.

West Africa Commission on Drugs. (2014). *Not Just in Transit: Drugs the State and Society in West Africa*. West Africa Commission on Drugs.

Wilkins, C., Sheridan, J., Adams, P., Russell, B., Ram, S. and Newcombe, D. (2013). The new psychoactive substances regime in New Zealand: a different approach to regulation. *Journal of Psychopharmacology,* 27(7): 584–9.

Wincup, E. (2014). Thoroughfares, crossroads and cul-de-sacs: drug testing of welfare recipients. *International Journal of Drug Policy*, 25(5): 1031–7.

Windle, J. (2015). A slow march from social evil to harm reduction: drugs and drug policy in Vietnam. In V. Felbab-Brown and H. Trinkunas (eds), *Improving Global Drug Policy: Comparative Perspective and UNGASS 2016*. Washington, DC: Brookings Institution.

Winstock, A. R. and Ramsey, J. D. (2010). Legal highs and the challenges for policy makers. *Addiction*, 105(10): 1685–7.

Wolfe, D. and Saucier, R. (2010). In rehabilitation's name? Ending institutionalised cruelty and degrading treatment of people who use drugs. *International Journal of Drug Policy,* 21(3): 145–8.

World Health Organization. (2012). *WHO Expert Committee on Drug Dependence: Thirty Fifth Report*. Geneva: World Health Organization.

World Health Organization. (2014). *Consolidated Guidelines on HIV Prevention, Diagnosis, Treatment and Care for Key Populations*. Geneva: World Health Organization.

Ysa, T., Colom, J., Albareda, A., Ramon, A., Carrion, M. and Segura, L. (2014). *Governance of Addictions: European Public Policies*. Oxford: Oxford University Press.

Appendix 1 Rates of drug use and drug-related harm

Country	*Drug Use Prevalence (last 12 months) WDR 2014*[1]	*Health Harms*[2] *HIV rate (IDU)* *HCV rate(IDU)* *Drug related mortality (rate per million)*
Australia	Cannabis, 10.3% Cocaine, 2.1% Amphetamine Type Stimulants (ATS), 2.1% Opioids, 3.4% Ecstasy, 3.0%	HIV rate: 1.2% HCV rate: 53% Drug related mortality (rate per million): 88.1
Colombia	Cannabis, 2.27% Cocaine, 0.81% ATS, 0.06% Opioids, 0.02%, Ecstasy, 0.28%	HIV rate: 1.9–3.8% HCV rate: no data Drug related mortality (rate per million): no data
New Zealand	Cannabis, 14.6% Cocaine, 0.6% ATS, 2.1% Opioids, 1.1% Ecstasy, 2.6%	HIV rate: 0.4% HCV rate: 50% Drug related mortality (rate per million): 21.7
Nigeria	Cannabis, 14.3% Cocaine, 0.7% ATS, 1.4% Opioids, 0.7% Ecstasy, no data	HIV rate: 4.2% HCV rate: no data Drug related mortality (rate per million): no data
Portugal	Cannabis, 2.7% Cocaine, 0.2% ATS, 0.2% Opioids, 0.29% Ecstasy, 0.3%	HIV rate: 4.9–16.5% HCV rate: 36.5% Drug related mortality (rate per million): 2.3
Sweden	Cannabis, 3.0% Cocaine, 0.5% ATS, 0.8% Opioids, 0.23% Ecstasy, 0.1%	HIV rate: 4.4% HCV rate: 55.7% Drug related mortality (rate per million): 57.6
UK (England and Wales)	Cannabis, 6.4% Cocaine, 1.9% ATS 0.7% Opioids, 0.76% Ecstasy, 1.3%	HIV rate: 1.2% HCV rate: 43% Drug related mortality (rate per million): 43.6
USA	Cannabis, 14.8% Cocaine, 2.3% ATS, 1.9% Opioids, 6.1% (prescription opioids 5.7%) Ecstasy, 1.2%	HIV rate: 9.0% amongst IDU HCV rate: 73.4% Drug related mortality (rate per million): 192.8
Vietnam	Cannabis, 0.3% Cocaine, no data ATS 0.22% Opioids, 0.53% Ecstasy, 0.22%	HIV rate: 13.4% HCV rate: 74.1% Drug related mortality (rate per million): 35.7

Notes:

[1]Drug use prevalence: taken from World Drug Report (2014) which refers to prevalence estimates from 2012 (or latest available). Annual prevalence rate (not lifetime).

[2]Harm indicators, taken from World Drug Report (2014) for consistency. We acknowledge that other data sources for specific countries may provide more recent findings, but for consistency have chosen the same source across all nine countries. We also acknowledge there are different harms that could have been looked at: e.g. social.

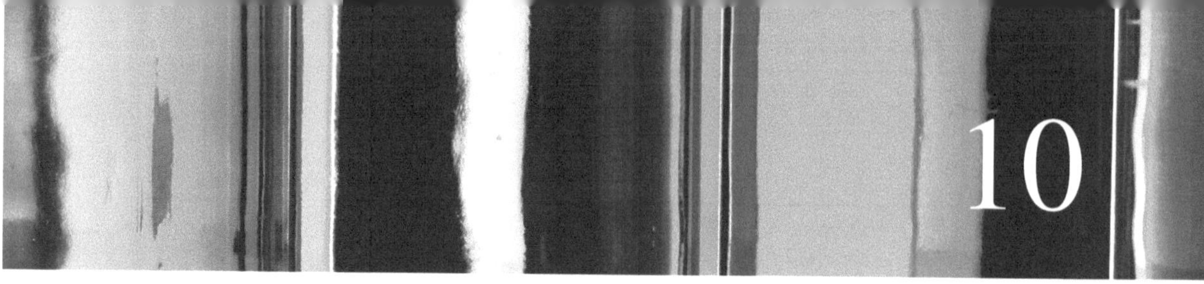

Alcohol Policy in Global Context

James Nicholls

INTRODUCTION

Alcohol has been a feature of human society for millennia; however, its consumption has never been evenly spread globally (Hames, 2012; Phillips, 2014). Both consumption and production of alcohol is higher in Europe than other world regions – a reflection of the long social and cultural history of alcohol in Europe (Anderson et al., 2012: 1; World Health Organization, 2014: 29). By contrast, consumption is low in the Middle East, North Africa and areas of the developing world where alcohol plays a less important role in cultural practices, is proscribed for religious reasons or where poverty or limited availability constrains use. There have been significant recent increases in alcohol consumption in China and the Far East, where urbanisation, an expanding middle class and targeted market expansion by established global producers have led to steep rises in the consumption of wine, beer and, in particular, spirits (World Health Organization, 2014).

Alcohol consumption is far less commonplace globally than it tends to appear from a western perspective. In 2014, while average annual consumption globally was 6.2 litres per person aged 15 or above, 61.7 per cent of the world's population in that age group had not drunk any alcohol at all in the preceding 12 months and 48 per cent are lifetime abstainers (World Health Organization, 2014: 33). Furthermore, 'the greater the economic wealth of a country, the more alcohol is consumed and the smaller the number of abstainers', with high-income countries having 'the highest per capita consumption and the highest prevalence of heavy episodic drinking among drinkers' (World Health Organization, 2014: xiv). Importantly, global regions with the highest levels of heavy episodic drinking are not always the same as those with highest overall consumption: in global data, 'there is no consistent association between total APC [adult per capita consumption] and the prevalence of HED [heavy episodic drinking] among drinkers' (World Health

Organization, 2014: 34). This highlights the variability of drinking patterns and behaviours across different countries – sometimes characterised as a distinction between 'wet' and 'dry' drinking cultures. In this characterisation, 'wet' cultures are those (such as in most Mediterranean regions) where drinking tends to occur regularly, with high overall levels but low prevalence of drunkenness, and consequently, fewer formal legislative controls. 'Dry' cultures are those where drinking is less regular, lower in absolute terms, but characterised by greater social acceptability of 'explosive' drunkenness – leading, in turn, to stricter regulatory efforts to curb alcohol harms (Room, 1989). While this binary framework is useful in broad, heuristic terms, it should be noted that the twentieth century was characterised by a high degree of convergence, with many 'dry' cultures adopting elements of routine drinking associated with 'wet' cultures, and – more recently – increased levels of binge drinking in many countries, such as France, conventionally seen as paradigmatically 'wet' (Järvinen and Room, 2007).

Alcohol has always been a popular drug in Europe and since the late middle ages its production has been increasingly industrialised and commercialised – making an ever-wider range of drinks available to consumers across different social classes (Kümin and Tlusty, 2002; Phillips, 2014). This culture of widespread consumption was exported to the Americas and colonies that were settled by Europeans from the sixteenth century onwards. However, many regions of the world retained, until recently, drinking cultures centred either around local, informal production or concentrated among social elites and special occasions (Hames, 2012). A key goal of global alcohol producers is to increase sales by promoting European styles of both routine and celebratory drinking in developing markets. This globalisation of European styles of drinking, driven by both cultural globalisation and the efforts of producers, poses significant problems regarding regulation. Should developing countries be prevented from adopting heavier-drinking cultures in order to protect public health? What constraints do governments across the world face when seeking to regulate an industry that is well-financed and highly resistant to legislative controls? What is the role of transnational policymaking in this context and what aspects of policy remain the proper domain of local governance reflecting local social and cultural contexts? According to the World Health Organization (WHO):

> Alcohol policies aim to minimize the health and social harms that arise from the use of alcohol. Since alcohol is not an ordinary commodity, these policies need to address market failures by seeking to deter children from using alcohol, protecting people who are not drinking from the harm drinking can cause, and providing all customers with information about alcohol's effects. (World Health Organization Europe, 2009: np)

Arguably, this is a narrow definition focussing only on the role of policy in tackling the negative consequences of alcohol consumption. Taken more broadly, alcohol policies – and policies relating directly or indirectly to alcohol – encompass a wide array of activities: ranging from the raising of state revenues through taxation to economic development at a local level through licensing and planning controls. Alcohol policies, as conceived by governments, are often designed to reduce harms – and most countries have clear policies on underage consumption, drink-driving and so forth – but also to support industry, employment and the rights of individuals to consume alcohol in ways that do not harm others. Indeed, alcohol policy development is very often a trade-off between the reduction of health and social order harms, consideration of economic impacts and the protection of personal freedom. Much policy discourse revolves around the relationship between these three factors, and is shaped by interpretations of evidence, political considerations and the interests of different stakeholders.

NATIONAL, REGIONAL AND GLOBAL ALCOHOL STRATEGIES

Historically, alcohol policy has been set at national and local levels. However, the World Health Organization has had a long-standing interest in alcohol issues, and from the early 1970s moved towards the adoption of the 'public health perspective' on alcohol policy that had been developed by Nordic researchers such as Kettil Bruun in the late 1960s. A key principle of public health perspectives on alcohol policy was to develop policies that operated across whole populations, rather than targeting subgroups of problematic drinkers *within* any given population. Public health policy advocacy was, from the start, international in scope: the first key articulation of this approach, *Alcohol Control Policies in Public Health Perspective* (Bruun et al., 1975), was a collaboration between the Finnish Foundation for Alcohol Studies and the Addiction Research Foundation of Ontario supported by the World Health Organization's European office, and subsequent iterations drew in researchers from across the globe (Edwards et al., 1994; Babor et al., 2010). A 1980 WHO expert committee report on alcohol problems endorsed both the analysis of alcohol harms at the core of the public health perspective and the kind of 'whole population' policy interventions on availability and pricing which public health advocates advanced (World Health Organization, 1980). The adoption of the public health perspective by the WHO created a key platform for this policy approach and also encouraged the development of large bodies of international comparative data on consumption, harms and policy impacts.

The WHO position on alcohol policy has been clarified in a series of policy statements and action plans. In 1993, the World Health Organization Regional Office for Europe published a European Alcohol Action Plan calling for focussed national policies aimed at reducing overall consumption in member states. In 1995, it formalised its call for the adoption of whole population-oriented national strategies with the publication of a European Charter on Alcohol. This outlined five ethical goals and ten 'strategies for action', including the development of national targets, restrictions on price and availability and further controls on alcohol marketing (World Health Organization Europe, 1993, 1995). In 2001, the Charter was reaffirmed with a special focus on the need to reduce alcohol consumption among young people (World Health Organization Europe, 2001). The European Action Plan was further updated in 2000 and in 2012, in each case maintaining calls for national alcohol strategies and the overall goal of reducing consumption across the population through policies targeted at price, availability and marketing as well as drink-driving and the wider adoption of screening and brief advice in primary care (World Health Organization Europe, 2000, 2012).

At the 58th World Health Assembly in 2005, the World Health Organization adopted a resolution calling for all member states to 'develop, implement and evaluate effective strategies and programmes for reducing the negative and social consequences of the harmful use of alcohol' (World Health Organization, 2005). Six years later, following a resolution at the 63rd World Health Assembly, the WHO published its *Global Strategy to Reduce the Harmful Use of Alcohol*. It called for greater international cooperation on the grounds that 'national and local efforts can produce better results when they are supported by regional and global action within agreed policy frames'. It also established objectives to raise global awareness and knowledge on alcohol harms, and to improve international partnerships and systems for developing policy advocacy (World Health Organization, 2011: 8). The Strategy calls for international action on alcohol pricing, availability and marketing, as well as the enforcement of laws on drink driving, better identification and treatment of at-risk drinkers, and more coordinated data-gathering. For its part, the WHO commits to provide leadership in the development of, and advocacy for, public health-oriented alcohol policies.

In Europe, there has been a long-term trend towards more restrictive alcohol policies in areas such as drink-driving and underage consumption (Anderson and Baumberg, 2006: 391). However, this has gone hand-in-hand with a trend towards economic liberalisation, which has tended to make alcohol more widely available and more affordable. Concerns over the impact of alcohol on society across Europe, as well as the activities of the WHO and advocacy groups, contributed to the development, in 2006, of the first EU-wide alcohol strategy (Commission of the European Communities, 2006); although this was viewed by many within the public health community as adopting approaches (such as industry partnerships and education campaigns) that were less effective than the supply-side controls favoured by the WHO and alcohol control advocates. In 2015, it was announced that the EU Alcohol Strategy, which had expired in 2013, would not be renewed. Nevertheless, there remain concerted calls from public health bodies across Europe for a revised Strategy to be adopted.

Recognition of the need for national and regional strategic approaches to alcohol policy is not confined to Europe. Regional strategies or plans of action have been adopted in the WHO Western Pacific Region, the Regional Committee for Africa and the Pan American Health Organization's Directing Council (World Health Organization, 2014: 24). However, the development of national strategies has been the source of controversy in some areas. For instance, there have been widespread claims that the development of national alcohol strategies in a number of sub-Saharan countries has been unduly influenced by major alcohol industry organisations including the brewer SABMiller (Babor et al., 2015). According to one study, the strategies produced by four African Governments (Lesotho, Malawi, Uganda and Botswana) were very similar in content to a document provided by SABMiller following a regional policy workshop (Bakke and Endal, 2010). The authors conclude that direct industry involvement in the development of national alcohol strategies in this region 'points to the likelihood that this was spurred by the new alcohol initiative at WHO in 2005. This may represent an attempt to establish policies on that continent before any WHO recommendations have the chance to influence the content of those policies' (Bakke and Endal, 2010: 27).

The move towards an approach based on regional strategies and international frameworks has very significant implications for alcohol policy development. In this context (as discussed in more detail below), the tension between public health and industry advocates has been heightened. At stake is the broad direction of global alcohol policy over the forthcoming decades, and for many, the choice appears to be between a laissez-faire approach that affords the alcohol industry maximal freedom at the cost of widespread social harms and a public health-oriented approach which places health promotion and risk-reduction at the heart of all policymaking, even where that may impinge on other personal freedoms. Whether the reality is quite that stark, given the enormous variations of policy and culture within countries, is less clear.

COMPARING ALCOHOL POLICIES BY COUNTRY

Alcohol policies vary considerably between countries, making it difficult to compare their impacts. At the time of writing, an international study to compare the impact of alcohol policies in different countries is underway, although cross-national findings remain to be published (Casswell et al., 2012). A number of researchers have, however, developed comparative scales against which to measure national policies in key areas, which can then be mapped against consumption and harm trends (see, e.g. Karlsson and Österberg, 2007; Babor et al., 2010: 243–8; Giesbrecht et al., 2013; Nelson et al., 2013; Naimi et al., 2014). Such studies generally score restrictive policies on availability, price and marketing highly while awarding lower scores to policies involving education, public awareness or voluntary trade agreements. In a 2012 analysis, Karlsson et al. divided the European area into four (Nordic, East, West and Southern Europe) and found that Nordic regions had both the most restrictive policies and some of the lowest levels of consumption – suggesting a relationship between the two. However, as Eisenbach-Stangl (2011) has pointed out, such scales tend to evaluate policies against an ideal strongly based on Nordic approaches, so it is perhaps to be expected that Scandinavian countries would achieve the highest scores [though recent American cross-state comparisons have found similar results (Erickson et al., 2014)]. Furthermore, while Southern Europe received the lowest policy score, it also had the second lowest level of consumption – suggesting that cultural factors are also key.

The role of cultural factors has been highlighted in a number of recent studies. One analysis of the consistent fall in alcohol consumption in Italy from the 1960s identified cultural changes as central to consumption trends in that country and concluded that 'alcohol policies had no role in drinking changes in Italy between 1960 and 1988, while they had a minor role in supporting the on-going decline thereafter' (Allamani et al., 2014b: 1660). Policy changes in Italy changes included the standardisation of VAT rates on all alcohol products in 1999, the introduction of a blood alcohol limit of 0.8 grams per litre for driving in 1988 and a further reduction to 0.5 in 2001, and new controls on the sale of alcohol at public events (Allamani et al., 2010). By contrast, in response to high and increasing levels of consumption, the Russian government introduced a suite of strict control policies in 2006. These included significant increases in licensing costs, tightened controls of production monitoring, a ban on unlicensed retail, and restrictions on where products above 15 per cent alcohol by volume (ABV) could be sold (Levintova, 2007). Subsequent analysis suggests the Russian policy intervention contributed to a steep decline in both alcohol poisoning and liver cirrhosis deaths (Pridemore et al., 2014). In Italy, then, gradual policy changes in the context of a cultural shift towards lower consumption made little apparent difference; in Russia sweeping changes in the context of very high consumption had a more dramatic effect.

International policy comparison is, therefore, complicated by the reality that alcohol policies operate within local drinking cultures, and, therefore, both reflect those cultures and have different effects depending on how those cultures shape existing drinking practices. As Bendtsen et al. put it, 'alcohol policies might be a response to adult drinking patterns or adult drinking patterns may influence the alcohol control policies' (2014: 1865). Nordlund (2014) notes that alcohol policies tend to be stricter in cultures traditionally more tolerant of heavy episodic drinking and public drunkenness, and vice versa. He proposes two ways of understanding the relationship between social norms and formal alcohol policies in different countries: first, a 'congruence hypothesis', suggesting that 'restrictive norms lead to restrictive policy and liberal norms lead to liberal policy', and second, a 'complementary hypothesis' in which 'the informal rules in some countries are very liberal so that alcohol policy must be restrictive in order to keep the alcohol problems at an acceptable level' (2014: 25–6). As Eisenbach-Stangl notes, there may also be a cultural bias here, as '"strict" controls are favoured in European cultures with less integrated alcohol consumption and – not accidentally – well-established alcohol research' (2011: 5).

The relationship between policy and culture is dynamic and often unpredictable: sometimes culture responds to policy, while at other times policy responds to changes in cultural norms. Furthermore, 'unplanned' variables (such as urbanisation or changing gender politics) appear to have a far higher correlation to changes in consumption patterns than alcohol policy changes (Allamani et al., 2012; Knibbe et al., 2014; Voller et al., 2014). The fact that this dynamic relationship cannot be easily reduced to a unidirectional causal process is, however, not a reason to sideline policy. While it is clear that 'neither imposed control policies nor changing socioeconomic factors exist in isolation' (Plant et al., 2014: 1586), policy is one of the few directly modifiable factors in this complex relationship. Therefore, whatever the limitations of policy impacts across different regions, it retains an important role in shaping behaviours and attitudes.

GLOBAL ALCOHOL POLICY: KEY INSTRUMENTS OF CONTROL

The alcohol market is regulated through a number of policy instruments, but these can be categorised according to a relatively limited number of areas:

- Availability: the retail accessibility of alcohol can be regulated through licensing, state monopolies or degrees of prohibition.
- Pricing: the costs of alcohol production and retail can be managed through taxation, import/export duties and statutory minimum retail prices.
- Marketing: many countries have regulations on where, how and in what forms alcohol can be advertised, whether alcohol companies can sponsor sports and other cultural events and what kinds of point-of-sale promotions may be used.
- Age: most countries have restrictions on the minimum purchase age for alcohol and the minimum age for alcohol consumption. Often these are the same, but in some case (as in the UK) they can differ widely.
- Drink-driving: restrictions on blood alcohol levels for driving exist in most countries, though they vary. There are also often restrictions on blood alcohol content for the use of other vehicles or machinery.

The remainder of this chapter will consider the first three of these instruments: availability, pricing and marketing controls. While consensus has largely been reached on the principles (if not the details) of controls on drink-driving and underage purchase, the remaining three remain the subject of intense debate as health advocates seek to promote control policies based on their greater restriction in the face of intense resistance from the alcohol industry.

Availability controls

Recent pan-European analysis found policies that increase the availability of alcohol are 'associated with increased consumption, especially at their initial introduction, in those countries that had a tradition of restrictive measures' (Allamani et al., 2014a). This accords with the general observation from international studies that increased availability is associated with increased consumption (Babor et al., 2010), while – looking at the reverse – there is 'slight evidence that on average introducing restrictive availability can be associated with decreasing consumption' (Baccini and Carreras, 2014: 1689). Cross-country comparisons highlight the fact that the impact of availability controls on consumption is mediated by existing drinking cultures, prevalence of different types of outlet and the degree to which policy changes represent a departure from existing practice. For instance, in regions of Africa with weak availability controls improved regulation may shift (rather than necessarily reduce) purchasing from informal suppliers – often women for whom brewing has historically provided a key source of income – to corporate brewers and retailers (Adelekan, 2008:

5). Importantly, any analysis of availability also needs to note that it is not a singular measure: 'availability' encompasses the general number of outlets across jurisdictions, changes in types of outlet (e.g. between bars and shops), density of outlets in specific areas and the hours during which retail is permitted (Holmes et al., 2014).

The most commonplace instrument for controlling the physical availability of alcohol is licensing. Licensing systems vary, but operate on the fundamental principle that the right to sell alcohol is constrained by the acquisition of a licence to do so from (usually) local authorities. Those authorities are empowered to either reject licence applications or to place conditions on applications that are accepted. While working within broadly similar frameworks – specifically regulating numbers of outlets in a given area, the hours of day during which alcohol sales are able to take place, and the conditions of sale in any given outlet – licensing systems can vary significantly between countries and, in federal systems such as the United States, Canada and Australia, between states and territories. Key variations tend to be whether there are instruments for limiting the density of outlets (such as the facility for considering 'overprovision' in Scottish licensing), whether there are fixed, staggered or zoned opening hours, whether there are requirements for server training and the extent to which licensing authorities are empowered to consider wider health or social harms in their decision-making. A further difference between jurisdictions is also whether off-sales (that is, sales in shops and supermarkets) fall within licensing controls at all. In Germany and Spain, for instance, only on-sales (that is, pubs, bars and so forth) are licensed.

Underpinning licensing is the principle that alcohol retail is a legitimate activity, albeit one that can only be carried out under conditions set by local authorities. Locally, the use of licensing conditions (which may include requirements regarding staff training, numbers of seats, use of CCTV, etc.) can lead to enormous variations in practice. The strictness of the conditions applied may vary by area and circumstance, as may the effectiveness of enforcement regimes (Valverde, 2003). Between national jurisdictions, differences tend to lie in the framework governing licensing practice: issues such as whether licensing authorities should disincentivise applications from particular types of outlets, what evidence they should consider or what role health harms should play in their considerations. In England and Wales, for instance, the only harms licensing authorities can consider are strictly limited to social disorder, child protection, public safety and public nuisance. In many Australian states and territories, by contrast, licensing authorities have a statutory obligation to consider how their decisions will contribute to the minimisation of alcohol-related harm more broadly – though requirements on other key issues, such as permitted trading hours, vary across the country (Davoren and O'Brien, 2014; Howard et al., 2014). The realities of local discretion, and the constant threat of legal challenge from alcohol retailers, means that such obligations are implemented in variable ways, demonstrating that within the broad principle of licensing different nuances and practice frameworks apply.

An alternative method for controlling physical availability is the establishment of state monopolies, such as exist in a number of Nordic countries as well as some American and Canadian states. In this instance, part or all of the wholesale and retail trades are owned by national or state companies. While state ownership of the wholesale trade has implications for revenue generation, it is through the ownership of retail outlets that both the extent and nature of availability can be controlled (Her et al., 1999). In most instances, monopolies are limited to the 'off' sale of alcohol being carried on through state-run outlets such as the 'system bolaget' in Sweden or the Liquor Control Board of Ontario (LCBO) outlets in Canada. Monopolies may cover all alcohol, or just specific beverages: in North America, for example, state monopolies vary between those covering wine and spirits or spirits-only and those covering wholesale only or both wholesale and retail outlets (Alcohol Research Group, 2011).

Studies comparing monopolies with licensed, private retail systems point to some consistent patterns in regard to market effects. The replacement of monopolies by licensed, private sales usually leads to a steep increase in the number of outlets; however, the effect on consumption and price has tended to be variable. A review by Her at al. (1999) found strong evidence of short-term increases in consumption following privatisation, but with this effect sometimes levelling off after a few years. However, a review by Hahn et al. found 'the privatization of retail alcohol sales was associated with a substantial increase in per capita sales of privatized beverages' (2012: 425). In the American examples, this was mostly driven by significantly increased wine sales that brought wine consumption in previously monopolised states closer to the national averages (Cook, 2012). Studies of privatisation in American states also found that while price may be expected to fall in a private market, countervailing factors (such as wages paid to shop workers, which tend to be higher in monopolies) means that, in most cases, prices actually rise – though revenues to the state often fall (Flanagan, 2003; Hahn et al., 2012). This may partially explain why the increased availability that follows privatisation does not lead to predictable increases in consumption.

The history of monopoly systems is an early example of transnational policy influence. Originally developed in the Swedish city of Gothenburg in the 1850s, the idea of local municipalities taking control of the alcohol trade aroused significant interest in the UK and went on to influence the activities of the Central Control Board (CCB), which was established in 1915 to oversee the liquor trade in the UK during World War 1 (Greenaway 2003; Nicholls, 2009; Duncan, 2014). In some areas, the CCB took control of the trade and introduced principles of salaried management and simple pub design based on Gothenburg principle. The work of the CCB in the UK would go on to influence the work of similar controls boards elsewhere, such as the LCBO, who sought to create an alcohol retail environment which, through design and regulation, would create a drinking culture based on rational refreshment rather than hedonistic pleasure (Malleck, 2013). While now limited mainly to Scandinavia, North America and Canada, the monopoly system remains a viable model of alcohol control – and one whose influence is bolstered by the fact that there is often a high concentration of alcohol research activity in areas where monopolies exist (especially where such research is funded by those monopolies).

Pricing controls

While the physical and temporal availability is an important driver of levels and patterns of consumption, a critical influence on consumption is the cost of alcohol to the consumer. Although estimates vary as to the precise degree of influence pricing changes have on purchasing patterns, the weight of evidence shows that alcohol consumers are responsive to price – though, importantly, one study of historical trends in 12 European countries 'was not able to find any relevance of price impacting on alcoholic beverage consumption' (Allamani et al., 2014a: 1707). Because alcohol is taxed at a number of points between production and consumption, this potentially gives governments leverage over the shape and scale of the alcohol market. However, alcohol taxation has, historically, rarely been used as a mechanism for shaping consumption trends; rather, it has tended to been used to ensure maximum revenue to the state from the alcohol trade. This has not meant universally high taxation, as the level of income generated per unit of alcohol needs to be balanced against the risk that excessive taxation will encourage illicit production or a black market in retail.

The complexity, and inconsistency, of alcohol taxation policies can be illustrated through an examination of taxation structures within the European Union. The European Union area contains the highest levels of per capita consumption in the world (though the very highest levels tend to be concentrated in eastern Europe and Russia). However, EU alcohol tax structures allow significant variation both within and between alcohol beverage categories, which makes efforts to use taxation as a means of reducing consumption especially difficult. For example, around half of EU countries do not levy any tax on wine – largely to protect national producers. Furthermore, where member states do tax wine, the level cannot vary between wine that is 1.2 per cent and 15 per cent ABV, therefore, precluding the use of tax incentives to produce lower alcohol products. By contrast, EU beer taxes are set by ABV so can be used to incentivise the production of beer with less alcohol content, especially as beer of less than 2.8 per cent ABV can be removed from tax entirely. Again, beer taxation levels vary enormously within the EU reflecting both local drinking cultures, the power of regional producers and levels of public and political concern around alcohol consumption (Cnossen, 2006; Österberg, 2011). Because changes to the key directives that govern alcohol taxation across the EU require unanimous agreement from member states, it is very unlikely that this variable (and now dated, as minimum thresholds were set in 1993) system will change.

Inconsistency in alcohol taxation systems is not unique to Europe. In Australia, beer and spirits are taxed by alcohol strength, but wine is taxed by retail value. The consequence of this is that higher strength wines can be taxed at a lower level if (as is the case with, for instance, cask wines) their retail price is lower. In effect, this incentivises the production of high-strength, mass-production cheap wine (Allen Consulting, 2011). The application of volumetric taxes (based only on volume of product), specific taxes based on alcohol content per litre or ad valorem taxes based on retail value (irrespective of strength) has profound implications for the prices consumers pay for alcohol of different strengths. Combined with the enormous range in levels of taxation applied even where the framework is the same (as is the case for beer taxation in Europe, for instance) this leads to relative alcohol prices varying significantly by country. In some instances, this can lead to issues of cross-border importation: in 2004, for example, Finland reduced its alcohol taxes to tackle cross-border importation from neighbouring states with lower tax levels (Mäkelä and Österberg, 2009). Similarly, very high taxes can encourage illicit alcohol production, which is currently estimated to account for around a quarter of all global alcohol consumption (World Health Organization, 2014: 30–1).

As is the case for most commodities, alcohol purchasing is price-responsive: as the price rises, sales tend to fall and vice versa. A key question, however, is how responsive it is and whether this applies the same way to different drinks and different sets of consumers. For instance, would a 10 per cent increase in the price of wine have the same effect as a 10 per cent increase on spirits? And do people who drink heavily respond in the same way to increases as people who only drink occasionally? For economists, this is a question of ‘price elasticity of demand’ (PED): the relative impact price changes have on particular products among particular sets of consumers. If changes in price are estimated to have no or relatively small effects on purchasing, then a product is said to be price ‘inelastic’; by contrast, if price changes have large effects on purchasing then the product is ‘elastic’. A key question for pricing policy research is whether, and to what extent, alcoholic beverages are elastic (Wagenaar at al., 2009; Fogarty, 2010; Sousa, 2014). As with all other alcohol policy questions, however, the way ‘people react to changes in alcohol prices will…be different in different countries and time periods, depending on the prevailing social, cultural and economic circumstances determining the role of alcoholic beverages in the society' (Österberg, 2011: 128).

As with policies discussed previously, the relationship between price and consumption is not uniform: rather it varies according to cultural and economic contexts. Where sudden and dramatic reductions in alcohol duties have been implemented, these have often been followed by spikes in consumption. For example, when Finland reduced its alcohol excise duty rates by a third, in 2004, it led to a consumption increase of around 10 per cent (Mäkelä and Österberg, 2009). A similar increase was found when wine and beer taxes were abolished in Hong Kong in 2008 (Chung et al., 2013). In Mediterranean countries, by contrast, where wine consumption was very high in the early part of the century, urbanisation and changing drinking trends have led to falls in wine-drinking and, in some cases, the substitution of wine for beer – which has a lower alcoholic content. In some parts of Europe, spirits consumption has increased considerably when its relative price has fallen. In Scotland, vodka sales are now far higher than 'traditional' whisky (Beeston et al., 2013). In Poland, spirits consumption fell between 1980 and 2000, but began to rise steeply during the 2000s – a shift that has been linked by one analyst to the effects of a 30 per cent cut in duties in imported spirits in 2002 (Zatoński, 2014).

Overall then, the relationship between pricing and consumption, as with availability is complex, varied and hard to predict at a global level. When analysed in detail, the levels of variability are significant with responses to price changes differing by income, patterns of consumption, nationality, region and preferred beverage. Nevertheless, when considered broadly, there is consensus among both the alcohol industry and alcohol control advocates that higher prices generally lead to a reduction in demand – even if this is not evenly spread across the population. Because alcohol industries generally aim to increase demand, while alcohol control advocates generally seek to reduce it, the two are largely at loggerheads over this issue.

Marketing controls

The alcohol industry has always been at the forefront of developments in marketing. The first trademark to be registered in the UK was the famous red triangle used to market Bass beer in 1876 (Cornell 2003: 152). In Ireland, Guinness first used the 'Brian Boru' harp on their bottles in 1862, thereby establishing an international brand association with Irish history and myth that persists to this day (despite stout being a beer style invented in London in the late eighteenth century). In 1930s America, Seagram were quick to respond to the repeal of Prohibition by marketing their whiskies as a source of responsible drinking (Jacobson, 2012). In the 2000s, alcohol manufacturers were quick to shift marketing spend to social media and quickly became some of the most successful brands on social network sites (Chester et al., 2010). Whether press, television, billboard or, more recently, social media marketing, the alcohol industry has consistently been at the vanguard of development and innovation.

While the claim is regularly made that alcohol marketing is aimed only at shifting brand allegiance within a static market, few seriously accept that the goal is not also to grow – or at the very least – sustain the market for alcohol (Nicholls, 2012a). Although increased profits from fewer sales can be achieved by the premiumisation of products in mature markets, it remains the case that in those regions well over 50 per cent of alcohol is consumed by those drinking at the highest levels, and most alcohol sold is at the cheaper end of the market (see, for example, Meier et al., 2009). Maintaining and expanding this capacity is critical, and marketing plays a fundamental role in supporting this. For this reason, alcohol control advocates seeking to reduce overall levels of consumption identify marketing (along with price and availability) as one of the three key areas for state regulation. Restrictions on marketing, so they argue, are essential to curbing or reducing alcohol use overall (Babor et al., 2010: 185–98). Therefore, there has been extensive international advocacy in recent years for greater controls on alcohol marketing, including global policies modelled on the UN's Framework Convention on Tobacco Control (Casswell and Maxwell, 2005; Casswell, 2012; Burns, 2013).

In a globalised media environment, alcohol marketing policy inevitably takes on an international dimension. This is especially the case in an era of digital communications, when viral marketing campaigns can easily achieve global reach and when social media allows for the line between official marketing and user-generated endorsements to become increasingly blurred (Nicholls, 2012b; McCreanor et al., 2013; Purves et al., 2015). Nevertheless, marketing restrictions tend to operate at a national level with only limited consistency across borders. This situation is complicated by the extensive use of voluntary, self-regulatory codes of marketing developed by alcohol industry bodies to prevent more formal modes of control. Some of these codes are transnational, especially where they are codes specific to individual companies, while others are applicable within single nations (see, for example, Diageo 2012; SABMiller, 2014).

Self-regulatory advertising codes developed by the alcohol industry follow a consistent pattern: placing restrictions on marketing that is aimed explicitly at children or that explicitly encourages irresponsible consumption. However, as underage purchasing is already illegal in most countries, codes targeting this merely reaffirm compliance with the spirit of the law. Furthermore, it has never been a convention that alcohol marketing explicitly advertises the fact that alcohol can get drinkers drunk: this has historically been avoided, and few examples exist where that convention has been broken (Dade, 2008). Hence, sceptics view self-regulatory codes as merely providing grounds for preventing stricter formal regulations that might restrict more fundamental marketing practices – such as striving to associate alcohol with all forms of celebration, encouraging alcohol consumption as part of a daily routine, linking alcohol with sport, music or other aspects of popular culture and linking alcohol brands with social success (Alcohol Concern, 2014).

The power of alcohol marketing on the global stage was clearly illustrated in the run-up to the 2014 Football World Cup in Brazil. In 2003, the Brazilian Government banned the sale of alcohol at football matches in an effort to curb violence. In 2012, however, FIFA demanded that the law be suspended for the duration of the World Cup. On a visit to stadiums under preparation, the General Secretary of FIFA stated that 'alcoholic drinks are part of the World Cup, so we're going to have them…the fact that we have the right to sell beer has to be part of the law' (BBC Online, 2012). It was clearly significant that Budweiser beer, produced by the transnational brewer AB-InBev, was one of the major sponsors of the competition (Gornall, 2014). Subsequently, the Brazilian Government succumbed and overturned the ban on alcohol in sports stadia. The success AB-InBev achieved in having national legislation overturned in order to facilitate alcohol marketing at a premier global sporting event illustrates how global alcohol, sports and media interests can even override national legislation when marketing is fundamentally threatened.

A contrary example, however, is the so-called *Loi Evin* passed in France in 1991. This banned alcohol adverts on television or in cinemas as well as any sponsorship of sporting or cultural events. Furthermore, it allowed adverts only to describe the main qualities of the product (such as origin and composition) and required health information to be included on all marketing messages (Regaud and Craplet, 2004). The actual effect of the *Loi Evin* remains unclear: it has not been systematically evaluated and while alcohol consumption has fallen since it was introduced, this is the continuation of a much longer-term trend (House of Commons Health Committee, 2010: 76). Nevertheless, while vehemently opposed by the alcohol industry, the *Loi Evin* has not been challenged at a transnational level and is not in breach of any international conventions. Unlike Brazil, which, despite being a fast-growing economy, remains a relatively small player on the global stage politically, France has been able to assert its national intentions in regard to alcohol marketing despite opposition from the industry. The *Loi Evin* provides one example of the extent to which national governments remain able, where they have the economic and political capacity, to establish strict controls on international alcohol marketing. However, the example of Brazil shows that such autonomy may, as yet, remain the preserve of the wealthier nations.

The precise mechanisms by which marketing affects behaviour are difficult to identify. It is especially difficult to demonstrate in a natural setting how a marketing message might lead to a direct change in behaviour. This is not necessarily because such effects do not exist, but because such effects are almost impossible to test in realistic environments. A much more likely effect is the reinforcement and 'cultivation' of attitudes towards alcohol that encourage its use (Hastings et al., 2005; Ruddock, 2013). Those cultural attitudes may include the assumption that non-drinking is abnormal; that alcohol is central to social pleasure; that it is the primary indicator of celebration and so forth. Two systematic reviews have provided evidence that exposure to advertising in youth is associated with a lower age of a first drink and higher levels of consumption once drinking begins (Anderson et al., 2009; Smith and Foxcroft, 2009); however, a 2014 Cochrane review of advertising bans found no 'clear effect either for or against banning or restriction of alcohol advertising' (Siegfried et al., 2014: 3). In reality, the evidence on the precise effects of alcohol marketing – despite numerous studies in a number of international settings – remains mixed. There is certainly evidence of some measurable effect among some populations, but searching for compelling scientific proof that a given marketing message changes behaviour may be chimerical. The best evidence is, most likely, the amount that producers and retailers are prepared to spend on marketing globally: their clear and unambiguous belief that marketing is at the heart of sales expansion may be circumstantial, but no less compelling for that.

GLOBAL CHALLENGES AND DEBATES

Despite having been at the forefront of developments in technology, logistics, retail and marketing for centuries, the alcohol industry has only recently become globalised. The development of transnational corporations such as AB-InBev, SABMiller and Diageo, and the amalgamation and incorporation of regional industries by those conglomerates, has created an environment in which alcohol policy increasingly works on a global level (Jernigan, 2009). By contrast, the alcohol control movement was one of the first social movements to adopt a global vision. The early temperance movement moved from America to Europe, via the UK, where developments such as total abstinence were created and exported back to America – and returned again in the form of prohibitionism (Nicholls, 2009). Not only were temperance ideas transatlantic from the 1820s onwards, the temperance movement as a whole became increasingly international through the nineteenth century and early twentieth centuries (Berridge, 2005). To give just one example, The Order of Good Templars – a temperance society founded in New York State in 1851 – was brought to the UK in 1868 and had, by the end of the century, established lodges in mainland Europe (especially Sweden),

Australia and New Zealand, South America, Africa and the Far East. Today, renamed the International Organisation of Good Templars (or IOGT International), it remains a key voice in global alcohol control advocacy and it is closely linked to leading advocacy groups such as the Global Alcohol Policy Alliance (Rutherford, n.d.; Fahey, 2003).

The local, national and global have, therefore, always intersected in alcohol policy debates. Historically, this involved local and national trade interests challenging policy ideas developed by increasingly transnational alcohol control advocacy organisations. Today, trade interests are increasingly a global affair: not only in the form of transnational producers, but also in the emergence of transnational trade defence organisations such as Spirits Europe, as well as international corporate social responsibility alliances such as the International Center for Alcohol Policies – renamed, in 2014, the International Alliance for Responsible Drinking. Despite fierce internal competition, the protection of key trade objectives – especially the prevention of restrictive national legislation that may create precedents internationally – has become a global issue. Similarly, alcohol control advocacy is increasingly characterised by the establishment of transnational coalitions such as the Global Alcohol Policy Alliance and Eurocare. These groupings allow coherent and consistent messages on key policy issues such as pricing, availability and marketing to be articulated in a range of forums by a number of closely associated bodies including the World Health Organization, which, especially through its European office, has been a strong ally of the alcohol control movement.

The increasing globalisation of alcohol policy debates has, to some degree, exacerbated a long-standing polarisation in perspectives between alcohol control advocates and alcohol industry bodies. This polarisation is, in many respects, inevitable as the aims of both groups are to a great extent incompatible. Alcohol control advocacy has always supported whole population policy interventions to reduce alcohol consumption; the alcohol industry has always supported minimal state regulation and the right to promote the consumption of its products. In the nineteenth century, the prohibition movement grew out of a belief that nothing less than radical intervention at national level could counter the power of the alcohol industry to protect its interests; today, it is argued that only strong state intervention to regulate price, availability and marketing can curb the power of the industry to skirt less intrusive forms of control. The interconnected nature of trade regulations, the key role of the EU in governing European policy, the role of bodies such as the World Trade Organization, the G8 and the G20 globally, and the dominating influence of multilateral trade agreements in constraining national governments, mean those battles increasingly take on a global character. Alcohol policy debates are now increasingly international and the question remains how best transnational bodies can act to support policymaking that is consistent and effective but also appropriate to the local contexts where it ultimately applies.

REFERENCES

Adelekan, M (2008) Non-commercial alcohol in sub-Saharan Africa. In *Noncommercial Alcohol in Three Regions*. Washington: ICAP, pp. 3–16

Alcohol Concern (2014) *Creating Customers: Finding New Ways and Places to Sell Alcohol, and New People to Buy It*. Cardiff: Alcohol Concern Cymru.

Alcohol Research Group (2011) *Alcohol Control Systems and the Potential Effects of Privatization*. Available at: http://www.usdrinksconference.com/assets/files/download/Privatization%20Pamphlet%20Final.pdf.

Allamani, A, Beccaria, F and Voller, F (2010) The puzzle of Italian drinking: trends in alcohol consumption, harms and policy: Italy, 1990–2010. *Nordic Studies on Alcohol and Drugs* 27, 465–78.

Allamani A, Voller F, Pepe V, Baccini M, Carreras G, Österberg E, Karlsson T, Lindeman M, Plant M, Knibbe R, Derickx M, Anderson P, Gual A, Matrai S, Elekes Z, Eisenbach-Stangl I, Guillemot J, Nordlund S, Øystein, S, Olsson B, Roumeliotis F, wiatkiewicz, Gmel G and Kuendig H (2012) Balance of power in alcohol policy: balance across different groups as a whole between societal changes and alcohol policy. In P Anderson, F Braddick, J Reynolds and A Gual (eds), *Alcohol Policy in Europe: Evidence from AMPHORA*. The AMPHORA project, pp. 32–42.

Allamani A, Pepe P, Baccini M, Massini G and Voller F (2014a) Europe. An analysis of changes in the consumption of alcoholic beverages: the interaction among consumption, related harms, contextual factors and alcoholic beverage control policies. *Substance Use and Misuse* 49: 1692–715.

Allamani A, Voller F, Pepe P, Baccini M, Massini G and Cipriani F (2014b) Italy between drinking culture and control policies for alcoholic beverages. *Substance Use and Misuse* 49: 1646–64.

Allen Consulting Group (2011) *Alcohol Taxation Reform Starting with the Wine Equalisation Tax*. Melbourne: Allen Consulting Group.

Anderson P and Baumberg B (2006) *Alcohol in Europe: A Public Health Perspective*. London: Institute of Alcohol Studies.

Anderson P, Braddick F, Reynolds J and Gual A (2012) *Alcohol Policy in Europe: Evidence from AMPHORA*. The AMPHORA project. Available at: http://www.amphoraproject.net/w2box/data/e-book/AMPHORA%20ebook.pdf.

Anderson P, de Bruijn A, Angus K, Gordon R and Hastings G (2009) Impact of alcohol advertising and media exposure on adolescent alcohol use: a systematic review of longitudinal studies. *Alcohol and Alcoholism* 44: 229–43.

Babor T, Caetano R, Casswell S, Edwards G, Giesbrecht N, Graha, K, Grube J, Gruenewald P, Hill L, Holder H, Romel R, Österberg E, Rehm J, Room R and Rossow R (2010) *Alcohol, No Ordinary Commodity: Research and Public Policy*, 2nd edn. Oxford: Oxford University Press.

Babor T, Robaina K and Jernigan D (2015) The influence of industry actions on the availability of alcoholic beverages in the African region. *Addiction* 110: 561–71.

Baccini M and Carreras G (2014) Analyzing and comparing the association between control policy measures and alcohol consumption in Europe. *Substance Use and Misuse* 49: 1684–91.

Bakke Ø and Endal D (2010) Alcohol policies out of context: drinks industry supplanting of government role in alcohol policies in sub-Saharan Africa. *Addiction* 105: 22–8.

BBC Online (2012) Brazil World Cup beer law signed by President Rousseff. *BBC News: Latin America and Caribbean*. Available at: http://www.bbc.co.uk/news/world-latin-america-18348012.

Beeston C, Reid G, Robinson M, Craig N, McCartney G, Graham L and Grant I (2013) *Monitoring and Evaluating Scotland's Alcohol Strategy: Third Annual Report*. Edinburgh: NHS Scotland.

Bendtsen P, Damsgaard M, Huckle T, Casswell S, Kuntsche E, Arnold P, de Looze M, Hofmann F, Hublet A, Simons-Morton B, ter Borgt T and Holstein B (2014) Adolescent alcohol use: a reflection of national drinking patterns and policy? *Addiction* 109: 1857–68.

Berridge V (2005) *Temperance: Its History and Impact on Current and Future Alcohol Policy*. York: Joseph Rowntree Foundation.

Bruun K, Edwards G, Lumio M, Mäkelä K, Pan L, Popham RE, Room R, Schmidt W, Skog O-J, Sulkunen P and Österberg E (1975) *Alcohol Control Policies in Public Health Perspective*. Helsinki: Finnish Foundation for Alcohol Studies.

Burns H (2013) Towards a global alcohol policy: current directions. In P Boyle, P Boffetta, A Lowenfels, H Burns, O Brawley, W Zato ski and J Rehm (eds), *Alcohol: Science, Policy and Public Health*. Oxford: Oxford University Press, pp. 395–406.

Casswell S (2012) Current status of alcohol marketing policy – an urgent challenge for global governance. *Addiction* 107: 178–85.

Casswell S and Maxwell A (2005) Regulation of alcohol marketing: a global view. *Journal of Public Health Policy* 26: 343–58.

Casswell S, Meier P, MacKintosh A, Brown A, Hastings G, Thamarangsi T, Chaiyasong S, Chun S, Huckle T, Wall M and You R (2012)

The International Alcohol Control (IAC) Study – evaluating the impact of alcohol policies. *Alcoholism: Clinical and Experimental Research* 36: 1462–7.

Chester J, Montgomery K and Dorfman L (2010) *Alcohol Marketing in the Digital Age*. Berkeley: Center for Digital Democracy and Berkeley Media Studies Group.

Chung VC, Yip BH, Griffiths SM, Yu EL, Kim JH, Tam WW, Wong AH, Chan IW and Lau JT (2013). The impact of cutting alcohol duties in drinking patterns in Hong Kong. *Alcohol and Alcoholism* 48: 720–28.

Cnossen S (2006). Alcohol taxation and regulation in the European Union. CESifo working paper 1831. Available at http://hdl.handle.net/10419/25866.

Commission of the European Communities (2006) *Communication from the Commission to the Council, the European Parliament, the European Economic and Social Committee and the Committee of the Regions: An EU Strategy to Support Member States in Reducing Alcohol Related Harm*. Brussels: European Commission.

Cook, P (2012) Alcohol retail privatization: a commentary. *American Journal of Preventive Medicine* 42: 430–2.

Cornell M (2003) *Beer: The Story of the Pint*. London: Headline.

Dade P (2008) *Drink Talking: 100 Years of Alcohol Advertising*. London: Middlesex University Press.

Davoren S and O'Brien P (2104) Regulating to reduce alcohol-related harm: liquor licensing and the harm minimisation test. In E Manton, R Room and M Thorn (eds), *Stemming the Tide of Alcohol: Liquor Licensing and the Public Interest*. Victoria: Foundation for Alcohol Research and Education, pp. 38–46.

Diageo (2012) *Diageo Marketing Code: Promoting Responsible Drinking*. Available at: http://www.diageo.com/en-row/NewsMedia/Pages/resource.aspx?resourceid=1287

Duncan R (2014) *Pubs and Patriots: The Drink Crisis in Britain During World War I*. Liverpool: Liverpool University Press.

Edwards G, Anderson P, Babor T, Casswell S, Ferrence R, Giesbrecht N, Godfrey C, Holder H, Lemmens P, Mäkelä K, Midanik L, Norström T, Romesjö A, Room R, Simpura J and Skog O-J (1994) *Alcohol Policy and the Public Good*. Oxford: Oxford University Press and WHO Europe.

Eisenbach-Stangl I (2011) *Comparing European Alcohol Polices: What to Compare?* Vienna: European Centre for Social Welfare and Policy Research. Available at: http://www.amphoraproject.net/w2box/data/AMPHORA%20Reports/Comparing_European_Alcohol_Policies.pdf.

Erickson D, Lenk K, Toomey T, Nelson T, Jones-Webb R and Mosher J (2014) Measuring the strength of state-level alcohol control policies. *World Medical and Health Policy* 6: 171–86.

Eurocare (2012) *Eurocare Recommendations for a Future EU Alcohol Strategy*. Brussels: Eurocare.

Fahey D (2003) Good Templars (IOGT). In D Blocker, D Fahey and I Tyrell I (eds), *Alcohol and Temperance in Modern History: An International Encyclopedia*. Santa Barbara: ABC-Clio, pp. 268–72.

Flanagan G (2003) *Sobering Result: The Alberta Liquor Retailing Industry Ten Years After Privatization*. Ottawa: Canadian Center for Policy Alternatives.

Fogarty J (2010) The demand for beer, wine and spirits: a survey of the literature. *Journal of Economic Surveys* 24: 428–78.

Giesbrecht N, Wettlaufer A, April N, Asbridge M, Cukier S, Mann R, McAllister J, Murie A, Pauley C, Plamondon L, Stockwell T, Thomas G, Thompson K and Vallance K (2013) *Strategies to Reduce Alcohol-related Harms and Costs in Canada: A Comparison of Provincial Policies*. Toronto: Centre for Addiction and Mental Health.

Gornall J (2014) World Cup 2014: festival of football or alcohol? *BMJ* 348: g3772.

Greenaway J (2003) *Alcohol and British Politics: A Study in Policy-making*. Houndsmills: Palgrave Macmillan,

Hahn R, Middleton J, Elder R, Brewer R, Fielding J, Naimi T, Toomey T, Chattopadhyay S, Lawrence B and Campbell CA (2012) Effects of alcohol retail privatization on excessive alcohol consumption and related harms: a community guide systematic review. *American Journal of Preventive Medicine* 42: 418–27.

Hames G (2012) *Alcohol in World History*. London: Routledge.

Harrison B. (1971) *Drink and the Victorians*. London: Faber and Faber.

Hastings G, Anderson S, Cooke E and Gordon R (2005) Alcohol marketing and young people's drinking: a review of the research. *Journal of Public Health Policy* 26: 296–311.

Her M, Giesbrech N, Room R and Rehm J (1999) Privatizing alcohol sales and alcohol consumption: evidence and implications. *Addiction* 94: 1125–39.

Holmes J, Guo Y, Maheswaran R, Nicholls J, Meier P and Brennan A (2014) The impact of spatial and temporal availability of alcohol on its consumption and related harms: a critical review in the context of UK licensing policies. *Drug and Alcohol Review* 33: 515–25.

House of Commons Health Committee (2010) *Alcohol: First Report of Session 2009–10, Vol. 1*. London: Stationery Office.

Howard S., Gordon R and Jones S (2014) Australian alcohol policy 2001–2013 and implications for public health. *BMC Public Health* 14: 848.

Järvinen, M and Room R (2007). Youth drinking cultures: European experiences. In M Järvinen and R Room R (eds), *Youth Drinking Cultures: European Experiences*. Aldershot: Ashgate, pp. 1–16.

Jacobson L (2012) Navigating the boundaries of respectability and desire: Seagram's advertising and the meaning of moderation after Repeal. *Social History of Alcohol and Drugs* 26: 122–46.

Jernigan D (2009) The global alcohol industry: an overview. *Addiction* 104(Suppl. 1): 6–12.

Karlsson T and Österberg E (2007) Scaling alcohol control policies across Europe. *Drugs: Education, Prevention and Policy* 14: 499–511.

Karlsson T, Lindeman M and Österberg E (2012) Does alcohol policy make any difference? Scale and consumption. In P Anderson, F Braddick, J Reynolds and A Gual (eds), *Alcohol Policy in Europe: Evidence from AMPHORA*. The AMPHORA project, pp. 15–23.

Knibbe RA, Derickx M, Allamani A and Massini G (2014) Alcohol consumption and its related harms in the Netherlands since 1960: relationships with planned and unplanned factors. *Substance Use and Misuse* 49: 1589–600.

Kümin B and Tlusty A (2002) *The World of the Tavern: Public Houses in Early Modern Europe*. Aldershot: Ashgate.

Levintova M (2007) Russian alcohol policy in the making. *Alcohol and Alcoholism* 42: 500–5.

McCreanor T, Lyons A, Griffin C, Goodwin I, Barnes H M and Hutton F (2013). Youth drinking cultures, social networks and alcohol marketing: implications for public health. *Critical Public Health* 23: 11–20.

Mäkelä P and Österberg E (2009) Weakening of one more alcohol control pillar: a review of the effects of the alcohol tax cuts in Finland in 2004. *Addiction* 104: 554–63.

Malleck D (2013) *Try to Control Yourself: The Regulation of Public Drinking in Post-Prohibition Ontario, 1927–44*. Toronto: UBC Press.

Meier P, Purshouse R and Brennan A (2009) Policy options for alcohol price regulation: the importance of modelling population heterogeneity. *Addiction* 105: 383–93.

Naimi TS, Blanchette J, Nelson TF, Nguyen T, Oussayef N, Heeren TC, Gruenewald P, Mosher J and Xuan Z (2014) A new scale of the US alcohol policy environment and its relationship to binge drinking. *American Journal of Preventive Medicine* 46: 10–16.

Nelson TF, Ziming X, Babor TF, Brewer RD, Chaloupka FJ, Grunewald PJ, Holder H, Klitzner M, Mosher JF, Ramirez RL, Reynolds R, Toomey TL, Churchill V and Naimie TS (2013) Efficacy and strength of evidence of ES alcohol control policies. *America Journal of Preventive Medicine* 45: 19–28.

Nicholls J (2009) *The Politics of Alcohol: A History of the Drink Question in England*. Manchester: Manchester University Press.

Nicholls J (2012a) The drip feed. *Points: The Blog of the Alcohol and Drugs History Society*, 3 May 2012. Available at: https://pointsadhsblog.wordpress.com/2012/05/03/the-drip-feed/.

Nicholls, J. (2012b) Everyday, everywhere: alcohol marketing and social media – current trends. *Alcohol and Alcoholism* 47: 486–93.

Nordlund S (2014) Popular norms, alcohol policy and drinking behaviour. In P Anderson, F Braddick, J Reynolds and A Gual (eds), *Alcohol Policy in Europe: Evidence from AMPHORA*. The AMPHORA project, pp. 24–31.

Österberg E (2011) Alcohol tax changes and the use of alcohol in Europe. *Drug and Alcohol Review* 30: 124–9.

Phillips R (2014). *Alcohol: A History*. Chapel Hill: University of North Carolina Press.

Plant M, Allamani A, Massini G and Pepe P (2014) Contextual determinants and alcohol control policies in the United Kingdom. *Substance Use and Misuse* 49: 1576–88.

Pridemore WA, Mitchell B, Chamlin M, Kaylen MT and Andreev E (2014) The effects of the 2006 Russian alcohol policy on alcohol-related mortality: an interrupted time series analysis. *Alcoholism: Clinical and Experimental Research* 38: 257–66.

Purves R, Stead M and Eadie D (2015) *'What Are You Meant to Do When You See It Everywhere?': Young People, Alcohol Packaging and Digital Media*. London: Alcohol Research UK.

Regaud A and Craplet M (2004) The 'Loi Evin': a French exception. *The Globe* 1&2: 33–6.

Room, R. (1989) Responses to alcohol-related problems in international perspective: characterizing and explaining cultural wetness and dryness. Presentation to 'La ricerca Italiana sulle bevande alcoliche nel confronto internazionale', Santo Stefano Belbo (CN), Italy, 22–23 September 1989. Available at: http://www.robinroom.net/response.htm.

Ruddock A (2013) *Youth and the Media*. London: Sage.

Rutherford D (n.d.) A noble past: history of the IOGT. Available at: http://www.iogt.us/iogt.php?p=35.

SABMiller (2014) *Policy on Commercial Communication*. Available at: http://www.sabmiller.com/docs/default-source/alcohol-policy/policy-on-commercial-communication-2014.pdf?sfvrsn=2.

Siegfried N, Pienaar DC, Ataguba JE, Volmink J, Kredo T, Jere M and Parry CDH (2014) Restricting or banning alcohol advertising to reduce alcohol consumption in adults and adolescents *The Cochrane Library* 11: CD010704.

Smith L and Foxcroft D (2009) The effect of alcohol advertising, marketing and portrayal on drinking behaviour in young people: systematic review of prospective cohort studies. *BMC Public Health* 9: 51.

Sousa J (2014) *Estimation of Price Elasticities of Demand for Alcohol in the United Kingdom. HMRC Working Paper 16*. London: HM Revenue and Customs.

Valverde M (2003) Police science, British style: pub licensing and knowledges of urban disorder. *Economy and Society* 32: 234–52.

Voller F, Maccari F, Pepe P and Allamani A (2014) Changing trends in European alcohol beverage drinking: selected social, demographic, economic factors, drinking's related harms and prevention control policies between the 1960s and 2000s. *Substance Use and Misuse* 49: 1515–30.

Wagenaar AC, Salois MJ and Komro KA (2009) Effects of beverage alcohol price and tax levels on drinking: a meta-analysis of 1003 estimates from 112 studies. *Addiction* 104: 179–90.

World Health Organization (1980) *Problems Related to Alcohol Consumption: World Health Organization Technical Report Series 650*. Geneva: World Health Organization.

World Health Organization (2005) *WHA58.26 Public Health Problems Caused by Alcohol*. Available at: http://www.who.int/substance_abuse/wha_resolution_58_26_public_health_problems_alcohol.pdf.

World Health Organization (2011) *Global Strategy to Reduce the Harmful Use of Alcohol*. Geneva: World Health Organization.

World Health Organization (2014) *Global Status Report on Alcohol and Health 2014*. Geneva: World Health Organization.

World Health Organization Europe (1993) *European Alcohol Action Plan*. Copenhagen: World Health Organization Europe.

World Health Organization Europe (1995) *European Charter on Alcohol*. Copenhagen: World Health Organization Europe.

World Health Organization Europe (2000) *European Alcohol Action Plan*. Copenhagen: World Health Organization Europe.

World Health Organization Europe (2001) *Declaration on Alcohol and Young People*. Copenhagen: World Health Organization Europe.

World Health Organization Europe (2009) *Evidence for the Effectiveness and Cost-Effectiveness of Interventions to Reduce Alcohol-Related Harm*. Copenhagen: World Health Organization Europe.

World Health Organization Europe (2012) *European Alcohol Action Plan to Reduce the Harmful Use of Alcohol 2012–20*. Copenhagen: World Health Organization Europe.

Zatoński W (2014) *Mind The Gap - Health and Inequality*. Presentation to Eurocare Annual Conference, Brussels, 27 November 2014.

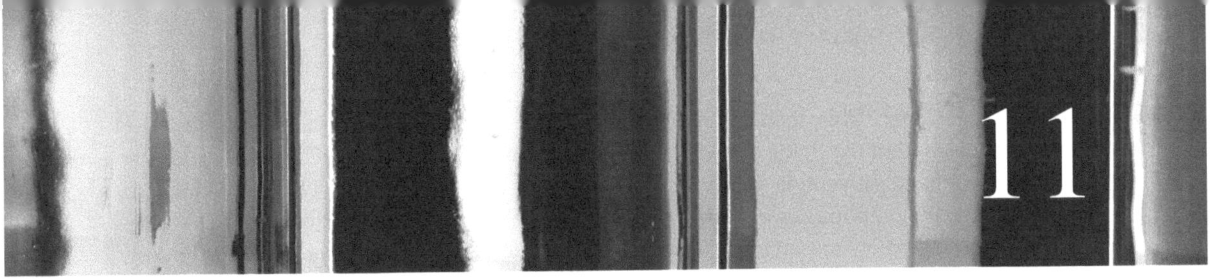

Drug Policy in Practice

Esben Houborg and Bagga Bjerge

INTRODUCTION

In this chapter, we present a *policy in practice* approach, which is an approach to analyze and understand drug policies that have gained increasing ground within the past decade amongst drug policy researchers. This approach is especially inspired by research within the fields of sociology and anthropology. While there is much research on how policies shape practice, there is less knowledge about policy *as* practice, which can answer questions about the kinds of activities policy making entails, and what policy makers do (cf. Freeman et al., 2011). We begin with briefly presenting how drug policies have most commonly been analyzed within the drug field. Subsequently, we go into details with the *policy in practice* approach, presenting three avenues of research in which drug policy researchers have applied this approach. First, *street-level bureaucrats: problematizing coherence and hierarchy*, a perspective that focuses on policy processes by examining the empirical, everyday practices of actors in the drug field. Second, a *policy network and governance* approach, which examines the interaction between a variety of different actors that come from state, market and civil society, and third, *policy and knowledge*, a perspective that critically scrutinizes the role of experts and expert knowledge in policy processes. Finally, we discuss the kinds of insights that the *policy in practice* approach may offer to the drug field as well as we aspire to sheet light on some of the 'complex "messiness" of policy making' (Freeman et al., 2011: 130), which can be traced in the drug policy field.

POLICY ANALYSIS IN THE DRUG FIELD

Studies of drug policy play an important part in how drug related issues are understood, discussed and managed both in public and amongst researchers. This includes a wide range of issues within the fields of drug control, drug treatment, prevention, harm reduction, and drug consumption, as well as across these fields. Drug policy researchers, Stevens and Ritter (2013), use Colebatch's (2002, 2006) distinction between three perceptions of policy that have been applied in the drug policy field: policy as 'authoritative choice', policy as 'structured interaction', and policy as 'social construction' (Colebatch, 2002, 2006) (see also Bjerge et al., 2013; Ritter, 2013; Lancaster et al., 2014).

The policy as 'authoritative choice' perspective perceives policy as a process through which political authorities reach the most rational solution to a pre-existing problem. This conception of public policy is closely associated with the institution of government as the center for decisions about how to handle particular issues, as having the capacity to enforce such decisions, and therefore to a large extent, determining collective action. Colebatch (2002, 2006) argues that this understanding of policy rests on three core assumptions: *instrumentality, hierarchy*, and *coherence. Instrumentality* means that policy is perceived as the pursuit of particular objectives and handling of clearly defined problems in a rational way, based on the best possible knowledge. Stevens (2007), therefore, calls it a rational-linear model of evidence based policy. *Hierarchy* means that the actors who decide on a policy are superior to the actors who carry the policies out. *Coherence* means that the different parts of the policy process from decision to implementation, are part of an organized whole.

Policy understood as 'structured interaction' includes how different actors such as private organizations (e.g. labor market organizations or business associations) are recognized as participants in the policy process, where they interact and negotiate the alignment of different agendas and interests.

Finally, policy as 'social construction' concerns how different actors (who do not necessarily represent recognized interests) get involved in, negotiate, and struggle over how to get things recognized as policy issues, how to define such issues, how to deal with them, and to what ends. This perspective has received increasing attention within drug policy research in recent years (e.g. Acevedo, 2007; Monaghan, 2008, 2010, 2011; Bancroft, 2009; Linnemann, 2013; Moore and Fraser, 2013; Lancaster, 2014; Lancaster and Ritter, 2014). From a *policy in practice* perspective, policy is perceived as social constructions, and it is a perspective that is clearly differentiated from the policy as 'authoritative choice' model. This means that the *policy in practice* perspective does not take its point of departure in particular models and ideas about what policy is and should be. Rather, the *policy in practice* perspective seeks to understand and explain policy on the basis on how policy is interpreted, negotiated, and implemented in, and between, different contexts.

POLICY IN PRACTICE: BUREAUCRATS, NETWORKS AND KNOWLEDGE

In the following sections we present three different approaches to the *policy in practice* perspective by using examples from the field of drug policy. To do this, we draw on the work by Laws and Hajer (2006), who have developed a categorization of policy approaches as an alternative to the formal and instrumental approaches in policy analysis outlined above. These categorizations involve (i) the practices of *street-level bureaucrats* and how these practices partake in shaping policy; (ii) the observation that policy is increasingly a matter of *governance* where different public and private actors and institutions interact and make policy; and (iii) the idea that rational policy making (*instrumentality*) on the basis of expert knowledge, is increasingly challenged in a risk society.

STREET-LEVEL BUREAUCRATS: PROBLEMATIZING COHERENCE AND HIERARCHY

Within sociology and anthropology, many studies have questioned a top-down conception of policy that rests on the key assumptions of *instrumentality, hierarchy* and *coherence* in relation to what policies are and how they work. One of the most important contributions to such a practice-oriented approach to policy analysis is Lipsky's (1980) work on so-called 'street-level bureaucrats'. This perspective has shown that when policies are implemented, they are influenced by the local context in which street-level bureaucrats work (see also Prottas, 1978). In their practices, street-level bureaucrats are influenced by a number of different things such as economic constraints, professional expectations, expectations from users, high work pressure competing moral positions, and norms and social relations in street-level bureaucracies (for example, police stations, social services, schools, etc.). In Lipsky's framework decisions, routines and the devices applied by street-level bureaucrats *become* the public policies they carry out (1980: xii). This means that to understand policy, it is necessary to study the actions, interpretations and strategies carried out by street-level workers in their everyday practices and the social and material conditions under which they are carried out.

Today, there is a growing amount of drug policy research literature about everyday practices in public institutions and how they affect policy – in practice – inspired by such an approach (Fraser and Valentine, 2008; Stevens, 2011a; Bjerge et al., 2014; Houborg and Frank, 2014). Many of these studies focus on how laws and regulations are interpreted, manipulated, and acted out in various ways in a given institutional context. That is, such approaches are inspired by literature that emphasizes relational and social constituent norms and logics as essential in the way actors act and make sense of their everyday practices (Goffman, 1963; Bourdieu, 1977; Meyer and Rowan, 1977; Moore, 1978; Herzfeld, 1992; Brunsson and Olsen, 1997). Though the degree of agency attributed to the individual actor in this literature varies, they all address the issue that (in a given social field, for example, a drug prevention organization) certain perceptions exist for what is perceived as 'right' and 'wrong', 'good' or 'bad' by the actors. That is, a more or less shared framework for how work is managed. Prior experiences, routines and traditions inform the actors' perceptions, as well as actual actions with regards to how they translate, adapt, or do not adapt to policies. This practice approach to policy analysis thus counters top-down explanations of policy and could rather be seen as a bottom-up approach to policy analysis by focusing on the practices of local actors as central to policy making. In this way, this approach also blurs the distinction between policy formulation and policy implementation (Freeman et al., 2011).

For example, a study of the bureaucratic management of local drug policies in Danish municipalities shows how economic cut downs and political opinions forces treatment organizations to prioritize some user groups more than others (Bjerge and Frederiksen, 2014). Though all citizens in need of treatment are guaranteed treatment services in Denmark (Socialministeriet, 2002; Pedersen and Nielsen, 2007), municipalities report that they have been forced to cut down services and focus primarily on young people because this group is perceived as the most resourceful and the most likely to quit using drugs. Applying the framework of Lipsky (1980), such policy can be regarded as 'creaming', which is a way to favor the most well-functioning citizens in street-level bureaucracies (ibid: 107). As a consequence, it is an ongoing challenge for these Danish employers to implement local drug policy strategies in a manner that ensures a reasonable level of service to the severely marginalized users in methadone treatment – especially because the political winds amongst policy makers in the drug field are blowing in a specific direction, or as a bureaucrat puts it: 'You know what our politicians say: the youth services! The youth services! The youth services! It's simply a political slogan' (Bjerge and Frederiksen, 2014: 73; our translation).

It would, however, be insufficient just to focus on the practices of front-line professionals. It is equally important to study the local practices of policy makers at other levels of the government structure (such as administrators and politicians), although access to these levels is often more difficult to achieve. An important example of such a study is Stevens' (2011b) investigation into how the British civil servants use 'evidence' in the making of national drug policy. The study shows that the use of evidence is highly complicated due to an overwhelming amount of inconclusive information, and much of this research is therefore not suitable for solving policy concerns. Instead, civil servants use evidence to 'create persuasive policy stories' (2011b: 237). That is, what civil servants believe will be politically acceptable policies are made claiming legitimacy in 'evidence', which Stevens highlights can, in fact, be used as a method of career advancement. In this way, civil servants are able to use certain bureaucratic techniques to manipulate their stories to 'fit' a system that has 'a distaste for uncertainty, complexity and contradiction'. (2011a: 247). Therefore, civil servants often do not use evidence that challenges the prevailing societal order of things or their own status. From this, the study asserts that the use of evidence in drug policy tends to support a specific way of considering and managing drug related issues, which is reproduced over and over again. To reach to such detailed, critical insights, it is important to expand the scope of more traditional drug policy approaches to include a focus on the everyday local practices, routines, values and strategies which different actors apply when drug policies are created and carried out.

Policy networks and governance

The approach to *policy in practice* discussed above, problematizes the assumptions of hierarchy and coherence in policy, but is itself mainly concerned with the everyday practices within public institutions. However, as noted by Laws and Hajer (2006), there is a second moment in the development of a *policy in practice* approach that problematizes the public institution as the main site for policy making and policy implementation. This approach moves beyond the public sector and the state as privileged sites for analyzing policy, in a development that sees a shift from a focus on the institution of *government* to practices of *governance* in policy research (Rhodes, 1996; Stoker, 1998). Here, policy understood as a purposeful collective action towards a particular issue is not associated with the institutional practices of government and the executive powers of the state, but with the way multiple actors who can come from different sectors of society (state, market and civil society) negotiate and organize collective action (Stoker, 1998; Kooiman, 2003). The point of departure here is that policy comes about through the *interaction* between a variety of different actors that come from state, market and civil society. Therefore, to study policy means to study this interaction and networks of actors from these different sectors and how they are formed in order to handle particular problems and issues (Kooiman, 2003). This approach to the study of policy in practice also studies how the state is 'hollowed out' from below (the local) and above (international) (Rhodes, 1994) and how the state itself works to develop policy networks (Colebatch, 2002).

Within the field of drug policy research, there have been a number of studies that have investigated how drug policy is negotiated between public and private stakeholder, both at the local and the national level. Kübler and Wälti (Kübler, 2001; Wälti and Kübler, 2003; Wälti et al., 2004) have conducted research into local drug policy in Switzerland, as well as carrying out comparative studies of local drug policy in different countries in Europe, where they found that policy, to an increasing extent, was made through public-private collaboration and networks. They also pointed out the danger that in the long run, the development of such 'new governance' could imply increasing state influence over civil society organizations. Some studies concluded that while the governance perspective certainly is relevant for understanding policy making and policy implementation within the field of drug policy, the state and its institutions still plays an important role in the field, both with regard to policy formulation (including legislation), and with regard to enforcing particular policies (Frank et al., 2008; Houborg and Frank, 2014; Zampini, 2014).

The governance literature is especially indebted to the writings of Foucault (Foucault, 1991; Dean, 1999; Rose, 1999). This literature takes its point of departure in Foucault's writings about a 'governmentalization' of the state that has been part of the development of the modern liberal state (Foucault, 2010). With the development of the modern liberal and capitalist society, the main objective of rule moved away from sovereign concern with controlling and defending territory, towards fostering and forming the health, wealth, and welfare of the population. This involves the development of modes of governing that involve both public and private institutions and the subjectification of individuals as self-governing subjects (Dean, 1999; Rose, 1999). O'Malley (1999, 2002), he has, for example, conducted several analyses on how drug policy articulates certain political rationalities that imply perceptions of drug users as particular kinds of subjects, targeted with specific kinds of social technologies. He has been particularly interested in the constitution of drug users as rational subjects within neo-liberal political rationalities.

Central to both the governance and the governmentality literature is the conception of policy as a social construction. What is being constructed from this perspective is the policy goals and the means to achieve them, but also the phenomenon that the policy seeks to address, that is, the policy problem (Houborg, 2008; Keane, 2009; Fraser & Moore, 2011; Bacchi, 2012; Lancaster et al., 2012). Both approaches thus break with the idea that the policy problem exists somewhat independently from the development of a policy towards it. Rather, they show how reality is constructed as something that requires collective action and is amenable to such action. Applying Kingdon (1984) and Duke et al. (2013) show how drug treatment in the UK was re-conceptualized and re-constituted in terms of 'recovery'. Fraser and Moore (2011), use Bacchi's (2009) conception of policy making through 'problematizations', to analyze Australian policy on methamphetamine. Keane (2002) has critically analyzed different discourses and models of addiction in relation to illicit drugs, alcohol, cigarettes, food, and sex, showing that addiction discourses are often associated with a medical rationality and a modernist notion of the autonomous individual.

It appears then, that the governance literature is mainly concerned with the interactions, negotiations and struggles between different actors in the development of collective action and governance networks. In addition, the governmentality literature is more concerned with the discourses or political rationalities that are articulated when problems are constructed and action is decided upon, as well as the social technologies that are developed. In line with this thinking, Dorn (1995) and Benoit (2003) have used the concept of 'policy space' as a way to analyze drug policy as part of the societal recognition, definition, and management of risks along with other policy areas. In this approach, the management of risk may be influenced by liberal, conservative, and social democratic ideologies. Benoit (2003) emphasizes political and institutional history in the area of welfare policy as an important factor behind the development of different drug policies. According to her, differences between perceiving drug problems as a collective responsibility or an individual responsibility influences the extent to which a drug policy emphasizes control of the individual and the welfare strategies directed at treating and compensating the individual. Dorn (1995) uses a welfare regime approach that distinguishes between social democratic, conservative, and liberal welfare policies to differentiate the governmental discourses that may affect the development of drug policies in different countries. That is, drug policies may, in different ways and to different degrees, articulate discourses that affect the way the risks, harms, and consequences associated with drug use are defined, recognized, and distributed. For example, the concept of policy space has been deployed to analyze how different political rationalities are articulated and negotiated in the historic development of drug policies in Denmark (Houborg and Bjerge, 2011).

Policy and knowledge

In the instrumental conception of policy, expert knowledge (evidence) is seen to provide the basis for a rational policy. However, just as institutions of government have increasingly been problematized by looking at the practices of governance, so has the role of the expert and expert knowledge also been problematized in policy analysis. There are different reasons for this. The first is the development of a risk society, characterized by the paradox that increasing knowledge does not create more certainty about how to act, but on the contrary, makes us increasingly aware of how little we know and how uncertain the conditions under which we act are (Beck, 2006; Callon et al., 2009). Cases where experts were not able to foresee important problems such as bovine spongiform encephalopathy (also known as mad cow disease) (Hinchliffe, 2001) or nuclear waste problems (Wynne, 2000), for example, produce particular suspicion about expert knowledge, but also mobilize lay people to engage in bringing about and contesting knowledge. In Latour's terms, fewer and fewer issues can be seen as settled non-contestable 'matters of fact', but become instead 'matters of concern' (Latour, 2004) characterized by being at the center of the production, deliberation, and contestation of knowledge of different kinds involving both experts and lay people (Epstein, 1997; Callon, 1999; Callon and Rabeharisioa, 2003). The second reason for the problematization of the traditional role of the expert and expert knowledge is research done in the field of science and technology studies, which has demonstrated that just as policy is shaped by the everyday practices of street-level bureaucrats, so is scientific knowledge shaped through scientific practice and the social and material conditions under which it takes place (Latour, 1987).

While the aforementioned approaches to the everyday making of policy in local practices, including the network and governance approach, are quite developed in drug policy research today, this third approach about a practice perspective on knowledge, expertise, and instrumentality is less developed. However, medical knowledge, and the ascendance of neuroscience in the epistemology of addiction in particular, has generated a social scientific interest in the constitution of such knowledge and the role it plays (Keane, 2008, 2009; Monaghan, 2008, 2010, 2011; Valentine, 2009; Campbell, 2010, 2011; Tieberghien and Decorte, 2013; Duke and Thom, 2014). In a study of addiction research in the USA, Campbell (2007) makes a detailed investigation of addiction research in practice and the epistemological assumptions upon which it has rested from the 1930s until the present. She shows the relationship between addiction research, drug policy, and a politics of knowledge where knowledge about the safe use of drugs has been held back by policy makers. Furthermore, Campbell highlights how some research has articulated a moral lexicon of addiction through which addiction has been represented as a disease of the will. Dehue (2002) was concerned with how a particular perception of what constituted 'evidence' influenced policy making, and more specifically, how randomized controlled trials (RCT) came to be the only relevant kind of knowledge that dominated Dutch political debates about the introduction of heroin-maintenance treatment (see also Bergmark and Hübner, this volume). Houborg (2012), in a similar way, conducted a case study of the relationship between science and politics in the Danish debate about heroin assisted treatment. This showed that a public debate about the epistemology in drug treatment research became an important topic. The same study also shows how drug users produced lay-knowledge by doing a survey about their experiences and attitudes towards substitution treatment as a way to bring a new kind of knowledge to the debate. These examples show that not only different kinds of knowledge, but also the way they are produced and their validity and relevance in relation to a policy problem, become topics for debate.

Today, when we study *policy in practice,* it is not only the taken for granted ideas about who the policy actors are, and what policy making *is* that has to be challenged, but also the similarly taken for granted ideas about what expertise and reliable knowledge is. In both cases, practice becomes the center for our attention, if we want to understand how collective action with the purpose of producing some sort of social order comes about.

CONCLUSION

The aim of this chapter has been to illustrate how a *policy in practice* approach, inspired by anthropological and sociological policy perspectives, can produce new and valuable knowledge in the drug policy field. First, this approach provides researchers with an analytical understanding of not only the content of drug policies or how they came about, but also how policies are implemented and reworked in the drug field. That is, studies applying this approach show that the outcome of policies are as much a result of the local setting, and actors involved in these settings, as they are a result of top-down decisions. Second, the *policy in practice* approach can be used to analyze dilemmas and contradictions in drug policy. Such dilemmas and contradictions are not necessarily known or thought of among policy makers, but become visible for actors affected by a given policy in their every day practices. The *policy in practice* approach can therefore also help to unfold contradictions that are not visible when studying policy documents, because such documents attempt to create an image of a coherent policy. For example, this could be various statements of a 'four pillar' drug policy where a non-problematic balance between law enforcement, drug treatment, prevention, and harm reduction is presented, but where studies of practice show serious contractions and conflicts between these different policy areas. To analyze contractions and discrepancies of policy by studying *policy in practice,* is not to write off policy making as what James Scott terms as the 'hubris of planners' (Scott, 1998: 247). This is an often raised critique, asserting that national as well as international politicians and policy planners are (totally) decoupled from practices when planning laws, strategies, and regulations, such as policing or drug treatment. Rather, discrepancies can be analyzed as a result of complex social realities and simplified pieces of policy, produced to accommodate political requirements for consensus and theoretical 'state of the art' (cf. Mosse, 2007: 460). Third, a *policy in practice* approach can show the experimental practices of frontline workers and institutions when they find that existing ways of thinking, talking, and acting do not work, or when they disagree with established drug policy (Houborg, 2010). Fourth, and following this point, a *policy in practice* approach can show that evidence-based methods and administrative guidelines frequently fall short when confronted with problems in practice in the drug field. Applying such an approach shows how deviance from guidelines and requirements can be analyzed as something other than unprofessional conduct, that is, as necessary, creative, and often experimental work to ensure that policies are implemented in ways that make sense in the everyday practices of, for example, drug treatment (Nielsen and Houborg, 2014, Bjerge, 2009). Finally, it is important to show how the validity and relevance of particular kinds of knowledge in the policy making process is established in practice, and becomes associated with particular kinds of policy.

REFERENCES

Acevedo, B. (2007). Creating the cannabis user. a post-structuralist analysis of the re-classification of cannabis in the United Kingdom (2004–2005). *International Journal of Drug Policy*, 18(3): 177–86.

Bacchi, C. (2009). *Analysing Policy: What's the Problem Represented To Be?* Frenschs Forest: Pearson Australia.

Bacchi, C. (2012). Why study problematizations? Making politics visible. *Open Journal of Political Science*, 2(1): 1–8.

Bancroft, A. (2009). *Drugs, Education and Society.* Cambridge: Polity Press.

Beck, U. (2006). Living in the world risk society. *Economy and Society*, 35(3): 329–45.

Benoit, E. (2003). Not just a matter of criminal justice: states, institutions, and North American drug policy. *Sociological Forum*, 18(2): 269–94.

Bjerge, B. (2009). *Mellem Vision Og Praksis: Strukturreformen, Rusmiddelbureaukrati Og New Public Management.* Copenhagen: Sociologisk Institut, Københavns Universitet.

Bjerge, B. and Frederiksen, K. S. (2014). Kommunernes mulighedsrum: Hvordan nås og fastholdes alkohol- og stofbrugere i den kommunale behandling? In M. Hesse, B. Thylstrup, M. U. Pedersen and K. F. Skovgaard (eds), *Misbrug and Behov – Organisering Af Indsats Og Behandling.* Aarhus: Center for Rusmiddelforskning, AU og Aarhus Universitetsforlag, pp. 44–64.

Bjerge, B., Houborg, E. and Frank, V. A. (2013). Drug policy research at the Centre for Alcohol and Drug Research. *Drugs: Education, Prevention and Policy*, 20(6): 443–50.

Bjerge, B., Nielsen, B. and Frank, V. A. (2014). Rationalities of choice and practicalities of care. *Contemporary Drug Problems*, 17(1): 74–87.

Bourdieu, P. (1977). *Outline of a Theory of Praxis.* Cambridge: Cambridge University Press.

Brunsson, N. and Olsen, J. P. (1997). *The Reforming Organization.* Bergen-Sandviken: Fagbokforlaget.

Callon, M. (1999). The role of lay people in the production and dissemination of scientific knowledge. *Science, Technology and Society*, 4(1): 81–94.

Callon, M., Lascoumes, P. and Barthe, Y. (2009). *Acting in an Uncertain World. An Essay on Technical Democracy.* Cambridge: The MIT Press.

Callon, M. and Rabeharisioa, V. (2003). Research 'in the wild' and the shaping of new social identities. *Technology in Society*, 25: 193–204.

Campbell, N. D. (2007). *Discovering Addiction. The Science and Politics of Substance Abuse Research.* Ann Arbor: The University of Michigan Press.

Campbell, N. D. (2010). Toward a critical neuroscience of 'addiction'. *Biosocieties*, 5(1): 89–104.

Campbell, N. D. (2011). The metapharmacology of the 'addicted brain'. *History of the Present*, 1(2): 194–218.

Colebatch, H. K. (2002). Government and governmentality: using multiple approaches to the analysis of government. *Australian Journal of Political Science*, 37(3): 417–35.

Colebatch, H. K. (2002). *Policy.* Buckingham: Open University Press.

Colebatch, H. K. (2006). Policy, models, and the construction of governing. In H. K. Colebatch (ed.), *The Work of Policy.* Oxford: Lexington Books, pp. 3–19.

Dean, M. (1999). *Governmentality. Power and Rule in Modern Society.* London: Sage.

Dehue, T. (2002). A Dutch treat: randomized controlled experimentation and the case of heroin-maintenance in the Netherlands. *History of the Human Sciences,* 15(2): 75–98.

Dorn, N. (1995). A European analysis of drug enforcement. In G. Estievenart (ed.), *Policies and Strategies to Combat Drugs in Europe.* Florence: Martinus Nijhoff Publishers, pp. 159–69.

Duke, K. and Thom, T. (2014). The role of evidence and the expert in contemporary processes of governance: the case of opioid substitution treatment policy in England. *International Journal of Drug Policy*, 25(5): 964–71.

Duke, K., Herring, R. Thickett, A. and Thom, B. (2013). Substitution treatment in the era of 'recovery': an analysis of stakeholder roles and policy windows in Britain. *Substance Use and Misuse* 48(11): 966–76.

Epstein, S. (1997). Activism, drug regulation, and the politics of therapeutic evaluation in the AIDS era: a case study of ddC and the 'surrogate markers' debate. *Social Studies of Science*, 27: 691–726.

Foucault, M. (1991). Governmentality. In G. Burchell, C. Gordon and P. Miller (eds), *The Foucault Effect. Studies in Governmentality.* London: Harvester Wheatsheaf, pp. 87–104.

Foucault, M. (2010). The birth of bio-politics: lectures at the college the France 1978–1979. Houndsmills: Macmillan.

Fraser, S. and Moore, D. (2011). Governing through problems: the formulation of policy on amphetamine-type stimulants (ATS) in Australia. *International Journal of Drug Policy*, 22(6): 498–506.

Fraser, S. and Valentine, K. (2008). *Substance and Substitution. Methadone Subjects in Liberal Societies.* Basingstoke: Palgrave Macmillan.

Freeman, R., Griggs, S. and Boaz, A. (2011). The practice of policy making. *Evidence and Policy*, 7(2): 127–36.

Goffman, E. (1963). *Stigma: Notes on the Management of Spoiled Identity.* New Jersey: Prentice-Hall Inc.

Herzfeld, M. (1992). *The Social Production of Indifference: Exploring the Symbolic Roots of Western Bureaucracy.* Chicago: University of Chicago Press.

Hinchliffe, S. (2001). Indeterminacy in-decisions. Science, policy and politics in the BSE (bovine spongiform encephalopathy) crisis. *Transactions of the Instituted of British Geographers, New Series*, 26(2): 182–204.

Houborg, E. (2008). Youth, drugs and the welfare state – constructing the Danish drug treatment system 1965–1972. In V. Asmussen, B. Bagga and E. Houborg (eds), *Drug Policy. History, Theory and Consequences.* Aarhus: Aarhus University Press, pp. 181–208.

Houborg, E. (2010). Regulating intoxication and disciplining pleasure. In T. Decorte and J. Fountain (eds), *Pleasure, Pain and Profit. European Perspectives on Drugs.* Pabst Science Publishers, pp. 83–100.

Houborg, E. (2012). The political pharmacology of methadone and heroin in Danish drug policy. *Contemporary Drug Problems*, 39(Spring): 155–92.

Houborg, E. and Frank, V. A. (2014). Drug consumption rooms and the role of governance and politics in policy processes. *International Journal of Drug Policy*, 25(5): 972–7.

Kingdon, J. (1984) *Agendas, Alternatives and Public Policies*, 1st edn. Boston: Little Brown.

Keane, H. (2002). *What's Wrong with Addiction?* Melbourne: Melbourne University Press.

Keane, H. (2008). Pleasure and discipline in the uses of Ritalin. *International Journal of Drug Policy*, 19(5): 401–9.

Keane, H. (2009). Intoxication, harm and pleasure: an analysis of the Australian National Alcohol Strategy. *Critical Public Health*, 19(2): 135–42.

Kooiman, J. (2003). *Governing as Governance.* London: Sage.

Kübler, D. (2001). Understanding policy change with the advocacy coalition framework: an application to Swiss drug policy. *Journal of European Public Policy*, 8(4): 623–41.

Lancaster, K. (2014). Social construction and the evidence-based drug policy endeavor. *International Journal of Drug Policy,* 25(5): 948–51.

Lancaster, K. and Ritter, A. (2014). Examining the construction and representation of drugs as a policy problem in Australia's National Drug Strategy documents 1985–2010. *International Journal of Drug Policy,* 25(1): 81–7.

Lancaster, K., Hughes, C. E., Chalmers, J. and Ritter, A. (2012). More than problem-solving: critical reflections on the 'problematisation' of alcohol-related violence in Kings Cross. *Drug and Alcohol Review*, 31(7): 925–7.

Lancaster, K., Ritter, A. and Colebatch, H. (2014). Problems, policy and politics: making sense of Australia's 'ice epidemic'. *Policy Studies*, 35(2): 147–71.

Latour, B. (1987). *Science in Action*. Cambridge: Harvard University Press.

Latour, B. (2004). *Politics of Nature. How to Bring the Sciences into Democracy*. Cambridge: Harvard University Press.

Laws, D. and Hajer, M. (2006). Policy in practice. In M. Moran, M. Rein and R. E. Goodin (eds). *The Oxford Handbook of Public Policy*. Oxford: Oxford University Press, pp. 409–24.

Linnemann, T. (2013). Governing through meth: local politics, drug control and the drift towards securitization. *Crime Media Culture*, 9(1): 39–61.

Lipsky, M. (1980). *Street-level Bureaucracy. Dilemmas of the Public Services*. New York: Russell Sage Foundation.

Monaghan, M. (2008). Appreciating cannabis: the paradox of evidence in evidence-based policy making. *Evidence and Policy: A Journal of Research, Debate and Practice*, 4(2): 209–31.

Monaghan, M. (2010). The complexity of evidence: reflections on research utilisation in a heavily politicised policy area. *Social Policy and Society*, 9(1): 1–12.

Monaghan, M. (2011). *Evidence Versus Politics: Exploiting Research in UK Drug Policy Making?* Bristol: Policy Press.

Meyer, J. W. and Rowan, B. (1977). Institutionalized organizations: formal structure as myth and ceremony. *The American Journal of Sociology*, 83(2): 340–63.

Moore, S. F. (1978). *Laws as Process. An Anthropological Approach*. London: Routledge and Kegan Hall.

Mosse, D. (2007). Is good policy unimplementable? Reflections on ethnography of aid policy and practice. In A. C. Jimenez (ed.), *The Anthropology of Organisations*. Aldershot: Ashgate, pp. 451–83.

Moore, D. and Fraser, S. (2013). Producing the 'problem' of addiction in drug treatment. *Qualitative Health Research*, 23(7): 916–23.

Nielsen, B. and Houborg, E. (2014). Socialt arbejde, behandling og omsorgens logik. misbrugsbehandling. B. Thylstrup, M. Hesse, M. U. Pedersen and K. Frederiksen (eds), *Organisering, Indsatser Og Behov*. Aarhus: Aarhus University Press, pp. 195–208.

O'Malley, P. (1999). Consuming risks: harm minimization and the government of 'drug-users'. In R. Smandych (ed.), *Governable Places. Readings on Governmentality and Crime Control*. Aldershot: Ashgate, pp. 191–213.

Pedersen, M. U. and Nielsen, M. K. (2007). *Behandlingsgaranti Og Ydelser I Dansk Stofmisbrugsbehandling*. Aarhus: Aarhus Universitet: Center for Rusmiddelforskning.

Prottas, J. M. (1978). The power of the street-level bureaucrat in public service bureaucracies. *Urban Affairs Review*, 13(3): 285–312.

Rhodes, R. (1994). The hollowing out of the state: changing the nature of the public service in Britain. *The Political Quarterly*, 65(2): 138–51.

Rhodes, R. (1996). The new governance: governing without government. *Political Studies*, 44(4): 652–67.

Ritter, A. (2013). How can and do empirical studies influence drug policies? Narratives and complexity in the use of evidence in policy making. *Drugs: Education, Prevention and Policy*, 20(3):169–74.

Rose, N. (1999). *Powers of Freedom. Reframing Political Thought*. Cambridge: Cambridge University Press.

Scott, J. (1998). *Seeing like a State: How Certain Schemes to Improve the Human Condition Have Failed*. New Haven: Yale University Press.

Socialministeriet (2002). *Behandlingsgarantien: § 85 I Serviceloven*. Copenhagen: Socialministeriet.

Stevens, A. (2007). Survival of the ideas that fit: an evolutionary analogy for the use of evidence in policy. *Social Policy and Society*, 6(1): 25–35.

Stevens, A. (2011a). *Drugs, Crime and Public Health*. Abingdon: Routledge.

Stevens, A. (2011b). Telling policy stories: an ethnographic study of the use of evidence in policy-making in the UK. *Journal of Social Policy*, 40(2): 237–55.

Stevens, A. and Ritter, A. (2013). How can and do empirical studies influence drug policies?

Narratives and complexity in the use of evidence in policy making. *Drugs: Education, Prevention and Policy*, 20(3): 169–74.

Stoker, G. (1998). Governance as theory: five propositions. *International Social Science Journal*, 50(155): 17–28.

Tieberghien, J. and Decorte, T. (2013). Understanding the science-policy nexus in Belgium: an analysis of the drug policy debate (1996–2003). *Drugs: Education, Prevention and Policy*, 20(3): 241–8.

Valentine, K. (2009). Evidence, values and drug treatment policy. *Critical Social Policy*, 29(3): 443–64.

Wynne, B. (2000). May the sheep safely graze? A reflexive view of the expert-lay knowledge divide. In S. Lash, B. Szerszynski and B. Wynne (eds), *Risk Environment and Modernity: Towards a New Ecology*. London: Sage, pp. 44–83.

Wälti, S. and Kübler, D. (2003). New governance and associative pluralism: the case drug policy in Swiss cities. *The Policy Studies Journal*, 31(4): 499–525.

Wälti, S., Kübler, D. and Papadopoulos, Y. (2004). How democratic is 'governance'? Lessons from Swiss drug policy. *Governance: An International Journal of Policy, Administration, and Institutions*, 17(1): 83–113.

Zampini, G. F. (2014). Governance versus government: drug consumption rooms in Australia and the UK. *International Journal of Drug Policy*, 25(5): 978–84.

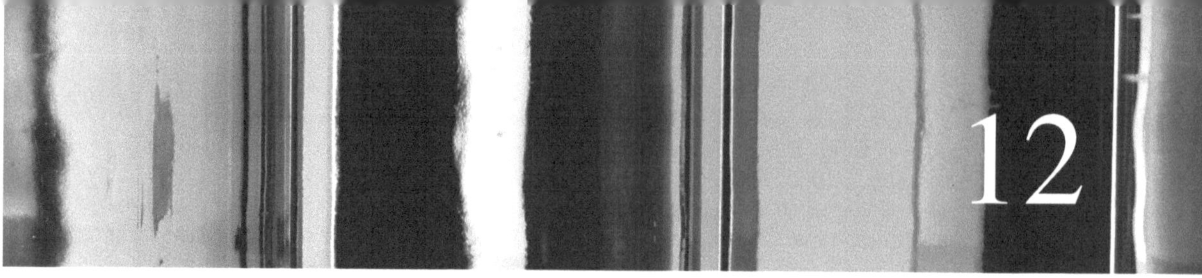

National Preventive Approaches to Tackle Alcohol Misuse

Elias Allara, Marica Ferri and Fabrizio Faggiano

INTRODUCTION

Prevention is the activity of public health dedicated to prevent the occurrence of pathological conditions and promote health (Last 2006). The value of prevention is particularly self-evident whenever the condition of interest is chronic, difficult to treat and significantly harmful to health (Ferri et al., 2015). In this chapter, we will make the case for prevention of alcohol misuse, which is broadly acknowledged as responsible for several medical, psychological, social and economic detrimental effects worldwide (Beaglehole et al. 2011; Shield et al. 2013; WHO 2014a). After providing a systematic overview of the most updated evidence base regarding preventive approaches tackling alcohol misuse, we will move to describing future perspectives and the possible implications of preventive approaches for national policymakers and health professionals.

DEFINITION AND CONSEQUENCES OF ALCOHOL MISUSE

Throughout this chapter, alcohol misuse or hazardous alcohol intake is defined as any 'maladaptive pattern of use indicated by […] continued use despite knowledge of having persistent or recurrent social, occupational, psychological or physical problem that is caused or exacerbated by the use [or by] recurrent use in situations in which it is physically hazardous' (WHO 2015).

A consolidated pathological pattern of alcohol misuse in adult life can deeply affect health and overall psychosocial functioning (Leshner 1997; Teesson et al. 2005; Concina et al. 2013; Shield et al. 2013). Heavy alcohol consumption is known to cause severe and life-threatening diseases such as alcohol dependence and other substance related disorders such as stroke, liver cirrhosis, pancreatitis and cancer (Shield et al. 2013). Alcohol misuse has also been linked to a number of conditions such as higher risk for assault, suicide, homicide, and behavioural and mental-health problems (WHO 2014a).

For the young or very young, alcohol misuse and alcohol use are generally considered synonymous. Early initiation to alcohol use has been associated with a greater risk of developing alcohol-related disorders, such as alcohol dependence and poisoning, with a 40 per cent estimated proportion of adult alcohol dependence in this early onset group (Grant and Dawson 1998), as well as with related harms including school drop-out, violence and injuries and behavioural and mental-health problems (Gruber et al. 1996; Grant et al. 2012), both in adolescence and in later adult life. However, it is worth noting that this relationship is mediated by early drunkenness while drinking small quantities of alcohol at an early age is in itself not related to adverse outcomes (Kuntsche et al. 2013). It has been argued that harmful alcohol effects are unlikely whenever children are used to drinking small amounts of alcoholic beverages in particular circumstances under parental supervision (Rolando et al. 2012).

It is therefore possible that definitions of alcohol misuse are not homogeneous in different studies. In this chapter, we will make explicit any deviations from the above mentioned definition of alcohol misuse.

THE NEED FOR PREVENTIVE APPROACHES IN ALCOHOL MISUSE

Prevention has historically been deemed a successful approach for tackling potentially life threatening conditions such as infectious diseases and cancer (Beaglehole et al. 2011). Traditional and highly effective preventive approaches, such as water sanitation, immunization programmes and population-based screening, have led to considerable improvements in population health of high income countries, and are currently being disseminated in middle income and low income countries (WHO Europe 2009, WHO 2014b, 2014c).

In previous years, some behaviours, such as alcohol misuse, smoking and improper diet, have been associated with a plethora of non-communicable diseases such as heart disease, stroke, cancer, diabetes and chronic respiratory disease, and their prevention is currently regarded as a priority at a global level (Beaglehole et al. 2011; US Department of Health and Human Services 2014). The UN High-Level Meeting on Non-Communicable Diseases in September 2011 identified five priority interventions – tobacco control, salt reduction, improved diets and physical activity, reduction in hazardous alcohol intake and essential drugs and technologies – which are regarded as fundamental strategies for tackling premature death and preventable morbidity and disability from non-communicable diseases (Beaglehole et al. 2011).

In this chapter, we will focus on one of such strategies – prevention of alcohol misuse. We feel that there are at least three reasons for which prevention of alcohol misuse appears reasonable and convenient.

First, the numerous consequences of excessive alcohol consumption described previously in this chapter suggest that efforts towards prevention are essential to avoid the development of potentially life threatening conditions.

Second, the need to prevent the misuse of alcohol is also highlighted by the considerably high prevalence of such risky behaviour among young people throughout the world (Bauman and Phongsavan 1999; WHO Europe 2009; WHO 2014a). Thirty-nine per cent of 15 to 16-year-old Europeans (Hibell et al. 2012) and 19 to 30 per cent of 12 to 18-year-old Canadians (Young et al. 2011) report binge drinking in the past month. Alcohol use and its consequences are now estimated to account for almost 4 per cent of the global burden of disease (WHO 2014a), and both adolescent binge-drinking and alcohol intoxication appear to be on the rise worldwide (WHO 2014a).

Third, to reduce the occurrence and cost of these health problems, preventive interventions need to be initiated before problems start to cause disability and vocational, educational and social harms (Spooner 2002). Prevention is getting even more compelling as the age of onset of alcohol use has been decreasing. In the US, initiation age has lowered since 1975, with youth now starting to drink at 12 years on average (Johnston et al. 2014).

In light of the above findings, early strategies to prevent alcohol misuse seem largely justifiable due to the harmful consequences of alcohol misuse, their considerable impact on global health and the apparent trend towards earlier initiation ages, which is more likely to result in worse prognosis.

GENERAL ORGANIZATIONS OF PREVENTION APPROACHES

Preventive strategies can act through different mechanisms and be focused on a wide range of targets. This section aims to provide an overview of the possible ways to organize prevention approaches and some of them will be used as a framework for later sections of this chapter.

Classical definitions

The classical categorization of prevention approaches, which arises from a work published by Hugh Leavell and E. Guerney Clark, is linked to the natural history of disease and divides preventive approaches into primary, secondary and tertiary prevention (Leavell and Clark 1979). This chapter will focus on primary prevention strategies tackling alcohol misuse with some considerations on secondary prevention interventions. A brief overview of tertiary prevention approaches is presented for reference purposes.

Primary prevention comprises all interventions that prevent a pathological condition from occurring, and emphasizes general health promotion, risk factor reduction, and other health protection measures (Last 2006; Faggiano et al. 2014a). The natural history of alcohol misuse comprises at least five stages according to the framework proposed by Bonomo and Proimos in 2005, which is based on the level of alcohol consumption (Bonomo and Proimos 2005): no use, experimentation, regular use, problem use and dependent use (Figure 12.1). Progression from earlier to more advanced stages does not occur necessarily and reversal is possible, although less common. Furthermore, it is also possible to observe a drinking pattern intermediate between experimentation stage and regular use, especially among adults, for example, whenever subjects drink occasionally although not for experimentation purposes. Individual drinking patterns can also shift between occasional and regular use, and sometimes even into problem use. The definition of primary prevention may be applied to different stages of the natural history of alcohol misuse: when the subject has not yet started to drink alcohol (first stage), with the general purpose to prevent alcohol misuse itself; or at any stage from experimentation to problem use (second to fourth stage), with the more specific aim to prevent the medical conditions and the psychosocial harms caused by alcohol misuse. In the latter case, primary prevention would comprise all actions aiming to eliminate alcohol misuse. This chapter will discuss primary prevention interventions focusing on the earliest stage, that is, aiming to prevent alcohol misuse before its onset, whereas approaches focusing on the later stages, that is, pursuing control of the harmful consequences of alcohol misuse, will be discussed in Chapter 13.

Secondary prevention is used after the disease has occurred, but before the onset of symptoms, and focuses on early detection and swift treatment of a pathological condition.

A common approach to secondary prevention is screening for pathological conditions, such as the Papanicolau test for the early detection of pre-cancerous or cancerous processes in the cervical canal of the uterus. Secondary prevention can be difficult in alcohol misuse, although in recent times some prevention programmes have started screening adolescents for character traits such as impulsivity and sensation seeking that are considered associated to predictors of possible later hazardous drinking behaviours (Castellanos-Ryan et al. 2011; Whelan et al. 2012; Conrod et al. 2013; Nees et al. 2012). This approach will be discussed in this chapter.

Tertiary prevention targets the person who already has symptoms of the pathological condition. It involves both therapeutic and rehabilitative measures once the disease is firmly established. Examples include the ongoing management of patients with chronic heart disease through medication, diet, exercise and periodic examination. Some interventions aiming to reduce the harms of the medical and socio-psychological consequences of excessive alcohol intake will be discussed in Chapter 13.

Institute of Medicine classification and later updates

A classification developed by the US Institute of Medicine is based on the level of risk and organizes prevention interventions in three categories: universal, selective and indicated interventions (Mrazek and Haggerty 1994). They can be thought as within the classical framework of primary prevention (described in the previous subsection), although some categories may present overlapping with secondary and tertiary prevention.

Universal prevention targets the whole population, interacting with the mechanisms present in the causal pathway from experimentation to disease and harms. In particular, it focuses on the ability to control stress and appropriately convey emotions, to relate with peers, to make decisions and to stand up to peer pressure.

Selective prevention targets specific groups and intervenes on their specific risk factors. Selective prevention interventions initially identify high-risk individuals – for example, in the case of alcohol misuse, those with pronounced character traits such as impulsivity and sensation seeking – and then involve them in the intervention, which usually comprises conveyance of techniques to address such specific character traits.

Indicated prevention acts at the individual level to prevent the development of a risk factor, to stop progression and diminish the frequency of substance use – and consequently to prevent dangerous substance use (Ferri and Bo 2013).

Selective interventions have the advantage of allowing limited resources to be used on those most at need. They also address individual needs of homogeneous risk groups and offer the opportunity to tailor interventions to the aetiological processes implicated in different risk profiles (Conrod et al. 2008, 2010). Selective prevention programmes are often overlooked due to their practical limitations. It is not only difficult to initially identify those individuals at greatest risk, but finding suitable, cost effective ways to screen and deliver interventions can also be challenging (Offord 2000). However, in recent years we have seen the development of selective school-based programmes such as 'Preventure', which are showing that these practical obstacles can be overcome (Conrod et al. 2013).

In addition to the categories of prevention proposed by the Institute of Medicine, the term '*environmental prevention*' has recently come into use to identify interventions that aim to 'alter the social, cultural, physical and economic environment in which individuals make their decisions about the use of drugs in order to reduce the prevalence of the use of psychoactive substances' (Burkhart 2011). Environmental interventions include regulatory actions to limit access to substances (e.g. taxation, sale and consumption restrictions), limit advertising and promote preventive media campaigns. Environmental measures are universal by definition, that is, they address the overall population and aim to reduce the effect of social pressure on alcohol misuse. They refer mainly to the social learning theory developed by Bandura (Bandura 1977) which was presented in Chapter 1. As alcohol related policies were covered in Chapter 9 and Chapter 10, this chapter will discuss only environmental prevention interventions, which are not related to implementation of policies or law enforcement, such as mass media campaigns for the prevention of alcohol misuse.

RISK AND PROTECTIVE FACTORS FOR ALCOHOL MISUSE

As mentioned previously, primary prevention focuses on reduction of risks factors and/or enhancement of protective factors (Hawkins et al. 1992; Spooner 2002). Risk factors are individual, group-specific or social characteristics that increase the likelihood of an individual developing a pathological condition (Arthur et al. 2002). As the exposure to risk factors increases, so does the likelihood of developing alcohol misuse problems (Newcomb 1995). Protective factors are characteristics, both at an individual or group level, which are known to reduce the likelihood of developing a particular risk behaviour (Arthur et al. 2002).

This section summarizes the risk and protective factors that have strong evidence to suggest that they precede alcohol misuse in adolescence. Risk and protective factors may be organized into two main categories: (i) biological and psychological individual factors (i.e. characteristics within individuals and their interpersonal environments that predispose to alcohol misuse) and (ii) environmental and contextual factors (i.e. broad societal and cultural factors).

Biological and psychological individual factors

From the 1990s onwards, biological determinants of alcohol misuse have been extensively studied, leading to a growing base of evidence that complements individual psychosocial factors (Volkow and Li 2007). Polymorphisms of genes encoding proteins involved in alcohol metabolism have been associated with clinical phenotypes of alcohol misuse. For example, alcohol dehydrogenase (ADH) is an enzyme that converts ethanol into the toxic intermediate acetaldehyde. Individuals presenting altered ADH alleles (e.g. ADH1B*2 and ADH1C*1 alleles) convert ethanol to acetaldehyde more rapidly, resulting in earlier onset of the unpleasant symptoms (due to acetaldehyde) that occur after alcohol consumption and which are likely to be protective against alcohol misuse. Lower frequencies of such protective alleles have been found among alcoholics than among non-alcoholics in East-Asian and European populations (Dick and Agrawal 2008). Polymorphisms of genes encoding proteins involved in neurotransmission – in particular in the processes of arousal, reward and memory – have been associated with alcohol misuse, although the mechanisms by which these genes may affect risk for alcohol misuse is not entirely clear (Hawkins et al. 1992; Lynskey et al. 2002; Volkow and Li 2007; Dick and Agrawal 2008).

Several psychological and interpersonal factors are also implicated with alcohol misuse. They include risk factors such as (i) temperament and personality traits (e.g. rebelliousness, non-conformity to traditional values and resistance to traditional authority, high tolerance for deviance, strong need for independence, sensation seeking trait, low harm-avoidance); (ii) attitudes (e.g. favourable attitudes to alcohol misuse and low perceived risks of alcohol misuse); and (iii) behavioural and emotional issues (e.g. early and persistent aggression, early conduct problems, adolescent delinquency, frequent drug use in late adolescence, depression, attention-deficit/hyperactivity disorder) (Hawkins et al. 1992; Scheier et al. 1997; Stockwell et al. 2004; Bonomo and Proimos 2005; Newton et al. 2012; Whelan et al. 2012). Protective factors include diverse characteristics such as an easy temperament in childhood, social and emotional competence, religious involvement, shy and cautious temperament, 'belief in natural order', social problem-solving skills and belief in own self-efficacy (Hawkins et al. 1992; Scheier et al. 1997; Stockwell et al. 2004; Newton et al. 2012).

Socio-contextual factors

Social influence is recognized to have a strong effect in determining behaviours in adolescents and theoretical models have widely acknowledged the influence of socio-contextual factors. In particular, the 'social norms theory' states that behaviour is influenced by incorrect perceptions ('perceived norm') of how the other members of social groups act (Perkins and Berkowitz 1986). Such a theory may play a significant role for alcohol misuse. Perception of alcohol misuse as a widespread and socially acceptable behaviour was found to be positively associated with prevalence of alcohol misuse (Newton et al. 2012; Concina et al. 2013).

In addition to perceived norms, the major environmental factors that influence alcohol misuse pertain to (i) peers (e.g. peer use of substance or poor social connections); (ii) family (e.g. familial attitudes that are favourable to the use of substances, parental modelling of substance misuse, poor or inconsistent parenting practices); and (iii) society (e.g. low parental socio economic status, living in a deprived neighbourhood) (Hawkins et al. 1992; Spooner 2002; Oetting and Lynch 2003; Loxley et al. 2004; Stockwell et al. 2004; Bonomo and Proimos 2005; Kuntsche and Jordan 2006; Ahern et al. 2008; Andersson 2014).

Implications for prevention interventions

The literature has identified a wide array of risk and protective factors for developing problem alcohol behaviour. However, it is unclear which risk factors or combinations of risk factors are more pertinent in impacting on adolescents' drug use. What we do know is that a greater risk of problem alcohol drinking is associated to a greater number of risk factors that persist and influence an individual over time (Hawkins et al. 1992; Loxley et al. 2004).

Initiation to alcohol misuse is determined by several individual factors and social pressures and it can hardly be tackled by a single intervention (Newton et al. 2012). In terms of developing effective and efficient prevention interventions, it seems sensible that interventions adopt a multi-component approach aimed at reducing risks and enhancing protective factors both at the individual and societal level, and take into account epidemiological studies on initiation age for alcohol experimentation (Hawkins et al. 1992; Spooner 2002; Bonomo and Proimos 2005; Newton et al. 2012).

EVALUATION OF PREVENTION INTERVENTIONS TACKLING ALCOHOL MISUSE

Advantages and challenges of evidence-based prevention

A number of official documents promote an evidence-based approach to prevention, which includes prevention of alcohol misuse (WHO Europe 2006; WHO Europe 2012; EMCDDA 2013). This is due to at least two reasons. First, and in contrast to common belief, prevention interventions are not just harmless or ineffective in the worst-case scenario. Increase in risk behaviours targeted by prevention programmes has been observed in interventions tackling risky behaviours such as substance misuse (Sloboda et al. 2009), as well as physical inactivity, early sexual intercourse and juvenile delinquency (Sallis et al. 1993; Kirby et al. 1997; Werch and Owen 2002; Petrosino et al. 2004). Second, resources are likely to be wasted if evidence of effectiveness is missing or not sought. Cochrane reviews on the prevention of risky behaviours (Faggiano et al. 2014d; Foxcroft and Tsertsvadze 2011a; Waters et al. 2011) show that effective interventions are in the minority of those evaluated by randomized studies. There is no reason to presume that non-evaluated interventions may be more effective than those that underwent rigorous evaluation.

However, evaluation of prevention interventions tackling alcohol misuse may present several challenges. Prevention interventions usually target psychological, social and organizational factors hypothesized to mediate the associations between intervention and alcohol misuse. Then, interventions are usually delivered as a complex combination of components (i.e. active ingredients targeting different mediators), both in terms of contents, activities, techniques and modes of delivery, which are usually poorly described. Less than 30 per cent of reports of randomized studies present a detailed description of the intervention allowing accurate replication and implementation, and fewer include descriptions of mechanisms of action (Riley et al. 2008; Michie et al. 2009). In addition, complex interventions, composed of several components, are usually evaluated together and that makes it difficult to disentangle the role of single ingredients on mediators and behavioural outcomes. The failure to conceptualize, define and describe intervention components and mediators restricts the potential for evaluation to add evidence about effective interventions and mechanisms of action. In addition, the effects of context are rarely recognized, reported or analysed.

Not knowing the reasons for which, and the context in which prevention interventions work limits knowledge about generalizability and optimization of interventions. It also increases the cost of implementation, as non-essential mediators and non-essential settings might be inappropriately targeted. In the section 'Future perspectives for prevention of alcohol misuse' we propose a possible solution to increase the supply of evidence based prevention interventions, which may improve the overall effectiveness of prevention interventions tackling alcohol misuse.

An evidence-based approach to organize prevention interventions

The previous section discussed some reasons for which careful appraisal of evaluation interventions might contribute positively to the development of effective and affordable strategies to tackle alcohol misuse. This section presents a framework that aims to classify prevention interventions according to their level of evidence, thus facilitating the identification of the best practices to prevent alcohol misuse in the current state of knowledge.

Prevention interventions may be classified according to the setting in which they are implemented, for example, family, school, communities and recreational settings. Such classification has the advantages of being oriented to practice and virtually independent on the background of the health professionals who are appointed to the choice and implementation of prevention interventions. This is particularly useful whenever it is necessary to disseminate the findings of prevention studies to a broad audience that is interested in knowing which interventions work best in a particular setting. At the time of writing, this is the classification approach chosen by the

Best Practice Portal (Ferri and Bo 2013) of the European Monitoring Centre for Drugs and Drug Addiction (EMCDDA), which is the European Union's leading agency for drugs prevention and monitoring. Although the EMCDDA focuses on alcohol only in the framework of poly-substance use and therefore the evidence on interventions for alcohol misuse might not be comprehensive, their system of classification of prevention interventions appears to flexibly balance completeness and intelligibility.

Within each target group, the EMCDDA Best Practice Portal organizes interventions by levels of evidence. The categories of effectiveness were created following those adopted by *BMJ Clinical Evidence* that were originally developed in the Cochrane Collaboration first editorial group for the publication '*A Guide to Effective Care in Pregnancy and Childbirth*' (Enkin et al. 2000).

The five levels of strength of evidence used within each target group are defined as follows (EMCDDA 2014):

1 *Beneficial.* Interventions for which precise measures of the effects in favour of the intervention are available from systematic reviews.[1] An intervention ranked as 'beneficial' is suitable for most contexts.
2 *Likely to be beneficial.* Interventions for which there is some evidence of effectiveness, that were shown to have limited measures of effect, that are likely to be effective but for which evidence is limited and/or those that are recommended with some caution in guidelines which have reliable methods for assessing evidence. An intervention ranked as 'likely to be beneficial' is suitable for most contexts, with some discretion.
3 *Trade-off between benefits and harms.* Interventions for which there is evidence of effects in favour of the intervention, but that showed some limitations or unintended effects which still need to be addressed.
4 *Unknown effectiveness.* Interventions for which there are not enough studies or where available studies are of low quality or with uncertain methodological rigour, making it difficult to assess whether they are effective or not. This category includes interventions for which more research should be undertaken.
5 *Evidence of ineffectiveness.* Interventions for which there is evidence of an effect in favour of no intervention or of a standard intervention.

OVERVIEW OF PREVENTION INTERVENTIONS TACKLING ALCOHOL MISUSE

Several preventive approaches have shown promise and are supported by a growing body of evidence. In this section we will focus on primary prevention of alcohol misuse and organize preventive approaches within primary prevention by following the EMCDDA classification by target groups and strength of evidence (as described previously). With regard to environmental interventions, only mass media campaigns for the prevention of alcohol misuse will be covered.

For prevention to be effective, it must be both relevant and developmentally appropriate (Dusenbury and Falco 1995; McBride 2003; Newton et al. 2012). It is argued that there are three periods during adolescence when the effects of prevention interventions targeting substance misuse can be optimized: the inoculation phase, the early relevance phase and the late relevance phase (Hawks et al. 2002; McBride 2003; Newton et al. 2012). The inoculation phase is the phase prior to initial experimentation with alcohol and corresponds to the earliest stage ('No use') described in Figure 12.1 (Bonomo and Proimos 2005). The early relevance phase occurs when most students are experiencing initial exposure to alcohol and corresponds to the second stage ('Experimentation') in Figure 12.1. Finally, the late relevance phase is a phase when the prevalence of alcohol misuse increases and the context of use changes, and corresponds to the third ('Regular use') and fourth ('Problem use') stages of Figure 12.1.

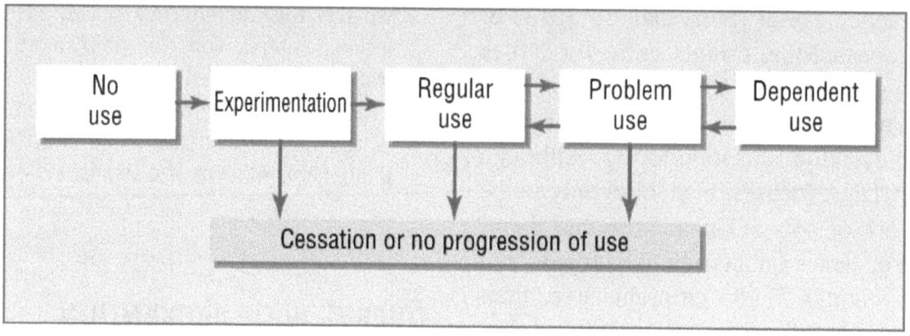

Figure 12.1 Trajectories of substance misuse

Source: (Bonomo and Proimos 2005).

Research has shown that there are a number of effective interventions that are implemented in the early relevance and late relevance phases (McCambridge and Strang 2004). They are generally indicated prevention interventions that target youth who have already started to use substances and experience related harms (Offord 2000).

As the goal of most prevention interventions is to prevent excessive uptake of alcohol, the inoculation stage is considered the most appropriate stage to intervene. It seems sensible that, due to the considerable number of individual and social factors associated with alcohol misuse, prevention interventions should intervene in all the settings in which preadolescents live, with particular regard to school, family, community and recreational settings. However, although such a holistic approach is conceptually sound, it is also resource intensive and not easily achievable. This section is thus organized to reflect the current situation, in which many prevention interventions are delivered exclusively in particular settings (Table 12.1).

Family

Many universal approaches based on knowledge, social norms or social competences have been shown to be ineffective (Faggiano et al. 2005; Foxcroft and Tsertsvadze 2011a). However, reviews have found evidence that school-based prevention can result in significant increases in knowledge about substances and improved attitudes towards substance use (Hansen 1992; Botvin 2000; Tobler et al. 2000; Botvin and Griffin 2007; Faggiano et al. 2008). Recent reviews of school-based universal prevention interventions have identified a number of effective programmes that incorporate a social influence and a social competence approach to prevention (Foxcroft and Tsertsvadze 2011a). These include the Life Skills Training programme (Botvin et al. 2001, 2003), the Unplugged programme (Faggiano et al. 2008, 2010), the Climate Schools programme (Newton et al. 2009, 2010) and the Good Behaviour Game (van Lier et al. 2009).

Newton et al. (2013) summarized the principles that have been associated with effective alcohol misuse prevention programmes in schools: being evidence based and theory driven; targeting risk factors for substance use and psychopathology; being developmentally appropriate; implemented prior to the onset of harmful patterns of use; integrated into a comprehensive health education curriculum; adopting a social influence or comprehensive approach; providing immediately- and youth-relevant content, use of peer interaction; sensitive to cultural and local attitudes; providing

Table 12.1 Preventive approaches organized by levels of evidence as proposed by the European Monitoring Centre for Drugs and Drug Addiction School

	School	*Family*	*Community*	*Recreational setting*	*Mass media*
Beneficial	• School-based programmes that implement the concepts of social influence and life skills • School-based interactive programmes • Multi-component prevention programmes	Multi-component prevention programmes	• Comprehensive approaches involving community, school and family and targeting high-risk youth • Mentoring for preventing alcohol use in young people	–	–
Likely to be beneficial	• School-based alcohol-specific prevention programmes • Standalone affective-focused interventions	Family-based prevention programmes	• Interactive programmes targeting vulnerable youth • Multi-component prevention programmes	–	Mass media campaigns to reduce drink driving
Unknown effectiveness	• Booster sessions • Multi-component versus single components programmes for alcohol misuse in young people • School-based generic prevention programmes tackling alcohol misuse • Standalone anti-alcohol peer-led programmes	Multi-component versus single components programmes for alcohol misuse in young people	• Anti-alcohol community interventions • Multi-component versus single components programmes for alcohol misuse in young people	Dedicated drink-driving programmes to change alcohol consumption	Standalone mass media campaigns for alcohol consumption
Ineffective	–	–	–	Educational interventions in recreational settings to influence attitudes and drinking behaviour	–

adequate initial coverage and continued follow-up in booster sessions; and delivered using interactive teaching approaches and within an overall framework of harm minimization. The authors (Newton et al. 2013) also argued that the main barriers to evidence-based prevention in schools are coverage, fidelity and quality when programmes are disseminated, some of which could be addressed through the use of new web-based technologies.

Nevertheless, specific programme formats or approaches cannot predict effectiveness, as even theoretically sound and well implemented interventions can be ineffective or even result in iatrogenic effects (Sloboda et al. 2009). Moreover, the addition of other components usually does not improve programme effectiveness (Faggiano et al. 2010), but once again with exceptions: a Dutch trial found effects on adolescents' alcohol use of a classroom-based general intervention only in the arm where a parent-information component was added (Koning et al. 2009). The combined intervention had long-term effects, mediated by self-control, parental rules and attitudes about alcohol use (Koning et al. 2011, 2012).

Beneficial interventions

School-based programmes that implement the concepts of social influence and life skills. One randomized controlled trial (RCT) with a sample size of N=7,079 provided evidence of 20 per cent lower odds of overall drunkenness [95% confidence interval (95%CI) 3% to 33%] and of 38 per cent lower odds of drunkenness (95%CI 9% to 53%) (Faggiano et al. 2010).

School-based interactive programmes implemented in schools with predominantly special population, were found in a meta-analysis of 207 studies (Tobler et al. 2000), in a re-analysis of the same set of studies (Roona et al. 2003) and in a further analysis of 15 studies (Porath-Waller et al. 2010) to be more effective than non-interactive programmes in reducing alcohol use or drink driving.

Multi-component prevention programmes. Interventions operating on different mediators and/or in different settings have shown in a systematic review (Foxcroft and Tsertsvadze 2011a) of 20 RCTs to be effective in reducing alcohol misuse in adolescents (12 of the 20 trials showed some evidence of effectiveness). One particular prevention programme showing promise in the field of adolescent drug and alcohol prevention, the Preventure Programme, recommends targeting four personality risk-factors for early-onset drinking or illicit drug use: hopelessness, anxiety-sensitivity, impulsivity and sensation-seeking. This school-based programme has now been shown to prevent alcohol and substance misuse in three separate trials across Canada and the United Kingdom (Conrod et al. 2013), and is based on a cognitive-behavioural and motivational approach. This intervention is associated with 50 to 60 per cent reduced drinking and binge-drinking rates over six months (Conrod et al. 2008), as well as two-year reductions in problem-drinking symptoms and illicit drug use in high risk youth (Conrod et al. 2010). A recent analysis of the two-year outcomes of the Adventure Effectiveness Trial showed that this targeted prevention programme produced 'herd' effects, in that the interventions indirectly resulted in less drinking behaviour in low risk youth who simply attended schools where interventions were delivered to high risk youth (Conrod et al. 2013). This prevention programme has been highlighted in a number of large reviews (Strang et al. 2012) as a promising prevention strategy and an alternative to universal approaches.

Interventions likely to be beneficial

School-based alcohol-specific prevention programmes targeting school-aged children up to 18 years of age have shown to be effective in a systematic review (Foxcroft and Tsertsvadze 2011b) of 53 RCTs in reducing alcohol misuse in adolescents ('statistically significant' outcomes in six out of 11 alcohol-specific trials).

Standalone affective-focused interventions aiming to increase decision making skills, compared to usual curricula and knowledge-focused interventions were found in a systematic review of 32 studies (29 RCTs and three population surveys, N= 46,539) (Faggiano et al. 2005) to be effective in improving decision making skills.

Interventions with unknown effectiveness

Booster sessions. A review of 29 reviews (McGrath et al. 2006) found evidence that booster sessions or similar extra components that aimed to reinforce the effects of a programme have a positive impact on the pre-specified outcomes. However, as the association between booster sessions and programme outcomes was not analysed statistically, the link should be treated as hypothetical.

Multi-component versus single components programmes for alcohol misuse in young people. There is little evidence that interventions with multiple components are more effective than interventions with single components as shown in a systematic review (Foxcroft and Tsertsvadze 2011a). Only one of the seven trials that assessed the additional benefit of multiple versus single component interventions clearly showed a benefit of components delivered in more than one setting.

School-based generic prevention programmes tackling alcohol misuse (not including life skills or social skills approaches, see above in the Beneficial subsection) have not provided sufficient evidence of effectiveness in a systematic review (Foxcroft and Tsertsvadze 2011b) of 53 RCTs in reducing alcohol misuse in adolescents (no evidence of programme effect in 24 out of 39 generic trials).

Standalone anti-alcohol peer-led programmes. There is evidence from a narrative review including results of one RCT (N=326) (Velleman 2009) that specific training given to young people in order to make them influence each other is not effective in reducing alcohol use and in increasing knowledge and attitudes towards alcohol.

Family

Comprehensive family-oriented prevention interventions proved to be effective in reducing alcohol misuse, as well as home visitation for disadvantaged families.

Beneficial interventions

Multi-component prevention programmes. Intervention delivered in more than one setting and/or operating on more than one mediator have shown in a systematic review (Foxcroft and Tsertsvadze 2011a) of 20 RCTs to be effective in reducing alcohol misuse in adolescents (12 of the 20 trials showed some evidence of effectiveness).

Interventions likely to be beneficial

Family-based prevention programmes (including development of parenting skills, parental support, nurturing behaviours, establishing clear boundaries or rules, parental monitoring, social and peer resistance skills, development of behavioural norms and positive peer affiliations) have shown to be effective in nine of the 12 RCTs analysed in a systematic review (Foxcroft and Tsertsvadze 2011c) in reducing alcohol misuse in adolescents, with persistence of effects over the medium and long term. An example of such type of intervention is the Strengthening Families Program (SFP), originally a selective programme for parents and children aged three to five, six to 11 and 12 to 16 in high-risk families, developed in 1983 in Utah, USA (Burkhart 2013). SFP was revised in 1992 into a shorter (and more universal) version (the Iowa SFP). In Europe, versions of the SFP are currently being implemented in Germany, Ireland, Greece, Spain, the Netherlands, Poland, Portugal, Slovenia, Sweden and the United Kingdom. The programme consists of parenting skills training, children's life skills training, and family life skills training, taught together in 14 two-hour group sessions preceded by a meal that includes informal 'family practice time' and group leader coaching.

Interventions with unknown effectiveness

Multi-component versus single components programmes for alcohol misuse in young people. See Section 'School', within the 'Interventions with unknown effectiveness' subsection.

Community

Comprehensive community based programmes were found more effective than interventions targeting community or school only in reducing alcohol misuse among high-risk young individuals.

Beneficial interventions

Comprehensive approaches involving community, school and family and targeting high-risk youth were found effective in a systematic review of 222 studies (14 systematic reviews; 103 RCTs; 52 controlled non-randomized studies; 18 controlled before-and-after studies; 35 before-and-after studies) (Jones et al. 2006) at preventing, delaying or reducing alcohol when compared with community-only programmes and school-community programmes targeting high-risk youth and in high-risk individuals when compared with low-risk individuals. There was no difference in effectiveness between 'school-community' programmes and 'community-only' programmes. No other significant differences were reported. One particular prevention programme showing promise in the field of adolescent drug and alcohol prevention, the Preventure Programme, described in the 'School' section, 'Beneficial interventions' subsection.

Mentoring for preventing alcohol use in young people. Mentoring, intended as a supportive relationship in which one person offers support, guidance and concrete assistance to the other, based on the sharing of experience and expertise without the mentor expecting personal gain, was found in a systematic review of three RCTs (Thomas et al. 2011) to reduce risk of alcohol use by 29 per cent compared to no intervention (95%CI 10% to 43%).

Interventions likely to be beneficial

Interactive programmes targeting vulnerable youth. Programmes offering strong behavioural life skills development content, emphasizing team-building, interpersonal communication methods and introspective learning approaches were found to be effective in a review of studies (Springer et al. 2004) in reducing 30-day alcohol use among vulnerable youth. Such programmes were based upon a clearly articulated and coherent theory, and provided quality contact with young people.

Multi-component prevention programmes. Interventions delivered in more than one setting and/or operating on more than one mediator have shown in a systematic review (Foxcroft and Tsertsvadze 2011a) of 20 RCTs to be effective in reducing alcohol misuse in adolescents: 12 out of 20 trials showed some evidence of effectiveness.

Interventions with unknown effectiveness

Anti-alcohol community interventions were analysed in a review of 29 reviews (McGrath et al. 2006) and some studies with no control groups suggested some reduction in alcohol use.

Multi-component versus single components programmes for alcohol misuse in young people. See Section 'School', within the 'Interventions with unknown effectiveness' subsection.

Recreational setting

Interventions with unknown effectiveness

Dedicated drink-driving programmes to change alcohol consumption. Programmes targeting drink-driving were found to have no impact on client behaviours in a systematic review (Jones et al. 2011). One low-quality RCT (N=575 clients) compared eight intervention premises, which promoted responsible drinking and placed breath analysis machines, with nine control premises, and revealed no significant differences in blood alcohol concentration.

Interventions with evidence of ineffectiveness

Educational interventions in recreational settings to influence attitudes and drinking behaviour. Educational interventions were found in a systematic review (Bolier et al. 2011) to have no effects on alcohol misuse and use of illicit drugs.

Mass-media

Mass-media campaigns associated with other interventions proved effective in reducing alcohol misuse, while no evidence of effectiveness was found for standalone mass-media campaigns in reducing alcohol misuse.

Interventions likely to be beneficial

Mass media campaigns to reduce drink driving were found to be effective in a narrative review (Wakefield et al. 2010) of four studies evaluating diverse mass media campaigns. Television advertisements to combat alcohol-impaired driving, in combination with supporting measures, have effects on reducing alcohol-impaired driving and alcohol-related accidents (Agostinelli and Grube 2002).

Interventions with unknown effectiveness

Standalone mass-media campaigns for alcohol consumption were found to be ineffective in a narrative review (Wakefield et al. 2010). In particular: (i) warnings on drink bottles as a standalone measure have no effect on alcohol consumption; (ii) the potential effects of media campaigns to reduce alcohol intake have generally been overshadowed by widespread unrestricted alcohol marketing strategies and by the view of drinking as a 'social norm'; and (iii) safe drinking campaigns sponsored by alcohol companies have been ineffective in changing drinking behaviour.

FUTURE PERSPECTIVES FOR PREVENTION OF ALCOHOL MISUSE

The field of prevention science is young and emerging, and the implications of delineating a science for the field of prevention are only recently appreciated (Faggiano et al. 2014a, 2014b). A number of international landmark events have taken place over the past two decades that are beginning to have a cumulative effect on the development of effective and evidence based prevention interventions addressing behavioural problems such as alcohol misuse. Such benchmarks include the establishment of the Society for Prevention Research (SPR) in the United States and the European Society for Prevention Research (EUSPR), and publication of works fostering the development of evidence based prevention interventions, such as the National Institute on Drug Abuse's Preventing Drug Abuse Among Children and Adolescents: A Research Guide (NIDA 2010), the European Drug Prevention Quality Standards (Brotherhood and Sumnall 2012; EMCDDA 2012), the SPR's Standards of Evidence and Knowledge (Flay et al. 2005) and the International Standards for Drug Use Prevention by the United Nations Office on Drugs and Crime (UNODC 2013).

The above mentioned documents underscore the importance of standardizing the criteria and processes for the development of evidence-based interventions, which might be useful to address the challenges of prevention evaluation discussed previously. Recent publications (Faggiano et al. 2014a, 2014b) propose a new framework to promote the implementation of effective prevention interventions tackling alcohol misuse and other risk behaviours (e.g. illicit drug use, physical inactivity, engagement in risky sexual behaviours, etc.). The outlined framework is based on existing systems for assessing the safety and effectiveness of medical drugs and devices, and on existing systems for optimising the evaluation of behavioural interventions (Collins et al. 2011). In most parts of the world, no prior evaluation is required for the implementation of prevention interventions, often leading to widespread dissemination of ineffective or harmful interventions and resulting in considerable harms to populations (Faggiano et al. 2014a, 2014b, 2014c). The proposed framework would incorporate as essential components: (i) the transparency of its decisions and (ii) the flexibility to adapt to heterogeneous interventions and replications. Similar to medicine approval systems, such approval process would be based on four consequential phases evaluating the effect of: single components (phase 1); combinations of components (phase 2); the final intervention, comprising only components found effective in the previous phases (phase 3); and the long term effects as well as the effects in different contexts (phase 4). Once phase 3 shows convincing results, the intervention would be approved for delivery to its target population. Such an evaluation and approval process may represent a unique opportunity for prevention targeting alcohol misuse, by strengthening the role and impact of prevention in times of limited economic resources, and for research, by promoting the robust evaluation of all promising prevention interventions and the identification of most effective components.

The above described approach would favour the identification of the socio-cultural and individual level factors that moderate the effects of prevention interventions and would ease trans-disciplinary and cross-cultural research efforts to produce effective interventions. Interventions might benefit even more than now from the continuing accrual of knowledge deriving from biomedical and psychosocial research such as the discovery of individual level psychological and biological characteristics that predispose or protect from alcohol misuse, and the identification of protective or hazardous socio-contextual factors. Such an integrated and personalized approach in primary prevention would target people who are healthy, resulting in possible risk for stigmatization that will need to be adequately addressed – for example, through proper counselling and communication. Possible approaches could comprise an active inclusion of subjects in the decisions about preventive strategies and a continued attention to preferences and values of individuals (Bradley and Kivlahan 2014), which are already becoming a current practice in the field of prevention and have an enormous potential for the improvement of health outcomes of people undertaking risk behaviours such as alcohol misuse.

IMPLICATIONS FOR NATIONAL DECISION MAKERS AND PUBLIC HEALTH PROFESSIONALS

Several preventive approaches, as well specific prevention programmes, have shown evidence of effectiveness. School-based programmes incorporating both social influence and social competence approaches, community based mentoring programmes and some mass-media campaigns have been found effective. Consistently with the complex aetiology of alcohol misuse, comprehensive multi-component programmes, for example, prevention programmes delivered in more than one setting, have shown evidence of effectiveness.

In general, information provision alone is not considered an effective strategy, whereas skills development programmes were found to prevent alcohol misuse. We feel that there may be at least four possible implications for national policymakers and public health professionals.

First, in addition to identifying effective interventions and approaches, there is also a need to develop the systems, such as training of deliverer and supply of intervention materials, required to extensively disseminate effective prevention interventions to all the target population.

Second, many current activities and proposals rely on an incomplete evidence base. Careful consideration should be given to all activities being implemented, including unintended effects and opportunity costs.

Third, wherever evidence of effectiveness is unclear, policies and interventions should be implemented only as part of sufficiently funded scientific research projects aiming to evaluate the effectiveness of such policies and intervention by using robust research methodologies.

Fourth, wherever evidence suggests that actions have iatrogenic effects, policymakers and public health professionals should attempt to modify actions that are not in line with good practice recommendations. Their choices can have considerable implications for the public's health and it seems sensible that national policymakers disinvest in harmful, ineffective, or non-evaluated approaches while switching public investments towards interventions that provide evidence of beneficial effects.

NOTE

1 The following study designs are considered: (i) randomized controlled trials in which the unit of randomization is an individual or a cluster (the school, community or geographical region); (ii) controlled trials without randomization allocating schools, communities or geographical regions; (iii) prospective cohort studies; (iv) interrupted time series; (v) controlled before-and-after studies.

REFERENCES

Agostinelli, G. and Grube, J.W. (2002). Alcohol counter-advertising and the media. A review of recent research. *Alcohol Research and Health*, 26(1): 15–21.

Ahern, J., Galea, S., Hubbard, A., Midanik, L. and Syme, S.L. (2008). 'Culture of drinking' and individual problems with alcohol use. *American Journal of Epidemiology*, 167(9): 1041–9.

Andersson, O. (2014). William Foote Whyte, Street Corner Society and social organization. *Journal of the History of the Behavioral Sciences*, 50(1): 79–103.

Arthur, M.W., Hawkins, J.D., Pollard, J.A., Catalano, R.F. and Baglioni Jr, A.J. (2002). Measuring risk and protective factors for substance use, delinquency, and other adolescent problem behaviors. The Communities That Care Youth Survey. *Evaluation Review*, 26(6): 575–601.

Bandura, A. (1977). *Social Learning Theory*. Englewood Cliffs: Prentice-Hall.

Bauman, A. and Phongsavan, P. (1999). Epidemiology of substance use in adolescence: prevalence, trends and policy implications. *Drug and Alcohol Dependence*, 55(3): 187–207.

Beaglehole, R., Bonita, R., Horton, R., Adams, C., Alleyne, G., Asaria, P., Baugh, V., Bekedam, H., Billo, N., Casswell, S., Cecchini, M., Colagiuri, R., Colagiuri, S., Collins, T., Ebrahim, S., Engelgau, M., Galea, G., Gaziano, T., Geneau, R., Haines, A., Hospedales, J., Jha, P., Keeling, A., Leeder, S., Lincoln, P., McKee, M., Mackay, J., Magnusson, R., Moodie, R., Mwatsama, M., Nishtar, S., Norrving, B., Patterson, D., Piot, P., Ralston, J., Rani, M., Reddy, K.S., Sassi, F., Sheron, N., Stuckler, D., Suh, I., Torode, J., Varghese, C., Watt, J., Lancet NCD Action Group and NCD Alliance. (2011). Priority actions for the non-communicable disease crisis. *Lancet*, 377(9775): 1438–47.

Bolier, L., Voorham, L., Monshouwer, K., van Hasselt, N. and Bellis, M. (2011). Alcohol and drug prevention in nightlife settings: a review of experimental studies. *Substance Use and Misuse*, 46(13): 1569–91.

Bonomo, Y. and Proimos, J. (2005). Substance misuse: alcohol, tobacco, inhalants, and other drugs. *BMJ (Clinical research ed.)*, 330(7494): 777–80.

Botvin, G.J. (2000). Preventing drug abuse in schools. *Addictive Behaviors*, 25(6): 887–97.

Botvin, G.J. and Griffin, K.W. (2007). School-based programmes to prevent alcohol, tobacco and other drug use. *International Review of Psychiatry (Abingdon, England)*, 19(6): 607–15.

Botvin, G.J., Griffin, K.W., Diaz, T. and Ifill-Williams, M. (2001). Preventing binge drinking during early adolescence: one- and two-year follow-up of a school-based preventive intervention. *Psychology of Addictive Behaviors*, 15(4): 360–5.

Botvin, G.J., Griffin, K.W., Paul, E. and Macaulay, A.P. (2003). Preventing tobacco and alcohol use among elementary school students through life skills training. *Journal of Child and Adolescent Substance Abuse*, 12(4): 1–17.

Bradley, K.A. and Kivlahan, D.R. (2014). Bringing patient-centered care to patients with alcohol use disorders. *JAMA*, 311(18): 1861–2.

Brotherhood, A. and Sumnall, H. (2012). *European Drug Prevention Quality Standards*. Lisbon: EMCDDA.

Burkhart, G. (2011). Environmental drug prevention in the EU. Why is it so unpopular? *Adicciones*, 23(2): 87–100.

Burkhart, G. (2013). *North American Drug Prevention Programmes: Are They Feasible in European Cultures and Contexts?* Lisbon: EMCDDA.

Castellanos-Ryan, N., Rubia, K. and Conrod, P.J. (2011). Response inhibition and reward response bias mediate the predictive

relationships between impulsivity and sensation seeking and common and unique variance in conduct disorder and substance misuse. *Alcoholism, Clinical and Experimental Research*, 35(1): 140–55.
Collins, L.M., Baker, T.B., Mermelstein, R.J., Piper, M.E., Jorenby, D.E., Smith, S.S., Christiansen, B.A., Schlam, T.R., Cook, J.W. and Fiore, M.C. (2011). The multiphase optimization strategy for engineering effective tobacco use interventions. *Annals of Behavioral Medicine*, 41(2): 208–26.
Concina, D., Giubertoni, A., Spina, P., Allara, E., Faggiano, F. and Avogadro Alcohol Group. (2013). Alcohol and the young: how does the press face the problem? *Epidemiology Biostatistics and Public Health*, 10(4): e8644-1–11.
Conrod, P.J., Castellanos, N. and Mackie, C. (2008). Personality-targeted interventions delay the growth of adolescent drinking and binge drinking. *Journal of Child Psychology and Psychiatry, and Allied Disciplines*, 49(2): 181–90.
Conrod, P.J., Castellanos-Ryan, N. and Strang, J. (2010). Brief, personality-targeted coping skills interventions and survival as a non-drug user over a 2-year period during adolescence. *Archives of General Psychiatry*, 67(1): 85–93.
Conrod, P.J., O'Leary-Barrett, M., Newton, N., Topper, L., Castellanos-Ryan, N., Mackie, C. and Girard, A. (2013). Effectiveness of a selective, personality-targeted prevention program for adolescent alcohol use and misuse: a cluster randomized controlled trial. *JAMA Psychiatry*, 70(3): 334–42.
Dick, D.M. and Agrawal, A. (2008). The genetics of alcohol and other drug dependence. *Alcohol Research and Health*, 31(2): 111–18.
Dusenbury, L. and Falco, M. (1995). Eleven components of effective drug abuse prevention curricula. *The Journal of School Health*, 65(10): 420–5.
EMCDDA (2012). *Guidelines for the Evaluation of Drug Prevention. A Manual for Programme Planners and Evaluators*. Lisbon: EMCDDA.
EMCDDA (2013). *European Drug Report*. Luxembourg: Publications Office of the European Union.
EMCDDA (2014). *Best Practice Portal: Prevention*. Available at: http://www.emcdda.europa.eu/best-practice/prevention (accessed 10 June 2014).
Enkin, M., Keirse, M., Neilson, J., Crowther, C., Duley, L., Hodnett, E. and Hofmeyr, J. (2000). *A Guide to Effective Care in Pregnancy and Childbirth*. Oxford: Oxford University Press.
Faggiano, F., Giannotta, F. and Allara, E. (2014a). Strengthening prevention science to ensure effectiveness of intervention in practice: setting up an international agenda. In Z. Sloboda and H. Petras (eds), *Defining Prevention Science*. Boston: Springer US, pp. 597–615.
Faggiano, F., Allara, E., Giannotta, F., Molinar, R., Sumnall, H., Wiers, R., Michie, S., Collins, L. and Conrod, P. (2014b). Europe needs a central, transparent, and evidence-based approval process for behavioural prevention interventions. *PLoS medicine*, 11(10): p. e1001740.
Faggiano, F., Concina, D., Molinar, R. and Allara, E. (2014c). [Primary prevention of cancer and cardiovascular diseases: an overview of scientific literature]. *Epidemiologia e Prevenzione*, 38(6 Suppl 2): 19–22.
Faggiano, F., Vigna-Taglianti, F.D., Versino, E., Zambon, A., Borraccino, A. and Lemma, P. (2008). School-based prevention for illicit drugs use: a systematic review. *Preventive Medicine*, 46(5): 385–96.
Faggiano, F., Minozzi, S., Versino, E., and Buscemi D. (2014d). Universal school-based prevention for illicit drug use. *The Cochrane Database of Systematic Reviews*, (12): CD003020.
Faggiano, F., Vigna-Taglianti, F.D., Burkhart, G., Bohrn, K., Cuomo, L., Gregori, D., Panella, M., Scatigna, M., Siliquini, R., Varona, L., van der Kreeft, P., Vassara, M., Wiborg, G., Galanti, MR. and EU-Dap Study Group (2010). The effectiveness of a school-based substance abuse prevention program: 18-month follow-up of the EU-Dap cluster randomized controlled trial. *Drug and Alcohol Dependence*, 108(1-2): 56–64.
Ferri, M., Ballotta, D., Carráb G., and Dias S. (2015). A review of regional drug strategies across the world: How is prevention perceived and addressed? *Drugs: Education, Prevention and Policy*, 22(5): 444–8.

Ferri, M. and Bo, A. (2013). EMCDDA best practice promotion in Europe: an internet based dissemination tool. *Adicciones*, 25(1): 3–6.

Flay, B.R., Biglan, A., Boruch, R.F., Castro, F.G., Gottfredson, D., Kellam, S., Mościcki, E.K., Schinke, S., Valentine, J.C. and Ji, P. (2005). Standards of evidence: criteria for efficacy, effectiveness and dissemination. *Prevention Science*, 6(3): 151–75.

Foxcroft, D.R. and Tsertsvadze, A. (2011a). Universal multi-component prevention programs for alcohol misuse in young people. *The Cochrane Database of Systematic Reviews*, (9): CD009307.

Foxcroft, D.R. and Tsertsvadze, A. (2011b). Universal school-based prevention programs for alcohol misuse in young people. *The Cochrane Database of Systematic Reviews*, (5): CD009113.

Foxcroft, D.R. and Tsertsvadze, A. (2011c). Universal family-based prevention programs for alcohol misuse in young people. *The Cochrane Database of Systematic Reviews*, (9): CD009308.

Grant, B.F. and Dawson, D.A. (1998). Age of onset of drug use and its association with DSM-IV drug abuse and dependence: results from the National Longitudinal Alcohol Epidemiologic Survey. *Journal of Substance Abuse*, 10(2): 163–73.

Grant, J.D., Scherrer, J.F., Lynskey, M.T., Agrawal, A., Duncan, A.E., Haber, J.R., Heath, A.C. and Bucholz, K.K. (2012). Associations of alcohol, nicotine, cannabis, and drug use/dependence with educational attainment: evidence from cotwin-control analyses. *Alcoholism, Clinical and Experimental Research*, 36(8): 1412–20.

Gruber, E., DiClemente, R.J., Anderson, M.M. and Lodico, M. (1996). Early drinking onset and its association with alcohol use and problem behavior in late adolescence. *Preventive Medicine*, 25(3): 293–300.

Hansen, W.B. (1992). School-based substance abuse prevention: a review of the state of the art in curriculum, 1980–1990. *Health Education Research*, 7(3): 403–30.

Hawkins, J.D., Catalano, R.F. and Miller, J.Y. (1992). Risk and protective factors for alcohol and other drug problems in adolescence and early adulthood: implications for substance abuse prevention. *Psychological Bulletin*, 112(1): 64–105.

Hawks, D., Scott, K. and McBride, N. (2002). *Prevention of Psychoactive Substance Use: A Selected Review of What Works in the Area of Prevention*. Geneva: Switzerland.

Hibell, B., Guttormsson, U., Ahlström, S., Balakireva, O., Bjarnason, T., Kokkevi, A. and Kraus, L. (2012). *The 2011 ESPAD Report*. Stockholm: The Swedish Council for Information on Alcohol and Other Drugs (CAN).

Johnston, L.D., O'Malley, P.M., Miech, R.A., Bachman, J.G. and Schulenberg, J.E. (2014). *Monitoring the Future National Survey Results on Drug Use: 1975–2013: Overview, key findings on adolescent drug use*, Ann Arbor: The University of Michigan.

Jones, L., Sumnall, H., Witty, K., Wareing, M., McVeigh, J. and Bellis, M. (2006). *A Review of Community-Based Interventions to Reduce Substance Misuse Among Vulnerable and Disadvantaged Young People*. Liverpool: Liverpool John Moores University.

Jones, L., Hughes, K., Atkinson, A.M. and Bellis, M.A. (2011). Reducing harm in drinking environments: a systematic review of effective approaches. *Health and Place*, 17(2): 508–18.

Kirby, D., Korpi, M., Barth, R.P. and Cagampang, H.H. (1997). The impact of the Postponing Sexual Involvement curriculum among youths in California. *Family Planning Perspectives*, 29(3): 100–8.

Koning, I.M., van den Eijnden, R.J., Engels, R.C., Verdurmen, J.E. and Vollebergh, W.A. (2011). Why target early adolescents and parents in alcohol prevention? The mediating effects of self-control, rules and attitudes about alcohol use. *Addiction*, 106(3): 538–46.

Koning, I.M., Verdurmen, J.E., Engels, R.C., van den Eijnden, R.J. and Vollebergh, W.A. (2012). Differential impact of a Dutch alcohol prevention program targeting adolescents and parents separately and simultaneously: low self-control and lenient parenting at baseline predict effectiveness. *Prevention Science*, 13(3): 278–87.

Koning, I.M., Vollebergh, W.A., Smit, F., Verdurmen, J.E., Van Den Eijnden, R.J., Ter Bogt,

T.F., Stattin, H. and Engels R.C. (2009). Preventing heavy alcohol use in adolescents (PAS): cluster randomized trial of a parent and student intervention offered separately and simultaneously. *Addiction*, 104(10): 1669–78.

Kuntsche, E. and Jordan, M.D. (2006). Adolescent alcohol and cannabis use in relation to peer and school factors. Results of multilevel analyses. *Drug and Alcohol Dependence*, 84(2): 167–74.

Kuntsche, E., Rossow, I., Simons-Morton, B., Bogt, T.T., Kokkevi, A. and Godeau, E. (2013). Not early drinking but early drunkenness is a risk factor for problem behaviors among adolescents from 38 European and North American countries. *Alcoholism, Clinical and Experimental Research*, 37(2): 308–14.

Last, J.M. (2006). *A Dictionary of Public Health*. New York: Oxford University Press.

Leavell, H.R. and Clark, E.G. (1979). *Preventive Medicine for the Doctor in His Community: An Epidemiologic Approach*. Huntington: Robert E. Krieger.

Leshner, A.I. (1997). Addiction is a brain disease, and it matters. *Science*, 278(5335): 45–7.

van Lier, P.A.C., Huizink, A. and Crijnen, A. (2009). Impact of a preventive intervention targeting childhood disruptive behavior problems on tobacco and alcohol initiation from age 10 to 13 years. *Drug and Alcohol Dependence*, 100(3): 228–33.

Loxley, W., Toumbourou, J.W., Stockwell, T., Haines, B., Scott, K., Godfrey, C., Waters, E., Patton, G., Fordham, R., Gray, D., Marshall, J., Ryder, D., Saggers, S., Sanci, L. and Williams, J. (2004). *The Prevention of Substance Use, Risk and Harm in Australia: A Review of the Evidence*. Canberra: Ministerial Council on Drug Strategy.

Lynskey, M.T., Heath, A.C., Nelson, E.C., Bucholz, K.K., Madden, P.A., Slutske, W.S., Statham, D.J. and Martin, N.G. (2002). Genetic and environmental contributions to cannabis dependence in a national young adult twin sample. *Psychological Medicine*, 32(2): 195–207.

McBride, N. (2003). A systematic review of school drug education. *Health Education Research*, 18(6): 729–42.

McCambridge, J. and Strang, J. (2004). The efficacy of single-session motivational interviewing in reducing drug consumption and perceptions of drug-related risk and harm among young people: results from a multi-site cluster randomized trial. *Addiction*, 99(1): 39–52.

McGrath, Y., Sumnall, H., McVeigh, J. and Bellis, M. (2006). *Drug Use Prevention Among Young People: A Review of Reviews*. London: National Institute for Health and Clinical Excellence.

Michie, S., Fixsen, D., Grimshaw, J.M. and Eccles, M.P. (2009). Specifying and reporting complex behaviour change interventions: the need for a scientific method. *Implementation Science*, 4: 40.

Mrazek, P.J. and Haggerty, R.J. (1994). *Reducing Risks for Mental Disorders: Frontiers for Preventive Intervention Research*. Washington, DC: National Academy Press for the Institute of Medicine, Committee on Prevention of Mental Disorders.

Nees, F., Tzschoppe, J., Patrick, C.J., Vollstädt-Klein, S., Steiner, S., Poustka, L., Banaschewski, T., Barker, G.J., Büchel, C., Conrod, P.J., Garavan, H., Heinz, A., Gallinat, J., Lathrop, M., Mann, K., Artiges, E., Paus, T., Poline, J.B., Robbins, T.W., Rietschel, M., Smolka, M.N., Spanagel, R., Struve, M., Loth, E., Schumann, G., Flor, H. and IMAGEN Consortium (2012). Determinants of early alcohol use in healthy adolescents: the differential contribution of neuroimaging and psychological factors. *Neuropsychopharmacology*, 37(4): 986–95.

Newcomb, M. (1995). Identifying high-risk youth: prevalence and patterns of adolescent drug abuse. In E. Rahdert, D. Czechowicz and I. Amsei (eds), *Adolescent Drug Abuse: Clinical Assessment and Therapeutic Intervention*. Rockville: National Institute on Drug Abuse, pp. 7–38.

Newton, N.C., Andrews, G., Teesson, M. and Vogl, L.E. (2009). Delivering prevention for alcohol and cannabis using the Internet: a cluster randomised controlled trial. *Preventive Medicine*, 48(6): 579–84.

Newton, N.C., Conrod, P., Teesson, M. and Faggiano, F. (2012). School-based alcohol and other drug prevention. In J. Verster, K. Brady, M. Galanter and P. Conrod (eds), *Drug Abuse and Addiction in Medical Illness:*

Causes, Consequences and Treatment. New York: Springer, pp. 545–60.

Newton, N.C., Teesson, M., Vogl, L.E. and Andrews, G. (2010). Internet-based prevention for alcohol and cannabis use: final results of the Climate Schools course. *Addiction*, 105(4): 749–59.

Newton, N.C., O'Leary-Barrett, M. and Conrod, P.J. (2013). Adolescent substance misuse: neurobiology and evidence-based interventions. *Current Topics in Behavioral Neurosciences*, 13: 685–708.

NIDA (2010). *Preventing Drug Use Among Children and Adolescents: A Research-Based Guide for Parents, Educators, and Community Leaders [Kindle Edition]*, 2nd edn. Bethesda: Children R the Future Publishing.

Oetting, E. and Lynch, R. (2003). Peers and the prevention of adolescent drug use. In Z. Sloboda and W. Bukoski (eds), *Handbook of Drug Prevention: Theory, Science and Practice*. New York: Kluwer Academic/Plenum Publishers, pp. 101–27.

Offord, D.R. (2000). Selection of levels of prevention. *Addictive Behaviors*, 25(6): 833–42.

Perkins, H.W. and Berkowitz, A.D. (1986). Perceiving the community norms of alcohol use among students: some research implications for campus alcohol education programming. *The International Journal of the Addictions*, 21(9–10): 961–76.

Petrosino, A., Turpin Petrosino, C. and John, B. (2004). 'Scared straight' and other juvenile awareness programs for preventing juvenile delinquency. *Campbell Systematic Reviews*, 9(5).

Porath-Waller, A.J., Beasley, E. and Beirness, D.J. (2010). A meta-analytic review of school-based prevention for cannabis use. *Health Education and Behavior*, 37(5): 709–23.

Riley, B.L., MacDonald, J., Mansi, O., Kothari, A., Kurtz, D., von Tettenborn, L. and Edwards, N. (2008). Is reporting on interventions a weak link in understanding how and why they work? A preliminary exploration using community heart health exemplars. *Implementation Science*, 3: 27.

Rolando, S., Beccaria, F., Tigerstedt, C. and Törrönen, J. (2012). First drink: what does it mean? The alcohol socialization process in different drinking cultures. *Drugs: Education, Prevention and Policy*, 19(3): 201–12.

Roona, M.R., Streke, A. and Marshall, D. (2003). No title. In T. P. Gullotta and M. Bloom (eds), *Encyclopedia of Primary Prevention and Health Promotion*. New York: Kluwer Academic/Plenum Publishers, pp. 1073–8.

Sallis, J.F., McKenzie, T.L., Alcaraz, J.F., Kolody, B., Hovell, M.F. and Nader, P.R. (1993). Project SPARK. Effects of physical education on adiposity in children. *Annals of the New York Academy of Sciences*, 699: 127–36.

Scheier, L.M., Botvin, G.J. and Baker, E. (1997). Risk and protective factors as predictors of adolescent alcohol involvement and transitions in alcohol use: a prospective analysis. *Journal of Studies on Alcohol*, 58(6): 652–67.

Shield, K.D., Parry, C. and Rehm, J. (2013). Chronic diseases and conditions related to alcohol use. *Alcohol research*, 35(2): 155–73.

Sloboda, Z., Stephens, R.C., Stephens, P.C., Grey, S.F., Teasdale, B., Hawthorne, R.D., Williams, J. and Marquette, J.F. (2009). The Adolescent Substance Abuse Prevention Study: A randomized field trial of a universal substance abuse prevention program. *Drug and Alcohol Dependence*, 102(1–3): 1–10.

Spooner, C. (2002). Public policy and the prevention of substance-use disorders. *Current Opinion in Psychiatry*, 15(3): 235–9.

Springer, J.F., Sale, E., Hermann, J., Sambrano, S., Kasim, R. and Nistler, M. (2004). Characteristics of effective substance abuse prevention programs for high-risk youth. *The Journal of Primary Prevention*, 25(2): 171–94.

Stockwell, T., Toumbourou, J.W., Letcher, P., Smart, D., Sanson, A. and Bond, L. (2004). Risk and protection factors for different intensities of adolescent substance use: when does the Prevention Paradox apply? *Drug and Alcohol Review*, 23(1): 67–77.

Strang, J., Babor, T., Caulkins, J., Fischer, B., Foxcroft, D. and Humphreys, K. (2012). Drug policy and the public good: evidence for effective interventions. *Lancet*, 379(9810): 71–83.

Teesson, M., Degenhardt, L., Hall, W., Lynskey, M., Toumbourou J.W. and Patton, G. (2005). Substance use and mental health in longitudinal perspective. In T. Stockwall, P.J. Gruenewald, J.W. Toumbourou and W. Loxley (eds), *Preventing Harmful Substance Use: The Evidence Base for Policy and Practice*. Chichester: John Wiley and Sons, pp. 43–52.

Thomas, R.E., Lorenzetti, D. and Spragins, W. (2011). Mentoring adolescents to prevent drug and alcohol use. *The Cochrane Database of Systematic Reviews*, (11): CD007381.

Tobler, N.S., Roona, M.R., Ochshorn, P., Marshall, D.G., Streke, A.V. and Stackpole, K.M. (2000). School-based adolescent drug prevention programs: 1998 meta-analysis. *The Journal of Primary Prevention*, 20(4): 275–336.

US Department of Health and Human Services (2014). *The Health Consequences of Smoking—50 Years of Progress. A Report of the Surgeon General*. Atlanta: US Department of Health and Human Services.

UNODC (2013). *International Standards on Drug Use Prevention*. Vienna: United Nations Office on Drugs and Crime.

Velleman, R. (2009). Alcohol prevention programmes: a review of the literature for the Joseph Rowntree Foundation (part two). In *Children, Young People and Alcohol: How They Learn and how to Prevent Excessive Use*. New York: Robert Rowntree Foundation.

Volkow, N. and Li, T. (2007). Treating and preventing abuse, addiction, and their medical consequences. In M. Tsuang, W. Stone, and M. Lyons (eds), *Recognition and Prevention of Major Mental and Substance Use Disorders*. Washington, DC: American Psychiatric Publishing Inc., pp. 263–96.

Wakefield, M.A., Loken, B. and Hornik, R.C. (2010). Use of mass media campaigns to change health behaviour. *Lancet*, 376(9748): 1261–71.

Waters, E., de Silva-Sanigorski, A., Hall, B.J., Brown, T., Campbell, K.J., Gao, Y., Armstrong, R., Prosser, L. and Summerbell, C.D. (2011). Interventions for preventing obesity in children. *The Cochrane Database of Systematic Reviews*, (12): CD001871.

Werch, C.E. and Owen, D.M. (2002). Iatrogenic effects of alcohol and drug prevention programs. *Journal of Studies on Alcohol*, 63(5): 581–90.

Whelan, R., Conrod, P.J., Poline, J.B., Lourdusamy, A., Banaschewski, T., Barker, G.J., Bellgrove, M.A., Büchel, C., Byrne, M., Cummins, T.D., Fauth-Bühler, M., Flor, H., Gallinat, J., Heinz, A., Ittermann, B., Mann, K., Martinot, J.L., Lalor, E.C., Lathrop, M., Loth, E., Nees, F., Paus, T., Rietschel, M., Smolka, M.N., Spanagel, R., Stephens, D.N., Struve, M., Thyreau, B., Vollstaedt-Klein, S., Robbins, T.W., Schumann, G., Garavan, H. and IMAGEN Consortium. (2012). Adolescent impulsivity phenotypes characterized by distinct brain networks. *Nature Neuroscience*, 15(6): 920–5.

WHO (2014a). *Global status report on alcohol and health 2014*. Geneva: Switzerland.

WHO (2014b). *Guidelines for the screening, care and treatment of persons with hepatitis C infection*. Geneva: Switzerland.

WHO (2014c). *Water Safety in Distribution Systems*. Geneva: Switzerland.

WHO (2015). Abuse (drug, alcohol, chemical, substance or psychoactive substance). Available at: http://www.who.int/substance_abuse/terminology/abuse/en/ (Accessed 26 June 2015).

WHO Europe (2006). *Gaining Health The European Strategy for the Prevention and Control of Noncommunicable Diseases*. Copenhagen, Denmark.

WHO Europe (2009). *Evidence for the Effectiveness and Cost-Effectiveness of Interventions to Reduce Alcohol-Related Harm*. Copenhagen, Denmark.

WHO Europe (2012). *Health 2020: A European Policy Framework Supporting Action Across Government and Society for Health and Well-Being*. Copenhagen: WHO Regional Office for Europe.

WHO, UNICEF and World Bank (2009). *State of the World's Vaccines and Immunization*, 3rd edn. Geneva: Switzerland.

Young, M.M., Saewyc, E., Boak, A., Jahrig, J., Anderson, B., Doiron-Brun, Y. and Clark, H. (2011). *Cross-Canada Report on Student Alcohol and Drug Use: Technical Report*. Ottawa: Canadian Centre on Substance Abuse.

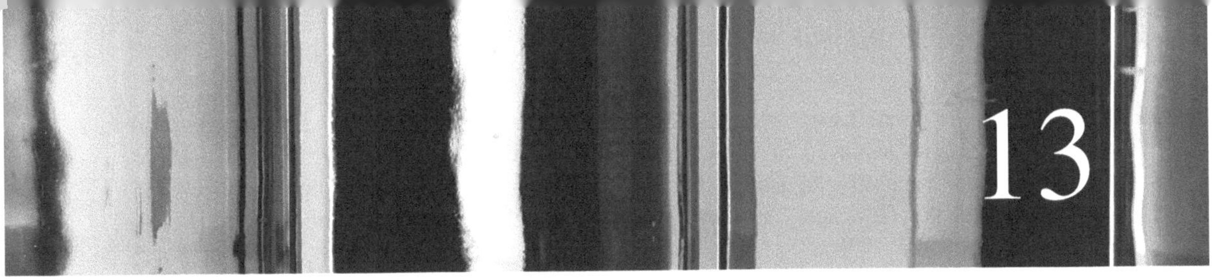

Community-Focused Approaches to the Prevention of Alcohol-Related Harms: From Past Experiences to Future Possibilities

Richard Midford and Anthony Shakeshaft

HISTORICAL CONTEXT

Community-focused prevention of alcohol problems goes back to the American Temperance Movement, which sprang up in the early years of the nineteenth century as a grassroots effort to make people aware of the threat that alcohol posed at home and at work (Cherrington, 1920; Holder, 1992). The foundation of the American Temperance Society in Boston in 1826 marked a transition to more organized, larger scale activity, and within 12 years, the Society claimed to have more than 8,000 local groups and over 1.5 million members (Merrill, 1988).

The Temperance Movement spread to Continental Europe, Britain and her colonies within a few years, but the message was taken up in different measure in different countries. The Movement was generally largest in English-speaking and Nordic countries, but there were also significant groups in some central and eastern European countries (Eriksen, 2003; Prestwich, 2003; Swiatkiewicz and Moskalewicz, 2003). At first, the Temperance Movement advocated moderation, but as it became more powerful, it became more prohibitionist, increasingly sought political influence and was less interested in working with individual communities. Alcohol was seen as the problem, and because it affected everybody, its use needed to be suppressed through public and political reforms, rather than relying on private and personal effort (Berridge, 2005).

The ever more prohibitionist Temperance Movement reached the peak of its influence in the first two decades of the twentieth century. A number of Nordic countries introduced prohibition, as did Canada and both Czarist Russia and the Soviet Union (Blocker, 2006; Sariola, 1954). During the First World War, Britain, Australia and New Zealand restricted the hours when alcohol could be sold (Grant and Serle, 1983; Jones, 1987). In the United States, the goal of the

Temperance Movement was national prohibition, which was achieved in 1919, when Congress passed enabling legislation, known as the Volstead Act (Blocker, 2006).

However, by the 1930s, support for prohibition had waned because of the associated rise in crime and corruption, and it was repealed in the United States and other previously prohibitionist countries (Pegram, 1998; Sariola, 1954). Prohibition was seen as a failure and this led to a reappraisal as to the cause of alcohol problems. In the immediate post prohibitionist era, emphasis on alcohol as a social issue decreased, and instead, attention focused on the individual drinker, who misused alcohol. The new view was that alcohol problems arose from the genetic and physiological make-up of the individual. Addiction concepts came back into fashion in the USA, with an emphasis on the 'sick individual' (Levine, 1978). This spread to Europe after the Second World War, helped by the expanding Alcoholics Anonymous movement. Individual disease and addiction were seen as the root of the problem, and accordingly, treatment became the response of choice (Blocker, 2006).

This 'medicalization' of alcohol and other drug problems has meant that, until relatively recently, the focus of prevention efforts has been on early identification and treatment of the addicted individual (Holder, 1992). In the early 1970s, an appreciation emerged in the public health area as to the wider health and social problems created by alcohol. This shift in emphasis from individual medical disorder to a broader view of alcohol problems has been important in recognizing the role of the community in both producing and responding to alcohol problems. The community produces particular alcohol problems, because of the way community life is organized and the community is an appropriate setting for preventing alcohol problems, because it is here that these problems are personally experienced.

The legitimacy of focusing prevention effort on the population as a whole was strengthened at this time through the work of Rose (1981, 1985) and Kreitman (1986). Rose argued very convincingly that while prevention, which concentrates on high risk individuals, leads to intervention appropriate for those individuals, its ability to reduce the burden of disease at the community level is small. Rose (1981) talked about this as the 'prevention paradox'. Kreitman (1986) explored this paradox in relation to alcohol use, and found that contrary to conventional wisdom, the majority of alcohol problems were caused by moderate rather than heavy, dependent drinkers, because they comprised such a large proportion of the drinking population. An additional consideration, raised by Holmila (2000a), is that curing the individual problem drinker will not result in a reduction in alcohol-related harm because the community dynamics, which caused these problems, are unchanged. In order to change the aggregate level of alcohol-related harm, changes have to occur at the community level.

Aguirre-Molina and Gorman (1996), in one of the first reviews of modern community-focused prevention approaches, stated that interventions based on this model had emerged as the most viable way of reducing the risk associated with alcohol use because they addressed the contributing contextual factors. In the 1990s, this form of prevention received substantial funding support in the USA and an increasing number of intervention programmes were undertaken. The results of 20 US-based community alcohol trials have been published since 1995, compared to two previously (Aseltine et al., 2008; Buka and Birdthistle, 1999; Chou et al., 1998; Clapp et al., 2005; Flynn et al., 2006; Gebhardt et al., 2000; Hingson et al., 1996, 2005; Holder et al., 2000; Klepp et al., 1995; Rowe, 1997; Schinke et al., 2000; Slater et al., 2006; Stevens et al., 1996; Treno et al., 2007; Wagenaar et al., 2000). The approach also began to receive strong state support in Finland and Sweden at this time because when these countries joined the European Union in 1995 they had to comply with the Union's one market policy and could no longer deal with population level alcohol problems through state control of availability (Holmila, 2000b; Leifman, 2001). The results of four Swedish (Andréasson et al., 2007; Rehnman et al., 2005; Stafström et al., 2006; Wallin et al., 2003, 2005) and two Finnish (Holmila, 1995, 2003) trials were published between 1995 and 2007. In this new environment of reduced state control, community-focused prevention emerged as the most promising alternative.

In addition to the US and Nordic trials during this period, four community-focused research projects were undertaken in New Zealand, led by the seminal Community Action Project (CAP), which sought to increase public support for preventive alcohol policy initiatives and moderate consumption norms (Casswell and Gilmore, 1989; Conway, 2002; Huckle et al., 2005, 2007). In Australia, the results of three community-focused projects have been published. The Community Mobilisation for the Prevention of Alcohol Related Injury (COMPARI) project in Western Australia focused on mobilising a regional city to comprehensively tackle the causes of local alcohol harm (Midford and Boots, 1999). A second trial evaluated the impact of community initiated alcohol sales and advertising restrictions in a remote community with high levels of harm (Midford et al., 2010). The results of a 20-community cluster randomized controlled trial (RCT), the Alcohol Action in Rural Communities (AARC) project, were published in 2014 (Shakeshaft et al., 2014).

In 1996, when community-focused alcohol prevention was gaining traction, a review by Gorman and Speer identified just eight controlled or time series studies that reported programme effects on alcohol related behaviour, and that of these eight, truly comprehensive programmes were the exception (Gorman and Speer, 1996). Since 1996, the results of only seven randomized trials of the effectiveness of community-action on alcohol have been published (Komro et al., 2008; Perry et al., 1996; Saltz et al., 2010; Schinke et al., 2000; Shakeshaft et al., 2014; Wagenaar et al., 2000; Wolfson et al., 2012), with only one, the AARC project, having a whole community focus (Shakeshaft et al., 2014). It would seem, then, that by the turn of the twenty-first century, the potential benefits of community-focused approaches to problematic alcohol use were well understood, but the processes of building the evidence-base and translating this knowledge into practice were still embryonic.

CONCEPTUALISING THE COMMUNITY APPROACH

The liberalization of alcohol markets in Finland and Sweden, as a consequence of joining the European Union, provides a distinct example of the state reducing its control in favour of individual consumer choice. However, Casswell (2000) suggested that this is not a unique, situation specific phenomenon, but rather part of a trend in Western countries over recent decades of lessening state control and growing consumer influence. This has made it increasingly difficult to deal with population level alcohol problems through state policies and regulations. In this new environment of reduced state involvement, the community emerges as alternative vehicle for taking action against these problems. The rationale for seeking to prevent alcohol-related harm at the community level is compelling in that alcohol is largely obtained and consumed within community contexts and the associated harms, such as car crashes, violence and property damage are borne collectively at the community level (Holder, 2000). Moreover, recent evidence clearly shows that rates of risky drinking and alcohol-related harms differ significantly between different communities (Breen et al., 2011, 2014; Czech et al., 2011). This means that communities are more likely than national or provincial governments to have a greater awareness as to the reality of the specific problems they face, a more direct knowledge of the particular needs of their members and a detailed understanding of local alcohol practices that need to change if problems are to be reduced. Unsurprisingly, then, community-action approaches have been shown to be highly acceptable to members of communities themselves (Czech et al., 2010).

There are powerful advantages to operating at the level of the whole community, where interventions seek to remove or ameliorate the underlying causes of problematic drinking. There is considerable potential for aggregate benefit because of the large numbers of individuals and harms involved. Also, changes in drinking behaviour are likely to be self-sustaining because the change establishes new community norms (Rose, 1985). Importantly though, the community has to be involved in decision-making, rather than just being the site for prevention initiatives. Thompson and Kine (1999) stressed the 'principle of ownership' in change, which means that effective and lasting change is most likely to occur when the people, who are affected, are part of the change process.

In one sense, community indicates a group of people living in close geographic proximity, as in a town or neighbourhood. In another sense, it can refer to social proximity, brought about by shared experience and heritage, as with an indigenous community or by a shared purpose, such as in a workplace or school. Here the community is viewed as catchment of people with common health risks, who may be targeted for a particular preventative health intervention. Catchment interventions tend to target at risk individuals with interventions that seek to improve their particular problematic health behaviour; for example, providing 'Quit' programmes for smokers. In this context, education campaigns, health promotion activities and social marketing can be effective. However, catchment programmes have limitations in preventing or reducing alcohol problems at the community level because drinkers identified as highly dependent, and therefore in need of intervention, only make up a small percentage of the community population, and as Kreitman (1986) discovered, they do not cause the majority of problems.

Holder (1998) and Thompson and Kinne (1999) articulated an alternate perspective of community. They considered that in functional terms, a community needs to be seen as a complex and enduring system of interacting components, such as health services, workplaces, volunteer groups and recreational facilities. The system is held together by some degree of community co-operation and consensus on common goals, norms and values. The system provides the context for all activities, including individual drinking behaviour, and produces certain outputs, including alcohol problems. Accordingly, greatest change is likely to be achieved by operating at the level of the overall community system. Here, change means not just influencing the operation of individual system components, such that they all coherently support safer drinking by individuals, but also systemic change, so that the structures and operation of the whole community are altered in a way that supports safer drinking. This approach does not emphasize working directly with problem drinkers to change their behaviour, rather, efforts are directed toward policy-makers, regulators, service agencies and others in positions to influence the environment in which problem drinking occurs. Local alcohol policy and regulation practices can be used to alter the community's social, economic or physical structures, and establish processes and priorities to reduce alcohol problems. Changes can include prioritising alcohol-related problematic behaviour such as public drunkenness, enforcing laws to prevent alcohol sales to underage or intoxicated persons, local restrictions on the sale of beverages particularly associated with problematic drinking, controlling location and density of alcohol outlets and ensuring server training for all licensed premises (Holder, 2000; Midford et al., 2010; Österberg, 1992; Stockwell and Gruenewald, 2004).

Within the broader community system, Holder (1998) identified interacting subsystems that are natural groupings of factors that research has shown to be important in the understanding of alcohol use and its regulation.

- Consumption subsystem – alcohol use as part of routine community life.
- Social norms subsystem – community values and social influences that affect drinking.
- Retail sales subsystem – alcohol availability and promotion.
- Formal regulation and control subsystem – rules, administration and enforcement.
- Legal sanctions subsystem – prohibitive uses of alcohol.
- Social, economic and health consequences subsystem – community identification of, and organized response to, alcohol problems.

A key issue in seeking to alter the operation of these subsystems, so their structure and operation supports safer drinking, is a partnership approach that involves a broad range of local community groups and individuals to bring about community-level change. The following are the key principles that underpin effective ecological change according to the system model (Holder, 2000):

- involve stakeholders and the community throughout the process;
- clearly define the alcohol problems to be tackled;
- identify a range of evidence-based interventions that are likely to be effective with the particular alcohol problems being targeted;
- identify indicators of change and monitor these indicators;
  - ensure high quality evaluation of programme goals;
  - adopt a multi strategy approach to the problems;
- proactively engage the media to gain community support for the interventions being undertaken;
- build on success to generate support for ongoing community prevention activity.

The system model elaborated by Holder (1998, 2000) is a useful heuristic because it takes into account the complexity and dynamics of how a community functions and the various elements that need to be influenced synergistically to change the ecology of drinking in a way that reduces problems. This understanding of the elements and process within a community system helps formulate strategies that are most likely to bring about change. Given its intuitive appeal, this approach has been endorsed by the World Health Organization, which similarly argues that all members of a community are responsible for action, precisely because the burden of alcohol harm is spread across multiple settings such as health services, policing, public spaces and workplaces (World Health Organization, 2010). It is unlikely that any prevention programme, whether it treats the community as a catchment or as a system, can completely eliminate local alcohol problems. However, understanding the community as an interactive system with a range of processes that contribute to alcohol problems means that the greater collective risk can be given the prominence it deserves as a focus for prevention efforts.

EVALUATION ISSUES

The RCT is generally considered the gold standard for measuring an intervention's effect, because it best equalizes biases and gives confidence that any differences between treatment and control are actually due to the intervention (Grossman and Mackenzie, 2005). However, given its clinical origins, usually with a focus on a single outcome of interest in a group of individual subjects, its limitations for measuring change at the community level need to be recognized. Logistically, randomized, community-focused alcohol trials are typically expensive and time consuming to conduct for a number of reasons, including that they require the availability of relatively large numbers of communities, a long time to engage, gain traction and have an impact with those communities and complicated ethics and consent processes. The results of randomized trials also typically have low generalizability because of the strict inclusion criteria and the need for standardized, strictly defined intervention protocols (Hawkins et al., 2007; Sanson-Fisher et al., 2007). In addition to logistical issues, there is likely to be considerable diversity within a community and an alcohol prevention programme with complex, multifaceted inputs. All of these elements will interact to produce different effects. Tones (1997) also noted that it is difficult to ensure comparability of communities allocated to the different study conditions, and it is '...all but impossible...; (Tones, 1997: i) to prevent other, unplanned inputs or treatment leakage to controls. The WHO European Working Group on Health Promotion Evaluation (1998), in its recommendations to policy makers considered that the use of RCTs is, in most cases, inappropriate, misleading and unnecessarily expensive when used to evaluate community health promotion programmes because these programmes are unlikely to be delivered in a standard manner.

While there is a substantial body of opinion that the RCT in an inappropriate or unworkable method for evaluating community health programmes, Rosen and colleagues considered that a properly designed RCT is a much better evaluation mechanism for answering specific questions about the efficacy of a community intervention than any of the alternatives (Rosen et al., 2006a). They suggested that there is a tendency to assume that all community health programmes are beneficial, so conducting research that includes a comparable control group is essential to check this preconception, and start from the premise that benefit is uncertain. They countered the argument of an RCT not being capable of dealing with complex multifaceted programmes by suggesting that even if the programme is complex it can be evaluated by a series of simple, well defined outcome measures. They also challenged the belief that an RCT is only useful when studying well defined groups of people under tightly controlled conditions. They cited a number of successful, randomized, controlled health trials, such as the Community Intervention Trial for Smoking Cessation (COMMIT) project and a hand washing intervention conducted with children in Jerusalem preschools that were aimed at the general population in normal community settings (COMMIT Research Group, 1995; Rosen et al., 2006b). In fact, they suggested that external validity, whereby the communities selected for study accurately represent the population of interest, may actually be higher in a community trial, than in a trial involving individuals, because of reduced volunteer bias. The selection and randomization at the community level also overcomes the concern that randomized, controlled trials focus on the individual, whereas health promotion is concerned primarily with community change. Cluster randomization, allows comparison at a community level, and if accompanied by multilevel modelling techniques, allows individual level data to be used to assess community wide interventions in a statistically efficient way. This is because the technique overcomes the problem of non-independence at the individual level (individuals from the same community are more likely respond in a similar manner, an effect called intra-class correlation).

There are cogent reasons to use a cluster randomized, controlled design to evaluate large scale, well-funded multi-community alcohol interventions, but for smaller scale projects, with fewer communities and limited funding, less expensive, less time consuming designs may be more appropriate. The quasi experimental design is an alternative to the RCT and it has been used in large community alcohol interventions, such as the Community Trials Project (CTP) (Holder, 2000). In this design, there is a concurrent control, but allocation to treatment or control conditions is done by the researcher or through self-selection by the community. It is often the most practical option where there are logistical and ethical complexities. Another experimental method is the time series design. This uses multiple observations before and after an intervention, which provides an assessment of trend over time. If the trend is stable before the intervention, but changes subsequently, the likelihood is that the change is related to the intervention. More common in health promotion research is the simple before and after trial. This is a basic way of testing whether an intervention has an effect, but the design has no capacity to account for the possibility that other factors, not related to the intervention, are responsible for the difference between the pre-test and post-test results.

Triangulation, which involves accumulating evidence from multiple sources, has been suggested by Tones (1997) as an alternative to the RCT because if data from different sources point in the same direction it is reasonable to assume the results achieved by an intervention are valid. This approach has received support from the WHO European Working Group on Health Promotion Evaluation (1998), who recommended a 'a multidimensional focus on the determinants of health' (p. 5). This expert group considered that the use of a wide range of qualitative and quantitative methods gives better understanding of the impact of a health promotion intervention. They outlined a number of principles that should be at the core of any evaluation.

- Participation – health promotion evaluations should involve those with a legitimate interest in the findings.
- Multiple methods – health promotion evaluations should draw on a variety of disciplines and use a broad range of information gathering procedures.
- Capacity building – health promotion evaluations should enhance the capacity of individuals, communities, agencies and governments to address important health promotion issues.
- Appropriateness – health promotion evaluations should take into consideration the complex nature of health promotion interventions and the long-term nature of their impact.

While the RCT is generally considered the superior research design in respect to questions about the effect of an intervention, other designs possess qualities that enable them to answer questions that go beyond efficacy (Ho et al., 2008). This suggests that a mixed methods design that combines different investigative approaches to suit the questions being asked is likely to produce a more comprehensive understanding of the phenomena being studied. In terms of evaluating a community-focused alcohol prevention trial, the mixed methods approach offers the potential to increase the reliability of data and validity of findings and to better understand the context, within which, and the processes by which, intervention effects are achieved.

A REVIEW OF RANDOMIZED COMMUNITY-FOCUSED ALCOHOL INTERVENTION EVALUATIONS

While the RCT has been held up as the gold standard, the evaluation issues discussed in the previous section highlight the complexity and limitations of conducting randomized evaluations of community-focused alcohol interventions. It is not surprising, therefore, that the results of only seven randomized trials of the effectiveness of alcohol community-action have been published to date (Komro et al., 2008; Perry et al., 1996; Saltz et al., 2010; Schinke et al., 2000; Shakeshaft et al., 2014; Wagenaar et al., 2000; Wolfson et al., 2012).

Of these seven randomized trials, six were based in the USA, and were focused explicitly on young people, rather than the whole community: the unit of randomization was schools or school districts in four trials (Komro et al., 2008; Perry et al., 1996; Schinke et al., 2000; Wagenaar et al., 2000) and university campuses in two trials (Saltz et al., 2010; Wolfson et al., 2012). These trials measured outcomes using a combination of self-reported data from students, parents/families and community members and alcohol purchase attempt outcomes. The only randomized trial that focused on reducing alcohol harms across the whole community was the Australian Alcohol Action in Rural Communities (AARC) project. This measured outcomes, using a combination of self-report data from randomly selected community members and a range of routinely collected data (alcohol-related crime, hospitalizations and traffic crashes) (Shakeshaft et al., 2014). The important features of these seven randomized trials are summarized in Table 13.1 and each trial is described in detail in the following pages.

Alcohol Action in Rural Communities (AARC) project

This cluster RCT engaged with 20 rural communities in New South Wales, Australia (Shakeshaft et al., 2014). The communities were selected on the basis of their population size (between 5,000 and 20,000). They were organized into pairs, matched on the proportions of males, young people and Aboriginal individuals in each community (these variables have been shown to be associated with disproportionately high rates of alcohol-related harm). One community in each pair was randomly allocated to the experimental condition.

The aims of AARC were to reduce risky alcohol consumption and harm across whole communities and to estimate the economic impact of community-action by conducting the first benefit–cost analysis. Thirteen interventions were implemented in each of the 10 experimental communities over a five-year period. A full description of the interventions is available elsewhere (Shakeshaft et al., 2012a), but can be summarized as a mix of:

- more effective use of alcohol-related data (engaging with communities, providing ongoing feedback to key stakeholders and media advocacy);
- targeting high-risk times, settings and individuals (Navarro et al., 2013), workplace safety, sports clubs, high schools and GP management of alcohol dependent individuals (Navarro et al., 2012);
- more frequent screening and early intervention (made available through the internet), GPs (Navarro et al., 2011), pharmacies, Aboriginal Medical Services (Clifford et al., 2013) and hospital emergency departments (Havard et al., 2012).

A total of 15 outcomes were reported (nine using routinely collected data and six using self-reported data). Of these, two were statistically significant in favour of the intervention: survey respondents in the experimental communities reported significantly lower average weekly consumption and lower levels of alcohol-related verbal abuse post-intervention, relative to respondents in the control communities. There were three outcomes of marginal statistical significance (≤0.01): alcohol-related street offences and the proportions of survey respondents who reported long-term and short-term risky drinking. The benefit-cost analysis showed the economic benefits outweighed the cost of the interventions (Shakeshaft et al., 2012b).

These outcomes could reflect three possibilities. First, it may be that community-action is most effective in reducing lower-levels of alcohol-related harm (i.e. harms that are not severe enough to be recorded in formal reporting datasets, such as police incidents and hospitalisations), which implies that a combination of community-action to target lower-level harms and tighter regulation to target more serious alcohol-related harms would further reduce harms. Second, they may reflect that different types of outcome data are susceptible to different levels of bias: it could be that self-report data are more likely to show a statistically significantly positive effect relative to routinely collected data. Third, given the routinely

Table 13.1 Summary of the seven published randomized community-focused alcohol intervention evaluations

Year	*Author Project*	*Country*	*Intervention focus*	*Evaluation design*	*Unit of randomization*	*Number of clusters*	*Outcomes*	*Statistically[1] or marginally[2] significant outcomes favouring intervention group*
2014	Shakeshaft et al. AARC	Australia	Whole community	Cluster RCT	Communities	20	• 6 self-report • 9 routinely collected	• Weekly average drinking[1] • Verbal abuse[1] • Weekly risky drinking[2] • Binge drinking[2] • Street offences[2]
2012	Wolfson et al. SPARC	USA	Universities	Cluster RCT	Universities	10	10 self-report	• Severe consequences due to one's own drinking[1] • Caused an alcohol-related injury to another person[1]
2010	Saltz et al. Safer California Universities	USA	Six settings in university campuses	Cluster RCT	University campuses	14	14 self-report	• Intoxication in two specific settings (last time in that setting and at least once a semester)[1] • Intoxication aggregated across all six settings (last time in that setting and at least once a semester)[1]
1996	Perry et al. Project Northland (Minnesota)	USA	Schools and related community groups	Cluster RCT	School districts	20	• 122 self-report • Purchase attempts	• 27 significant outcomes; 25 in favour of the intervention group[1] • Most differences between intervention and controls groups <5%.
2008	Komro et al. Project Northland Chicago	USA	Schools and related community groups	Cluster RCT	Study units	22 (comprising 61 schools)	• 18 self-report • Purchase attempts	• Home-based programs reduced alcohol, marijuana and tobacco use combined[1] • Ability to purchase alcohol by buyers who looked under age[2]
2000	Wagenaar et al. CMCA	USA	City and school district	Cluster RCT	City and school districts	15	• 22 self-report • 4 observed	Of the 26 individual outcomes: • Self-reported provision of alcohol to youth by 18 to 20 year olds[1] Aggregating individual scores: • Practices of on-sale alcohol outlets[1] • Behaviour of 18 to 20 year olds[1] • Practices of off-sale alcohol outlets[2]
2000	Schinke et al. Native American youth	USA	Schools	Cluster RCT	Schools	27 schools in 10 reservations	• 16 self-report	Smokeless tobacco use[1] Alcohol use[1] Cannabis use[1]

[1]Where $p \leq 0.05$. [2]Where $p \leq 0.1$.

collected data showed small to moderate effectiveness and high levels of uncertainty (wide 95% confidence intervals), it may be that the study had insufficient power to detect any true intervention effectiveness as statistically significant because of the limited sample size of 20 communities, or that the intervention 'dose' varied across communities. These possibilities highlight the practical and methodological difficulties of conducting community-focused RCT intervention research.

Study to Prevent Alcohol Related Consequences (SPARC)

This cluster RCT was conducted with universities in North Carolina (Wolfson et al., 2012). The 10 participating universities were classified as small (≤6,000 undergraduate students) or large, and more ready (≥2.2 on the readiness survey scale) or less ready, and then grouped into one of four cells: small and more ready (n=2); small and less ready (n=2); large and more ready (n=4); and large and less ready (n=2). Within each cell, universities were randomly allocated to the intervention (n=5) or control (n=5) condition.

The aim of SPARC was to reduce high-risk drinking and alcohol-related consequences among university students. A community organization group was established on each campus, which comprised four university employees with student support responsibilities and a full-time organizer. This group selected and implemented interventions through five specific processes:

- Assessment – data from existing sources and a college drinking survey were used to develop a comprehensive picture of alcohol use and harms on each campus.
- Coalition building – a coalition was formed on each campus comprising staff, students and community members. One-on-one meetings were also organized between stakeholders and coalition members, which replicated a strategy used by one of other RCTs, the Communities Mobilising for Change on Alcohol (CMCA) project.
- Strategic planning – literature review identified a matrix of the best and most promising interventions, and each campus was required to select strategies from at least three of four areas: (i) alcohol availability; (ii) harm minimization; (iii) social norms; and (iv) alcohol price and marketing.
- Action – coalitions implemented their strategic plans.
- Sustainability – SPARC organizers and coalitions sought: university funding for a 'safe rides' programme; meetings with top and middle level campus administrators to promote long-term support; new grant funds; discussions with a local non-profit agency to incorporate SPARC into their mission.

The impact of the intervention strategies was measured by the implementation of a student survey at four time points, using a repeated, cross-sectional design. A random sample of 1,200 undergraduate students (stratified by stage of study) was invited to complete the survey at each of the four data collection time points. Ten individual outcomes were measured, grouped into three categories: (i) high-risk drinking; (ii) alcohol-related consequences; and (iii) alcohol-related injuries. A key innovation of this study was that it measured the extent to which students were likely to have been exposed to the intervention elements (or 'dose'), using an Environmental Strategy Implementation Survey. There were two statistically significant main effects in favour of the intervention campuses: a reduction in severe consequences due to one's own drinking and a reduction in having caused an alcohol-related injury to another person due to one's own drinking. The 'dose' measure identified a significant relationship between the likely extent of exposure to intervention elements and two outcomes: interpersonal consequences due to others' drinking and having caused an alcohol-related injury to another person due to one's own drinking. These results led the authors to conclude that the SPARC approach can reduce problems associated with high-risk drinking, provided interventions are implemented with commitment and intensity.

Safer California Universities study

This cluster RCT involved university campuses in California (Saltz et al., 2010). Fourteen campuses met the inclusion criteria and consented (eight from the University of California and six from the California State University system). The campuses were stratified by university system and allocated to matched pairs, based on campus drinking behaviour determined by a baseline survey. Campuses within each matched pair were then randomly allocated to either the intervention or control condition.

The aim of this study was to reduce rates of intoxication in the intervention, relative to control campuses. The intervention focused on off-campus parties because student survey data showed that these were associated with high rates of alcohol-related problems. The intervention comprised three law enforcement strategies (roadside driving under the influence checks; police compliance checks of sales to minors and party patrols to enforce local and state laws regarding provision of alcohol to minors and disturbing the peace), complemented by heightened publicity through various communication channels (e.g. newspapers, websites, emails, brochures) to increase awareness of the law enforcement operations. In addition, each campus pushed for the implementation of an additional fine on party hosts if police cited the same address twice in a designated time period. The goal was to implement the interventions over two years, with a focus on the first eight to 10 weeks of the teaching year.

A student survey was used to measure the impact of the intervention strategies at four time points (fall semesters in 2003 to 2006). A random sample of 2,000 undergraduate students per school was invited to complete the survey in 2003, followed by 1,000 students per school in 2004 to 2006. Outcomes were reported separately for six settings (Greek party, dorm party, campus event, off-campus party, bar/restaurant, outdoor setting), of which two were targets of the intervention, and two measures of intoxication (intoxicated in one of those settings at least once in a semester, being intoxicated the last time when in one of those settings). In addition to those 12 individual outcomes, the impact of the intervention was also reported for both measures of intoxication (at least once a semester and last time in that setting) aggregated across all settings. In total, therefore, there were 12 outcomes across six settings and two outcomes aggregated across all settings (n=14 outcomes). A statistically significant benefit in favour of the intervention campuses was reported for the two of the six settings that were targeted (off-campus parties and bars/restaurants) and for both measures of intoxication (at least once a semester and last time in that setting) and for the outcomes aggregated across all settings. There was some evidence that higher levels of implementation were associated with intervention effects. This trial suggests that a community mobilization approach can reduce the frequency of intoxication among university students in some off-campus settings and that the effect of interventions is positively related to the extent to which they are implemented.

Project Northland (Minnesota)

This comprised a cluster RCT of school districts in northeast Minnesota (Perry et al., 1996). The 24 school districts were combined into 20 (the four small districts were combined with nearby districts), blocked by size (small, medium, large, very large) and then randomly allocated to either the intervention (n=10) or control (n=10) condition.

The aim of Project Northland was to prevent adolescent alcohol use. It comprised a multi-component intervention in which different programme elements targeted the same cohort of students over three years. The intervention involved strategies for schools (education programmes, behavioural curricula, peer participation), parents (education programmes and family activities) and community task-force activities.

- Schools – home-work based activity books were completed by students in sixth grade with their parents and later displayed at an 'evening fair'. Seventh grade activities focused on an eight-week, peer-led classroom curriculum and a peer participation programme. Eighth grade activities included the continuation of some seventh grade programmes, commencement of a new eight-session classroom curriculum and a theatre production.
- Parents – in sixth grade, parents participated in homework based activity books with their teenagers, and received information on adolescent alcohol use (Northland Notes for Parents), as well as participating in the 'evening fair'. Seventh grade parents received four booklets that included prescriptions for parents and activities for them to complete with their teenagers, as well as new issues of Northland Notes for Parents. Eighth grade activities included new issues of Northland Notes for Parents, facilitating student group meetings and participating in interviews and meetings organized by students to discuss alcohol issues.
- Community task forces – these were established while students were in sixth grade. Membership comprised community members, government officials, law enforcement personnel, youth workers, health professionals and clergy. Seventh grade activities included developing resolutions (e.g. enactment of local ordinances requiring responsible beverage service training) and the initiation of a gold card programme where businesses provided discounts to students who pledged to be alcohol and drug free.

The impact of the intervention strategies was measured using four methods: (i) student survey; (ii) a phone survey of parents in half the households of the class of 1998 cohort; (iii) alcohol purchase attempts by young buyers; and (iv) alcohol retailer telephone surveys. The student survey was administered to sixth grade students in 1991 (baseline), then repeated for the same students in the spring of 1992 (sixth grade), 1993 (seventh grade) and 1994 (eighth grade). Outcomes were categorized into two broad groups: drug and alcohol use or tendency to use, peer influence, self-efficacy and perceived access scores (nine outcomes); and drinking norms, family communication and functional measures (reasons not to use alcohol) (16 outcomes). The first nine outcomes were analysed separately for three groups (all students, those not using alcohol at baseline and those who were using alcohol at baseline) at all three follow-up time points, meaning there were 81 individual outcomes examined. The second group of 16 outcomes were only analysed for all students at different combinations of follow-up time points, resulting in 41 individual outcomes examined. In total, then, 122 individual possible outcomes were examined. Of these, 27 were statistically significant and all but two were in favour of the intervention group. For the drug and alcohol use or tendency to use, peer influence, self-efficacy and perceived access outcomes, there were no statistically significant effects for students who reported alcohol use at baseline. Most statistically significant outcomes were modest (less than 5 per cent difference between the intervention and control groups). This study provides modest evidence that the intervention had some impact on the outcomes measured, although the majority were not statistically significant and the main impacts were for students who had not commenced alcohol use at baseline.

Project Northland Chicago

This was a cluster RCT of schools and their communities in Chicago (Komro et al., 2008). The 61 eligible and participating schools were organized into 22 study units, of which 10 (29 schools) were randomized to the intervention and 12 (32 schools) to the control condition.

The aim of Project Northland Chicago was to reduce alcohol and other drug use, risk factors for alcohol and other drug use, and positively impact on growth rates (or trajectories) for both alcohol and other drug use and associated risk factors. The three intervention components essentially replicated those Project Northland Minnesota:

- School – six to 10 sessions per year of peer-led classroom curricula.
- Family – four home-based sessions per year with parents/families, including other educational, school and community activities.
- Community – peer leadership and youth-planned community-service projects and neighbourhood change.

The impact of the intervention strategies was measured using three methods: (i) student survey; (ii) parent and community leader surveys; and (iii) alcohol purchase attempts. A total of 19 outcomes were identified: eight based on the student surveys; seven on the parent surveys; three on the community leader surveys; and one on the alcohol purchase attempts. The student surveys (n=8 outcomes) comprised three main outcomes (students' drug use, students' alcohol use and students' alcohol intentions) and five intermediate outcomes (norms supportive of use, perceived outcomes supportive of use, self-efficacy, parental involvement and extent of access to alcohol). There was no statistically significant difference in favour of the intervention, relative to the control group on any outcome, although a greater participation in the home programmes was significantly related to lower growth in drug use over time. This study provides no evidence that the intervention had an effect on students' drug or alcohol use, their risk factors for drug or alcohol use or their alcohol intentions, relative to prevention as usual in the control schools.

Communities Mobilising for Change on Alcohol (CMCA)

This cluster RCT involved communities in Minnesota and Western Wisconsin (Wagenaar et al., 2000). Communities were defined as a city and its associated school district. Fifteen eligible and consenting communities were organized into matched pairs (and one triplet) based on state, presence of a residential college or university, population size and the results of the baseline alcohol purchase attempt survey. One community from each pair or triplet was randomly allocated to the intervention condition (n=7) and the remainder to the control condition (n=8).

The aims of CMCA were to reduce youth access to alcohol and to modify young people's drinking behaviours. The interventions were implemented in the school districts and were specifically designed to:

- reduce the number of alcohol outlets that sell to young people;
- reduce the availability of alcohol to young people from non-commercial sources, such as parents, siblings and older peers;
- reduce community tolerance of underage drinking and adult provision of alcohol to young people.

A key intervention component in this trial was undertaking 1,518 one-on-one meetings with community leaders and members to help improve mutual understanding, build relationships and to identify individuals for the core leadership group A thorough review of alcohol control policies, procedures and enforcement practices was undertaken and media advocacy efforts resulted in a substantial increase in media coverage of alcohol issues in the experimental communities.

The impact of the interventions was measured using four data sources: (i) school-based surveys; (ii) telephone surveys of 18 to 20 year olds; iii) alcohol purchase attempts by people who appeared to be under-age; and (iv) telephone surveys of alcohol outlet owners and managers. A total of 26 outcomes were derived from these four data sources, grouped into four overall measures: (i) off-sale purchasing; (ii) on-sale purchasing; (iii) 18 to 20 year olds; and (iv) high school students. Aggregating individual outcome scores within these four overall measures showed a statistically significant improvement for on-sale purchasing and for 18 to 20 year olds. Of the 26 individual outcome measures, the only statistically significant result was a 17 per cent reduction in self-reported provision of alcohol to youth by 18 to 20 year olds. The authors concluded that CMCA demonstrates the feasibility of mobilising communities and that its potential benefits warrant further development. Most innovatively, CMCA illustrates the potential capacity for community-action approaches to engage with alcohol retailers to implement supply reduction strategies, in addition to demand and harm reduction strategies.

Preventing substance use among Native American youth

This cluster RCT involved Native American youth from 10 reservations in North and South Dakota, Idaho, Montana and Oklahoma (Schinke et al., 2000). Within these communities, the interventions engaged with third, fourth and fifth grade students in 27 tribal and public schools. The aim of this trial was prevent alcohol, smoking and cannabis use. The 27 schools were randomly allocated to one of three intervention conditions.

- Skills training – This comprised 50-minute sessions over 15 weeks that involved instruction, modelling and rehearsal of cognitive-behaviour therapy (CBT) skills associated with substance abuse prevention. The CBT based intervention was culturally tailored to Native American values, legends and stories, and took account of the everyday realities of Native American youth. It was delivered by group leaders and slightly older peers. Two 50-minute booster sessions were also provided semi-annually.
- Skills training and community involvement – in addition to skills training, this component mobilized Native American constituents (families, teachers, school counsellors, residents, law enforcement officials and commercial establishments frequented by youth) to participate in substance abuse prevention activities, including media releases about the benefits of substance abuse prevention efforts for Native American youth. The two semi-annual booster sessions were also provided to students in this treatment arm.
- Control – students in schools in the control condition received no intervention.

The impact of the interventions was measured using self-report surveys (with saliva samples as a bogus pipeline). There were four behaviours (cigarette smoking, smokeless tobacco, alcohol use and cannabis use) measured at four post-intervention time points (6, 18, 30 and 42 months), giving a total of 16 possible outcomes. Five statistically significant impacts were identified. At 30 months follow up, those in the skills training group reported less smokeless tobacco use than those in both other comparison groups and those in the skills training group reported less alcohol use that those in the control group. At 42 months follow up, the two statistically significant effects reported at 30 months were maintained and a third significant effect emerged: those in the skills training group reported less cannabis use that those in the control group. These results suggest that community involvement did not provide any additional benefit to the youth skills training alone.

A REVIEW OF KEY NON-RANDOMIZED COMMUNITY-FOCUSED ALCOHOL INTERVENTION EVALUATIONS

As outlined in the 'Evaluation Issues' section, there are valid reasons to consider that the non-randomized trial, in in its various forms, may offer the best option for evaluating community-focused alcohol interventions in many circumstances. Indeed, non-randomized trials have made a valuable contribution to the body of research on community-focused alcohol interventions, even if they cannot provide the same level as confidence that the reported outcomes are a consequence of the intervention. The results of key evaluations that have helped shape the research in this field are briefly summarized.

Community Action Project (CAP)

This New Zealand trial was one of the first non-US trials of a community-action approach (Casswell and Gilmore, 1989). It organized six New Zealand cities into three groups: two cities received an intervention comprising of an alcohol-focused community organizer and media campaign, two cities received an intervention of a media campaign only and two acted as no intervention controls. The community organizers worked with local organizations to focus on alcohol availability (including the promotion of non-alcoholic beverages), advertising and some pricing policies. The media campaign focused on reducing heavy drinking by young men. It found support for control policies on advertising and availability, and that price held steady in the treatment communities but dropped in the reference communities. The perception of alcohol being essential to entertaining and as being relatively innocuous decreased significantly in the community-action cities.

Community Mobilisation for the Prevention of Alcohol Related Injury (COMPARI)

This Australian trial involved two rural communities in Western Australia (one intervention, one control) (Midford and Boots, 1999). It comprised a combination of 22 intervention components, grouped into five domains: networking and support; community development; alternate options in health education; health marketing; and policy institutionalization. It found a significant downward trend in per capita alcohol consumption in the intervention community, relative to the control community and relative to non-rural communities generally in Western Australia, both of which showed an upward trend in consumption. It also found no change in a proxy measure of alcohol harm, the rate of weekend night accident and emergency department presentations in the intervention community, compared to an increase in the control community. An unusual outcome of this project was that the approach was sustained in the intervention community for more than 10 years.

Community Trials Project (CTP)

This quasi-experimental US trial selected three experimental communities in California and South Carolina on the basis of their pre-existing interest in reducing alcohol harm and having a sufficient population to identify the effect of interventions (Holder et al., 2000). These communities were then pair matched with non-intervention controls. The project implemented and evaluated a combination of five intervention strategies: community mobilisation; encouraging responsible beverage service; limiting access to alcohol to reduce underage drinking; increasing local enforcement of drinking and driving laws; and using zoning restrictions to limit access to alcohol. It found reductions in the following self-reported outcomes: a 6 per cent reduction in alcohol consumed per drinking occasion; a 49 per cent reduction in 'having had too much to drink'; and a 51 per cent reduction in self-reported occasions of driving while over the legal limit. It also found reductions in alcohol-related harm, including a 10 per cent reduction in night-time injury road accidents, a 6 per cent reduction in road accidents where the driver had been drinking and a 43 per cent reduction in assault injuries that resulted in at least a one-night hospital stay. At the time, CTP was the largest and most rigorous community alcohol prevention trial.

The Swedish six-community alcohol and drug prevention trial

This Swedish trial, in a similar manner to the US CTP, employed a quasi-experimental approach (Hallgren and Andréasson, 2013). It recruited six intervention communities across Sweden on the basis that they were willing, and had the capacity, to increase local level alcohol and drug prevention efforts. Six demographically matched control communities were then selected for comparison. Intervention communities selected their preferred interventions from a menu of evidence-based options and were provided with training and support to implement their choices. Young people were the focus of most selected interventions, including parental education and training, and school-based interventions. Other interventions selected included responsible beverage service (RBS), prevention of drunk driving and screening and brief intervention in primary health care settings. All six intervention communities received support to mobilize community resources effectively. The main outcomes of interest were changes in youth drinking and alcohol-related hospitalizations. The impact of the trial on three additional factors frequently associated with hazardous drinking by young people was also measured: parental provision of alcohol; adult attitudes towards youth drinking; and the perception by young people as to the availability alcohol. The study reported no statistically significant differences between the intervention and control communities, which the authors attributed to the selection by communities of strategies with little evidence of effect.

A SUMMARY INTERPRETATION OF OUTCOMES FROM COMMUNITY-FOCUSED ALCOHOL INTERVENTION EVALUATIONS

A number of key features can be summarized from the results of community-focused alcohol intervention evaluations published to date.

A clear focus on young people rather than communities generally

With the single exception of the AARC project, randomized trials have focused on young people, with the unit of randomization and the focus of the interventions either schools or university campuses. This could reflect evidence about the nature of alcohol-related harm (e.g. that alcohol-related harms are most prevalent among young people or that there is clear evidence about the benefits of delaying the initiation to alcohol use) or it may be a logistical consideration (e.g. that it is easier to engage, implement interventions and measure outcomes among well-defined and more accessible, sub-populations within communities). An examination of the relatively less stringent, non-randomized trials may provide some support for the argument that randomized trials focus on young people in education settings because they are logistically easier to conduct: three of the four non-randomized trials summarized above are community-wide, rather than focused on young people. This suggests that schools and university campuses are easier to engage in randomized trials and, conversely, whole communities are easier to engage in non-randomized trials.

Whatever the reasons, most of the most methodologically stringent evidence, to date, has been derived from the six out of seven randomized trials that focused on young people in school or university campus settings. To make this point in the reverse, AARC is the only randomized trial to date that has focused on the assessing the impact on a whole community of interventions that were implemented across a range of settings. Simply because of this, its contribution to the evidence base is proportionately greater.

Use of a system-model, rather than a catchment, approach

While the original Project Northland (Perry et al., 1996). was undertaken just prior to Holder's 1998 articulation of the application of a systems approach to community-focused alcohol interventions (Holder, 1998), all seven randomized trials can be characterized as taking a system-level, rather than a catchment-level approach, in the sense that they all engaged with a range of community stakeholders to deliver at least some of the intervention components. This finding most likely reflects the increased recognition in the late 1990s as to the importance of engaging simultaneously with different community elements if adopting this model. However, given the complexity, level of funding and long timeframes that are typical of randomized, systems-level alcohol interventions, it is not surprising that the trials were few and far between: one in 1996 (Perry et al., 1996), two in 2000 (Schinke et al., 2000; Wagenaar et al., 2000) and four since 2008 (Komro et al., 2008; Saltz et al., 2010; Shakeshaft et al., 2014; Wolfson et al., 2012).

The system-model approach, adopted to greater or lesser degrees in both the randomized and non-randomized trials summarized previously, highlights an important shift away from only targeting demand or harm reduction strategies at individuals within communities to a more ecological or public health type approach, which also acknowledges the relationship between supply-side control strategies and levels of alcohol consumption and harm in a community. In terms of operationalizing the need for supply-side controls, most of these trials attempted to engage with alcohol retailers, parents and older peers to reduce the supply of alcohol to young or underage drinkers and three of the randomized trials specifically measured alcohol purchase attempts as an outcome (Komro et al., 2008; Perry et al., 1996; Wagenaar et al., 2000).

Few statistically significant effects are reported, and those that are reported appear skewed towards lower level harms

The general pattern of results from the seven community prevention RCTs was that statistically significant benefits were achieved for a minority of outcomes. Across all seven trials, a total of 222 outcome measures were defined, of which a statistically significant outcome in favour of the intervention group was reported for 41 (18 per cent) of outcomes. This low level of effect is also reflected in the non-randomized trials. For example, the one non-randomized trial focusing on young people, the Swedish six-community alcohol and drug prevention trial, reported not one statistically significant difference between groups (Hallgren and Andréasson, 2013). It is also consistent with a previous review of interventions aimed at reducing underage drinking (Wagenaar et al., 2006).

One interpretation of this pattern of results is that community-action is only likely to be effective with a small number of outcomes. In addition to a small number of effects, it may be that community action interventions are most effective in reducing lower-level alcohol related harms that may be relatively easier to shift. The AARC trial, for example, reported statistically significant improvements on self-reported rates of verbal abuse and average weekly alcohol consumption, but no impact on binge drinking and the negative consequences of alcohol consumption that were severe enough to require police or hospital intervention (Shakeshaft et al., 2014).

An alternative explanation for the apparent superior impact of community-focused programmes on lower-level alcohol harms may lie in the self-report methodology: of the four studies that used a measure other than self-report, none found a statistically significant effect (AARC found no impact on routinely collected data outcomes and the three studies that used alcohol purchase attempts reported no significant effects) (Komro et al., 2008; Perry et al., 1996; Shakeshaft et al., 2014; Wagenaar et al., 2000). The significant effects on self-reported outcomes, and the absence of significant effects on non-self-reported outcomes, could be a further indication that community-action only reduces lower-level harms (i.e. those that do not require formal intervention by authorities). However, there could be methodologically-related bias in self-reported data, or the combination of community-action interventions most likely to significantly impact on relatively serious alcohol-harms is yet to be evaluated using a randomized trial.

Effects may not be generalizable to different communities

As noted earlier, the strict inclusion criteria, typical of randomized trials, can limit the external validity, or generalizability, of the results obtained in the intervention communities to other communities. The Northland projects, for example, implemented essentially the same intervention in rural communities in Minnesota and in Chicago; reporting a significant impact in favour of the intervention communities on 27 of 122 individual possible outcomes in Minnesota (Perry et al., 1996), but no significant impacts in Chicago (Komro et al., 2008). The conclusion of the Chicago trial researchers that a successful intervention in one community will not necessarily work in another is an important insight for community action approaches for at least two reasons. First, from a methodological perspective, an advantage of randomized trials is that they typically consider the impact of interventions averaged across multiple communities, which means the results are less prone to the influence of communities at extreme ends of the alcohol harm continuum (i.e. those with either relatively high or low baseline rates of alcohol-related harm). Consequently, caution needs to be exercised in relation to single community and non-randomized evaluations because they are susceptible to findings unique to a particular community Second, from a practical perspective, it suggests a need to develop interventions that are targeted to the specific alcohol-related problems in a community, rather than applying the same interventions to all communities irrespective of their baseline differences. Descriptive analyses from the AARC project, for example, identified statistically significantly different baseline rates of alcohol-related crime, alcohol-related traffic crashes and rates of risky drinking across the 20 communities involved in that project (Breen et al., 2011, 2014; Czech et al., 2010, 2011). Tailoring specific intervention strategies to the particular alcohol-related harms and drinking patterns in different communities does raise the question about how to achieve standardization in interventions that are tailored to individual communities, but Craig and colleagues indicate that complex, mixed method evaluation designs provide one mechanism for addressing the problem (Craig et al., 2008).

Little evidence of sustainability

A clear issue in relation to published community-focused alcohol trials to date is the extent to which the interventions are sustainable beyond the life of the evaluation component of the programme. The only trial to actively consider and report on this issue is the COMPARI project (Midford et al., 2005). In their analysis, the researchers explored the issue of what makes a community-focused programme sustainable by conducting interviews with 23 community informants subsequent to the intervention research phase. This unique analysis identified key components related to sustainability: a culture of intersectoral collaboration on alcohol issues; better use of resources; higher levels of treatment referral; and 'strong acknowledgement that the local committee was crucial in sustaining the project' (Midford et al., 2005: 3).

It was also noted that over time, the community-focused approach increasingly emphasized individual prevention through education and training, which may reflect the difficulty of maintaining true community mobilization and a sense of collective responsibility.

The other trials summarized here have tended to approach the issue of sustainability by encouraging communities to take more control over selecting the interventions that are most appropriate for their community and/or engaging with existing service providers to implement the selected interventions. This is consistent with the concept of complex interventions that emphasize community led action rather than have researchers pre-specify which interventions ought to be implemented in each community (Craig et al., 2008). It also provides a practical basis for sustainability because it can engender a greater sense of local community ownership over the interventions. However, in light of what occurred in the Swedish six-community trial, care needs to be taken that the chosen interventions are strongly backed by evidence of effect (Hallgren and Andréasson, 2013).

Little evidence about whether community-focused interventions are a good economic investment

Even if outcome results are modest, community trials can still represent a good investment in economic terms if the costs of their implementation are outweighed by the benefits of the outcomes they achieve. Although Holder (2000) identified the need for cost effectiveness analyses in prevention over a decade ago, there have only been two attempts to weight the economic costs against outcomes achieved in community-focused intervention trials, both of which relate to whole of community trials, as opposed to those focused on schools or university campuses: the CTP trial by Holder and colleagues and the AARC trial by Shakeshaft and colleagues (Holder et al., 2000; Shakeshaft et al., 2012b)

Holder et al. (2000) conducted what was, by their own admission, a relatively simple cost-effectiveness analysis on the distal effects of the drinking and driving outcome in the CTP trial, which was only one measure of the project's impact. They identified a net economic benefit valued at US$2,032,590, or US$2.88 in savings for every US$1 invested in the CTP trial. Shakeshaft et al. (2012b) performed a comprehensive benefit-cost analysis as part of the AARC trial, using the outcomes based on the routinely collected data (traffic crashes, crime and hospitalizations) and the value that households place on reducing risky drinking and alcohol-related harm in their community. They also identified a net economic benefit in the experimental communities, relative to the control communities, estimated at between $1.37 and $1.75 for every $1 invested in the AARC interventions.

CONSIDERATIONS FOR THE FUTURE

The community-focused research reviewed in this chapter provides evidence that changing the community environment can reduce alcohol use and associated problems in the young and adult populations of the intervention communities. While researchers have not identified which particular combination of environmental strategies is most effective and economically efficient in preventing alcohol related problems, the studies conducted to date suggest that it is important to consider which environmental strategies are most likely to be best matched to the targeted outcome and population. Results from the CMCA study provide an illustration of this. CMCA was effective in reducing alcohol use among 18 to 20 year olds, but not among high school students, and a possible explanation is that the CMCA communities focused on sales from licensed alcohol premises, which were more commonly used by the older age group to source alcohol (Toomey and Lenk, 2011; Wagenaar et al., 1999, 2000).

Communities may have limited guidance about specific environmental strategies. However, they can draw on a range of studies to guide their efforts. A number of studies have identified particular settings and situations where alcohol environmental changes are needed, such as at alcohol outlets, community festivals and sporting events where the likelihood of sales to underage or obviously intoxicated patrons is high (Lenk et al., 2006; Perry et al., 1996; Toomey and Lenk, 2011). Other studies have determined how specific strategies can be applied to best effect; for example, alcohol compliance checks were found to be effective if implemented at least three monthly (Wagenaar et al., 2005).

While the best path for future community-focused alcohol prevention is that defined by past research, Toomey and Lenk (2011) and Czech and colleagues (Breen et al., 2011, 2014; Czech et al., 2010, 2011) considered that research has left many questions unanswered. Three of these are fundamental to designing more effective interventions in the future.

- Which individual or combinations of environmental interventions are most effective in reducing problematic alcohol use?
- Would the addition of individual-focused interventions improve the effect of environmental measures?
- Why do some communities seem more resistant to alcohol harms than others and how can researchers better understand the characteristics of these communities in order to leverage this when developing environmental interventions?

A fourth, broader question, raised by the findings from AARC project is whether community action alone is the best way to address local level alcohol problems (Shakeshaft et al., 2014). The most effective community interventions involve substantial systemic change, and the effects, when achieved, are few, and generally involve lower-level harms. The interventions to achieve these changes are also lengthy, difficult to implement and expensive. In contrast, studies of jurisdiction level alcohol policies have found that change in a single alcohol policy, such as raising the legal drinking age to 21, which occurred in many US states during the 1970s and 80s, have substantially reduced a range of alcohol related problems (DeJong and Blanchette, 2014).

Shakeshaft and colleagues indicated that legislative strategies, such as pricing control, restrictions on availability and drink driving laws are broadly effective, while the community action trials to date have typically achieved benefit within a subset of harms (Shakeshaft et al., 2014). This comparison highlights the limitations of community-focused action, but as Thompson and Kinne (1999) stressed, local ownership is important in community change. This means community involvement has to be considered a key component in a multi-faceted approach to initiating, undertaking and sustaining measures to reduce the problems associated with the use of alcohol. In practice, legislative controls are required to set the general alcohol framework at a national or jurisdictional level, while community-action approaches allow targeting of specific problem drinking patterns and harms within defined populations. One of the great challenges for future research is determining a balance between these two approaches that is optimally effective, acceptable to communities and economically efficient.

REFERENCES

Aguinis, H., Pierce, C. A. and Quigley, B. M. (1993). Conditions under which a bogus pipeline procedure enhances the validity of self-reported cigarette smoking: a meta-analytic review. *Journal of Applied Social Psychology*, 23(5): 352–73.

Aguirre-Molina, M. and Gorman, D. M. (1996). Community-focused approaches for the prevention of alcohol, tobacco, and other drug use. *Annual Review of Public Health*, 17(1): 337–58.

Andréasson, S., Sjöström, E. and Bränström, R. (2007). A six-community prevention trial to reduce alcohol and drug use-related problems in Sweden: planning and early findings. *Substance Use and Misuse*, 42(12–13): 2017–27.

Aseltine, R. H., Schilling, E. A., James, A., Murray, M. and Jacobs, D. G. (2008). An evaluation of national alcohol screening day. *Alcohol and Alcoholism*, 43(1): 97-103.

Berridge, V. (2005). *Temperance Its History and Impact on Current and Future Alcohol Policy.* York: Joseph Rowntree Foundation.

Blocker Jr, J. S. (2006). Did prohibition really work? Alcohol prohibition as a public health innovation. *American Journal of Public Health*, 96(2): 233–43.

Breen, C., Shakeshaft, A., Sanson-Fisher, R., D'Este, C., Mattick, R. and Gilmour, S. (2014). Identifying individual- and population-level characteristics that influence rates of risky alcohol consumption and harm in communities. *Australian and New Zealand Journal of Public Health*, 38(1): 60–5.

Breen, C., Shakeshaft, A., Slade, T., Love, S., D'Este, C. and Mattick, R. P. (2011). Do community characteristics predict levels of alcohol-related crime? *Alcohol and Alcoholism*, 46: 464–70.

Buka, S. L. and Birdthistle, I. J. (1999). Long-term effects of a community-wide alcohol server training intervention. *Journal of Studies on Alcohol*, 60(1): 27-36.

Casswell, S. (2000). A decade of community action. *Substance Use and Misuse*, 35(1–2): 55–74.

Casswell, S. and Gilmore, L. (1989). An evaluated community action project on alcohol. *Journal of Studies on Alcohol and Drugs*, 50(4): 339–46.

Cherrington, E. H. (1920). *The Evolution of Prohibition in the United States of America.* Westerville: American Issue Press.

Chou, C. P., Montgomery, S., Pentz, M. A., Rohrbach, L. A., Johnson, C. A., Flay, B. R. and MacKinnon, D. P. (1998). Effects of a community-based prevention program on decreasing drug use in high-risk adolescents. *American Journal of Public Health*, 88(6): 944–8.

Clapp, J. D., Johnson, M., Voas, R. B., Lange, J. E., Shillington, A. and Russell, C. (2005). Reducing DUI among US college students: Results of an environmental prevention trial. *Addiction*, 100(3): 327-34.

Clifford, A., Shakeshaft, A. and Deans, C. (2013). Training and tailored outreach support to improve alcohol screening and brief intervention in Aboriginal Community Controlled Health Services. *Drug and Alcohol Review*, 32(1): 72–9.

COMMIT Research Group. (1995). Community Intervention Trial for Smoking Cessation (COMMIT): I. Cohort results from a four-year community intervention. *American Journal of Public Health,* 85(2): 183–92.

Conway, K. (2002). Booze and beach bans: turning the tide through community action in New Zealand. *Health Promotion International*, 17(2): 171–7.

Craig, P., Dieppe, P., Macintyre, S., Michie, S., Nazareth, I. and Petticrew, M. (2008). Developing and evaluating complex interventions: the new Medical Research Council guidance. *BMJ*, 337: a1655.

Czech, S., Shakeshaft, A. P., Breen, C. and Sanson-Fisher, R. W. (2010). Whole-of-community approaches to reducing alcohol-related harm: what do communities think? *Journal of Public Health*, 18(6): 543–51.

Czech, S., Shakeshaft, A., Sanson-Fisher, R. and Breen, C. (2011). The development and application of a proxy measure of alcohol-related traffic crashes for rural communities. *Accident Analysis and Prevention*, 43(6): 2160–5.

Dejong, W. and Blanchette, J. (2014). Case closed: research evidence on the positive public health impact of the age 21 minimum legal drinking age in the United States. *Journal of Studies on Alcohol and Drugs*, 17: 108–15.

Eriksen, S. (2003). Denmark. In J. S. Blocker, D. M. Fahey and I. R. Tyrrell (eds), *Alcohol and Temperance in Modern History.* Oxford: ABC Clio, pp. 192–4.

Flynn, B. S., Worden, J. K., Bunn, J. Y., Dorwaldt, A. L., Dana, G. S. and Callas, P. W. (2006). Mass media and community interventions to reduce alcohol use by early adolescents. *Journal of Studies on Slcohol*, 67(1):66-74.

Gebhardt, T. L., Kaphingst, K. and DeJong, W. (2000). A campus-community coalition to control alcohol-related problems off campus: An environmental management case study. *Journal of American College Health*, 48(5): 211-5.

Gorman, D.M. and Speer P.W. (1996). Preventing alcohol abuse and alcohol-related problems through community interventions: a review of evaluation studies. *Psychology and Health*, 11(1): 95–131.

Grant, D. and Serle, G. (1983). *The Melbourne Scene 1803–1956*. Sydney: Hale & Iremonger.

Grossman, J. and Mackenzie, F. J. (2005). The randomized controlled trial: gold standard, or merely standard? *Perspectives in Biology and Medicine*, 48(4): 516–34.

Hallgren, M. and Andréasson, S. (2013). The Swedish six-community alcohol and drug prevention trial: effects on youth drinking. *Drug and Alcohol Review*, 32(5): 504–11.

Havard, A., Shakeshaft, A. P., Conigrave, K. M. and Doran, C. M. (2012). Randomized controlled trial of mailed personalized feedback for problem drinkers in the emergency department: the short-term impact. *Alcoholism: Clinical and Experimental Research*, 36(3): 523–31.

Hawkins, N. G., Sanson-Fisher, R. W., Shakeshaft, A., D'Este, C. and Green, L. W. (2007). The multiple baseline design for evaluating population-based research. *American Journal of Preventive Medicine*, 33(2): 162–8.

Hingson, R., McGovern, T., Howland, J., Heeren, T., Winter, M. and Zakocs, R. (1996). Reducing alcohol-impaired driving in Massachusetts: the Saving Lives Program. *American Journal of Public Health*, 86(6): 791–7.

Hingson, R., Zakocs, R., Heeren, T., Winter, M., Rosenbloom, D. and DeJong, W. (2005). Effects on alcohol related fatal crashes of a community based initiative to increase substance abuse treatment and reduce alcohol availability. *Injury Prevention*, 11(2): 84–90.

Ho, P. M., Peterson, P. N. and Masoudi, F. A. (2008). Evaluating the evidence is there a rigid hierarchy? *Circulation*, 118(16): 1675–84.

Holder, H. D. (1992). What is a community and what are implications for prevention trials for reducing alcohol problems? In H. D. Holder and J. M. Howard (eds), *Community Prevention Trials for Alcohol Problems*. Westport: Praeger, pp. 15–33.

Holder, H. D. (1998). *Alcohol and the Community: A Systems Approach to Prevention*. Cambridge: Cambridge University Press.

Holder, H. D. (2000). Community prevention of alcohol problems. *Addictive Behaviors*, 25(6): 843–59.

Holder, H. D., Gruenewald, P. J., Ponicki, W. R., Treno, A. J., Grube, J. W., Saltz, R. F., Voas, R. B., Reynolds, R., Davis, J., Sanchez, L., Gaumont, G. and Roeper, P. (2000). Effect of community-focused interventions on high-risk drinking and alcohol-related injuries. *The Journal of the American Medical Association*, 284(18): 2341–7.

Holmila, M. (1995). Community action on alcohol: experiences of the Lahti Project in Finland. *Health Promotion International*, 10(4): 283–91.

Holmila, M. (2000a). Lessons learned about the community initiatives in preventing alcohol and drug-related harm. In K. Elmeland (ed.), *Lokalt Alkohol-Och Drogforebyggande Arbete I Norden*. Helsingfors: Nordiska namnden for alkohol-och drogforskning (NAD), pp. 67–73.

Holmila, M. (2000b). The Finnish case: community prevention in a time of rapid change in national and international trade. *Substance Use and Misuse*, 35(1–2): 111–23.

Holmila, M. (2003). The evaluation of the Metropolitan project; process and causality. *Nordisk Alkohol and Narkotikatidskrift*, 20: 81–90.

Huckle, T., Conway, K., Casswell, S. and Pledger, M. (2005). Evaluation of a regional community action intervention in New Zealand to improve age checks for young people purchasing alcohol. *Health Promotion International*, 20(2): 147–55.

Huckle, T., Greenaway, S., Broughton, D. and Conway, K. (2007). The use of an evidence-based community action intervention to improve age verification practices for alcohol purchase. *Substance Use and Misuse*, 42 (12–13): 1899–914.

Jones, S. G. (1987). Labour, society and the drink question in Britain, 1918–1939. *The Historical Journal,* 30(1): 105–22.

Klepp, K. I., Kelder, S. H. and Perry, C. L. (1995). Alcohol and marijuana use among adolescents: long-term outcomes of the Class of 1989 Study. *Annals of Behavioral Medicine*, 17(1): 19-24.

Komro, K. A., Perry, C. L., Veblen-Mortenson, S., Farbakhsh, K., Toomey, T. L., Stigler, M. H., Jones-Webb, R., Kugler, K., Pasch, K. E. and Williams, C. L. (2008). Outcomes from a randomized controlled trial of a multi-component alcohol use preventive intervention for urban youth: Project Northland Chicago. *Addiction*, 103(4): 606–18.

Kreitman, N. (1986). Alcohol consumption and the Preventive Paradox. *British Journal of Addiction,* 81(3): 353–64.

Leifman, H. (2001). Homogenisation in alcohol consumption in the European Union. *Nordic Studies on Alcohol and Drugs*, 18(English Supplement): 15–30.

Lenk, K. M., Toomey, T. L. and Erickson, D. J. (2006). Propensity of alcohol establishments to sell to obviously intoxicated patrons. *Alcoholism: Clinical and Experimental Research*, 30(7): 1194–9.

Levine, H. G. (1978). The discovery of addiction: changing conceptions of habitual drunkenness in America. *Journal of Studies on Alcohol,* 39(1): 1347–70.

Merrill, J. L. (1988). The Bible and the American Temperance Movement: text, context, and pretext. *Harvard Theological Review*, 81(2): 165.

Midford, R. and Boots, K. (1999). COMPARI: Insights from a three year community-focused alcohol harm reduction project. *Australian Journal of Primary Health – Interchange*, 5(4): 46–58.

Midford, R., Young, D., Chikritzhs, T., Playford, D., Kite, E. and Pascal, R. (2010). The effect of alcohol sales and advertising restrictions on a remote Australian community. *Drugs: Education, Prevention and Policy*, 17(1): 21–41.

Midford, R., Wayte, K., Catalano, P., Gupta, R. and Chikritzhs, T. (2005). The legacy of a community mobilisation project to reduce alcohol related harm. *Drug and Alcohol Review*, 24(1): 3–11.

Navarro, H., Shakeshaft, A., Doran, C. and Sanson-Fisher, R. (2011). The potential cost-effectiveness of general practitioner delivered brief intervention for alcohol misuse: evidence from rural Australia. *Addictive Behaviors,* 36(12): 1191–8.

Navarro, H. J., Shakeshaft, A., Doran, C. M. and Petrie, D. J. (2012). The cost-effectiveness of tailored, postal feedback on general practitioners' prescribing of pharmacotherapies for alcohol dependence. *Drug and Alcohol Dependence*, 124(3): 207–15.

Navarro, H., Shakeshaft, A., Doran, C. and Petrie, D. (2013). A multi-strategy community approach to reduce alcohol-related violent crime incidents: a cost-benefit analysis. *International Journal of Environmental Research and Public Health,* 10(11): 5490–506.

Österberg, E. (1992). Effects of alcohol control measures on alcohol consumption. *Substance Use and Misuse*, 27(2): 209–25.

Pegram, T. R. (1998). *Battling Demon Rum: The Struggle for a Dry America, 1800–1933*. Chicago: Ivan R. Dee.

Perry, C. L., Williams, C. L., Veblen-Mortenson, S., Toomey, T. L., Komro, K. A., Anstine, P. S., McGovern, P. G., Finnegan, J. L., Forster, J. L., Wagenaar, A. C. and Wolfson, M. (1996). Project Northland: outcomes of a communitywide alcohol use prevention program during early adolescence. *American Journal of Public Health*, 86(7): 956–65.

Prestwich, P. E. (2003). France, Temperance. In J. S. Blocker, D. M. Fahey and I. R. Tyrrell (eds), *Alcohol and Temperance in Modern History.* Oxford: ABC Clio, p. 251.

Rehnman, C., Larsson, J. and Andréasson, S. (2005). The beer campaign in Stockholm–Attempting to restrict the availability of alcohol to young people. *Alcohol*, 37(2): 65–71.

Rose, G. (1981). Strategy of prevention: lessons from cardiovascular disease. *British Medical Journal (Clinical Research ed.)*, 282(6279): 1847-51.

Rose, G. (1985). Sick individuals and sick populations. *International Journal of Epidemiology*, 14(1): 32–8.

Rosen, A.L., Manor, O., Engelhard, D. and Zucker, D. (2006a). In defense of the randomized controlled trial for health promotion research. *American Journal of Public Health,* 96(7): 1181–6.

Rosen, L., Manor, O., Engelhard, D., Brody, D., Rosen, B., Peleg, H., Meir, M. and Zucker, D. (2006b). Can a handwashing intervention make a difference? Results from a randomized controlled trial in Jerusalem preschools. *Preventive Medicine*, 42(1): 27–32.

Rowe, W. (1997). Changing ATOD norms and behaviors: a Native American community commitment to wellness. *Evaluation and Program Planning*, 20(3): 323–33.

Saltz, R. F., Paschall, M. J., McGaffigan, R. P. and Nygaard, P. M. (2010). Alcohol risk management in college settings: the safer California universities randomized trial. *American Journal of Preventive Medicine*, 39(6): 491–9.

Sanson-Fisher, R. W., Bonevski, B., Green, L. W. and D'Este, C. (2007). Limitations of the randomized controlled trial in evaluating population-based health interventions. *American Journal of Preventive Medicine*, 33(2): 155–61.

Sariola, S. (1954). Prohibition in Finland, 1919–1932; its background and consequences. *Quarterly Journal of Studies in Alcohol*, 15(3): 477–90.

Schinke, S. P., Tepavac, L. and Cole, K. C. (2000). Preventing substance use among Native American youth: three-year results. *Addictive Behaviors*, 25(3): 387–97.

Shakeshaft, A., Doran, C., Petrie, D., Breen, C., Havard, A., Abudeen, A., Harwood E, Clifford A, D'Este C, Gilmour S, Byrnes, J., Navarro, H. J. and Sanson-Fisher R. (2012a). The Alcohol Action in Rural Communities (AARC) Project. *Working with Communities to Select, Implement and Measure the Impact of Strategies to Reduce Alcohol-Related Harm*. Deakin: Foundation for Alcohol Research and Education. Retrieved 3 July 2014 from http://www.fare.org.au/research-development/featured-research/alcohol-action-in-rural-communities/

Shakeshaft, A., Doran, C., Petrie, D., Breen, C., Havard, A., Abudeen, A., Harwood, E., Clifford, A., D'Este, C., Gilmour, S. and Sanson-Fisher, R. (2012b). *Alcohol Action in Rural Communities (AARC) Project: Detailed description of the interventions and their costs (Monograph No. 64)*. Sydney: National Drug and Alcohol Research Centre. Retrieved 3 July 2014 from https://ndarc.med.unsw.edu.au/sites/default/files/ndarc/resources/Mono.64.pdf

Shakeshaft, A., Doran, C., Petrie, D., Breen, C., Havard, A., Abudeen, A., Harwood, E., Clifford, A., D'Este, C., Gilmour, S. and Sanson-Fisher, R. (2014). The effectiveness of community action in reducing risky alcohol consumption and harm: a cluster randomized controlled trial. *PLOS Medicine*, 11(3): e1001617.

Slater, M. D., Kelly, K. J., Edwards, R. W., Thurman, P. J., Plested, B. A., Keefe, T. J., Lawrence, F. R. and Henry, K. L. (2006). Combining in-school and community-based media efforts: reducing marijuana and alcohol uptake among younger adolescents. *Health Education Research*, 21(1): 157-67.

Stafström, M., Östergren, P. O., Larsson, S., Lindgren, B. and Lundborg, P. (2006). A community action programme for reducing harmful drinking behaviour among adolescents: the Trelleborg Project. *Addiction*, 101(6): 813–23.

Stevens, M., Mott, L. and Youells, F. (1996). Rural adolescent drinking behavior: three year follow-up in the New Hampshire substance abuse prevention study. *Adolescence*, 31(121): 159–66.

Stockwell, T. and Gruenewald, P.J. (2004). Controls on the physical availability of alcohol. In N. Heather and T. Stockwell (eds), *The Essential Handbook of Treatment and Prevention of Alcohol Problems*. New York: John Wiley & Sons Ltd, pp. 213–34.

Swiatkiewicz, G. and Moskalewicz, J. (2003). Poland. In J. S. Blocker, D. M. Fahey and I. R. Tyrrell (eds), *Alcohol and Temperance in Modern History*. Oxford: ABC Clio, pp. 482–6.

Thompson, B. and Kinne, S. (1999). Social change theory. applications to community health. In N. Bracht (ed.), *Health Promotion at the Community Level: New Advance*, 2nd edn. Thousand Oaks: Sage Publications, pp. 29–46.

Tones, K. (1997). Beyond the randomized controlled trial: a case for 'judicial review'. *Health Education Research*, 12(2): i–iv.

Toomey, T. L. and Lenk, K. M. (2011). A review of environmental-based community interventions. *Alcohol Research and Health*, 34(2): 163–6.

Treno, A. J., Gruenewald, P. J., Lee, J. P. and Remer, L. G. (2007). The Sacramento Neighborhood Alcohol Prevention Project: outcomes from a community prevention trial. *Journal of Studies on Alcohol and Drugs*, 68(2): 197–207.

Wagenaar, A., Erikson, D. J., Harwood, E. M. and O'Malley, P. M. (2006). Effects of state coalitions to reduce underage drinking: a national evaluation. *American Journal of Preventive Medicine*, 31(4): 307–15.

Wagenaar, A.C., Gehan, J. P., Jones-Webb, R., Toomey, T. L., Forster, J. L., Wolfson, M. and Murrary, D. M. (1999). Communities mobilizing for change on alcohol: lessons and results from a 15 community randomized trial. *Journal of Community Psychology*, 27(3): 315–26.

Wagenaar, A. C., Murray, D. M., Gehan, J. P., Wolfson, M., Forster, J. L., Toomey, T. L., Perry, C. L. and Jones-Webb, R. (2000). Communities mobilizing for change on alcohol: outcomes from a randomized community trial. *Journal of Studies on Alcohol and Drugs*, 61(1): 85–94.

Wagenaar, A. C., Toomey, T. L. and Erickson, D. J. (2005). Preventing youth access to alcohol: outcomes from a multi-community time-series trial. *Addiction*, 100(3): 335–45.

Wallin, E., Norström, T. and Andréasson, S. (2003). Alcohol prevention targeting licensed premises: a study of effects on violence. *Journal of Studies on Alcohol and Drugs*, 64(2): 270–7.

Wallin, E., Gripenberg, J. and Andréasson, S. (2005). Overserving at licensed premises in Stockholm: effects of a community action program. *Journal of Studies on Alcohol and Drugs*, 66(6): 806–14.

Wolfson, M., Champion, H., McCoy, T. P., Rhodes, S. D., Ip, E. H., Blocker, J. N., Martin, B. A., Wagoner, K. G., O'Brien, M. C., Suffin, E. L., Mitra, A. and Durant, R. H. (2012). Impact of a randomized campus/community trial to prevent high-risk drinking among college students. *Alcoholism: Clinical and Experimental Research*, 36(10). 1767–78.

WHO European Working Group on Health Promotion Evaluation (1998). *Health Promotion Evaluation: Recommendations to Policy-Makers*. Copenhagen: WHO Regional Office for Europe.

World Health Organization. (2010). *Global Strategy to Reduce the Harmful Use of Alcohol.* Geneva: World Health Organization. Retrieved 3 July 2014 from http://www.who.int/substance_abuse/alcstratenglishfinal.pdf?ua=1

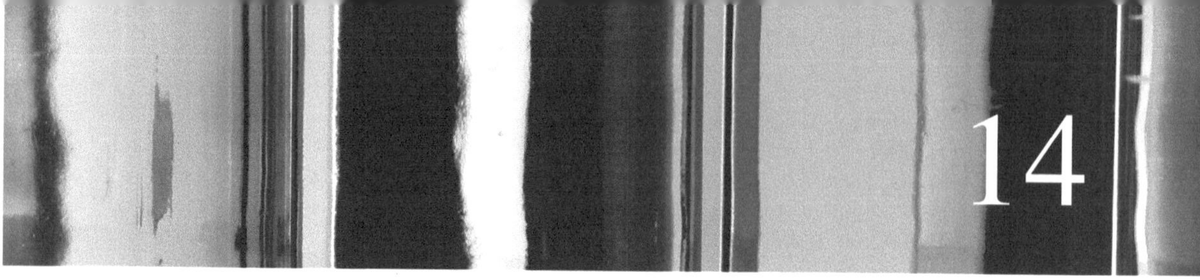

14

Bridging Harm Reduction and Recovery

Heino Stöver

INTRODUCTION

Harm reduction (HR) has become an acknowledged and central principle in drug policy and drug services. Focusing first on illicit drugs, nowadays it has also been expanded to include work with users of alcohol, tobacco, etc. It has become part of public health strategies to reduce the adverse effects of certain behaviours: The definition of harm reduction by the International Harm Reduction Association[1] also includes legal drugs: '"Harm Reduction" refers to policies, programmes and practices that aim primarily to reduce the adverse health, social and economic consequences of the use of legal and illegal psychoactive drugs without necessarily reducing drug consumption. Harm reduction benefits people who use drugs, their families and the community' (IHRA 2010). Harm reduction is a strategy that is:

- complementary to demand reduction;
- focused on the consequences of certain types of behaviour and not on behaviour as such;
- realistic and pragmatic;
- non-prejudicing, non-judgemental aiming at the reduction of problems.

(see Stornach 2003).

If harm reduction is understood in a broad sense then it is being applied in many ways already: being allowed to use alcohol to a limited extent when driving (0.5 per mille in most European countries), warnings against health damages (on cigarette boxes and bottles containing alcohol) or safety advice regarding potentially risky behaviour in many other areas of everyday life (e.g. use of seat belts, protective road barriers etc.).

In the area of illicit drugs, harm reduction has turned out to be a proven, effective and cost effective (Wilson et al. 2015) key strategy to prevent drug-related overdoses and the transmission of infectious disease and has now become an integral part of health policy (Kimber et al. 2010; Rhodes and Hedrich 2010), as the Global State of Harm Reduction states:

> In the few places where harm reduction has been implemented to sufficient scale and quality, it has had a significant impact in reducing HIV transmission. The core harm reduction package endorsed by the Joint United Nations Programme on HIV/AIDS (UNAIDS), the United Nations Office on Drugs and Crime (UNODC) and the World Health Organization (WHO) is vital for global responses to the epidemic. (IHRA 2015: 10)

However, the harm reduction approach has been, and still is being, controversially discussed and at times stands in opposition to abstinence based treatment measures (Room 2010: 108). Metaphors such as prolongation of dependence, complicity of dependent persons and capitulation before dependence are very popular and widespread. Despite the fact that there is no evidence that HR contributes to the initiation or prolongation of drug use, the HR perspective is controversial (Rhodes and Hedrich 2010).

This chapter will look at relevant debates and discussions on harm reduction including the content, limits and future of this approach. Recently, 'recovery' has been suggested as a new approach, which promises to overcome some of the pitfalls of harm reduction. The chapter will touch briefly on this development and link harm reduction with recovery. Harm reduction can be seen as a first step in a longer process of recovery rather than as an alternative to becoming drug free.

ABSTINENCE AS A TOTALITARIAN CONCEPT

In the field of drug use and drug services, the public, as well as professional debate, has focussed mainly on abstinence as the key element and the ultimate goal. Alcoholics Anonymous (AA) and other self-help organizations adhere strictly to this goal as the one and only. For many alcohol dependent persons this has become the message contributing to their survival and AA has proved to be the most successful self-help group in the world. The demand for abstinence is a clear straightforward message, there is no doubt about it, it is a strategy of 'either – or'. The popular, and for many years also professional, perception of dependence on drugs has been based on the process of 'doing addiction' (Stanton Peele), addiction as a construction of human helplessness and pharmacological super power. The only way to regain personal power was to abstain from the pharmacological dominance of psychotropic substances. Any goal lying in between abstinence and addiction has not been accepted or acknowledged – neither professionally nor in the general population. And this perception of dependence has been implemented in everyday constructions of dependence. Everyone on the street would recommend total abstinence to people dependent on any drug. But moreover, on a professional level it has been incorporated into internationally accepted professional definitions of dependence and classification (ICD-10 and DSM-V).

People becoming sober, people recovered were seen as 'heroes' and evidence of the concept that the only healthy way to deal with drugs is to abstain. Any behaviour in between, any controlled drinking pattern has been seen as leading again, and directly, back into relapse and spoiling the proper goal of abstinence. Consequently, for a long time the goal of 'controlled drinking' as an additional therapeutic goal was discredited as a false and even dangerous message. However, more recent and modern perceptions and understandings of the dynamics of alcohol consumption patterns include the goal of 'controlled drinking', especially for people who were 'problem drinkers' rather than 'dependent drinkers' (Davies et al. 1956; Edwards 1985; Thom 1999). Understanding of alcohol consumption theory generated new ways of measuring alcohol consumption, which resulted in a continuum of no problem to problem to dependent drinking and opened up the possibility of a range of goals. Led by clinical psychologists and others critical of the 'disease' concept and the total abstinence goal, this led to a wider view of what constituted appropriate interventions in the alcohol field (Heather and Robertson 1985).

However, for many years, still evident in the public view and partly embedded even in professional thinking, there is a sort of linearity associated with the perception of dependence – any other goal but abstinence leads more or less directly back into dependence. 'Rock bottom' was seen as the turning point, and partners, families, relatives and also professionals and law enforcement agencies were invited to put pressure on dependent people in order to reach this point by increasing suffering.

Abstinence can be understood as a totalitarian concept, it dominated the whole discussion and practice around dependence and (severe long-term) drug taking for many years. Often the debate about this concept has been led very emotionally and morally. Abstinence orientation is a concept of purity and clarity; it gets spoilt with interim messages and compromises. It includes going for it all or for nothing. However, social-psychologically, this perception of dependence was working successfully and still is quite vivid in our society and might be valid for many people facing severe problems with their drug habits. And indeed, abstinence might be, and is, the survival goal for many people.

However, abstinence as the sole and ultimate goal has been doubted by some professionals and self-help movements since the early eighties of the last century. It was the HIV virus affecting people using opioids intravenously and often sharing needles and other equipment, which greatly changed the standard approach towards drug dependence.

Until the mid-eighties the strategy of 'either quit or die' was a deterrent to many users who may have wanted to access treatment and the drug services were unable to contact those clients who were unable to fulfil the rigid requirements. The appearance of HIV/AIDS in the drug using population changed the situation dramatically: now there was an urgent need to get into contact with opiate users despite their current dependence in order to convey key messages ('safer use' and 'safer sex') and to deliver harm reduction tools (such as needles and syringes, condoms, methadone, etc.) (Stöver and Schäffer 2014).

DEVELOPMENTS IN THE ACCEPTANCE OF HARM REDUCTION STRATEGIES

For the above mentioned reasons, professionals, as well as people in the wider community, mistrusted the necessity of delivering harm reduction measures: fears of prolonging dependency, stabilizing people in their habit, sending the wrong messages and spoiling the ultimate goal. Also harm reduction was, and in parts of the world still is, suspected of triggering people into unhealthy behaviour, for example, drug use or sexual intercourse. The inherent assumption is that delivering realistic, detailed and pragmatic advice and information about safer drug use or safer sex would encourage people to overcome their 'natural' fears more easily and would tempt them to experiment. The condom or the needle/syringe programme would have the inherent power to change people's behaviour. In short, harm reduction was suspected of attracting more, and young and inexperienced people, into an unhealthy life style or habit.

However, there are some developments that contributed to the necessity of differentiation in dealing with drug dependence, drug treatment and working in the huge 'grey' area between abstinence and dependence. Apart from life threatening scenarios such as infectious diseases (HIV/AIDS, hepatitis and other STIs), there was also the necessity of accepting the fact that becoming abstinent might be a very long process for many people, and most people need several attempts to reach this final goal, if they reach it at all. Those not reaching this goal at once, or at all, need support in order to survive, that is, to survive in a healthy and decent way and to the highest attainable degree of quality of life. This means that small steps have a value, not necessarily linked to the ultimate goal – small steps can be acknowledged and seen as a goal by themselves.

Furthermore, societal circumstances have changed quite dramatically over the last 30 years. Differentiations, heterogeneity, pluralisation of living conditions and individualization of life styles have become key drivers of change. 'One size fits all' programmes, messages and advice no longer reach the whole target group. Therefore, the concept of abstinence also has lost much of its monolithic dimension. Control over intoxicant use has become a key area of concern of studies and investigations, which means that the ultimate goal of stopping potentially damaging behaviour altogether is no longer the primary goal, but aiming at users gaining more power and developing more responsibility have become goals either on the way to abstinence or as goals in themselves.

Controlled consumption patterns, intermittent using patterns and harm reduction strategies, now more reflect the differentiated living conditions of people with problematic drug use patterns. In addition, the pluralistic status of modern Western society is mirrored in a differentiation of health behaviour and targets; drug use expresses these developments.

Studies have shown that focusing on abstinence alone with no preventive strategies for lapse and relapse would be too risky (Strang et al. 2008). The WHO (2010) has calculated that approximately 20 per cent of drug-related deaths are caused by forced abstinence in therapeutic institutions or custodial settings. Therefore, additional strategies need to be in place in order to avoid drug-related emergencies.

As with many other areas in health policy, Western democracies are addressed to the 'educated citizen', who is able to make informed choices and personal decisions and choose behavioural patterns that contribute to increased health. The background in health policies is that a learning strategy is much more persuasive and effective than a control strategy to be developed for, and applied by, citizens. This is relevant also for drug users. The success in decreasing incidence rates of HIV-infections is due to the learning achievements of users plus the easy availability of protective materials (condoms, needles and syringes). In most Western European countries, HIV-incidence rates have declined dramatically over the past 20 years. 'In settings where comprehensive harm reduction has been implemented, HIV rates among people who inject drugs are low – in some cases, almost negligible' (Furnish 2015: 4). Instead, HIV is increasing among people who inject drugs (PWID) in countries that do not apply harm reduction strategies (such as Russia; Dutta et al. 2013).

PROBLEMS AND CHALLENGES IN THE IMPLEMENTATION OF HR

Harm reduction strategies are targeting drug users of illicit drugs as well as society at large. This includes the fact that many harm reduction measures are responses to the damages caused by clandestine life style in subcultures and repressive drug policy, rather than caused by the drug of choice itself. Although harm reduction is now part of many national and European drug programmes, it is still far from being introduced in all settings where drug users are living (See Chapter 29, this Handbook).

Opioid substitution treatment

Opioid dependence is recognized by the major global health organisations, including the WHO and UNODC, as a chronic relapsing brain disorder, for which the most effective intervention is opioid maintenance treatment (OMT) combined with psychosocial therapy (WHO 2009). Although this harm reduction oriented treatment approach is generally supported all across Europe, many specific aspects of treatment provision differ across national boundaries (Goulão and Stöver 2012)

For example, variations exist between countries with respect to the level of access to treatment (both in the community and in prisons), medication options available to patients, whether doses of medications are individualized or standardized, whether psychosocial counselling is mandatory or even available, the use of control measures, such as supervised dosing, and the availability of treatment guidelines and physician training. Even the predominant setting of treatment differs between countries, with some (e.g. Greece, Italy, Spain, Portugal, Norway) preferring management in specialist clinics and others (e.g. France) delivering opioid substitution treatment (OST) within the normal primary care setting. Other countries, such as Germany and the UK, have a hybrid model combining primary care and a specialized setting (Duke and Thom 2014).

The implication of such variability in opioid dependence management remains unclear. Previous literature suggests that patient populations in different European countries are relatively similar demographically and that treatment variation is therefore probably due to system-level factors such as treatment goals, policy and structure rather than patient variables. How treatment is structured, organized and delivered may be influenced by political objectives, religious and cultural values, financial considerations, available resources, public attitudes and stigma toward addiction, all of which vary widely across Europe. This variability in treatment approaches distinguishes OST from the treatment of other chronic diseases (e.g. diabetes, hypertension) that typically have a more consistent pattern of treatment delivery (Beccaria et al. 2013).

The European Quality Audit of Opioid Treatment (EQUATOR) analysis (Fischer and Stöver 2012) suggests that current systems of opioid-dependence treatment in Europe may be failing to achieve optimal outcomes in a substantial subset of patients. In general, opioid-dependent patients report high rates of cycles in and out of opioid maintenance treatment (OST), past misuse or diversion of their medication and continued on-top heroin use despite being prescribed OST. Building on evidence from this analysis of variable treatment delivery across Europe, these findings suggest that greater treatment benefits could be achieved by optimizing treatment structures as well as available interventions (Benyamina and Stöver 2012)

Currently, there is a wide range of reasons for users remaining outside treatment, and potentially changing the conditions that patients are required to meet to enter or remain in treatment may improve access. It is important to find ways of making treatment more acceptable to patients and users. Factors that could improve patients' willingness to enter or remain in treatment include reducing the preconditions of treatment (e.g. relaxing dose supervision or urine-testing requirements). It is important to note that supervised dosing can play a role in ensuring the safety of treatment, especially during the early stages of therapy. However, once feasible, unsupervised dosing is likely to maximize the chances of recovery, as individuals who need to attend fewer clinic appointments may be able to return to a more normal life and potentially be able to work. Unsupervised dosing is also less costly than supervised dosing, which may be important in those countries suffering budgetary pressures. Thus, strategies are needed that correctly balance the need for supervision without overly restricting patient access and retention. Where available, abuse-deterrent formulations of OST medications can be used to minimize the likelihood of misuse and minimize the need for supervision. For example, in the case of methadone, most practitioners consider that, to limit abuse, it is best to use diluted liquid solutions rather than methadone tablets because the former are less readily abused. In the case of buprenorphine, using the abuse-deterrent formulation containing naloxone can reduce the likelihood of parenteral misuse. Even though the buprenorphine-naloxone combination is the preferred formulation in some clinical guidelines (e.g. in Denmark and the US), many countries continue to favour the use of mono-buprenorphine, most probably because it is generic. Providing the safest treatment options in a GP-based setting may offer a better balance between an open-access, less stigmatized environment, while managing concerns about diversion and misuse, thus potentially improving patients' willingness to enter and remain in treatment. What is certain is that delivering all treatments in exactly the same way, in exactly the same settings, does not take advantage of the inherent advantages of certain medication formulations over others; neither does it take into account that some treatment options may be more suitable than others for particular patients or patients at particular stages of their opioid-dependence.

Evidence from long-term studies of heroin users indicates that opioid dependence is a chronic relapsing condition (Office of National Drug Control Policy 2012). Thus, many patients may cycle between treatment and relapse. A key aim in the treatment of opioid dependence is to maximize treatment retention, thus potentially maximizing long-term remission or recovery. Paradoxically, patient satisfaction with current OST medication was found to be high in this study, suggesting that dissatisfaction with treatment is unlikely to be the driver for patients cycling between treatment and relapse. Based on the variable rates of prior OMT per country, a more likely explanation is that entry into, or retention within, treatment is influenced by the different way in which medications are used and the different treatment structures that apply in each country (Dale-Perera et al. 2012).

The aspirations of patients entering treatment are to either stabilize or stop their drug use, to enter a path towards a 'normal' life. Although treatment can offer this potential, many patients are failing to achieve some of the most basic goals of treatment. For example, a substantial proportion of patients continue to use illicit drugs on top of, and/or misuse, their OST medication. As shown in the current analysis (Benyamina and Stöver 2012), patients appear to be uninformed of their OST options, which may reduce the likelihood of success of each new treatment episode. Patients seem to be consulting their uninformed peers rather than healthcare professionals for information on OST options, and communication between patients and physicians about treatment choices may be suboptimal. In addition, aspects of treatment delivery, such as the level of supervised dosing and the stigma of regularly attending a specialist clinic, may be a barrier to entering or remaining in treatment. These findings suggest that healthcare professionals and policymakers should review whether their current treatment system is delivering the desired outcomes for patients and public health (Benyamina and Stöver 2012).

Needle and syringe programmes

Over the last 30 years, many programmes have been implemented worldwide in order to facilitate the access of intravenous drug users to sterile injection equipment. Data have shown the positive effects of contributing substantially to the drop in new HIV cases. However, there is still a huge gap geographically between high and middle/low income countries. In high income countries, there is almost a 24 hour, seven-day a week accessibility to clean injection equipment via free available automats (such as Germany, where in more than 120 cities, there are 180 automats delivering approximately half a million packages with several syringes and needles each), whereas in other parts of the world, needles are only accessible via pharmacies – if at all. The needle has become the major symbol for harm reduction. Historically, at the beginning of the eighties, the needle became the symbol of health damage and social ruin. Handing out syringes was interpreted as contributing to the stabilization of addiction. However, the learning process in the media, and also in the general population, was that other unintended damages could be successfully avoided, and that if clean needles were not available, PWID would have been put at great risk to themselves, partners and friends.

Prison-based needle and syringe programmes

People in prisons are disproportionally affected by drug dependence, blood-borne-virus-infections (e.g. HIV, HBV/HCV, STIs) and other diseases (e.g. mental health problems and alcohol misuse) as compared to the population outside of prison. Risk behaviour (such as sharing drugs/syringes or unprotected sexual contacts) before and during imprisonment are increasing threats to their health status and a challenge for public health in general. Despite the research evidence demonstrating the need and effectiveness of harm reduction programmes in prisons (UNODC 2015), and the multiple international guidelines recommending their implementation, politicians, prison staff and professionals in many countries are still resistant to implementing these essential public health measures. The implementation of harm reduction measures, such as needle/syringe exchange, condom distribution and OST in prison, lags far behind the availability and accessibility of these interventions outside of prisons (See Chapter 29, this Handbook).

While community-based needle and syringe programmes (NSP) have been implemented in 82 countries (Mathers et al. 2010), in 2013, only eight countries around the world reported having NSP in prisons. The first prison needle and syringe programme (PNSP) was established in Switzerland in 1992; 25 years later, despite the evidence (Stöver and Nelles 2003) of their feasibility, PNSP have been established in only nine countries, often on a pilot basis for a limited time and in a limited number of prisons.

The history of PNSPs demonstrates that needle exchange projects can be successfully implemented in jurisdictions that are relatively well resourced and financed (Switzerland, Germany, Spain), as well as in countries in economic transition that operate with significantly less funding and infrastructural supports (Moldova, Kyrgyzstan). Successful programmes took into account not only institutional size, security level or structure of the particular prison in which a programme was started, but also the needs of the prisoner population. Once transmission risks have been recognized as a severe threat to the health of prisoners, staff, families and partners by the representatives of the penitentiary system, prisons have shown flexibility and creativity by designing and implementing a PNSP adapted to the needs of the particular population and institutional set-up in an institution (UNODC et al. 2012).

Prevention of overdose-related deaths (including provision of naloxone take home)

Overdose is the leading cause of death among (injecting) drug users. Overall, the number of overdose deaths has declined in Europe in recent years; however, some countries still report an increase. Regarding the rate of drug-induced deaths per million populations, exceptionally high levels are found in Estonia and to a lesser extent in Norway, whereas all south European countries show rates below the EU average (13 deaths/million population). Men account for the vast majority of drug-induced deaths in all countries equally (Teles et al. 2014).

Opioids, especially heroin, are the most common drugs implicated in overdose death, accounting for three quarters of drug-induced deaths in Europe. In some countries, opioids are involved in more than 90 per cent of overdose deaths, whereas in a few countries less than half of drug-induced deaths are related to opioid use. Other non-opioid substances that are commonly involved in overdose are cocaine, amphetamines, benzodiazepines and to some extent new psychoactive substances (Teles et al. 2014).

The prevalence of HIV and AIDS among injecting drug users in Europe has decreased significantly during the 2000s. It has been suggested (Teles et al. 2014) that this decline, on the one hand, is largely attributable to the increased availability of prevention, treatment and harm reduction services, and on the other hand, associated with the decrease in injecting drug use in recent years. Nonetheless, compared to 2010, more new HIV cases were reported in 2011, thus indicating an increase after years of decline. Rising numbers of HIV-positive injecting drug users are especially seen in Greece and Romania, but some other countries, located in eastern and south Europe, have also experienced a rise in HIV infections in recent years. Estonia, the country with the highest rate of drug-induced death is also top of the list when it comes to the rate of newly diagnosed drug-related HIV infections, followed by Latvia and Lithuania. Furthermore, Latvia and Estonia are the countries with the highest incidence of AIDS among injecting drug users (Teles et al. 2014: 38).

The differences between the countries regarding the prevalence of HIV and AIDS and the extent to which the virus affects injecting drug users can be largely attributed to the variation and discrepancy in harm reduction measures. On the one hand, implementation of harm reduction responses very early in the HIV epidemic (in countries such as the Netherlands or the United Kingdom) seems to have led to a stable and relatively low national HIV and AIDS prevalence among drug injectors. On the other hand, in countries where harm reduction responses were implemented later in the HIV epidemic (e.g. in Spain or Portugal), and thus at a time when a large proportion of drug injectors was already infected, are still high, though decreasing prevalence rates are found. In contrast, several eastern European countries, where harm reduction services are very limited or not available are seeing growing numbers of HIV and AIDS cases.

Levels of viral hepatitis, especially hepatitis C, remain disproportionately high among injecting drug users in Europe, with some countries reporting a prevalence rate of more than 60 per cent. While data suggest a downward trend in HCV infections in some countries, other nations still see an increase. This seems to be especially true for younger drug injectors. Other infectious or non-infectious diseases, as well as other causes of deaths (trauma, suicide etc.), also appear to play a significant role in mortality related to drug use, although systematically collected data is rarely available. The data presented results from a European inquiry on models of preventing avoidable deaths: *Essentials and Recommendations on Opioid Overdose* (Teles et al. 2014).

In order to further investigate and understand the mechanisms behind drug related mortality, especially with regards to the remaining high death rates among illicit drug users in Europe, more detailed, systematic and comparable research is needed. This especially applies to a more sufficient and regular data collection in European countries, which would not only contribute to an improved understanding and clearer picture of the phenomenon but would also facilitate a trend analysis in a more efficient, timely manner.

As a non-selective opioid antagonist, naloxone is an effective antidote for opioid overdose that rapidly reverses the opioid effects, such as respiratory depression.

The objective of naloxone administration is to restore normal spontaneous breathing but not necessarily fulfil arousal (McDonald and Strang 2015). Currently, there is no recent evidence of serious adverse effects caused by this substance and its utilization is satisfactorily safe. It is not possible to overdose with naloxone and no pharmacological effect exists in the absence of opioids. Thus, the benefits of using naloxone surpass the eventual minor existing risks (e.g. allergic reactions; Bazazi et al. 2010). Naloxone efficacy and relevance is recognized by its inclusion on the WHO's Model List of Essential Medicines.

Once this substance has a quick effect on opioid inhibition, the induction of severe withdrawal symptoms after its administration in an overdose situation can take place. There are reports that evidence the fear of withdrawal symptoms as one of the potential obstacles to PUD use of naloxone if drug users possess it (Worthington et al. 2006). Also, as naloxone has a short half-life (about 30 to 90 minutes), while the majority of opioids have a longer one, it is possible to see a return of overdose symptoms, and the administration of a second antagonist dose can be required in those cases. The return to a new life-threatening overdose after naloxone wears off seems to be a rare situation, even if some degree of intoxication can occur again (Vilke et al. 2003). Naloxone's profile in terms of short lasting effect has been used several times by laypersons as an argument against the use of this substance for overdose reversal. Although it is stressed that, similar to procedures occasionally performed by emergency personnel, if the layperson possesses a second dose of naloxone, it can be applied, if needed (Strang et al. 2013). Also, if preconceptions regarding naloxone's profile are impeding its distribution, there is the suggestion that alternative substances with a longer-acting opiate antagonist, such as Nalmefene, can be considered in its place (Strang et al. 2013). In fact, there are still today, passionate debates regarding the effective use of naloxone for reversing overdose, that is, without the re-occurrence of overdose symptoms and without the induction of, and hard to tolerate, withdrawal symptoms (that can potentially lead the person to use drugs again). Among the practical concerns, there is a problem in evaluating if the administration of naloxone in two separate doses is a good option for managing an overdose situation. In fact, this is a question even more pertinent when we talk about overdoses with long-acting opioids (e.g. methadone), that are more challenging to manage and may require repeated administrations of naloxone (UNODC 2013). In any case, implementing monitoring practices by medical staff after naloxone administration and overdose reversal is fundamental, the current suggestion being that there should be periods of observation after naloxone administration, which must be extended in cases where long-acting opioids are involved.

Currently, in most European countries, naloxone administration is still permitted exclusively by medical staff, and at the same time, its access depends on medical prescription. In the UK, naloxone was legally approved in 2005 to be administered by anyone with the purpose of saving a life. The restricted access to naloxone is currently a great obstacle that legally impedes non-medical services that are in a great position to respond to overdose situations (e.g. outreach teams) by possessing a store of naloxone and using it in emergency situations. To overcome the legal constrains, in some US states (e.g. Massachusetts), a prescription model of 'standing order' is being used, allowing trained non-medical staff to distribute naloxone without the provider's presence. Current prescription practices also constrain the wider provision of naloxone to drug users and/or family/network, despite the recognition of this approach's great potential for reducing drug-induced deaths.

Presently, across Europe, only seven countries have initiatives of peer to peer/take home naloxone distribution – Denmark,

Germany, Italy, Romania, UK, and more recently, Estonia and Norway (this last with nasal naloxone) (even though the overdose prevention programmes that include the distribution of naloxone date back to the 90s). But, with the exception of the UK case (more precisely Scotland and Wales, where large distribution of naloxone is done by specialized drug services), national programmes are not implemented, and distribution is made on a small/moderate scale. An exception in terms of prescription requirements of naloxone kits comes from Italy, were the substance is distributed over the counter in pharmacies (although, few data are available about the extent to which this is routinely done).

Arguments frequently put forward for circumscribing the power of naloxone administration by medical staff include the probability that the layperson may not apply the intervention appropriately, may perform non-sterile administration, may provoke damages associated with injection (if administered by this route) and may face ethical issues regarding medication administration to persons unable to give consent (and without professional regulation). Many of these questions can be responded to by the provision of naloxone that is administered intramuscularly and the delivery of emergency doses in pre-filled syringes (Strang et al. 2013). Pre-filled syringes with naloxone are licenced in some contexts (e.g. recently approved in UK) making it possible to solve potential insufficient interventions, but it continues to be an unlicensed medical product in other countries, even in the ones that provide take home naloxone (e.g. Estonia). Although naloxone is manufactured in several different administration formulations, such as intramuscular, intravenous, subcutaneous and most recently, intranasal, the first one, besides being easy to administer, may be more suitable for drug users as it provides a slower onset and an extended effect, possibly minimizing withdrawal symptoms. In the last few years, the intranasal modality has also received a lot of attention, as it can be seen as a more user-friendly option (including by non-drug users and family member for whom injection can be scary). In some countries, the intranasal option is already listed as an essential medicine, but its use, as a substitute for the intramuscular one, is not currently consensual because more studies are needed to evaluate its effectiveness. Furthermore, taking into account the differences in prices between both (intramuscular being cheaper), cost-effective comparisons are needed in order to assess the advantages of making the intranasal modality available.

Additional issues that arise regarding the wider distribution of naloxone for drug users and their families/network concern the possible use of this antagonist as a 'safety net' (i.e. a security for consuming more or taking more risks). The few studies dedicated to understanding to what extent this is a real risk, found that only a residual percentage of drug users affirm that they would consume more if they possess naloxone (6 per cent; Strang et al. 1996). Moreover, a small scale study showed a decrease in heroin use following overdose prevention training with naloxone distribution (Seal et al. 2005). Other arguments stress that if the drug user possesses naloxone, there is a risk that calling emergency services in an overdose situation becomes a second line intervention, contributing both to failure to avoid drug-induced deaths and to drug users' detachment from health services. Although evidence shows that drug users see naloxone administration as the second action to take after calling emergency services and do not perceive the first action as a substitute for the second (Lagu et al. 2006). In fact, many of the arguments used against naloxone administration by non-medical personnel and distribution to drug users do not find support in the literature. In addition to myths linked to this issue, political concerns can also lie behind some of those arguments, especially in countries with prohibitionist approaches to drug consumption, as there is a misgiving that supporting this harm reduction measure can mistakenly be viewed as synonymous with drug use connivance.

What can be concluded at this point, is that although naloxone is recognized as a highly effective and safe intervention in opioid overdose, its availability continues to be strongly constrained and community-based interventions (e.g. peer distribution, family provision) still raises resistance and faces practical challenges. Thus, making naloxone available, not only in an enlarged number and type of services, but mostly in homes and in the pockets of drug users and their families/network is the goal of the extensive advocacy movements that, in line with scientific evidence, state that this is a necessary measure to finding a practical solution to overdose deaths. Also, and although we cannot attribute a price to a life, the cost-effectiveness is politically relevant and evidence shows that naloxone distribution to drug users is likely to be cost-effective (Coffin and Sullivan 2013). 'In some countries, legislative reform may be needed to allow the low-threshold provision of naloxone, but the measure is regarded as a low-cost approach that can empower healthcare workers and people who use drugs to save lives' (EMCDDA 2013. In addition, naloxone market issues, related to supply and demand that can influence naloxone costs and, consequently, its access, must be discussed more seriously between governments and pharmaceutical companies. Fluctuations in prices are visible across different countries around the globe, frequently influenced by the different political positioning around naloxone.

In the UN resolution for promoting measures to prevent drug overdose, in particular opioid overdose (resolution 55/7, 2012), we can read that it is necessary to 'understanding that opioid overdose treatment, including the provision of opioid receptor antagonists such as naloxone, is part of a comprehensive approach to services for drug users and can reverse the effects of opioids and prevent mortality', and taking this in consideration, member states should 'include effective elements for the prevention and treatment of drug overdose, in particular opioid overdose, in national drug policies (…) and to share best practices and information on the prevention and treatment of drug overdose, in particular opioid overdose, including the use of opioid receptor antagonists such as naloxone' (UNODC et al. 2012: 2).

Finally, the 2014 WHO Guidelines represent a paradigm shift in the treatment of opioid overdose (WHO 2014). Whereas, historically, naloxone has been administered only by medically trained hospital and ambulance staff, the guidelines place naloxone in the hands of non-medical first responders.

It is important to note that the WHO Guidelines state that take-home naloxone recipients need to be trained in the administration of the antidote. In fact, beyond distribution of naloxone kits, take-home naloxone programs typically cover training in overdose awareness, emergency response (calling an ambulance, correct use of naloxone) and training in recovery position and rescue breathing. Calling an ambulance is a crucial aspect of community-based overdose management: medical supervision following naloxone administration is necessary, as naloxone has a relatively short half-life of 60 to 90 minutes, and overdose victims can dip back into unconsciousness once the antagonist wears off.

Drug consumption rooms

By providing healthcare to drug users while they consume in hygienic and safer conditions, drug consumption rooms (DCR) can potentially perform a double role in overdose prevention, contributing to reduce both occurrences and deaths.

Although a number of facilities provide areas for consumption via several routes (smoked, snorting, free-basing and chasing the dragon),[2] they traditionally target the specific group of those who inject in the streets and face situations of severe marginalization: degraded heath, long-term use, risky patterns of use including poly-drug consumption, detachment from drug services, poor housing and living conditions and lack of a hygienic place for consuming. Obviously, these conditions pose individual and social risk factors for overdose occurrence, and DCR can have a role in responding to them through interventions with immediate, middle and long term outcomes (Hedrich 2004).

In the sphere of preventing overdose occurrence, a long-term impact of these facilities can potentially be obtained by promoting access to a range of protective social, healthcare and drug treatment services. Also, by reducing consumption in open scenes (which besides individuals, benefits communities in health and security issues) and offering a non-judgemental and dignified space for consuming, they can have an effect on reducing the stigma surrounding drug use and overdose. By providing this judgement-free environment to people at risk in the consumption moment, DCRs become favourable settings for delivering training in overdose prevention, recognition and response to their clients and providing naloxone training and kits. This approach can promote the reduction of risky behaviours not only within the facilities, where the overdose risk assessment and tailor-made advice on safer use is delivered by staff, but beyond them, where empowered clients can assess their own risk and act in accordance.

Conversely, DCRs have a role in preventing drug-induced deaths, through providing supervision by socio-medical staff, particularly skilled in safe consumption, capable of recognizing and properly responding to an overdose emergency. If this situation occurs, professionals can offer proper intervention following the first signs, which can not only avoid deaths but can also minimize potential damages/morbidities associated with the episode. If located close to open drug scenarios, they can also be key-resources when overdoses take place in the surrounding territory (Hedrich 2004). An example of this comes from the DAVE's facility, in the surroundings of Madrid, where staff responded to four times as many emergencies in the open drug scene than within the room (Hedrich 2004).

Even if the benefits of DCR in reaching specific groups and reducing morbidity and mortality are largely accepted, currently, it is merely possible to find a classification of this harm reduction response as 'likely to be beneficial', in the EMCDDA best practice portal (updated in 2013). Concerning drug-related deaths, and although there are some favourable results, we face a lack of evidence, at review-level, about the efficacy of DCR with regard to this indicator (Hedrich et al. 2010).

However, research on DCR suffers from several methodological challenges considering the logic of local, micro-environmental and law enforcement interventions (e.g. availability of treatment and harm reduction services; police actions). Causal relationships between DCR interventions and fluctuations in drug-related/induced deaths are hard to establish and the majority of existing studies rely on the record of overdoses occurring within the facilities (lack of conclusive studies at population level). In addition, it is still difficult to comprehend to what extent DCRs can really prevent overdose occurrences.

Presently, it is suggested that a circumstantial risk factor for overdose occurrence is injecting in public places, where the possibility of testing the sample's strength is restricted and the injection is frequently rushed for fear of arrest in countries with more punitive law enforcement policies (Kerr et al. 2006). Furthermore, public injection is more frequent amongst the most vulnerable drug users, namely the homeless, something that combines circumstantial and individual risk factors for overdose. Therefore, 'those who inject in public space are caught in a dilemma – needing both privacy and exposure in the event of an overdose' (Fitzgerald et al. 2004; Dovey et al. 2001: 319). DCRs can be a suitable solution for responding to this dilemma, offering a space where users do not inject alone or accompanied by strangers, and have sufficient time and safety to consume in a less risky way. In fact, it has been shown that DCRs can effectively reach street users at higher risk for overdose, with self-reports and observations reporting a reduced risk for these episodes, especially for those attending the facilities regularly (Hedrich et al. 2010). Rates of emergency in Europe (data from Switzerland, Spain and Germany), that mostly involve heroin overdoses with intravenous consumption, have been shown to be low, varying from 0.5 (minimum in Switzerland) to 3.5 (maximum in Germany); (Hedrich 2004). Besides, the reduced number of overdoses in these facilities, reports from a German study suggest that they tend to be less severe than those happening on the street (Happel and Steinmetz 2001). Also, from the thousands of overdoses occurring in DCRs over time, there are no reports of fatal outcomes (Poschadel et al. 2003; Förster and Stöver 2014), which is particularly noteworthy when weighed up against the thousands of injections in this context. The response to overdose occurrences is not homogeneous among the several facilities, but commonly they provide oxygen and naloxone, administered by trained professionals.

Taking into account this and other suggestions, the implementation of DCR in European countries (especially the ones dealing with intravenous consumption) is now recommended in the most recent guidelines specifically directed to overdose prevention (Frisher and Stöver 2012). However, less than a dozen countries have invested in implementing them. In this field, the creation of supervised structures of consumption with the intention of preventing fatal and non-fatal overdoses along with other harms, started almost 30 years ago in Switzerland. Currently, there are 88 facilities (see Table 14.1), spread mostly through northern Europe (Denmark, Germany, Luxemburg, Netherlands, Norway, Switzerland) and present in Spain and Greece.

They are mostly integrated (i.e. part of a wider network of services: for example, Madrid) and a few specialized (i.e. exclusively consumption room; for example, Frankfurt; Hedrich 2004). The data gathered from each of these experiences are encouraging, suggesting a positive impact in a range of indicators, including in drug-induced deaths. Some examples are in Germany, where no drug-induced deaths have been registered since 1994 in these facilities (Schatz and Nougier 2012); in Switzerland, drug-related deaths (including overdoses) decreased from 353 to 193, although a causal relationship cannot be established with DCR; in Spain, there was a decrease in overdose deaths from 1,833 in 1991 to 773 in 2008 (Schatz and Nougier 2012); in Norway, low emergency (overdose) rates were found and increased access to overdose responses by professionals was reported (Schatz and Nougier 2012); in Luxembourg, reports gave a count of 1,025 overdoses deaths successfully avoided (Skretting and Olsen 2008; Schatz and Nougier 2012); in the Netherlands, a significant shift of consumption route occurred in DCR clients – only 10 per cent used intravenously, which is a risk factor for overdose (Havinga and Van Der Poel 2011, as cited in Schatz and Nougier 2012); and in Denmark, although a good situation assessment is not currently available, it is admitted in the 2013 National report that DCR could have made a contribution to the dramatic reduction of drug-induced deaths verified in the country's south region.

Table 14.1 Eighty-eight drug consumption rooms (DCRs) have been set up in Europe (2014)

Country	*No. of DCRs*
Switzerland	13
Netherlands	30
Germany	24
Spain	13
Luxembourg	1
Norway	1
Denmark	5
Greece	1

Source: Stöver and Schäffer (2014).

In the EMCDDA best practice portal, some of the facilities installed in these countries are highlighted for their good practice (e.g. ABRIGADO, Luxembourg).

Although congruent in the positive outcomes reported, practices and policies implemented in these facilities vary between and within countries, facing different challenges according to the national policies. Some of the differences are as follows: in Germany (except in Hamburg) and Luxembourg, where clients in OST are not eligible to use the majority of rooms while in the rest of the countries they are; residency restrictions are imposed in Switzerland, Netherlands, and in some rooms in Germany, but not in Spain; Norway is the only country that simply allows heroin consumption; checks by police in the DCR registration process exist only in the Netherlands; user passes are required in some facilities in each of those countries, with the exception of Spain; no show for several weeks causes pass revocation in the Netherlands; and new or occasional PWID are not admitted in Germany (Hedrich 2004; Schatz and Nougier 2012). In legal terms, some of the countries that introduced DCR, or intend to do so in the future, face the need to adjust specific laws. Namely, they need to decriminalize drug consumption within the rooms and regulate them in cases where their broad drug policies criminalize drugs purchase. This is the case in Germany, Denmark, Luxembourg, Norway and Switzerland. In Germany, for example, DCR clients must possess user cards to avoid prosecution, especially when the facilities are far from drug markets.

In addition to those experiences, several other initiatives for the implementation of DCR were developed across Europe (e.g. Belgium, France, Italy, UK), with no tangible results achieved so far. Portugal, for example, established the legal basis for these facilities in 2001, but only recently a project is being considered with the possibility of being installed in Lisbon. In fact, although some conquests have been made, DCR continues to raise some controversy among countries and public opinion, displaying a range of popular arguments to oppose them: DCR can 'normalize' and validate the use of drugs; new consumers (with no dependence or using another routes of consumption) can be attracted by the good conditions of these places; facilities can become drug trafficking spots; and they can dissuade people from seeking treatment. None of these concerns, however, is sustained by evidence; on the contrary, it refutes them (Hedrich 2004; Hedrich et al. 2010).

Putting this together, the spread and effectiveness of DCR across Europe will depend on the removal of the numerous barriers discussed above. Among them, there is the lack of political will and sustained commitment, manifested in the absence of funding and consecutive rejection of proposals. On the contrary, where DCRs are seen as one piece of the puzzle in the national harm reduction policy and when they are implemented as part of a comprehensive drug policy model, successful evolution of those facilities, as well as the optimization of their outcomes, is expected (Houborg and Frank 2014)

Strategies to shift from intravenous to heroin inhalation use

Intravenous drug use has been predominantly practiced since illegal heroin use became known in Germany in the early 1970s. The available data suggests that the risk of accidental overdose when smoking heroin is substantially reduced compared to injecting a substance of unknown purity and quality. Moreover, the risk of transmitting HIV, Hepatitis B or C via blood contact is considerably reduced when smoking heroin rather than when injecting it intravenously. In spite of the significant strain on the lungs and the respiratory tract caused by smoking, it can be concluded that inhalation use – measured by the indicators 'overdose' and 'viral infections' is considerably less dangerous than intravenous use.

A recent research project ('SMOKE IT!' in Germany) studied to what extent a change of consumption method can be supported by making new equipment for drug use available. Participants in drug consumption rooms received 'SMOKE-IT!' packs that contained new heroin smoking foils, as well as information about inhalation drug use. The vast majority of the 165 respondents favoured using the foils from the 'SMOKE-IT!' packs (82.5 per cent). The survey showed that two-thirds of the sample used the SMOKE-IT foils for inhaling instead of injecting. Almost six out of 10 said that smoking was healthier than injecting; 35 per cent of participants named the reduced risk of a hepatitis or HIV infection as a particularly important factor. A third of the respondents used the smoking foils to avoid the danger of an overdose.

Targeted media and personal intervention in association with the dispensation of attractive drug use equipment can motivate opiate users to change their method of drug use. The main reason for inhalation use is that it is significantly less dangerous, measured by the indicators 'overdose' and 'viral infections'. All drop-in centres should expand their syringe-exchange services to include the dispensation of smoking foils. (Stöver and Schäffer 2014)

There are many more examples of harm reduction strategies in the field of illicit drug use: heroin prescription Verthein et al. 2013, drug checking (developed in Austria,[3] Switzerland, Netherlands, Catalonia, etc.), safer use of crack/cocaine (Krawczyk et al. 2015), cannabis (Hall/Fischer 2010), HCV prevention – a challenge for evidence-based harm reduction (Hickman 2010), new psychoactive substances (Grund et al. 2010), etc. However, the harm reduction method has been expanded to other fields of licit drug use, as well as prevention.

EXPANSION OF HARM REDUCTION STRATEGIES TO OTHER AREAS OF HEALTH

'Harm reduction' has turned out to be an effective and efficient public health strategy that is dealing with pragmatic goals and which accepts the behaviour of individuals without judging it or conveying prejudices which might lead to stigmatizing effects, discrimination and exclusion.

The harm reduction philosophy and strategy have been expanded to other areas of health challenges, such as alcohol consumption, tobacco smoking, overeating, etc. The adoption of harm reduction measures in relation to tobacco began only a few years ago (Gartner et al. 2010), alcohol harm reduction has a long tradition and is a core feature of alcohol policy in many countries (Robson and Marlatt 2006; Herring et al. 2010). The harm reduction approach has also been a leading aspect in the development of public health interventions in relation to cannabis (Hall and Fischer 2010) and recreational and stimulant drug use (Fletcher et al. 2010; Grund et al. 2010). Finally, it had been expanded to the creation of settings, with regards to prisons (Stöver 2015).

HARM REDUCTION A STAND-ALONE OR BRIDGE TO OR PART OF RECOVERY PROGRAMMES?

In the early years of harm reduction, initiatives were implemented as standalone, not connected with abstinence-based drug services at all. In the meantime, this has changed substantially, because drug users in low threshold services, on the one hand, seek more therapeutic support, and on the other hand, the therapeutic institutions have to integrate harm reduction measures such as opioid substitution programmes, naloxone programmes, etc. to avoid adverse effects of their intervention. Therefore, depending on regions and institutions, there are more or less connections between low and high threshold drug services trying to bridge the gap between service levels.

As mentioned earlier, OST has always been a controversial topic. As part of a raft of harm reduction measures to address the HIV crisis, it gained wide support and application and, in some countries, became a key part of treatment responses for drug dependence (Beccaria et al. 2013). However, around the beginning of this century, controversy regarding the evidence for OST as an effective treatment increased, there was an ideological shift away from harm reduction and proponents of abstinence approaches gained a stronger voice in policy discourse. The shift came initially from the USA where a 'recovery advocacy movement' had been gaining ground during the 1990s (White 2007a), which was concerned with recovery from alcohol as well as drug problems. It should be noted that recovery is not a new concept. It has a long history stemming from the nineteenth century temperance and recovery movements (Yates and Malloch 2010). However, according to White (2007a), the new wave of recovery advocacy was a reaction against the perceived professionalization and commercialization of addiction treatment and disengagement from the process of addiction recovery located in grass-roots communities. Linked also to evidence of a process of re-stigmatization and criminalization of AOD problems, White (2007a: 696) argues that

> trends inside the treatment industry and shifts in broad cultural attitudes and social policies set the stage for a new politicized coalition of recovering people and their families and visionary addiction treatment professionals.

The emergence of new grass-roots recovery advocacy organisations, the development of a national network of agencies and recovery projects, provision of 'seed money' for local groups, support for peer based recovery services and financial support from a number of sources underpinned the early evolution of the new movement. Its goals were broad, aiming to counter negative public views of AOD problems, promote laws and social policies to support recovery and improve the quality of services, and, importantly for subsequent debates, 'portray alcoholism and addictions as problems for which there are viable and varied recovery solutions' (White 2007a: 698). At the same time, White (2007b) recognized that the shift towards a recovery paradigm was happening without any clear definition of 'recovery'. Noting that recovery as an organizing concept (for policy and practice) poses financial and ideological threats to existing treatment systems and professional roles, White observed that the growth of recovery institutions, agencies and specialists, setting up in competition with the establishment, posed a threat to the integrity of the movement and highlighted the importance of having a clear definition to guide future development (White 2007b: 230). His proposed definition emphasized the *experience* of recovery and the *process* of recovery:

> Recovery is the experience (a process and a sustained status) through which individuals, families, and communities impacted by severe alcohol and other drug (AOD) problems utilize internal and external resources to voluntarily resolve these problems, heal the wounds inflicted by AOD-related problems, actively manage their continued vulnerability to such problems, and develop a healthy, productive, and meaningful life. (White 2007b: 236)

The drive to build a consensus definition led to the Betty Ford Institute Consensus Panel (2007) that involved a group of researchers, policy makers, clinicians and members of the recovering community: they held a conference to discuss the definition of recovery and how it could be measured. White was a member of the Panel, as well as Dr Thomas McLellan, the Deputy Director of the White House Office of National Drug Control Policy from 2009 to 2010.

They defined recovery as 'a voluntarily maintained lifestyle characterised by sobriety, personal health and citizenship' (Betty Ford Institute Consensus Panel 2007: 222). Sobriety was, therefore, identified as a key issue in recovery.

The process by which the recovery advocacy movement crossed the Atlantic and arrived in the UK is documented by Wardle (2012). Harm reduction, according to Wardle, had undergone a transformation from 'its inception as vigorous, innovative public health model to its mature form as a strategic, top–down tool of risk management and crime reduction' (Wardle 2012: 295). In other words, it had moved away from its earlier grass-roots radical, public health approach towards a pragmatic, stigmatized form of harm reduction that promoted the expansion of methadone maintenance as a treatment to reduce crime. This, and the growing numbers remaining in the services and receiving methadone maintenance over long periods, opened the door to the influence of the American experience. A further influence came from the mental health field. By 2008, recovery had become a key organizing principle underlying mental health services in the UK, Australia, New Zealand and the USA (Shepherd et al. 2008) and had a considerable impact on the *Essential Care* report from the Scottish Advisory Committee on Drug Misuse (SACDM 2008). This report set out the principles of service provision for people with substance use problems but, as in the mental health field, adopted a broad definition of recovery and did not specify any particular outcome goal. Learning from the recovery movement in the United States was spread by key recovery advocates, such as William White, travelling to Britain to help to formulate and broker recovery ideas and support stakeholders involved in the recovery movement. White was hailed as an effective 'policy entrepreneur' (Duke et al. 2013; Duke and Thom 2014), an inspiration for recovery leaders in the UK who, in turn, went on to bring recovery ideals to Australia. This international shift did not take place in other European countries, possibly because other factors were lacking. Taking the UK as an example, along with the challenge to what was seen as an increasingly 'institutionalized' version of harm reduction by around 2005, new research indicated that many drug users said they favoured a drug free treatment goal (McKeganey et al. 2004) and, although the details of the research suggested a more nuanced interpretation, this was used to argue in favour of abstinence by a growing group of stakeholders that included abstinence based therapeutic communities and services. When the media took up the issue, arguing that drug users were failing to exit treatment, a very public debate ensued. An eventual influence on policy was manifest in a shift towards accepting the language of recovery and in government action to carve agreement between the opposing parties by setting up an expert working group that included stakeholders from a range of different professional backgrounds and ideological positions. The report from the expert group supported the continuing use of methadone as a treatment approach, as part of a full range of interventions within a recovery-orientated treatment system (Duke et al. 2013). The established harm reduction approach remains in place; however, there is no doubt that both from a policy and a practice point of view, the concept and language of 'recovery' has become established and has had an impact on approaches to commissioning and planning of drug treatment services in the UK.

The recovery movement as it has emerged and grown over the last few years, has posed a challenge to the established harm reduction movement and to the evidence that has underpinned policy and practice based on harm reduction principles. The debates have revealed deep-seated and long-standing ideological differences and competition for resources and support in the treatment field. While the new recovery movement aims to bring back grass-roots involvement, White

(2007a: 230) argues that there are innumerable threats to the promises of the recovery paradigm.

Recovery as an organizing concept poses financial and ideological threats to existing social institutions and professional roles that have been granted cultural authority to manage AOD problems. The recovery paradigm is spawning alternative institutions (e.g. recovery advocacy organizations, peer-based recovery support centres) and roles (e.g. recovery coaches, personal recovery assistants, recovery support specialists) that are challenging treatment institutions and competing with them for status and financial resources. Through this process, the recovery concept risks reification, commodification, commercialization and overextension.

CONCLUDING REMARKS

More than 30 years ago, the concept of harm reduction was developed as a counter concept against the dominance of solely abstinence-oriented drug services and drug policies. It has been developed since then and shown its impact on public health, especially in the early years in the field of illicit drug use. The successes of harm reduction strategies have led to a wide acceptance and acknowledgement and finally integration into European, Australian and Canadian drug strategies and action plans.

Harm reduction has undergone a huge process of transformation from an innovative public health model to its mature form as a strategic, top–down tool of risk management (and crime reduction). However, the expansion of the harm reduction philosophy and methods into other areas of public health and drug services/policies (alcohol, tobacco, etc.) needs to be discussed. Partly because the same controversies show up as in earlier times with opioid users and the needle exchange programmes. However, examples mentioned here (e.g. alcohol, tobacco, e-cigarettes (Stimson, Thom, Costall et al. 2014) and cannabis indicate that harm reduction is a promising approach to add to existing strategies in coping with dependencies. Harm reduction is supposed to be a valuable approach in itself, but needs more connection and interaction with abstinence-based drug services in order to identify and strengthen pathways of recovery.

The established harm reduction approaches remain in place; however, from both ends – abstinence and harm reduction – a better and deeper sustainable cooperation and alignments of concepts is needed in order to enhance the chances of stabilization and recovery.

NOTES

1 Now called Harm Reduction International (HRI).
2 Luxembourg, counting with a 'blow room' functioning as a pilot project; Netherlands, taking into account that 90 per cent of the clients consume by this route; Spain; Switzerland, Germany and Denmark (Schatz and Nougier 2012; Schäffer and Stöver 2014).
3 www.checkyourdrugs.at/aktuelles/ (accessed 8 August 2015).

REFERENCES

Bazazi, A. R., Zaller, N. D., Fu, J. F. and Rich, J. D. (2010). Preventing opiate overdose deaths: Examining objections to take-home naloxone. *Journal of Health Care for the Poor and Underserved*, 21(4): 1108–13.

Beccaria, F., Einstein, S. and Thom, B. (eds) (2013). Stakeholders in substitution treatment in six European countries. *Substance Use and Misuse* (special issue), 48 (11).

Benyamina, A. and Stöver, H. (2012). Barriers to treatment access and informed patient choice in the treatment of opioid dependence in Europe. *Heroin Addiction and Related Clinical Problems*, 14 (4): 65–80.

Betty Ford Institute Consensus Panel (2007). What is recovery? A working definition from the Betty Ford Institute. *Journal of Substance Abuse Treatment*, 33: 221–8.

Coffin, P. O. and Sullivan, S. D. (2013). Cost-effectiveness of distributing naloxone to heroin users for lay overdose reversal. *Annals of Internal Medicine*, 158(1) : 1–9.

Dale-Perera, A., Goulão, J. and Stöver, H. (2012). Quality of care provided to patients receiving opioid maintenance treatment in europe: results from the EQUATOR survey. *Heroin Addiction and Related Clinical Problems* 14(4) : 23–38.

Dovey, K., Fitzgerald, J. and Choi, Y. (2001). Safety becomes danger: dilemmas of druguse in public space. *Health and Place*, 7: 319–31.

Davies, D. L., Shepherd, M. and Myers, E. (1956). The two years prognosis of 50 alcohol addicts after treatment in hospital. *Quarterly Journal of Studies on Alcohol*, 17: 485–502.

Duke, K., Herring, R., Thickett, A. and Thom, B. (2013). Substitute prescribing in the era of 'recovery': an analysis of stakeholder roles and policy windows in Britain. *Substance Use and Misuse*, 48 (11): 966–76.

Duke, K. and Thom, B. (2014). The role of evidence and the expert in contemporary processes of governance: the case of opioid substitution treatment policy in England. *International Journal of Drug Policy*, 25: 964–71.

Dutta, A., Wirtz, A., Stanciole, A., Oelrichs, R., Semini, I., Baral, St., Pretorius, C., Haworth, C., Hader, S., Beyrer, C. and Cleghorn, F. (2013). *The Global HIV Epidemics Among People Who Inject Drugs*. Washington, DC: The World Bank.

EMCDDA.(2013): Annual Drug Report

Edwards G. (1985). Paradigm shift or change in ownership? The conceptual significance of D.L. Davie's classic paper. *Drug and Alcohol Dependence*, 15: 19–35.

Fischer, G. and Stöver, H. (2012). Assessing the current state of opioid-dependence treatment across Europe: methodology of the European Quality Audit of Opioid Treatment (EQUATOR) project. *Heroin Addiction and Related Clinical Problems*, 14(3): 5–70.

Fitzgerald, J., Dovey, K, Dietze, P., Rumbold, G. (2004): Health outcomes and quasi-supervised settings for street injecting drug use. *International Journal of Drug Policy,* 15 (4): 247–257

Fletcher, A. Calafat, A., Pirona A., and Olszewski, D., (2010). Young people, recreational drug use and harm reduction 357. Harm reduction: evidence, impacts and challenges. EMCDDA Monograph, Lisbon/Portugal

Förster, St. and Stöver, H. (2014). *Auswertung der Frankfurter Konsumraumdokumentation, 1. Halbjahr 2013. Dokumentationszeitraum 01.01. – 30.06.2013*. Kurzbericht. Frankfurt am Main: ISFF. Available from http://www.frankfurt-university.de/fachbereiche/fb4/forschung/forschungsinstitute/isff/forschungsprojekte/dokumentation-drogenkonsumraeume.html (accessed 30 November 2015).

Furnish, D. (2015): Foreword. In: The Global State of Harm Reduction 2014 http://www.ihra.net/files/2015/02/16/GSHR2014.pdf (accessed 08 May 2016)

Gartner, C. Hall, W. (2010). Harm reduction policies for tobacco users. International Journal of Drug Policy. March 2010 Volume 21, Issue 2, Pages 129–130. DOI: http://dx.doi.org/10.1016/j.drugpo.2009.10.008.

Goulão, J., Stöver, H. (2012). The profile of patients, out-of-treatment users and treating physicians involved in opioid maintenance treatment in Europe. *Heroin Addiction and Related Clinical Problems*, 14(4): 7–22.

Grund, J. P., Coffin, P., Jauffret-Roustide, M., Dijkstra, M., de Bruin, D. and Blanken, P. (2010). The fast and the furious – cocaine, amphetamines and harm reduction In T. Rhodes and D. Hedrich (eds), *EMCDDA Monographs: Harm Reduction: Evidence, Impacts and Challenges*. Lisbon: European Monitoring Centre for Drugs and Drug Addiction, pp. 191–234.

Hall, W.; Fischer (2010). Harm reduction policies for cannabis. Harm reduction: evidence, impacts and challenges. EMCDDA Monograph,

Happel, H. V. and Steinmetz, J. (2001). Überdosierungen im Konsumraum. In akzept e. V. *Gesellschaft mit Drogen - akzeptanz im Wandel*. Münster: Kongreßbericht Berlin.

Hedrich, D., Kerr, T. and Dubois-Arber, F. (2010). Drug consumption facilities in Europe and beyond. In T. Rhodes and D. Hedrich (eds), *EMCDDA Monographs: Harm Reduction: Evidence, Impacts and Challenges*. Lisbon: European Monitoring Centre for Drugs and Drug Addiction, pp. 305–32.

Herring R., Thom B., Beccaria, F., Kolind, T. and Moskalewicz, J. (2010). Alcohol harm reduction in Europe. In T. Rhodes and D. Hedrich (eds), *EMCDDA Monographs: Harm Reduction: Evidence, Impacts and Challenges*. Lisbon: European Monitoring Centre for Drugs and Drug Addiction, pp. 275–304.

Hickmann, M. (2010). HCV prevention — a challenge for evidence-based harm reduction. Harm reduction: evidence, impacts and challenges. EMCDDA Monograph.

Houborg, E. and Frank, V.A. (2014). Drug consumption rooms and the role of politics and governance in policy processes. *International Journal of Drug Policy*, 25(5): 972–7.

International Harm Reduction Association (IHRA) (2010). *What is Harm Reduction?* Available from: http://www.ihra.net/what-is-harm-reduction.

International Harm Reduction Association (IHRA) (2015). *Global State of Harm Reduction Report*. Available from: http://www.ihra.net/global-state-of-harm-reduction.

Heather N. and Robertson I. (1985). *Problem Drinking: The New Approach*. Harmondsworth Penguin Books.

Hedrich, D. (2004). *European Report on Drug Consumption Rooms*. Lisbon: European Monitoring Centre for Drugs and Drug Addiction.

Kimber, J., Palmateer, N., Hutchinson, S., Hickman, M., Goldberg, D. and Rhodes, T. (2010). Harm reduction among injecting drug users – evidence of effectiveness. In T. Rhodes and D. Hedrich (eds), *EMCDDA Monographs: Harm Reduction: Evidence, Impacts and Challenges*. Lisbon: European Monitoring Centre for Drugs and Drug Addiction, pp. 115–64.

Kerr, T., Small, D., Moore, D. and Wood, E. (2006). *Insight into Insite*. Supervised Injecting/Insite. Available from: http://uhri.cfenet.ubc.ca/content/view/57/92/.

Krawczyk, N., Linhares, C., Filho, V. and Bastos, F.I. (2015). The interplay between drug-use behaviors, settings, and access to care - a qualitative study exploring attitudes and experiences of crack cocaine users in Rio de Janeiro and São Paulo, Brazil. *Harm Reduction Journal*, 12: 24.

Lagu, T., Anderson, B. J. and Stein, M. (2006). Overdoses among friends: drug users are willing to administer naloxone to others. *Journal of Substance Abuse Treatment*, 30(2): 129–33.

Mathers, B., Degenhardt, L., Ali, R., Wiessing, L., Hickman, M., Mattick, R. P., Myers, B., Ambekar, A. and Strathdee, S. A. (2010). HIV prevention, treatment and care for people who inject drugs: a systematic review of global, regional and national coverage. *Lancet*, 375(9719): 1014–28.

McDonald, R. and Strang, J. (2015). Saving lives with pre-supply of naloxone – from concept to coordinated care. In: A. Dichtl and H. Stöver (eds), *Naloxon – Überlebenshilfe im Drogennotfall*. Frankfurt: Fachhochschulverlag, p. 9.

McKeganey, N. P., Morris, Z., Neale, J. and Robertson, M. (2004). What are drug users looking for when they contact drug services: abstinence or harm reduction. Drugs: *Education, Prevention and Policy*, 11(5): 423–35.

Office of National Drug Control Policy (2012). *Medication-Assisted Treatment for Opioid Addiction. Healthcare Brief. Office of National Drug Control Policy Executive Office of the President*. www.WhiteHouse.gov/ONDCP.

Poschadel, S., Höger, R., Schnitzler, J. and Schreckenberg, D. (2003). *Evaluation der Arbeit der Drogenkonsumräume in der Bundesrepublik Deutschland. Schriftenreihe des Bundesministeriums für Gesundheit und Soziale Sicherheit*. Bd. 149. Baden-Baden: Nomos.

Rhodes, T. and Hedrich, D. (eds) (2010). Harm reduction among injecting drug users – evidence of effectiveness. In T. Rhodes and D. Hedrich (eds), *EMCDDA Monographs: Harm Reduction: Evidence, Impacts and Challenges*. Lisbon: European Monitoring Centre for Drugs and Drug Addiction, pp. 115–64

Robson, G.; Marlatt, G.A. (2006). Harm reduction and alcohol policy. International Journal of Drug Policy July 2006 Volume 17, Issue 4, p 255–376 Harm reduction and its application to alcohol policy Edited by Godfrey Robson, Alan Marlatt

Room, R. (2010). The ambiguity of harm reduction – goal or means, and what constitutes harm? In T. Rhodes and D. Hedrich (eds), *EMCDDA Monographs: Harm Reduction: Evidence, Impacts and Challenges*. Lisbon:

European Monitoring Centre for Drugs and Drug Addiction, pp. 108–14.

Schatz, E. and Nougier, M. (2012). *IDPC Briefing Paper - Drug Consumption Rooms: Evidence and Practice*. Available from: http://dx.doi.org/10.2139/ssrn.2184810.

Schäffer, D. and Stöver, H. (2014). *Drug Consumption Rooms in Europe: Models, Best Practice and Challenges*. Available from: http://bdoc.ofdt.fr/index.php?lvl=notice_display&id=75084.

Scottish Advisory Committee on Drugs Misuse (SACDM) (2008). *Essential Care. A Report on the Approach Required to Maximise Opportunity for Recovery from Problem Substance Use in Scotland*. Edinburgh: Scottish Advisory Committee on Drugs Misuse.

Shepherd, G., Boardman, J. and Slade, M. (2008). *Making Recovery a Reality Policy Paper*. London: Sainsbury Centre for Mental Health.

Stimson G.V., Thom B. and Costall P. (2014). Disruptive innovations: the rise of the electronic cigarette. *The International Journal of Drug Policy*, 25(4): 653–5.

Stöver, H. and Schäffer, D. (2014): SMOKE IT! Promoting a change of opiate consumption pattern – from injecting to inhaling. *Harm Reduction Journal*, 11: 18.

Stornach, B. (2003). Alcohol and harm reduction. In E Buning, M Gorgulho, A. G. Melcop and P. O'Hare (eds), *Alcohol and Harm Reduction. An Innovative Approach for Countries in Transition*. Amsterdam: International Coalition on Alcohol and Harm Reduction, pp. 27–33.

Seal, K. H., Thawley, R., Gee, L., Bamberger, J., Kral, A. J., Ciccarone, D. and Edlin, B. R. (2005). Naloxone distribution and cardiopulmonary resuscitation training for injection drug users to prevent heroin overdose death: a pilot intervention study. *Journal of Urban Health*, 82 (2): 303–11.

Stöver, H. and Nelles, J. (2003). Ten years of experience with needle and syringe exchange programmes in European Prisons. *International Journal of Drug Policy*, 14(5–6): 437–44.

Stöver, H. (2015). *Global Overview of the Transfer of Harm Reduction into Prisons. Drug Users in Prison: Interventions to Reduce Harm and Enable Recovery. Presentation First European Conference on Addictive Behaviours and Dependencies*. Lisbon/Portugal, 24 September 2015.

Strang, J., Darke, S., Hall, W., Farrell, M. and Ali, R. (1996). Heroin overdose: the case for take-home naloxone. *British Medical Journal*, 312(7044): 1435–6.

Strang, J., Manning, V., Mayet, S., Best, D., Titherington, E., Santana, L. and Semmler, C. (2008). Overdose training and take-home naloxone for opiate users: Prospective cohort study of impact on knowledge and attitudes and subsequent management of overdoses. *Addiction*, 103(10): 1648–57.

Strang, J., Bird, S. M. and Parmar, M. K. B. (2013). Take-home emergency naloxone to prevent heroin overdose deaths after prison release: rationale and practicalities for the N-ALIVE randomized trial. *Journal of Urban Health*, 90(5): 983–96.

Teles, S., Moura, H., Pinto, M., Oliveira, J. M., Rodrigues, C., Bernard, C. and Stöver, H. (2014). *Preventing Avoidable Deaths: Essentials and Recommendations On Opioid Overdose*. Available from: http://www.eurohrn.eu/images/stories/pdf/publications/study_report_euroHRN_II.pdf

Thom B. (1999). *Dealing with drink. Alcohol and Social Policy, From Treatment to Management*. London: Free Association Press: pp. 142–6.

Yates R. and Malloch M. S. (2010) The road less travelled? A short history of addiction recovery. In R Yates and M S Malloch (eds), *Tackling Addiction. Pathways to Recovery*. London: Jessica Kingsley Publisher, pp. 26–42.

Vilke, G. M., Sloane, C., Smith, A. M. and Chan, T. C. (2003). Assessment for deaths in out-of-hospital heroin overdose patients treated with naloxone who refuse transport. *Academic Emergency Medicine*, 10(8): 893–6.

Wardle, I. (2012). Five years of recovery: December 2005 to December 2010 – from challenge to orthodoxy. *Drugs: Education, Prevention and Policy*, 19 (4): 294–8.

White, W. L. (2007a) Addiction recovery: its definition and conceptual boundaries. *Journal of Substance Abuse Treatment*, 33: 229–41.

White, W. L. (2007b). The new recovery advocacy movement in America. *Addiction*, 102: 696–703.

UNODC, ILO and UNDP (2012). *HIV Prevention, Treatment And Care In Prisons And Other Closed Settings: A Comprehensive Package Of Interventions. A Policy Brief.* Vienna: UNODC.

United Nations Office on Drugs and Crime (UNODC). (2013). *Opioid Overdose: Preventing And Reducing Opioid Overdose Mortality.* Discussion paper UNODC/WHO 2013. Vienna: UNODC. Available from: from http://www.unodc.org/docs/treatment/overdose.pdf

United Nations Office on Drugs and Crime (UNODC). (2015). *A Handbook for Starting and Managing Needle and Syringe Programmes in Prisons and Other Closed Settings.* Vienna: UNODC. Available from: http://www.unodc.org/documents/hiv-aids/publications/Prisons_and_other_closed_settings/ADV_COPY_NSP_PRISON_AUG_2014.pdf

Verthein U, Bonorden-Kleij K, Degkwitz P, Dilg C, Köhler W, Passie T, Soyka M, Tanger S, Vogel M, Haasen C. (2008). Long-term effects of heroin-assisted treatment in Germany. *Addiction*, 2008; 103: 960–6.

WHO (2009). *Guidelines for the Psychosocially Assisted Pharmacological Treatment of Opioid Dependence.* Geneva: WHO. Available from: http://www.who.int/substance_abuse/publications/opioid_dependence_guidelines.pdf

WHO (2010). *Prevention of Acute Drug - Related Mortality in Prison Populations During the Immediate Post-Release Period Immediate Post-Release Period.* Geneva: WHO. Available from: http://www.rsat-tta.com/Files/Prison_Mortality.pdf.

WHO (2014). *Community Management of Opioid Overdose.* Geneva: WHO. Available from: http://apps.who.int/iris/bitstream/10665/137462/1/9789241548816_eng.pdf?ua=1&ua=1.

Wilson, D. P., Shattock, A. J. and Fraser-Hurt, N. (2015). The cost-effectiveness of harm reduction. *International Journal of Drug Policy,* 26(Suppl. 1): S5–11.

Worthington, N., Piper, T. M., Galea, S. and Rosenthal, D. (2006). Opiate users' knowledge about overdose prevention and naloxone in New York City: a focus group study. *Harm Reduction Journal*, 3: 19.

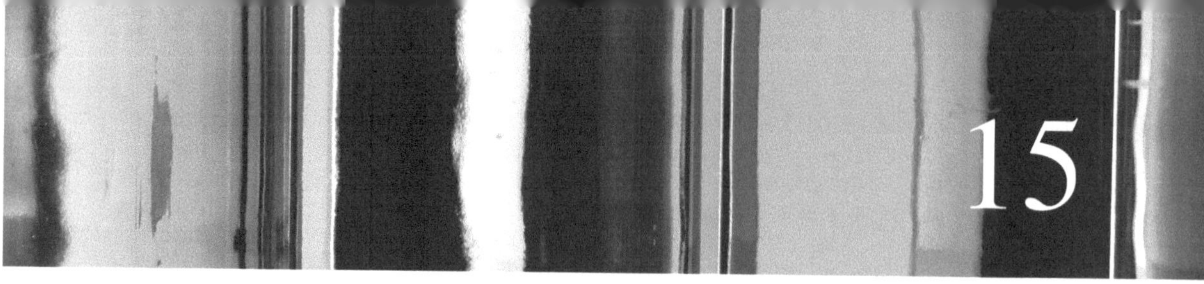

The Treatment Response: Systemic Features, Paradigms and Socio-Cultural Frameworks

Harald Klingemann and Jessica Storbjörk

CURE, CARE OR CONTROL? A TIMELINE OF SOCIETY'S DEFINITIONS AND RESPONSES TO ALCOHOL AND OTHER DRUG PROBLEMS

The problem of conformity and deviance represents a major axis concerning the analysis of social systems and social control (Parsons, 1951: 250–1). The response of society to behaviours considered and labelled as 'deviant' – in this case, various types of addictive behaviours – is shaped by normative expectations and images of the social problem at hand. The handling of addiction and addiction treatment systems as social institutions can be considered as a specific case (Mäkelä, 2001) and will vary according to the framing of the problem as a form of delinquency, disease or social care issue. Along these lines, Mäkelä and Säilä (1987) have pointed out the following functions of the management of alcohol-related problems (and hence, other substance-related problems): the treatment of alcohol-related medical complications, the provision of material services and spiritual comfort or harm reduction and the manipulation of drinking and the control of disruptive behaviour. The relative importance of these aspects of 'cure', 'care' or 'control' will depend on changing societal beliefs and socio-cultural factors varying from society to society. In general, framings of substance use problems, and the treatment thereof, are quite stable but can be changed. For instance, legal pressures and explicit coercive treatment exists but may be replaced by indirect forms of social control (Klingemann et al., 1992: 289; Weisner et al., 2010; see 'Coercion and treatment ultimatums: ethical challenges'). Since 2010, starting with a fundamentally different drug strategy approach (HM Government, 2010), a recovery discourse has come to dominate UK drug policy and treatment, implying a shift from a strong focus on harms and crime-reduction to a focus on support for drug users to choose recovery, become drug-free and reintegrated – a rhetorical change from punishment to treatment (Duke, 2013; Hunt and Stevens, 2004).

However, the institutionalisation of the societal response to addiction problems, as the expression 'treatment system' conveys, represents only a specific stage in the historical development of societal interventions. Taking alcohol treatment systems as the historically older example, the origins of today's highly developed treatment systems in central and northern Europe and North America can be traced back to strong social moral movements, such as the American National Temperance Society (NTS), the Blue Cross and the Good Templars, fighting the abuse of alcoholic beverages and the 'spirits or rum plague' in the late nineteenth Century (Blocker et al., 2003; Fahrenkrug, 1984; Klingemann et al., 1992). The early American social activists and physicians already marked a certain shift from moral to medical conceptualizations of 'inebriety'. Consequently, 'concerns about alcohol problems and the elevation of sobriety as a social value spawned…a multi-branched field of addiction treatment' (White, 2002: 1087). Its strong lay element, for example, visitor commissions claiming abstinence pledges at the homes of problem drinkers (see example of Switzerland; Klingemann, 1986: 265) and the general moral claims, were gradually replaced by increasing professionalization and medicalization, although with great differences between countries, as a comparison between the American and the Swiss treatment systems illustrates. Different from European countries, faith-based treatment programmes still play a central role in the United States (Klingemann et al., 2013). The high religiosity in the United States is mirrored to some extent in the treatment provisions, suggesting that the treatment response is embedded in the general socio-cultural makeup of countries.

Finally, epidemiological data, which became available in the 1970s (see Smart, 2007) challenged the disease model by showing the variability of drinking patterns over time and the relevance of problem drinking in addition to revealing the low coverage of treatment interventions (Klingemann and Bergmark, 2006). The focus of high threshold treatment systems on the most severe cases was increasingly questioned and put into perspective by these findings and its latent ideological function revealed. In addition, per capita consumption and problem drinkers became targets of alcohol policy following the theoretical work of Ledermann (1964) claiming a link of per capita consumption in societies and alcohol-related problems. More recently, restrictive alcohol and drug policies targeting entire populations have been challenged, and we can see a shift towards more focus on the control of individual problem substance-users who cannot manage in a consumer society, hence a renewed interest in treatment (Sulkunen, 2009). Taken together, these understandings point to necessary changes for matching the treatment response to the continuum of addictive behaviour. At present, however, well-formed treatment systems are mostly matters for the Western world, whereas many developing countries struggle with low access to treatment and building a system from scratch.

These introductory remarks on the historical background and socio-cultural variability of different societies' response to addiction as a disease or a social problem set the scene for an overview of the paradigms, analytical concepts and empirical approaches guiding and characterizing treatment systems. The chapter starts out with a review of approaches for classifying and defining treatment systems. These models serve as frameworks for treatment planning and monitoring strategies. The related steering policies of treatment systems from an administrative or clinical perspective are highlighted by reviewing the role of (i) evidence-based approaches, (ii) systemic features such as combined versus segregated service provision and (iii) the implementation of non-voluntary treatment linked to the criminal justice system. This Weberian 'ideal type' of top-down treatment systems rational planning is put into perspective by the more flexible and open market perspective conceptualized as part of New Public Management (NPM). Evidence on the treatment gap, a review of clients' needs and treatment seeking, complement this bottom-up approach. Furthermore, treatment-mapping strategies, such as expert surveys and case studies as well as dynamic diffusion approaches depicting innovation processes and barriers to change within treatment systems, also show the limits of these models in practice. Finally, results from an expert survey in 14 countries illustrate the interaction and development of key treatment systems characteristics over time. Taken together, this chapter focuses on a juxtaposition of the rational narrative of treatment system planners and policy makers and the empirical and normative perspectives in socio-cultural and politically diverse societies.

ATTEMPTS OF TREATMENT PLANNING, CONCEPTUALIZATION AND CLASSIFICATION OF 'TREATMENT SYSTEMS'

Most Western countries aim for an accessible and cost-efficient addiction treatment system that will relieve the harms of substance abuse to individuals, families and communities. Systems researchers argue that we must turn our gaze from the effectiveness of single treatment *methods*, which have been the main target of treatment research for decades, to a holistic approach studying the impact of varying treatment *systems*, and that the system is more than the mere sum of discrete treatment technologies (Babor, 2015). However, research has so far been unable to provide evidence concerning which type of system best helps reduce problems on the individual or population level. This is one of the goals of current treatment systems research (Babor, 2015, see Pedersen et al., 2004), together with other 'pressing topics' such as needs assessment, system mapping and monitoring (including measurement of effectiveness) and comparative analyses (Babor et al., 2008). In fact, due to the great diversity in treatment organization across and within countries, research has difficulties even trying to portray and compare treatment systems. Despite, or perhaps because of the quite fragmented and arbitrary emergence of treatment systems over the last 200 years (which accelerated after the Second World War) and the overall lack of coherency, there are several attempts to create theoretical models for how to organize treatment systems. Policy-makers and system administrators in well-developed (or 'mature'; Babor and Poznyak, 2010, below) systems are committed to both higher level *strategic* planning regarding the system's goals and visions and the *technical,* operational and allocative planning (Ritter et al., 2014). However, as stressed in the section 'Treatment system research: mind the gaps in treatment systems resistant to change!', systems are difficult to change and existing institutions serve as important barriers to radical change (e.g. Duke, 2013; Pierson, 2000).

Definitions

The planning and study of treatment systems requires useful operational definitions of what we mean by 'treatment' and by 'system'. The definitions forwarded vary in terms of the dimensions stressed. Some definitions are loose categorical descriptions referring to either an ad-hoc collection of services in a geographical area and/or the sharing of some characteristics such as financing (Bergmark, 2010). Babor et al. (2008) identified key components (resources, tasks and linking elements) and suggest that a treatment system is an arrangement of facilities, programmes and personnel providing care that is designed to function and accomplish key tasks in a coordinated way. Such an arrangement includes linkages between different levels of specialized care and linkages to other types of services. They expand the definition by adding in policy determinants central for the structural resources available for treatment (Babor et al., 2008). Other definitions more generally emphasize that 'system' 'refers broadly to those social structures and processes that have the function of alcohol treatment and in a narrower sense, the interconnection of different treatment units or agencies, chains of treatment and referral channels' (Klingemann et al., 1992: 4). Thus, linkages and interconnections (or a 'discrete entity composed of interrelated parts') (Bergmark, 2010: 566) are central yet difficult to capture and treatment may either be conceptualized with references to *functions* or *intentions*. Hence, aspects and activities that function as treatment may be broader than activities aimed at providing treatment and intended treatment may not always work as intended.

Conceptual frameworks and treatment planning in context

The goals of theorizing and planning treatment systems are manifold and entail *equity* (regarding access), *efficiency* (the most appropriate mix of services and successful outputs) and *economic* (cost-efficiency) goals (Babor et al., 2008). To this list we can add *accessibility* – as concerns geography, culture and language – and *acceptability* or legitimacy of services (Eagar et al., 2001). In practice, these planning efforts meet resistance when models must be pragmatically adapted to the local context and pre-exceeding cultural, political, financial and legal conditions – that is, trade-offs. Treatment planners also lack accurate assessments of (unmet) needs, reliable data on service use and the performance of current services, as well as the planning and functioning of neighbouring health or welfare systems. In addition, conflicting goals and planning at the local, regional or national levels may occur (Ritter et al., 2014). Consequently, treatment systems are often fragmentary and lack overall coordination (Babor, 2015) and the character of a system depends more on the images of addiction (see section 'Cure, care or control? A timeline of society's definitions and responses to alcohol and other drug problems') and perceptions of such problems' importance than on consumption patterns, resources or treatment needs (Klingemann et al., 1992, 1993).

It is difficult to find suitable definitions and there is no generally accepted conceptual framework for addiction treatment systems (Rush, 2010). Some influential concepts and models have been *continuum of care* or the related *core-shell* and *stepped care* approaches. Continuum of care understands problem severity as a continuum and refers to the mix of services that clients are expected to pass through sequentially depending on acuity, severity and complexity (see Babor, 2015; McGonigle et al., 1992; Rush, 2010). In the core-shell model developed in the 1970s, intake assessment, referral and case management occur in the core. The service user is thereafter assigned to a certain treatment – theoretically located in the shell – that matches the needs (Glaser et al., 1978). Similarly, stepped care implies that the least intensive and intrusive level of care is chosen after an initial assessment. If needed, the service user can step up or down if a service proves inappropriate (Breslin et al., 1998). These models focus on addiction care and have to a large extent become subsumed under the broader treatment systems and public health perspectives that include linkages to other support systems (health, social, etc.) where people not seeking specialized addiction services may find the help they need due to co-occurring problems (Rush, 2010). Thus, a broader perspective is needed to grasp how a 'system' can make an impact at the population level. Such a perspective must recognize that many people resolve their problems without formal help (Klingemann et al. 2010) and that most people in the general population who suffer from addiction problems have less severe acuity, chronicity and complexity (degree of co-occurring conditions) compared to a smaller number with the highest need for specialized or intensive care. The less severe can be treated in integrated services or handle their problems within the informal community (see Rush, 2010).

Such a broad approach was first implemented by the Institute of Medicine (IOM) (1990), which promoted early interventions. More recent examples are the *tiered model* and the *public health* approach to addiction treatment systems. The tiered framework acknowledges the *chronic care model*, which addresses the need for repeated and continuing measures for those with more severe substance problems, similar to the treatment of chronic conditions such as diabetes (Babor, 2015). The tiered model was first developed for addiction treatment in the UK in the early 2000s (National Treatment Agency, 2002; Rush, 2010). The model, advanced in Canada as an integrated approach (Rush, 2010), has five tiers: Tier 1 refers to health promotion and prevention targeting the general population; Tier 2 includes early intervention and is directed towards people at risk; Tier 3 consists of treatment and support for people with identified problems; Tier 4 comprises more intensive services and specialized care, including residential care; and Tier 5 refers to highly specialized care for individuals with complex problems (Rush, 2010; Rush et al., 2013).

The optimal treatment system from the public health perspective (Babor et al., 2008; Babor, 2015) requires (i) health and welfare policies as well as more specific addiction treatment policies and funding arrangements that facilitate the system's governance and monitoring. These policies determine (ii) structural resources such as infrastructure, staff and programmes, and (iii) system qualities in terms of accessibility/equity, economy (cost-effectiveness), efficiency (appropriate mix of services) and integration. These determinants (policies, structural resources and qualities) are theorized to contribute to the effectiveness of services on both the individual and population level by reducing the burden of addiction (deaths, disease and morbidity) – that is, population impact. The outcome can be moderated by factors such as population characteristics and drinking and drug use (sub)cultures – that is, the system must match its citizens and their needs (Babor et al., 2008; Babor, 2015). It is clear, however, that there will always be system boundaries between different parts such as specialized addiction care and primary care (Babor et al., 2008).

Including low and mid-income countries, there are attempts, driven by the World Health Organization (WHO), to classify the development and improve and monitor systems internationally. For example, the WHO-SAIMS (Substance Abuse Instrument for Mapping Services) classifies systems into four levels ranging from minimal development to limited, modest and mature (Babor and Poznyak, 2010). The European Monitoring Centre for Drugs and Drug Addiction (EMCDDA, 2013) is also trying to set up a coherent framework for measuring treatment systems and finding important dimensions for characterizing addiction treatment systems.

To conclude, we can recall that the development of treatment systems has been fragmented, arbitrary and culture-bound and that interconnectedness is difficult to achieve, conceptualize and measure. The implementation of strategic conceptual models is difficult and planning may not always change everyday work. It has, for example, been recognized that the tiered framework 'admittedly…[is] an "ideal vision" that needs to be tested against the vagaries of community implementation' (Rush, 2010: 632) and that the core-shell model was never realized in practice (Glaser, 2001). The literature often assumes that a well-planned and integrated system (see the section 'A combined and integrated versus a specialized and segregated approach?') is beneficial to the service users and such planning may avoid clients falling through the system's cracks. However, given the stigma attached to substance abuse (Lloyd, 2013; Room, 2005, 2006), we can ask whether such a system may actually be undesirable from a service user point of view if negative attitudes contribute to suboptimal health care for these patients (van Boekel et al., 2013) or if the substance users for other reasons wish to keep their addiction problems from societal agencies. Considering service user involvement and client choice, service users may 'benefit from a greater variety of choices between agencies, and may lose options if the agencies become more "joined up" and rationalized into a system sharing client information between agencies' (Room, 2010: 578). A more fragmented system may offer more choices (Wiseman, 1970).

THE MARKET PERSPECTIVE

The previous section points to rationality as the basis for conceptualizing and planning the system – a 'dream of rationality' (Bergmark, 2010: 567). However, Bergmark argues that addiction treatment systems are not products of rationality and that the focus should instead be on crucial features such as the market aspect as a linking mechanism, and that the system should be considered as a treatment market (Bergmark, 2010). The market perspective is usually conceptualized as part of NPM, which has entered public administration and health and welfare services. NPM has, among other things, created demands for greater efficiency, lowered costs and market-inspired solutions such as contracting-out services in purchaser-provider models and facilitating competition based on tendering processes (Hood, 1995; Pollitt and Bouckaert, 2011; Pollitt and Sorin, 2011). Accompanying these tendencies are various means of control, auditing and the (experienced) need to steer and monitor systems (Power, 1997), including a focus on outcomes and statistical reporting of activities in NPM (Hansen Löfstrand, 2012).

NPM has had a major impact in countries such as the UK, USA, Australia and in smaller countries such as Sweden, and the market aspect is an important attribute of many health, welfare and addiction treatment systems (Bergmark, 2010; Pollitt and Sorin, 2011; Stenius, 1999). The contracting-out of services may also have other roots, such as the idealism regarding governments partnering with non-profit grassroots agencies, which led to the contracting-out of services in the USA in the 1980s (Room, 2010; Weisner and Room, 1984). Regardless of the rationale for imposing competition into the addiction treatment system, we can conceptualize the market perspective as the antithesis to the system approach in the previous section as the contracting-out of services and competition between agencies work against efforts to increase linkages and collaboration (Bergmark, 2010; Room, 2010). However, as stated by Room, financing may be crucial but it is not the sole determinant of systems that are highly guided by (i) ideology, images of addiction and conceptualizations of suitable responses (see sections 'Cure, care or control? A timeline of society's definitions and responses to alcohol and other drug problems' and 'How much (little) do we know about AOD (Alcohol and other drug) interventions: three treatment mapping strategies'); (ii) the professions and institutions handling addictions (see section 'Cure, care or control? A timeline of society's definitions and responses to alcohol and other drug problems'); and (iii) the social standing and power position of the service users (Room, 2010). The last point draws attention to substance users seldom living up to market ideas of self-managing customers (Bjerge, 2012; Gingrich, 2011) and the fragmented demands of NPM. The purchaser of care is separated from the service user creating a situation where it is the needs and views of the purchasers, and not the preferences of the consumers, that constitute treatment demands (Bergmark, 2010;

Gingrich, 2011). In addition, NPM appears to introduce or escalate a de-professionalization and re-distribution of power away from professionals and towards high-ranking bureaucrats negotiating contracts and purchasing treatment (Bjerge, 2012; Burton and van den Broek, 2009; Christensen and Lægreid, 2011; Evetts, 2009; Gingrich, 2011; Power, 1997). Such a development is consistent with the implementation of evidence-based treatment guidelines in well-developed systems (Davies, 2003; Rehm et al., 2013) (see the section 'The search for the best treatment modalities and the quest for evidence').

The research base of the NPM effects in public services is thin, especially when it comes to addiction treatment systems and outcomes at the service user level (Hull and Ritter, 2014; Pollitt and Sorin, 2011). The few existing reports show some improved performances (Pollitt and Sorin, 2011), positive experiences (McLellan et al., 2008), reduced waiting lists and increased capacity use (Hull and Ritter, 2014; McLellan et al., 2008). Nevertheless, there are few signs of improved outcomes for the treated (Hull and Ritter, 2014; Humphreys and McLellan, 2011; Pedersen et al., 2011) and there are indications of unintended consequences such as the following: prevention of preconditions for effective care (Bjerge, 2012; Nesvåg and Lie, 2010); gaming of the system (Bjerge, 2012; Lu and Ma, 2006); encouragement of fragmented care provision and the undermining of care in less profitable cases where there are multiple needs – 'creaming' and cherry picked clients (Hansen Löfstrand, 2012; Kaukonen and Stenius, 2005; Moore and Fraser, 2013); and cost-increasing effects (Christensen and Lægreid, 2011; Drechsler, 2005; Dunleavy et al., 2006; Pollitt et al., 2007; Stenius, 2011). NPM has also been found to streamline services, hence creating a less variable system (Bjerge, 2012; Stenius, 2011), which may limit client choice (see 'The search for the best treatment modalities and the quest for evidence'). It is, despite of the research shortage, clear that the market perspective changes incentives and the functioning of the system, as well as challenges interconnectedness and linkages.

SPECIFIC ISSUES

A combined and integrated versus a specialized and segregated approach?

The extent to which a system is to be characterized as a combined and integrated system or a specialized and segregated system refers to the joint handling of various substances and to the integration of addiction treatment with other service sectors. The use of the term 'prevention and treatment of substance use disorders' assumes that the treatment system addresses the whole range of addictive behaviours and problems (alcohol, illicit drugs, tobacco, etc.) under one umbrella, which is also suggested by, for example, the tiered and public health models. In practice, the societal response to various addiction problems and related policies can be characterized on a *continuum* reaching from fully integrated to entirely addiction-specific segregated approaches. Communalities in terms of national policies and strategies, the service sector and dominant professions (e.g. medical versus socio-therapeutic; professional versus lay people), financing sources (public funds, health insurers, out-of-pocket) and similar treatment methods as well as objectives (e.g. abstinence, substitution, reduction) and joint client monitoring systems, can be used to assess the degree of addiction service provision integration in a country.

The debate concerning the *pros and cons* of an integrated versus specialized approach, points to factors promoting or impeding a certain treatment response. The issue can be illustrated by an early debate in the *British Journal of Addiction* (Pittman, 1967) with Raistrick (1988) pleading for a combined approach similar to the rationale of emergency rooms, that is, observing similarities in relapse patterns across specific types of addictions. The focus shifts from the type of licit or illicit drug in question to commonalities in patient profiles. Pittman counters that 'because of the social, cultural and legal perceptions that individuals have of alcohol and other drugs… these differential mind sets make effective programming for both groups in the same service difficult' (Pittman, 1988: 871, 1989). He furthermore points out the discrepancy in treatment goals, which includes moderation and substitution in the case of drug treatment but abstinence when alcoholism is treated (Pittman, 1988: 872). *The former assumption* about emotional blocks hindering integration trends has been more specifically addressed by Bergmark (1998), who explored, based on data from 19 countries, the relationship between the degree of system integration and the focus on drugs or alcohol as serious problems. According to Roizen (1993), the merging of systems could consequently be influenced by increasing the perceived seriousness of alcohol problems ('drug-ification' of alcohol), de-escalating drug problems ('alcoholization of drug problems'), emphasising a pragmatic middle ground (e.g. integrated primary prevention) or by adopting a public health approach (downgrading drugs as a problem, non-moralistic interventions, establishing alcohol and tobacco use as public health problem) (Roizen, 1993: 8). The latter assumption, which claims differing treatment objectives as barriers to treatment integration, has been empirically addressed by research on controlled drinking and harm reduction policies in the alcohol field. Studies on the acceptance of moderate alcohol use as treatment goal (Klingemann 2016) support the assumption of an increasing convergence. Further indicators, in some countries, are the establishment of wet places similar to drop-ins and injection rooms in the field of illicit drugs (Muckle et al. 2012).

Another system *determinant* is the 'seniority' of the systems, and the question of when they emerged can play a role in their organizational relationship and willingness to change. Typically, specialized alcohol treatment systems emerged much earlier than programmes for illicit drug use with the HIV and drug problems becoming virulent only in the 1960s and 1970s. However, contrary to Europe and North America, treatment for alcohol-related disorders in Asia has been only recently established – for example, virtually non-existent in China before the 1990s (Tang et al., 2012: 563) and struggling for governmental recognition as a specialized system as is the case in Korea (Jeek Wook et al., 2013). The integration issue is not on the agenda here.

Furthermore, it can be assumed that other organizational factors, such as more general public policies to *merge or centralize* hospitals and health services, will have an impact on the integration dynamic in the addiction treatment sector (e.g. Nesvåg and Lie, 2010; Wahlbeck, 2010). Arguments in favour of integration policies tend to gain ground by pointing at the contradiction between polydrug *use* and comorbidity while at the same time drawing attention to the persistence of services organized separately as substance-related. It has been highlighted that it may be less stigmatizing to seek help for addiction problems within general health care than in a specialized addiction unit. Contrarily, acknowledging the increasing *heterogeneity* of clients (with an even broader spectrum after the adoption of the DSM-V) might be used as an argument for a differentiated and specialized treatment response.

Another aspect of integration that may or may not imply the integration of various substances is the increasing integration of addiction treatment and mental health, health care or social welfare, often targeting cost-containment and driven by the acknowledgement of co-morbidities. Thus far, very limited evidence on the *effects* of integration policies in practice is available. As Wahlbeck states when referring to integration with health care: 'integration of addiction treatment is based on a surprisingly weak evidence base…we need more longitudinal data examining the effects of reforms' (Wahlbeck, 2010: 701). Likewise, we need more knowledge regarding whether treatment approaches are 'diluted' or abandoned in favour of approaches shared by the dominant professional group in combined treatment teams, that is, addiction medicine competing with social work and social-therapeutic practice (see Tammi and Stenius, 2014).

It should be kept in mind at this point that the integration issue appears to be a *policy debate* for rich countries that can afford treatment and develop highly specialized treatment systems (Morisano et al., 2014: 15). The WHO Atlas survey in 147 countries shows that fewer than half of the countries have a specific budget allocated for the treatment of substance use disorders. Specialized treatment services for alcohol use disorders are reported by 35 per cent of the countries and for drug use disorders in 52 per cent. Mental health services are the most common treatment setting for alcohol use disorders (35 per cent) (Atlas on substance use, 2010: X).

Finally, the positioning of integrated approaches within public health policies, general addiction policies and national action plans calls for further analysis. A comparative study by Zobel and colleagues from 19 European countries that explored their declared efforts to integrate various levels of addiction policies showed that only with respect to juveniles were joint approaches actually implemented (Zobel et al., 2004: 54–7).

The search for the best treatment modalities and the quest for evidence

The dominance and implications of evidence-based practices (EBP) in/for addiction treatment systems call for an introductory exposition but the topic is fully covered by Bergmark and Hübner (Chapter 35 this Handbook). As stated in 'Attempts of treatment planning, conceptualization and classification of "treatment systems"', the search for effective treatment interventions has long dominated treatment research. There is by now a significant amount of treatment outcome literature that has been reviewed at several points. These suggest treatment techniques that can help people overcome substance use problems (e.g. Berglund et al., 2003). The EBP quest is highly understandable: we want to receive, provide and pay for high quality treatments that have been proven effective ('quality' is also a central feature of NPM; see the section 'The market perspective') and we assume that practices grounded in evidence are better than those based on faith, tradition, etc. Therefore, reviews of the outcome research are increasingly being translated into EBP guidelines, which seek to be implemented in the majority of more developed addiction treatment systems (Rehm et al., 2013); this may change the allocation of resources and treatment provided. Yet, we have little knowledge about what works regarding the implementation of research into practice (Moore et al., 2011) – there are several examples of how the implementation of EBP/guidelines have led to little change in actual practices – and the development towards EBP has been criticized for several reasons.

A first line of critique refers to deficiencies in the interpretation of the outcome literature, reviews and compilation of guidelines. Scientists have put forward the randomized controlled trial – usually studying 'pure' rather than 'typical' service users and providing the highest evidence regarding causal effects – and, as a consequence, EBP guidelines may not generalize to real world patients, that is, problems regarding *external validity* (Humphreys et al., 2005; Orford, 2006; Poikolainen, 2002; Storbjörk, 2014a). The hegemonic treatment outcome research has also been claimed to *de-contextualize treatment* by assuming that psychosocial therapies follow the same logic as pharmacological treatments. Hence, it ignores the role of contextual and other important factors in change processes (Orford, 2006):

> Formal 'treatment' sometimes plays a small or large part in the extended, multi-influenced process, but when it does it is construed most appropriately, not as a technical input, but rather as a special example of the many influences [interpersonal and social processes occurring in people's lives] to which a person will be exposed. (Orford, 2006: 653)

Another limitation is that of the 'Dodo bird verdict', that is, psychotherapies and addiction treatments, which regardless of their specific components and underlying theories, produce equivalent outcomes (Luborsky et al., 2002; Rosenzweig, 1936). Roughly speaking, equally large percentages of patients do better, worse or do not change their substance use regardless of which type of EBP is used. This provides support in favour of the dodo bird verdict being valid also within the addiction treatment field – such evidence is provided in comprehensive studies such as project MATCH (Allen et al., 1997), the UK Alcohol Treatment Trial (UKATT; Orford et al., 2006) and COMBINE (Anton et al., 2006) (see Bergmark, 2008). A radical but perhaps fair conclusion is that the search for effective treatment methods is by now futile. 'We are, I believe, now facing a crisis regarding treatment research in the substance misuse field, and a paradigm shift is called for' (Orford, 2006: 653; see also Bergmark, 2008).

Another line of critique concerns the service user perspective that potentially may be in conflict with EBP. The original model of evidence-based medicine integrated and gave equal weight to (i) the use of current best available research evidence; (ii) the integration of individual clinical expertise; and (iii) service user preferences and choices (Sackett et al., 1996). Voices have been raised claiming that client preferences in practice draw the short straw while scientific evidence is given considerable weight. It should not be assumed that (potential) service users will always appreciate us finding the best solution for them, thereby eliminating any choice for them. Hence, EBP has sometimes and somewhat in contradiction to Sackett's model come to be a conflict between research/evidence and service user involvement, which is another strong tendency across the world (elaborated by Bjerge et al., in Chapter 30, this volume). Reconnecting to NPM and the market perspective (see the section 'The market perspective') that splits the 'customer' into purchaser and a generally stigmatized and powerless service user, also implies that patients are not in a good bargaining position concerning what services are offered to or pressed on them (Room, 2010). Orford (2006) suggests that clients' choice is given far greater weight than professional allocation rules.

Coercion and treatment ultimatums: ethical challenges

There is vast literature on the importance of motivation for successful treatment outcomes. Paradoxically, social control is widely used to push people into treatment for the sake of the individual or for (significant) others. Such informal, formal and legal pressures also have a much wider scope and penetration than the legislated compulsory care (civil commitments and criminal justice legislation) that still exists in many countries (Israelsson and Gerdner, 2012). For example, compulsory care is rare in Sweden but close to one-fifth of those entering treatment 'voluntarily' report coming in order to avoid coercive care (Storbjörk, 2012). The general long-term trend is that compulsory care, civil commitments in particular, is being abandoned or has fallen into disuse in well-developed countries because of low effectiveness and for the sake of safeguarding human rights (Hall et al., 2012, 2013; Israelsson and Gerdner, 2012). Recently however, there is a slight increase in coerced addiction care stemming from the criminal justice system, and compulsory and ethically questionable detention is on the rise in some countries such as in Cambodia, China, Thailand and Vietnam (Hall et al., 2012; UNODC, 2010; Xiao et al., 2015). In fact, legally coerced treatment – treatment as an alternative to criminal justice sanctions – is widespread internationally (e.g. Australia, Austria, Canada, Germany, Ireland, New Zealand, South Africa, UK, US, etc.) and in some countries it is growing. There is some support for the effectiveness of drug courts in reducing recidivism (Mitchell et al., 2012; Wilson et al., 2006) and for reduced substance use after other types of court-mandated or quasi-compulsory treatment (Uchtenhagen et al., 2008; McSweeney et al., 2007; UNODC, 2010). There are some methodological concerns but studies indicate that such treatment is at least as good as voluntary treatment. However, referral source does not necessarily correspond well with service users' perceptions of coercion, which may be of greater importance for outcomes (Wild et al., 1998). For example, those diverted to treatment may be highly motivated to participate and change.

It is reasonable to claim that an important part of entry into addiction treatment consists of (social) pressures, or more extreme ultimatums and coercive measures. For example, Weisner et al. (2010) have shown the importance of various family, welfare, employment and legal ultimatums regarding entry into US addiction treatment, and Storbjörk (2012) has reported corresponding pressures regarding entry into the Swedish comprehensive addiction treatment system with universal, although means-tested, coverage (Klingemann and Hunt, 1998; Klingemann et al., 1992). Self-choice co-exists with threats of consequences, such as going to jail or loss of job/welfare benefits/romantic partner unless you go to treatment. In fact, in a review by Wild (2006), it was concluded that some US reviews find that coercion 'works', whereas other reviews point to inconclusive findings or methodological problems. His conclusion is that 'proliferation of social control tactics to facilitate addiction treatment is a world-wide social experiment without a compelling evidence-base on its utility' (Wild, 2006: 46). The consequences of such social control/coercion are still unclear (Hall et al., 2012, 2013). The US National Institute on Drug Abuse (NIDA, 2012) claims that treatment does not need to be voluntary to be effective (Article 11). Sanctions from family, employment and/or the criminal justice system can increase entry and retention and thereby secure the ultimate success of treatment (NIDA, 2012). Nevertheless, there are only a few studies that longitudinally study the relationship between different types of entry pressures and outcomes (see Wild et al., 2006) and, as an example, Storbjörk (2012) found that informal, formal and legal treatment entry pressures were generally associated with poorer treatment outcomes among alcohol misusers.

To conclude, coercion is frequently involved in entering addiction treatment systems and the evidence-base is still unclear. Most of the literature on coerced treatment is on legal coercion or about ethical considerations rather than empirical reports (Wild et al., 2002). Apart from arguments regarding individual autonomy and human rights, if (social) pressures to enter treatment are associated with poorer treatment outcomes (e.g. Storbjörk, 2012), the implication would be to promote less enforced treatment entries and paternalistic principles. It is, however, not only the well-being and rights of the individual substance user that is in focus in discussing treatment systems. Treatment is often legitimized by utilitarian principles. In this line of reasoning, it is the interests of the community (to secure peace and order), the family (to be protected from physical, social, moral and economic harms) and the public (to be protected from the economic burden of abuse) that need to be protected from the harms of misuse (Nilssen, 2005). For example, acknowledging people that have been hurt by the substance user and trying to straighten out the past are integral parts of the influential 12-step treatment. Recently, the international research community has started to investigate harms to others caused by substance use (WHO, 2014). It remains to be seen if and how this new interest may change the view of the individual substance user and the importance of the utilitarian principles of the treatment systems. This change is similar to a development in the UK (Hunt and Stevens, 2004) in the early 2000s when focus shifted from health effects on the individual substance user to harms on the community and social level, which promoted more coercive care.

'Mind the gap' and clients' needs

When characterizing treatment systems, system qualities such as accessibility, economy and efficiency are seen as major components of an optimal treatment system (Babor, 2015). More specifically, needs assessment studies try to identify the gap between existing services and population needs and provide information concerning which development level a given system has reached (Babor, 2015; Babor and Poznyak 2010: 706, 707). As a recent example, under the umbrella of the Alcohol Measures for Public Health Research Alliance (AMPHORA) project, a study in six countries (Austria, Italy, Germany, Spain, Switzerland and England) has been launched that aims at measuring the need for alcohol treatment services (Room, 2011). Conceptual and methodological problems impeded the development of a standardized approach. The treatment gap refers to the basic concepts of 'need' and 'access', and the gap between these two is referred to as the Prevalence Service Utilization Ratio (PSUR; Drummond et al., 2011: 33). Several approaches have been used to define and measure treatment needs: Babor conceptualizes 'treatment need' as 'the number of people in a geographic region who meet criteria for dependence or harmful use, and who would benefit from treatment but do not access it' and adds that 'the numbers of "unmet need" are likely to be greater than the number of "demand for treatment" as "unmet need" includes those people who do not perceive the need for, or do not desire any treatment' (Babor, 2015). To identify empirically the treatment gap, it is most common to refer to population survey data and compare the problem population with the number of people receiving any kind of treatment. The model by Rush (1990) is based on proxy measures of prevalence (mortality rates, local projections of national survey, average level of consumption) (Rush, 1990: 51). Expert opinion on treatment needs and gaps in services and necessary improvements by service providers are additionally used (e.g. the Australian ACT Medicare Local Needs Assessment Overview).

These approaches are, however, very limited, focusing on a top-down provider view without measuring treatment needs directly among potential clients. Using the treatment market as a frame of reference, Bergmark observes: 'It is not the preferences of the consumer that constitute the demand in such a market, but its construction of the needs of the clients by the purchaser that represents the demand' (Bergmark, 2010: 569). Consequently, specific treatment needs, in conflict with the prevailing treatment philosophy (e.g. controlled consumption and harm reduction versus abstinence; quality of life versus consumption-oriented outcomes) tend not to be taken into consideration when calculating the treatment gap and are not considered as legitimate. This point is exemplified by surveys in the US with a 12-step abstinence oriented system, which show that reduction and control of consumption as outcomes were preferred by alcohol dependent individuals without treatment exposure (Dawson et al., 2005).

The attempt to develop a standardized instrument for service needs assessment, which would be universally applicable, seems to come at the expense of a differentiated view, which also accommodates social-cultural specificities. As Room comments on the Amphora project: 'I am less convinced by the project's apparent assumption that a culture-free definition of need for treatment can be found' (Room, 2011: vi). A more fundamental bias is potentially related to the assumption that 'addicts' cannot make informed decisions, implying a paternalistic concept of 'objective needs' (Bergmark, 2010: 569). Alternative approaches to need-based improvements of the treatment response would include a broader analysis of various treatment barriers based on both treated and untreated populations. Self-change research in particular provides insight in the role of the treatment continuum in the change process from addiction (DiClemente, 2007; Klingemann et al., 2010).

HOW MUCH (LITTLE) DO WE KNOW ABOUT AOD INTERVENTIONS: THREE TREATMENT MAPPING STRATEGIES

The empirical mapping and description of treatment systems is typically based on data from national monitoring/client systems, expert surveys and epidemiological studies. The availability and validity of these data vary greatly and the lack of reliable information about the interplay of actors in the system, even in rich countries, and the non-use of available information (e.g. from monitoring systems; Stern et al., 2009) might reflect various stakeholder positions profiting from such a strategic ignorance (Heimer, 2012; McGoey, 2012a, 2012b). This questions the feasibility and relevance of standardized instruments (e.g. the WHO-SAIMS; Babor, 2015) claiming to examine broad treatment system issues. Consequently, and as described below, more pragmatic approaches have been adopted by collecting rather basic information from as many countries as possible ('expert survey approach') or by providing a more in-depth analysis of systems within a small sample of countries mostly different in terms of treatment philosophies and socio-cultural makeup ('expert case study approach'). The latter approach has been complemented by attempts to capture the dynamic aspect of innovations in open treatment systems including international policy adoption ('dynamic diffusion approach').

Expert survey

The 'expert survey approach' used by supranational organizations such as the WHO and the EMCDDA relies on a network of institutionally based informants, which serve as local observers. A recent example is the WHO ATLAS-SU project survey in 147 countries (representing 88 per cent of the world population) collecting information about treatment and prevention with a special focus on low- and middle income countries. The questionnaire was completed in 2008 by national focal points. The country profiles included information about administration and financing of treatment services, sectors and settings, availability, coverage and capacity and treatment system organization. The dominant role of nongovernmental organizations and self-help groups is a key finding with 70 per cent of the surveyed countries indicating NGO as being active in the rehabilitation field and 60 per cent reporting that ex-addicts provide formal addiction care. Faith-based NGOs are important in richer countries, whereas traditional healers are found in low-income countries. Only 48 per cent of all countries devised national standards of addiction care. The availability of specific treatment types varies significantly between regions (Atlas on substance use, 2010: xii–xiv). The ATLAS-SU survey, even though limiting the data request to a few basic pieces of information and providing support to the regional data providers, once again shows a socio-cultural bias in the perceived importance of addiction and the willingness to invest in inventories: Response rates varied by WHO region and were highest in South-East Asia and Europe (91 per cent and 83 per cent, respectively) and lowest in the Americas and Western Pacific (58 per cent and 54 per cent, respectively) (Atlas on substance use, 2010: 4, 5). Open-ended questions on the organization of the treatment system were often answered in a cursory way (e.g. 'integrated with general health care') without providing more detailed information.

Following a similar approach, EMCDDA produces drug treatment profiles for the 27 EU Member States, and Turkey and Croatia as Candidate Countries, providing a description of the national context: overall drug treatment system and organization; description of monitoring systems; current treatment demand data; and availability and provision of treatment services as well as references and additional resources. Data are compiled with the assistance of the Reitox national focal points network. EMCDDA treatment data collection has been updated recently, in order to provide an comprehensive overview of drug treatment in the European countries covering treatment demand, provision, and treatment structure and organisation. The revision of tools and procedures aimed towards improved comparability across EU countries; improved estimates of the treatment population; advanced treatment analysis (of clients' profile and interventions and planning tools and targeted dissemination (EMCDDA, 2013:19). The limitation to EU and drugs only restricts its practical relevance but allows for the elaboration of more detailed treatment system mapping than the global ATLAS-SU survey.

The rationale for this type of treatment system mapping is to provide standardized and comparable data for policymakers and service planners who 'need reliable information from across an increasingly broad range of service providers to correctly assess the capacity of the treatment response, determine access barriers and support investment decisions' (EMCDDA, 2013:4). However, these expectations have not been met so far as acknowledged by EMCDDA (2013: 16). Conceptual issues limit the validity of this approach such as a provider oriented view, lack of differentiation by treatment objectives, and a treatment demand measure that excludes a direct assessment of clients' needs (see the section '"Mind the gap" and clients' needs'). No empirical support is available for the extent to which this kind of data is accessed and used by policy makers, administrators and service providers in decisions affecting the treatment system.

Expert case study

The expert case study approach pursues a broader in-depth analysis of treatment systems focusing on socio-historical aspects, retrospective views of the development of the treatment response, estimates of future trends, and most importantly, treatment philosophies and societal images of addiction, as frameworks for the systems. Based on expert networks and reviews of the literature, this perspective uses a mixed-method framework combining 'country system stories' (e.g. culture specific dynamics) and quantitative information (e.g. client loads or number and type of services).

Expert case studies are scarce, given the considerable efforts and funding required. The project International Studies in the Development of Alcohol Treatment Systems (ISDATS) was launched in 1987 by the description of the legal framework of alcohol treatment in six countries (Klingemann and Takala, 1987) followed by a comprehensive study of treatment systems in 16 countries. The study aimed at providing an account of treatment systems by tracing their evolution and highlighting the relative impact of economic, political, legal, medical and ideological factors on the evolution of the systems (Klingemann et al., 1992: 2). A key finding was that 'the attention paid to alcoholism treatment seems to depend more on cultural and political traditions than on clearly defined treatment needs or total economic resources' (Klingemann et al., 1992: 298). A test of this tentatively supported hypothesis over time along with changing parameters would allow for more insight into the evolution of systems from a more holistic perspective (for a summary of the study, see Klingemann et al., 1993). This, however, is not within the limits of a static expert survey approach.

A twin study on drug treatment systems in 20 countries (International Study of the Development of Drug Treatment Systems – ISDRUTS), again aimed at a description of the functioning of treatment systems in general within their socio-cultural context, was based on a network of 47 contributors/key informants, whereby the study linked the treatment systems to leitmotivs in country groups such as 'the experimental countries' (England, Switzerland, Netherlands) or 'drug prohibition and the abstinence paradigm' (USA, Canada, Sweden, Finland). It additionally added topical chapters on finances, gender and system integration and included comments on the country group reports by external interdisciplinary teams (Klingemann and Hunt, 1998). This represented from a qualitative methodology a strengthening of the expert case study approach and its practical relevance to 'enable…health planners and administrators, and treatment professionals to place the development of their own countries' treatment systems in a wider context and to examine the extent to which that development shares common structural features with that of other countries and other cultures' (Klingemann and Hunt, 1998: xv).

Such a holistic, comparative approach has also been used to assess the socio-cultural impact on assumingly identical interventions or treatment schemes across different treatment systems. Mäkelä et al. (1996) analysed Alcohol Anonymous (AA) as a mutual help movement in eight societies and could conclude that 'there are important variations in AA practices in different societies…these differences reflect the surrounding culture and society…cultural differences in the interaction styles and personal expressiveness influence what goes on in and around AA meetings in different places' (Mäkelä et al. 1996: 239). Whereas the spiritual aspect of AA blends in with strong religious orientations in the US, and faith-oriented treatment programmes in general, this is not necessarily the case in other countries (Klingemann et al., 2013).

Dynamic diffusion

The dynamic diffusion approach has been adopted to characterize change and communication processes within treatment systems on various levels in terms of policy, innovation development and the adoption of new practices. Rogers developed a comprehensive model of diffusion processes of innovations, which has been influential. It conceptualizes 'diffusion' as 'the process through which an innovation is communicated through certain channels over time among the members of a social system' (Rogers, 1983; Rogers, 2002: 990).

This model has been used to study the natural diffusion of new types of drug use and consumption patterns (overview see Ferrence, 2001). The gap between research and practice and the transfer of evidence-based approaches, such as the dissemination of research-based treatments for addiction counsellors (Garner, 2009; Herie and Martin, 2002; Miller et al., 2006), evidence-based addiction medication (Heinrich and Cummings, 2014) and the diffusion of prevention programmes (Rogers, 2002), have been explored within this framework on the facility, regional and national level. This network approach opens a broader perspective beyond the national boundaries approaching policy adoption processes and the exchange/flow of treatment interventions, models and philosophies from a global, multilateral perspective. Different from Rogers' approach,

Mäkelä conducted a cross-national structural analysis of the social and cultural preconditions associated with the strength of AA in 132 countries, showing that 'by 1986, the diffusion of AA had definitely moved beyond the cultural confines of the Anglo-Saxon and Protestant world. Long lasting activities had been typically established in all wealthy, non-Communist, non-Islamic countries' (Mäkelä, 1991: 1412). Mäkelä highlights the blocking of AA for political reasons (Mäkelä, 1991: 1406, 1996: 239), thereby implicitly referring to the 'compatibility' criteria in Roger's model, which 'is the degree to which an innovation is perceived as being consistent with the existing *values*, past experiences and needs of potential developers' (Rogers, 2002: 990; highlighted by author). Klingemann and Klingemann's (1999) analysis of the estimated chances for the adoption of controversial heroin prescription programmes in 19 countries in the aftermath of the Swiss vote rejected referendum 'Youth without drugs' in 1997 outlines endogenous and exogenous factors influencing the perceived chances to implement a heroin trial. Interaction and modelling between experimental countries and status quo countries is characterized by political power games and influence (Klingemann and Klingemann, 1999).

Finally, indirectly related to the study of the potential change of treatment systems, and its 'benchmarking' from an international perspective, is research on the attitudes of treatment providers and images of addiction in the general population concerning the changeability and therefore 'treatability' of substance use disorders. Roughly comparable studies from several countries have more specifically analysed the acceptance of treatment objectives other than abstinence, notably of controlled drinking by treatment providers (Dawe and Richmond, 1997; Klingemann and Rosenberg, 2009; Luquiens et al., 2011; Rosenberg and Davis, 2014; Rosenberg and Melville, 2005; Rosenberg et al., 1996, 2013; Klingemann 2016). Differences in the acceptance of broader treatment outcomes have implications for the makeup of the treatment programmes and for the attractiveness of programmes among potential service users. Even though these studies do not focus on communication and diffusion processes between programmes and professional groups, their findings can be used as change potential indicators for the supply side in the treatment system. The 'Images of addiction' survey is part of the international collaborative project Addiction and Lifestyles in Contemporary Europe: Reframing Addictions Project (ALICE-RAP, WP 3, see: http://blogs.helsinki.fi/imagesofaddiction/). The popular images of nine different addictions in five European countries (Poland, Norway, Germany, Finland, and Sweden) were investigated and provided data on the perceived chances for treatment success, self-change and the severity of various types of addictive behaviours.

CURRENT TRENDS AND CHANGES: A BRIEF EXPERT SURVEY IN 14 COUNTRIES

The theoretical framework presented so far facilitates the characterization of the treatment response in a given country. Nevertheless, the empirical mapping of treatment systems follows a more pragmatic logic and consequently, as shown above, it provides – with a considerable time lag – only limited insight into the dynamics and functioning of treatment systems in practice. To highlight some current trends and issues, and to illustrate the theoretical issues and dimensions drawing upon current developments, a brief expert mail-survey in 14 countries was conducted for this chapter in the spring to summer of 2014 by the authors asking for a rapid assessment of the 'hottest issues': 'the validity of the Atlas-SU survey country profile information' (see the section 'How much (little) do we know about AOD interventions: three treatment mapping strategies'), 'the funding environment' and 'future trends'.

Experts who had participated in follow-ups of ISDATS or ISDRUTS and were still active in the field were approached. The sample was complemented with additional experts known to the authors (see Expert survey box).

EXPERT SURVEY 2014: PARTICIPANTS

Special thanks to the country experts for taking their time to participate in this survey; however, full responsibility concerning the interpretations falls with the authors: (Australia) L. Berends; (China) Liu Tieqiao; (Canada) R. Jesseman, R. Notarandre, B. Rush and W.J. Skinner; (Denmark) M.U. Pedersen and B. Thylstrup; (England) S. MacGregor; (Finland) O. Kaukonen and K. Stenius; (Hungary) Z. Elekes; (Iceland) H. Ólafsdóttir; (Netherlands) D. van de Mheen; (Norway) A. Skretting; (Poland) G. Swiatkiewicz; (Sweden) A. Bergmark; (Switzerland) F. Moggi; (USA) K. Humphrey and M. Sobell.

Obviously the interpretations based on this country convenience sample cannot be generalized. From the analysis of the country feedback emerge the following tentative conclusions and dynamic perspectives:

- Supporting the results of early treatment mapping (i.e. ISDATS and ISDRUTS), changes in the treatment systems are mainly influenced by **general political changes and changes in the health care systems**, and to a much lesser extent, by the burden of addictive behaviour: The most prominent example is the US health reform with transformative policies since January 2014 (among others the Affordable Care Act) that put addiction treatment on an equal level with other medical conditions and will lead to increased demand and treatment provisions. In Hungary, liberalization policies have led to a rollback in harm reduction policies and a cut of treatment capacity despite an increasing number of alcoholics, the shutdown of leading research and treatment institutions in 2007 to 2008 and the implementation of penal code modifications in 2013, eliminating training programmes for first-time offenders (also the Australian, Icelandic and UK systems are facing financial challenges and cuts). Even seemingly non-reversible trends, such as the decrease of coercion, cannot be taken for granted and are subject to political forces (e.g. coercive treatment is introduced for those repeatedly taken into police custody for alcohol problems in the Northern Territory, Australia). As mentioned above, in England, changes from Labour to Conservative governments have changed the makeup of policies and treatment strategies. A rebalancing from pragmatic harm reduction and drug treatment in favour of alcohol has occurred. At the same time, a new emphasis on moral and social approaches can be observed, underlining the personal responsibility and burden of marginal populations on the welfare budget. Politically strengthened right wing parties in Switzerland are trying to implement guilt concepts demanding that hospitals should charge parents of young acutely intoxicated binge drinkers. Examples of aftermaths concerning health care and local government reformations are found in the Nordic countries. Addiction treatment in Norway (Nesvåg and Lie, 2010) and Finland (Tammi and Stenius, 2014) has faced and faces centralization, whereas treatment in Denmark has been decentralized (Bjerge, 2012). These comprehensive reforms were by-products of larger reforms and were not driven by arguments specific to addiction treatment. As an anomaly that proves the rule, an independent centralization reform proposal – not tied to an overarching reform – regarding Swedish addiction treatment was turned down in 2013 (Storbjörk, 2014b).
- A strong **integration dynamic** is under way regarding AOD with other health/welfare systems. Most common is the integration of Mental Health Care and addiction treatment, but the full implementation into the general public health care systems is also a perspective adopted. An example is Switzerland, which turned towards a public health approach. This tendency is facilitated by attempts to medicalize treatment and to diffuse addiction-related pharmaceutics, for example, in Poland. Fear or processes of **medicalization**

are also reported in Denmark, Finland, Norway, Poland, Sweden and Switzerland. Other examples of integration efforts are found in Finland (integration with mental health initiated in 2009), Canada (more collaboration with mental health and primary care is anticipated), Iceland and the Netherlands (anticipated integration with primary health care).

- The abstinence paradigm in treatment in terms of zero-tolerance has been softened and complemented by **alternative legitimate outcomes and treatment and harm-reduction modalities**. In the USA, as the Medicaid code covers providers and physicians for screening and brief interventions and referral for treatment (SBRIT), the focus has shifted on reduction of use and non-abstinence (Humphreys and Frank 2014). Harm reduction measures, in a first phase limited to 'experimental countries' (e.g. Switzerland and the Netherlands), have by now gained ground in most countries, although with different speed and with alcohol harm reduction only slowly 'catching up' with drug use. More specifically, heroin prescription, needle exchanges, supervised injection facilities and opioid overdose prevention by Naloxone have become more prevalent and easier to defend in the debate. However, there is always a debate before installing such facilities, as exemplified by the cases of Canada and Norway. Supervised Injection Facilities have been at the centre of political controversy in Canada due to its reliance on federally-issued exemptions, failed renewals and court cases. Moreover, heroin prescription has been debated and opposed for some years in Norway. As concerns other countries in our survey, Australia belongs to countries with a longer tradition of harm reducing interventions, whereas China (driven by an HIV epidemic), England, Finland, Iceland and even Sweden – with its strong reliance on prohibition – are advancing in these respects.
- A higher sensitivity to the **treatment gap in** terms of outreach and new treatment approaches becomes evident. The perspective, however, is oriented towards *groups with specific needs* such as young people, women, trauma victims. Aboriginal people, individuals with dual diagnoses and treatment naive, and often socially integrated people with the beginning of alcohol problems. A bias in most treatment systems in terms of not investing resources according to the burden of diseases persists when comparing licit and illicit drug use. Political consensus across the political spectrum can be easily reached when emphasizing measures for young people and women, whereas men's health and specific treatment needs, as well as the situation of older adults, are topics only reluctantly addressed. There are, however, countries that swim against the tide and openly prioritize more marginalized users. For example, Denmark is actively trying to reach the most excluded, vulnerable and often older drug users and, like Norway, invests in the prevention of drug overdoses. Iceland has opened an outreach programme for injecting drug users.
- Increased **efforts to control, increase effectiveness and 'systemize'** treatment systems can be observed on several levels: Firstly, efforts to **monitor addiction** and treatment have been intensified in many countries, documenting problem trends and treatment efforts. Participation in these *monitoring* systems tends to be mandatory and imposed by funding sources. Secondly, in many countries, **NPM** has been adopted and applied to addiction treatment. An interesting example is Finland, which was anticipated to turn into one big market in which five regions would purchase care from local providers, a development that would include annual performance target negotiations and performance evaluations of the local providers. However, the reform was put on hold until after the 2015 election. Thus, this development implies quality indicators/control, diffusion of guidelines, attempts to standardize treatment according to EBP and outcome-evaluation (e.g. Australia, Canada, Denmark, Finland, Netherlands, Norway, and Sweden). However, monitoring, performance measurements, and guidelines – tools for steering and controlling systems – can also be found independent of the presence of NPM, for example, in Canada with a low degree of marketization and competition. More systemic views have been replaced by **result oriented perspectives** where England stands out as an interesting example as payment by results contracts, emphasizing treatment completion and successful exit from treatment regardless of treatment technique, are being adopted. Likewise, Australia focuses on outcomes. In Iceland, marketization is low and no performance measurement system has been adopted. Neither does Poland have performance

measurements or quality controls. Thirdly, changes in the power distribution/task between central and regional authorities are seen as a strategy to steer treatment; as described above, centralization tendencies can be observed in the Nordic countries. However, the impact is uncertain as federalist countries such as Canada, Australia and Switzerland show that the political power in health matters belongs to the provinces/regions. An exception is China, which decentralized drug treatment and shifted it to the local level 2008.

From a more general perspective, the 14 reports demonstrate a high degree of reformation, considerable complexity and broad diversity of treatment provisions *within* each country. Consequently, this represents a high barrier to any general model construction and planning.

TREATMENT SYSTEM RESEARCH: MIND THE GAPS IN TREATMENT SYSTEMS RESISTANT TO CHANGE!

Room forwarded the concept of the 'two worlds of alcohol problems' (Room, 1977) to highlight the difference between the focus on clinical populations and a more general epidemiological perspective. Those not accessing treatment have been the subject of self-change research, which has shown that most people quit or control their problem behaviour on their own (Klingemann et al., 2010). Yet, the interface between the two worlds has only slowly been acknowledged. Attempts to put the treatment gap on the agenda are still characterized by a top down approach assuming illiterate addicted populations, which should be reached for their own good. For pragmatic, but also ideological reasons, empirical needs assessment approaches are often based on crude indirect methods and do not give a voice to potential customers in their specific socio-cultural environments. Consequently, the quest for the *best* treatment organization and the *best* treatment methods/modalities that are universally valid belongs to a 'third world of planners' and at best provides 'ideal types' in the sense of Max Weber (see also Rush, 2010: 632). The adoption of the market model in practice was therefore to be expected. We can conclude that the crisis in the addiction treatment systems is characterized by a widening gap between the two (three) worlds of alcohol problems (Klingemann and Bergmark, 2006) with epidemiological studies as an eye opener (Smart, 2007). A first step to empirically assess the conditions for a more adequate treatment response is to overcome the static view of treatment systems and have a look at factors, often outside the treatment system, which promote or impede change. It is thus clear by now that there are a range of 'non-specific' or 'common factors' that, regardless of the specific treatment technique, help produce good outcomes (Bergmark, 2008; Messer and Wampold, 2002: Wampold and Imel, 2008). Hence, the perceived importance of treatment as a response to perceived addiction problems should perhaps be downplayed somewhat.

Why don't continents move? Why don't people (treatment systems) change?

A reformulation of Prochaska and Prochaska's (1999) transtheoretical model points to the observation that addiction treatment systems tend to evolve slowly over a long period of time, and concepts such as 'path dependency' (Pierson, 2000) have been put forward to explain such permanency. It implies a tendency towards preserving existing arrangements – the status quo. Interests, conceivable options and decisions are limited by past decisions, even though previous circumstances no longer apply. Solutions and work models may survive despite the fact that the original problem has faded away and organizations find reasons to survive in a changing environment.

Overall, research on the rationale, process, promoting and hindering factors, and outcomes of treatment system reforms, are neglected areas of research (Wahlbeck, 2010). There are plenty of examples of how evidence-based interventions have not been translated into practice in treatment systems across the world. We can mention how opiate maintenance treatment (methadone and buprenorphine) and needle-exchange programmes for long were strongly limited and regulated in Sweden, despite the solid evidence-base, because they did not fit into the prohibitionist drug policy (Johnson and Hagström, 2005; Tryggvesson, 2012). Another example is the growing scientific support for controlled drinking or moderation as treatment goals (Dawson et al., 2005; Sanchez-Craig et al., 1984) and how this idea has been opposed (Sobell and Sobell, 2011) because it conflicts with the ideology of the strong AA movement and previous beliefs, which is well-rooted in the loss of control dimension of the dependence concept, that alcoholics cannot stop drinking once they have started.

Addiction treatment system reforms are often made without considering the implications for the population; there appears to be little scientific evidence behind reforms (Babor et al., 2008), and such efforts seem to have little impact on treatment outcomes (Humphreys and McLellan, 2011; Pedersen et al., 2011). The scarce research indicates that major organizational changes to treatment systems are driven more by circumstances other than scientific findings concerning the effectiveness of the imposed model (Room, 1998, Rosenqvist and Stenius, 1986). For example, comprehensive reforms of addiction treatment systems are often by-products of larger reforms concerning the overarching structure and not driven by problems or arguments specific to addiction care (MacGregor, 2013; Sabatier, 1998) (see Nordic examples in 'Current trends and changes: a brief expert survey in 14 countries'). Debates and reforms are foremost guided by ideological, political and economic considerations – often *claiming* to be research-oriented. Policy processes and controversies may be more driven by overarching narratives and value differences than by technical deficiencies or scientific evidence, especially when it comes to social policy and sciences, and areas such as substance abuse for which the evidence-base is quite scarce (Kübler, 2001; MacGregor, 2013; Tieberghien and Decorte, 2013; Weible, 2007; Weiss, 1979). Belgian (Tieberghien and Decorte, 2013) and UK (MacGregor, 2013) studies of drug policy show how overarching narratives of drugs play a dominant role in policymaking. Science may be used, either as ammunition to promote a certain course of action or as subordinate to other types of information and competing values, interests and electoral considerations – a tension between science and values.

REFERENCES

Allen, J. P., Mattson, M. E., Miller, W. R., Tonigan, J. S., Connors, G. J., Rychtarik, R. G. Townsend, M. (1997). Matching alcoholism treatments to client heterogeneity: Project MATCH post treatment drinking outcomes. *Journal of Studies on Alcohol*, 58(1): 7–29.

Anton, R. F., O'Malley, S. S., Ciraulo, D. A., Cisler, R. A., Couper, D., Donovan, D. M., Gastfriend, D.R., Hosking, J.D., Johnson, B.A., LoCastro, J.S., Longabaugh, R., Mason, B.J., Mattson, M.E., Miller, W.R., Pettinati, H.M., Randall, C.L., Swift, R., Weiss, R.D., Williams, L.D., Zweben A. and COMBINE Study Research Group (2006). Combined pharmacotherapies and behavioral interventions for alcohol dependence. The COMBINE study: a randomized controlled trial. *JAMA*, 295(17): 2003–17.

Atlas on substance use (2010). *Resources for Prevention and Treatment of Substance Use Disorders*. Geneva: World Health Organization.

Babor, T. F. (2015). Treatment systems for population management of substance use disorders: requirements and priorities from a public health perspective. In N. El-Guebaly and A. Uchtenhagen (eds), *Textbook of Addiction*

Treatment: International Perspectives. Milan: Springer-Verlag Italia, pp. 1214–27.
Babor, T. F. and Poznyak, V. (2010). The World Health Organization substance abuse instrument for mapping services. Rationale, structure and functions. *Nordic Studies on Alcohol and Drugs,* 27(6): 703–11.
Babor, T. F., Stenius, K. and Romelsjö, A. (2008). Alcohol and drug treatment systems in public health perspective: mediators and moderators of population effects. *International Journal of Methods in Psychiatric Research,* 17(1): 50–9.
Berglund, M., Thelander, S. and Jonsson, E. (eds) (2003). *Treating Alcohol and Drug Abuse: An Evidence Based Review*. Weinheim and Cambridge: Wiley-VCH.
Bergmark, A. (1998). The relationship between alcohol and drug treatment systems. In H. Klingemann and G. Hunt (eds), *Drug Treatment Systems in an International Perspective. Drugs, Demons and Delinquents*. Thousand Oaks: Sage Publications, pp. 298–307.
Bergmark, A. (2008). On treatment mechanisms – what can we learn from the COMBINE study? *Addiction,* 103(5): 703–5.
Bergmark, A. (2010). On the idea of treatment systems. *Nordic Studies on Alcohol and Drugs,* 27(6): 565–73.
Bjerge, B. (2012). Structural reforms as New Public Management policy: three dilemmas in Danish substance misuse treatment. In M. Hellman, G. Roos and J. von Wright (eds), *A Welfare Policy Patchwork: Negotiating The Public Good in Times of Transition*. Helsinki: Nordic Centre for Welfare and Social Issues (NVC), pp. 181–201.
Blocker, J. S., Fahey, D. M. and Tyrell, I. R. (eds) (2003). *Alcohol and Temperance in Modern History: An International Encyclopedia.* Santa Barbara: ABC-Clio.
Breslin, C., Sobell, M., Sobell, L., Cunningham, J. A., Sdao, J. K. and Borsoi, D. (1998). Problem drinkers: evaluation of a stepped care approach. *Journal of Substance Abuse,* 10(3): 217–32.
Burton, J. and van den Broek, D. (2009). Accountable and countable: Information management systems and the bureaucratization of social work. *British Journal of Social Work*, 39(7): 1326–42.
Christensen, T. and Lægreid, P. (2011). Complexity and hybrid public administration – theoretical and empirical challenges. *Public Organization Review*, 11(4): 407–23.
Davies, B. (2003). Death to critique and dissent? The policies and practices of new managerialism and of 'evidence-based practice'. *Gender and Education*, 15(1), 91–103.
Davis, A. K. and Rosenberg, H. (2013). Acceptance of non-abstinence abstinence goals by addiction professionals in the United States. *Psychology of Addictive Behaviors,* 27(4): 1102–9.
Dawe, S. and Richmond, R. (1997). Controlled drinking as a treatment goal in Australian alcohol treatment agencies. *Journal of Substance Abuse Treatment,* 14(1): 81–6.
Dawson, D. A., Grant, B. F., Stinson, F. S., Chou, P. S., Huang, B. and Ruuan, W. J. (2005). Recovery from DSM-IV alcohol dependence: United States, 2001–2002. *Addiction,* 100(3): 281–92.
DiClemente, C. C. (2007). Mechanisms, determinants and processes of change in the modification of drinking behavior. *Alcoholism-Clinical and Experimental Research,* 31(10): 13–20.
Drechsler, W. (2005). The re-emergence of 'Weberian' public administration after the fall of New Public Management: the central and eastern European perspective. *Administrative Culture,* 6: 94–108.
Drummond, C., Gual, A., Goos, C., Godfrey, C., Deluca, P., Von Der Goltz, C., Gmel, G., Scafato, E., Wolstenholme, A., Mann, K., Coulton, S. and Kaner E. (2011). Identifying the gap between need and intervention for alcohol use disorders in Europe. *Addiction,* 106(1): 31–6.
Duke, K. (2013). From crime to recovery: the reframing of British drug policy. *Journal of Drug Issues*, 43(1): 39–55.
Dunleavy, P., Margetts, H., Bastow, S. and Tinkler, J. (2006). New Public Management is dead – long live digital-era governance. *Journal of Public Administration Research and Theory*, 16(3): 467–94.
Eagar, K., Garrett, P. and Lin, V. (2001). *Health Planning: Australian Perspectives*. Crows Nest: Allen and Unwin.
EMCDDA. (2013). *EMCDDA Treatment Strategy*. Lisbon: European Monitoring Centre for

Drugs and Drug Addiction. Available from: www.emcdda.europa.eu/system/files/publications/735/Treatment_strategy_413394.pdf (Accessed 12 April 2016).

Evetts, J. (2009) New professionalism and New Public Management: changes, continuities and consequences. *Comparative Sociology*, 8(2): 247–66.

Fahrenkrug, W. H. (1984). *Alkohol, Individuum und Gesellschaft. Zur Sozialgeschichte des Alkoholproblems in den USA*. Frankfurt/Main: Campus.

Ferrence, R. (2001). Diffusion theory and drug use. *Addiction,* 96(1): 165–73.

Garner, B. R. (2009). Research on the diffusion of evidence-based treatments within substance abuse treatment: a systematic review. *Journal of Substance Abuse Treatment,* 36(4): 376–99.

Gingrich, J. R. (2011). *Making Markets in the Welfare State: The Politics of Varying Market Reforms*. Cambridge: Cambridge University Press.

Glaser, F. (2001). Journal interview – Conversation with Frederick B. Glaser. *Addiction*, 96(12): 1709–23.

Glaser, F. B., Greenberg, S. W. and Barrett, M. (1978). *A Systems Approach to Alcohol Treatment*. Toronto: Alcohol Research Foundation.

Hall, W., Babor, T. F., Edwards, G., Laranjeira, R., Marsden, J., Miller, P., Obot, I., Petry, N., Thamarangsi, T. and West, R. (2012). Compulsory detention, forced detoxification and enforced labour are not ethically acceptable or effective ways to treat addiction. *Addiction* 107(11): 1891–3.

Hall, W., Babor, T. F., Laranjeira, R., Marsden, J., Miller, P., Obot, I., Petry, N., Thamarangsi, T. and West, R. (2013). Compulsory detention in addiction treatment. Response. *Addiction,* 108(3): 650–1.

Hansen Löfstrand, C. (2012). Homelessness as politics and market. In B. Larsson, M. Letell and H. Thörn (eds), *Transformations of the Swedish welfare state: From Social Engineering to Governance*. New York: Palgrave Macmillian, pp. 247–61.

Heimer, C. A. (2012). Inert facts and the illusion of knowledge: strategic uses of ignorance in HIV clinics. *Economy and Society*, 41(1): 17–41.

Heinrich, C. J. and Cummings, G. R. (2014). Adoption and diffusion of evidence-based addiction medications in substance abuse treatment. *Health Services Research,* 49(1): 127–52.

Herie, M. and Martin, G. W. (2002). Knowledge diffusion in social work: a new approach to bridging the gap. *Social Work,* 47(1): 85–95.

HM Government (2010). *Drug Strategy 2010: Reducing Demand, Restricting Supply, Building Recovery: Supporting People to Live a Drug Free Life*. London: HM Government.

Hood, C. (1995). The 'New Public Management' in the 1980s: variations on a theme. *Accounting Organizations and Society,* 20(2–3): 93–109.

Hull, P. and Ritter, A. (2014). *The Potential Role of Pay-For-Performance in Alcohol and Other Drug Treatment Funding: A Literature Review*. Sydney: Drug Policy Modelling Program, National Drug and Alcohol Research Centre, UNSW.

Humphreys, K. and McLellan, A.T. (2011). A policy-oriented review of strategies for improving the outcomes of services for substance use disorder patients. *Addiction,* 106(12): 2058–66.

Humphreys, K., Weingardt, K. R., Horst, D., Joshi, A. A. and Finney, J. W. (2005). Prevalence and predictors of research participant eligibility criteria in alcohol treatment outcome studies, 1970–1998. *Addiction*, 100(9): 1249–57.

Humphreys, K. and Frank, R.G. (2014). The affordable care act will revolutionize care for substance use disorders in the United States. *Addiction*, 109: 1957–8.

Hunt, N. and Stevens, A. (2004). Whose harm? Harm reduction and the shift to coercion in UK drug policy. *Social Policy and Society,* 3(4): 333–42.

Institute of Medicine (IOM) (1990). *Broadening the Base of Treatment for Alcohol Problems*. Washington, DC: National Academy Press.

Israelsson, M. and Gerdner, A. (2012). Compulsory commitment to care of substance misusers: international trends during 25 years. *European Addiction Research,* 18(6): 302–21.

Jeek Wook, K., Lee, B. C., Tae-Cheon, K. and Ihn-Geun, C. (2013). The current situation of treatment systems for alcoholism in Korea. *Journal of Korean Medical Science,* 28(2): 181–9.

Johnson, B. and Hagström, B. (2005). The translation perspective as an alternative to the policy diffusion paradigm: the case of the Swedish methadone maintenance treatment. *Journal of Social Policy*, 34(3): 365–88.

Kaukonen, O. and Stenius, K. (2005). Universalism under re-construction: from administrative coercion to professional subordination of substance abusers. In N. Kildaland and S. Kuhnle (eds), *Normative Foundation of the Welfare State. The Nordic Experience*. London and New York: Routledge, pp. 130–48.

Klingemann, H. (1986). Control or cooperation – lay help and professional intervention in alcohol problems in Switzerland. *Zeitschrift für Soziologie,* 15(4): 259–77.

Klingemann, H. and Bergmark, A. (2006). The legitimacy of addiction treatment in a world of smart people. *Addiction,* 101(9): 1230–7.

Klingemann, H. and Hunt, G. (eds) (1998). *Drug Treatment Systems in an International Perspective: Drugs, Demons and Delinquents.* London: Sage Publications.

Klingemann, H. and Klingemann, H. D. (1999). National treatment systems in global perspective. *European Addiction Research,* 5(3): 109–17.

Klingemann, H. and Rosenberg, H. (2009). Acceptance and therapeutic practice of controlled drinking as an outcome goal by Swiss alcohol treatment programmes. *European Addiction Research,* 15(3): 121–7.

Klingemann, H., Schlaefli, K. and Steiner, M. (2013). 'What do you mean by spirituality? Please draw me a picture!' Complementary faith-based addiction treatment in Switzerland from the client's perspective. *Substance Use and Misuse,* 48(12): 1187–202.

Klingemann, H., Sobell, M. B. and Sobell, L. C. (2010). Continuities and changes in self-change research. *Addiction,* 105(9): 1510–8.

Klingemann, H. and Takala, J. P. (1987). International studies of the development of alcohol treatment systems – a research agenda for the future. *Contemporary Drug Problems*, 14(1): 1–13.

Klingemann, H., Takala, J. P. and Hunt, G. (eds) (1992). *Cure, Care or Control: Alcoholism Treatment in Sixteen Countries.* Albany: State University of New York Press.

Klingemann, H., Takala, J. P. and Hunt, G. (1993). The development of alcohol treatment systems: an international perspective. *Alcohol Health and Research World,* 17(3): 221–7.

Klingemann, J. (2016). Acceptance of Reduced-Risk Drinking as a Therapeutic Goal within the Polish Alcohol Treatment System. *Alcohol and Alcoholism*, 51(4): 436–441.

Kübler, D. (2001). Understanding policy change with the advocacy coalition framework: an application to Swiss drug policy. *Journal of European Public Policy,* 8(4): 623–41.

Ledermann, S. (1964). *Alcool, Alcoolisation, Alcoolism*, Vol. 2. Paris: PUF.

Lloyd, C. (2013). The stigmatization of problem drug users: a narrative literature review. *Drugs: Education, Prevention and Policy,* 20(2): 85–95.

Lu, M. and Ma, C. T. (2006). Financial incentives and gaming in alcohol treatment. *Inquiry*, 43(1): 34–53.

Luborsky, L., Rosenthal, R., Diguer, L., Andrusyna, T. P., Berman, J. S., Levitt, J. T., Seligman, D.A. and Krause, E. D. (2002). The dodo bird verdict is alive and well – mostly. *Clinical Psychology: Science and Practice,* 9(1): 2–12.

Luquiens, A., Reynaud, M. and Aubin, H. J. (2011). Is controlled drinking an acceptable goal in the treatment of alcohol dependence? A survey of French alcohol specialists. *Alcohol and Alcoholism,* 46(5): 586–91.

Mäkelä, K. (1991). Social and cultural preconditions of Alcoholics-Anonymous (AA) and factors associated with the strength of AA. *British Journal of Addiction,* 86(11): 1405–13.

Mäkelä, K. (2001). Conversation with Klaus Mäkelä. *Addiction,* 96(10): 1393–403.

Mäkelä, Klaus, Ilkka Arminen, Kim Bloomfield, Irmgard Eisenbach-Stangl, Karin Helmersson Bergmark, Noriko Kurube, Nicoletta Mariolini, Hildigunnur Ólafsdóttir, John H. Peterson, Mary Phillips, Jürgen Rehm, Robin Room, Pia Rosenqvist, Haydée Rosovsky, Kerstin Stenius, Grazyna Swiatkiewicz, Bohdan Woronowicz and Antoni Zielinski (eds) (1996). *Alcoholics Anonymous as a Mutual-Help Movement. A Study in Eight Societies*. Madison: The University of Wisconsin Press.

Mäkelä, K. and Säilä, S. L. (1987). The distribution of alcohol-related overnight stays among different authorities in Finland, 1960–1980. *Contemporary Drug Problems,* 14(1): 125–36.

MacGregor, S. (2013). Barriers to the influence of evidence on policy: are politicians the problem? *Drugs: Education, Prevention and Policy*, 20(3): 225–33.

McGoey, L. (2012a). Strategic unknowns: towards a sociology of ignorance. *Economy and Society,* 41(1): 1–16.

McGoey, L. (2012b). The logic of strategic ignorance. *British Journal of Sociology,* 63(3): 533–76.

McGonigle, J. J., Krouk, M., Hindmarsh, D. and Campano-Small, C. (1992). Understanding partial hospitalization through the continuity-of-care model. *International Journal of Partial Hospitalization*, 8(2): 135–40.

McLellan, T., Kemp, J., Brooks, A. and Carise, D. (2008). Improving public addiction treatment through performance contracting: the Delaware experiment. *Health Policy*, 87(3): 296–308.

McSweeney, T., Stevens, A., Hunt, N. and Turnbull, P. J. (2007). Twisting arms or a helping hand? Assessing the impact of 'coerced' and comparable 'voluntary' drug treatment options. *British Journal of Criminology*, 47(3): 470–90.

Messer S. and Wampold, B. (2002). Let's face facts: common factors are more potent than specific therapy ingredients. *Clinical Psychology: Science and Practice*, 9(1): 21–5.

Miller, W. R., Sorensen, J. L., Selzer, J. A. and Brigham, G. S. (2006). Disseminating evidence-based practices in substance abuse treatment: a review with suggestions. *Journal of Substance Abuse Treatment,* 31(1): 25–39.

Mitchell, O., Wilson, D. B., Eggers, A., & MacKenzie, D. L. (2012). Assessing the effectiveness of drug courts on recidivism: A meta-analytic review of traditional and non-traditional drug courts. *Journal of Criminal Justice*, 40(1), 60–71.

Moore, D. and Fraser, S. (2013). Producing the 'problem' of addiction in drug treatment. *Qualitative Health Research*, 23(7): 916–23.

Moore, G., Redman, S., Haines, M. and Todd, A. (2011). What works to increase the use of research in population health policy and programme: a review. *The Policy Press*, 7(3): 277–305.

Morisano, D., Babor, T. F. and Robaina, K. A. (2014). Co-occurrence of substance use disorders with other psychiatric disorders: implications for treatment services. *Nordic Studies on Alcohol and Drugs,* 31(1): 5–25.

Muckle, W., Muckle, J., Welch, V., and Tugwell, P. (2012). Managed alcohol as a harm reduction intervention for alcohol addiction in populations at high risk for substance abuse. *Cochrane Database of Systematic Reviews* (12).

National Treatment Agency for Substance Misuse (2002). *Models of Care for Treatment of Adult Drug Misusers. Update*. London: National Treatment Agency for Substance Misuse.

National Institute on Drug Abuse (NIDA) (2012). *Principles of Drug Addiction Treatment: A Research-Based Guide*, 3rd edn. Washington, DC: National Institute on Drug Abuse.

Nesvåg, S. and Lie, T. (2010). The Norwegian substance treatment reform: between New Public Management and conditions for good practice. *Nordic Studies on Alcohol and Drugs*, 27(6): 655–66.

Nilssen, E. (2005). Coercion and justice: a critical analysis of compulsory intervention towards adult substance abusers in Scandinavian social law. *International Journal of Social Welfare*, 14(2): 134–44.

Orford, J. (2006). Is treatment-matching dead? Comments on Bühringer. *Addiction*, 101(5): 653–4.

Orford, J., Hodgson, R., Copello, A., John, B., Smith, M., Black, R., Fryer, K., Handforth, L., Alwyn, T., Kerr, C., Thistlethwaite, G., Slegg, G. and UKATT Research Team (2006). The clients' perspective on change during treatment for an alcohol problem: qualitative analysis of follow-up interviews in the UK alcohol treatment trial. *Addiction*, 101(1): 60–8.

Parsons, T. (1951). *The Social System*. London and New York: Collier-Macmillan The Free Press.

Pedersen, M. U., Hesse, M. and Bloomfield, K. (2011). Abstinence-orientated residential rehabilitation of opioid users in Denmark: do changes in national treatment policies affect treatment outcome? *Scandinavian Journal of Public Health*, 39(6): 582–9.

Pedersen, M. U., Vind, L., Milter, M. and Grönbaek, M. (2004). *Alkoholbehandlingsindsatsen i Danmark – Semmenlignet med Sverige*. [The alcohol treatment efforts in Denmark – compared with Sweden.] Aarhus: Centre for Rusmiddelforskning.

Pierson, P. (2000). Path dependence, increasing returns, and the study of politics. *American Political Science Review*, 94(2): 251–67.

Pittman, D. J. (1967). Rush to combine – sociological dissimilarities of alcoholism and drug abuse. *British Journal of Addiction*, 62(3–4): 337–43.

Pittman, D. J. (1988). The combined approach – a comment. *British Journal of Addiction*, 83(8): 871–3.

Pittman, D. J. (1989). The combined approach – a response. *British Journal of Addiction*, 84(4): 444–5.

Poikolainen, K. (2002). A nice try that fails: the Swedish Council on Technology Assessment in HealthCare (SBU) evaluation of the effect of treatment of alcohol and drug problems: the epidemiologist's view. *Alcohol and Alcoholism*, 37(5): 416–18.

Pollitt, C. and Bouckaert, G. (2011). *Public Management Reform: A Comparative Analysis: New Public Management, Governance and the Neo-Weberian State*. Oxford: Oxford University Press.

Pollitt, C. and Sorin, D. (2011). *The Impacts of the New Public Management in Europe: A Meta-Analysis*, COCOPS Work Package 1, Deliverable 1.1. Rotterdam: COCOPS.

Pollitt, C., van Thiel, S. and Homburg, V. (2007). New Public Management in Europe. *Management Online Review*, 1–6.

Power, M. (1997). *Audit Society: Rituals of Verification*. Oxford: Oxford University Press.

Prochaska, J. O. and Prochaska, J. M. (1999). Why don't continents move? Why don't people change? *Journal of Psychotherapy*, 9(1): 83–102.

Raistrick, D. (1988). The combined approach – still an important debate. *British Journal of Addiction*, 83(8): 867–9.

Rehm, J., Rehm, M., Hannu, A., Allamani, A., Aubin, H., Bühringer, G., Daeppen, J. B., Frick, U., Gual, A. and Heather, N. (2013). Alcohol dependence treatment in the EU: a literature search and expert consultation about the availability and use of guidelines in all EU countries plus Iceland, Norway, and Switzerland. *The International Journal of Alcohol and Drug Research*, 2(2): 53–67.

Ritter, A., Hull, P., Berends, L. and Chalmers, J. (2014). *Planning Processes for Alcohol and Other Drug Treatment in Australia*, Working Paper No 9. Sydney: Drug Policy Modelling Program, National Drug and Alcohol Research Centre, UNSW. Available from: http://dpmp.unsw.edu.au/project/review (Accessed 13 April 2016)

Rogers, E.M. (1983). *Diffusion of Innovations*. New York: Free Press.

Rogers, E. M. (2002). Diffusion of preventive innovations. *Addictive Behaviors*, 27(6): 989–93.

Roizen, R. (1993). *Merging Alcohol and Illicit Drugs: A Brief Commentary on the Search for Symbolic Middle Ground*. Paper presented at the International Conference on Alcohol and Drug Treatment System Research, Toronto, Canada.

Room, R. (1977). Measurement and distribution of drinking patterns and problems in general populations. In G. Edwards, M. M. Gross, M. Keller, J. Moser and R. Room (eds), *Alcohol-Related Disabilities*. Offset Publication No. 32. Geneva: World Health Organization, pp. 61–87.

Room, R. (1998). Mutual help movement for alcohol problems in an international perspective. *Addiction Research and Theory*, 6(2): 131–45.

Room, R. (2005). Stigma, social inequality and alcohol and drug use. *Drug and Alcohol Review*, 24(2): 143–55.

Room, R. (2006). Taking account of cultural and societal influences on substance use diagnosis and criteria. *Addiction*, 101(Suppl. 1): 31–9.

Room, R. (2010). Alcohol and drug treatment systems: what is meant, and what determines their development. *Nordic Studies on Alcohol and Drugs*, 27(6): 575–9.

Room, R. (2011). Building a pan-European alcohol policy research competence. *Addiction*, 106(Suppl. 1): v–vi.

Rosenberg, H. and Davis, A. K. (2014). Differences in the acceptability of non-abstinence goals by type of drug among American substance abuse clinicians. *Journal of Substance Abuse Treatment*, 46(2): 214–18.

Rosenberg, H. and Melville, J. (2005). Controlled drinking and controlled drug use as outcome goals in British treatment services. *Addiction Research and Theory,* 13(1): 85–92.

Rosenberg, H., Devine, E. G. and Rothrock, N. (1996). Acceptance of moderate drinking by alcoholism treatment services in Canada. *Journal of Studies on Alcohol,* 57(5): 559–62.

Rosenqvist, P. and Stenius, K. (1986). Nya målgrupper för alkoholistvården. [New target groups for alcohol treatment.] *Alkoholpolitik – Tidskrift för Nordisk Alkoholforskning*, 3(4): 215–19.

Rosenzweig, S. (1936). Some implicit common factors in diverse methods of psychotherapy. *American Journal of Orthopsychiatry*, 6(3): 412–15.

Rush, B. (1990). A systems-approach to estimating the required capacity of alcohol treatment services. *British Journal of Addiction,* 85(1): 49–59.

Rush, B. (2010). Tiered framework for planning substance use service delivery systems: origins and key principles. *Nordic Studies on Alcohol and Drugs*, 27(6): 617–36.

Rush, B. R., Tremblay, J., Fougere, C., Behrooz, R., Perez, W. and Fineczko, J. (2013). *Development of a Needs-Based Planning Model for Substance Use Services and Supports in Canada: Final Report*. Toronto: Centre for Addiction and Mental Health.

Sabatier, P.A. (1998). The advocacy coalition framework: revisions and relevance for Europe. *Journal of European Public Policy*, 5(1): 98–130.

Sackett, D. L., Rosenberg, W. M., Gray, J. A., Haynes, R. B. and Richardson, W. S. (1996). Evidence based medicine: what it is and what it isn't. *BMJ*, 312(7023): 71–2.

Sanchez-Craig, M., Annis, H. M., Bronet, A. R. and MacDonald, K. R. (1984). Random assignment to abstinence and controlled drinking: Evaluation of a cognitive-behavioral program for problem drinkers. *Journal of Consulting and Clinical Psychology*, 52(3): 390–403.

Smart, R. G. (2007). Natural recovery or recovery without treatment from alcohol and drug problems as seen from survey data. In H. Klingemann and L. C. Sobell (eds), *Promoting Self-Change from Addictive Behaviors – Practical Implications for Policy, Prevention and Treatment*. New York: Springer, pp. 59–72.

Sobell, M. B. and Sobell, L. C. (2011). It is time for low-risk drinking goals to come out of the closet. *Addiction*, 106(10): 1715–17.

Stenius, K. (1999). *Privat Och Offentligt I Svensk Alkoholistvård: Arbetsfördelning, Samverkan Och Styrning Under 1900-Talet.* [Private and public in Swedish alcoholism treatment: division of labour, co-operation and management principles during the 20th century.] Lund: Arkiv.

Stenius, K. (2011). Market forces do not solve the problems. *Addiction*, 106(2): 2067–71.

Stern, S., von Stokar, T., Trageser, J. and Thomas, R. (2009). *Evaluation Act-Info*. Zürich: INFRAS.

Storbjörk J. (2012). On the significance of social control: treatment-entry pressures, self-choice and alcohol and drug dependence criteria one year after treatment. *International Journal of Social Welfare*, 21(2): 160–73.

Storbjörk J. (2014a). Implications of enrolment eligibility criteria in alcohol treatment outcome research: generalizability and potential bias in 1 and 5 year outcomes. *Drug and Alcohol Review,* 33(6): 604–11.

Storbjörk J. (2014b). Stakeholders' arguments for and against moving Swedish substance abuse treatment to the health care system: how a fat reform proposal became a thin government bill. *Nordic Studies on Alcohol and Drugs*, 31(1): 81–110.

Sulkunen P. (2009). *The Saturated Society: Governing Risk and Lifestyles in Consumer Culture*. Los Angeles: Sage.

Tammi, T. and Stenius, K. (2014). Capabilities for handling complex substance abuse problems and its relationship to the treatment system: using the DDCAT instrument to explore local treatment systems in Finland. *Nordic Studies on Alcohol and Drugs,* 31(1), 45–58.

Tang, Y. L., Hao, W. and Leggio, L. (2012). Treatments for alcohol-related disorders in China: a developing story. *Alcohol and Alcoholism,* 47(5): 563–70.

Tieberghien, J. and Decorte, T. (2013). Understanding the science-policy nexus in Belgium: an analysis of the drug policy debate (1996–2003). *Drugs: Education, Prevention and Policy*, 20(3): 241–8.

Tryggvesson K. (2012). Sprutbyte – visst, bara de slutar med droger. Svenska myndigheters och politikers hantering av rena sprutor till narkomaner. [Needle-exchange–of course, they just have to stop using drugs. On Swedish authorities' and policy-makers' handling of clean needles to drug users.] *Nordic Studies on Alcohol and Drugs*, 29(5): 519–40.

Uchtenhagen, A., Stevens, A., Berto, D., Frick, U., Hunt, N., Kerschl, V., McSweeney, T., Puppo, I., Santamaria, A., Schaaf, S., Steffan, E., Gegenhuber, B., Turnbull, P. and Werdenich, W. (2008). Evaluation of therapeutic alternatives to imprisonment for drug-dependent offenders. Findings of a comparative European multi-country study. *Heroin Addiction and Related Clinical Problems*, 10(2): 5–10.

United Nations Office on Drugs and Crime (UNODC) (2010). *From Coercion to Cohesion: Treating Drug Dependence Through Health Care, Not Punishment*. Discussion paper. Vienna: UNODC.

Van Boekel, L., Brouwers, E., van Weeghel, J. and Garretsen, H. (2013). Stigma among health professionals towards patients with substance use disorders and its consequences for healthcare delivery: systematic review. *Drug and Alcohol Dependence*, 131(1–2): 23–35.

Wahlbeck, K. (2010). Moving towards integrated addiction treatment systems. *Nordic Studies on Alcohol and Drugs*, 27(6): 699–702.

Wampold, B. and Imel, Z. (2008). The importance of treatment and the science of common factors in psychotherapy. In S. Brown and R. Lent (eds), *Handbook of Counselling Psychology*, 4th edn. Hoboken: John Wiley & Sons, pp. 249–62.

Weible, C. M. (2007). An advocacy coalition framework approach to stakeholder analysis: understanding the political context of California marine protected area policy. *Journal of Public Administration Research and Theory*, 17(1): 95–117.

Weisner, C., Hinman, A., Lu, Y., Chi, F. W. and Mertens, J. (2010). Addiction treatment ultimatums and U.S. health reform: a case study. *Nordic Studies on Alcohol and Drugs*, 27(6): 685–98.

Weisner, C. and Room, R. (1984). Financing and ideology in alcohol treatment. *Social Problems*, 32(2): 167–88.

Weiss, C. H. (1979). The many meanings of research utilization. *Public Administration Review*, 39(5): 426–31.

Wild, C., Newton-Taylor, B. and Alletto, R. (1998). Perceived coercion among clients entering substance abuse treatment: structural and psychological determinants. *Addictive Behaviors*, 23: 81–95.

Wild, T. C. (2006). Social control and coercion in addiction treatment: towards evidence-based policy and practice. *Addiction*, 101(1): 40–9.

Wild, T. C., Cunningham, J. A. and Ryan R. M. (2006). Social pressure, coercion, and client engagement at treatment entry: a self-determination theory perspective. *Addictive Behaviors*, 31(10): 1858–72.

Wilson, D. B., Mitchell, O. and MacKenzie, D. L. (2006). A systematic review of drug court effects on recidivism. *Journal of Experimental Criminology*, 2: 459–87.

Wild, T. C., Roberts, A. and Cooper, E. L. (2002). Compulsory substance abuse treatment: an overview of recent findings and issues. *European Addiction Research*, 8(2): 84–93.

Wiseman, J. P. (1970). *Stations of the Lost: The Treatment of Skid Row Alcoholics*. Englewood Cliffs: Prentice-Hall.

White, W. L. (2002). Addiction treatment in the United States: early pioneers and institutions. *Addiction*, 97(9): 1087–92.

World Health Organization (WHO) (2014). *Global Status Report on Alcohol and Health*. Geneva: World Health Organization. Available from: http://www.who.int/substance_abuse/publications/global_alcohol_report/msb_gsr_2014_1.pdf?ua=1 (Accessed 7 July 2014).

Xiao, S., Yang, M., Zhou, L. and Hao, W. (2015). Transition of China's drug policy: problems in practice. *Addiction*, 110: 193–4.

Zobel, F., Ramstein, T. and Arnaud, S. (2004). Les interventions publiques nationales en matière d'abus de substances et de dépendences. In Institut Universitaire de Medicine Sociale et Préventive (eds), *Raisons de Santé*, Vol. 101. Lausanne: IUMSP.

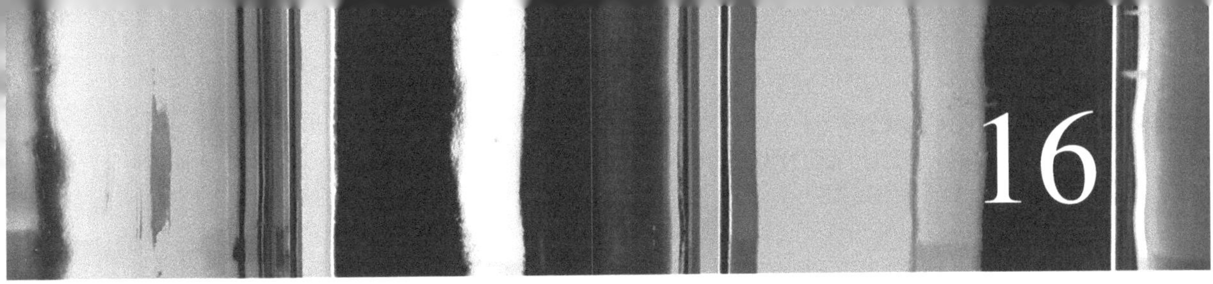

Matching Patients to Treatments or Matching Interventions to Needs?

Morten Hesse, Birgitte Thylstrup and Anette Søgaard Nielsen

INTRODUCTION

Although recovery from alcohol and drug abuse and dependence without formal treatment is quite common (Cunningham and Breslin, 2004), some patients may benefit from treatment interventions. First, early identification and intervention may reduce harm to oneself and others. Second, offering qualified treatment options seems relevant if some patients have tried to change alcohol or drug habits on their own several times without success.

Although some treatments have shown to be ineffective in the long-term (Roth and Fonagy, 1998), there is still no treatment that is known to be superior to other kinds of treatment for any type of substance use disorder (SUD). This has led some observers to think in terms of the 'dodo bird verdict', that is, all treatments are equally effective (Sellman, 2010), a statement that strongly simplifies what we know about addiction and its treatment (Carroll and Rounsaville, 2010).

In healthcare in general, personalized treatment has been a significant trend since the late twentieth century (Ginsburg et al., 2011), and the idea that when treating a patient other factors besides the diagnosis should be considered in a structured evidence-based fashion is gaining increasing support. Whilst the idea that a patient is more than his/her diagnosis may be as old as the idea of medical treatment itself, this approach is only recently beginning to merge with the ambition to ensure a science-based approach to treatment. In the field of medicine, this movement has focused primarily on molecular genetics to identify potential drugs that can be effective or harmful in treating a particular patient. However, in the field of psychiatry in general and substance use disorders in particular, personalized medicine is also an approach to psychotherapy.

THE HETEROGENEITY OF INDIVIDUALS WITH ALCOHOL AND DRUG USE DISORDERS

To a certain degree, drug and alcohol problems are social problems. However, people with substance use disorders are heterogeneous in many respects and vary in terms of social background, gender, age, intelligence, mood, attitude to their drug or alcohol use, the level of social support, the severity of their drug problems, and a wide range of other individual characteristics (Burnam and Watkins, 2006). These differences have prognostic significance: patients whose lives are functioning better have a later onset of substance use or externalizing problems, and patients who abuse fewer substances and have a less frequent family history of drug and alcohol problems are more likely to recover (e.g. Moss et al., 2010). Moreover, the relevance of possible psychiatric comorbidity has also received a great deal of attention (e.g. Grant et al., 2004), for instance, the fact that personality disorders predict specific treatment outcomes for specific patients (Jansson et al., 2009). However, other patient differences may be as important as their individual characteristics. Patients may differ in terms of their goals for treatment and perceived treatment needs, for instance, patients who have suffered fewer consequences from their substance use, those who have fewer non-drinking people in their social network, those who are young, or those who are enrolling in treatment for the first time are less likely to have a goal of total abstinence than patients with the opposite characteristics (DeMartini et al., 2014).

The heterogeneity within the substance abusing patient population and the difficulty in identifying a particular successful treatment approach for the patient population as a whole, has long led researchers to conclude that 'one size does not fit all'. Instead, the hypothesis that some treatments would be more attractive and effective in targeting specific patient groups than others has been put forward (Gibbon et al., 2010). Thus, many treatment institutions aim at offering a varied menu of treatment options that match the individual patient.

MATCHING TREATMENT TO PSYCHO-SOCIAL CHARACTERISTICS

In the alcohol and drug field, matching treatment to the patients' psycho-social characteristics has mainly consisted of attempts to match specific psychological characteristics to specific treatment interventions, models, or treatment structures. In the alcohol field in particular, studies have found that specific factors seem to affect treatment outcomes differentially in various treatment models, such as neuropsychological functioning, psychopathology, strategies in thinking, meaning seeking, self-efficacy, confidence, social functioning, prior Alcoholics Anonymous involvement, readiness to change drinking behavior, and cognitive flexibility (Longabaugh and Wirtz, 2001). These findings led to the idea to conduct a large trial to test the various matching hypotheses; the first major study, Project MATCH, was carried out in the 1990s (see also Chapter 35, this volume). In Project MATCH, 952 outpatients and 774 aftercare patients were randomized into one of three treatments: motivational enhancement therapy (MET), cognitive-behaviorally oriented coping skills therapy (CST), and 12-step facilitation (TSF). The MET is a low-intensity treatment consisting of only four sessions, in which patients are given feedback on their drinking habits, based on assessment results. After this, the therapist guides the patient through identifying discrepancies, for example, discrepancies between one's own perception of control over drinking and evidence of control, or between personal values and behavior when drinking and not drinking. Thus, a central aim of the sessions is to resolve ambivalence towards change and to strengthen commitment to positive change. The CST is a 12-session cognitive-behavioral treatment that is based on identifying high-risk situations for drinking or situations in which drinking is used to cope with experienced problems, developing alternative coping skills for high-risk situations and problem solving in collaboration between the patient and the therapist (Kadden et al., 1995). The TSF is a 12-session introduction to the Twelve Steps program of Alcoholics Anonymous that focuses mainly on the first three steps (accepting one's own powerlessness over drinking, surrendering control, and asking others for help) (Nowinski et al., 1999).

The idea behind Project MATCH was to identify patient characteristics that could predict success within these three different treatment models, and to test variables that had already shown evidence of being relevant matching variables. On a more conceptual level, the idea was that specific approaches to treatment would result in better outcomes, because the fit between patient characteristics and treatment characteristics would be superior to the 'one size fits all' approach. Consequently, it was hypothesized that matching patients to treatment would result in better outcomes than random treatment assignment. For instance, it was predicted that patients with higher levels of alcohol dependence would fare best with the TSF treatment, as the main message in this treatment approach would hypothetically match the patients' sense of powerlessness to control his or her drinking. It was also predicted that a higher intensity of treatment would result in better outcomes with patients with higher alcohol involvement, as these patients were less likely to change drinking habits without continuous and intensive support, and that patients with worse cognitive functioning would need a higher intensity of treatment over a longer period of time. In contrast, it was predicted that patients with high levels of anger would benefit from less confrontational and intensive treatments, and that patients with greater interest in religion would fare better with the TSF treatment because of its references to a higher power.

The failure to reject the null hypothesis in Project MATCH implied that the three treatments were equally effective for a wide range of patients suffering from alcohol use disorder. Drinking and negative consequences declined regardless of which treatment the patients received, even prior to treatment and at treatment entry (Babor, 2008). Of the 16 predicted matches, only one was supported by the findings in Project MATCH: patients with low psychiatric severity fared better with the TSF compared to the other two treatments (Allen et al., 1997b). A secondary analysis of an additional 17 pre-specified matches showed that patients who scored high on alcohol dependence fared better with the TSF, patients who scored low on alcohol dependence fared better with the CBT, and that patients with high levels of anger fared better with the MET (Allen et al., 1997a). Additionally, the low-intensity treatment (MET) did not produce poorer overall outcomes compared to the other two treatments, although it only consisted of four sessions compared to the 12 sessions in the other two interventions.

As a pragmatic attempt to test the matching effect and in order to test the main effects of two forms of treatment, the United Kingdom Alcohol Treatment Trial (UKATT) was carried out in the UK a few years later. In this study, MET was compared to a new treatment approach, Social Behaviour and Network Therapy (SBNT). The SBNT addresses both the patient's social behavior and functioning and involves his or her social network. More than 700 patients were randomized in the UKATT trial, and as was found in Project MATCH, the patients improved considerably during the outpatient treatment period in both treatment groups. As substantial reductions in alcohol consumption and better mental health were reported in both groups, and none of the matching hypothesis could be confirmed, the UKATT failed to even confirm any of the few findings from Project MATCH (Heather et al., 2008).

The question is why did so few matching variables predict outcomes in the two high quality trials? The project findings were surprising for several reasons. First, there were good conceptual reasons to accept most of the matching hypotheses. Also, the treatments in both studies were highly discriminable from each other (Carroll et al., 1998), had substantial empirical support, and the constructs used in the studies were assessed with well-validated instruments. Taking these factors into account, it awakened considerable surprise when both Project MATCH and UKATT demonstrated that so few matching effects were statistically significant and that the model lacked substantial explanatory power.

ASSESSMENT REACTIVITY: PATIENT BEHAVIOR AND REACTION TO TREATMENT

One possible explanation for the unexpected conclusions of the matching effects studies is that the very substantial assessments carried out before and after treatment had an effect that outweighed the effects of most of the matching variables or even the treatment itself. It is not surprising that a study that aims at testing 33 different matching hypotheses requires a rather lengthy assessment of various patient characteristics, such as motivation to change, cognitive functioning, and sociopathy. It is very likely that the thorough baseline assessment, which lasted for an average of eight hours, as well as the five follow-up waves, resulted in a substantial amount of patient contact during the course of the study, which in itself would produce marked effects. In support of this explanation is the fact that in the outpatient group in Project MATCH, very substantial reductions in use had already occurred in the time between the baseline assessment and the first treatment session (Allen et al., 1997b). This, and the fact that a new comprehensive assessment was undertaken in the study every three months, supports the hypothesis of assessment reactivity; that a large amount of assessment supports patient focus on specific problems in and of itself, thus promoting change, and in these two studies, a change in drinking behavior. Research conducted after Project MATCH has supported the assessment reactivity hypothesis in both outpatient and student samples, for example, a randomized study on 975 students with hazardous drinking showed that even only 10 minutes of assessment reduced their problems with alcohol 12 months later (Kypri et al., 2007). Although research literature within this field is still limited, and at this point only includes a few high-quality trials of adequate size, evidence is building that patients who are randomly assigned to be assessed more regularly, or more comprehensively or both, are more likely to fare better after treatment, and to participate and engage more quickly in further treatment and intensive treatment interventions (Maisto et al., 2007).

The next logical question is whether assessment reactivity will have an impact on treatment versus no treatment comparisons. A study by Hester and colleagues compared the difference between no-treatment and brief computer-delivered intervention (CDI) to reduce heavy drinking and alcohol-related problems in college students. In all, 144 students were randomized to either the CDI or an assessment-only control group with follow-ups at one and 12 months. Compared to the condition at baseline assessment for both the experimental and control groups, the mean between-groups effect sizes difference at follow-up averaged 0.34 and 0.36 at one and 12 months, respectively, a small effect size according to a generally accepted criterion. However, when only a minimal baseline assessment was conducted in the control group, the difference rose to 0.82, which is a large effect size (Hester et al., 2012). The amount of time needed to conduct the pre-treatment assessment was not provided by the authors, but the assessment was definitely less comprehensive than the assessment in Project MATCH. The findings provide strong evidence for the fact that significant and meaningful differences emerge as the result of including assessment in research and evaluation studies. Although UKATT involved far less assessment than Project MATCH, reducing the risk of assessment reactivity, UKATT also failed to show any significant matching effects (Heather et al., 2008). Still, far less use of assessment certainly does not mean that the amount of assessment in UKATT was minimal; whilst certainly shorter than the eight-hour assessment for Project MATCH, UKATT still had three hours of assessment prior to treatment entry, as well as two follow-up waves. Given that Clifford and colleagues found statistically and clinically meaningful effects from brief follow-up interviews (Clifford et al., 2007; Maisto et al., 2007), and that Kypri and colleagues found small but significant effects of a very brief follow-up assessment over 12 months later (Kypri et al., 2007), and that a fairly brief assessment in the study of Hester and colleagues may radically attenuate control and experimental differences (Hester et al., 2012), these findings cannot rule out the likelihood of finding meaningful matching effects. However, it remains possible that studies focusing on single matches, using much shorter baseline assessment packages and fewer follow-up waves, will provide a much larger power to detect relevant and significant matching effects.

THE TREATMENTS: SIMILARITIES, DIFFERENCES AND OTHER ASPECTS

While differences in treatment interventions were discriminated well in the Project MATCH and the UKATT, there were also certain similarities. In both projects, all treatments, including the MET, were highly structured. Studies have shown that highly structured treatment interventions that involve formal assessment as well as the development, monitoring and review of individual plans for patient care, reduce the heterogeneity of the treatment intervention and the error in assessing matches between patient characteristics and treatment models (i.e. Gastfriend and McLellan, 1997; Latimer et al., 2000a, 2000b). But what if the level of structure is an important matching characteristic in and of itself? What if subgroups of individuals with substance use disorders benefit more from treatment that is either high or low on structure? Some studies published shortly after Project MATCH suggest that this may be the case. For example, patients with drug use disorders (DUD), who have depressive symptoms, and patients with high levels of so-called 'learned helplessness' in particular, seem to benefit from high levels of structure with a directive therapist, whereas patients low on learned helplessness seem to benefit more from a less structured treatment (Gottheil et al., 2002; Thornton et al., 2003).

That the structure plays a significant role is also supported by the fact that the compliance rate in Project MATCH was very high, and probably was related to the high rate of structured follow-up assessments, and the relatively short treatment period. In comparison, a Danish randomized controlled trial in an outpatient alcohol treatment institution randomized 150 consecutive patients to either low or high structured treatment (Nielsen et al., 1998). The low structured treatment was based on methods from psychoanalytical theory including willingness to discuss problems related to the alcohol abuse rather than the alcohol abuse itself, whereas the highly structured treatment was based on a written contract with formulated treatment goals, focusing on the alcohol abuse itself as well as detailed routines for developing coping strategies and evaluating progress. For both treatment conditions, the treatment period was longer (up to one-year) than in Project MATCH. Also, the study only involved baseline and follow-up assessments at one and two years after starting in treatment, in order to let the treatment process progress with as little disruption as possible. Inspired by the findings of an old study by McLachlan (1972), the Danish study used the patients' individual conceptual levels as a matching variable, that is, a schema that provides the basis by which the individual relates to the environmental events that he or she experiences (Harvey et al., 1961). It is assumed that the conceptual level spreads across a low to high continuum, involving the patient's attitude to the environmental structure, norms, and authorities, and his or her ability to solve conflicts (Harvey et al., 1961). The Danish study showed how matching the treatment structure to the conceptual level of the patients increased compliance and decreased the drop out from treatment (Nielsen et al., 1998). Thus, matching the treatment structure to the patients' conceptual levels did not affect outcome among the patients who stayed in treatment, but prevented dropouts and made more patients stay in treatment, thus increasing the likelihood for a better outcome (Carlson and Gabriel, 2001; Walker, 2009; Zhang et al., 2003).

COMMON FACTORS IN TREATMENTS

Another question raised by Project MATCH in particular is whether the treatments that were studied differed from each other significantly. While the treatment approaches in Project MATCH were clearly discriminable, important process indicators of treatment were not. For instance, all participants received a high level of exposure to their study treatments, and the intended difference in treatment dose between MET and the two more intensive treatments was achieved. As would be expected, Alcoholics Anonymous involvement was significantly higher for participants assigned to TSF versus the other treatments, and the treatments did not differ in the utilization of other non-study treatments. Non-specific aspects of treatment, such as the therapist's skillfulness and the quality of the therapeutic alliance, were comparable across treatment models (Carroll et al., 1998). However, individual variation and common factors that have little to do with treatment models and interventions may account for much of the observed change, a fact that is supported by much earlier treatment research (Brunette et al., 2004; Cleary et al., 2008; Graham et al., 2004; Meier et al., 2005). For instance, in Project MATCH, patients who scored relatively high in self-efficacy for maintaining abstinence at baseline had a rather good prognosis regardless of their relationship with the therapist, whereas patients who scored low on self-efficacy improved their prognosis dramatically if they were able to build a strong relationship with their therapist (Ilgen et al., 2006). The findings suggest that patients who need the support of a therapist may benefit regardless of the treatment model as long as they are able to build a good rapport with the therapist. This supports studies on the predictive value of the quality of the treatment rapport, that is, the predictive value of the patient's assessments of the treatment alliance (Horvath and Symonds, 1991), and of the therapist's ability to build a good rapport (Najavits et al., 2000; Siqueland et al., 2000; Thylstrup and Hesse, 2008). Likewise, the Danish study on patient-treatment matching demonstrated that patients with a relatively low conceptual level engaged more in treatment if treated by a therapist with a high conceptual level, while patients that showed a high conceptual level seemed to be able to engage in treatment of the therapist's conceptual level (Nielsen et al., 2000).

EXCLUSION CRITERIA IN STUDIES

Another relevant discussion point of the results in Project MATCH and UKATT is the high number of patients who were excluded from study participation, particularly in Project MATCH. For instance, Humphreys and Weisner have shown how the inclusion and exclusion criteria in research studies result in patient samples that differ considerably from patients in clinical practice (Humphreys and Weisner, 2000). Also, an analysis by Bühringer of deficits in research studies suggested that certain major design aspects of Project MATCH and other research studies, such as stringent patient exclusion criteria and low treatment dosage, minimize the chances of detecting patient-treatment interactions relevant for outcome (Buhringer, 2006). The patient exclusion rate in Project MATCH was indeed high (61 percent) for the sake of internal validity. However, when the research is streamlined by excluding a large proportion of patients during the assessment procedure at study intake, the variance in hypothetically relevant patient characteristics is also reduced considerably, affecting both the chances of detecting patient-placement information and the external validity of the study (Buhringer, 2006).

SUMMARY OF THE TWO MAJOR MATCHING STUDIES IN THE ALCOHOL FIELD

Both the Project MATCH and UKATT were large randomized clinical trials that had the statistical power to detect small effects. Nevertheless, the two major matching studies conducted in the alcohol field have been inconclusive to date, and have not helped us come closer to understanding whether matching particular patient characteristics to particular treatment models would improve care. Findings from studies on matching treatment to psycho-social characteristics imply that the best treatment we can provide to individuals with alcohol or drug problems involves a qualified, confident, and empathic counsellor, who believes in his/her own treatment approach as well as in the patient's ability to improve. However, as always in science, the failure to reject the null hypothesis does not automatically lead to the acceptance of the null hypothesis. Rather, the null hypothesis is always consistent with an infinite number of alternative explanations (for example, the experiment or measurement failed). Importantly, it has been suggested that future research should improve the theoretical and methodological basis for detecting other relevant patient-treatment interactions, and should stimulate research on other major treatment factors, such as specific treatment modules, site and setting, and time in treatment (extensiveness and intensity), as well as other relevant service components (Buhringer, 2006). Moreover, given the accumulating evidence that patients respond positively to baseline and follow-up assessment, it is also very likely that the comprehensive assessment needed to test a range of matching hypotheses is too effective in itself at positively changing drinking or drug use behavior, so that the actual treatment makes only an incremental difference.

WHERE DO WE GO FROM HERE? PERSPECTIVES ON MATCHING

An alternative way to test the matching hypothesis is to assess particular patient challenges and implement treatments that specifically address those challenges. That is, tailoring and adapting treatment interventions so they address current patient concerns as well as concerns that may arise as treatment progresses. This approach is sometimes referred to as 'enhanced services' or 'integrated care', and as far back as the early 1990s, well-designed studies supported the efficacy of enhanced treatment services (McLellan et al., 1993). One way forward may be to design very specific treatment strategies to reach very specific patient goals, the so called flexible treatment packages.

These treatment packages may come in the form of ongoing involvement by on-site or off-site services, such as when substance abuse treatment services offer linkage to treatment for infection with HIV or hepatitis C viruses, or in the form of time-limited approaches to specific patient problems over specific periods of time. Some, but not all, of these kinds of interventions may be evaluated meaningfully in terms of changes in substance use, but in certain cases substance use outcomes may be a distal, or even irrelevant outcome (McLellan et al., 2005, 2007). In some cases, regardless of whether treatment for infection with HIV or hepatitis C viruses has any impact on alcohol or drug use, the intervention may be extremely important for the patient's general physical health and overall well-being. In other cases, it is reasonable to state that the ultimate outcome should be reductions in substance use when linking patients to substance abuse treatment services, even if the ultimate outcome depends on the quality of the services that the patients have been offered (Hesse et al., 2007). Several studies that have tested specific psychotherapies and pharmacological treatments for specific conditions comorbid with substance use disorders have found that evidence-based treatment does not always need to focus exclusively on substance use outcomes in order to be helpful. For instance, antidepressant medication has been found to both reduce depressive symptoms and drug and alcohol use (Nunes and Levin, 2004), and psychotherapies for depression have been shown to reduce both as well (Hesse, 2009; Hunter et al., 2012; Watkins et al., 2011), whereas the same is not true of psychotherapies for anxiety (Hesse, 2009; Hunter et al., 2012; Watkins et al., 2011). The effect of the pharmacological treatments may be that by treating the depression or the anxiety, the patient becomes more capable of receiving treatment for his or her substance use disorder, as suggested by Nielsen and colleagues (Nielsen et al., 2000). Also, Safren and colleagues designed a treatment that addressed depressive symptoms and non-adherence to HIV treatment in a group of people who were HIV-positive, had serious depressive symptoms, and were in treatment for intravenous drug use. During treatment, significant gains were made in terms of treatment adherence to antiviral medication and depressive symptoms, and the gains in terms of depressive symptoms were retained at follow-up (Safren et al., 2012).

These examples emphasize that evidence-based treatment does not always need to focus exclusively on substance use outcomes, and that other patient concerns may be at least as important as the substance use. A more needs-based approach may target several problems related to the substance disorder and extend beyond the current standard of an acute care format, in which the expectation is that fixed amounts of medications or durations of treatment result in reductions in substance use and improvements in overall living conditions. One approach that falls under the flexible treatment package is the chronic care perspective advocated by McLellan and colleagues, in which treatment is provided for indeterminate periods, evaluated during the course of treatment, and may involve a form of continuing-care (McLellan et al., 2005). Another important concern is that, in some instances, patients who are not currently undergoing treatment may become the target of treatment (Thiesen and Hesse, 2010). For obvious reasons, the approach to treating patients who do not turn up at the clinic differs from the approach toward treating patients who do. For instance, Zanis and colleagues designed and tested an outreach counselling intervention for patients who had been discharged one-year earlier in the hope of helping them re-enroll in treatment. In the study, they identified patients who had died, patients who no longer needed treatment, and patients who needed treatment but were not receiving any at the time, and their study findings indicate that the outreach model brings more benefit to the patients as compared to the standard referral (Zanis et al., 1996). Another approach to reach out-of-treatment patients is through their close relatives. Several studies have tested a program called Community Reinforcement And Family Training (CRAFT) (Meyers et al., 1998; Roozen et al., 2010; Smith et al., 1998). The CRAFT program is based on behavior therapy, and encourages family members to support treatment entry, reinforce behaviors that are incongruent with drug or alcohol use through praise and appreciation (e.g. when the patient participates in family activities while sober), withholding attempts at negative reinforcement (e.g. scolding the patient for using substances), and taking steps to prevent family violence. The model has been tested against other models for family involvement, including the Johnson Institute Intervention (in which family members confront the patient with the consequences of the drug use), as well as Al Anon-based counselling (in which family members are encouraged to disengage from the patient until he or she agrees to enter treatment and accept a goal of total abstinence), and has been shown to be superior in terms of enrolment in treatment and reduction in substance use (Fals-Stewart and Birchler, 2001; O'Farrell and Fals-Stewart, 2001). What is important to emphasize is that the 'matching' is not a question of matching a psychotherapeutic treatment model to specific patient characteristics, but involves addressing the patient's living situation in general, such as cases in which the patient does not show up at the clinic door or does not have a supportive social network.

ALLOCATING OUTPATIENT PATIENTS TO LEVELS OF CARE

While there is evidence that matching effects do not occur when attempts are made to match patients to specific treatment modalities and contents, there may be some evidence that patients can be matched to treatment intensity. For example, patients with a high level of alcohol related problems seem to benefit more from intensive treatment (McKay et al., 2002), as did patients with a chaotic substance use and lifestyle and severe psychiatric problems (i.e. McLellan et al., 1983; Weisner et al., 2000). If matching patients to different treatment intensities is justified, the challenge is how to match them to the appropriate level of care in routine practice. In recent decades, researchers and clinicians have been working on developing allocation guidelines, for example the Patient Placement Criteria of the American Society of Addiction Medicine. The aim of these guidelines is to rethink how to engage people in treatment using six dimensions in the assessment procedure: intoxication, physical and mental health, readiness to change, relevance of relapse prevention, and recovery environment (Mee-Lee et al., 2013). However, the predictive value of following these guidelines and the degree of improvement of treatment outcomes is limited (Magura et al., 2003). Another example is the Stepped Care model, which defines the 'good level of care' as treatment in which the intensity and quality is monitored and assessed on a regular basis, and decisions on whether to intensify or de-intensify treatment are based on ongoing evaluations and perceived relevance to the individual patient situation (Bower and Gilbody, 2005; Sobell and Sobell, 2000).

Given the relative lack of empirically-based allocation guidelines, adapting a pragmatic approach for allocating alcohol dependent patients to appropriate levels of care seems worthwhile. Such pragmatic approaches are currently under development. In the Netherlands, Merkx and colleagues assess the predictive validity of guidelines for allocating outpatients to different levels of care in routine alcohol outpatient treatment facilities, based on the hypothesis that patients matched to the recommended level of care show better outcomes (Merkx et al., 2011). However, the study still has difficulty showing effect, which may be due in part to the diversity of the study sample, the need to adjust the algorithm for allocating patients, the need to increase differences in the intensity between the levels of care, and the need to improve the fidelity to the treatment manuals (Merkx et al., 2011). Nevertheless, the findings from the study still leave questions regarding the relevance of the effectiveness of the matching hypothesis undetermined. So far, there still seems to be a discrepancy between the evidence and the relevance of the matching hypothesis. National health authorities, social service administrations, and health insurance companies are still waiting for answers in their effort to avoid a mismatch between patients and treatments that may lead to the undertreatment or overtreatment of some patients with adverse treatment effects and wasted resources.

CHOOSING MATCHING VARIABLES

Another highly important reason for not yet being able to develop matching models between patient attributes and specific treatment models may be that the choice of patient characteristics is either wrongly chosen or wrongly defined. Until this point, most research on matching has been carried out in the field of alcohol treatment and has concentrated on studying 'objective' patient characteristics, such as drinking pattern, duration of the excessive drinking periods, drinking symptoms, and other characteristics related to alcohol consumption, in order to find the best way of matching patients to optimal treatment. The prioritization of these characteristics is based on the assumption that they correspond well with the aim of the treatment, yet this may be an oversimplified way to approach what treatment is actually about. Obviously, research in the field of substance abuse treatment requires the use of certain criteria for defining alcohol and drug problems and disorders, including loss of control, social impairment, and risky use or pharmacological dependence (APA, 2013). However, these criteria cannot mirror all of the dynamics that are involved in problems related to substance use disorders. The rather few qualitative studies that have been carried out on the patients' subjective perceptions of their problems and treatment needs indicate that the 'objective' symptoms or patient characteristics measured in quantitative studies may cover diverse subjective experiences (Nielsen, 2003). As drinking and drug behavior differ significantly between cultures and subcultures, the perceived problems and treatment needs are also very likely to vary between individuals (Nielsen, 2003).

It is probable that the heterogeneity in patients' perceptions of their individual characteristics, symptoms and other so-called 'objective' variables explains in part why research on treatment matching has shown rather disappointing results so far. Insight into the patient's particular situation may suggest treatment approaches that are not readily apparent from the clinical data alone. Not only should the patient's present circumstances and experience be taken into account, but also his or her past experience, as it is from this platform that he or she makes the decision whether to engage in treatment or not. Perhaps it is time to include a new matching criteria in studies on treatment matching, namely how the patients themselves experience their alcohol and drug use disorder. An inclusion of such criteria would contribute not only to our understanding of which patient needs the treatments should meet and match, but may also improve the way we address the patient's readiness to change (Prochaska and DiClemente, 1982) and collaborate with him or her during the process in determining the optimal form of treatment (Thylstrup, 2011; Ware et al., 2008).

CONCLUDING COMMENTS

Although it has proven difficult to identify matching variables that support treatment effect, it still makes clinical sense to match treatment to patient needs. In our view, the concept 'one size does not fit all' is as valid for substance abuse treatment as it ever was. As predicted by the Project MATCH research group, there may be slight differences between approaches to treatment that suit some patients better than others, but if there are, the studies have failed as of yet to identify the differences, and it remains to be established whether any one treatment is more qualified than others. In summary, it seems that the relevance of matching criteria differs from what we have believed to be relevant until now. Does this mean that we simply need individual custom-made treatments rather than matching evidence based treatments to the individual? Perhaps we do need a more individualized approach than what is practiced at the moment. However, there is no reason that such an approach should not use relevant knowledge from evidence-based treatment research and involve relevant assessment procedures as well as ongoing monitoring and evaluation. As these efforts have been shown to support the quality of treatment, they should be part of a standard treatment routine, as long as it does not disregard the individual patient's experiences, needs, and hopes for the future. The next logical step in the search to find a suitable and knowledge-driven method of allocating patients to treatments may be to provide evidence-based interventions that can help the patients improve in terms of their most salient concerns. This includes offering flexible treatment packages that are based on an ongoing involvement and collaboration with the patient, addressing other patient concerns in addition to the substance use, such as physical and mental health problems, housing, employment, family problems, and providing linkage to, and collaboration with, other relevant services. What we propose is that a 'new' match that involves a shared decision making process and allows the treatment provider to use his or her knowledge and expertise while simultaneously supporting the patient in choosing the treatment package that best suits his or her current life situation. Furthermore, we suggest that future addiction treatment research investigate potentially relevant factors further.

While individual patient characteristics are essential for meeting patient needs in substance use treatment, matching these needs with treatment allocation is also determined by a broad range of other factors. This includes the selection of site, setting and duration of treatment, the intensity of interventions, and choice of specific treatment components, as well as patient involvement, patient-therapist interaction, shared decision making, and social support. Not only are these factors important, but they may hold the keys to better our understanding of the usefulness of patient matching methods and their effect.

REFERENCES

Allen, J. P., Anton, R. F., Babor, T. F., Carbonari, J., Carroll, K. M., Connors, G. J. and Zweben, A. (1997a). Project MATCH secondary a priori hypotheses. *Addiction,* 92(12): 1671–1698.

Allen, J. P., Mattson, M. E., Miller, W. R., Tonigan, J. S., Connors, G. J., Rychtarik, R. G. and Townsend, M. (1997b). Matching alcoholism treatments to client heterogeneity: Project MATCH posttreatment drinking outcomes. *Journal of Studies on Alcohol,* 58(1): 7–29.

APA. (2013). *Diagnostic and Statistical Manual of Mental Disorders*, 5th edn. Arlington: American Psychiatric Association.

Babor, T. F. (2008). Treatment for persons with substance use disorders: mediators, moderators, and the need for a new research approach. *International Journal of Methods in Psychiatric Research,* 17(Suppl. 1): S45–9.

Bower, P. and Gilbody, S. (2005). Stepped care in psychological therapies: access, effectiveness and efficiency. Narrative literature review. *The British Journal of Psychiatry,* 186: 11–17.

Brunette, M. F., Mueser, K. T. and Drake, R. E. (2004). A review of research on residential programs for people with severe mental illness and co-occurring substance use disorders. *Drug and Alcohol Review*, 23(4): 471–81.

Buhringer, G. (2006). Allocating treatment options to patient profiles: clinical art or science? *Addiction,* 101(5): 646–52.

Burnam, M. A. and Watkins, K. E. (2006). Substance abuse with mental disorders: specialized public systems and integrated care. *Health Affairs (Millwood),* 25(3): 648–58.

Carlson, M. J. and Gabriel, R. M. (2001). Patient satisfaction, use of services, and one-year outcomes in publicly funded substance abuse treatment. *Psychiatric Services,* 52(9): 1230–6.

Carroll, K. M. and Rounsaville, B. J. (2010). Perhaps it is the Dodo Bird verdict that should be extinct. *Addiction,* 105(1): 18–20.

Carroll, K. M., Connors, G. J., Cooney, N. L., DiClemente, C. C., Donovan, D. M., Kadden, R. R. and Zweben, A. (1998). Internal validity of project MATCH treatments: discriminability and integrity. *Journal of Consulting and Clinical Psychology,* 66(2): 290–303.

Cleary, M., Hunt, G. E., Matheson, S., Siegfried, N. and Walter, G. (2008). Psychosocial treatment programs for people with both severe mental illness and substance misuse. *Schizophrenia Bulletin,* 34(2): 226–8.

Clifford, P. R., Maisto, S. A. and Davis, C. M. (2007). Alcohol treatment research assessment exposure subject reactivity effects: Part I. Alcohol use and related consequences. *Journal of Studies on Alcohol and Drugs,* 68(4): 519–28.

Cunningham, J. A. and Breslin, F. C. (2004). Only one in three people with alcohol abuse or dependence ever seek treatment. *Addictive Behaviors,* 29(1): 221–3.

DeMartini, K. S., Devine, E. G., DiClemente, C. C., Martin, D. J., Ray, L. A. and O'Malley, S. S. (2014). Predictors of pretreatment commitment to abstinence: results from the COMBINE study. *Journal of Studies on Alcohol and Drugs,* 75(3): 438–46.

Fals-Stewart, W. and Birchler, G. R. (2001). A national survey of the use of couples therapy in substance abuse treatment. *Journal of Substance Abuse Treatment,* 20(4): 277–83; discussion 285–6.

Gastfriend, D. R. and McLellan, A. T. (1997). Treatment matching - theoretic basis and practical implications. *Medical Clinics of North America,* 81(4): 945–66.

Gibbon, S., Duggan, C., Stoffers, J., Huband, N., Vollm, B. A., Ferriter, M. and Lieb, K. (2010). Psychological interventions for antisocial personality disorder. *Cochrane Database of Systematic Reviews,* (6): CD007668.

Ginsburg, G. S., Staples, J. and Abernethy, A. P. (2011). Academic medical centers: ripe for rapid-learning personalized health care. *Science Translational Medicine,* 3(101): 101cm27.

Gottheil, E., Thornton, C. and Weinstein, S. (2002). Effectiveness of high versus low structure individual counseling for substance abuse. *American Journal on Addictions,* 11(4): 279–90.

Graham, H. L., Copello, A., Birchwood, M. J., Mueser, K. T., Orford, J., McGovern, D., Atkinson, E., Maslin, J., Preece, M., Tobin, D. and Georgiou, G. (2004). *Cognitive-Behavioural Integrated Treatment (CBIT): A Treatment Manual for Substance Misuse in People with Severe Mental Health Problems.* Chichester: Wiley & Sons Ltd.

Grant, B. F., Stinson, F. S., Dawson, D. A., Chou, S. P., Ruan, W. J. and Pickering, R. P. (2004). Co-occurrence of 12-month alcohol and drug use disorders and personality disorders in the United States: results from the National Epidemiologic Survey on Alcohol and Related Conditions. *Archives of General Psychiatry,* 61(4): 361–8.

Harvey, O., J., Hunt, D. and Schroder, H. M. (1961). *Conceptual Systems and Personality Organization.* New York: Wiley.

Heather, N., Copello, A., Godfrey, C., Heather, N., Orford, J., Raistrick, D. and UKATT Research Team (2008). UK Alcohol Treatment Trial: client-treatment matching effects. *Addiction,* 103(2): 228–38.

Hesse, M. (2009). Integrated psychological treatment for substance use and co-morbid anxiety or depression vs. treatment for substance use alone. A systematic review of the published literature. *BMC Psychiatry,* 9: 6.

Hesse, M., Vanderplasschen, W., Rapp, R., Broekaert, E. and Fridell, M. (2007). Case management for persons with substance use disorders. *Cochrane Database of Systematic Reviews,* (4): CD006265.

Hester, R. K., Delaney, H. D. and Campbell, W. (2012). The college drinker's check-up: outcomes of two randomized clinical trials of a computer-delivered intervention. *Psychology of Addictive Behaviors,* 26(1): 1–12.

Horvath, A. O. and Symonds, B. D. (1991). Relation between working alliance and outcome in psychotherapy: a meta-analysis. *Journal of Counseling Psychology,* 38: 139–49.

Humphreys, K. and Weisner, C. (2000). Use of exclusion criteria in selecting research subjects and its effect on the generalizability of alcohol treatment outcome studies. *American Journal of Psychiatry,* 157(4): 588–94.

Hunter, S. B., Watkins, K. E., Hepner, K. A., Paddock, S. M., Ewing, B. A., Osilla, K. C. and Perry, S. (2012). Treating depression and substance use: a randomized controlled trial. *Journal on Substance Abuse Treatment,* 43(2): 137–51.

Ilgen, M., Tiet, Q., Finney, J. and Moos, R. H. (2006). Self-efficacy, therapeutic alliance, and alcohol-use disorder treatment outcomes. *Journal of Studies on Alcohol,* 67(3): 465–72.

Jansson, I., Hesse, M. and Fridell, M. (2009). Influence of personality disorder features on social functioning in substance-abusing women five years after compulsive residential treatment. *European Addiction Research,* 15(1): 25–31.

Kadden, R., Carroll, K., Donovan, D., Cooney, N., Monti, P., Abrams, D. and Hester, R. (eds) (1995). *Cognitive Behavioral Coping Skills Therapy Manual: A Clinical Research Guide for Therapists Treating Individuals with Alcohol Abuse and Dependence*, Vol. 3. Rockville: NIAAA.

Kypri, K., Langley, J. D., Saunders, J. B. and Cashell-Smith, M. L. (2007). Assessment may conceal therapeutic benefit: findings from a randomized controlled trial for hazardous drinking. *Addiction,* 102(1): 62–70.

Latimer, W. W., Newcomb, M., Winters, K. C. and Stinchfield, R. D. (2000a). Adolescent substance abuse treatment outcome: the role of substance abuse problem severity, psychosocial, and treatment factors. *Journal of Consulting and Clinical Psychology,* 68(4): 684–96.

Latimer, W. W., Winters, K. C., Stinchfield, R. and Traver, R. E. (2000b). Demographic, individual, and interpersonal predictors of adolescent alcohol and marijuana use following treatment. *Psychology of Addictive Behaviors,* 14(2): 162–73.

Longabaugh, R. and Wirtz, P. W. (2001). Matching hypotheses. In R. Longabaugh and P. W. Wirtz (eds), *Project MATCH Hypotheses: Results and Causal Chain Analyses*, Vol. 8. Rockville: National Institute on Alcohol Abuse and Alcoholism, pp. 4–17.

Magura, S., Staines, G., Kosanke, N., Rosenblum, A., Foote, J., DeLuca, A. and Bali, P. (2003). Predictive validity of the ASAM Patient Placement Criteria for naturalistically matched vs. mismatched alcoholism patients. *American Journal on Addictions,* 12(5): 386–97.

Maisto, S. A., Clifford, P. R. and Davis, C. M. (2007). Alcohol treatment research assessment exposure subject reactivity effects: Part II. Treatment engagement and involvement. *Journal of Studies on Alcohol and Drugs*, 68(4): 529–33.

McKay, J. R., Donovan, D. M., McLellan, T., Krupski, A., Hansten, M., Stark, K. D. and Cecere, J. (2002). Evaluation of full vs. partial continuum of care in the treatment of publicly funded substance abusers in Washington State. *American Journal on Drug and Alcohol Abuse,* 28(2): 307–38.

McLachlan, J. F. C. (1972). Benefit from group therapy as a function of patient-therapist match on conceptual level. *Psychotherapy: Theory, Research and Practice,* 9(4): 317–23.

McLellan, A. T., Arndt, I. O., Metzger, D. S., Woody, G. E. and O'Brien, C. P. (1993). The effects of psychosocial services in substance abuse treatment *JAMA,* 269(15): 1953–9.

McLellan, A. T., Chalk, M. and Bartlett, J. (2007). Outcomes, performance and quality - what's the difference? *Journal of Substance Abuse Treatment,* 32: 331–40.

McLellan, A. T., Luborsky, L., Woody, G. E., O'Brien, C. P. and Druley, K. A. (1983). Predicting response to alcohol and drug abuse treatments. Role of psychiatric severity. *Archives of General Psychiatry,* 40(6): 620–5.

McLellan, A. T., McKay, J. R., Forman, R., Cacciola, J. and Kemp, J. (2005). Reconsidering the evaluation of addiction treatment: from retrospective follow-up to concurrent recovery monitoring. *Addiction,* 100(4): 447–58.

Mee-Lee, D., Shulman, G. D., Fishman, M. J., Gastfriend, D. R. and Miller, M. M. E. (2013). *The ASAM Criteria: Treatment Criteria for Addictive, Substance-Related, and Co-Occurring Conditions*, 3rd edn. Carson City: The Change Companies.

Meier, P. S., Barrowclough, C. and Donmall, M. C. (2005). The role of the therapeutic alliance in the treatment of substance misuse: a critical review of the literature. *Addiction,* 100(3): 304–16.

Merkx, M. J., Schippers, G. M., Koeter, M. W., Vuijk, P. J., Oudejans, S. C., Stam, R. K. and van den Brink, W. (2011). Guidelines for allocating outpatient alcohol abusers to levels of care: predictive validity. *Addictive Behaviors,* 36(6): 570–5.

Meyers, R. J., Miller, W. R., Hill, D. E. and Tonigan, J. S. (1998). Community reinforcement and family training (CRAFT): engaging unmotivated drug users in treatment. *Journal of Substance Abuse,* 10(3): 291–308.

Moss, H. B., Chen, C. M., and Yi, H. I. (2010). Prospective follow-up of empirically derived alcohol dependence subtypes in wave 2 of the National Epidemiologic Survey on Alcohol And Related Conditions (NESARC): recovery status, alcohol use disorders and diagnostic criteria, alcohol consumption behavior, health status, and treatment seeking. *Alcoholism: Clinical and Experimental Research,* 34(6): 1078–83.

Najavits, L. M., Crits-Christoph, P. and Dierberger, A. (2000). Clinicians' impact on the quality of substance use disorder treatment. *Substance Use & Misuse,* 35(12–14): 2161–90.

Nielsen, A. S. (2003). Alcohol problems and treatment: the patients' perceptions. *European Addiction Research,* 9(1): 29–38.

Nielsen, B., Nielsen, A. S. and Wraae, O. (1998). Patient-treatment matching improves compliance of alcoholics in outpatient treatment. *Journal of Nervous and Mental Diseases,* 186(12): 752–60.

Nielsen, B., Nielsen, A. S. and Wraae, O. (2000). Factors associated with compliance of alcoholics in outpatient treatment. *Journal of Nervous and Mental Diseases,* 188(2): 101–7.

Nowinski, J., Baker, S. and Carroll, K. (1999). *Twelve Steps Facilitation Therapy Manual: A Clinical Research Guide for Therapists Treating Individuals with Alcohol Abuse and Dependence*, Vol. 1. Rockville: NIAAA.

Nunes, E. V. and Levin, F. R. (2004). Treatment of depression in patients with alcohol or other drug dependence: a meta-analysis. *JAMA,* 291(15): 1887–96.

O'Farrell, T. J. and Fals-Stewart, W. (2001). Family-involved alcoholism treatment. An update. *Recent Developments in Alcoholism,* 15: 329–56.

Prochaska, J. O. and DiClemente, C. C. (1982). Transtheoretical therapy: toward a more integrative model of change. *Psychotherapy: Theory, Research and Practice,* 19(3): 276–88.

Roozen, H. G., de Waart, R. and van der Kroft, P. (2010). Community reinforcement and family training: an effective option to engage treatment-resistant substance-abusing individuals in treatment. *Addiction,* 105(10): 1729–38.

Roth, A. and Fonagy, P. (eds) (1998). *What Works for Whom?: A Critical Review of Psychotherapy Research*, 1st edn. New York: Guilford Press.

Safren, S. A., O'Cleirigh, C. M., Bullis, J. R., Otto, M. W., Stein, M. D. and Pollack, M. H. (2012). Cognitive behavioral therapy for adherence and depression (CBT-AD) in HIV-infected injection drug users: a randomized controlled trial. *Journal of Consulting and Clinical Psychology,* 80(3): 404–15.

Sellman, D. (2010). The 10 most important things known about addiction. *Addiction,* 105(1): 6–13.

Siqueland, L., Crits-Christoph, P., Barber, J. P., Butler, S. F., Thase, M., Najavits, L. and Onken, L. S. (2000). The role of therapist characteristics in training effects in cognitive, supportive-expressive, and drug counseling therapies for cocaine dependence. *Journal of Psychotherapy Practice and Research,* 9(3): 123–30.

Smith, J. E., Meyers, R. J. and Delaney, H. D. (1998). The community reinforcement approach with homeless alcohol-dependent individuals. *Journal of Consulting and Clinical Psychology,* 66(3): 541–8.

Sobell, M. B. and Sobell, L. C. (2000). Stepped care as a heuristic approach to the treatment of alcohol problems. *Journal of Consulting and Clinical Psychology,* 68(4): 573–9.

Thiesen, H. and Hesse, M. (2010). Biological markers of problem drinking in homeless patients. *Addictive Behaviors,* 35(3): 260–2.

Thornton, C. C., Patkar, A. A., Murray, H. W., Mannelli, P., Gottheil, E., Vergare, M. J. and Weinstein, S. P. (2003). High- and low-structure treatments for substance dependence: role of learned helplessness. *American Journal of Drug and Alcohol Abuse,* 29(3): 576–84.

Thylstrup, B. (2011). Numbers and narratives. *Nordic Studies on Alcohol and Drugs,* 28(5–6): 471–86.

Thylstrup, B. and Hesse, M. (2008). Substance abusers' personality disorders and staff members' emotional reactions. *BMC Psychiatry,* 8: 21.

Walker, R. (2009). Retention in treatment–indicator or illusion: an essay. *Substance Use & Misuse,* 44(1): 18–27.

Ware, N. C., Hopper, K., Tugenberg, T., Dickey, B. and Fisher, D. (2008). A theory of social integration as quality of life. *Psychiatric Services,* 59(1): 27–33.

Watkins, K. E., Hunter, S. B., Hepner, K. A., Paddock, S. M., de la Cruz, E., Zhou, A. J. and Gilmore, J. (2011). An effectiveness trial of group cognitive behavioral therapy for patients with persistent depressive symptoms in substance abuse treatment. *Archives of General Psychiatry,* 68(6): 577–84.

Weisner, C., Mertens, J., Parthasarathy, S., Moore, C., Hunkeler, E. M., Hu, T. and Selby, J. V. (2000). The outcome and cost of alcohol and drug treatment in an HMO: day hospital versus traditional outpatient regimens. *Health Services Research,* 35(4): 791–812.

Zanis, D. A., McLellan, A. T., Alterman, A. I. and Cnaan, R. A. (1996). Efficacy of enhanced outreach counseling to reenroll high-risk drug users 1 year after discharge from treatment *American Journal of Psychiatry,* 153(8): 1095–6.

Zhang, Z., Friedmann, P. D. and Gerstein, D. R. (2003). Does retention matter? Treatment duration and improvement in drug use. *Addiction,* 98(5): 673–84.

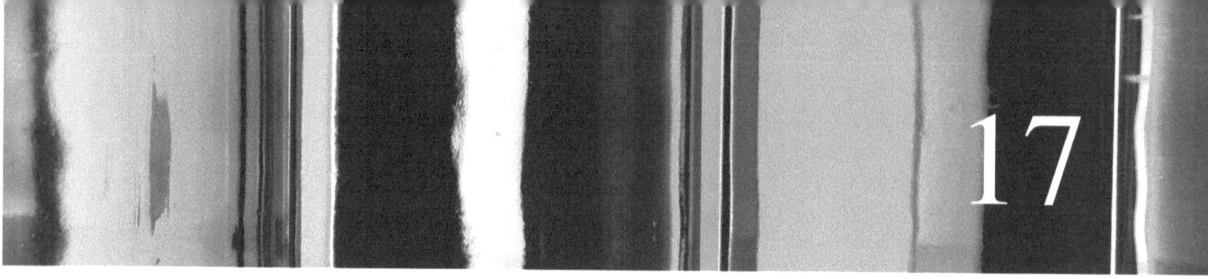

17

Workforce Development and Professionalization

Anna Nelson

INTRODUCTION

Problems associated with substance use have been noted for centuries and those who have supported and worked alongside the people, families and communities experiencing these problems have an interesting and largely unwritten history. This chapter examines some of this history of the alcohol and other drug (AOD) workforce, and then takes a more detailed look at contemporary approaches to addiction workforce development in Europe, the USA, the United Kingdom and Australia. A recurrent theme related to a general health and human services workforce shortages is also identified. A more in-depth look is provided of New Zealand's addiction workforce development in the form of a case study and key considerations for the future of addiction workforce development internationally are identified.

THE EARLY WORKFORCE

Many of the people who initially worked with people with problematic substance use,[1] or as they were known historically 'drunken inebriates', came from religious, spiritual or philanthropic groups. During the early 1700s, countries that had alcohol and other substance related problems (including opium and laudanum) often largely perceived them to be a moral failing. Even when genuine medical concerns were raised and the term 'addiction' was first proffered as a term that described 'an overwhelming desire to drink alcohol' in the nineteenth century, the medical profession still favoured a combination of both medical treatment and moral enlightenment to treat this 'disease' (Bennett and Holloway, 2005).

Before there was any formal training to work with people with alcohol and other drug problems, and before there was an expectation that such work should be funded by the state, groups with various religious affiliations demonstrated a strong commitment to this area. Prior to any conceptualisation of 'addiction' and the establishment of evidence based interventions, religious, spiritual and philanthropic groups (mostly voluntary) offered some of the only forms of support, treatment and intervention for people with problematic substance use.

Even as the medical profession became more interested in the problem of 'inebriety', comparing it to that of the 'insane', they nonetheless endorsed the need for partnership with these groups.

> The disease of inebriety resembles in many particulars the disease of insanity, and it is as much the duty of the Christian, the philanthropist, and the Statesman to establish homes for the treatment of the inebriate, as they have acknowledged it to be their duty to sustain asylums for the care of the insane. (Kerr, 1888: 33))

By the late 1880s, however, the role of medicine had become more prominent in the care and cure of the 'inebriate' and there were calls for a move away from moral and religiously based cures that were seen as ineffective. While religious groups, as well as medicine and science, continue major roles in understanding and treating the problems related to addiction, the workforce has grown, expanded and acquired new skills and capabilities to meet emerging challenges, issues and complexities.

WHAT IS WORKFORCE DEVELOPMENT?

The expanded focus on the capability and capacity of the workforce has become known as 'workforce development'. While historically the term workforce development has been used to describe a variety of activities undertaken by governments and organizations around the world (Jacobs and Hawley, 2009), the term is used in contemporary contexts to describe simultaneous consideration of individual, organization and systems approaches to developing a workforce that is fit for purpose (Jacobs and Hawley, 2009). Jacobs and Hawley propose a broad economic definition:

> Workforce development is the coordination of public and private sector policies and programs that provides individuals with the opportunity for a sustainable livelihood and helps organizations achieve exemplary goals, consistent with the societal context. (Jacobs and Hawley, 2009: 12)

However, when a specific workforce, such as that located within the AOD sector is concerned, more precise definitions can be applied. Australia's National Centre for Education and Training on Addiction (NCETA) have led the way in providing definitions of workforce development in the AOD context. Roche and Pidd cite NCETA's (2002) definition of workforce development as:

> A multi-faceted approach which addresses the range of factors impacting on the ability of the workforce to function with maximum effectiveness in responding to alcohol and other drug related problems. Workforce development should have a systems focus. Unlike traditional approaches, this is broad and comprehensive, targeting individual, organisational, and structural factors, rather than just addressing education and training of individual mainstream workers. (Roche and Pidd, 2010: 2)

WORKFORCE PLANNING

Workforce planning is an important part of any organizational strategic plan and it is an integral component of workforce development. It ensures services are equipped with the right number of people, with the right skills and attitudes, doing the right work at the right time, at the right costs and with the right work output (WHO, 2010). Workforce planning assists organizations to plan for the future, anticipate change, manage the workforce, meet business goals and provide high quality and consistent services (Te Pou o Te Whakaaro Nui, 2014). Workforce planning maps service design with the required workforce and analyses workforce capability and capacity.

INTERNATIONAL HEALTH WORKFORCE TRENDS

The relatively recent broader conceptualisation of workforce development occurred in parallel with the international recognition that we do not have enough people with the right skills in the health workforce to meet current demands worldwide. The World Health Organization (WHO) (2011a) has described the health workforce as being in a state of global crisis. WHO estimate that there is a shortage of 2.4 million doctors, nurses and midwives worldwide and that millions of people in low and medium income countries have little or no access to health care. This concern extends beyond actual numbers of health staff to include their education, competency, skills and experience to adequately meet the needs of the people they serve. WHO maintain that there should be a focus on 'the accessibility, acceptability, quality and productivity of the health workforce, placing equity at the centre of the agenda' (WHO, 2014: iv).

By 2022, Organisation for Economic Co-operation and Development (OECD) countries will be facing a health workforce shortfall of somewhere in the region of 22 to 29 per cent (Figure 17.1; from KPMG, 2013: 16):

> Disconnects still exist between health services and educational and workforce planning, contributing to inefficiencies and misalignment in training, deployment and uptake into the workforce. Limited capacity for human resource management

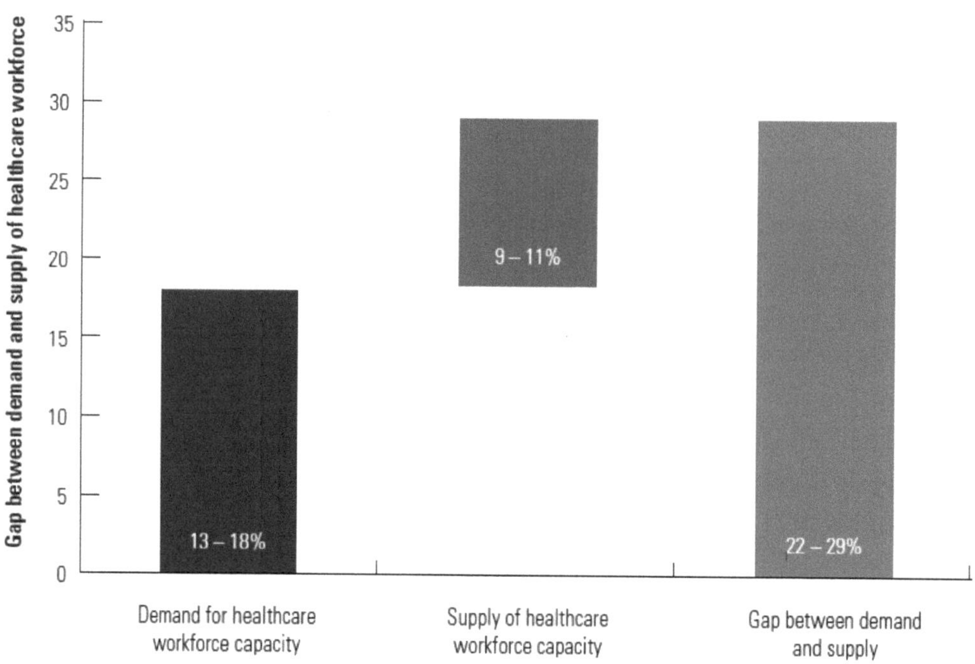

Figure 17.1 Gap between demand for, and supply of, healthcare workforce capacity by the year 2022

Source: OECD data. Analysis: KPMG (2013).

at the national, provincial and facility levels, limited cross-sectoral and multi-stakeholder involvement and other underlying, constraining health system factors all contribute to the difficulties countries have in following through on policy-level commitments, and implementing strategies and plans. (World Health Organization, 2012: 8)

While the main emphasis of the WHO health workforce agenda and other international health workforce policy is on physical health and midwifery, there has also been an international focus on mental health human resources and workforce development. This is significant as in some parts of the world the addiction workforce sits within the wider mental health sector, in other countries, these two sectors are seen as very distinct. There are specifically concerns about the lack of mental health nurses, psychiatrists, social workers and occupational therapists globally. While the mental health workforce data is not broken down into specialisms, parallels may be drawn from this information about the addiction workforce, which in some countries make up a small part of the wider mental health workforce (WHO, 2011b; Morris et al., 2012).

INTERNATIONAL ADDICTION WORKFORCE DEVELOPMENT

Higher income and OECD countries have had the advantage of being sufficiently well resourced to focus on AOD workforce development. For many countries around the world (for example, many African countries), their primary effort is on building a physical health care workforce which takes priority over mental health and addiction services and workforce development.

The following section looks at some examples of addiction workforce development in a variety of countries. They are presented here as an illustration of the different approaches taken to addressing contemporary workforce development challenges.

Australia

Australia has made a significant contribution to our understanding of workforce development initiatives that help to build the capacity and capability of the mainstream alcohol and other drug workforce. As early as 2001, Roche had described workforce development in an AOD workforce context in the following way:

At the most general level, workforce development includes policies, guidelines, management support and supervision and the legitimisation of initiatives through organisational and structural supports. Its primary aim is to facilitate and sustain developments in the AOD workforce. It does this at different levels, targeting structural, organisational and individual factors. (Roche, 2001. 6–7)

For many, this represented a paradigm shift in thinking about workforce development. It posited that workforce development involved much more than just education and training of the AOD sector and examined the components that shaped the functions and efficiency of the workforce.

In 2010, NCETA (Roche and Pidd, 2010) suggested an overarching model of workforce development for the AOD sector in Australia. This model comprised five levels, each of which should, they recommend, be addressed in any workforce development strategy:

- Systems
- Organizations
- Workplaces
- Teams
- Individuals

They identified different levels and components associated with workforce development in the AOD sector and provided an associated visual representation (see Figure 17.2).

In 2010, NCETA identified two main AOD workforces:

1 Those who were specialist in the AOD field.
2 Generalist health, social care and wider workforces who might come into contact with people experiencing problematic substance use (Roche and Pidd, 2010).

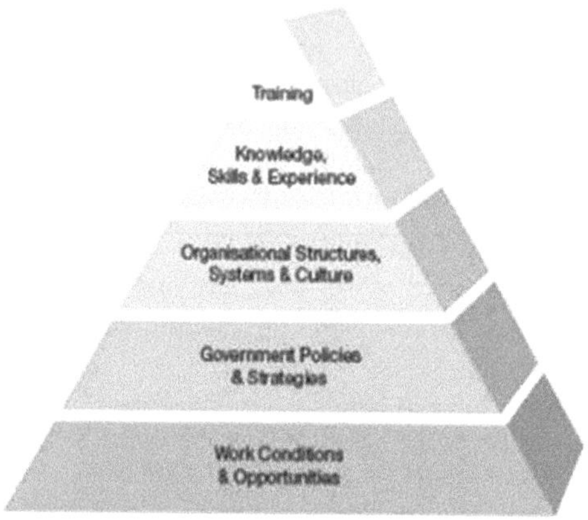
Training
Knowledge, Skills & Experience
Organisational Structures, Systems & Culture
Government Policies & Strategies
Work Conditions & Opportunities

Figure 17.2 The different levels and components of workforce development (Roche and Pidd, 2010: 29)

The first group might include the nurses, doctors, counsellors, social workers, psychotherapists and psychologists who work in speciality addiction services. Taking a human services systems approach, the second group of the AOD workforce might include health professionals, the police, teachers, probation officers, social service social workers, youth workers, bar staff and clergy (among others). Each component part of the workforce requires different interventions at each of the five levels in the workforce development model presented.

According to NCETA's more recent work (NCETA, 2013: 3–4) there have been three phases of workforce development in Australia to date and a clear direction for future work:

- Phase 1. Individual worker focus
- Phase 2. The AOD internal systems focus
- Phase 3. A human services systems approach

NCETA suggests that while the AOD systems approach was an improvement on an individual worker focus, the recognition that AOD interventions can be used to support people across the broader human services workforce spectrum is of paramount importance.

Australia's National Alcohol and Other Drug Workforce Development Strategy, 2015 to 2018

In 2015, Australia's Intergovernmental Committee on Drugs released Australia's National Alcohol and Other Drug Workforce Development Strategy developed by NCETA. This strategy supports Australia's National Drug Strategy and identifies key strategic areas that require action to enhance the capacity and capability of Australia's AOD workforce. In line with the National Drug Strategy, the workforce development Strategy has a focus on supporting an AOD workforce that is sustainable and capable of meeting future challenges, innovation and reform, and works to prevent and minimize alcohol and other drug related harm across the domains of supply, demand and harm reduction (Intergovernmental Committee on Drugs, 2015).

The strategy identifies 12 key outcome areas. These are to:

1. understand the specialist AOD prevention and treatment workforce;
2. create a sustainable specialist AOD prevention and treatment workforce by addressing recruitment and retention issues;
3. match roles with capabilities;
4. enhance capacity to cater for older AOD clients as well as those with co-and multiple morbidities and other complex needs;
5. improve child and family sensitive practice;
6. improve consumer participation in AOD service provision, policy and planning;
7. increase the capacity of the workforce to respond appropriately to AOD issues among Aboriginal and Torres Strait Islander peoples;
8. increase the capacity of the workforce to respond appropriately to AOD issues among culturally and linguistically diverse (CALD) groups;
9. increase the capacity of the workforce to respond appropriately to AOD issues among lesbian, gay, bisexual, transgender and intersex individuals;
10. enhance the capacity of generalist health, community, welfare and support services workers to prevent and reduce AOD harm;
11. continue to develop the criminal justice workforce to prevent and reduce AOD harm;

> 12 promote the ability of the education sector to prevent and reduce AOD harm responsibility for implementing the actions outlined in the Strategy is shared by all governments, recognizing that jurisdictions face different challenges and will undertake actions in line with their own priorities, timing and resources (Intergovernmental Committee on Drugs, 2015: iv).

The strategy also expands on the broad human services focus that NCETA has previously advocated and clearly articulates tiers of activity involving different specialist and generalist workforces (see Figure 17.3). This Strategy will provide Australia with strategic direction for future AOD workforce development and builds strongly on the work that NCETA has already done. It identifies key areas of development specific to the Australian context, as well as providing clear direction for AOD workforce development internationally.

United States of America

In 2013, the Substance Abuse and Mental Health Services Administration (SAMHSA) reported to the United States Congress on the nation's substance abuse and mental health workforce issues. That report requested by the Senate Appropriations Committee Subcommittee on Labor, Health and Human Services, Education and Related Agencies (LHHS-ED) built on and followed a number of other workforce development reports by SAMSHA (2006a, 2006b, 2007). The Committee requested the report due to concerns about:

> The growing workforce crisis in the addictions field due to high turnover rates, worker shortages, an aging workforce, stigma and inadequate compensation. The Mental Health Parity and Addiction Equity Act and the Patient Protection and Affordable Care Act are anticipated to increase the number of individuals who will seek substance use disorder services and may exacerbate current workforce challenges. (SAMHSA, 2013: 1)

The changes that are likely to result from the Patient Protection and Affordable Care Act (known as Obama Care) and the Mental Health Parity and Addiction Equity Act will increase the number of people who are eligible for health care coverage for mental health and addiction issues through Medicaid

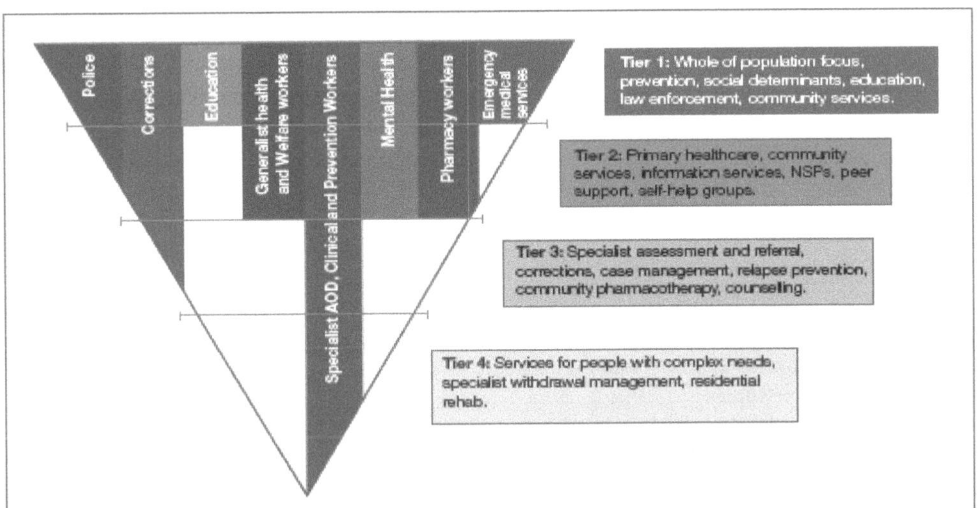

Figure 17.3 Tiers of activity in which different occupational groups make their contribution to reducing AOD-related harm

and health insurances exchanges. It is estimated that up to 38 million more Americans will be covered by health insurance as a result of these changes and that as many as 11 million of these may have serious mental illness, psychological distress and or a substance use disorder (SAMSHA, 2011). These legislative changes coupled with increased mental health and addiction screening in primary care, a large number of veterans returning from overseas deployments in the armed services and initiatives to reduce the prison population are likely to put enormous strain on the addiction workforce throughout the USA.

Workforce crisis signalled

SAMHSA (2013) identified a number of specific concerns facing the addiction workforce in the USA that, combined with the likely increase in people wanting to access services, appears to signify a potential addiction workforce crisis. Concerns over the ethnic composition of the workforce, in contrast to the over representation of African Americans who are recipients of services requires any workforce development initiatives to focus on recruitment and retention of ethnic minorities as well as the provision of training in cultural competence (SAMHSA, 2013). Requisite education levels for substance abuse counsellors is lower than for those working as mental health counsellors and 45 states do not require any college degree to qualify to work as a substance abuse counsellor. Other workforce concerns include:

- High turnover of staff
- Worker shortages
- An ageing workforce
- Inadequate compensation (salary rates)
- Recruitment and retention
- Lack of workforce data
- Prejudice about mental illness and addiction (SAMHSA, 2013: 9)

Previous USA workforce development initiatives include an emphasis on technology and knowledge transfer and training in evidence based practices and recruiting a diverse workforce and integrating primary and behavioural health care. Further workforce development strategies or approaches identified in the SAMHSA (2013) report include:

- Promoting cross training to enhance capabilities for working with co-occurring problems and complex needs
- Focussing on recruiting a diverse workforce to meet the needs of ethnic minorities, children and adolescents, 'geriatric' patients and those living in rural areas
- Increasing the numbers of people and families with a lived experience in the workforce
- Disseminating and promoting the adoption of evidence based practices, including supervision
- Encouraging and disseminating behavioural health core competencies for primary and other health care workforces
- Providing training and education on recovery-orientated care and recovery principles
- Developing standardized workforce data collection (SAMHSA, 2013: 20–1)

Addiction Technology Transfer Centers (ATTC) were set up in 1993 in 14 regional centres to provide a mechanism by which to strengthen and support the addiction workforce in all 50 states. These centres appear to have taken a more individualistic approach to workforce development with a focus on knowledge transfer, evidence based practice, skill building and practice change, clinical supervision and supporting emerging leaders. In 2012, the ATTC centres produced the first USA workforce survey (Ryan et al., 2012) that provided an overview of the characteristics and workforce development needs of the addiction workforce.

SAMHSA also sponsors a number of other initiatives that have incorporated workforce development elements, for example Partners for Recovery, which works to address workforce development, leadership development, cross-systems collaboration and destigmatisation in the USA.

It appears, however, that a much needed holistic and systemic approach to workforce development that addresses the workforce concerns raised by SAMHSA (2013) will be required across all 50 states in the USA if the potential crisis is to be alleviated.

Europe

The European Union (EU) as a collective looks to have a broad emphasis on the general physical health workforce and it has prioritized increasing the numbers of nurses and doctors in line with WHO recommendations. The EU are concerned about difficulties in recruiting and retaining health care staff and recognize that there will be a labour shortage due to both an ageing general population and an ageing health care workforce (European Commission, 2012).

A WHO report co-funded by the European Commission in 2008, does however, address mental health workforce development issues across much of the European region and was used as a baseline against which progress could be measured towards the vision and milestones in the Mental Health Declaration for Europe (WHO, 2005). The declaration stated the following workforce development actions:

- Design recruitment and education and training programmes to create a sufficient and competent multidisciplinary workforce (2005: 3)
- Include mental health in the curricula of all health professionals and design continuous professional education and training programmes for the mental health workforce (2005: 5)
- Encourage the development of specialized expertise within the mental health workforce to address the specific needs of groups such as children, young people, older people and those with long-term and severe mental health problems (2005: 5)

While it does not specifically mention the addiction workforce, some insight can be gained from the 2008 report focussing on mental health. The report recognizes the challenges involved in achieving a multidisciplinary workforce that is prepared to deliver timely and effective interventions to people requiring treatment for mental health problems.

The 2008 WHO report suggested that workforce development strategies that focus on these recognized challenges help to provide solutions, and investigated workforce development strategies in 42 different countries. Of these, only 18 (less than half) had workforce development strategies in place. For example, while the Netherlands did have many higher education training programmes, and competencies, these were not coordinated at a national level and the Netherlands had no mental health workforce development strategy or programme (WHO, 2008). Of those countries that did have some mental health workforce development strategies in place, for the most part, they took an individualized approach and focussed on education and training, the movement of personnel (migration) and increasing the numbers of personnel. The report concluded that:

> The most striking observations...are the variation in staff numbers, differences in education and the lack of reliable information available from countries in many areas. Surprisingly, at a time of reform and rapid change in the numbers, composition and competencies of the workforce, in combination with ubiquitous concern about recruiting adequate numbers of staff members, fewer than half the countries in this survey have produced a mental health workforce strategy. (WHO, 2008: 110)

Since 2008, there looks to have been no further progress reports, although some individual countries may have developed their own workforce development strategies information on this was difficult to locate.

United Kingdom

In England, the National Drug Treatment Agency (NTA, now part of Public Health

England) and the Drug Strategy Directorate (part of the Home Office) published the Joint National Treatment Agency and Drug Strategy Directorate: Workforce Development Plan for the Substance Misuse Field (Home Office, 2006). This document sets out a conceptual framework, that built on work completed by Healthwork UK in 2001, and was aimed at providing support to local partnerships workforce planning activities. It also outlined a programme of work and milestones to meet the workforce development requirements of the substance misuse field. Workforce shortages to meet the needs of the national drug strategy at the time were identified as a risk, and an across government approach taken (NTA and Drug Strategy Directorate, 2006).

The NTA and Drug Strategy Directorate's workforce development plan made it clear that its success depended on substance misuse knowledge and skills being embedded in mainstream health and social care service provision, as well as increasing the capacity and competence of those in the specialist substance misuse field. In earlier work by Healthwork UK (2001), it had been estimated that there were approximately 4 million workers who required some knowledge of substance misuse. This acknowledgment, in line with work from other countries in the UK, was a recognition that issues related to addiction can and do manifest in a variety of ways, and that people will present to a variety of different services for support.

This workforce development plan aimed to:

- be a workforce planning and development resource to local partnerships, commissioners, managers and individual practitioners;
- encourage the development of local and regional workforce strategies that will:
    - increase the workforce capacity in the substance misuse field
    - improve the substance misuse competence of generic and specialist practitioners working with adults and children and young people in the substance misuse field
    - develop leadership and managerial skills across the workforce;
- provide a conceptual framework of the substance misuse workforce;
- outline the core competence required by those working in the substance misuse field;
- outline how to improve integration and skills sharing with mainstream structures (NTA and Drug Strategy Directorate, 2006: 5).

In 2009, the NTA published further workforce development guidance in relation to the Adult and Integrated Drug Treatment Service (IDTS) drug treatment plan 2010/2011 (NTA, 2009). This guidance reflected the need for local partnerships to consider the workforce needs of their substance misuse workforce in order to deliver the treatment requirements of their service users. The focus was aimed at individualized competency (including for support staff and managers) that is evidence based and accredited as well as recruitment of new entrants and internships in the substance misuse field.

The need for strategic leadership at a national and local level in relation to substance misuse workforce development was acknowledged in the paper 'Supporting the development of Scotland's Alcohol and Drug Workforce' [The Convention of Scottish Local Authorities (COSLA) and The Scottish Government, 2010], which sets out a range of responsibilities for COSLA, NHS Health Scotland, Scottish Drugs Recovery Consortium, Alcohol Focus Scotland, NHS Education Scotland, Scottish Training on Drugs and Alcohol and others. The paper recognized that the substance misuse workforce in Scotland is drawn from a wide range of sectors including health, education, social work and the voluntary sector (COSLA and the Scottish Government, 2010: 1). In 2008, NHS Health Scotland completed a service user consultation on their views of the workforce development needs and requirements of the Scottish substance misuse workforce which provided valuable insight. Service users who participated identified that the training and development needs of staff included attitudes (empathy and respect) and developing basic interpersonal and motivational interviewing skills as well as understanding and working with the social determinants of health. The main service delivery criticism focused on stigmatising attitudes, especially towards drug users (NHS Health Scotland, 2008: 3).

The Scottish plan is also one of first workforce development plans internationally that specifically identify those with a lived experience of addiction as a crucial element to the substance misuse workforce:

> The workforce will learn from and value the service user, who is an expert by experience-and enable them to lead satisfying, hopeful and contributing lives. It is likely that the more traditional 'workforce' will be joined by people in recovery themselves, recruited because of their lived experience of addiction. Contributing as peer mentors and supporters of those in recovery, they must also be skilled and trained to become an effective part of the alcohol and drug 'workforce'. (NHS Health Scotland, 2008: 1–2)

This plan also focussed on the development of competence, skills and expertise to more adequately address the needs of service users with substance misuse related problems from a recovery and wellbeing focussed approach and mapped learning priorities for a variety of 'levels' of workers (ranging from the wider workforce, through to general practitioners and specialist workers). Scotland's recovery focussed approach has implications for the substance misuse workforce that may previously have been used to working within a harm reduction framework that was more health focussed. While there are a number of definitions of 'recovery', Scotland's recovery focussed approach proposes that:

> Recovery is a process through which an individual is enabled to move-on from their problem drug use towards a drug-free life and become an active and contributing member of society. Moving to an approach that is based on recovery will mean a significant change in both the pattern of services that are commissioned and in the way that practitioners engage with individuals. (Scottish Government, 2008: vi)

In 2011, the Welsh Government reviewed and updated its Substance Misuse Workforce Development Plan 2011 to 2014. There was clear attention given to the specialist drug and alcohol workforce as well as generic workers who may have a substance misuse role (for example teachers and police officers). The priority workforce development areas set out in this plan were partnerships, skills and competence development and performance management and workforce planning. Monitoring of the plan, which links to the National Core Standards for Substance Misuse Services in Wales document, was via the Substance Misuse Advisory Regional Teams (SMARTs) performance management system. The plan was also supported through the on-going development of the workforce development website (www.susbstancemisuseworkforce-wales.org) (Welsh Government, 2011).

In Northern Ireland, workforce development is a key part of the National Strategic Direction for Alcohol and Drugs, Phase 2 – 2011 to 2016 [The Department of Health, Social Services and Public Safety (DHSSPS), 2011]. One of its overarching long term objectives is to 'develop a competent and skilled workforce across all sectors that can respond to the complexities of alcohol and drug use and misuse' (DHSSPS, 2011: 36). They directed the strategy at both generalist and specialist workforces. It prioritizes skills development and competence, with access to supportive training and agreed protocols for inter-service working and cooperation. It outlines both short to medium term outcomes and goals, as well as some longer term outcomes. Long-term outcomes include:

- Development of a training framework, which ensures that skill development (an individual's development of competency as defined by the occupational standards), is evidenced to a quality standard that is recognized throughout the UK.
- Dissemination of Drug and Alcohol National Occupational Standards (DANOS) across Northern Ireland.
- Improved competence and capacity of the alcohol and drug misuse, and wider, workforce (DHSSPS, 2011: 58).

The workforce development plans across the four countries in the United Kingdom, while different in some respects, all have the following themes in common:

- The workforce includes specialists as well as other health, education and social care practitioners
- The focus is aimed at skills development and competence of the workforce
- Inter-service partnership and cooperation are integral

Each plan was also linked to the UK's Drug and Alcohol National Occupational Standards (DANOS) and the relevant qualifications framework with an emphasis on the development of career pathways to improve recruitment and retention. DANOS covers most of the substance misuse related tasks and activities relevant to the field in the form of occupational standards that are broken down into elements and competency components. Substance misuse workers need to provide evidence that they have met the competencies and can complete the tasks specified. Substance misuse workers should also be covered by a code of practice and ethics (like that of the Federation of Drug and Alcohol Professionals – FDAP) and receive regular supervision (FDAP, 2012).

Other organizations that provide workforce development support for the substance misuse sector in the UK include Skills for Health, the Substance Misuse Skills Consortium and the National Skills Academy and as well as a number of education providers.

Summary

The workforce development approaches taken by the countries overviewed here all recognize the importance of the addiction workforce, but have evolved in a variety of ways. Australia, led by NCETA and supported by governmental mandate, present a clear model for AOD workforce development that recognizes the importance of five component levels (systems, organizations, workplaces, teams, individuals). This model is also partially recognized within the strategies from the countries in the UK. This approach to workforce development sanctions initiatives to be undertaken at a variety of levels and does not rely solely on increasing individual capability or knowledge and skills. This is essential in supporting systems and culture change that is required to meet shifting demands.

Most of the countries represented here have recognized the need to see the addiction workforce more broadly than just addiction treatment specialists. This broad conceptualization of what constitutes the addiction workforce needs to be integrated within a systemic approach to workforce development that will include, at its core, the importance of partnership and collaboration within health and across the social care, justice and education sectors.

ADDICTION WORKFORCE DEVELOPMENT: AN AOTEAROA[2] NEW ZEALAND CASE STUDY

Aotearoa New Zealand's workforce historically was primarily comprised of Christian and philanthropic volunteers who supported a moral failing perspective in regard to people who experienced problematic substance use. By the late 1880s, the issue of problematic substance use (mainly alcohol) had started to become the domain of the medical practitioner, as science tried to make sense of the 'disease'. Often people were 'treated' alongside those with mental health problems in psychiatric hospitals that historically had reputations for heavy handed custodial care (Crawford, 2008).

In New Zealand today, Christian-based social services continue to be involved in supporting the needs of people and their families and whānau[3] experiencing distress as a result of problematic substance use, as do a range of other non-governmental organizations (NGOs) and state health services. The correctional system also continues to play a role in identifying and treating people.

Queen Mary Hospital (built in 1916) in Hanmer Springs in New Zealand's South Island had historically rehabilitated returned service men from the First World War, as well as patients with tuberculosis, 'alcoholism' and women with 'nervous disorders' using the natural hot pools that were clustered around the hospital (Crawford, 2008). In the 1970s, Queen Mary Hospital began treating people with alcohol and other drug related problems, offering a therapeutic residential programme which was the first of its kind in the country. From 1979 to 1987, it also offered AOD counsellor training courses funded in the main by the Alcoholic Liquor Advisory Council (ALAC). A range of professionals came for training or induction, including probation officers from the southern region, who needed skills in working with people with AOD related problems (T. Huriwai, personal communication, April 2014).

A large part of this workforce has always been people with their own lived experience of addiction related problems in 'recovery' wanting to continue giving support to their peers. Peer support has historically been provided in self-support or mutual aid groups [e.g. Alcoholics Anonymous (AA)] or by people training and becoming qualified to deliver 'professional' services within the health and social care system. This has offered an alternative to moral and/or medical interventions, from the perspective of someone who has 'been there'.

ALAC (it later became known as the Alcohol Advisory Council of New Zealand, which is now part of the Health Promotion Agency), was integral in building an addiction workforce in New Zealand. Set up in 1976 by the New Zealand Government, its core task was 'the encouragement and promotion of moderation in the use of liquor, the discouragement and reduction of the misuse of liquor, and the minimisation of the personal, social, and economic harm resulting from the misuse of liquor' under the Alcohol Advisory Council Act (1976). As part of its remit to minimise alcohol related harm, it was an integral part of many addiction services since inception, and worked to support the growth of the addiction workforce.

In the early 1990s, workforce development in mental health was identified within the National Mental Health Strategy, which comprised three documents:

- 'Looking Forward: Strategic Directions for Mental Health Services' (Ministry of Health, 1994)
- 'Moving Forward: The National Mental Health Plan for More and Better Services' (Ministry of Health, 1997)
- 'Blueprint for Mental Health Services in New Zealand: How Things Need to Be' (Mental Health Commission, 1998).

Workforce planning and development were recognized as fundamental to the success of these policies and their goals of producing more and better mental health services. Workforce development activity was defined in a further three key strategic documents (Ministry of Health, 2002: 8). Although not the primary focus of these strategies, the need for addiction workforce development was visibly established within these documents.

- 'Towards Better Mental Health Services: The Report of the National Working Party on Mental Health Workforce Development' (Ministry of Health, 1996) identified seven overarching strategies – retention and recruitment, communication with the education sector, increased investment in training, research, destigmatization, provider responsibility, management practice and organizational change.
- 'Developing the Mental Health Workforce: The report of the National Mental Health Workforce Development Co-ordinating Committee' (Mental Health Commission and Ministry of Health, 1999) identified five strategies – competencies development, organizational effectiveness, child and youth, Māori and Pacific peoples.

- 'Tuutahitia te Wero, Meeting the Challenges: Mental Health Workforce Development Plan 2000 to 2005' (Health Funding Authority, 2000) detailed 11 goals, which included strengthening and developing the Māori workforce, child/tamariki and youth/rangatahi workforce and Pacific workforce and developing generic skills training. This document also outlined that workforce development was any 'initiative that influences entry to and exit from the mental health and addiction sector, movement within the sector, education, training, skills, attitudes, rewards and the associated infrastructure' (2000: 1)

Much of the work in the AOD workforce development area was undertaken by the Alcohol and Drug Treatment Workforce Development Advisory Group, which had been set up in early 1999 by ALAC to assist in the development and implementation of workforce initiatives aimed at improving responses to people experiencing alcohol problems (ALAC, 2001). This group initiated and guided the development of the first Practitioner Competencies for Alcohol and Drug Workers in Aotearoa – New Zealand (ALAC, 2001). This in turn lead to the establishment of a sector led organization to manage the competencies: The Drug and Alcohol Practitioners Association Aotearoa New Zealand (dapaanz, now known as the Addiction Practitioners' Association, Aotearoa New Zealand).

In 2001, the Ministry of Health published 'A National Strategic Framework for Alcohol and Drug Services'. This strategy was aimed specifically at 'increasing the capacity of the specialist alcohol and drug treatment sector, both in terms of service delivery and workforce. Workforce development is fundamental to the sector becoming better equipped to meet the ever increasing demands' (Ministry of Health, 2001: iii). This strategic framework identified workforce capacity objectives and targets that included having at least 50 per cent of the employed addiction workforce with specialist post graduate alcohol and drug qualifications by July 2002 (a target set in 'Moving Forward', Ministry of Health, 1997). The desired outcomes relating to the alcohol and other drug workforce were:

- A culturally responsive workforce
- A trained and competent workforce
- A recognized career pathway (Ministry of Health, 2001: 41)

One of the recommendations from this strategic framework was the development of a national alcohol and other drug workforce development group. This group was to be specifically tasked with the development of a coordinated and targeted response to the issues facing the alcohol and other drug treatment workforce. This recommendation saw the beginnings of what was to become Matua Raki, the national addiction workforce development centre.

In 2002, the Mental Health Workforce Development Programme (MHWDP) and the Mental Health Research and Development Strategy Programme (MHRDS) were established with initial funding by the Ministry of Health and sat within the Health Research Council. These programmes were subsequently moved under the Wise Trust umbrella and renamed as Te Pou o Te Whakaaro Nui. As the original name suggested, the programmes focussed specifically on mental health research, development and workforce.

In 2002, the Ministry of Health published Mental Health (Alcohol and other Drugs) Workforce Development Framework. The recommendations in that framework saw the establishment of the Māori mental health workforce development centre, Te Rau Matatini, as well as the infant, child and youth mental health workforce development organization within the University of Auckland (The Werry Centre). That document also provided a framework for workforce development based on five strategic imperatives (Figure 17.4):

1 Workforce development infrastructure
2 Organizational development
3 Recruitment and retention
4 Training and development
5 Research and evaluation

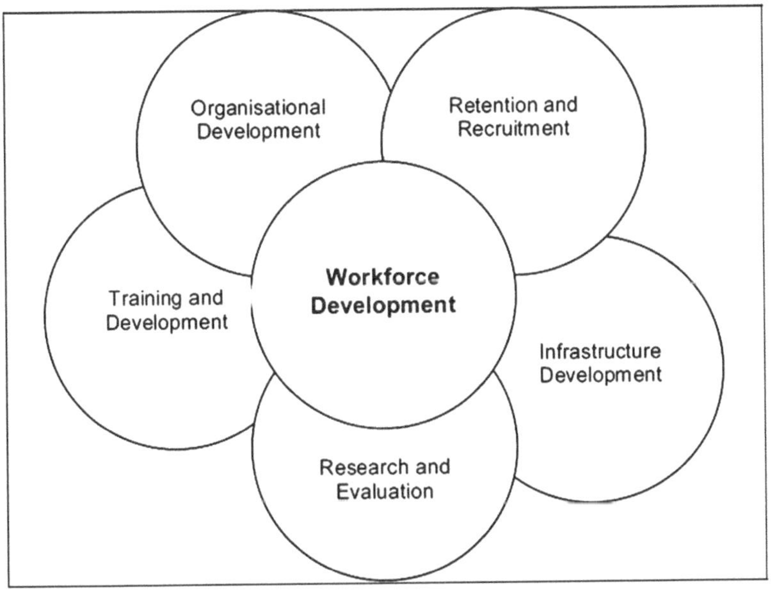

Figure 17.4 The five strategic imperatives for Mental Health Workforce Development (Ministry of Health, 2002: 16)

The framework was to become the structure upon which the workforce programmes, which had now been established (the Mental Health Workforce Development Programme, Matua Raki, Te Rau Matatini and The Werry Centre),[4] would be expected to work towards.

Matua Raki-the National Addiction Workforce Development Centre

In 2004, the Ministry of Health contracted the National Addiction Centre [formally the National Centre for Treatment Development (Alcohol, Drugs and Addiction)] at the University of Otago, Christchurch School of Medicine, to develop and host a National Addiction Treatment Workforce Development Programme. The National Addiction Centre was established by ALAC in 1996 as a resource for the alcohol and other drug treatment field in New Zealand.

The programme that was developed was eventually given the name Matua Raki. The name Matua Raki symbolises the characteristics of the addiction treatment sector and those within it. The characteristics of passion, commitment and excellence were often used to describe the sector and when considered in relation to the Māori legend of the journey of Tane to the heavens for knowledge, there was resonance. The metaphor of Matua Raki, or the 'highest heaven' symbolises this passion, commitment and pursuit of excellence shown by the addiction sector. The underscored k denotes the Kāti Mamoe dialect and recognizes the original location of the programme in the South Island of New Zealand.

At the time of writing, Matua Raki sits within Te Pou o te Whakaaro Nui, and has its main office in Wellington, the capital city in New Zealand. With a small team of people with extensive knowledge of working in the addiction sector, and with firm relationships within the sector they work across projects that include those with a focus on:

- Advanced practice addiction nurses
- Best practice implementations (guidelines and best practice advice)
- Co-existing problems ('dual diagnosis')
- Children of Parents with Mental Illness and or Addiction (COPMIA)
- Cultural competency (especially Māori responsiveness)
- Māori addiction workforce
- Early intervention
- Pacific addiction workforce
- Professional development (a suite of trainings)
- Supporting the peer and consumer workforces
- Therapeutic communities
- Implementing the Substance Addiction (Compulsory Assessment and Treatment) Act

This programme of work is based on priorities outlined in current policy and strategy including 'Towards the Next Wave of Mental Health and Addiction Services and Capability: Workforce Survey Review' (Health Workforce New Zealand, 2011) and 'Rising to the Challenge: The Mental Health and Addiction Service Development Plan' (Ministry of Health, 2012). Each project aims to address each of the five workforce development strategic imperatives, as they relate to current needs and context. Sometimes, infrastructure and organizational imperatives are the focus, at other times, resources and training for the practitioners on the ground are provided. For more information and examples of Matua Ra<u>k</u>i's work, see www.matuaraki.org.nz.

The Māori addiction workforce

The 1970s and 1980s brought about important changes in the way Aotearoa New Zealand saw itself, and the way the public sector delivered services to New Zealanders. The public sector began to talk about a bicultural New Zealand, and describe the Treaty of Waitangi[5] as the country's founding document. Government departments began to adopt the idea that the languages, cultures and traditions of both Māori and Pākehā[6] should be officially recognized by the state. Aotearoa New Zealand is now seen by many as a bi-cultural country; the indigenous tangata whenua[7] Māori and others who are non-Māori. While a number of different ethnicities live in Aotearoa New Zealand, Māori are given special respect and authority as the first people of this land.

Special mention needs to be made regarding the development of the Māori addiction workforce in Aotearoa, who have a similar yet varied history to that of the 'mainstream' addiction workforce. The Māori addiction sector, like the rest of the sector has been strongly influenced by those with their own lived experience of addiction related harm. In the early 1980s, it was clearly recognized that although Māori were experiencing addiction related harm (at higher levels than for the non-Māori population) they were not accessing or being seen by addiction treatment services. This led to the recognition that for addiction services to be more accessible and appropriate for Māori that either addiction services needed to be more culturally competent or that these services required cultural support staff. In 1991, ALAC established a number of Māori development roles around the country that began developing community based workers and kaumātua and kuia[8] who could mentor and support AOD workers (Cave et al., 2008).

Over the years, this vision for a collective Māori voice that could advocate for Māori interventions (Cave et al., 2008) has grown and developed to include specialized Māori addiction training and education, specialized Māori addiction treatment services, Māori practitioner competencies and a Māori addiction workforce development strategy. Coupled with this, there is now a very clear expectation that all non-Māori addiction practitioners are culturally competent to provide an appropriate service to Māori and their whānau.

DAPAANZ (ADDICTION PRACTITIONERS ASSOCIATION AOTEAROA NEW ZEALAND)

The first version of the Practitioner Competencies for Alcohol and Drug Workers in Aotearoa New Zealand was published by ALAC in 2001. It was drafted with support from the Alcohol and Drug Treatment Workforce Development Advisory Group and consulted on with those in the sector. Following development of these competencies dapaanz (originally the Alcohol and Drug Practitioners Association Aotearoa New Zealand) was established as the professional body representing addiction treatment practitioners in New Zealand. Anyone with an interest in addiction treatment is eligible for membership of dapaanz, and experienced and qualified practitioners and supervisors can apply to be 'registered'. Dapaanz's first Code of Ethics was developed in 2002 and updated in 2005 but with a constant emphasis on competence and professionalism. In 2011, the competencies were reviewed and updated to include competencies for the wider addiction workforce (including the gambling and smoking cessation workforces) and the association changed its name to the Addiction Practitioners Association Aotearoa New Zealand.

Matua Raki and dapaanz work closely together and in partnership with the other mental health and addiction workforce development centres in New Zealand to build the capacity and capability of the mental health and addiction workforces. While the main focus of the five workforce centres [the Mental Health Workforce Development Programme and Matua Raki (within Te Pou o Te Whakaaro Nui), Te Rau Matatini, Le Va and The Werry Centre] has been on the specialist mental health and addiction workforces, attention has also more recently been given to other workforces in the health, social care, justice and education space that may also work with people with mental health distress or problematic substance use.

SUMMARY

Around the world, there has been clear acknowledgement of the lack of health workforce to meet the requirements of our populations. In parallel to this mental health and addiction workforce development has also been a focus for some countries that recognize the need in this particular area.

While each country outlined in this chapter has taken a different approach to addiction workforce development, some important common themes emerged that are clearly important components of any workforce development strategy. These include that:

- the workforce includes addiction specialists and all other workforces who may meet and work with people with problematic substance use;
- there is a focus on competence and skill development of practitioners;
- there is an emphasis on collaboration and partnership within health and across other sectors (social care, justice, education).

Nonetheless, there are considerable disparities in the visibility, importance and content of addiction workforce development strategy internationally. Below are some of the key elements that need to be considered in any addiction workforce development strategy or programme. Some of these are apparent in the countries covered in this chapter and in the case study on New Zealand, while others are new and emerging areas for consideration.

Key considerations for addiction workforce development

- A systems wide approach must be taken that addresses infrastructure and organizational change as well as individual skill development
- A workforce development and planning approach must be seen as an integral part of the development of any organizational planning

- Support and promotion of the support and peer workforces, as well as 'professional' or 'clinical' workforces, needs to be undertaken
- Consideration needs to be given to service users, families and communities experiencing problematic substance use as part of the 'natural workforce' that may also require development
- The stigma associated with being part of the addiction workforce should be addressed to encourage recruitment and pay parity
- The collection of consistent high quality workforce data is imperative
- Work with education providers to ensure addiction is covered in a variety of core qualifications (e.g. social work) needs to be undertaken
- Cultural competence across the addiction workforce should be seen as a core skill
- Recognizing and engaging in collaboration and partnership is important within and across sectors and professions
- Offering inter-professional workforce development opportunities is important
- Consideration needs to be given to the integration of workforce development initiatives that cover alcohol, other drugs and other addiction related problems (for example, gambling)
- Preparing the workforce for changes resulting from innovation and technology will be crucial

Addiction workforce development needs to build the capability and capacity of the sector to meet addiction related needs at a community level. It should recognize that the workforces that support people who may have problematic substance use and their families and whānau are wide and varied, requiring broad responses. While addiction workforce development may require further professionalization and a raising of standards in line with emerging complexities, this must not be done at the expense of peer and support services that have often provided a backbone for the workforce throughout history.

An addiction workforce would ideally be made up of a variety of people with a variety of backgrounds, lived experience and education in order to meet the complex and diverse needs of the people they serve. This workforce should be supported by sound infrastructure, legislation and organizational commitment to providing quality addiction supports to service users, family and whānau.

NOTES

1 Please note a variety of language is used throughout this chapter to describe addiction/problematic substance use/substance misuse/substance abuse/AOD problems to depict the different approaches to research, policy, diagnosis and workforce development around the world in the language most preferred by each country.
2 Aotearoa is the Māori word for New Zealand.
3 Whānau refers to an extended family and/or community of people traditionally connected by a common ancestor but in contemporary times can be connected through a common 'cause or purpose'.
4 Aotearoa New Zealand now also has a Pacific health workforce development centre, Le Va.
5 The Treaty of Waitangi is an agreement, in Māori and English, that was made between the British Crown and about 540 Māori rangatira (chiefs) in Waitangi in 1840.
6 Term used to describe New Zealanders who are 'of European descent'.
7 People of the land.
8 Leaders and elders.

REFERENCES

Alcohol Advisory Council of New Zealand (2001) *Competencies for Alcohol & Drug Workers in Aotearoa -New Zealand.* Occasional Publication 13. The Alcohol and Drug Treatment Workforce Development Advisory Group. Wellington: ALAC.

Bennett, T. and Holloway, K. (2005) *Understanding Drugs, Alcohol and Crime.* Maidenhead: Open University Press.

Cave, T., Roberston, P., Pitama, S. and Huriwai, T. (2008) *He Tētē Kura: Māori Addiction Treatment 1980–2008.* Christchurch: Matua Raki

COSLA & the Scottish Government (2010) *Supporting the development of Scotland's alcohol and drug workforce* Available from http://www.gov.scot/Resource/Doc/254429/0110090.pdf (Accessed 21 April 2016)

Crawford, R. (2008) *Too Good to Last – The Death of a Caring Culture. Queen Mary Hospital: The Therapy of Addictions. Hanmer Springs, 1972–1991*. Hanmer Springs: Sunbeam Publishers.

DHSSPS (2011) *New Strategic Direction for Alcohol and Drugs. Phase 2 2011-2016. A Framework for Reducing Alcohol and Drug Related Harm in Northern Ireland.* Available from file:///C:/Users/nelsona/Downloads/NI_New%20Strategic%20Direction%20for%20Alcohol%20and%20Drugs%20Phase%202_2011-2016.pdf (Accessed 21 April 2016)

European Commission (EC) (2012) *Commission Staff Working Document on an Action Plan for the EU Health Workforce*. Strasbourg: EC. Available from: http://ec.europa.eu/health/workforce/docs/staff_working_doc_healthcare_workforce_en.pdf (Accessed 7 June 2014).

Federation of Drug and Alcohol Professionals (FDAP) (2012) *Developing Standards of Practice in the Drugs and Alcohol Workforce: A Practical Guide from the Federation of Drug and Alcohol Professionals*. Available from: http://www.fdap.org.uk/documents/Vision%20thing%20practitioners%20&%20managers.pdf (Accessed 8 July 2014).

Home Office (2006) *Joint National Treatment Agency and Drug Strategy Directorate; Workforce Development Plan for the Substance Misuse Field.* Available from: http://www.drugsandalcohol.ie/19462/1/2006_Joint_workforcedevelopmentplan.pdf (Accessed 21 April 2016)

Health Funding Authority (2000) *Tuutahitia te Wero, Meeting the Challenges: Mental Health Workforce Development Plan 2000–2005*. Wellington: Health Funding Authority.

Healthwork UK (2001) *A Competent Workforce to Tackle Substance Misuse. An Analysis of the Need for Occupational Standards in the Drug and Alcohol Sector*. Manchester: Healthwork UK.

Health Workforce New Zealand (2011) *Towards the Next Wave of Mental Health & Addiction Services and Capability: Workforce Service Review Report.* Available from https://www.health.govt.nz/system/files/documents/pages/mental-health-workforce-service-review.pdf (Accessed 21 April 2016)

Intergovernmental Committee on Drugs (2015) *National Alcohol and Other Drug Workforce Development Strategy 2015–2018*. Available from: http://www.nationaldrugstrategy.gov.au/internet/drugstrategy/Publishing.nsf/content/naodwds2015-18 (Accessed 16 September 2015).

Jacobs, R. and Hawley, J. (2009). Emergence of workforce development: definition, conceptual boundaries, and implications. In R MacLean and D. Wilson (eds), International Handbook of Education for the Changing World of Work Bridging Academic and Vocational Learning. Amsterdam: Kluwer, pp. 2537–52.

Kerr, N. (1888) *Inebriety: its etiology, pathology, treatment, and jurisprudence*. Available from https://archive.org/details/66640570R.nlm.nih.gov (Accessed 21 April 2016)

KPMG (2013) *An Uncertain Age: Reimagining Long Term Care in the 21st Century.* Available from: http://www.kpmg.com/Global/en/IssuesAndInsights/ArticlesPublications/an-uncertain-age/Documents/an-uncertain-age-v4.pdf (Accessed 6 January 2015).

Mental Health Commission. (1998) *Blueprint for Mental Health Services in New Zealand: How things need to be*. Wellington: Mental Health Commission.

Mental Health Commission and Ministry of Health (1999) *Developing the Mental Health Workforce: The report of the National Mental Health Workforce Development Co-ordinating Committee*. Wellington: Mental Health Commission.

Ministry of Health (1994) *Looking Forward: Strategic Directions for Mental Health Services*. Wellington: Ministry of Health.

Ministry of Health (1996) *Towards Better Mental Health Services: The Report of the National Working Party on Mental Health Workforce Development*. Wellington: Ministry of Health.

Ministry of Health (1997) *Moving Forward: The National Mental Health Plan for More and Better Services*. Wellington: Ministry of Health.

Ministry of Health (2001) *A National Strategic Framework for Alcohol and Drugs Services*. Wellington: Ministry of Health.

Ministry of Health (2002) *Mental Health (Alcohol and other Drugs) Workforce*

Development Framework. Available from http://www.moh.govt.nz/moh.nsf/Files/MentalHealthWorkforceDevelopmentFramework/$file/MentalHealthWorkforceDevelopmentFramework.pdf (Accessed 21 April 2016)

Ministry of Health (2012) *Rising to the Challenge 2012-2017: The mMental Health and Addiction Service Development Plan*. Available from http://www.health.govt.nz/publication/rising-challenge-mental-health-and-addiction-service-development-plan-2012-2017 (Accessed 21 April 2016)

Morris, J., Lora, A., McBain, R. and Saxena, S. (2012) Global mental health resources and services: a WHO Survey of 184 Countries. *Public Health Reviews*, 34(2).

National Centre for Education and Training on Addiction (NCETA) (2002) *Submission to the Intergovernmental Committee on Drugs (IGCD)*. Adelaide: NCETA, Flinders University.

National Centre for Education and Training on Addiction (NCETA) (2013) *A Literature Review to Support the Development of Australia's Alcohol and Other Drug Workforce Strategy*. Adelaide: NCETA, Flinders University.

National Treatment Agency for Substance Misuse (NTA) (2009) *Workforce Development Drug Treatment, Reintegration and Recovery in the Community and Prisons Adult Plans 2010/11*. Available from: http://www.nta.nhs.uk/uploads/workforce_supplementary_2010_11.pdf (Accessed 1 August 2014).

NHS Health Scotland (2009 and 2011) *Seeking Service Users Views: Workforce Training and Development Requirements 2008*. Glasgow: NHS Health Scotland.

Roche, A. and Pidd, K. (2010) *Alcohol and Other Drugs Workforce Development Issues and Imperatives: Setting the Scene*. National Centre for Education and Training on Addiction (NCETA). Adelaide: NCETA, Flinders University.

Roche, A. (2001) What is this thing called workforce development? In A. Roche and J. McDonald (eds), *Systems, Settings, People: Workforce Development Challenges for the Alcohol and other Drugs Field*. Adelaide: NCETA, Flinders University, pp. 5–22.

Ryan, O., Murphy, D. and Krom, L. (2012) *Vital Signs: Taking the Pulse of the Addiction Treatment Workforce, A National Report-Executive Summary*. Missouri: ATTC National Office, University of Missouri-Kansas City. Available from: http://www.attcnetwork.org/documents/VitalSignsReport.pdf (Accessed 7 June 2014).

Scottish Government (2008) *The Road to Recovery: A new approach to tackling Scotland's drug problem* Available from http://www.gov.scot/Publications/2008/05/22161610/0 (Accessed 21 April 2016)

Substance Abuse and Mental Health Services Administration (SAMHSA) (2006a) *Report to Congress: Addiction Treatment Workforce Development*. Rockville: SAMSHA.

Substance Abuse and Mental Health Services Administration (SAMHSA) (2006b) *Strengthening Professional Identity: Challenges of the Addiction Treatment Workforce*. Rockville: SAMSHA.

Substance Abuse and Mental Health Services Administration (SAMHSA) (2007) *An Action Plan for Behavioural Health Workforce Development*. Rockville: SAMSHA.

Substance Abuse and Mental Health Services Administration (SAMHSA) (2011) *Results from the 2010 National Survey on Drug Use and Health: Summary of National Findings*. Rockville: SAMSHA.

Substance Abuse and Mental Health Services Administration (SAMHSA) (2013) *Report to Congress on the Nation's Substance Abuse and Mental Health Workforce Issues*. Available from: http://store.samhsa.gov/shin/content/PEP13-RTC-BHWORK/PEP13-RTC-BHWORK.pdf (Accessed 23 June 2014).

Te Pou o Te Whakaaro Nui (2014) *Getting it Right: Workforce Planning Approach*. Available from: http://www.tepou.co.nz/library/tepou/getting-it-right-a-workforce-planning-approach (Accessed 7 January 2015).

Welsh Government (2011) *Substance Misuse Workforce Development Plan 2011–2014* Available from: http://www.substancemisuseworkforcewales.org/resources/publications/?lang=en (Accessed 8 July 2014).

World Health Organization (WHO) (2005) *WHO European Ministerial Conference on Mental Health Facing the Challenges, Building Solutions*. Helsinki: WHO. Available from: http://www.euro.who.int/__data/assets/

pdf_file/0008/88595/E85445.pdf (Assessed 7 July 2014).

World Health Organization (WHO) (2008) *Policies and Practices for Mental Health in Europe-meeting the challenges*. Geneva: WHO. Available from: http://www.euro.who.int/en/publications/abstracts/policies-and-practices-for-mental-health-in-europe.-meeting-the-challenges (Accessed 7 June 2014).

World Health Organization (WHO) (2010). *Workload Indicators of Staffing Need: User's Manual*. Geneva: World Health Organization Press.

World Health Organization (WHO) (2011a) *Transformative Scale Up of Health Professional Education: An Effort to Increase the Number of Health Professionals and to Strengthen Their Impact on Population Health*. Geneva: WHO. Available from: http://www.who.int/hrh/resources/transformative_education/en/ (accessed 20 June 2014).

World Health Organization (2011b) *Mental Health Atlas 2011*. Geneva: WHO.

World Health Organization (2012) *Human Resources for Health: Action Framework of the Western Pacific Region 2011–2015*. Available from: http://www.wpro.who.int/hrh/documents/HRH_Action_Framework.pdf (Accessed 31 July 2014).

World Health Organization (2014) *A Universal Truth: No Health Without a Workforce*: Geneva: WHO.

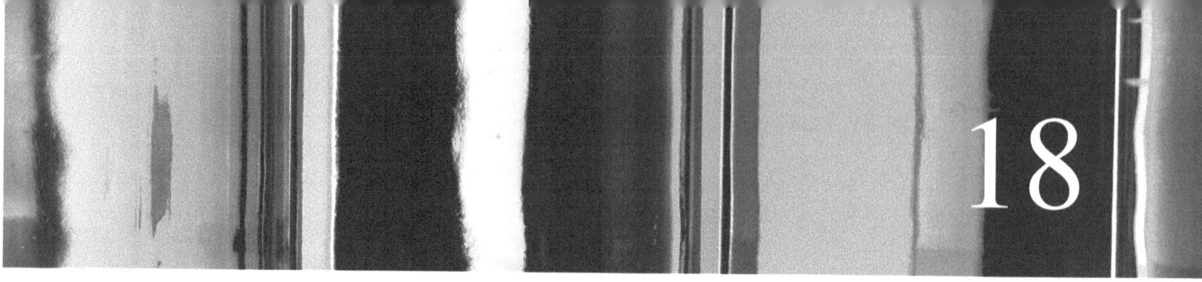

18

Reflecting on Intoxication

Geoffrey Hunt and Vibeke Asmussen Frank

Every society on Earth is a high society. (Jay 2010: 9)

The universal need for liberation from the restrictions of mundane existence is satisfied by experiencing altered states of consciousness. (Rudgley 1993: 3)

INTRODUCTION

These statements about the universal desire for intoxication and the pleasurable features of intoxication may seem surprising given recent concerns about binge drinking and intoxication, especially among young people, where an increase in youthful drunken behavior has grabbed the attention of researchers, the media, and public officials. 'Drinking to intoxication' is viewed by the authorities, according to Helen Keane as 'the most harmful of alcohol-related behaviors with a significant negative impact on individual and community safety and well-being' (Keane 2009: 135). This attitude to drinking and intoxication is widespread and many other examples from the UK, the USA, Australia, Denmark, and other European countries can be easily found. Overall, this concern would seem to suggest that agreement exists on the notion that intoxication, either from alcohol or from other mind-altering substances, is, by definition, physically harmful and socially and morally problematic. As Becker noted 'the goal of artificially inducing a change in one's consciousness is considered by many to be immoral' (1967: 164) and the desire to seek intoxication 'is at best tolerated and is often stigmatized or even criminalized when it is associated with the use of intoxicant drugs' (Yardley 2012: 1).

This approach to intoxication as a problematic activity is, however, not shared by all researchers, especially anthropologists, sociologists, and cultural historians, many of whom have sought to examine the role and meaning of intoxication not from a problem perspective but instead sought to explain why it is that so many people of different ages, from totally different social backgrounds, in so many different cultures, at so many different times in history, should seek to alter their state of consciousness. Intoxication, here defined as the use of substances to alter consciousness, has featured as a 'universal human theme' from the early Bronze Age's affinity with alcohol to the Neolithic period's cultural use of cannabis and the classical epoch's rituals with opium to youthful fascination with dance drugs such as ecstasy (Rudgley 1993; Walton 2001; Weil 1972). A distinguishing feature of intoxicants across time and place is the pleasure and enjoyment associated with the consumption experience – the chemical and physiological reactions and the users' interaction with others in particular milieus. Pleasurable descriptions of altered states – happiness, freedom, euphoria – from psychoactive drugs have been recorded since prehistoric times (Rudgley 1993). Furthermore, the deliberate pursuit of intoxication through opium by writers within the romantic period, for example, Coleridge, De Quincy, Byron and Walter Scott, gave them not merely pleasure but also opened up for them new avenues of poetic inspiration. 'Opium for De Quincy…offered dreams that money can buy…and allowed transport to the realms of imagination' (Boon 2002: 37).

The purpose of this paper is to examine some of the key elements that researchers have identified as important in researching intoxicants and intoxication, while avoiding a health or social problem perspective. More specifically, following in the tradition of Rudgley (1993), Walton (2001), and Sulkunen (2002), this paper is intended to provide and discuss important themes and issues relevant for studying intoxication in a socio-cultural, contextual, situated, and comparative way. The intention of the paper is to examine the 'embeddedness of culture in social practice' (Sherratt 1995: 2), thereby producing an understanding of intoxication within the relationships between culture, consumption, and society. We will do so by exploring both the classic and contemporary research on the subject, introducing those perspectives that emphasize a sociological or anthropological approach.

Prior to commencing this paper, we would like to begin by making some preliminary statements. In examining the available research on intoxication, an obvious division exists that separates those researchers that focus on alcohol intoxication and drunkenness from those who concentrate solely on illicit drug intoxication. Researchers, who have focused on intoxication within its entirety, are in the minority. To note this characteristic may be unsurprising given the sharp divide that exists between drug and alcohol research in general, as well as between legal and illegal intoxicants. However, for the purposes of this paper, and following writers such as Goodman et al. (1995), Herring et al. (2013), Rudgley (1993), Walton (2001), and Withington and McShane (2014), we will deal with intoxicants in general, although at different sections of the paper we will use empirical studies that will focus more specifically on alcohol or on illicit drugs respectively. Also, where applicable, we have used empirical examples taken from a number of studies conducted by one of the authors in San Francisco.[1] In the rest of the paper, we will examine four themes – culture, sociability, and social settings; post-modernism, youthful intoxication and meaning; gender and intoxication; and finally, controlling and calibrating intoxication. These themes are critical for a socio-cultural perspective on intoxication, and have been highlighted by a number of researchers since the 1940s.

CULTURE, SOCIABILITY, AND SOCIAL SETTING

Early anthropological and sociological theories of intoxication sought primarily to understand the role of intoxication in different societal contexts and the norms that influenced the resulting behaviors (Sulkunen

2002). Some of these early theorists analyzed the different functions of intoxication from both alcohol and drugs in different non-industrialized societies and sought to develop a perspective on intoxication at the societal level, thereby identifying universal characteristics. Drugs, particularly of a psychoactive nature, appeared to possess mystical or magical qualities, and mind altering substances were intimately connected and integrated into community life, enriching daily life as well as enhancing spirituality. La Barre's (1938) study is among the first to document the rituals and beliefs associated with peyote use among Native American tribes. Others have similarly looked at psychedelic use, long revered for their religious, social and medicinal qualities (Dobkin De Rios 1990; Grob 2002). Bourguignon's (1973) meta-analysis of anthropological works on hallucinogens and altered states of consciousness among 'other worldly' locales – especially in the Americas and Africa – suggests the following:

> Altered states of consciousness occur in all human societies...frequently embedded into religious patterns of belief and ceremonial, with varying degrees of ritualization...also ritualized in a secular context. Ritualization maybe thought of as an imposition of order, a bringing under social and ideological control of what are potentially disruptive psychological states and forces. (Bourguignon 1973: 21)

Early anthropologists, such as Horton (1943), argued that alcohol intoxication was also a societal mechanism for reducing tension, alleviating anxiety and fear in the face of uncertainty. This perspective was utilized by many other anthropologists, for example, Szwed (1966), who examined the ways in which drinking was used by residents of a Newfoundland parish to reduce tension and conflict at political meetings. If antagonistic behavior occurred, it could be excused later on the grounds that an individual just could not hold his liquor (Szwed 1966). Also, Lemert (1958), in his work on the Northwest Coast Indians, argued that intoxication was a direct reaction to the disintegration of their traditional culture through contact with the culture of the white men. While some of these early theories have been largely discarded, partly because of critiques of functionalist theory,[2] they did emphasize the importance of seeking explanations at the social level rather than at any individual level. So, although the state of intoxication is an individual or psychological component of drinking, it is nevertheless 'inextricably conjoined with the social and collective part of drinking practices' (Partanen 1991: 223). As Marshall argues, 'the pharmacological effects of alcohol on human beings make people feel different than when they haven't imbibed. The meanings given to this experience, that is, how one interprets these feelings and orders his or her experience, are provided by the culture in which one is participant' (Marshall 1983: 200).

This latter element is extensively detailed in the 'pathbreaking' but now somewhat neglected book, *Drunken Comportment*, by MacAndrew and Edgerton. Published in 1969, and using a wide range of comparative ethnographic material and examining different types of drunken comportment, they showed that 'over the course of socialization, people learn about drunkenness what their society "knows" about drunkenness; and accepting and acting upon the understandings thus imparted to them, they become the living confirmation of their society's teachings' (1969: 88) and highlighted the ways in which drunken behavior varies from one culture to another and within individual cultures through time. From compiling this material, they argued that drunken behavior is primarily a matter of socio-cultural learning and while it may differ from behavior that was acceptable when sober, it nevertheless remained within 'certain culturally sanctioned limits' (Partanen 1991: 224). Their book emphasized the importance of the culturally defined nature of intoxication: 'the way that people comport themselves when they are drunk is determined not by alcohol's toxic assault upon the seat of moral judgment, conscience or the like but by what their society makes of and imparts to them concerning the state of drunkenness' (MacAndrew and Edgerton 1969: 165). The significance of their seminal work was to establish the view that the interpretations that individuals make of intoxication is only partially shaped by the chemical or pharmacological effects of the substance (Paton-Simpson 1996). That intoxication is not solely the result of the pharmacological qualities of the substance, but instead is also dependent upon the combination of the substance itself, the mind-set of the user, and the social setting in which the substance is used was also explored by Zinberg (1984) in his research on intoxication from illicit drugs. Zinberg based his research on the pioneering work of Howard Becker (1953), whose now classic paper on 'Becoming a Marihuana user', highlighted the importance of having to learn from others how to become intoxicated within particular settings or contexts when using psycho-active substances for the first time, thereby emphasizing the social nature of intoxication.

This crucial role of alcohol and psychoactive drugs in sociable interactions in many diverse societies and cultures has led researchers to argue that intoxicants operate as 'a medium of sociability'. For example, Partanen argues that 'drinks delineate and articulate a world in which the expression of sociability becomes possible; they provide material and symbolic means for the achievement of a heightened sense of sociability' (Partanen 1991: 221; see also Douglas 1987). Heightening sociability through the use of substances has also been noted by researchers in the drug field. For example, ecstasy can produce, as Jackson has noted, 'a temporary and partial dip in the feeling of fear and anxiety which suffuse much of our social experiences' (Jackson 2004: 64). Because norms of appropriate social and personal behavior and notions of privacy are transformed, people often became much more eager to interact with others and willing to share their personal thoughts and feelings. This openness in turn can lead users to bond more closely with friends and partners. A characteristic also noted by researchers who have studied the cultures and effects of marijuana use (Becker 1967; Orcutt 1975; Warner et al. 1999). Changes in notions of social boundaries can also result in a diminution in the perception of social distance between people. Spencer describes this process as 'the abolition of difference and the creation of a sense of "communion"' (Spencer 1985: 154, cited in Malbon 1999).

As in the case of drinking and drug use, the experience of intoxication is also viewed as being intimately tied up with commensality, with trust and reciprocity (Kneale 2003). The importance of commensality or sociability can be seen if we consider the answers provided by our young respondents in the study on the dance scene in San Francisco. Many of the respondents described their intoxication, whether from alcohol or illicit drugs, including ecstasy, mushrooms, and marijuana, as a central feature in their socializing with their friends. For many of the young people interviewed, using alcohol and drugs and becoming intoxicated was not only a social activity, it was an activity that they undertook purposefully in order to become more sociable (cf. Yardley 2012). Throughout their interviews, they emphasized that using either drugs or alcohol and becoming intoxicated allowed them to have more confidence and more easily relate to others. Intoxicants allowed them to relax, de-stress, be more open, or to be more one's real self. When asked about their drinking or their drug use, they noted a desire to lose control and become 'wasted', while nevertheless emphasizing the appropriate setting in which getting wasted should take place. Hence, not only was sociability emphasized, but also, as Zinberg noted, the social context, in which either substance was consumed, was also portrayed as fundamental to the whole experience. The intricate relationship between intoxication, sociability, and setting has been documented in such diverse settings as Greek symposiums (Osborne 2014), alehouses (Clark 1983), African Beer Gardens (Wolcott 1974), Mexican cantinas (Palafox 2001), Amazon rain forests (Dobkin de Rios 1969), or kava ceremonies in Tonga (Jay 2010). The emphasis on the importance of the social group and the social setting in determining acceptable intoxicated behavior was a critical finding both in the work of MacAndrew and Edgerton, and that of Zinberg (1984), and is still important today in research on drug and alcohol consumption.

While these early studies of intoxication have pointed towards the importance of situating the experiences of intoxication within in a wider socio-cultural context, many of these studies, and especially those in anthropology, focused on non-industrialized societies or in the case of drug research primarily on drug using sub-cultures. However, more recently, partly as a result of changes in leisure practices and youth cultures, researchers have begun to examine contemporary attitudes towards intoxication and especially intoxicated behavior by young people within the nighttime economy (Chatterton and Hollands 2003; Hayward and Hobbs 2007; Miles 2000).

POST-MODERNISM, YOUTHFUL INTOXICATION, AND MEANING

Early theories of the sociable role of intoxication are somewhat mirrored in more contemporary theories of youthful intoxication put forward by sociologists and cultural criminologists. Recently, researchers have explained youthful intoxication in terms of its role in the society within an analysis of changing societal conditions, including changes in youth cultures. Measham and Brain (2005) have argued that this shift in 'cultures of intoxication' can only be understood if it is situated in the changes that are occurring at the macro, meso, and micro levels that influence contemporary youth drinking and drug using patterns. At the macro- or societal level, researchers such as Beck (1992) and Furlong and Cartmel (1997) have identified changes occurring in post-modern or post-industrial society over the last 20 years that have led to a new situation for young people. 'Relationships with family and friends, experiences in education and the labour market, leisure and lifestyles and the ability to become independent young adults' (Furlong and Cartmel 1997:1) have all altered significantly. As a result of the weakening of traditional sources of social differentiation based on social class and communities, as noted by Furlong and Cartmel (1997) and Miles (2000), young people today are viewed 'as attempting to find self-fulfillment and ways of identifying with other young people through the consumption of goods' (Furlong and Cartmel 1997: 61). This increased commodification of youth culture (Brain et al. 2000), has led to manufacturers deliberately marketing commodities to young people and manipulating youthful liminal drives (Hayward and Hobbs 2007).

At the meso-level, researchers have emphasized the marked changes within the nighttime economy and the redevelopment and rejuvenation of the inner urban areas into zones that provide 'highly structured provision for hedonistic economic activity' (Hayward and Hobbs 2007: 451; see also Hadfield 2009) in which alcohol is central. Nightlife activities are an integral part of young people's consumption and their lifestyle (Chatterton and Hollands 2003) and consumption and leisure activities have become 'important in the process of self-production' (Riley et al. 2010: 35; see also Measham and Moore 2009). At the micro- or individual and/or group level, researchers have argued that young people today are experiencing the paradox existing in the post-industrial consumer society where they feel, at the same time, both ontologically insecure and over-controlled (Hayward and Hobbs 2007: 447; see also Garland 2001). Given these developments, young people seek intoxication not only for the 'inherent excitement of the alcoholic or drug rush' (Hayward and Hobbs 2007: 447) but their desire for 'determined intoxication' (Measham 2008) is a way of experiencing self-actualization and self-expression, thereby seizing some sense of control over their lives. They are 'exercising individual rights to pleasure, hedonism or escapism' (Riley et al. 2010: 37).

Given these changes, the desire to discover new and exciting forms of consumption can be seen in contemporary leisure practices that are increasingly associated with elements of the novel, the extraordinary, and the transcendental. The need to transcend or transgress (Presdee 2000) the normal or the mundane has been noted by other writers, such as Cohen and Taylor (1992) and Lyng (2005) who examined the increasing need for leisure activities to be out-of-the-ordinary, and to have the potential of disrupting or breaking the routine of life. Emotionally exciting activities 'offset the suffocation of an over controlled alienated existence within the mundane reality of modern life' (O'Malley and Mugford 1994: 206). The search for new and exciting experiences, or as Campbell (1989) calls it, 'the ceaseless consumption of novelty' (Campbell 1989: 205) and 'the endless emergence of new wants' (O'Malley and Mugford 1991: 57) create a vital demand for the consumption of new commodities including mind-altering substances (Reith 2005). For example, many of the respondents in the study of the dance scene in San Francisco used ecstasy as a catalyst for creating new possibilities in how they perceived and related to themselves and the world around them. The experience on ecstasy and the opportunity to experience life and interactions with others outside of everyday norms and expectations uncovered a way of being that respondents had previously not experienced or had not been aware of, but which they found pleasing and preferable.

Given the desires to seek new identities through the consumption of new commodities (Miles 2000), plus the desire to discover new thrills to overcome the mundane, then it is obvious why, for example, ecstasy and other mind altering substances would have such a widespread appeal for young people, especially within the exciting, transgressive, and pleasurable context of the dance scene and its electronic music (Hunt and Evans 2008). As O'Malley and Mugford have noted 'in such a cultural milieu...illicit and even dangerous drug taking as a leisure activity appears as an intelligible form of the normatively sanctioned search for the extraordinary' (O'Malley and Mugford 1991: 57). Entering the extraordinary, removed the raver or clubber 'from the "normal" times, spaces and social relations of their everyday lives' (Malbon 1999: 83). Other writers have also argued that the desire for intoxication within the night-time economy can be seen as the continuation of the carnival tradition in which the traits of transgression, danger, and disorder have become increasingly regulated and commercially sponsored (Presdee 2000). Using the work of Bakhtin (1984), Presdee argues that carnival was a time when 'the pleasures of the body were foregrounded, in opposition to the dominant and accepted values of restraint and sobriety' (Presdee 2000: 38). Carnival permits transgression and allows the world to be turned 'upside down'. This transgression or transformation of the everyday within raves inspiring 'pleasure, excitement, exhilaration and desire' (Lupton 1999: 167) were central and fundamental features of both alcohol and ecstasy's appeal for young people, and have been an important focus of study in more contemporary research on intoxication.

While we have here similar arguments to explain intoxication, as the early theorists put forward, either at the level of coping with anxiety or ontological insecurity, contemporary theories have sought to explain youthful intoxication with an analysis of societal change at different analytical levels of society. Focusing specifically on young people is significantly different to much of the early anthropological work, which had little or nothing to say about intoxication among young people. Moreover, as Sulkunen (2002) has noted, while sociologists and anthropologists have traditionally considered the norms, function, and role of intoxication, researchers today have sought to examine the meaning of intoxication for the individuals involved. Instead of concentrating solely on the functional uses of intoxication, they have examined what it is about intoxication that makes the desire for an altered consciousness meaningful.

GENDER AND INTOXICATION

Traditionally, women's intoxication has been stigmatized and women who drink to intoxication are seen as not 'respectable' (Fillmore 1984; Griffin et al. 2009; Skeggs 1997). The norms surrounding intoxicated women have evolved in recent decades, although women's intoxication is still typically viewed more negatively than men's (de Visser and McDonnell 2012; Griffin et al. 2009; Leyshon 2005; Measham and Østergaard 2009). As Simonen (2011) has noted, historically, women have been disregarded in the world of intoxication and intoxication was viewed primarily as a characteristic of a masculine environment. Important early anthropological and sociological work emphasized the extent to which drinking and intoxication are male-dominated activities, which both enforce and enhance gender divisions within the society. Alcohol use, misuse, and intoxication have long been associated with men and masculinity (Hunt et al. 2005; Mullen et al. 2007; Peralta 2007; Peralta 2008; Peralta et al. 2010), For example, within many cultures, to drink is to be masculine and to drink heavily and become intoxicated is to be even more masculine (Guttmann 1996; Messerschmidt 1997; Peralta 2007). Intoxicated behavior is acceptable or normative in certain contexts because it works to affirm masculinity and male solidarity (Connell and Messerschmidt 2005; Dunning et al. 1988; Hunt et al. 2005; Peace 1992; Skeggs 1997). In this way, excessive drinking and intoxication by young men needs no further explanation – they are just being men (Østergaard 2007). In contrast, until very recently, there has been a relative underdevelopment of research on women and intoxication and especially around issues of intoxication and potential pleasure. In fact, research on women and pleasure has more often than not been viewed as 'disreputable pleasures' (Ettorre 2007; O'Malley and Valverde 2004). This neglect is even more surprising given the extent to which young people today, both men and women, are involved in what Parker and colleagues have referred to as the 'leisure-pleasure landscape' (Parker et al. 1998: 25).

The role of women within intoxication research was primarily defined in the role of controlling men's drinking and intoxication. However, this is not to suggest that all research has overlooked the issue of female intoxication, especially as a major public issue. For example, Charles Booth writing in the early 1900s in his nine-volume report the 'Life and Labour of the London Poor' (1970), noted that while drunkenness had declined, drinking had increased and this could be laid at the feet of women. Much of this work pointed the finger at women as the cause for many of the social ills of society.[3] More recently, the issue of female intoxication has returned to the public spotlight, where the seeming increase in public intoxication by women has become a pertinent issue again given much attention in the public media. In the UK media, female intoxication has been associated with an increase in 'laddette' cultures, in which young women have been demonized by the tabloid press (Jackson 2006). According to one news' report, a laddette is defined 'as mouthy and always up for a laugh, she can smoke eight fags at once and drink all her weekly alcohol units in two hours' (Ridley 2004, cited in Jackson 2006). A few contemporary researchers have begun to examine female intoxication not solely as an example of a growing public health and social order problem or as yet a further example of the increasing parity between male and female drinking patterns and consumption. Instead, some researchers have begun to consider the extent to which, although the behavior may appear similar, the meaning of intoxication for women is different from that of men. In other words, contemporary feminist researchers have begun to examine female intoxication as another example of new ways of accomplishing femininity and an attempt to develop what Measham in her article 'Doing Gender, Doing Drugs' (2002) argued for: an examination of the effects of alcohol or drugs on the performance or accomplishment of gender: '[d]rug use is not just mediated by gender, but, far more significantly, drug use and the associated leisure, music, and style cultures within which drug use is located are themselves ways of accomplishing a gendered identity' (Measham 2002: 335). Measham argued that it is not just that gender influences the substances people use (e.g. men and women have different rates of drug use or prefer different substances), but that drug use itself conveys meaning about one's gender identity. This theme was further pursued by Waitt and colleagues (2011), who argued that becoming intoxicated from alcohol allowed women to perform gender differently and engage in different gender performances. Drinking to intoxication and losing control may allow young women to escape the demands of living in a post-modern society. This approach leads us to examine drinking and intoxication in relation to both *masculinities* and *femininities* as situated, social accomplishments. However, given the changing nature of what some writers (Griffin et al. 2013; McRobbie 2009) have referred to as post-feminism culture which calls on young women 'to enact "excessive" or "hyper-sexual" forms of femininity' (authors' emphasis) (Griffin et al. 2013: 186) coupled with what Brain et al. (2000) have called a 'new alcohol order', and new cultures of intoxication, young women's relationship to normative ideas of acceptable alcohol consumption has changed (Hutton et al. 2013; Waitt et al. 2011). Young women today have to negotiate notions of acceptable femininity while intoxicated as well as managing elements of risk and uncertainty. Hence, as both Griffin et al. (2013) and Waitt et al. (2011) have emphasized, the attempt of young women to engage in post-feminist notions of freedom and sexual empowerment within contemporary cultures of intoxication may be a precarious path to negotiate, and attempting to navigate these competing, and often contradictory discourses, young women face 'an impossible space to occupy' (Griffin et al. 2013: 186).

CONTROLLING AND CALIBRATING INTOXICATION

An emerging area of research is what could be described as the 'range of intoxication' or 'calibrated intoxication', that is, the extent to which individual drinkers or drug users decide, though not always successfully, the degree to which they will become intoxicated. This more calculated approach to intoxication has been called by a number of contemporary researchers – a 'controlled loss of control' (Measham 2004a; see also Beck and Rosenbaum 1994). For example, in their study of youthful drinking in Italy, Beccaria and Guidoni (2002) argue that their respondents identified a 'threshold' between becoming 'tipsy' and getting drunk. A similar threshold existed for respondents we interviewed in the dance scene in San Francisco, who distinguished between being 'buzzed' and being drunk. To achieve this buzz, some respondents noted that it was important not to become intoxicated too often: 'Like you can't do it too much…Like doing too much it takes away…the buzz'. While these characteristics would suggest that the type of intoxication sought after was based on not consuming too much, respondents also emphasized the importance of drinking enough to reach the desired level. Drinking moderately was not sufficient. For many, intoxication was not an unfortunate side-effect of drinking, but a primary goal. This aim was true for many respondents and illustrates what Measham and Brain (2005) called 'determined drunkenness'. Respondents did not wish to remain in control when intoxicated, they wanted to get 'wasted'.

A number of researchers have noted that controlling intoxication is not solely about controlling the intake, it is also about utilizing different substances to manage the intensity of intoxication (Forsyth 1996; Hammersley et al. 1999; Solowij et al. 1992). Certain drugs are used to increase or diminish the effects of others. In examining issues of controlled or calibrated intoxication, we do not wish to suggest that intoxication is always the result of decision-making processes that are calculated and rational, but instead merely to note the extent to which to becoming intoxicated may involve some decision-making processes and is not only done with little or no forethought or is decided on the spur of the moment (Mayock 2005).

One significant element of controlling and calibrating intoxication is related to the importance of planning intoxication within the constraint of the night-out. Although MacAndrew and Edgerton (1969) coined the phrase 'time-out' to suggest the ways in which being intoxicated allowed the drinker or drug user to step outside normally acceptable ways of behaving, few researchers have examined the impact or experience of intoxication on notions of time. And yet it is apparent that time becomes manipulated or modified by intoxication either in terms of seeming to stop time and allowing for time to be experienced, modifying linear time or creating a sense of elasticity (Yardley 2012).[4] However, in spite of this ability to interrupt notions of linear time, many of our respondents emphasized the idea of temporal organization. Their narratives dealt with issues on how intoxication had to dovetail with the constraints of the night-out. A sense of linear, chronological, and fixed notion of time oscillated around using drugs to fit with the timing of the nighttime economy. Although 'intoxication...enjoys an immunity to the clock' (Yardley 2012: 66), young people tailored their bouts of intoxication to fit in with the constraints that operated around their leisure activities. Dance events and attending clubs occur mainly at the weekend, which is viewed as a highly symbolic period where individuals can experience 'a cathartic release from the working week' (Measham 2004a: 321; see also Hayward 2002). The weekend is a 'time-out from weekday pressures' (Measham 2004b: 210) in which the pursuit of hedonism takes place albeit within a structured environment. Malbon (1999), in his work on clubs and dance events, also noted the extent to which dance activities typically revolve around set beginnings and endings as venues are increasingly governed by strict licensing restrictions, which dictate the duration of the event. Given these time restrictions, attendees must co-ordinate their drug taking and alcohol consumption and resulting intoxication to occur within specified time boundaries. Although many of the young people interviewed in our research on the dance scene in San Francisco consumed both drugs and alcohol both before and after the event, the majority organized their substance use to dovetail with the timing of the night out, taking ecstasy, for example, just before they gained entry to the club to ensure that the intoxication effects peaked when they were inside; furthermore, consumption began at home with pre-drinking, followed by taking ecstasy at the club or event to provide energy for dancing, followed by marijuana or ketamine taken after the club had closed, usually at home. The respondents also described a series of decisions made about the type of drugs to use, the combinations, and the sequences to be employed in order to achieve not only a certain form of intoxication, but also to ensure that the effects dovetailed with the predetermined time parameters of the evening. Respondents believed that certain substances and certain combinations were inherently time-sensitive and that synchronizing the timing of when to consume specific drugs was an essential factor in maximizing the pleasure of intoxication and managing any potential risks. Respondents applied a combination of timed-use techniques to control the effects, taking additional substances at different times in order to both prolong or 'maintain' the high and avoid negative interactions that might arise from combining different substances.

These constraints suggest an interesting paradox between the attempts to achieve a sense of timelessness or a certain kind of 'time-out', through consuming drugs or alcohol, while attempting to accomplish this experience within pre-determined time-constraints. Thus, in spite of variations in drug effects or attempts to rid themselves of the pressures of time, many of the respondents in our San Francisco study described their experiences within a linear notion of time synchronized to fit the time restrictions of the event or the night-out. Unlike their counterparts in the late 1960s and 1970s (Young 1971), young substance users today have not dropped out from society but instead are intent on enjoying themselves and their drugs within the societal confines of the acceptable time-out period at the end of the week (see also Gusfield 2003). For contemporary drug and alcohol users, the weekend has become the acceptable time when a 'controlled loss of control' (Measham 2004a) can take place. In such circumstances, while seeking a state of intoxication, they plan their drug using practices to fit their available leisure time and would therefore seem willing to attain this experience within the acceptable parameters as defined by society.

CONCLUSION

Intoxicating substances are a fact of life and are inherently social substances. Since the development of fruit for fermentation into alcohol to 'the development of a range of mind-altering and mood-altering substances that keyed into brain chemistry' (Bancroft 2009: 175), the seeking of intoxication has been a constant feature of human life. We have not only become adapted to use drugs but also have adapted plants to encourage their psychoactive properties. The drive for intoxication has been developed and worked on in many different historical periods and in many different cultures, and it is therefore clear that the topic of intoxication is eminently worthy of sociological, anthropological, and historical investigation. However, what is also sociologically interesting is the fact that the boundaries between acceptable and unacceptable intoxication are constantly changing and, as we have noted, these changes are determined by changing societal norms and values. Intoxication is inherently and constantly a social practice governed by changing social and cultural norms and values.

In considering some of the key elements that have been explored in studying intoxicants and intoxication, we believe that it is appropriate to end this paper by considering the contemporary situation and examine briefly the emerging research on intoxication and embodiment as well as briefly considering the development of new pharmaceutical drugs – often referred to as lifestyle medicines or lifestyle drugs and the issue of intoxication (Flower 2004; Moldrup 2004). Viewing intoxication from an embodiment perspective is developing, and this perspective focus on the embodied, sensorial, and affective dimensions of intoxication, rather than the socio-cultural meanings of intoxication (Jayne et al. 2010). While studies focusing on this perspective are emerging within club studies and research on the nighttime economy (e.g. Bøhling 2014; Hubbard 2005; Jayne et al. 2010), this perspective still needs to be further explored within other kinds of settings, situations, and contexts where intoxication takes place and within different kinds of social groups.

In terms of the latter emerging research area – lifestyle medicine – Bancroft has called this a new form of intoxication 'functional intoxication' (2009: 147), intoxication that is sought after and allowable but in a targeted medicalized form. Instead of seeking for a state of intoxication in overcoming the mundane and seeking the unusual, Bancroft suggests that we are moving away from substances as pleasure and instead emphasizing the use of intoxicants to change and modify the self in the world. The aim today is to alter, manage, and enhance an individual's efficacy in the social world and exhibit a more successful identity. Dispassionate drugs used to modify the self into the rhythms of modern life and blunt the edge of stresses and strains.

These contemporary drugs are conceived as medicines to intervene at the boundary between health and illness with the specific aim of enhancing lifestyle (Quintero 2012). Researchers have also noted the extent to which pharmaceutical companies are marketing potential diseases, based on encouraging individuals to consider previously defined personal problems as potentially medical treatable problems. 'A raft of new semi-medicinal pharmaceuticals in development, which in theory will make us work harder, feel more sociable concentrate better, keep us awake' (Bancroft 2009: 6). Given these developments, it would appear that a new form of chemical intoxication is developing and that we as a society are not prepared to walk away from it, but, in fact, are enthusiastically embracing it.

NOTES

1 For a further discussion of the methodology used and the sample interviewed see Fazio et al. (2010), Hunt et al. (2007, 2010, 2011) and Moloney et al. (2008).
2 For a further discussion, see Coser (1977) and Holmwood (2005).
3 For a further discussion on inebriate women at the turn of the twentieth century, see Hunt et al. (1989).
4 For a further discussion of intoxication from hashish and non-linear time see Boothroyd's discussion (2006) of Walter Benjamin.

REFERENCES

Bakhtin, M. (1984). *Rabelais and His World*. Bloomington: Indiana University Press.

Bancroft, A. (2009). *Drugs, Intoxication and Society*. Cambridge: Polity Press.

Beccaria, F. and Guidoni, O.V. (2002). Young people in a wet culture: functions and patterns of drinking. *Contemporary Drug Problems*, 29(Summer): 305–34.

Beck, U. (1992). *Risk Society: Towards a New Modernity*. London: Sage Publications.

Beck, J. and Rosenbaum, M. (1994). *Pursuit of Ecstasy: The MDMA Experience*. Albany: State University of New York Press.

Becker, H.S. (1953). Becoming a marijuana user. *American Journal of Sociology*, 59: 235–42.

Becker, H.S. (1967). History, culture and subjective experience: an exploration of the social bases of drug-induced experiences. *Journal of Health and Social Behavior*, 8(3): 163–76.

Bøhling, F. (2014). Crowded contexts: on the affective dynamics of alcohol and other drug use in nightlife spaces. *Contemporary Drug Problems*, 41(3): 361–92.

Boon, M. (2002). *The Road of Excess: A History of Writers on Drugs*. Cambridge: Harvard University Press.

Booth, C. (1970). *The Life and Labour of the People of London*. New York: AMS Press.

Boothroyd, D. (2006). *Culture on Drugs: Narco-cultural Studies of High Modernity*. Manchester: Manchester University Press.

Bourguignon (1973). *Religion Altered States of Consciousness and Social Change*. Columbus: Ohio State University Press.

Brain, K., Parker, H. and Carnwath, T. (2000). Drinking with design: young drinkers as psychoactive consumers. *Drugs: Education, Prevention and Policy*, 7(1): 5–20.

Campbell, C. (1989). *The Romantic Ethic and the Spirit of Modern Consumerism*. Oxford: Basil Blackwell Ltd.

Chatterton, P. and Hollands, R. (2003). *Urban Nightscapes: Youth Cultures, Pleasure Spaces and Corporate Power*. London: Routledge.

Clark, P. (1983). *The English Alehouse 1200–1830*. Harlow: Longman House.
Cohen, S. and Taylor, L. (1992). *Escape Attempts: The Theory and Practice of Resistance to Everyday Life*. New York: Routledge.
Connell, R.W. and Messerschmidt, J.W. (2005). Hegemonic masculinity: rethinking the concept. *Gender and Society*, 19: 829–59.
Coser, L. (1977) *Masters of Sociological Thought: Ideas in Historical and Social Context*, 2nd edn. Fort Worth: Harcourt Brace Jovanovich.
de Visser, R. and McDonnell, E.J. (2012). 'That's OK. He's a guy': a mixed-methods study of gender double-standards for alcohol use. *Psychology and Health*, 27: 618–39.
Dobkin de Rios, M. (1990). *Hallucinogens: Cross-Cultural Perspectives*. Prospect Heights: Waveland Press.
Douglas, M. (1987). *Constructive Drinking: Perspectives on Drink from Anthropology*. Cambridge: Cambridge University Press.
Dunning, E., Murphy, P. and Williams, J. (1988). *The Roots of Football Hooliganism*. New York: Routledge, Kegan Paul.
Ettorre, E. (2007). *Revisioning Women and Drug Use: Gender, Power, and the Body*. Houndmills: Palgrave Macmillan.
Fazio, A., Joe-Laidler, K., Moloney, M. and Hunt, G. (2010). Gender, sexuality, and ethnicity as factors of club drug use among Asian Americans. *Journal of Drug Issues*, 40(2): 405–32.
Fillmore, K.M. (1984). 'When angels fall': women's drinking as a cultural preoccupation and as reality. In S.C. Wilsnack and L.J. Beckman (eds), *Alcohol Problems in Women: Antecedents, Consequences, and Intervention*. New York: The Guilford Press, pp. 7–36.
Flower, R. (2004). Lifestyle drugs. *Trends in Pharmacological Sciences*, 25(4): 182–5.
Forsyth, A.J.M. (1996). Are raves drug supermarkets? *International Journal of Drug Policy*, 7(2): 105–10.
Furlong, A. and F. Cartmel (1997). *Young People and Social Change: Individualization and Risk in Late Modernity*. Buckingham: Open University Press.
Garland, D. (2001). *The Culture of Control: Crime and Social Order in Contemporary Society*. Chicago: The University of Chicago Press.
Goodman, J., Lovejoy, P.E. and Sherratt, A. (eds) (1995). *Consuming Habits: Drugs in History and Anthropology*. London: Routledge.
Griffin, C., Bengry-Howell, A., Hackley, C., Mistral, W. and Szmigin, I. (2009). 'Every time I do it I absolutely annihilate myself': loss of self-consciousness and loss of memory in young people's drinking narratives. *Sociology*, 43: 457–76.
Griffin, C., Szmigin, I., Bengry-Howell, A., Hackley, C. and Mistral, W. (2013). Inhabiting the contradictions: Hypersexual femininity and the culture of intoxication among young women in the UK. *Feminism and Psychology* 23(2): 184–206.
Grob, C.S. (ed.) (2002). *Hallucinogens: A Reader*. New York: Jeremy P. Tarcher/Putnam.
Gusfield, J.R. (2003 [1987]). Passage to play: rituals of drinking time in American society. In M. Douglas (ed.), *Constructive Drinking. Perspectives on Drink from Anthropology*. London: Routledge, pp. 73–90.
Guttmann, M.C. (1996). *The Meaning of Macho: Being a Man in Mexico City*. Berkeley: University of California Press.
Hadfield, P. (ed.) (2009). *Nightlife and Crime: Social Order and Governance in International Perspective*. Oxford: Oxford University Press.
Hammersley, R., Ditton, J., Smith, I. and Short, E. (1999). Patterns of ecstasy use by drug users. *British Journal of Criminology*, 39(4): 625–47.
Hayward, K. (2002). The vilification and pleasures of youthful transgression. In J. Muncie, G. Hughes and E. McLaughlin (eds), *Youth Justice: Critical Readings*. London: Sage Publications, pp. 80–93.
Hayward, K. and D. Hobbs (2007). Beyond the binge in 'booze Britain': market-led liminalization and the spectacle of binge drinking. *The British Journal of Sociology*, 58(3): 437–56.
Herring, J, Regan, C., Weinberg, D. and Withington, P. (2013). *Intoxication and Society: Problematic Pleasures of Drugs and Alcohol*. Houndsmill: Palgrave MacMillan.
Holmwood, J. (2005) Functionalism and its critics. In A. Harrington (ed.), *Modern Social Theory: An Introduction*. Oxford: Oxford University Press, pp. 87–109.
Horton, D. (1943). The functions of alcohol in primitive societies: a cross-cultural study.

Quarterly Journal of Studies on Alcohol, 4: 199–320.

Hubbard, P. (2005). The geographies of 'going out': emotion and embodiment in the evening economy. In J. Davidson, L. Bondi and M. Smit (eds), *Emotional Geographies*. Aldershot: Ashgate, pp. 117–34.

Hunt, G. and Evans, K. (2008). 'The great unmentionable': exploring the pleasures and benefits of ecstasy from the perspectives of drug users. *Drugs: Education, Prevention and Policy*, 15(4): 329–49.

Hunt, G., Evans, K. and Kares, F. (2007). Drug use and the meanings of risk and pleasure. *Journal of Youth Studies*, 10(1): 73–96.

Hunt, G., Mellor, J. and Turner, J. (1989). Wretched hatless and miserably clad: women and inebriate reformatories from 1900–1913. *The British Journal of Sociology*, 40(2): 244–70.

Hunt, G. Moloney, M. and Evans, K. (2010). *Youth, Drugs, and Nightlife: Pleasures, Risks, and Identity.* Abingdon: Routledge.

Hunt, G., Moloney, M. and Fazio, A. (2011). Embarking on large-scale qualitative research: Reaping the benefits of mixed methods in studying youth, clubs and drugs. *Nordic Studies on Alcohol and Drugs*, 28(5/6): 433–52.

Hunt, G.P., MacKenzie, K. and Joe-Laidler, K. (2005). Alcohol and masculinity: the case of ethnic youth gangs. In T.M. Wilson (ed.), *Drinking Cultures: Alcohol and Identity*. Oxford: Berg, pp. 225–54.

Hutton, F., Wright, S. and Saunders, E. (2013). Cultures of intoxication: young women, alcohol and harm reduction. *Contemporary Drug Problems*, 40(4): 451–80.

Jay, M. (2010). *High Society: The Central Role of Mind-Altering Drugs in History, Science and Culture*. Rochester: Park Street Press.

Jayne, M.G., Valentine, G. and Holloway, S.L. (2010). Emotional, embodied and affective geographies of alcohol, drinking and drunkenness. *Transactions of the Institute of British Geographers*, 35(4): 1–15.

Jackson, C. (2006). Wild girls: an exploration of 'ladette' cultures in secondary schools. *Gender and Education*, 18(4): 339–60.

Jackson, P. (2004). *Inside Clubbing: Sensual Experiments in the Art of Being Human*. Oxford: Berg Publishers.

Keane, H. (2009). Intoxication, harm and pleasure: an analysis of the Australian National Alcohol Strategy. *Critical Public Health*, 19(2): 135–42.

Kneale, J. (2003). *Drunken Geographies: Mass-Observation's Studies of 'A Social Environment...Plus Alcohol', 1937–48*. London: Leisure and Visual Culture Conference, Roehampton University of Surrey, Centre for Cultural Research in Sport.

La Barre, W. (1938). *The Peyote Cult.* Oklahoma: University of Oklahoma Press.

Lemert, E.M. (1958). The use of alcohol in three Salish tribes. *Quarterly Journal of Studies on Alcohol*, 19: 90–107.

Leyshon, M. (2005). 'No place for a girl': rural youth, pubs, and the performance of masculinity. In J. Little and C. Morris (eds), *Critical Studies in Rural Gender Issues*. Aldershot: Ashgate, pp. 104–22.

Lupton, D. (ed.) (1999). *Risk and Sociocultural Theory: New Directions and Perspectives*. New York: Cambridge University Press.

Lyng, S. (ed.) (2005). *Edgework: The Sociology of Risk-Taking*. New York: Routledge.

MacAndrew, C. and Edgerton, R.B. (1969). *Drunken Comportment: A Social Explanation*. Chicago: Aldine.

Malbon, B. (1999). *Clubbing: Dancing, Ecstasy and Vitality*. New York: Routledge.

Marshall, M. (1983). 'Four hundred rabbits': an anthropological view of ethanol as a disinhibitor. In R. Room and G. Collins (eds), *Alcoholism and Disinhibition: Nature and Meaning of the Link (National Institute on Alcohol Abuse and Alcoholism Research Monograph No. 12)*. Rockville: National Institute on Alcohol Abuse and Alcoholism, pp. 186–204.

Mayock, P. (2005). 'Scripting' risk: young people and the construction of drug journeys. *Drugs: Education, Prevention and Policy*, 12(5): 349–68.

McRobbie, A. (2009) *The Aftermath of Feminism: Gender, Culture and Social Change*. Thousand Oaks: Sage.

Measham, F. (2002). 'Doing gender' – 'Doing drugs': conceptualising the gendering of drugs cultures. *Contemporary Drug Problems*, 29(2): 335–7.

Measham, F. (2004a). The decline of ecstasy, the rise of 'binge' drinking and the persistence of pleasure. *Probation Journal: The Journal of Community and Criminal Justice*, 51(4): 309–26.

Measham, F. (2004b). Play space: historical and socio-cultural reflections on drugs, licensed leisure locations, commercialisation and control. *International Journal of Drug Policy,* 15: 337–45.

Measham, F. (2008). The turning tides of intoxication: young people's drinking in Britain in the 2000s. *Health Education*, 108(3): 207–22.

Measham, F. and Brain, K. (2005). 'Binge' drinking, British alcohol policy and the new culture of intoxication. *Crime, Media, Culture* 1: 262–83.

Measham, F. and Moore, K. (2009). Repertoires of distinction: exploring patterns of weekend polydrug use within local leisure scenes across the English night time economy. *Criminology and Criminal Justice*, 9(4): 437–64.

Measham, F. and Østergaard, J. (2009). The public face of binge drinking: British and Danish young women, recent trends in alcohol consumption and the European binge drinking debate. *Probation Journal*, 56: 415–34.

Messerschmidt, J.W. (1997). *Crime as Structured Action: Gender, Race, Class, and Crime in the Making,* Thousand Oaks: Sage Publications.

Miles, S. (2000). *Youth Lifestyles in a Changing World*. Philadelphia: Open University Press.

Moldrup, C. (2004) The use of the terms 'lifestyle medicines' or lifestyle drugs. *Pharmacy World and Science*, 26(4): 193–6.

Moloney, M. Hunt, G. and Evans, K. (2008). Asian American identity and drug consumption: from acculturation to normalization. *Journal of Ethnicity in Substance Abuse*, 7(4): 376–403.

Mullen, K., Watson, J., Swift, J. and Black, D. (2007). Young men, masculinity and alcohol. *Drugs: Education, Prevention and Policy*, 14: 151–65.

O'Malley, P. and Mugford, S. (1991). The demand for intoxicating commodities: Implications for the 'War on Drugs'. *Social Justice*, 18(4): 49–75.

O'Malley, P. and Mugford, S. (1994). Crime, excitement and modernity. In: Barak, G. *Varieties of Criminology: Readings from a Dynamic Discipline*. Westport, CT: Praeger. Pp189–211.

O'Malley, P. and Valverde, M. (2004) Pleasure, freedom and drugs: the uses of 'pleasure' in liberal governance of drug and alcohol consumption. *Sociology,* 38: 25–42.

Orcutt, J.D. (1975). Social determinants of alcohol and marijuana effects: a systematic theory. *The International Journal of the Addictions*, 10(6): 1021–33.

Osborne, R. (2014). Intoxication and sociality: the symposium in the ancient Greek world. In P. Withington and A. McShane (eds), *Cultures of Intoxication. Past and Present Supplement 9*. Oxford: Oxford University Press, pp. 34–60.

Østergaard, J. (2007). Mind the gender gap? When boys and girls get drunk at a party. *Nordic Studies on Alcohol and Drugs*, 24: 127–48.

Palafox, R.A. (2001). Cantinas and drinking in Mexico. In I. De Garine and V. De Garine. *Drinking: Anthropological Approaches*. New York: Berghahn Books. Pp.169–180.

Parker, H., Aldridge, J. and Measham, F. (1998). *Illegal Leisure: The Normalization of Adolescent Recreational Drug Use*. London: Routledge.

Partanen, J. (1991). *Sociability and Intoxication: Alcohol and Drinking in Kenya, Africa, and the Modern World*. Helsinki: The Finnish Foundation for Alcohol Studies.

Paton-Simpson, G. (1996). The varied meanings of drinking and intoxication – a review. *Contemporary Drug Problems*, 23: 221–58.

Peace, A. (1992). No fishing without drinking: the construction of social identity in rural Ireland. In D. Gefou-Madianou (ed.), *Alcohol, Gender and Culture*. New York: Routledge, pp. 167–80.

Peralta, R. (2007). College alcohol use and the embodiment of hegemonic masculinity among European American men. *Sex Roles*, 56: 741–56.

Peralta, R.L. (2008). 'Alcohol allows you to not be yourself': toward a structured understanding of alcohol use and gender difference among gay, lesbian, and heterosexual youth. *Journal of Drug Issues*, 38(2): 373–99.

Peralta, R.L., Steele, J.L., Nofziger, S. and Rickles, M. (2010). The impact of gender on binge drinking behavior among U.S. college students attending a Midwestern university: an analysis of two gender measures. *Feminist Criminology*, 5(4): 355–79.

Presdee, M. (2000). *Cultural Criminology and the Carnival of Crime*. London: Routledge.

Quintero, G. (2012) *'They Can Get Your Teen Just as High': The Social Construction of Recreational Pharmaceutical Use as a Drug Problem*. Paper presented at the Society for Applied Anthropology, Baltimore.

Reith, G. (2005). On the edge: drugs and the consumption of risk in late modernity. In S. Lyng (ed.), *Edgework: The Sociology of Risk-Taking*. New York: Routledge, pp. 227–45.

Ridley, J. (2004) 27 faces of women, *The Daily Mirror*, 19 March, p. 6. Available from: www.mirror.co.uk/news/allnews/tm_objectid=14067588&method=full&siteid=50143&headline=27-faces-of-women-name_page.html (accessed 26 August 2004).

Riley, S., Morey, Y. and Griffin, C. (2010). The 'pleasure citizen': Analyzing partying as a form of social and political participation. *Young*, 18(1): 33–54.

Rudgley, R. (1993). *Essential Substances: A Cultural History of Intoxicants in Society*. New York: Kodansha International.

Sherratt, A. (1995). Introduction: peculiar substances. In J. Goodman, P.E. Lovejoy and A. Sherratt (eds.), *Consuming Habits: Drugs in History and Anthropology*. London: Routledge, pp. 1–10.

Simonen, J. (2011). In control and out of control. The discourse on intoxication among young Finnish women in the 1980s and 2000s. *Nordic Studies on Alcohol and Drugs*, 28(2): 131–47.

Skeggs, B. (1997). *Formations of Class and Gender*. London: Sage Publications.

Solowij, N., Hall, W. and Lee, N. (1992). Recreational MDMA use in Sydney: a profile of 'ecstasy' users and their experiences with the drug. *British Journal of Addiction*, 87(8): 1161–72.

Sulkunen, P. (2002). Between culture and nature: intoxication in cultural studies of alcohol and drug use. *Contemporary Drug Problems*, 29(2): 253–76.

Szwed, J.F. (1966). Gossip, drinking, and social control: consensus and communication in a Newfoundland parish. *Ethnology*, 5(4): 434–41.

Waitt, G., Jessop, L. and Gorman-Murray, A.W. (2011). 'The guys in there just expect to be laid': embodied and gendered socio-spatial practices of a 'night out' in Wollongong, Australia. *Gender, Place and Culture*, 18(2): 255–75.

Walton, S. (2001). *Out of It: A Cultural History of Intoxication*. London: Hamish Hamilton.

Warner, J., Weber, T. and Albanes, R. (1999). 'Girls are retarded when they're stoned'. Marijuana and the construction of gender roles among adolescent females. *Sex Roles*, 40(1–2): 25–43.

Weil, A.T. (1972). *The Natural Mind*. Boston: Houghton Mifflin.

Withington, P. and McShane, A. (2014). *Cultures of Intoxication. Past and Present, Supplement 9*. Oxford: Oxford University Press.

Wolcott, H.F. (1974). *The African Beer Gardens of Bulawayo: Integrated Drinking in a Segregated Society*, Monograph, No. 10. New Brunswick: Rutgers Centre of Alcohol Studies.

Yardley, T. (2012). *Why We Take Drugs: Seeking Excess and Communion in the Modern World*. London: Routledge.

Young, J. (1971). *The Drugtakers: The Social Meaning of Drug Use*. London: Judson, McGibbon and Kee.

Zinberg, N.E. (1984). *Drugs, Set, and Setting: The Social Bases of Controlled Drug Use*. New Haven: Yale University Press.

19

Identity, Friendship and Sociality

Thomas Thurnell-Read

INTRODUCTION

This chapter explores how drug and alcohol consumption relates to identity, friendship and sociality and starts with the observation that the conditions under which drugs and alcohol are consumed are inescapably socially defined. Even solitary consumption takes place in the context of societal expectations that often construct normative boundaries separating acceptable from unacceptable styles and settings of use. Indeed, a particularly fruitful strand of work in the social sciences has been to foreground the social context of intoxication and drunkenness as being integral to understanding the motivations, subjective experiences and identities of users (Jayne et al., 2006; Hunt et al., 2010). While this growing body of research does not seek to undermine valued explanations of pathology, addiction and an array of physical and psychological harms that might arise from drug and alcohol use, they do, as this chapter will demonstrate, bring to the fore the inescapably social nature of alcohol and drug use analysis.

Since the 1990s, academic research on drug taking and drinking cultures have made a turn towards the inclusion of the social context in explanations of why the consumption of such substances might be seen as pleasurable and desired by those who participate in spite of prohibition, regulation and wider long-standing discourses of risk and harm. As such, the social pleasures and potential benefits of drug use have long been, and in many ways still remain, 'the great unmentionable' of drug and alcohol research (Hunt and Evans, 2008). These benefits can be found in the immediate moment through feelings of camaraderie, intimacy and mutual support (e.g. Niland et al., 2013), as well as in the longer term by building lasting group loyalties and through shared experiences that lay the foundations for future narrations of identity and group belonging (Blackshaw, 2003).

This move has taken place in spite of what, in many countries, has amounted to an intensification of media and policy discourses that position alcohol and drugs as a societal problem to be blamed on the moral failures of individuals (Plant and Plant, 2006; Taylor, 2008). Against this backdrop, social science scholars working on drink and drugs have trod a precarious path in seeking to acknowledge the pleasurable, socially positive, features of intoxication. One feature of this move has been to find order in the apparent chaos of heavy 'binge' drinking and to explore how the consumption of alcohol sustains complex rituals that unite the individual with the group. Both Tomsen (1997) and Campbell (2000), for example, highlight in their work how the apparent disorder and disarray of drinking settings, while disparaged by external commentators, contains its own internal logic that gives rise to social pleasures for participants and for the display and performance of identity and belonging. Likewise, in their influential paper, Measham and Brain (2005) demonstrate that through 'determined drunkenness' aspects of drinking, previously conceptualised as negative or risky, emerged as desired aspects of the drinking experience, integral to the sense of fun, playfulness and release desired by young drinkers. In these and other examples to be explored below, a challenge presented to the researcher has been both a methodological and epistemological one; how can the experience of collective drug use or heavy alcohol consumption by adequately captured and analysed in order to reveal and give due recognition to pleasurable aspects of either drinking or drug taking that are often embodied in complex ways? Similarly, how might these pleasures and benefits be presented whilst still giving due regard to the potential and actual harms of substance (mis)use?

In this sense, the 1990s is identifiable as a seminal decade in work on drug and alcohol use in the social sciences and signalled a new willingness to break from simplistic discourses of deviance and pathology borne solely by the individual by instead foregrounding the significance of friendship, relaxation, excitement, fun and playfulness. Notably, it was the emergence of the rave scene and clubbing in Britain and the USA around this time that prompted a number of studies of ecstasy use where exactly these concerns were brought to prominence (Thornton, 1995; Saunders, 1996; Parker et al., 1998; Malbon, 1999). The strength of these studies, perhaps made possible by the relative novelty of ecstasy both as a substance and as a topic of academic research, was that drug use was a prominent but integrated feature of overlapping concerns of friendship, social relations and embodied feelings of well-being, trust and communality. As such, Malbon (1999: 3) observed that the experience of clubbing was 'constituted through the practices, imaginations and emotions of the clubber themselves' rather than abstracted and often moralising media or public order discourses. Markedly, as Parker et al. (1998: 7) noted, ravers and ecstasy users came from different social classes and from both sexes, making blanket condemnation of pathology more difficult.

There has also been a move towards a more complex explanation of how individuals might become integrated into social groups where drug or heavy alcohol use is a prominent feature. The past dominance of a narrative of 'peer pressure' emphasising a descent or indoctrination into a 'deviant' subcultural or lifestyle has been challenged. While the role of the peer group has long been associated with decisions to use certain substances, this has often been framed as a 'peer pressure' scenario involving initiation into a deviant lifestyle (Foster and Spencer, 2013). As such, the most accomplished work on drink and drugs from this period 'tends to concentrate on the theoretical goal of moving beyond pathologizing alcohol consumption in order to present the everyday social relations and cultural practices bound up with drinking' (Jayne et al., 2006: 453). Pilkington (2007: 222) has argued convincingly for the need to address the more complex nature of drug and alcohol use within friendship groups by suggestion that 'the friendship group is thus better understood as providing a set of reference points underpinned by bonds of emotionality and mutual accountability about acceptable and unacceptable drug use and a secure and supportive environment in which to enact the ensuring drugs decisions'. Similarly, Cullen seeks to problematise the uncritical peer pressure model and instead give full understanding of 'a wider process of reciprocity, and the construction and negotiation of individual and group gendered, classed and generational identities' (Cullen, 2010: 493). Emerging from this critical process is a vibrant field of research – although not one without limitations, some of which will be addressed in the concluding section – where a range of contemporary studies are revealing insights into the intimate lives of individuals and groups who drink alcohol or take drugs for pleasure and for a number of distinctly social benefits (Griffin et al., 2009; Vander Ven, 2011).

The chapter therefore argues that the consumption of drugs and alcohol is inherently social and relational and best analysed not as an isolated and problematic behaviour of disparate, possibly deviant, individuals but as a social practice constituted and (re)formed by and through friendships, groups and spontaneously formed acquaintances. This is not to say that the individual can or should fade from analytical view. Rather, it is to suggest that a wealth of scholarship now demonstrates the value of giving due regard to the pleasures, emotions and feelings that animate much drug and alcohol use at its core, which we might locate at the intersection of individual and group identities. As such, when one participant in Chatterton and Holland's (2002: 109) study of nightlife in British cities explains that 'it's great to be in one of those groups. It feels really powerful in a horrible sort of way…you are accepted you know' it speaks of the considerable social function of alcohol to bind the individual to the group and to produce an array of emotions and feelings such as acceptance, belonging and power.

The chapter aims to offer a review of recent research that has intensified the centrality of identity, friendship and sociability to understandings of drug and alcohol use. Following this brief introduction, the chapter will examine the role played by the consumption of drugs and alcohol in constructions of individual, group and national identity. In particular, the case of the consumption of the stimulant khat amongst Somalis in East Africa (Beckerly and Nuur, 2005; Carrier, 2005) and within the European Somali diaspora (Griffiths et al., 1997; Osman and Söderbäck, 2011), will be used to demonstrate the complicated interplay of substance and identity which intersects gender, ethnicity, social class, nationality, age and familial facets of identity construction. The following section will then draw on a range of recent empirical studies to pinpoint some of the ways in which alcohol and drug use are constituted socially. The section will highlight eight different, yet often overlapping, features of the sociality that emerges from and around drug and alcohol consumption. In concluding, the chapter brings these themes together to reflect on the importance of understanding the embodied, affective and – at times what can only problematically be called – positive aspects of drug and alcohol use.

IDENTITY

Rather than pre-empt the work undertaken elsewhere in this volume (for instance, see Chapter 23, 24 & 25 this Handbook), this section will aim to illustrate how drug and alcohol use are in numerous ways important constituents of the identities of those who consume them and, further, that these identities are constructed and negotiated within the settings and practices of their consumption. Rather than attempt to delineate and separate examples of how alcohol and drug use might relate to, for example, gender, sexuality, social class or ethnicity, I will here aim to illustrate how alcohol and drug consumption can be bound up with intersecting and overlapping facets of personal, group and national identity. As such, two recent studies, both of which focus on practices of drinking alcohol as an integral part of sports participation, illustrate how identity is performed and negotiated through alcohol consumption within specific social settings.

In Joseph's ethnographic study of older Caribbean men's alcohol consumption at cricket grounds in Canada we see how 'drinking at the cricket ground is central to their aged, gendered, classed and national identities' (Joseph, 2012: 161). Here, Caribbean migrants bring with leisure practices, principally the specific sport of cricket and a particular style of public ritualised drinking, which are reconfigured in the diaspora as potent markers of ethnic identity. Additionally, while the cricket ground itself is coded as a specifically masculine social space, with women and children being typically excluded, the drinking of alcohol functions as a means of performing masculinity and, further still, a specifically aging masculinity. Indeed, many of the older men might have had the transition from active participant to relatively less active spectator, brought on by age and diminishing physical capacities, eased by the consumption of alcohol as a substitute activity and a replacement means to publically display their masculinity.

Similarly, Fletcher and Spracklen (2013) illustrate how the importance placed on post-match drinking of alcohol in British cricket clubs constructed lines of inclusion and exclusion for British Muslim male cricket players. Thus, while British Muslim players might be fully engaged participants of the sport itself they are, by their religious prohibition of alcohol consumption, excluded from participation in the wider social life of the club. While some aspects of 'Britishness' and 'masculinity' are accessible through participation in the sport, others are inaccessible due to the social significance placed on (heavy) alcohol consumption in underlying the dominant sporting white masculine identity. Again, we see how alcohol can play a vital constitutive role in the construction and negotiation of identity. As is addressed below, alcohol can bind the individual to a group as much as it can exclude others.

Similar interplay and intersection of identities can be observed in the growing body of research into the use of khat as a recreational drug within certain sections of the Somali community. Khat, also known as miraa, is the leaf of a plant grown in eastern Africa, which is chewed by users for its mild narcotic effects. Khat might have a medicinal use, cultural use in ceremonies, a social use in leisure spaces and a functional use during work, for instance, by providing lorry drivers with the stamina and attentiveness required for long trips (Carrier, 2007). Notably, these effects are seen as distinctly social:

> Chewers report an immediate emotional effect of euphoria, which increases the sense of well-being and can facilitate social interaction. Indeed, khat seems to greatly exacerbate the chewers' urge to express themselves, albeit at the expense of their listening skills. The initial stage of a typical khat-chewing session is therefore characterized by a din of voices, with all attendant speaking excitedly and at the same time. (Anderson et al., 2007: 14)

As with other drugs, learning to consume khat and appreciate its effects, as well as mitigate against its negative impacts, can be seen as a social process. As Carrier (2007: 7) states, 'one learns to appreciate miraa's effects in the company of friends, one learns terms for miraa that have strong cultural resonances, and chewing sessions have great social significance' (Carrier, 2007: 7).

Khat use has become closely associated with Somalis both in East Africa and within the Somali diaspora in Europe (Beckerly and Nuur, 2005). With khat use entering Europe with East African Migrants, the production and distribution of the substance now amounts to a global supply chain (Anderson et al., 2007). In this context, there are suggestions that khat use is heightened amongst

Somali communities in Europe and takes on an increased significance as a marker of cultural identity and becomes the focus of community sociability, at least for men (Griffiths et al., 1997; Carrier, 2005). Similarly, in their study of khat use amongst Somalis in Sweden, where the substance has been prohibited though nonetheless still extensively used since 1989, Osman and Söderbäck (2011: 216) noted how khat was seen as 'a medium for cultural and community cohesiveness' that benefited individual users by facilitating conversation, relaxation and bonding. The sociable setting of khat use would provide a stage for the discussion of topics ranging from football, community gossip, to job opportunities and news of the latest weddings 'back in Somalia' (Carrier, 2005). Indeed, chewing khat provides migrants, and their offspring, with 'tangible links to Africa' (Carrier, 2005: 15).

A further layer of complexity can be added to this brief description by noting the gendered nature of khat consumption. While khat is consumed by both Somali men and women, the latter are more likely to do so within the confines of the home as opposed to the more public setting of the 'mafrish', a café-like setting in which men consume khat and secondary services such as tea are provided. Further, several studies have noted that Somali women more likely to engage in prevention and to position excessive khat use as a threat to families and community cohesion (Osman and Söderbäck, 2011; Nordgren, 2013). Indeed, perhaps the loudest call for the prohibition of khat in the UK (which came into force in June 2014) has been its perceived negative impact on the employment chances of young Somali men where there is a fear that while khat might usefully fill the spare time enforced by unemployment, it also inhibits social mobility and integration.

Khat is therefore by turns depicted as both a benefit and a threat to the individuals and the community in terms of maintaining culture and binding individuals, through their everyday habits and practices, to the community but also, at the same time, often perceived as a threat and a danger. As with the studies by Joseph (2012) and Fletcher and Spracklen (2013) discussed at the start of the section, looking at the case of khat consumption illustrates a number of themes central to the focus of this chapter. First, the benefits of khat are largely defined as being social and as encouraging sociability through candid talk and conviviality. Pushing beyond this, we see how khat use is framed by wider constructions of identity in relation to ethnicity, gender and social class. Again, we see that there is no straightforward way to disaggregate these components of personal and group identity. Rather we must locate drug or alcohol use within these intersecting strands of identity. It is through the social interaction that is a central feature of drug and alcohol consumption that identity is negotiated and performed.

FRIENDSHIP, BONDING AND SOCIABILITY

Having explored the ways in which alcohol and drug use are entwined with complex constructions and performances of identity, the remainder of this chapter will now consider more specifically how this relates to sociality in the form of friendship, interpersonal bonding and intimacy. While studies have established that there is a long history of links between drinking rituals (Wilson, 2005), popularity and social acceptance (for example, Balsa et al., 2010), a more detailed account may be offered as to how this sociality plays out in practice. The section draws on the considerable array of empirical studies that have, in the last decade or so, brought to the fore the social nature of drug and alcohol consumption and, in particular, the role of peer groups, friendships and bonding rituals. While previous studies might have sought to isolate individual users, there is now more acceptance of how substance use is 'intricately woven into friendship' (Foster and Spencer, 2013: 224). To understand this, we must explore the affective aspects of drug use within friendships that cultivate feelings of trust, belonging and intimacy.

Recent years have seen young people become the focus of much research on the role of alcohol consumption. In recent work in New Zealand by Niland et al. (2013: 531, original emphasis) it is noted that for young people drinking can be understood as 'a shared *social* practice that is pleasurable and undertaken within friendships'. Likewise, a review of over 80 studies of young people's motivations to consume alcohol found a common narrative based around sociability and drinking as a means to relax and bond with friends (Kuntsche et al., 2005). Such studies have highlighted how, in numerous ways, it is remiss to attempt an understanding of drug or alcohol use without paying due attention to interpersonal relationships and the relational interactions they give rise to and support. While by no means intended as an exhaustive list, I shall here outline eight ways in which drug and alcohol consumption encourages, facilitates or in other ways plays a prominent role in friendships, bonding rituals and, most generally, sociality.

Spaces and times suitable for sociality to take place

Alcohol and drug use can have a significant influence on the time and location of social interaction and both the formation and maintenance of friendships. Indeed, much drinking can be highly ritualistic in nature (Beccaria and Sande, 2003), bringing people together at specified times and in particular places. Wolburg and Treise (2004) noted in their study of heavy drinking in North America that alcohol played an important ritual function in designating times and locations for collective drinking. As such, certain bars would be associated with particular styles and intensities of drinking, with particular drinking partners and with particular activities such as watching either live or televised sports matches. Social drinking was also found to be temporally structured with key moments being marked by the coming together of friends and acquaintances to share in a Friday night drinking session to mark the end of the working week or, for students, occasions such as the end of the midterm examination season.

It should also be worth noting that these spaces are often heavily gendered (e.g. Leyshon, 2008; Waitt et al., 2011). Crawford (2009), for instance, observes that the convergence of sport and alcohol provide places where the consumption of both sport and alcohol becomes a highly gendered collective activity. Women may be overtly or implicitly excluded. As Driessen has observed in relation to the Spanish taverns in Andalusia, drinking spaces can be seen as 'a social context for the creation and maintenance of friendship and the celebration of masculinity' (Driessen, 1992: 73). Similarly, Campbell (2000) suggests that in New Zealand the rural pub has long been a stage upon which a particular masculinity is enacted through ritualistic and, notably, collective public drinking practices.

These themes are well identified in Anne Allison's (1994) ethnographic study of Japanese 'hostess clubs', where paid female staff serve all male groups of officer workers and 'play the part' of 'hostess' by pouring drinks, laughing at jokes and helping the customers to 'feel like a man'. The hostess plays out a role that functions to support the identity of both individual customers and the collective group. Through her interaction with the group, through serving alcohol and encouraging drunken disinhibition, she works to literally 'create a group' (Allison, 1994: 65) out of the individual workers. Such complex social interactions belie any easy distinctions between individual/collective and causation based explanations. Alcohol, in particular, provides the space and time for this coming together of disparate individuals.

Shared experiences brought about by substance consumption

Perhaps the most prominent quality linking alcohol and drug use to sociability and friendship is that consumption can be a shared activity that is conducted rarely by individuals alone but by groups. Indeed, a key feature of Measham and Brain's (2005) influential discussion of 'determined drunkenness' is that achieving a state of advanced intoxication is, in and of itself, a desired and ritualistic activity for many young people. It has recently been noted that 'for young people, the pleasures of drinking tend to be shared ones' (Brown and Gregg, 2012: 361). Further still, a range of secondary activities commonly pursued as part of drug or alcohol consumption offer shared experience though which individuals might bond and form social ties. Playing or watching sport, dancing, talking, gambling or playing card and dice games are all sociable activities that frequently take place alongside the consumption of alcohol. This sense that alcohol can be a pleasurable enhancement to social situations and leisure activities in allowing people to share pleasurable experiences together is readily exploited in industry marketing and is most apparent in the 'buddy' or 'best mates' narrative identifiable in numerous beer commercials and marketing campaigns (Wolburg and Treise, 2004).

While this theme can often emerge from the accounts of research participants in a rather matter-of-fact way, a good example being the oft used phrase 'having a laugh with friends' (Parker et al., 1998: 157), it is in itself an insight which necessitates further unpacking. In both stag parties (Thurnell-Read, 2012) and bachelorette parties (Montemurro and McClure, 2005), while the drinking of alcohol is one of the main activities pursued by the group, a range of secondary activities are also pursued. Drinking games, for example, provide a common group focus, a competitive activity, encourage involvement and 'foster a low-key and enjoyable atmosphere' where 'inhibitions tend to be reduced, facilitating a sense of friendship and camaraderie' (Borsari, 2004: 36). Many such drinking games also have as a specific feature of making individuals, or the entire group, drink more quickly and in greater quantities than they might otherwise.

While this is often a positive and directly desired element of the substance use, risks and dangers either of the substances themselves or, more commonly, those which the situation in which intoxication takes place gives rise to can foster displays of care and protection between friends. A recent study by MacLean and Moore (2014) of young people's drinking experiences in Australia observed that while the urban environment presented risks, most notably through interpersonal violence, those risks also in some ways proved beneficial in that friendships were strengthened around a mutual need for friends to protect and support each other.

Stories upon which status can be built and future bonding based

While alcohol or drug use provides a shared experience through which friends and acquaintances can bond, the social implications of this are not solely limited to the moment of consumption. Indeed, several recent studies have illustrated how the incidents of the night of heavy drinking provide stories which circulate between friends long after the event (Sheehan and Ridge, 2001; Griffin et al., 2009). The telling of drinking stories can therefore support the status of the individual but also work to build and sustain group loyalty. As Fry observes 'story-telling reinforced the value of drinking experiences beyond the individual's experience creating a greater sense of cohesion, intimacy and bonding with peers' (Fry, 2011: 68). Similarly, in their study of young Danish tourist's narrations of drinking escapades in a Bulgarian holiday resort, Tutenges and Sandberg (2013: 542) noted the importance of this collective nature of drinking stories that were 'not a long recital performed by one single person' but 'constructed collaboratively and proceeded in a flow of statements, questions, pauses for thought and finally, laughter that dissipated the tension'. Being part of, and party to, these stories and their telling therefore represents a significant social tool for cementing friendships and group identity.

Notably, the narration of drinking stories takes on a normative quality where appropriate ways of drinking and behaving whilst drunk are expressed, negotiated and standardised. Such narratives may, however, form an alternative account where spontaneity, irreverence and risk taking are valorised. For instance, Hackley et al. (2013), turning the literary analysis of Mikhail Bakhtin to focus group recollections of young British people's drinking stories, explore the carnivalesque qualities of narratives of drunkenness and intoxication. Such accounts are characterised by satirical laughter, the spectacle of surreal or unusual events and the subversion of social order, rules and roles.

Further still, the emergence of social media has provided a new inflection to this centrality of drinking stories to collective experiences and recollections of intoxication. Thus, in recent years, there are indications that sites such as Facebook and Twitter are allowing a boarder circle of friends and acquaintances to share in drinking via vicarious consumption of drunkenness (Brown and Gregg, 2012; Niland et al., 2013).

Sharing substances as a symbolic marker of friendship

Through their commodity value, drugs and alcohol can take on a symbolic quality and a social function where their exchange can communicate friendship and reciprocity between individuals and within groups. So to, amongst clubbers the sharing of drugs such as ecstasy and 'poppers' as well as other commodities, such as chewing gum and bottled water, when clubbing symbolises a wider sense of sociability and openness (Moore and Miller, 2005). This might be heightened when bonding centres around prohibited substances, the very act of sharing drugs together can itself affirm feelings of trust and support between friends (Foster and Spencer, 2013). Social groups might place ritualistic importance on the buying of 'rounds' of drinks, ensuring that all group members receive and consume specific drink at specific moments and, further still, that all group members drink at the same time and aim to achieve similar levels of intoxication. During British premarital stag tours in eastern European cities, it is common for drinks to be bought from a communal fund or 'kitty' to which all group members have contributed (Thurnell-Read, 2012).

In their study of 44 drug users in Florida, USA, Belackova and Vaccaro identified sharing and reciprocity to be central to marijuana use between peers, where 'the decision to share marijuana is a symbolic gesture that is selectively made to enact and affirm a friendship identity between two or more people' (Belackova and Vaccaro, 2013: 296). Further, non-reciprocating friends were found to be at risk of being cut out of the peer circle. A similar symbolic value of substance sharing was noted by Cullen in her study of young women's smoking practices in Britain. She noted that 'young women, via the sharing and exchange of cigarettes, performed and produced a range of ways of "doing girl" to secure their place within their friendship groups' (Cullen, 2010: 492).

Easing of pressures and social anxieties and brought on by social situations and interactions

In numerous studies, both alcohol and various drugs have been shown to give those who consumer them a feeling of confidence or easing of general social anxieties. Noting that many studies of young women's drinking have tended to overplay or at least take for granted the apparent centrality of intimacy to drinking amongst female friends, Stepney (2013) instead reminds us that alcohol plays a role in easing social anxiety and facilitating 'small talk'. There is also some evidence that, for many young men, alcohol consumption is seen to boost social confidence, particularly in relation to talking to and 'picking up' women (de Visser and Smith, 2007).

While the ability of alcohol to bestow confidence, or so called 'Dutch courage', upon those who consume it has a long cultural lineage, we might here focus on how that confidence allows individuals to partake in particular social settings and, within those settings, to play certain social roles appropriately. As such, two recent studies of drinking amongst American students (Vander Ven, 2011; Chrzan, 2013) have found that alcohol allowed students to negotiate competing demands of balancing high academic achievement with a rich social life. Students used alcohol consumption not only to unwind after class, following assessments and at the end of term but to manage their self-identity and the transformation between a studious, academic role and an extrovert and sociable identity. In both cases, the highly sociable atmosphere of the college campus, for many, seemed to necessitate alcohol consumption in order to live up to expected social norms relating to being a fun, confident and sociable and to ease feelings of anxiety or timidity.

Deindividualisation

While it is clear that alcohol and drug use can play an important role for individuals in the constitution of their personal identity, a striking feature of many studies in this field is the prominence of discourses of deindividualisation and group identity formation. Thus, alcohol or drug use might offer a way for an individual to 'open up', to be more sociable and to be less self-orientated. American college students attending spring break celebrations in costal resorts across America and the Caribbean have been shown to drink more alcohol and to be more likely to experiment with drugs or partake in risky behaviours such as unprotected sex by entering a state of 'situational disinhibition' (Josiam et al., 1998; Sönmez et al., 2006). The situation, and the expected 'script' of spring break hedonism, allow the participant to let go of individual concerns or inhibitions.

Similarly, ecstasy is specifically associated with increased empathy, making users more communicative and less self-orientated (Saunders, 1996) and has been shown to bring on a feeling of openness and to make users feel less judgmental and less self-conscious (Hunt and Evans, 2008). In Thornton's (1995) study, a reoccurring theme amongst clubbers was that the effects of taking ecstasy, in combination with the visual and aural spectacle of the night club, allowed participants to 'lose' themselves in the music and experience (Thornton, 1995).

More recently, a number of studies have noted that heavy drinking amongst young people might increasingly be seen as a means of release from pressures to construct and present a coherent and disciplined individual identity to the world in contemporary societies. The 'passing out stories' of young British drinkers have been explored, revealing the evident pleasure taken as 'a sort of "time out" from the world of rational civilized individual subjectivity and self-control' (Griffin et al., 2009: 471). Indeed, the ability and willingness to let go of oneself appears to be a new demand on many young people where the public display of self-destructive drinking is a sought after and intended element of the experience of intoxication (Thurnell-Read, 2011; Brown and Gregg, 2012). Thus, through drunkenness and intoxication individuals are able to show to friends and the wider world that they do not take themselves too seriously and are willing to perform a lack of restraint that seems to bear increasingly cultural stock in a wider atmosphere of individualisation (see Smith, 2014).

Group cohesion and solidarity

While drugs and alcohol might be used by individuals as a means of opening up and becoming more sociable and gregarious, a further theme emerging from many studies is that consumption of alcohol or drugs can make groups, clubs and social circles more coherent and defined. Such has been observed in a number of different contexts. Drinking games and rituals in Norway and Italy carry the social function of 'cementing friendships and developing a community spirit' and 'enhancing group conformity' (Beccaria and Sande, 2003: 104), while drinking alcohol is important for establishing solidarity amongst young gang members in the San Francisco Bay area (Hunt et al., 2005). Zhou et al. identified collective drinking of alcohol as an important feature of sports team participants where alcohol was commonly used to foster 'a sense of camaraderie and cohesion' (Zhou et al., 2014: 288). Indeed, participation in some social clubs or groups may expressly necessitate alcohol consumption. For example, Dempster's (2011) research at a British university found that sports teams in particular often treated alcohol consumption as a prerequisite of membership, although interestingly such conformity to expected excesses of student drinking was also cited as a sign of weakness by others.

Again, the premarital stag and bachelorette party are occasions where group cohesion is expected and where alcohol is seen as a primary facilitator of developing a collective identity for the group (Montemurro and McClure, 2005; Thurnell-Read, 2011, 2012). As noted above, all members of the group may be required to drink specific drinks at specific times. Further still, there is an implicit understanding at such events that all group members will drink alcohol and that, to some extent, all group members will become active participants in drunken activities and incidents.

Boundary marking and exclusion

Strong social groups frequently operate to assert relatively fixed boundaries and, often, involve the visible and overt exclusion of others. Further, a subtler process of distinction, where in-group members frame their individual or collective identity in relation to real or perceived out-groups, may be apparent. This might include marking boundaries between different types of users of the same substance, between users of different substances or between users and non-users. For example, in Thornton's (1995) study, British clubbers made common reference to a perceived mainstream from which they set themselves apart. Here, the musical taste, styles of dress and modes of behaviour of others were all invoked in contrast to those of the clubbers themselves. However, it was in the differences between intoxicants of choice that notably formed a dividing line, with clubbers framing their use of ecstasy in opposition to the heavy drinking of alcohol seen in the more mainstream British night-time leisure venues. Similarly, emerging from the more recent work of Hunt et al. (2010: 193, 198) on club based drug taking amongst American young people, many clubbers readily expressed anti-alcohol views where drunk individuals were perceived by clubbers as anti-social in being 'pushy' and 'volatile', while drugs such as MDMA were represented as more social in encouraging conviviality, playfulness and sociability.

Friendship groups over time may change with particular individuals, prompted by their drug usage, leaving one social group to join another (see Pilkington, 2008). As identified above in the work by Fletcher and Spracklen (2013), those who abstain, for any of a number of reasons, might find certain social roles or opportunities inaccessible to them. Even for those who do partake, difference in stances towards particular drugs or intensities of use may mean that friendship groups may be drawn and fractured by divergent attitudes to drug use and practice (Parker et al., 1998). Amongst a group that readily defines their sociality around drinking of alcohol, non-drinkers might be seen to not 'fit in' with the group identity and, as such, be conspicuously marginalised (Niland et al., 2013).

CONCLUSION

This chapter has sought to highlight the complex ways in which drug and alcohol consumption, and the feelings, experiences, activities and settings involved, play a significant role in the construction of identity and in sociability between individuals and within groups. By way of conclusion, this final section reflects on the relational, embodied nature of this sociality fostered by alcohol and drug consumption. It argues that a nuanced understanding of the sociality implicit in much substance use is integral to current and future developments in the field.

In the second section of the chapter, I have attempted to draw out some of the ways in which sociality is played out during drug and alcohol consumption. However, it is also interesting to note that across many of these studies the manner in which participants refer to this sociality is tellingly epigrammatic. In many of the empirical studies discussed, reference to fun, 'having a laugh' and 'hanging out' (Waitt and Warren 2008), indicate both the complexity and, somewhat contradictory, the banality of drug and alcohol consumption. Rather than vague, ill-defined, descriptors, such terms, in their brevity, indicate the self-evident and taken for granted nature of the social benefits of alcohol and drug use as they appear to those who actually use them. In these accounts, an emphasis on being 'in the movement' and an appeal to fun and good times with close friends speaks of the affective and embodied nature of the experience of intoxication.

In their use, alcohol and drugs play an important role in mediating between individual and group identity. It is precisely this duel function, a loss of self on the one hand and the collectively of sociability on the other, that many users find appealing and, it is worth adding, that government backed law and order and health interventions find so problematic to engage with. Intoxication redefines sociality and relationships between individuals, groups and society. We have seen that individuals pursue intoxication as a means of letting go and of losing themselves, that by transgressing social rules and strictures of social control, individuals can bond in groups (Griffin et al., 2009). In my own work on stag tourism (Thurnell-Read, 2011, 2012), alcohol was revealed to provide a vital role in allow individuals to 'let go' and 'cut loose', in doing so becoming part of a group while at the same time, often but not always, flagrantly flouting many wider conventions of social propriety.

In terms of methodology, it is also worth noting that a number of the studies referenced in this chapter employ qualitative methods, involving either ethnographic forms of participant-observation or in-depth semi-structured interviews with individuals or friendship groups in which participants are encouraged to freely elaborate their own accounts of drug and alcohol consumption. Such methodologies have implications for the types of knowledge that can be generated about drink and drugs and the experience of those who consumer them. The empirical proximity that these research undertakings have the potential to achieve allows for a greater understanding of the sense of the extraordinary and altered states that intoxication can give rise to. As Shelia Henderson argues in her discussion of gendered aspects of 1990s rave drug use, 'a whole host of visual, aural and oral stimuli brought crowds of diverse young people together in a sensual social space on a grand scale' (Henderson,

1999: 40). Such studies have shown that drug and alcohol consumption is a social, emotive, affective and embodied activity. Again, the evident need to give due attention to this complexity, and to the subjective and qualitative aspects of drug and alcohol use, suggests that the advances of recent decades need to continue in order to develop a fuller picture of the nature of drug and alcohol use across a range of social and cultural contexts.

As Cameron Duff has argued (2011, 2013; Chapter 39, this volume), there is a need to move beyond overly reified accounts of substance use and instead to work towards understandings of 'assemblages' that place alcohol (or drugs) as active actors in affective networks encompassing users and substances but also bodies, settings, objects and practices. Indeed, while the turn towards the social and the sociable during the 1990s allowed for rich qualitative insights and a move away from simplistic accounts of pathologised 'problem' drug and alcohol use, it seems the current direction of the field of research might further enhance our understanding by deploying exactly the theoretical frameworks that Duff proposes and that have the potential to allow for even more holistic analyses to be made.

Not wishing to overplay the progress of this field of research, it is worth acknowledging a number of areas that remain relatively underexplored. As no doubt this overview demonstrates, a significant proportion of contemporary research in this field focuses on young people. Perhaps because their identity is seen to be more 'in process' and their social networks, friendships and bonding rituals more in flux and open to adaptation, the drinking and drug taking practices of young adults and adolescents make for enticing research subjects. However, how sociality and identity relate to alcohol and drug consumption in later life or, for that matter, within the family, remain underexplored and largely untheorised (a notable exception being the 2011 book of Jayne et al. exploring alcohol across three generations of the same families). Similarly, the spectacular nature of public displays of drunkenness, or the equally spectacular setting of the rave or nightclub, means that more mundane spaces in which drinking and drug use take place are, again, conspicuously overlooked. Thus, consumption in the home remains methodologically difficult to access.

The fact that our understanding of drug and alcohol consumption remains wedded to conceptualisations of leisure also means that little research has been conducted into drug and alcohol use within the work place. Interestingly, widespread media coverage of comments by British Professor David Nutt linking the global financial crisis with the bravado and risk taking culture brought on by cocaine use of investment bankers in New York and London (Williams, 2013), perhaps provides clues as to future directions the social sciences might take in understanding the social uses of drugs and alcohol consumption. While the college campus, the local high street bar, pub or club on a Saturday or the sports ground club house all provide vibrant examples of the roles played by drugs and alcohol in the construction, performance and maintenance of identity, the social and the sociable extend into spaces, times and practices that have still not been the subject of sustained academic inquiry.

REFERENCES

Allison, A. (1994) *Nightwork: Sexuality, Pleasure, and Corporate Masculinity in a Tokyo Hostess Club*. Chicago: University of Chicago Press.

Anderson, D., Beckerleg, S., Hailu, D. and Klein, A. (2007) *Khat Controversy: Stimulating the Debate on Drugs*. Oxford: Berg.

Balsa, A.I., Homer, J.F., French, M.T. and Norton, E.C. (2010) Alcohol use and popularity: social payoffs from conforming to peers behavior, *Journal of Research on Adolescence*, 21(3): 559–68.

Beccaria, F. and Sande, A. (2003) Drinking games and rite of life projects: a social comparison of

the young people's use of alcohol during the rite of passage to adulthood in Italy and Norway. *Young*, 11(2): 99–119.
Beckerly, S. and Nuur, S. (2005) A view from the refugee camps: new Somali khat use in Kenya. *Drug and Alcohol Today*, 5(3): 25–7.
Belackova, V. and Vaccaro, C.A. (2013) 'A friend with weed is a friend indeed': understanding the relationship between friendship identity and market relations among marijuana users. *Journal of Drug Issues*, 43(3): 289–313.
Blackshaw, T. (2003) *Leisure Life: Myth, Masculinity and Modernity*. London: Routledge.
Borsari, B. (2004) Drinking games in the college environment: a review. *Journal of Alcohol and Drug Education*, 48(2): 29–51.
Brown, R. and Gregg, M. (2012) The pedagogy of regret: Facebook, binge drinking and young women. *Continuum: Journal of Media and Cultural Studies*, 26(3): 357–69.
Campbell, H. (2000) The glass phallus: pub(lic) masculinity and drinking in rural New Zealand. *Rural Sociology*, 65(4): 562–81.
Carrier, N. (2005) Under any other name: the trade and use of khat in the UK. *Drugs and Alcohol Today*, 5(3): 14–16.
Carrier, N. (2007) *Kenyan Khat: The Social Life of a Stimulant*. Boston: Brill.
Chatterton, P. and Holland, R. (2002) Theorising urban playscapes: producing, regulating and consuming youthful nightlife city spaces. *Urban Studies*, 39(1): 95–116.
Chrzan, J. (2013) *Alcohol: Social Drinking in Cultural Context*. New York: Routledge.
Crawford, G. (2009) Consuming sport, consuming beer: sport fans, scene, and everyday life. In L.A. Wenner and S.J. Jackson (eds), *Sport, Beer, and Gender: Promotional Culture and Contemporary Social Life*. Bern: Peter Lang, pp. 279–98.
Cullen, F. (2010) 'Two's up and poncing fags': young women's smoking, practices, reciprocity and friendship. *Gender and Education*, 22(5): 491–504.
de Visser, R. and Smith, J.A. (2007) Young men's ambivalence towards alcohol. *Social Science and Medicine*, 64(2): 350–62.
Dempster, S. (2011) I drink, therefore I'm man: gender discourses, alcohol and the construction of British undergraduate masculinity. *Gender and Education*, 23(5): 635–53.
Driessen, H. (1992) Drinking on masculinity: alcohol and gender in Andalusia. In D. Gefou-Madianou (ed.), *Alcohol, Gender and Culture*. Oxford: Routledge, pp. 71–9.
Duff, C. (2011) Reassembling (social) contexts: new directions for a sociology of drugs. *International Journal of Drug Policy*, 22(6): 404–6.
Duff, C. (2013) The social life of drugs. *International Journal of Drug Policy*, 24(3): 167–72.
Fletcher, T. and Spracklen, K. (2013) Cricket, drinking and exclusion of British Pakistani Muslims? *Ethnic and Racial Studies*, 37(8): 1310–27.
Foster, K. and Spencer, D. (2013) 'It's just a social thing': drug use, friendship and borderwork among marginalized young people. *International Journal of Drug Policy*, 24(3): 223–30.
Fry, M.L. (2011) Seeking the pleasure zone: understanding young adult's intoxication culture. *Australian Marketing Journal*, 19(1): 65–70.
Griffin C., Bengry-Howell, A., Hackley, C., Mistral, W. and Szmigin, I. (2009) Every time I do it I absolutely annihilate myself': loss of (self-) consciousness and loss of memory in young people's drinking narratives. *Sociology*, 43(3): 457–76.
Griffiths, P., Gossops, S., Wickenden, S., Dunworth, J., Harris, K. and Lloyd, C. (1997) A transactional pattern of drug use: qat (khat) in the UK. *The British Journal of Psychiatry*, 170: 281–4.
Hackley, C., Bengry-Howell, A., Griffin, C., Mistral, W., Szmigin, I. and Hackley, R. (2013) Young adults and 'binge' drinking: a Bakhtinian analysis, *Journal of Marketing Management*, 29(7): 933–49.
Henderson, S. (1999) Drugs and culture: the question of gender. In N. South (ed.), *Drugs: Cultures, Controls and Everyday Life*. London: Sage pp. 36–48.
Hunt G. and Evans, K. (2008) 'The great unmentionable': exploring the pleasures and benefits of ecstasy from the perspective of drug users. *Drugs*, 15(4): 329–49.
Hunt, G., MacKenzie, K. and Joe-Laidler, K. (2005) Alcohol and masculinity: the case of ethnic youth gangs. In T.W. Wilson (ed.), *Drinking Cultures: Alcohol and Identity*. Oxford: Berg pp. 225–54.

Hunt, G., Moloney, M. and Kristen, E. (2010) *Youth, Drugs, and Nightlife*. New York: Routledge.

Jayne, M., Holloway, S. and Valentine, G. (2006) Drunk and disorderly: alcohol, urban life and public space. *Progress in Human Geography*, 30(4): 451–68.

Jayne, M., Valentine, G. and Holloway, S.L. (2011) *Alcohol, Drinking, Drunkenness: (Dis) orderly Spaces*. Farnham: Ashgate.

Joseph, J. (2012) Around the boundary: alcohol and older Caribbean-Canadian men. *Leisure Studies*, 31(2): 147–63.

Josiam, B.M., Hobson, J.S.P., Dietrich, U.C. and Smeaton, G. (1998) An analysis of the sexual, alcohol and drug related behavioural patterns of students on spring break, *Tourism Management*, 19(6): 501–13.

Kuntsche, E., Knibbe, G. and Engels, R. (2005) Why do young people drink? A review of drinking motives. *Clinical Psychology Review*, 25(7): 841–61.

Leyshon M (2008) 'We're stuck in the corner': young women, embodiment and drinking in the countryside. *Drugs: Education, Prevention and Policy*, 15(3): 276–89.

MacLean, S. and Moore, D. (2014) 'Hyped up': assemblages of alcohol, excitement and violence for outer-suburban young adults in the inner-city at night. *International Journal of Drug Policy*, 25(3): 378–85.

Malbon, B. (1999) *Clubbing: Dancing, Ecstasy and Vitality*. London: Routledge.

Measham, F. and Brain, K. (2005) Bing drinking, British alcohol policy and the new culture of intoxication. *Crime, Media and Culture*, 1(3): 262–82.

Montemurro, B. and McClure, B. (2005) Changing gender norms for alcohol consumption: social drinking and lowered inhibitions at bachelorette parties. *Sex Roles*, 52(6): 279–88.

Moore, K. and Miller, S. (2005) Living the high life: the role of drug taking in young people's lives. *Drugs and Alcohol Today*, 5(2): 29–32.

Niland, P., Lyons, A.C., Goodwin, I. and Hutton, F. (2013) 'Everyone can loosen up and get a bit of a buzz on': young adults, alcohol and friendship practices. *International Journal of Drug Policy*, 24(6): 530–7.

Nordgren, J. (2013) The moral entrepreneurship of anti-khat campaigners in Sweden – a critical discourse analysis. *Drugs and Alcohol Today*, 13(1): 20–7.

Osman, F. and Söderbäck, M. (2011) Perceptions of the use of khat among Somali immigrants living in Swedish society. *Scandinavian Journal of Public Health*, 39(2): 212–19.

Parker, H., Aldrige, J. and Measham, F. (1998) *Illegal Leisure: The Normalization of Adolescent Recreational Drug Use*. Hove: Routledge.

Pilkington, H. (2007) Beyond 'peer pressure': rethinking drug use and 'youth culture'. *International Journal of Drug Policy*, 18(3): 213–24.

Plant, M. and Plant, M. (2006) *Binge Britain: Alcohol and the National Response*. Oxford: Oxford University Press.

Saunders, N. (1996) *Ecstasy: Dance, Trance and Transformation*. San Francisco: Quick American Archives.

Sheehan, M. and Ridge, D. (2001) 'You become really close…you talk about the silly things you did, and we laugh': the role of binge drinking in female secondary students' lives. *Substance Use and Misuse*, 36(3): 347–72.

Smith, O. (2014) *Contemporary Adulthood and the Night-Time Economy*. London: Palgrave Macmillan.

Sönmez, S., Apostolopoulosb, Y., Yuc, C. H., Yangd, S., Mattilae, A. and Yue, L. (2006) Binge drinking and casual sex on spring break. *Annals of Tourism Research*, 33(4): 895–917.

Stepney, M. (2013) British women's experiences of drinking alcohol: dynamics of emotional proximity and distance. *Emotion, Space and Society*, 10: 105–12.

Taylor, S. (2008) Outside the outsiders: media representations of drug use. *Probation Journal*, 55(4): 369–87.

Thornton, K. (1995) *Club Cultures: Music, Media and Subcultural Capital*. Cambridge: Polity.

Thurnell-Read, T. (2011) 'Off the leash and out of control': masculinities and embodiment in eastern European stag tourism. *Sociology*, 45(6): 977–91.

Thurnell-Read, T. (2012) 'What happens on tour': the premarital stag tour, homosocial bonding and male friendship. *Men and Masculinities*, 15(3): 249–70.

Tomsen, S. (1997) A top night: social protest, masculinity and the culture of drinking violence. *British Journal of Criminology*, 37(1): 90–102.

Tutenges, S. and Sandberg, S. (2013) Intoxication stories: the characteristics, context and implications of drinking stories among Danish Youth. *International Journal of Drug Policy*, 24(6): 538–44.

Vander Ven, T. (2011) *Getting Wasted: Why College Students Drink Too Much and Party Too Hard*. New York: New York University Press.

Waitt, G. and Warren, A. (2008) 'Talking shit over a brew after a good session with your mates': surfing, space and masculinity. *Australian Geographer*, 39(3): 353–65.

Waitt, G., Jessop, L. and Gorman-Murray, A. (2011) 'The guys in there just expect to be laid': embodied and gendered socio-spatial practices of a 'night out' in Wollongong, Australia. *Gender, Place and Culture*, 18(2): 255–75.

Williams, R. (2013) Financial meltdown was caused by too many bankers taking cocaine, says former government drugs tsar Prof David Nutt. *The Sunday Times*, 15 April 2013.

Wilson, T. (2005) *Drinking Cultures*. New York: Berg.

Wolburg, J. and Treise, D. (2004) Drinking rituals among the heaviest drinkers: college student binge drinkers and alcoholics. In C. Otnes and T. Lowrey (eds), *Contemporary Consumption Rituals: A Research Anthology*. Mahwah: Lawrence Erlbaum. pp. 3–20.

Zhou, J., O'Brien, S. and Heim, D. (2014) Alcohol consumption in sportspeople: the role of social cohesion, identity and happiness. *International Review of Sociology of Sport*, 49(3–4): 278–93.

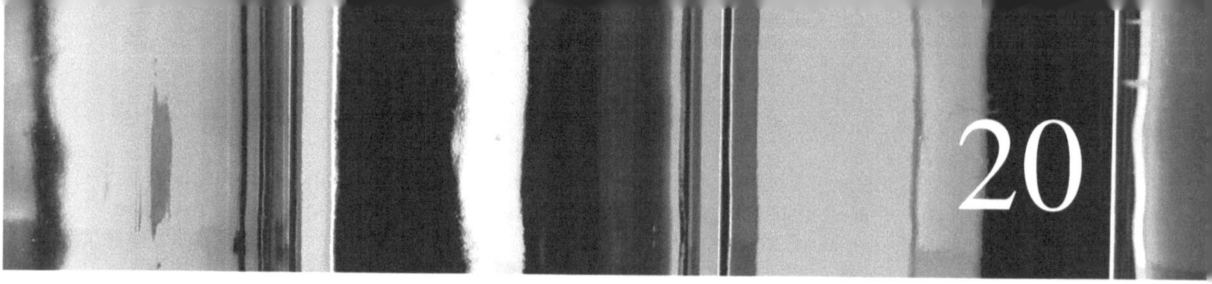

20

Consumption and Context

Mark Jayne, Gill Valentine
and Sarah L. Holloway

INTRODUCTION

Research focused on consumption and context has been an important theoretical and empirical driver of drug and alcohol research across the social sciences.[1] In this chapter we begin with a review of studies that have focused on drug and alcohol consumption with reference to contexts such as supranational, national and regional scales. The chapter then considers foundational characteristic of research that considers class, gender, age, ethnicity and so on with reference to spaces and places around the world. In reviewing these bodies of literature, we argue that despite generating rich and detailed findings with regards to consumption researchers have tended to under-theorise context.

In doing so, we advance arguments outlined in Chapter 8 in order to highlight how researchers have overwhelmingly failed to pursue understanding of connections, mobilities, similarities, differences and relationalities between case studies (including consideration of policy transfer, legislation, planning, design and policing strategies, everyday drug and alcohol production and consumption cultures and so on) and have tended to consider space and place as a passive backdrop, rather than as an active constituent to the topic being researched (Jayne et al., 2008; DeVerteuil and Wilton, 2009). To that end, we unpack writing on 'the city', 'the countryside' and 'the home' in order to highlight how theorists have offered more critical accounts of the context of drug and alcohol consumption. The paper then turns to literature focused on more-than-representational theory that focuses on practices relating to drug and alcohol consumption and how human and nonhuman formations are enacted or performed in ways that elude an epistemological focus on representation alone (see Thrift, 2004). We also introduce writing on 'assemblages', which draws on post-structuralist writing to highlight how research into the context of drug and alcohol consumption should look beyond 'static arrangements or a set of parts, whether organized under some logic or collected randomly, but to processes of arranging, organizing, fitting together … where assemblage is a whole of some sort that expresses some identity and claims to a territory' (McCann and Ward, 2011: 12). In doing so, we highlight fruitful avenues for research to advance understanding of consumption and context in drug and alcohol research.

CONSUMPTION AND CONTEXT: WHY GEOGRAPHY MATTERS

There is a voluminous amount of writing that addresses how drug and alcohol consumption are differentially and discursively constructed in specific spaces and places. There is also a significant body of writing concerning national, regional or local alcohol consumption related to legislation, initiatives and policies, as well as work that draws on large scale transnational statistical reports and cross-cultural surveys. There is also now a long tradition of large transnational surveys and projects that measures alcohol consumption around the world (e.g. ECAS, 2002; ESPAD, 2003; WHO, 2004). Similarly, there are now numerous national and transnational surveys of drug consumption and investigations of policy and practice (Public Health England, 2013; UNODC, 2014; The White House, 2014).

Theorists have also investigated the relationship between context, drug taking and drinking patterns and identity, and lifestyle and forms of sociability in a large number of different locations around the world: including community tolerance of drug use in Columbia and Guatemala (Mcllwaine and Moser, 2004); drug taking and dancing in a gay nightclub in Sydney, Australia (Slavin, 2004); and violence and moral economy of homeless heroin addicts in San Francisco (Bourgois, 1998). Other work has considered alcohol consumption and gender in India (Chatterjee, 2003), drinking and young people in Vietnam (Thomas, 2002) and masculinity and identity in Newcastle-upon-Tyne (Nayak, 2003).

While such examples of drugs and alcohol research are generally underpinned by studies of specific space and places, researchers have nonetheless tended to undertheorise *spatialities* that constitute the topics at hand. Indeed, there has been a failure to formulate research agendas that also offer the opportunity to pursue a more integrated understanding of how interpenetration of political, economic, social, cultural and spatial elements impact on drug and alcohol consumption at particular spatial scales in either theoretical and empirical terms. For example, while much research focuses on drug and alcohol consumption at national or local levels, often pursuing comparisons between different contexts, research has generally tended to shy away from making connections, describing similarities or differences and relationalities between case studies. This has also ensured a lack of theoretical arguments that translate beyond specific people and spaces and places, other than dialectical approaches that consider drug and alcohol consumption as either a criminal/social/medical problem or as a social or cultural practice. While there have been some attempts to conjoin these issues via a focus on transnational, national and local levels (for example, Holder, 2000; Harrison, 1996; Jones, 1987), there has been little success in developing perspectives that translate beyond the empirical evidence generated in specific contexts.

Moreover, even when research offers a useful antidote to general approaches, a number of weaknesses can be identified. For example, research has focused on specific contexts and people via study of consumption, identity, lifestyle and forms of sociability, research has focused on gender differences and drinking patterns (Plant, 1997; Ettorre, 1997; Harnett et al., 2000; Waterson, 2000), masculinity, femininity and ethnicity (Shaikh and Nax, 2000), drinking amongst various black and minority ethnic groups and so on (Stivers, 2000; Share, 2003). In these studies, however, location, context and the relationships between the people and places tend to be considered as a peripheral issue. Such limitations are perhaps best evidenced by the lack of attempt to join up, to compare or contrast research in different contexts.

CONSUMPTION AND CONTEXT: SPACE, PLACE AND IDENTITY

It is nonetheless small-scale, generally ethnographic research that has arguably generated the most productive dialogue regarding critical approaches to understanding drug and alcohol consumption and context. Key foundational elements to this work have been to address context as relational, with the spaces and places being studied not considered as passive backdrops but active constituents to the practices and processes being studied. Such work focuses, for instance, on the mundane 'things' that make up our everyday life; a focus on the interpenetration of spatial scales (e.g. the body, the home, the street, the pub, the city, neighbourhoods, the countryside, the urban, nations and so on); and consideration of the ways in which drug and alcohol consumption is constituted by constellations of social relations in diverse spaces and places (Thrift, 2005).

Indeed, theorists have begun to move beyond generalised depictions, to show that far than being homogenised, drug and alcohol consumption is varied and constructed through diverse practices, experiences and contexts by different social groups who have a variety of experiences. Studies have sought to connect the general and specific ways in which broad political, economic, social cultural and spatial practices and processes relating to drug and alcohol consumption play out in different ways, at different times and for different people in different spaces and places.

The city

For example, 'the city', has been a particularly important focus for research on drug and alcohol consumption and context. Over the past 30 years, many cities have reinvented themselves as sites of consumption (Hannigan, 1998; Jayne, 2006). This has been bound up with political and socio-cultural change associated with Fordism, Post-Fordism and neo-Fordism (Kumar, 1995), changes in the local state and the rise of the entrepreneurial city (Hall and Hubbard, 1996) and a decline in extractive and industrial manufacturing and a move towards a more service based, cultural and 'symbolic' economy, which includes the support of leisure and the night-time economy (Jayne, 2005). Work has usefully concluded that urban nightlife is constructed through a number of contradictory tendencies towards both deregulation and (re)regulation and the twin imperatives of fun and disorder (Malbon, 1999; Chatterton and Hollands, 2003; Hobbs et al., 2003). On the one hand, during the weekends and evenings, city streets host large number of revellers intent on having fun, spending money, drinking alcohol, taking drugs and dancing. This is an economy of pleasure, and the '24-hour city' becomes the vehicle for economic growth, profit generation and entrepreneurialism. However, while the financial success of the night-time economy has stimulated further demand for its deregulation, the night-time continues to be heavily influenced by concerns for tighter regulation, social control and zoning, due to lingering moral panics and fear of violence and disorder.

In arguing for a more sophisticated understanding that does not homogenise alcohol consumption at night, Latham (2003) suggests that such general depictions of urban life lack understanding of day-to-day uses of space. In summary, scratching the surface appearance of urban transformation allows depiction not of a homogenised, purified set of spaces and experiences but something more complicated and contested. Latham's (2003) ethnographic study of two streets in Auckland, New Zealand uncovers a public culture that is underpinned by tolerance diversity and creative energy, with a mixing of post-industrial lifestyles, sexually polymorphous and industrial male public cultures that inhabit hotels and pubs, a mixing of vernacular and gentrified, and a convivial ecology, which can be seen to spill into the streets generating 'new solidarities and new collectivities' and a greater sense of belonging (Latham, 2003: 1719). Edensor (2006) also highlights how in the city of Port Louis in Mauritius, the Keg and Marlin pub allows ethic and social mixing and Hunt et al. (2005) suggest that gangs of ethnic young men drinking on the streets of San Francisco offer economically, cultural and spatially marginalised people the opportunity to visibly contribute to urban street life. Similarly, Altay (2008) describes 'Minibars' that emerge around and between buildings in Ankara, Turkey, where not being able to afford bars and clubs, young people take advantage of pavements, low masonry walls 'to hang out' and drink alcohol. Such writing highlights how drinking and drunkenness and drug taking can be considered in terms of the connectivities and belonging generated in public space, and as being grounded in pleasures, enjoyment and 'riskyness' of heterogeneous groups of people mixing in city spaces in ways that perhaps would not be acceptable, to them or city authorities, if the mediating factor of the consumption of alcohol in bars, pubs and other establishments was not present to enabled drinkers to claim to be active citizens.

The countryside

Writing that considers drugs and alcohol in the context of rural areas, although less voluminous than writing on the city, has sought to engage with the political, economic, social, cultural and spatial practices and processes that constitute ideological constructions of the context of 'the countryside'. In broad terms, the rural landscape is commonly portrayed as an idyllic place to grow up (Short, 1991; Bunce, 1994). This imagining of the rural has as Kraack and Kenway (2002: 146) describe both 'aesthetic and moral components'. The aesthetic component refers to the way that 'the rural' is commonly understood to be a picturesque, natural physical environment, characterised by trees, fields and open space. The moral component alludes to the way that rural communities are stereotyped as close-knit, harmonious environments, where residents can live out a simple/pure existence free from the stress, dangers and corruptions of urban life such as drug taking and alcohol related violence and disorder (Valentine et al., 2007).

For example, anthropological studies that focus on rural areas in 'developing countries' have considered the relationship between the 'natural rhythms' of agricultural production and related constructions of masculinity and femininity. Men and women's relationship to farming via discourses of fertility and physical strength have been investigated in terms of the social rules that circulate around alcohol. Where drunkenness for men is celebrated as loosening everyday conscious states in order to make men more productive farmers, women's connection to nature is expressed through menstruation and childbirth. Around these stories, the times, amounts and types of drinks ascribed to gendered roles and rules have been considered (see Gefou-Madianou, 1992; De Garine and De Garine, 2001). Moreover, in studies in rural Africa and Europe writers have investigated the symbolic role of alcohol in terms of fertility. De Garine's (2001) study of tribal life in Cameroon presents a distinction between the role of beer in rituals and everyday life, where masculinity is constructed via different levels of drunkenness for different occasions when men can become drunk so that – 'he walks from the right to left, falls down, sometimes vomits and fights'. In a similar vein, Papagaroutfali (1992) describes how gender differences are played out in celebratory drinking practices in contemporary rural Greece where Ouzo is considered as a 'manly' drink, whereas women are supposed to favour fruit-flavoured liqueurs or 'sipping' beer and wine diluted with soft drinks.

Elsewhere in Europe, gendered drinking has been shown to be bound up with specific rural contexts. Abad (2001) shows that in Spain, at different times of the year, men drink throughout the day in public spaces in order to assure the fertility of the land and to ensure a productive harvest. In contrast, women are only allowed to consume alcohol in public on feast days, or in secret while on trips to nearby towns. The relationship between gender and agricultural tradition is also present in the work of Bianquis-Gasser (1992), who in discussing the French region of Alsace, shows how drinking practices change at different points of the agricultural calendar. Alcohol consumption is associated with 'men's affairs', where men drink as a sacrament, often in cellars likened to a chapel – cold, vaulted, silent and dark. To achieve immortality men must drink deeply – they must lose their everyday conscious state, their mundane awareness. Women gain this status through childbirth and men by making and drinking wine. The relationship between productivity is also considered by Peace (1992), who focuses on drinking and rural identity in Ireland. In this case, men's substantial drinking takes place in a small number of bars frequented by fishermen, where dramas and sagas around competitive fishing practices unfold. The men constantly move between bars in order to ensure the possibility of conversational encounters, to support camaraderie and to facilitate conflict. Such movement is important not only in terms of social cohesion but also in terms of securing work opportunities. In a similar vein, Campbell (2000) considers the performativity of gender in Rural New Zealand, depicting 'conversational cockfighting' and disciplines of 'being able to hold your drink' – describing the pub as the last bastion of male camaraderie. Other theorists have considered the intersection of alcohol consumption *and* drug taking amongst a diverse range of social groups in countries such as Spain, Vietnam, USA and Australia (Cronk and Sarvela, 1997; Okumura et al., 2002; Reilly et al., 2002; Alvarez et al., 2006).

Writing has also focused on intersections of class, gender, age and ethnicity as key to understanding drug and alcohol consumption in rural areas. For example, the role of men in pub life is also shown by Leyshon (2005) to be central to assertions of rural masculinity and marginalisation in the face of the restructuring of the countryside. Heley (2008) also talks about the shifting terrain of rural pubs – and describes how newcomers have tried to (re)create the typical English gentlemen (New Squires) that involves a nostalgic fiction of provincial bygone age, ales 'off the wood', tankards on the shelf and dominance of an area of the pub known as 'the office' previously colonised by local framers, which is now a destination of choice for this new collective, aware of the historic role of this private bar. In a similar vein, Wolcott's (1974) work on African beer gardens in Bulawayom, Mars (1987) study of Newfoundland longshoremen and Hensen's (1983) study of bars in Catalonia shows how 'freezing out' techniques making people feel uncomfortable and assert particular masculine identities. Such writing is thus focused on considering constructions of hegemonic masculinity and how idealised local rural identities are legitimised around alcohol consumption. This is taken further by Leyshon (2005, 2008) who describes the binaries of masculinity and femininity and the trading of insults such as 'drinking like a girl' in rural England. Leyshon (2005) consider bodily drinking performances and the ways in which gatherings of men were exclusive, hierarchical, homophobic and sexist, where men consume large amounts of alcohol without seeming drunk and by visibly and loudly occupying specific spaces in the pub.

Research has also focused on restructuring of the rural economy in terms of class conflict. In the UK, Hunt and Satterlee (1986) argue that that while 'the pub' can be a place where social groups occupy the same space, social barriers are also consolidated in these spaces. In particular, Hunt and Satterlee discuss the impact of urban life on the countryside via industrial re-structuring and middle-class incomers. Drawing on research in a Cambridgeshire village with seven pubs, the research shows how alcohol can enhance social solidarity as well as entrenching social demarcation and division. Working-class pubs were described as being the neighbourhoods' social centre, where round buying in intimate groups, or the pooling of money and drinking with offspring and kin were commonplace. Working class pubs re-affirmed a cohesion that already existed, and incomers, if they lived on the 'right' estate would be gradually accepted, but as they did not have a shared knowledge or historical connections with the locality and the pub, they were never fully accepted. In contrast, drinking in middle-class pubs are shown to be focused on good fellowship and of being part of the 'right-set' of people. Within this process of forging 'belonging', Hunt (1991) describes particular discourses of public/private drinking and also 'civilizing' ideas that the working-class could learn from the middle-class drinking practices.

The home

More recent writing has also focused on the home as a site of drug and alcohol consumption, highlighting the importance of ideology in obscuring domestic drug taking and drinking (Blunt and Dowling, 2006). While city centre binge drinking and drug taking challenges the civility of our streets, domestic drinking can accrue cultural capital to an individual when it is characterised as part of a cultured domestic lifestyle or considered as constituents of ways to unwind; acting as good hosts by making others feel welcome in their home and so on. In this way, the contemporary geographical imaginary of drug taking/binge drinking as a city centre problem (Kneale and French, 2008), when set against the positive spatial discourses surrounding the meaning of home (Laurie et al., 1999; Blunt and Dowling, 2006), works to 'hide' harmful/hazardous domestic drinking and drug taking. In effect, binge drinking (and associated drug cultures), although technically referring to periods of episodic heavy alcohol consumption, has come in cultural terms to mean dangerous drinking by uncouth youth in the streets, and often labelled as 'the British disease'. As a result, many of those who consume high levels of alcohol and drugs in very different domestic circumstances continue to regard their own practices as unremarkable and feel unwarrantedly insulated from concern (Holloway et al., 2008).

CONSUMPTION AND CONTEXT: MORE-THAN-REPRESENTATION AND ASSEMBLAGES

In this final section we consider a small but growing interest in more-than-representation and assemblage thinking as key theoretical tools that seek to develop new ways to critically interrogate the context of drug and alcohol consumption. For example, more-than-representational theory shows us that by working from the viewpoint that '[q]uestions about how emotions are embodied and located merit further elaboration in the context of typical and less typical everyday lives' (Davidson et al., 2005: 5), in parallel with studies that investigate affect as 'a sense of push in the world…a notion of broad tendencies and lines of force' (Thrift, 2004: 60). Theorists have made significant progress in advancing understanding of how embodied emotions and affect are intricately connected to specific contexts and practices.

Our own work has focused on emotions, embodiment and affect in order to consider people's experience of drinking in cities at night, with empirical research showing that respondents talked in detail about the ways in which alcohol, drinking and drunkenness offers both a sense of 'belonging' and allows relationships with friends and strangers based on an ethic of 'transformation' and 'care' that is underpinned by sociability and social interaction in crowded commercial areas such as bars, pubs and clubs and public spaces such as streets and squares (Jayne et al., 2010). While there are social differences and unequal power relations bound up in such emotional, embodied and affective geographies, our research shows that that there are also similarities and connectivities that bind drinkers together as a 'counter public' enabling interaction with people, space and place in a way that is intimately (dis)connected from sober experiences.

It is in the context of these findings that the long-standing use of selective statistics by politicians and policy makers that have come to inform popular discourses depicting cities in terms of high levels of violence and disorder that can clearly be seen to be out of line with the majority of peoples' experiences of alcohol consumption and urban life. In these terms, the continued evocation of city centres as drunken, violent and out of control in order to underpin policy and planning is highly problematic. Such visions of violent and disorderly cities can be clearly associated with moral judgments around embodied, emotional and affective drunkenness that while not being unlawful are considered as unsavoury, uncouth, un-feminine and so on. In these terms, public campaigns that target, for example, the perpetrators of violence, rather than 'criminalising' generalised groups of drinkers, for example, young people/women would be more culturally legible for young drinkers (also see Jayne et al., 2010, 2016). We thus follow the argument of Waitt et al. (2010) that in order to resonate with drinkers, progressive alcohol campaigns should not stigmatise excessive alcohol consumption but rather offer more salient measures to warn against potential problematic experiences associated with alcohol consumption that relate to the way that, for example, young women already conceive of their own 'big night out' (e.g. in terms of an 'ethics' of personal and group safety). In a similar vein, Bunton and Coveney (2011) ague that sustained theoretical and empirical attention must be applied to considering the embodied and emotional pleasure of taking drugs in public spaces and commercial spaces (also see Cooperstock 1971).

Indeed, such writing highlights how drugs and alcohol are consumed by people because they offer unique and explicit connection both 'within' and 'outside' (with the city itself) the body allowing people to become 'subjects which are caught and situated as bodies with radiating ripples and circuits of feeling, intensity, response and sensation … [via] flows that wrap into and fold out of our bodies' (Dewsbury 2011: 21). In particular, drugs and alcohol allows drinkers to experience, negotiate and perform shifting emotions (over a few minutes, hours and longer time periods), including subjectivities that are multiple, emergent diverse and complex, bound up with bodily sensations and affective experiences that are challenging, at times unpredictable, fun, sad and often un-rememberable 'intoxicated geographies'.

Recent work has also focused more specifically on the human and non-human 'assemblages' that constitute the context of drug and alcohol consumption. Drawing on post-structuralist writing of Latour (2005) and Deleuze and Guattari (1988), writing on networks, practices and spaces speak 'not to static arrangement or a set of parts, whether organized under some logic or collected randomly, but to processes of arranging, organizing, fitting together'. Towards that end, geographical writing on alcohol, drinking and drunkenness has begun to engage with such assemblage thinking (see for example, Jayne et al., 2010; Shaw, 2010, 2014, 2015;

Waitt et al., 2010; Bohling, 2014, 2015; Jayne and Valentine 2015b) in response to the challenge of Jayne et al. (2010) to understanding alcohol, drinking and drunkenness with regards to:

> Individual and collective emotional and embodied experiences of different types of alcohol consumption at different times and in different places and spaces and how they are affected by, and may affect a range of different relations, including embodied identities (age, ethnicity, gender, sexuality, etc.), emotional and embodied state (e.g. hunger, thirst, sadness, excitement, etc.), varying neurological responses to alcohol, social mixing, personal interaction, atmosphere (how sounds, smells, etc. affect the transpersonal circulation of moods and feelings), non-human materialities e.g. the taste and viscosity of different drinks and drinks containers (glasses, bottles etc.), and the physical layout of different commercial venues or public spaces (e.g. opportunities to sit, stand, move, dance, availability of toilet facilities, the proximity of other bodies, etc.). (Jayne et al., 2010: 548–9)

Moreover, writing on spatialities of drug consumption and context is also pursuing this fruitful research agenda, highlighting the importance of understanding the interpenetrations of human and non-human actors in effecting bodies and spaces (Malins, 2004, 2014; Duff 2014; Fraser et al., 2014). Race (2009, 2014, 2015), for example, has focused on the relationships between drugs and queer identity, including investigation of the interpenetration of 'real life' and 'virtual worlds' constructed through assemblages of mobile apps, online dating, fantasy adventure and the use of methamphetamine in sexual activity, facilitated online but which usually takes place in the home. Malins et al. (2008) have also theorised bodies, risks and urban spaces with reference to women injecting drugs by focusing on alley ways, stairwells, toilets, parks, restaurants and 'performances' and assemblages of people and things. Taking such arguments with regards to consumption and context in new directions, Williams (2016) considers the disjuncture between drug taking in public and domestic spaces and the context and role of worship and spirituality in an institutional religious space of Pentecostal drugs rehab practices. Vitellone (2010, 2015) has traced the spatialities of 'techno-sociology' of habit, habitus, discourse and the materialities and affective registers of syringe use. Such work responds to Duff's concern that 'critical discussions of the problem of context are surprisingly rare in drug policy debate' and highlights how studies assemblages of space, embodiment and practice are well placed to begin to offer more fruitful understanding of the 'the sheer complexity of context' with regards to alcohol and drug consumption (Duff, 2007: 503).

CONCLUSION

In this chapter we have highlighted a large amount of academic and policy related research focusing on the context of drug and alcohol consumption. Tracing out the genealogy of theoretical and empirical trajectories highlights work that is concerned in mapping how diverse drugs and alcohol consumption is undertaken by different social groups, in different spaces and places around the world. In doing so, such research has addressed the shifting terrain of the differential and discursive construction of the pleasures and dangers of how, when, why and for whom drug and alcohol consumption is considered as 'problematic' or in need of political, policy or police and legislative intervention. At its best, writing addresses context with regards to progressive and critical engagement with political, economic, social and cultural practices and processes and considers space and place not as passive backdrops but are active constituents. This includes studies of 'materialities' and 'representations' of mundane 'things' and offering insights into constellations of social relations, as well highlighting similarities, differences and relationalities of the body, the home, the street, the pub, the city, neighbourhoods, the countryside, the urban, nations and so on. Recent research into assemblages of embodiment, emotion and affect has further advanced this project and in doing so has opened up new fruitful avenues for researchers to advance theoretical and empirical understanding of the complex relationships between drug and alcohol consumption and context.

NOTE

1 This paper draws on, updates and advances previous arguments made in Jayne et al. (2010, 2011a, 2011b) and Jayne and Valentine (2015b).

REFERENCES

Abad, L. C. (2001) 'Gender and drink in Aragon, Spain', In I. de Garine and V. De Garine (eds), *Drinking: Anthropological Approaches*. New York: Bergham Books, pp. 144–57.

Alvarez, F. J., Queipo, D., Del Rio, M. C. and Garcia, M. C. (2006) 'Patterns of drug use by young people in rural community of Spain', *Addiction*, 84(6): 647–52.

Altay, C. (2008) 'Possibilities of reconfiguration: sustaining creative use in urban space', *Urban Design*, 108: 34–6.

Bianquis-Gasser, I. (1992) 'Wine and men in Alsace, France', In I. de Garine and V. De Garine (eds), *Drinking: Anthropological Approaches*. New York: Bergham Books, pp. 101–7.

Blunt, A. and Dowling, R. (2006) *Home*. London: Routledge.

Bohling, F. (2014) 'Crowded contexts: on the affective dynamics of alcohol and other drug use in nightlife spaces', *Contemporary Drug Problems*, 41: 361–92.

Bohling, F. (2015) 'Alcoholic assemblages: exploring fluid subjects in the night-time economy', *Geoforum*, 58: 132–42.

Bourgois, P. (1998) 'The moral economies of homeless heroin addicts: confronting ethnography, HIV risk, and everyday violence in San Francisco shooting encampments', *Substance Use and Misuse*, 33(11): 2323–51.

Bunce, M. (1994) *The Countryside Ideal: Anglo-American Images of Landscape*. London: Routledge.

Bunton, R. and Coveney, J. (2011) 'Drug's pleasure', *Critical Public Health*, 21(1): 1–14.

Campbell, H. (2000) 'The glass phallus: pub(lic) masculinity and drinking in rural New Zealand', *Rural Sociology*, 65(4): 562–81.

Chatterjee, P. (2003) 'An empire of drink: gender, labour and the historical economies of alcohol', *Journal of Historical Sociology*, 16(2): 183–208.

Chatterton, P. and Hollands, R. (2003) *Urban Nightscapes: Youth Culture, Pleasure Spaces and Corporate Power*. London: Routledge.

Cooperstock, R (1971) 'Sex differences in the use of mood-modifying drugs: an explanatory model', *Journal of Health and Social Behavior*, 12(3): 238–44.

Cronk, C. E. and Sarvela, P. D. (1997) 'Alcohol, tobacco, and other drug use among rural/small town and urban youth: a secondary analysis of the monitoring the future data set', *American Journal of Public Health* 87(5): 760–4.

Davidson, J., Smith, M. and Bondi, L. (eds) (2005) *Emotional Geographies*. Aldershot: Ashgate.

De Garine, I (2001) 'Drinking in Northern Cameroon amongst the Masa and Muzey', In I. De Garine, I. and V. De Garine (eds), *Drinking: Anthropological Approaches*. New York: Bergham Books, pp. 51–65.

De Garine, I. and De Garine, V. C. (eds) (2001) *Drinking: Anthropological Approaches*. New York: Bergham Books.

Deleuze, G. and Guattari, F. (1988) *A Thousand Plateaus*, trans. B. Massumi. London: Atlhone Press.

DeVerteuil, G. and Wilton, R. D. (2009) 'The geographies of intoxicants: from production and consumption to regulation, treatment and prevention', *Geography Compass*, 3(1): 478–94.

Dewsbury, J. D. (2011) 'The Deleuze-Guattarian assemblage: plastic habits', *Area*, 43(2): 148–53.

Duff, C. (2007) 'Towards a theory of drug use contexts: space, embodiment and practice', *Addiction Theory and Research*, 15(5): 503–19.

Duff, C. (2014) *Assemblages of Health: Deleuze's Empiricism and the Ethology of Life*. London: Springer.

Edensor, T. (2006) 'Caudan: domesticating the global waterfront', In D. Bell and M. Jayne (eds), *Small Cities: Urban Experience beyond the Metropolis.* London: Routledge, pp. 205–16.

Ettorre, E. (1997) *Women and Alcohol: A Private Pleasure or Public Problem?* London: The Women's Press.

ECAS (2002) *European Comparative Alcohol Study 1998–2001*. Brussels: European Union.

ESPAD (2003) *European Schools Project on Alcohol and Drugs 1995–2003*. Brussels: European Union.

Fraser, S., Moore, D. and Keane, H. (2014) *Habits: Remaking Addiction*. London: Palgrave Macmillan.

Gefou Madianou, D. (1992) *Alcohol, Gender and Culture*. London: Routledge.

Hall, T. and Hubbard, P. (1996) 'The entrepreneurial city: new urban politics, new urban geographies', *Progress in Human Geography,* 20: 153–74.

Hannigan, J. (1998) *Fantasy City: Pleasure and Profit in the Postmodern Metropolis*. London: Routledge.

Hansen, E. C. (1983) 'Drinking to prosperity: the role of bar culture and coalition formation in the modernization of the Alto Panádes', in J.C. Aceves (ed). *Economic Transformaton and Steady State Values: Essays in the Ethnography of Spain*. Flushing, NY: Queens College, pp 42–51.

Harnett, R., Thom, B., Herring, R. and Kelly, M. (2000), 'Alcohol in transition: towards a model of young men's drinking styles', *Journal of Youth Studies*, 3(1): 61–77.

Harrison, L. (ed.) (1996) *Alcohol Problems in the Community*. London: Routledge.

Heley, J. (2008) 'Rounds, range rovers and rurality: the drinking geographies of a New Squirarchy', *Drugs: Education, Prevention and Policy,* 15(3): 315–21.

Hobbs, D., Hadfield, P., Lister, S. and Winslow, S. (2003) *Bouncers: Violence and Governance in the Night-time Economy*. Oxford: Oxford University Press.

Holder, H. D. (2000) 'The supply side initiative as an international collaboration to study alcohol supply, drinking and consequences: current knowledge, policy issues and research opportunities', *Addiction*, 95(4): S416–63.

Holloway, S. L., Jayne, M. and Valentine, G. (2008) '"Sainsbury's is my local": English alcohol policy, domestic drinking practices and the meaning of home', *Transactions of the Institute of British Geographers,* 33: 532–47.

Hunt, G. (1991) 'The middle class revisited: eating and drinking in an English village', *Western Folklore*, 50: 401–20.

Hunt, G. P, Mackenzie, K and Joe-Laidcr, K. (2005), 'Alcohol and masculinity: the case of ethnic youth gangs', in T. M. Wilson, (ed), *Drinking Cultures*. Oxford: Berg, pp 225–254.

Hunt, G. and Satterlee, S. (1986) 'The pub, the village and the people', *Human Organisation*, 54(1): 62–74.

Jayne, M. (2006) *Cities and Consumption*. London: Routledge.

Jayne, M. and Valentine, G. (2016) 'Alcohol-related violence and disorder: new critical perspectives', *Progress in Human Geography*, 40(1): 67–87.

Jayne, M., Valentine, G. and Holloway, S. L. (2008) 'Geographies of alcohol, drinking and drunkenness: a review of progress', *Progress in Human Geography*, 32(2): 243–59.

Jayne, M., Valentine, G. and Holloway, S. L. (2010) 'Emotional, embodied and affective geographies of alcohol, drinking and drunkenness', *Transactions of the Institute of British Geographers,* 35(4): 540–54.

Jayne, M., Valentine, G. and Holloway, S. L. (2011a) 'What use are units? Critical geographies of alcohol policy', *Antipode,* 44(3): 828–46.

Jayne, M., Valentine, G. and Holloway, S. L. (2011b) *Alcohol, Drinking, Drunkenness: (Dis)Orderly Spaces.* Aldershot: Ashgate.

Jones, S. G. (1987) 'Labour, society and the drink question in Britain', *The Historical Journal*, 30(1): 105–22.

Kneale, J. and French, S. (2008) 'Mapping alcohol: health, policy and the geographies of problem drinking in Britain', *Drugs: Education, Prevention and Policy,* 15: 233–49.

Kraack, A. and Kenway, J. (2002) 'Place, time and stigmatised youthful identities: Bad Boys in Paradise', *Journal of Rural Studies,* 18: 145–55.

Kumar, K. (1995) *From Post-Industrial to Post-Modern Society*. Blackwell: Oxford.

Latham, A. (2003) 'Urbanity, lifestyle and making sense of the new urban cultural economy: notes from Auckland, New Zealand', *Urban Studies*, 40(9): 1699–724.
Latour, D. (2005) *Reassembling the Social: An Introduction to Actor–Network Theory*, Oxford: Oxford University Press.
Laurie, N., Dwyer, C., Holloway, S. L. and Smith, F. M. (1999) *Geographies of New Femininities*. Harlow: Addison Wesley Longman.
Leyshon, M. (2005) 'No place for a girl: rural youth pubs and the performance of masculinity', In J. Little and C. Morris (eds), *Critical Studies in Rural Gender Issues*. Aldershot: Ashgate, pp. 104–22.
Leyshon, M. (2008) '"We're stuck in the corner": young women, embodiment and drinking in the countryside', *Drugs: Education, Prevention and Policy*, 15(3): 267–89.
Malbon, B. (1999) *Clubbing: Dancing, Ecstasy and Vitality*. London: Routledge.
Malins, P. (2004) 'Body–space assemblages and folds: theorizing the relationship between injecting drug user bodies and urban space', *Media and Cultural Studies*, 18(4): 21–36.
Malins, P. (2014) *Machinic Assemblages: Deleuze, Guattari and an Ethico-Aesthetics of Drug Use*. Available from: http://www.janushead.org/71/Malins.pdf?origin=publication_detail.
Malins, P., Fitzgerald, J. L. and Threadgold, T. (2008) 'Spatial "folds": the entwining of bodies, risks and city spaces for women injecting drug users in Melbourne's Central Business District', *Gender, Place and Culture*, 13(5): 509–27.
Mars, G. (1987) 'Longshore drinking, economic security and union politics in Newfoundland', in M. Douglas (ed.) *Constructive Drinking: Perspectives on Drinking from Anthropology*. Cambridge: Cambridge University Press, pp. 91–101.
McCann, E. and Ward, K. (2011) *Mobile Urbanism: City Policymaking in the Global Age*. Minnesota: University of Minnesota Press.
Mcllwaine, C. and Moser, C. (2004) 'Drugs, alcohol and community tolerance: an urban ethnography from Colombia and Guatemala', *Environment and Urbanization*, 16(2): 49–62.
Nayak, A. (2003) 'Last of the "real Geordies"? White masculinities and the subcultrual response to deindustrialisation', *Environment and Planning D: Society and Space*, 21: 7–25.
Okumura, J., Wakai, S. and Umenai, T. (2002) 'Drug utilisation and self-medication in rural communities in Vietnam', *Social Science and Medicine*, 54(12): 1875–86.
Papagaroutfali, E. (1992) 'Uses of alcohol amongst women: games of resistance, power and pleasure', In D. Gefou-Madianou (ed.), *Alcohol, Gender and Culture*. London: Routledge, pp. 48–70.
Peace, A. (1992) '"No fishing without drinking": the construction of social identity in rural Ireland', In D. Gefou-Madianou (ed.), *Alcohol, Gender and Culture*. London: Routledge, pp. 167–80.
Plant, M. (1997) *Women and Alcohol: Contemporary and Historical Perspectives*. London: Free Association Books.
Public Health England (2013) *Drug Statistics from the National Drug Treatment Monitoring Study*. London: Public Health England.
Race, K (2009) *Pleasure Consuming Medicine: The Queer Politics of Drugs*. Durham: Duke University Press.
Race, K. (2014) 'Complex events: drug effects and emergent causality', *Contemporary Drug Problems*, 41(1): 301–34.
Race, K. (2015) '"Party and play": online hook-up devices and the emergence of PNP practices amongst gay men', *Sexualities*, 18(3): 253–75.
Reilly, D., Didcott, P., Swift, W.,and Hall, W. (2002) 'Long-term cannabis use: characteristics of users in an Australian rural area', *Addiction*, 93(6): 837–46.
Shaikh, Z. and Nax, F. (2000) *A Cultural Cocktail: Asian Women and Alcohol Misuse*. Warks: Aldgate Press.
Share, P. (2003) *A Genuine 'Third Place'? Towards an Understanding of the Pub in Contemporary Irish Society*. Paper Presented at the 30th SAI Annual Conference, Cavan, 26 April.
Shaw, R. (2010) 'Neoliberal subjectivities and the development of the night-time economy in British cities', *Geography Compass*, 4: 893–903.
Shaw, R. (2014) 'Beyond night-time economy: affective atmospheres of the urban night', *Geoforum*, 51: 87–95.

Shaw, R. (2015) '"Alive after five" constructing the neoliberal night in Newcastle-upon-Tyne', *Urban Studies*, 52(3): 456–70.

Short, J. (1991) *Imagined Country: Society, Culture and Environment*. London: Routledge.

Slavin, S. (2004) 'Drugs, space, and sociality in a gay nightclub in Sydney', *Journal of Contemporary Ethnography*, 33(3): 265–95.

Stivers, R. (2000) *Hair of the Dog: Irish Drinking and its American Stereotype*. New York: Continuum.

The White House (2014) *National Drug Control Strategy*. Washington, DC: The White House.

Thomas, M. (2002) 'Out of control: emergent cultural landscapes and political change in urban Vietnam', *Urban Studies*, 39(9): 1611–24.

Thrift, N. (2004) 'Intensities of feeling towards a spatial politics of affect', *Geografiska Annaler Series B Human Geography*, (86B)1: 57–78.

Thrift, N. (2005) 'Space: the fundamental stuff of geography' in S. L. Holloway, S. Rice and G. Valentine (eds.), *Key Concepts in Geography'*. London: Sage, pp 95–108.

Unites Nations Office of Drugs and Crime (UNODC) (2014) *World Drugs Report*. Vienna: UNODC.

Vitellone, N. (2010) 'Just another night in the shooting gallery? The syringe, space and affect', *Environment and Planning D: Society and Space*, 29(1): 867–80.

Vitellone, N. (2015) 'Syringe sociology', *The British Journal of Sociology*, 66(2): 373–90.

Waitt, G., Jessop, A. and Gormely-Murray, A. (2010) 'The guys in there just expect to be laid? Place, drinking cultures and young women', *Gender, Place and Culture*, 18(2): 255–75.

Waterson, J. (2000) *Women and Alcohol in Social Context: Mothers Ruin Revisited*. Palgrave: London.

Williams, A. (2016) 'Spiritual landscapes in rehab: Pentecostal worship, belief and embodiment', *Emotion, Space and Society*, doi:10.1016/j.emospa.2015.12.001.

Wolcott HF. (1974), *African beer gardens of Bulawayo: Integrated drinking in a segregated society*. New Brunswick, NJ: Rutgers Center of Alcohol Studies.

World Health Organisation (WHO) (2004) *Global Status Report: Alcohol Policy*. Stockholm: World Health Organisation.

PART III

Controversies and New Approaches in Social Science Drug and Alcohol Studies

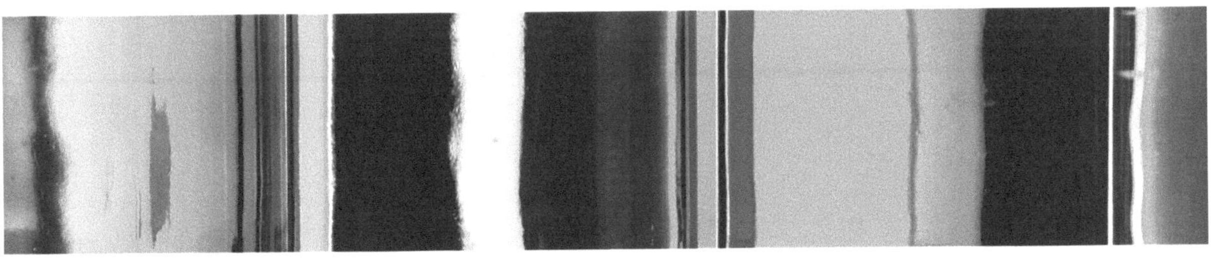

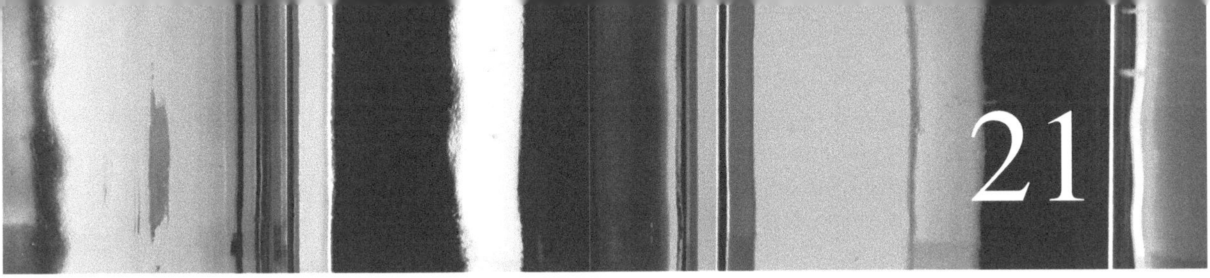

21

Addiction: Critical Reflections on a Debated Concept

Helen Keane

INTRODUCTION

Why do some people continue to drink heavily when alcohol is causing major problems in their lives? Why do smokers struggle to quit despite a strong desire to do so, and why do they so often relapse? Why are illicit drug users prepared to risk imprisonment in order to access their drugs? Addiction is a core concept in the drug and alcohol field because of its ability to provide an explanatory response to such questions. It provides a reason for seemingly irrational behaviour by positing the existence of some kind of force or drive that overpowers the individual will, compelling people to act in ways counter to their own interests and even their own desires.

Thus, from a critical perspective, addiction can be thought of as a specific set of ideas and practices that attempts to shape varied drug and alcohol problems into an abstract and unified entity: a disorder of compulsion located in the self. From this view, 'addiction' and 'the addict' are created and culture-bound categories rather than natural types and the medical and scientific project of identifying the universal truth of addiction is in fact part of the process by which the phenomenon itself is brought into being. Given this constitutive process, it is not surprising that despite its best efforts, addiction science has been unable to stabilise addiction into a single clear-cut entity. While a particular model may have scientific dominance at any one time, different conceptualisations are put into practice in different locations (clinics, laboratories, courts, schools and so forth) and prior understandings continue to circulate and exert an influence.

One key feature of the addiction concept is its relationship to levels of substance use deemed heavy or excessive. On one hand, in an everyday sense, the addict is assumed to be someone who consumes too much – drinks too heavily or uses drugs daily in ever-increasing amounts. The stories of addiction presented in the media and in texts such as the *Big Book* of Alcoholics Anonymous (1976) usually feature accounts of prodigious binges and levels of use that shock the 'normal' viewer or reader. However, the diagnostic criteria for addiction found in the two major medical classification systems (the DSM and the ICD) do not include an item explicitly about how much the individual is consuming (WHO, 1992; APA, 2013). Instead, as is discussed later, the focus is on 'maladaptive' use and a sense of loss of control over behaviour.

In contrast, screening tests developed to quickly identify and measure substance use problems include direct questioning about consumption. For example, the Fast Alcohol Screening Test begins with 'How often do you have eight or more drinks on one occasion?' The Fagerstrom Nicotine Dependence Questionnaire (which explicitly aims to measure tobacco addiction) includes the questions 'How soon after waking do you smoke your first cigarette?' and 'How many cigarettes do you smoke a day'? And while both tests include other questions about experiences of harm and personal conflict, it is the responses to questions about levels of consumption that have been found to have the most predictive power (Hodgson et al., 2003; Borland et al., 2010). In addition, public health campaigns that provide guidelines for safer versus risky drinking emphasise numbers of drinks per day (or per session) (see for instance: National Health and Medical Research Council, 2009).

Recently, some alcohol researchers have responded to the fluctuating nature of definitions of addiction by arguing that all that is in fact required to define substance use disorders is 'heavy use over time' (Rehm et al., 2014). Their view is that it is prolonged heavy substance use that produces the changes in the brain now identified as the source of compulsion as well as accounting for the majority of physical, psychological and social harms associated with addiction. Thus, the concept of addiction is in some sense redundant, at least when making decisions about prevention and treatment of substance use problems. In addition, reconceptualising substance use disorders in terms of heavy use would avoid the 'culturally relative arbitrary definitions' of loss of control and personal and social failure that are embedded in assessments of addiction (Rehm et al., 2014). While this argument does reveal some of the strangeness of attempting to identify problem substance use without directly assessing actual consumption, it does not solve the problem of how 'heavy use' itself is to be evaluated in an objective and non-culturally specific way. But more importantly for the purpose of this chapter, it does not acknowledge the centrality of notions of disordered will and eroded self-control to the meaning and experience of addiction. The alienation from the self, inner conflict and 'unfreedom' embedded in the category addiction has been vital to its success and power as a hybrid medical/moral concept (Keane, 2005).

While this chapter is focused on addiction as a debated concept, it should be remembered that addiction is not just an explanation or a discursive frame. It also captures a powerful embodied experience of loss of control over consumption, linked to a sense of loss of control over one's life (Weinberg, 2002, 2011). While much of the social science literature on addiction has addressed addiction as a socially constructed category that acts to pathologise and regulate behaviour that deviates from social norms, recent work has also emphasised the importance of recognising addiction as a lived phenomenon incorporating biological, personal, cultural and social elements (Fraser and Valentine, 2008; Kushner, 2010). Indeed, one of the questions a critical approach to addiction raises is the nature of the relationship between the complex social realities of drug use (which includes experiences of loss of control) and the expert and lay discourses which form these realities into stable and bounded categories (Moore, 1992).

This dual aspect of addiction comes to the fore when considering the treatment programmes and other strategies which aim to cure, help and/or punish the addicted.

Addiction promotes intervention into the conduct of others or the conduct of oneself. The different techniques applied to the addicted individual, from 12-step programmes to pharmacological regimes, become part of the addiction experience and promote particular understandings of compulsive desire (Moore and Fraser, 2006; Fraser and Valentine, 2008; Carr, 2010). It is not just that the kinds of treatment applied depend on how addiction is conceived, but that the treatment itself constitutes the nature of the problem. For example, if recovery from addiction is seen as requiring complete abstinence from all mood-altering substances, this suggests a more pervasive and deep-seated problem from one that can be ameliorated through more modest changes in consumption patterns.

The most authoritative models of addiction are medical and scientific. There is a long history of different scientific disciplines and medical specialties attempting to identify the essential characteristics of compulsive and excessive drinking and drug use (Campbell, 2007). Debate and disagreement about the nature of addiction and dependence characterise the field, as well as a history in which the key agents of addiction have changed from pharmaceutical properties to neurotransmitters. This is not to deny that certain models and actors can achieve dominance through a combination of scientific, technical and political networks (Vrecko, 2010b). Currently, the dominant scientific paradigm is of addiction as 'a chronic, relapsing brain disease' caused by dysfunction in neural reward systems (NIDA, 2007). According to this model, the powerful action of psychoactive drugs on the neurotransmitter dopamine causes the disordered behaviour of the addict, but crucially, other non-substance related activities such as eating, having sex, gambling and playing video games can produce the same effects (Potenza, 2008; Olsen, 2011; APA, 2013). Therefore, addiction science now supports an expanded category of addiction that is not confined to problems of drug and alcohol use. However, as this chapter goes on to discuss, drugs as a legal and social category remain central to understandings of addiction. And despite the scientific and institutional authority of the brain disease model and the rhetoric of progress produced by neurogenetic research, there are limits to its influence (Courtwright, 2010).

One of these limits is found in the tradition of conceptualising and operationalising addiction as a psychiatric disorder. In the American Psychiatric Association's Diagnostic and Statistical Manual of Mental Disorders (DSM), addiction is constituted as a disorder characterised by impaired control over substance use and continued use despite harm (APA, 2013). Unlike the brain disease model, the DSM model was developed as a diagnostic tool and is based on a list of observable or reportable symptoms. It aims to describe addiction in terms of its appearance, rather than provide an explanatory account of its development. However, its influence goes far beyond the clinical as it has been the standard model used in medical, epidemiological and clinical research.[1] In the most recent edition of the manual, DSM-5, published in 2013, important changes were made to the substance-related disorder categories, which are discussed in some detail later in this chapter. But despite acknowledging the important advances in addiction neuroscience that had taken place since the previous edition, the manual retained its descriptive approach to diagnosis, leading some prominent critics to question its relevance and credibility (Parker, 2010; Insel, 2013).

Addiction science and its language of compulsion, chemical imbalances and craving have become enmeshed in our everyday thinking and talking about consumption, compulsion and excess (Campbell, 2007: 1). But self-help traditions of acting on problems of alcohol and drug consumption have also had a substantial cultural influence, not only on public understandings of addiction but on drug treatment and policy (especially in the United States). In particular, Alcoholics Anonymous (AA) and its view of the alcoholic as powerless over drink has played a large role in establishing and spreading the idea of addiction as a disease (Reinarman, 2005).

However, the AA understanding of the disease of addiction is quite different from medical disease models. For AA, alcoholism encompasses a profound spiritual and moral malaise that must be addressed through the process of recovery, an open-ended project of work on the self. There has been a recent resurgence of professional and research interest in recovery as a paradigm for drug treatment, most notably reflected in the adoption of sobriety, wellbeing and empowerment as goals in UK drug policy (White, 2007; Duke, 2012). This twenty-first century refiguring of recovery to reflect neo-liberal ideals of the productive healthy citizen demonstrates the continuing relevance and appeal of moral responses to the problem of addiction.

This chapter will first briefly review the critical scholarship that examines addiction as a culturally and historically specific concept connected to ideals of self-control, autonomy and productivity. It will then examine the two most influential contemporary understandings of addiction, the brain disease model and the DSM model. The chapter does not attempt to provide a comprehensive review of these models, rather it aims to highlight some key themes and points of tension.

ADDICTION, SELF-CONTROL AND FREEDOM

Historical and sociological reflection on addiction has become a small but flourishing sub-field of scholarship (Fraser et al., 2014). Central to this body of work are studies that reveal the way addiction as an explanatory concept based on 'loss of control' becomes possible and meaningful only in particular historical and cultural locations (Levine, 1978; Room, 1985; Berridge, 1999; Reinarman, 2005). Much of this work has been deeply influenced by the ideas of Foucault, examining how addiction operates as a powerful therapeutic and political discourse, which classifies, normalises and disciplines subjects (Valverde, 1998; Bourgois, 2000; Fraser and Valentine, 2008; Keane, 2009).

Histories of the concept of addiction generally begin with the shift from pre-modern views of excessive drinking and drunkenness as wilful immoral conduct to the modern notion of alcoholism as a 'disease of the will' (Valverde, 1998). In his influential article 'The Discovery of Addiction', Harry Levine (1978) argued that in eighteenth century America, drunkenness, even habitual drunkenness, was regarded as natural and normal. People were assumed to drink to excess because they enjoyed it and chose to indulge in a pleasurable sin. Levine argues that addiction as a disease of the will came to make sense only when self-control became a vital individual and social value with the rise of the middle class in the nineteenth century.

In a series of articles spanning four decades, Robin Room has developed this socio-historical approach into a multidimensional understanding of addiction as a concept and experience that is enmeshed with systems of globalisation, industrialisation and commercialisation (Room, 1985, 1998, 2001, 2003). He has highlighted the centrality of failures of will to the diagnosis of addiction. For example, in the DSM and other medical models, alcohol dependence is not identified simply through the amount a person drinks, but through symptoms such as routinely drinking more than he or she intended to or repeated unsuccessful efforts to cut down (2003; see APA, 2013 and WHO, 1992). Underlying these criteria is the belief that the individual exercise of self-discipline is the key to a successful and meaningful life. As Room (1985) notes, addiction links loss of control over drinking or drug use with loss of control over the project of life in general.

This earlier work on addiction highlighted its roots in the eighteenth and nineteenth century constitution of the citizen as a productive worker. However, addiction has gained a new salience in the context of neo-liberalism and late capitalism, where consumption has become a prime site for the expression of values of freedom, autonomy, creativity and choice. As Gerda Reith has observed, in affluent societies addiction proliferates as a 'consumer pathology', a disorder that turns the 'sovereign consumer' on its head: 'transforming freedom into determinism and desire into need' (Reith, 2004: 286). Addiction in Reith's account is a classic Foucauldian discourse, a mode of governance that acts through rather than against individual freedom. She highlights the almost infinite ability of neo-liberal addiction discourse to produce new disordered identities such as pathological gamblers, bulimics, shopping addicts and internet addicts as 'unfreedom' is identified within expanding sites of consumption.

Toby Seddon (2010) has developed a similar argument about the enmeshment of addiction and understandings of freedom, although one more grounded in historical analysis of drug prohibition and regulation. Seddon argues that liberal conceptions of freedom have been mutually constitutive with understandings of the problem of drugs, as both developed in different phases over the past two centuries. He presents addiction as a quintessentially capitalist concept, connected to the circulation of drugs as a global commodity. Thus, transformations in capitalism can be linked to changes in the concept of addiction. The contemporary valorisation of consumerism co-exists with the idea of certain forms of disordered, repetitive consumption as a public menace.

While these critical accounts of the concept of addiction provide a crucial 'big picture' view of its historical and contemporary meanings and operation, they necessarily overlook the specificities of different models of addiction and their mobilisation in different contexts and locales. There are some seemingly irresolvable tensions that exist both within and between contemporary approaches to addiction, as the following discussion demonstrates.

HIJACKED BRAINS

In 1997, Alan Leshner, the then head of the US National Institute on Drug Abuse (NIDA) declared that 'addiction is a brain disease' (Leshner, 1997). He stated that scientific advances over the previous two decades had shown that repeated drug use changes brain structure and function in long lasting ways, so that the 'addicted brain' is fundamentally different from the 'non-addicted brain' (Leshner, 1997, 2001). It is these changes that produce the compulsive drug craving, seeking and use (and subsequent harmful consequences) that are the essence of addiction. Since then, the NIDA model of addiction as a 'chronic, relapsing, brain disease' has become firmly established as the dominant scientific paradigm of addiction (Vrecko, 2010b; Campbell, 2012).

The central player in this enactment of addiction is the 'neural reward system', which is damaged by long-term drug consumption. The explanatory narrative that has been distilled from the complex science of drugs and reward is a simple one, enhanced by the appeal of evolutionary logic. The story is that the brain's reward system evolved in order to reinforce 'survival relevant natural goals' such as searching for food, eating and sex (Hyman, 2005). Specifically, these activities produce pleasure via the release of the neurotransmitter dopamine, which binds 'the hedonic properties of a goal to desire and to action' (Hyman, 2005). Addictive drugs are able to 'hijack' this reward system because they act in a similar way to natural rewards and produce an artificially intense and rapid positive response (Robinson and Berridge, 2003). The brain adapts to the presence of a drug and synapses and circuits are remodelled, further increasing the reinforcing effects of the drug. Drugs become the highest motivational priority and other goals and relationships are abandoned (Leshner, 2001: 76).

Identifying addiction as a brain disease produces it as a fundamentally biological phenomenon. Visual representations have been central to this localisation of addiction in the inner neurological space of the individual (Keane, 1999; Dumit, 2004). PET scans, which show addiction as a particular pattern of colour contrasted with the different pattern that denotes the 'healthy brain', have become a feature not only of research articles but of educational material and public health campaigns warning of the dangers of drug use. But these vivid images of localisation are combined with an expansionary understanding of the biological that enables 'brain processes' to incorporate all relevant aspects of psychological and social experience, from memory, mood and affect to intention, risk-taking and self-perception. In the brain disease model, social and cultural features are acknowledged, often in phrases such as 'addiction is not just a brain disease' (Leshner, 1997: 46). But they are either relegated to the vague background realm of 'environmental influences' or refigured as effects of disordered brain chemistry. For example, the propensity of teenagers to experiment with drugs and their vulnerability to addiction is explained as a consequence of incomplete development of brain regions and different forms of neuroadaptation (Volkow and Li, 2004).

The biologisation of addiction is vividly demonstrated in NIDA scientists Volkow and Li's account of 'the neurobiology of behaviour gone awry'. They employ a brain/heart analogy to install a robustly organic vision of addiction:

> Drug addiction is a disease of the brain, and the associated abnormal behavior is the result of dysfunction of brain tissue, just as cardiac insufficiency is a disease of the heart and abnormal blood circulation is the result of dysfunction of myocardial tissue. (Volkow and Li, 2004: 963)

The brain/heart analogy is supported by an illustration that symmetrically juxtaposes PET scans of a healthy brain and an addicted brain and PET scans of a healthy heart and a heart damaged by a heart attack. The caption instructs readers in the following:

> [To] note the decreased glucose metabolism in the OFC (orbitofrontal cortex) of the addicted person and the decreased metabolism in the myocardial tissue in the person with a myocardial infarct. Damage to the OFC will result in improper inhibitory control and compulsive behaviour, and damage to the myocardium will result in improper blood circulation. (Volkow and Li, 2004: 964)

The echoing of terms and phrases (decreased metabolism, damage to the X will result in improper Y) produces addiction as a physiological rather than psychological phenomenon, as incontrovertible, concrete and physically present in the body as heart disease. Nevertheless, Volkow and Li shift from terms such as 'improper inhibitory control' to 'aberrant behaviour', producing brain disease as a biological reality that can be linked to the deviant conduct of the addict in a cause and effect relationship. In this way, the brain is *not* like the heart, it can be read as equivalent to the self – a disordered brain equals a disordered self and a disordered life. Thus, the brain disease model reiterates traditional notions of the addict as a particular kind of person with an out of control existence, but with the addition of a powerful 'neuroscience of difference' in which the addict's deviance from the norm is deeper and longer lasting than the observable signs of disorder (Buchman et al., 2010).

Advocates of the brain disease model have argued that because it contradicts the traditional view of addicts as lacking in will power or strength of character it will undermine the stigma of the condition. They suggest that recognising addiction as an illness requiring medical treatment will lead to a more enlightened and humane response to drug problems (Leshner, 1997; Volkow and Li, 2004). Setting aside their questionable optimism about the effects of designating something a mental illness, the assertion that the addict is a different kind of human being, and has become so as a result of choices about consumption, is at odds with these claims (Buchman et al., 2010). The brain disease model with its metaphor of hijacking produces addicts' 'aberrant behaviour' as evidence of otherness, rather than responses to the particular circumstances and predicaments of individual lives.

However, there is an instability in this neurological discourse of reward and compulsion. The molecular style of thought found in the brain disease model has the potential to destabilise as well as reinforce the difference of the addict (although not because it constitutes addiction as a disease). Because it is the affinity between drugs and the brain that explains why people take psychoactive substances and why some find it impossible to stop, the narrative of the hijacked brain is in part a normalising account of addiction. It suggests that human brains have an inherent capacity for addiction. For example, in a report on the neuroscience of substance use, the World Health Organization describes the action of substances in the brain as part of 'the common biological inheritance shared by all humans' and states that substance dependence is 'a disorder that could affect any human being' rather than a sign of weakness (WHO, 2004: 242, 248). Sociologist Nikolas Rose has emphasised the normalising potential of such neurochemical explanations, arguing that they construct the problem of addiction as a correctible error rather than a deep, resistant and pervasive pathology (Rose, 2003, 2007). In his view, neurochemistry renders addiction an anomaly rather than an abnormality and thereby promises to lift the moral weight that characterises earlier disease models.

In addition, the emphasis on the common dopaminergic effects of psychoactive substances at least brings into question the socio-legal categorisation of psychoactive substances into useful medications, legal substances and illicit drugs. From a neuroscientific perspective, it is unclear why some drugs are subject to international control while others are readily available on prescription or for sale in the supermarket. Moreover, the brain disease model suggests that the pleasure of drugs is not qualitatively different from rewards such as food, sex and social interaction, because these experiences are all mediated through dopamine. Drugs are harmful precisely because they are enough like healthy and natural pleasures to act as substitutes for them.

Thus, the increasing recognition of behavioural addictions as 'genuine' addictions (as in the DSM-5) is another effect of the neuroscientific discourse of addiction. Despite the notion of drugs as 'hijackers' of the brain, the dopamine hypothesis supports the existence of non-drug compulsions that are as powerful and potentially harmful as drug dependence. There is no reason why intensely rewarding activities such as gambling, sex and eating highly palatable food should not share the capacity to overload and restructure the brain through pleasure (Shaffer et al., 2004; Pelchat, 2009). In this expanded form, addiction can be re-imagined as a problem of the majority rather than confined to a marginalised minority (Sussman et al., 2011). It is a problem that can develop from activities that are not only morally neutral but positively valued and encouraged.

Nevertheless, the disruptive potential of the brain disease model is constrained by the other entrenched medical, social and legal assemblages that constitute and regulate drugs and drug use. While the NIDA endorsed model of addiction theoretically supports the existence of non-drug addictions, publications by its scientists retain their focus on 'drugs of abuse' and their pernicious neural, psychological and social effects (Hyman and Malenka, 2001; Volkow and Li, 2004; NIDA, 2007). Moreover, as historian David Courtwright points out (2010), the brain model has achieved cultural prominence as a scientific theory without undermining prohibitionist drug policy in the United States. Indeed, US policy towards illicit drug use became more not less punitive as the brain disease paradigm came to the fore in the 1980s and 1990s (Courtwright 2010: 140).

DSM: SUBSTANCE USE (AND OTHER ADDICTIVE) DISORDERS

One of the early aims expressed for the DSM-5 revision was the incorporation of neuroscientific and genetic research (such as the research into neural reward and compulsion) into its disease categories. The ultimate goal was to produce a pathophysiologically-based psychiatric nosology more akin to that of other branches of medicine (Charney et al., 2002; Hyman, 2007). However, this aim remained unfulfilled as the biomarkers of mental illness continued to remain elusive and their discovery subject to seemingly endless deferral (Schuckit, 2012). Thus, in the DSM-5, addiction is described in the opening paragraph of the relevant chapter as a dysfunction of neural circuits, but the diagnosis of the disorder remains based on the subjective evaluation of feelings and reported experiences.

Nevertheless, despite this continuity with earlier editions, the DSM-5 has installed a new version of addiction as a medical syndrome: substance use disorder (SUD) (see Table 21.1 for opioid use disorder, which is one of the SUDs and illustrates the generic SUD criteria) (APA 2013). SUD replaced the two disorders of substance dependence and substance abuse that were found in the DSM-IV, the former representing an addictive drug disorder, the latter harmful drug use without the features of dependence or impaired control (APA, 2000). Substance use disorder is a rather ungainly entity with 11 heterogeneous criteria, combining all but one of the DSM-IV substance abuse items and all of the DSM-IV substance dependence items.

Table 21.1 DSM-5 opioid use disorder criteria

A. A problematic pattern of opioid use leading to clinically significant impairment or distress, as manifested by at least two of the following, occurring within a 12-month period:

1) Opioids are often taken in larger amounts or over a longer period than was intended.
2) There is a persistent desire or unsuccessful efforts to cut down or control opioid use.
3) A great deal of time is spent in activities necessary to obtain the opioid, use the opioid, or recover from its effects.
4) Craving or a strong desire or urge to use opioids.
5) Recurrent opioid use resulting in a failure to fulfill major role obligations at work, school or home.
6) Continued opioid use despite having persistent or recurrent social or interpersonal problems caused or exacerbated by the effects of opioids.
7) Important social, occupational, or recreational activities are given up or reduced because of opioid use.
8) Recurrent opioid use in situations in which it is physically hazardous.
9) Continued opioid use despite knowledge of having a persistent or recurrent physical or psychological problem that is likely to have been caused or exacerbated by the substance.
10) Tolerance, as defined by either of the following:
    a. A need for markedly increased amounts of opioids to achieve intoxication or desired effect.
    b. A markedly diminished effect with continued use of the same amount of the opioid.

Note. This criterion is not considered to be met for those taking opioids solely under appropriate medical supervision.

11) Withdrawal, as manifested by either of the following:
    a. The characteristic opioid withdrawal syndrome (refer to Criteria A and B of the criteria set for opioid withdrawal).
    b. Opioids (or a closely related) substance are taken to relieve or avoid withdrawal symptoms.

Note. This criterion is not considered to be met for those individuals taking opioids solely under appropriate medical supervision.

While the brain disease model unifies different manifestations of addiction with a single causal narrative of dysfunction, SUD can hardly be said to represent a single disorder. The disjunctive nature of diagnosis in the DSM combined with the existence of 11 criteria means that there are numerous possible manifestations of SUD, which may not share any common symptom. Moreover, the threshold for diagnosis is low: the presence of any two or three symptoms indicates mild substance use disorder, four or five symptoms moderate substance use disorder and six or more severe substance use disorder. This approach to diagnosis ensures that individuals with a wide variety of problems can be treated under contemporary health management systems, but it does raise the question of whether the attribution of disease is plausible in all cases. In the case of alcohol, for example, high levels of consumption are normative features of the leisure activities of groups such as students and young people (Measham and Brain, 2005). It seems quite likely that a high percentage of young drinkers could easily achieve a diagnosis of SUD, but is this individual attribution of pathology a useful approach to youth drinking patterns?

One feature that the DSM has in common with the brain disease model is the attempt to produce a generic model of addiction applicable across a range of substances, whatever their effects, legal and social status or route of administration. In the DSM-5, the SUD criteria can be applied to 10 different substance categories to produce entities such as alcohol use disorder, opiate use disorder and tobacco use disorder. However, this generalising approach produces some strange constructions that paradoxically highlight the differences between different forms of substance use. For example, given that any level of smoking is assumed to be physically harmful, how can criterion eight, recurrent use in physically hazardous situations, be effectively evaluated in tobacco use disorder? This criterion was devised to capture behaviour such as driving under the influence of alcohol or operating machinery while high and hardly makes sense in relation to smoking.

Before examining the SUD diagnostic criteria in more detail, it is important to note that the DSM is a diagnostic manual and the process of diagnosis involves establishing medical authority over a condition and its treatment. It is not the subject (nor his or her family or friends) who is able to judge the nature of their problem, but the external and clinical gaze of the expert. The technical rationality of the DSM, with its checklists of numbered criteria and precise specifications of inclusion and exclusion aims to make psychiatric diagnosis as objective and reliable as possible (Kirk and Kutchins, 1992).

Nevertheless, for the SUD, as in many of the mental disorders, introspection and self-report is a crucial part of the diagnostic process. Some of the symptoms (such as withdrawal) may be exhibited by the patient, others (such as employment problems) may be a matter of record, but others are based on feelings, self-perception, intentions, forms of desire and aspects of cognition. For example, criterion one asks whether the substance is taken in larger amounts than intended, criterion two asks the subject whether there is a 'persistent desire' to cut down or control substance use and criterion nine asks whether substance use is continued *despite knowledge* of problems caused by the substance (emphasis added). As Room et al. (1996) have noted, such items assume a post-Enlightenment and reflective 'modern self' who stands outside of feelings and sensations and is able to evaluate and describe subjective states from an external viewpoint.

What is the clinician specifically identifying when he or she diagnoses SUD? The DSM-5 states that the 'essential feature' of substance use disorder is 'a cluster of cognitive, behavioral and physiological symptoms indicating that the individual continues using the substance despite significant *substance-related problems*' (APA, 2013: 483, emphasis added). As is the case in most medical models, this enactment of addiction places harm at the centre of the disorder. Specifically, a causal link must be established between drug use and various negative physical, psychological and social effects that are assembled into the entity 'substance-related problems'. As Mariana Valverde (1998) has observed, medical accounts of addiction demand a lot of work from the notion of harm, as it appears to promise an objective measure of dysfunction. Harm suggests that the problem is not the subjective and normative issue of excess (drinking or consuming more than is acceptable) but the consequences of the drinking or using and the subject's recognition of these consequences.

But the evaluation of harm is not a straightforward technical exercise, let alone the evaluation of use despite knowledge of harm. The criteria of occupational, educational and social harm (numbers five and six) assume certain middle-class norms of lifestyle, such as a structured routine of employment in which intoxication and/or absenteeism will result in economic loss and downward mobility. It assumes a social life that is external to drinking and drug use, rather than enmeshed with it. The notion of physical or psychological problems being caused by the substance (criterion nine) is also complicated by social context. For example, in highly marginalised populations, such as the homeless injecting drug users studied by Bourgois and Schonberg (2009), harmful drug use is in one sense highly visible. However, Bourgois and Schonberg stress the structural nature of the extreme social and physical suffering experienced by these users, which is over-determined by poverty, unemployment, incarcerations, dysfunctional social services and interpersonal violence as well as chronic drug and alcohol use. Giving up alcohol and drugs would not by itself ameliorate these conditions of existence. Indeed, it could produce isolation from social networks. Moreover, many of the harms are not caused directly by persistent drug use, but by the legal status of heroin and the prohibitionist policies that have been enacted to control its use. By isolating individual patterns of substance use from particular social worlds and identifying them as the primary cause of suffering, the category of substance dependence acts to obscure these other elements of reality.

Two of the diagnostic criteria equate addiction with the mismanagement or misuse of time. These criteria rely on and reproduce culturally specific understandings of time as a commodity or resource and a socially specific context in which other more important and rewarding activities are in competition with substance use (Room, 2003). Criterion three specifies that a 'great deal of time' is spent obtaining and using the substance or recovering from its effects, which requires a judgement about how much time is too much. For some, a weekly debilitating hangover could be a clear sign of excess and disorder, for others, an unremarkable feature of the weekend routine. As noted earlier, criterion seven identifies harm in relation to the giving up of 'important social, occupational or recreational activities' because of substance use. The manual gives the example that 'the individual may withdraw from family activities and hobbies in order to use the substance' (APA, 2013: 483). Embedded in this example, and the criterion itself, is a hierarchical ranking of pleasures, in which family life and wholesome pursuits (assumed to be accessible and appealing to all) are placed above solitary consumption or the wrong sort of friends. Failure to order one's priorities in this way is designated a sign of disorder.

In addition to use despite harm, a central element of the notion of addiction is loss of control or compulsion. The addict is someone whose choices and actions are no longer truly voluntary because addictive desire is both qualitatively and quantitatively distinct from normal desire. Indeed, it could be argued that harm has achieved its centrality in models of addiction because it is a way of identifying the compulsion that makes addiction a 'different state of being' than non-addiction.

The addict's persistent repetition of self-damaging behaviour is interpreted as the sign of compromised autonomy, or to use older language, a diseased will (Valverde, 1998). The three DSM criteria (one, two and four) that attempt to identify the existence of loss of control directly do not use the moralised and scientifically outmoded language of freedom of will but they both identify a conflict within the self that bears the traces of this history. For example, craving or a 'strong desire' to use the substance (criterion four) signifies the strength of the forces directing the addict's behaviour, emphasising that addiction is outside normal experiences of desire, attachment and habit. Craving links this pathological intensity with a particular kind of problematic object, such as illicit drugs, implying that they produce an inherently different kind of desire.

Another crucial element in the conversion of the ideas of self-control and deficiencies of will into a medical category is the existence of physiological dependence on the substance, as manifested by the existence of tolerance (criterion 10) and withdrawal (criterion 11). Indeed, until the late twentieth century, it was the existence of physical dependence on a substance such as alcohol or heroin which was regarded as the proof of genuine addiction. The delirium tremens of the alcoholic and sweating and cramps of the heroin addict were read as vivid signs of the physical otherness of the true addict. But by the 1990s, the influence of neuroscience made the privileging of physiological dependence and questions about which substances and activities are genuinely addictive seem outmoded (WHO Expert Committee on Drug Dependence, 1993). Neuroscientific knowledge of drug actions and reward mechanisms located the brain as the source of all aspects of addiction, from withdrawal symptoms to craving to the power of particular places, people and things to provoke relapse in a former addict. The shift away from physiological dependence as the pre-eminent indicator of addiction was also the result of increasing concern about drugs, such as cocaine, which did not have a clear-cut withdrawal syndrome.

Thus, in the DSM-5, tolerance and withdrawal have been moved from the top to the bottom of the list of SUD criteria. Moreover, these criteria are explicitly not to be counted towards diagnosis if they occur in those taking medications such as opiates and antidepressants under medical supervision. This normalising of drug dependence when it occurs as a result of medical treatment demonstrates the continuing role played by models of addiction in constructing boundaries between legitimate and illegitimate drug use. It also reveals the limits of the ability of neuroscience to shift the ethical and moral framework of addiction. If, as the brain disease model suggests, neural reward pathways are fundamentally altered by prolonged drug use, and this is the essence of addiction, it is unclear why the symptoms experienced by opiate dependent pain patients (for example) should be interpreted differently from the same symptoms experienced by opiate dependent street addicts (Bell and Salmon, 2009; Keane and Hamill, 2010).

However, the DSM-5 has opened up the category of addiction to non-substance or behavioural addictions, citing the neuroscience of reward as the justification for this move. The manual states that problem gambling belongs with substance-related disorders because 'gambling behaviors activate reward systems similar to those activated by drugs abuse' (APA, 2013: 481). However, pathological gambling (renamed gambling disorder) is the only non-drug addiction included. Other conditions proposed for inclusion, such as internet gaming disorder, hypersexuality and obesity, were excluded because of insufficient research (although internet gaming disorder was included in the chapter of the manual for conditions requiring further research) (APA, 2013).

The establishment of behavioural addictions in the DSM-5 makes theoretically possible a phalanx of new mental disorders based on failures of will and self-control, many related to everyday activities. As discussed earlier, the brain model of addiction is one of the drivers of this expansionary approach to addiction (Vrecko, 2010a: 40). The broader cultural trend towards the valorisation of consumption and freedom (and consumption *as* freedom) should also be recognised as an environment that supports the proliferation of addiction (Sedgwick, 1992; Reith, 2004).

However, while gambling disorder is grouped with substance disorders in the manual, it is still constituted as different from these conditions because its object of addiction is not a drug. The substance use disorders are in a subsection titled 'Substance-Related Disorders' and they are listed alphabetically from alcohol use disorder to tobacco use disorder. Gambling disorder follows in its own section, a section titled 'Non-Substance-Related Disorders', and while some of its diagnostic criteria related to loss of control are similar to those of the substance disorders, terms such as withdrawal and tolerance are not used. And gambling disorder retains specific and unique criteria, such as gambling while distressed, relying on others for money and chasing one's losses, which mark it out as different from alcohol and drug addictions.

The point to be made here is that while the brain disease model focuses on the disrupted reward system that it views as underlying all addictive behaviour, it still constitutes drugs of abuse as the sources of disorder, via the narrative of hijacking. In contrast, the DSM-5 retains an object-focused approach in which each addictive object (alcohol, opiates, tobacco, gambling and so on) has its own designated disorder. However, it continues to divide these disorders according to a drug/non-drug binary, and therefore, reinforces the existence of 'drugs' as a particularly problematic and powerful category of things. In this way, the radical potential of neuroscientific discourse to challenge categories of normal and pathological forms of desire and consumption is forestalled.

In summary, the DSM model of addiction, now called substance use disorder, produces addiction as a mental disorder in which a pattern of repeated and compulsive substance use produces significant physical, psychological and social harm. SUD assembles diverse elements such as harms, risk, misuse of time, loss of self-control, pathological desire and biological disturbance into the condition of addiction and locates it within the individual. However, the identification and evaluation of harm is not an objective or technical exercise as it involves judgments about what a meaningful and productive life looks like. In addition, harm does not exist in a vacuum but emerges from interactions between individual behaviour and the social.

CONCLUSION

From the critical perspective adopted in this chapter, addiction can be thought of as a specific set of ideas and practices that attempts to shape varied drug and alcohol problems into an abstract and unified entity: a disorder of compulsion located in the self. In this context, 'addiction' and 'the addict' are culture-bound categories rather than natural types, and the medical and scientific project of identifying the universal truth of addiction is in fact part of the process by which the phenomenon itself is brought into being. This chapter examined two influential contemporary models of addiction, the chronic, relapsing brain disease model that dominates addiction science and the category of substance use disorder found in the DSM-5. Both versions reveal the way ideas of aberrant behaviour, harm and loss of control produce addiction as an entity located within the individual. Both can also be considered expansive models of addiction in their loosening of the connection between drugs and addiction. But while the recognition of behavioural addictions in neuroscientific accounts and the DSM have the potential to normalise compulsive attachments as part of human existence, drug use continues to be understood as an inherently suspect form of consumption.

ACKNOWLEDGMENTS

This entry incorporates material previously published in a chapter of the book *Habits: Remaking Addiction* by Suzanne Fraser, David Moore and Helen Keane (Palgrave Macmillan, 2014). It is reproduced with the permission of Palgrave Macmillan.

NOTE

1 The WHO International Classification of Diseases (ICD-10) also contains a widely used diagnostic model of substance dependence that is similar to the DSM model (World Health Organization, 1992). However, while the ICD-10 is often used by governments in official coding, the DSM is more commonly used by mental health professionals and in research.

REFERENCES

Alcoholics Anonymous (1976) *The Big Book*, 3rd edn. New York: Alcoholics Anonymous World Services.

American Psychiatric Association (APA) (2000) *Diagnostic and Statistical Manual of Mental Disorders DSM-IV-TR*, 4th edn, text revision. Washington, DC: American Psychiatric Press.

American Psychiatric Association (APA) (2013). *Diagnostic and Statistical Manual of Mental Disorders DSM-5*, 5th edn. Washington, DC: American Psychiatric Press.

Bell, K. and Salmon, A. (2009) 'Pain, physical dependence and pseudoaddiction: redefining addiction for "nice" people?', *International Journal of Drug Policy*, 20(2): 170–8.

Berridge, V. (1999) *Opium and the People: Opiate Use and Drug Control Policy in Nineteenth and Early Twentieth Century England*. London: Free Association Books.

Borland, R., Yong, H.H., O'Connor, R.J., Hyland, A. and Thompson, M.E. (2010) 'The reliability and predictive validity of the heaviness of smoking index and its two components: findings from the International Tobacco Control Four Country study', *Nicotine and Tobacco Research*, 12(S1): S45–50.

Bourgois, P. (2000) 'Disciplining addictions: the bio-politics of methadone and heroin in the United States', *Culture, Medicine and Psychiatry*, 24(2): 165–95.

Bourgois, P. and Schonberg. J. (2009) *Righteous Dopefiend*. Berkeley: University of California Press.

Buchman, D., Iles, J. and Reiner, P. (2010) 'The paradox of addiction neuroscience', *Neuroethics*, 4(2): 65–77.

Campbell, N. (2007) *Discovering Addiction: The Science and Politics of Substance Abuse Research*. Ann Arbor: University of Michigan Press.

Campbell, N. (2012) 'Medicalization or biomedicalization: does the diseasing of addiction fit the frame?' In J. Netherland (ed.), *Critical Perspectives on Addiction*. New York: Emerald, pp. 3–25.

Carr, E. (2010) *Scripting Addiction: The Politics of Therapeutic Talk and American Sobriety*. New Jersey: Princeton University Press.

Charney D., Barlow D., Botteron K., Cohen J., Goldman D., Gur R., Lin K.M., López J., Meador-Woodruff J., Moldin S., Nestler E., Watson, S. and Zalcman, S. (2002) 'Neuroscience agenda to guide development of a pathophysiologically based classification system', In D. Kupfer, M. First and D. Regier (eds), *A Research Agenda for DSM-V*. Washington, DC: American Psychiatric Association, pp.31–84.

Courtwright, D. (2010) 'The NIDA brain disease paradigm', *BioSocieties*, 5(1): 137–47.

Duke, K. (2012) 'From crime to recovery: the reframing of British drugs policy?' *Journal of Drug Issues*, 20(10): 1–17.

Dumit, J. (2004) *Picturing Personhood: Brain Scans and Biomedical Identity*. Durham: Duke University Press.

Fraser, S. and Valentine, k. (2008) *Substance and Substitution: Methadone Subjects in Liberal Societies*. Basingstoke: Palgrave Macmillan.

Fraser, S., Moore, D. and Keane, H. (2014) *Habits: Rethinking Addiction*. Basingstoke: Palgrave Macmillan.

Hodgson, R., John, B., Abbasi, T., Hodgson, R., Waller, S., Thom, B., and Newcombe, R. (2003) 'Fast screening for alcohol misuse', *Addictive Behavior*, 28(8): 1453–63.

Hyman, S. (2005) 'Addiction: a disease of learning and memory', *The American Journal of Psychiatry*, 162(8): 1414–22.

Hyman, S. (2007) 'Can neuroscience be integrated into the DSM-V?' *Nature Reviews Neuroscience*, 8: 725–32.

Hyman, S. and Malenka, C. (2001). 'Addiction and the brain: the neurobiology of compulsion and its persistence', *Nature Reviews Neuroscience*, 2: 695–703.

Insel, T. (2013) 'Transforming diagnosis', *National Institute of Mental Health: Director's Blog*. Available from: http://www.nimh.nih.gov/about/director/2013/transforming-diagnosis (Accessed 4 July 2013).

Keane, H. (1999) 'Adventures of the addicted brain', *Australian Feminist Studies*, 14(29): 63–76.

Keane, H. (2005) 'Addiction and the bioethics of difference', In M. Shildrick and R. Mykitiuk (eds), *Ethics of the Body: Postconventional Challenges*. Cambridge: MIT Press, pp. 91–112.

Keane, H. (2009) 'Foucault on methadone: beyond biopower', *International Journal of Drug Policy*, 20(5): 450–52.

Keane, H. and Hamill, K. (2010) 'Variations in addiction: the molecular and the molar', *BioSocieties*, 5(1): 52–69.

Kirk, S. and Kutchins, H. (1992) *The Selling of DSM: The Rhetoric of Science in Psychiatry*. New York: Aldine de Gruyter.

Kushner, H. (2010) 'Toward a cultural biology of addiction', *BioSocieties*, 5(1): 8–24.

Leshner, A. (1997) 'Addiction is a brain disease, and it matters', *Science*, 278(5335): 45–6.

Leshner, A. (2001) 'Addition is a brain disease', *Issues in Science and Technology*, XVII(3): 75–80.

Levine, H.G. (1978) 'The discovery of addiction: changing conceptions of habitual drunkenness in America', *Journal of Studies on Alcohol*, 39(1): 143–74.

Measham, F. and Brain, K. (2005) 'Binge drinking, British alcohol policy and the new culture of intoxication', *Crime, Media, Culture*, 1(3): 262–83.

Moore, D. (1992) 'Deconstructing "dependence": an ethnographic critique of an influential concept', *Contemporary Drug Problems*, Fall: 459–91.

Moore, D. and Fraser, S. (2006) 'Putting at risk what we know: reflections on the drug-using subject in harm reduction', *Social Science and Medicine*, 62(12): 3035–47.

National Health and Medical Research Council (2009) *Australian Guidelines to Reduce Health Risks from Drinking Alcohol*. Canberra: Commonwealth of Australia.

National Institute on Drug Abuse (NIDA) (2007) *Drugs, Brains, and Behavior: The Science of Addiction*. Bethesda: National Institutes of Health.

Olsen, C. (2011) 'Natural rewards, neuroplasticity, and non-drug addictions', *Neuropharmacology*, 61(7): 1109–22.

Parker, C. (2010) 'Psychiatric diagnosis and DSM-5: Maps to nowhere', *CorePsych Blog*. Available from: http://www.corepsych.com/2010/02/psychiatric-diagnosis/ (Accessed 10 August 2013).

Pelchat, M. (2009) 'Food addiction in humans', *The Journal of Nutrition*, 139(3): 620–2.

Potenza, M. (2008) 'The neurobiology of pathological gambling and drug addiction', *Philosophical Transactions of the Royal Society B*, 363(1507): 3181–9.

Rehm, J., Marmet, S., Anderson, P., Gual, A., Kraus, L., Nutt, D.J., Room, R., Samokhvalov, A.V., Scafato, E., Trapencieris, M., Wiers, R.W. and Gmel, G. (2014) 'Defining substance use disorders: do we really need more than heavy use?' *Alcohol and Alcoholism*, 48(6): 633–40.

Reinarman, C. (2005) 'Addiction as accomplishment: the discursive construction of disease', *Addiction Research and Theory*, 13(4): 307–20.

Reith, G. (2004) 'Consumption and its discontents', *British Journal of Sociology*, 55(2): 283–300.

Robinson, T. and Berridge, K. (2003) 'Addiction', *Annual Review of Psychology*, 54: 25–53.

Room, R. (1985) 'Dependence and society', *British Journal of Addiction*, 80(2): 133–9.

Room, R. (1998) 'Alcohol and drug disorders in the international classification of disease: a shifting kaleidoscope', *Drug and Alcohol Review*, 17(3): 305–17.

Room, R. (2001) 'Governing images in public discourse about problematic drinking', In N. Heather, T. Peters and T. Stockwell (eds), *Handbook of Alcohol Dependence and Alcohol-Related Problems*. Chichester: John Wiley & Sons, pp. 33–45.

Room, R. (2003) 'The cultural framing of addiction', *Janus Head*, 6(2): 221–34.

Room, R., Janca, A., Bennett, L., Schmidt, L. and Sartorius, N. (1996) 'WHO cross-cultural applicability research on diagnosis and assessment of substance use disorders', *Addiction*, 91(2): 199–220.

Rose, N. (2003) 'The neurochemical self and its anomalies', In R. Ericson and A. Doyle (eds), *Risk and Morality*. Toronto: University of Toronto Press, pp. 407–37.

Rose, N. (2007) *The Politics of Life Itself: Biomedicine, Power, and Subjectivity in the Twenty-First Century*. New Jersey: Princeton University Press.

Schuckit, M. (2012) 'Editorial in reply to the comments of Griffith Edwards', *Journal of Studies on Alcohol and Drugs*, 73(4): 521–2.

Seddon, T. (2010) *A history of Drugs: Drugs and Freedom in the Liberal Age*. London: Routledge.

Sedgwick, E. (1992) 'Epidemics of the will', In J. Crary and S. Kwinter (eds), *Incorporations*. New York: Zone Books.

Shaffer, H., LaPlante, D., LaBrie, R., Kidman, R., Donato, A., and Stanton, M. (2004) 'Toward a syndrome model of addiction', *Harvard Review of Psychiatry*, 12(6): 367–74.

Sussman, S., Lisha, N. and Griffiths, M. (2011) 'Prevalence of the addictions: a problem of the majority or the minority?' *Evaluation and the Health Professions*, 34(1): 3–56.

Valverde, M. (1998) *Diseases of the Will: Alcohol and The Dilemmas of Freedom*. Cambridge: Cambridge University Press.

Volkow, N. and Li, T. (2004) 'Drug addiction: the neurobiology of behaviour gone awry', *Nature Reviews Neuroscience*, 5: 963–70.

Vrecko, S. (2010a) '"Civilizing technologies" and the control of deviance', *BioSocieties*, 5(1): 36–51.

Vrecko, S. (2010b) 'Birth of a brain disease: science, the state and addiction neuropolitics', *History of Human Sciences*, 23(52): 52–67.

Weinberg, D. (2002) 'On the embodiment of addiction', *Body and Society*, 8(4): 1–19.

Weinberg, D. (2011) 'Sociological perspectives on addiction', *Sociology Compass*, 5(4): 298–310.

White, W. (2007) 'Addiction recovery: its definition and conceptual boundaries', *Journal of Substance Abuse Treatment*, 33(3): 229–41.

WHO Expert Committee on Drug Dependence (1993) *WHO Expert Committee on Drug Dependence: 28th Report*, WHO Technical Report Series 836. Geneva: World Health Organization.

World Health Organization (WHO) (1992) *The ICD-10 Classification of Diseases and Related Health Problems*. Geneva: World Health Organization.

World Health Organization (WHO) (2004) *Neuroscience of Psychoactive Substance Use and Dependence*. Geneva: World Health Organization.

22

Learning to Live with 'Big Fat Words'? An Exploration of the Dominant Concepts Applied to Problem Drug and Alcohol Use

Shane Butler and Paula Mayock

INTRODUCTION

At the 28th International Congress on Alcohol and Alcoholism, which was held in Washington in 1968, amidst a series of relatively mundane presentations on specific aspects of alcohol-related problems, one controversial paper by two prominent Nordic sociologists, Nils Christie and Kettil Bruun, presented a scathing and fundamental critique of the conceptual framework that underpinned research and policy on alcohol and illicit drugs at this time (Christie and Bruun, 1969). They argued that the language in which these concepts were presented was emotionally charged and devoid of the clarity and precision one might expect of discourse that purported to be scientific and to offer a rational basis for public policy on alcohol and other psychoactive substances. They commented particularly on the split at research and policy levels between alcohol and illicit drugs: 'huge conferences gather to discuss questions of alcohol and alcoholism, while quite different conferences gather to discuss drugs or narcotics' (1969: 65). As Christie and Bruun saw it, research on illicit drugs was primarily concerned with clarifying how and why these were 'bad drugs', while research in the alcohol field – guided by the then popular disease concept of alcoholism – was focused on identifying the negative attributes of alcoholics, who were considered to be 'bad users' of what was essentially a good drug. And these sociologists were also struck by the emotional intensity with which these two propositions were commonly expressed: 'sometimes, the insistence that "alcoholism *is* sickness" or "marihuana *is* a narcotic" is so strong that it seems as if life and death were at stake' (emphasis in original) (1969: 66).

In addition to commenting on what they perceived to be the scientific shortcomings of the dominant conceptual approaches to alcohol and drug issues, Christie and Bruun also sought to explain why such conceptual confusion and imprecision should have gone largely unchallenged: 'why, then, is so much energy put into big, fat words without very much content, and why are these words in general so uncritically received by eagerly awaiting consumers?' (1969: 68). Continuing the metaphor, they went on to explain the survival of these big fat words in terms of the ideological function they served in western society – as 'grease in the social machinery' (1969: 72): by which they meant that by putting a spurious scientific gloss on debate about these issues and ignoring the inherent interest group conflicts and clashing value systems, the concepts preserved the political status quo. In relation to illicit drugs, which were generally referred to as 'narcotics', the conceptual framework did not challenge the international prohibitionist system, or offer succour to those who might see drug use as a fundamental human right or campaign for the legalisation of drugs that were illegal under this system. Similarly, the conceptual framework did not challenge the orthodoxy of the disease concept by suggesting that alcohol created risk for all its consumers rather than for a minority of 'bad' drinkers; and as long as the disease concept remained unchallenged, there was no justification for tighter control systems which might create conflict between the state and the drinks industry, threaten employment and revenue generation, and, perhaps most significantly, antagonise the voting public.

Christie and Bruun did not confine themselves to an explanation of the societal functions served by these concepts, but declared themselves to be enemies of 'big fat words'; and they advocated what they saw as a more honest style of public debate and policy making, based upon clear differentiation between scientific knowledge and value judgement:

> Within our field, technical problems which call for technical advice, and ethical problems which call for political decisions, where we all have a voice, are usually interwoven. Conceptual refinement is one way of giving to the experts what belongs to them, and to us all the decision on ethics which belong to all of us. (Christie and Bruun, 1969: 72)

This chapter, written almost half a century after this well-known critique, is an attempt to trace the fate of these big fat words – *that illicit drugs are bad* and *that alcoholism/addiction is a disease* – in the intervening years and to explore the extent to which Christie and Bruun's 'conceptual refinement' has come to be the norm in popular and policy discourse on the topic of drug and alcohol problems. The chapter will first look at the evolving history of the concept of psychoactive drug use as deviance, a concept that reflects the view that those who use drugs of this kind ought to be – and perhaps usually are – aware of the moral evils entailed in this practice; the chapter will then look at historical shifts in the concept of addiction as disease. In each of these explorations, attention will also focus on how or whether the policy process has achieved the Christie and Bruun ideal of policy transparency, particularly insofar as it relates to a clear differentiation between value-neutral research findings and value judgements.

DRUG USE AS DEVIANCE

Wars on drugs

Within the wider discipline of sociology, with its preoccupation with social order, the study of behaviour that threatens such order by its disregard for culturally shared rules or norms has long been a major focus of attention. Behaviour of this kind has been conventionally described as *deviance*, and those who show disregard for generally accepted norms are referred to as *deviant*. It is the concept of illicit drug use as deviance that has provided the main ideological underpinning for the system of international drug controls that evolved during the twentieth century and which, from its establishment in 1948, has driven the work of the United Nations (UN) on this issue (Bewley-Taylor, 2001). These international policy developments have been implicitly based on the idea of consensus amongst the populations of UN member states as to the evil of illicit drugs and the undesirability of using such 'narcotics' for hedonistic or recreational purposes. It is assumed that the 'drug problem' has an objective existence, verified by scientific research that confirms the health and behavioural risks associated with such drug use. However, anti-drug measures have been consistently presented in the kind of emotional and moralistic language of which Christie and Bruun disapproved, with illicit drug use assumed to run counter to dominant value systems and to constitute such an obvious social and moral evil that it deserves to be prohibited and to have severe criminal justice sanctions attaching to the production, trade and, to a lesser extent, use of these drugs. A utopian, 10-year scheme based on the slogan 'A Drug-Free World – We Can Do It' was proclaimed by the United Nations General Assembly Special Session as recently as 1998 (Pryce, 2012: 126–7). At international level, anti-drug campaigns have been characterised by a high degree of hyperbole, not least through the common use of the American metaphor of a *war on drugs* – a metaphor that gained currency during the presidency of Richard Nixon in the early-1970s and subsequent to Christie and Bruun's denunciation of big fat words.

However well-established it may be or however much it continues to be reflected in domestic legislation of UN member states, international drug prohibition has rarely been without its critics over the past half-century. One of the more obvious points of criticism, and one that featured centrally in Christie and Bruun's critique, was the difficulty in explaining in purely rational terms why the use of some mind-altering drugs (such as cannabis, cocaine or heroin) should be automatically categorised as deviance while the use of alcohol (and to a lesser degree other licit drug, such as caffeine or tobacco) is not. Distinctions of this kind between 'good' and 'bad' drugs have evolved historically over the past two centuries (Berridge, 2013), perhaps not entirely in an arbitrary way but certainly not on the basis of scientific evidence concerning their relative potentials for risk. The libertarian anti-psychiatrist, Szasz (1975), argued that conventional distinctions between psychoactive drugs largely reflected the extent to which various drugs had been incorporated into cultural rituals or 'ceremonials'; on this basis, for instance, we can understand that it is much easier in Western countries to demonise new drugs such as cannabis or cocaine than to demonise alcohol, the use of which is firmly engrained in the culture of these societies. Most importantly, Szasz was insistent that science played no serious role in this process and that to expect pharmacologists to distinguish between good drugs and bad drugs was tantamount to expecting them to distinguish between tap water and holy water.

If we look at the sociological literature on the application of the deviance concept to illicit drug use over the past half-century or so, what emerges is that sociologists have generally adopted a critical, relativistic approach to this subject – an approach that in policy terms has been subversive of the war on drugs perspective. Howard Becker, an American sociologist, was one of the early researchers to challenge the positivistic notion that 'deviance' had an objective existence that had been discovered and validated by science. Instead, he coined the term 'moral entrepreneur' as part of his wider argument that deviance or social problems were 'constructed' by moral crusaders who succeeded in imposing their own beliefs and value systems on society. For Becker 'deviance is *not* a quality of the act the person commits, but rather a consequence of the application by others of rules and sanctions to an "offender"' (Becker, 1963: 9); and, as he saw it, drug users were simply people who did not accept societal rules about drug use. Becker also challenged conventional ideas about the evils inherent in illicit drug use and the alleged power of these drugs to enslave new users. He did this in the first instance by showing that, contrary to the idea that cannabis ('marihuana') use was immediately pleasurable and habit forming, novice users had to be taught by more experienced users how to smoke this drug, how to recognise its effects and how to enjoy these effects.

During the 1970s and 1980s, British sociologists writing from a 'new deviancy' perspective developed this critique of conventional views of drug use as deviancy. Focusing particularly on media representations of drug use, they argued that: (i) populist representations of the 'drug problem' tended to ignore socioeconomic factors, which were frequently correlated with more risky styles of drug use, while simultaneously tending towards the creation of a 'moral panic' – that is, exaggerating the threat that drug use posed to public order and morality; and (ii) such stereotypical and absolutist images of drug users, operating both at the level of public attitudes and through their influence on health and criminal justice service provision, led to 'deviancy amplification' – that is, they compounded the process of social exclusion and marginalisation experienced by drug users (Cohen, 1972; Young, 1987).

While the study of deviance is no longer a major sub-specialisation within sociology (Sumner, 1994), sociologists have continued to study drug issues and, to a large extent, have continued to publish research that is highly critical of positivistic notions of drug use as deviance. American sociologists have been critical, for instance, of media coverage and official policy responses to the use of crack cocaine during the 1980s and 1990s on the basis that the dominant reaction to crack was one which exaggerated its addictive and criminogenic potential, while ignoring the racial and socioeconomic factors that created vulnerability for some of its users (Reinarman and Levine, 2004). However, perhaps the best known and most controversial research on this topic has been a longitudinal study of drug use by adolescents and young adults in the north-west of England, which began as a five-year study of secondary school students but which continued to track research subjects over a 14-year period until their late-twenties (Parker et al., 1998; Aldridge et al., 2011). It should be emphasised that this longitudinal research was conducted with a 'normal' or socially stable sample of young people rather than with a clinic or treatment sample, but what emerged most clearly from its quantitative data was that illicit drug use was neither a minority behaviour nor a behaviour that was deemed deviant or morally unacceptable by most of this cohort of research subjects. The researchers constructed a theoretical framework, usually referred to as the 'normalisation' hypothesis, around these findings: the essence of this framework being that young people largely ignore legal and popular cultural strictures in relation to illicit drug use, and instead make decisions about use or non-use based on their own evolving individual and collective awareness of the risks attached to such drug use. The researchers also argued that illicit drug use by young people was not reflective of a wider rejection of societal norms and that most young drug users were otherwise quite conventional, if not conservative, in their attitudes and behaviours. The normalisation thesis was accused of exaggerating the degree to which young people retained 'agency' in relation to drug decision making, while simultaneously underestimating the influence of structural factors in this process (e.g. Shiner and Newburn, 1997, 1999). Nonetheless, the length of the follow-up period and the strength of the empirical findings provide compelling support for the fact that substantial numbers of otherwise conventional and well-functioning young people do not accept the notion of illicit drug use as deviance or moral evil.

Science and policy making

If we wish to look at an initiative that attempted to take such critical views of conventional drug policy out of the academic sphere and into the realm of practical politics, it is instructive to look at the experience of the British psychopharmacologist, David Nutt. In 2008, Professor Nutt was appointed as chairman of the Advisory Council on the Misuse of Drugs (ACMD), a statutory body charged with responsibility for offering scientific advice to government on drug policy. In the spirit of Christie and Bruun (albeit without reference to this by now ancient sociological diatribe), Nutt had consistently promoted the idea that drug policy should primarily reflect scientific evidence as to the risks associated with drug use rather than moralism or popular prejudices. He was critical of the British classification system (e.g. Nutt et al., 2007) in which drugs were assigned to one of three classes – A, B and C – ostensibly on the basis of their harmfulness, and he was critical of what he perceived to be the ignoring of scientific advice where politicians believed such advice to be electorally unpopular. Nutt believed, for instance, that because alcohol was a legal drug, policy makers consistently underplayed alcohol-related harms, just as they exaggerated harms associated with cannabis because cannabis was illegal. When Nutt, playfully but quite rationally, demonstrated that more harms stemmed from horse riding ('equasy') than from use of the illicit drug ecstasy (Nutt, 2009), he was deemed by the political establishment to have gone too far and was asked to resign as chair of the ACMD. Following this effective dismissal from his role as chief scientific advisor on drugs to the British government, Nutt published a book – '*Drugs Without the Hot Air*' – in which he further elaborated his criticisms of the spurious scientific basis of British and international drug policies (Nutt, 2012). Nutt may, therefore, be seen as a scientist whose preference for research evidence rather than big fat words brought him into conflict with politicians, the ultimate decision makers in drug policy.

Harm reduction and recovery

The widespread use of harm reduction practices (that is health service interventions that are aimed at reducing harms stemming from drug use where drug users either cannot or will not become abstinent) from the 1980s onwards, indicates that many health service providers pragmatically acknowledged the difficulties involved in delivering services based solely on abstinence or 'drug-free' models of care (e.g. Rhodes and Hedrich, 2010). However, the introduction of harm reduction practices (such as needle and syringe exchange schemes, opioid substitution prescribing or medically-supervised injection facilities) based upon public health considerations into jurisdictions that were still formally signatory to the UN drug conventions might readily have been construed as challenging the international prohibitionist regime or, even perhaps, as supporting the view that citizens of liberal democracies should have the freedom to use any psychoactive drug of their choice. Some advocates of harm reduction (e.g. Hunt, 2004) argued that its introduction should occur in the context of a strong human rights perspective on drug use that would explicitly challenge UN orthodoxy. Others, however (e.g. Reinarman, 2004), championed the 'virtues of ambiguity': by which was meant the introduction of harm reduction practices in a relatively covert way, with little or no public debate or official announcement, and certainly without reference to drug use as a human right – so as to minimise the risk of attack from defenders of the prohibition regime. Jurisdictions that opted for ambiguity, rather than creating open debate and being led by public opinion on these complex issues (such as was the case in Ireland; Butler and Mayock, 2005), obviously cannot be seen as satisfying the Christie and Bruun ideal of policy transparency previously discussed.

The widespread adoption of harm reduction strategies in healthcare interventions into problem drug use during the 1980s had been largely prompted by public health fears of the transmission of HIV/AIDS between needle-sharing drug injectors – and through sexual contact into the non-drug-using population. Twenty years later, however, medical advances had transformed AIDS from a short-term, fatal condition into a chronic but manageable condition, and this undoubtedly contributed during the first decade of the new millennium to the international resurgence at policy and popular cultural level (e.g. Scottish Government, 2008; Best, 2012) of the concept of 'recovery': a concept that arguably represents an ideological return to fundamentalist abstinence or 'war on drugs' beliefs rather than any new technological advance in addiction treatment. Debate about the relative merits of recovery versus harm reduction has been polarised and acrimonious, displaying features of emotional intensity comparable to those that annoyed Christie and Bruun in 1968; and the debate has not been marked by a clear differentiation between science and ideology (e.g. Best et al., 2010; Peele, 2012). Methadone maintenance has been particularly prone to attack by critics of harm reduction, with prescribers – implicitly at least – accused of preventing patients from recovering by keeping them 'parked' on indefinite methadone scripts even when they wish to become drug free (e.g. McKeganey et al., 2004). A specific example of tension between scientific and political perspectives on methadone maintenance may be discerned in the relationship between British politicians and the Advisory Council on the Misuse of Drugs in the context of the governmental request – in late 2014 – for a review of the possibility of imposing time limits on this form of opiate substitution treatment (ACMD, 2014). Whether the concept of 'recovery' is a scientific development or merely some latter-day version of Christie and Bruun's 'big fat words' is a moot point.

DRUG ADDICTION AS DISEASE

The other dominant concept highlighted by Christie and Bruun is that of addiction or, specifically, of addiction as disease. In contrast with the deviance concept that attributes responsibility for their drug use and related problems to those deemed to have chosen to use psychoactive drugs, proponents of the addiction concept see problem drug use primarily as involuntary or compulsive behaviour. Addiction is usually seen as a medical condition characterised by loss of control – or at least diminished control – so that victims of this condition are unable to abstain from drug use even in the face of clear evidence of serious negative consequences associated with their drug use. There are two main and related implications of the addiction concept. The first is that addicts cannot be held responsible for having this condition and, to some extent at least, must also be regarded as having diminished responsibility for the social and behavioural problems stemming from it. The second is that public policy responses to addiction based on moralism are ineffective and that priority should be given to health service responses aimed at the treatment and rehabilitation of addicts.

Addiction as a social construct

Historical and social scientific research on the addiction concept is largely agreed that this idea emerged in Europe and North America from the late eighteenth century onwards (Levine, 1978; Room, 2003). Generally, such research does not support the view that the 'discovery' of addiction was an essentially technical or scientific process; instead, it tends to see addiction as a social construct – explicable in relation to the social, cultural, political and economic circumstances in which it was created and developed, rather than as the product of value-free scientific endeavour (e.g. Reinarman, 2005). Much of early addiction theory and its associated practices was concerned with alcohol, and with the practical issue of how society might best deal with the behavioural difficulties created by people variously referred to as 'habitual drunkards', 'inebriates' or 'dipsomaniacs'. Specialist 'inebriate asylums' or 'inebriate reformatories', which operated as an institutional alternative to prisons and lunatic asylums, were established on both sides of the Atlantic in the late-nineteenth century. However, as Valverde

(1998) has spelt out, these specialist institutions were not unambiguously based on a medical model of care provision for their inmates; they neither viewed addiction to alcohol as a disease of the body nor as a disease of the mind, but instead favoured the idea that it was a 'disease of the will'; and management of the inebriate asylums tended to be more reflective of a religious temperance than a medical scientific ethos. Edwards (2000) commented summarily that 'inebriate reformatories, which had been established in America and Britain as the tangible product of "inebriety is a disease" never made much of a contribution to solving the drink problem. They were closed or put to other uses' (2000: 96). And two decades into the twentieth century, these institutions had virtually disappeared.

Disease concept of alcoholism

The first full flowering of this addiction as disease notion, originating during the 1930s in post-Prohibition USA, was what is commonly referred to as the 'disease concept of alcoholism' (Jellinek, 1960). Essentially, this concept proposed that for the vast bulk of its consumers, alcohol was a relatively harmless product and that alcohol-related problems only affected a small proportion of drinkers who had a particular vulnerability – akin to an allergy – to this legal and commonly-used drug. This latter group of drinkers, it was claimed, suffered from the disease of alcoholism and as such deserved to be treated in a non-moralistic way through the provision of healthcare treatment and rehabilitation services (Room, 1978); the corollary of this disease concept was that public policy measures aimed at regulating or limiting consumer access to alcohol were unnecessary and unjustified. Its advocates presented the disease concept as a new, scientific approach to the understanding of alcohol problems that made previous policy controversies and ideological conflicts between 'wets' and 'drys' redundant. Although the World Health Organisation (WHO) used its prestige and influence to promote the disease concept internationally between 1950 and 1970, from the early-1970s onwards, it quietly dropped it, replacing it with a public health model of alcohol problems – the main tenets of which were diametrically opposed to those of the disease concept. This public health approach, which has been developed and refined over the succeeding decades, identified alcohol's toxicity, addictiveness and capacity to intoxicate as features that pose risk to all its consumers and not just to those with biological or psychological predispositions to alcohol problems: all summarised in the description of alcohol as 'no ordinary commodity' (Babor et al., 2010). The public health perspective had little interest in service provision for 'alcoholics', and instead, advocated the use of alcohol control strategies aimed at reducing total societal consumption levels. It is also important to note that Alcoholics Anonymous (AA), which was founded in the USA in 1935 and is commonly assumed to have the disease concept of alcoholism as a central plank of its activities (e.g. Peele, 1995), uses the language of disease as metaphor and bases its suggested programme of recovery on spirituality rather than on medical science. Kurtz (2002), a historian of AA, acknowledged that most AA members speak of their problems in terms of disease, but argued that 'the use of that vocabulary no more implies deep commitment to the tenet that alcoholism is a disease in some technical medical sense than speaking of sunrise or sunset implies disbelief in a Copernican solar system' (2002: 6).

In summary, it would now be generally agreed that the emergence of the disease concept of alcoholism is best understood as a social construct from an era in American history where Prohibition was perceived to have failed and from a political culture that had grown weary of ongoing conflicts about alcohol policy. It was not, despite the claims of its early proponents, a scientific or evidence-based development but rather a form of 'big fat words', which served an ideological function in a state which had legalised alcohol following a period of alcohol prohibition.

While the disease concept may be credited with reducing the stigma attached to alcoholism treatment within health service systems, it contributed little or nothing to enhancing the technical efficacy of treatment interventions; indeed, its opponents argue that from a public health viewpoint it may have been positively harmful insofar as it promoted the idea that risk was mainly related to inherited, individual predisposition rather than population drinking habits. Conversely, critics of the public health approach to alcohol challenge the scientific basis of this approach and see it as a form of neo-temperance ideology; and, generally, attempts to have a public health approach to alcohol enshrined in public policy have been marked by ongoing conflict between proponents of this approach and the drinks industry (e.g. Peele, 2010). If we apply the 'big fat words' approach to the public health slogan that alcohol is 'no ordinary commodity', then perhaps the main criticism of this slogan is not so much that it exaggerates the risk attached to consumption of this drug as that it ignores the unique pleasures which are also associated with drinking.

The disease concept no longer commands scientific respect or policy acceptance in the developed world, but it might be foolish to assume that it exerts no influence in popular cultural terms. As Room (2001) has argued: 'The alcohol experience suggests that old discourses rarely die; they go out of fashion or they go underground as being "politically incorrect", but there are still elements of them extant in the culture in which they once flourished' (2001: 41).

Brain disease model of addiction

The most recent version of the addiction as disease model, which has been promoted since the mid-1990s, has its base in advances in the neurosciences and in genetics and is presented for public and political consideration in terms of a simple claim that 'addiction is a brain disease' (e.g. Leshner, 1997; Volkow and Li, 2004). Scientists who promote this model of addiction as a chronic, relapsing disease use PET and fMRI scans to illustrate the neural correlates of addictive craving, arguing that addiction essentially consists of a 'hijacking' of the brain's reward circuits – so that sufferers find it difficult, if not impossible, to abstain from drug use, despite their awareness of the personal and social costs of such drug use. Advocates of this brain disease model of addiction, as did their predecessors who promoted the disease concept of alcoholism half a century earlier, believe that its acceptance can lead to a reduction in the public stigmatisation and criminalisation of addicts and, ultimately, to the development and widespread use of effective medical interventions. However, sceptics – who include both behavioural scientists and medically-trained psychiatrists (e.g. Hall and Carter, 2013; Satel and Lilienfield, 2013) – see this exclusive focus on the brain as reductionist and as generally exaggerating the importance of brain function in its explanation of a phenomenon which has obvious psychosocial correlates. Its critics argue that the 'hijacked brain' perspective overstates the degree to which addicts lose all capacity to make choices about abstinence, while underestimating their capacity for recovery, with or without formal healthcare intervention. Social science critics also express concern lest futuristic policy expectations based upon high-technology, clinical interventions into individual 'hijacked brains' might undermine public health strategies – such as population-based alcohol strategies – stemming from social science research (Midanik and Room, 2005). In any event, the brain disease model has not as yet resulted in any radically new pharmacological interventions, and ethical and other misgivings about controversial innovations in the form of neurosurgery (such as 'deep brain stimulation') for intractable addictions (Carter and Hall, 2011) make it unlikely that this will be a major area of clinical development in the immediate future.

In concluding this summary of what is by now more than two centuries of the addiction as disease concept, it is clear that this concept remains contested and that the medical approach has not succeeded in supplanting the moral approach to such an extent that problem drug users are invariably regarded as sick people rather than as 'moral degenerates'. Legal systems, for instance, have not accepted that addicts are suffering from a brain disease that absolves them of responsibility for crimes, which, it is argued, are the result of their addiction (Morse, 2011). Furthermore, despite the scientific rhetoric of the brain disease model of addiction and its associated promise of technological 'breakthroughs' in addiction treatment, no such clinical advances have as yet materialised. And, as was made clear in the debate concerning the relative merits of the words 'addiction' and 'dependence' in the revised Diagnostic and Statistical Manual of the American Psychiatric Association (e.g. Keane et al., 2011; Room, 2011), the process of sharpening and refining substance use disorders within diagnostic systems is still fraught with value conflicts and terminological confusion.

DISCUSSION

Christie and Bruun's (1969) 'big fat words' seem broadly comparable to what Robin Room has referred to as 'governing images' (Room, 1978, 2001). As Room defines this phenomenon, 'a governing image or discursive formation gathers together a broad field in terms of a single frame of understanding, often summarized in a few shorthand phrases. It is thus always an imperfect fit to the reality it seeks to cover…' (Room, 2001: 40). Whether we refer to them as big fat words or governing images (and the latter seems much less pejorative), it seems clear that these largely competing concepts – one moralistic and the other medical – still retain their dominance 50 years after Christie and Bruun's outburst on this topic. They are clearly an 'imperfect fit' in the sense that there is no cultural consensus on the evils of psychoactive drugs and the deviance of those who use them, just as there is no scientific consensus on the validity of conceptualising people who develop drug-related problems as having the disease of addiction. Each concept in its own way, however, may be seen as representing a partial truth: psychoactive drug use (in all its varieties) is inherently risky to health and social order and, across cultures, religious faiths and age groups, there are varying degrees of concern with – if not downright rejection of – such drug use. Similarly, even in the absence of scientific certitude and dramatic breakthroughs in treatment technologies, societal management of problem drug users through healthcare rather than through criminal justice systems has an understandable appeal for many.

It should perhaps be reiterated that Christie and Bruun did not argue prescriptively for one conceptual model rather than another but rather – in Shakespearean terms – wished a plague on both houses. What they really called for was 'conceptual refinement', a phrase used to refer to a transparent debate and policy-making process in which conventional scientific findings are clearly differentiated from value systems and ethical beliefs. These sociologists understood that most members of the public would neither have the desire nor the capacity to engage in scientific research into drug issues, but argued that the public deserved to be given research evidence free from bias of all descriptions. Conversely, Christie and Bruun accepted that public discourse and public policy making in relation to psychoactive drugs was heavily bound up with ethical judgements and value systems, and that – regardless of their scientific competence – all members of the public who wished to do so should be allowed to contribute to the public policy process on the basis of their own values and ethical beliefs.

What the review presented here of developments over the past 50 years suggests is that the aspiration to disentangle scientific evidence and political/ideological elements of the psychoactive drug debate has made relatively little progress. While the concepts may have changed somewhat, the overall tone of the drug debate is still as heated and emotionally charged as it was in the late-1960s. The earnestness, for example, with which proponents of the brain disease model of addiction present their case has much in common with the zeal of earlier pleadings that 'alcoholism is a disease'; and the evangelical style with which the 'recovery' movement is promoted is not dissimilar to the military rhetoric of the 'war on drugs'. In brief, big fat words would still appear to be the order of the day.

The Christie and Bruun ideal of conceptual refinement may be seen as reflecting, however implicitly, a rational public policy model, and what has changed in the intervening half century is that considerably more sociological scrutiny has been devoted to the policy process. Much of this research has focused on the interface between research and policy, effectively demolishing the idea that the policy process is a rational, linear affair in which policy makers are primarily influenced by research evidence (Weiss, 1977, 1986). Research that has focused specifically on the alcohol/drug policy process has broadly been in line with that on the wider public policy process in that it confirms that the way in which politicians – the ultimate policy makers – are selective and discriminating in how they use research evidence in reaching decisions in contentious and highly politicised policy areas (e.g. Monaghan, 2010; MacGregor, 2013; Stevens and Ritter, 2013). In light of this more subtle and complex analysis of the policy process, it is possible to understand how politicians see research findings as just one element to be considered alongside media representation of, and public opinion on, the issues involved, as well as the impact of lobby groups of varying influence on decision making on these issues. This allows us to understand, for instance, how apparently solid research evidence that public health would be enhanced by implementing strategies (such as price increases, reduced availability at retail level and greatly restricted advertising and promotional campaigns) based on the 'no ordinary commodity' slogan are largely ignored by government – as public health strategies of this kind are likely to be viewed as paternalistic and unpopular by the electorate, besides which, they clash with neoliberal consumerist ideologies and bring government into conflict with the drinks industry. Similarly, it allows us to understand how governments may contribute to discourse on the importance of 'recovery' and the evils of keeping patients 'parked' on long-term methadone even in the face of research reports which challenge this perspective.

In conclusion, discourse on alcohol and drug problems has not achieved the type of clarity and rationality that Christie and Bruun hoped for, but still remains mired in big fat words. Today's social scientists may, however, be more accepting of this situation: neither believing that the policy process is, or should be, an essentially rational business, and perhaps less disturbed by big fat words.

REFERENCES

Aldridge, J., Measham, F. and Williams, L. (2011) *Illegal Leisure Revisited: Changing Patterns of Alcohol and Drug Use in Adolescents and Young Adults*. London: Routledge.

Advisory Council on the Misuse of Drugs (ACMD) (2014) *Time Limiting Opioid Substitution Therapy*. London: Advisory Council on the Misuse of Drugs.

Babor, T., Caetano, R., Casswell, S., Edwards, G., Giesbrecht, N., Graham, K, Grube, J., Hill, L., Holder, H., Homel, R., Livingston, M., Osterberg, E., Rehm, J., Room, R. and Rossow, I. (2010) *Alcohol: No Ordinary Commodity – Research and Public Policy.* 2nd ed. Oxford: Oxford University Press.

Becker, H. (1963) *Outsiders: Studies in the Sociology of Deviance*. New York: The Free Press.

Berridge, V. (2013) *Demons: Our Changing Attitudes to Alcohol, Tobacco and Drugs.* Oxford: Oxford University Press.

Best, D., Bamber, S., Battersby, A., Gilman, M., Groshkova, T., Honor, S., McCartney, D., Yates, R. and White, W. (2010) 'Recovery and straw men: an analysis of the objections raised to the transition to a recovery model in the UK addiction services', *Journal of Groups in Addiction and Recovery,* 5: 264–88.

Best, D. (2012) *Addiction Recovery: A Movement for Social Change.* Brighton: Pavilion Publishing.

Bewley-Taylor, D. (2001) *The United Nations and International Drug Control, 1909–1997.* London: Continuum.

Butler, S. and Mayock, P. (2005) '"An Irish solution to an Irish problem": Harm reduction and ambiguity in the drug policy of the Republic of Ireland', *International Journal of Drug Policy,* 16: 415–22.

Christie, N. and Bruun, K. (1969) 'Alcohol problems: the conceptual framework' In M. Keller and T. Coffey (eds), *Proceedings of the 28th International Congress on Alcohol and Alcoholism* (Vol. 2). Highland Park: Hillhouse Press, pp. 65–73.

Carter, A. and Hall, W. (2011) 'Proposals to trial deep brain stimulation to treat addiction are premature', *Addiction,* 106: 235–37.

Cohen, S. (1972) *Folk Devils and Moral Panics: The Creation of the Mods and the Rockers.* London: MacGibbon and Kee.

Edwards, G. (2000) *Alcohol: The Ambiguous Molecule.* London: Penguin.

Hall, W. and Carter, A. (2013) 'Anticipating possible policy uses of addiction neuroscience research', *Drugs: Education, Prevention and Policy,* 20: 249–57.

Hunt, N. (2004) 'Public health or human rights: what comes first?', *International Journal of Drug Policy,* 15: 231–37.

Jellinek, E. (1960) *The Disease Concept of Alcoholism.* New Haven: Hill House Press.

Keane, H., Moore, D. and Fraser, S. (2011) 'Addiction and dependence: making realities in the DSM', *Addiction,* 106: 875–7.

Kurtz, E. (2002) 'Alcoholics Anonymous and the disease concept of alcoholism', *Alcoholism Treatment Quarterly,* 20: 5–40.

Leshner, A. (1997) 'Addiction is a brain disease, and it matters', *Science,* 278: 45–57.

Levine, H.G. (1978) 'The discovery of addiction: changing conceptions of habitual drunkenness in America', *Journal of Studies on Alcohol,* 39: 143–74.

MacGregor, S. (2013) 'Barriers to the influence of evidence on policy: are politicians the problem?', *Drugs: Education, Prevention and Policy,* 20: 225–33.

McKeganey, N., Morris, Z., Neale, J. and Robertson, M. (2004) 'What are drugs users looking for when they contact drug services: abstinence or harm reduction?', *Drugs: Education, Prevention and Policy,* 11: 423–35.

Midanik, L. and Room, R. (2005) 'Contributions of social science to the alcohol field in an era of biomedicalization', *Social Science and Medicine,* 60: 1107–16.

Monaghan, M. (2010) 'The complexity of evidence: reflections on research utilisation in a heavily politicised policy area', *Social Policy and Society,* 9: 1–12.

Morse, S. (2011). 'Addiction and criminal responsibility' In J. Poland and G. Graham (eds), *Addiction and Responsibility.* London: The MIT Press, pp. 159–99.

Nutt, D., King, L., Saulsbury, W. and Blakemore, C. (2007) 'Developing a rational scale for assessing the risks of drugs of potential misuse', *Lancet,* 369: 1047–53.

Nutt, D. (2009) 'Equasy – An overlooked addiction with implications for the current debate on drug harms', *Journal of Psycholpharmacology,* 23: 3–5.

Nutt, D. (2012) *Drugs Without the Hot Air: Minimising the Harms of Legal and Illegal Drugs.* Cambridge: UIT.

Parker, H., Aldridge, J. and Measham, F. (1998) *Illegal Leisure: The Normalization of Adolescent Recreational Drug Use.* London: Routledge.

Peele, S. (1995) *Diseasing of America: How we Allowed Recovery Zealots and the Treatment Industry to Convince us we are Out of Control.* Lexington: Lexington Books.

Peele, S. (2010) 'Alcohol as evil – temperance and policy', *Addiction Research and Theory,* 18: 374–82.

Peele, S. (2012) 'AA and abstinence as prevention techniques', *Drugs: Education, Prevention and Policy,* 19: 284–90.

Pryce, S. (2012). *Fixing Drugs: The Politics of Drug Prohibition.* Houndmills: Palgrave Macmillan.

Reinarman, C. (2004) 'Public health and human rights: the virtues of ambiguity', *International Journal of Drug Policy,* 15: 239–41.

Reinarman, C. (2005) 'Addiction as accomplishment: the discursive construction of disease', *Addiction Research and Theory,* 13: 307–20.

Reinarman, C. and Levine, HG (2004) 'Crack in the rearview mirror: deconstructing drug war mythology', *Social Justice,* 31: 182–99.
Rhodes, T. and Hedrich, D. (2010) *Harm Reduction: Evidence, Impacts and Challenges.* Lisbon: European Monitoring Centre on Drugs and Drug Addiction.
Room, R. (1978) *Governing Images of Alcohol and Drug Problems: The Structure, Sources and Sequels of Conceptualizations of Intractable Problems.* PhD dissertation. Berkeley: University of California.
Room, R. (2001) 'Governing images in public discourse about problematic drinking' In N. Heather, T. Peters and T. Stockwell (eds), *International Handbook of Alcohol Dependence and Problems.* Chichester: John Wiley, pp. 33–45.
Room, R. (2003) 'The cultural framing of addiction', *Janus Head,* 6: 221–34.
Room, R. (2011) 'Substance use disorders – a conceptual and terminological muddle', *Addiction,* 106: 879–82.
Satel, S. and Lilienfield, S. (2013) *Brainwashed: The Seductive Appeal of Mindless Neuroscience.* New York: Basic Books.
Scottish Government (2008) *The Road to Recovery: A New Approach to Tackling Scotland's Drug Problem.* Edinburgh: Scottish Government.
Shiner, M. and Newburn, T. (1997) 'Definitely, maybe not: the normalization of recreational drug use amongst young people', *Sociology,* 31: 511–29.
Shiner, M. and Newburn, T. (1999) 'Taking tea with Noel: the place and meaning of drug use in everyday life' In N. South (ed.), *Drugs: Cultures, Controls and Everyday Life.* London: Sage, pp. 139–59.
Stevens, A. and Ritter, A. (2013) 'How can and do empirical studies influence drug policies? Narratives and complexity in the use of evidence in policy making', *Drugs: Education, Prevention and Policy*, 20: 169–74.
Sumner, C. (1994) *The Sociology of Deviance: An Obituary.* Buckingham: Open University Press.
Szasz, T. (1975). *Ceremonial Chemistry: The Ritual Persecution of Drugs, Drug Addicts and Pushers.* London: Routledge and Kegan Paul.
Valverde, M. (1998). *Diseases of the Will: Alcohol and the Dilemmas of Freedom.* Cambridge: Cambridge University Press.
Volkow, N. and Li, T. (2004) 'Drug addiction: the neurobiology of behaviour gone awry', *Nature Reviews Neuroscience,* 5: 963–70.
Weiss, C. (1977) *Using Social Research in Public Policy Making.* Lexington: Heath.
Weiss, C. (1986) 'The many meanings of research utilization', In M. Bulmer (ed.), *Social Science and Social Policy.* London: Allen Unwin, pp. 31–40.
Young, J. (1987) 'Deviance', In P. Worsley (ed.), *The New Introducing Sociology.* Harmondsworth Middlesex: Penguin, pp. 407–450.

NILS CHRISTIE[1] (1928–2015)

Dangerous words

Words are important carriers of meaning. Self-evidently useful. Also, highly specialized words are necessary in specific situations. The surgeon needs a special tool, fast. The carpenter high up on the ladder calls for tools which only other carpenters know the words for and can deliver quickly. Or the physicist needs to use a word, understandable only to the few. The philosopher or the social scientist may believe they have the same need for special words.

But then some people want to use words only to show off, especially if the words indicate that the users are of high social status. Or the users get so used to the specialized words that they use them thoughtlessly outside the narrow group. Then what happens is that all those outside the group become like deaf people.

Words, therefore, can be dangerous tools. Let me say something about words which are especially dangerous.

The first kind of dangerous words are those created *before experience*; either experience acquired personally, or experience coming from immersing oneself in the phenomenon or the thinking which the word conveys. The word 'concept' means to grip.[2] But if there is nothing to grip, if there are no events or thoughts inside the concept, then the concept will, after all, be empty. One can easily learn words like democracy or representative government, and also accept that Norway is an example of such a country. But if one wants to use the words, one soon discovers that these are words without any precise content. But exactly because of their ambiguity they can be well suited to blur disagreements and hereby create peace in the country. Drug is also one of the big multifarious words – a word that, because of its lack of precision, allows nicotine users and alcohol users to get on with their activities in peace.

As a consequence of this way of thinking, people should not learn to use, and especially not write, these kinds of words before they know a lot about other things.

Maybe one should not learn to write before one is very knowledgeable, preferably through personal experience. As a university teacher I still try to stop students using big words. I try to say: forget the words, tell me concretely what it is about, give me descriptions, episodes, do role play, but do not use the big words before they are filled up with meaning – and maybe even not then. Imperialism, democracy, capitalism, psychopathy, recidivism, intensive treatment, debility, unemployment. ... Yes, exactly unemployment, this simple word which people still use. Unemployment. What a false message. As if unemployment existed. Our society is full of tasks, work which should be done, people who need help. It is not work but salary which is lacking. Paid unemployment is the right word. But that word directs attention towards a problem of distribution and not to the presumed problem, the unemployed.

Other kinds of harmful words are the *monopolized*. These are the profession's own words. They are to a large extent created to symbolize power; the white coats of the health personnel with the stethoscope in the breast pocket is language, in the same way as the Latin they often use when they are describing us. Lawyers have their gowns and their words; and pedagogues, too, have their specialized words - dyslexia is one of their valued words. Anomie and stratification are among the favourite words of sociologists. These are the properties of the professionals. Laymen will discover this if they steal the words, try to employ them for their own aims. Client really means the person who comes when the master whistles. Have mercy on the client who talks back using the words of the master.

A third kind of harmful words, of special interest in normal social gatherings, are the *imperialistic*. Here I think of the words which, in a way, supersede all other words in talking about a person. 'The murderer' is such a word. Or 'the safe cracker'. Or 'the drug addict'. But people are not murderers, safe crackers or drug addicts all the time. They are much more than that. Nice, helpful, unclean, maybe nicely dressed, good at singing, generous, lying, obscene towards ladies, knowledgeable, good at looking after chickens. The existence of imperialistic words probably relates to types of society. In places where people only know each other a little, one personal characteristic can easily be seen as encompassing all of the person. Craig Calhoon (1995) introduces the concept of categorical identities in contrast to more complex understandings of total human beings or networks of concrete social relations. My own image of the last one is the old-fashioned settlement or village communities where people appear as wholes, types, where we know many aspects of each individual, and hence one sole characteristic will seldom get a foothold. People are so multiple; understanding needs a novel about each of them. Such novels are built through continuous oral retellings in these societies. This is in contrast to the city-societies of strangers, where one characteristic can become the dominant label exactly because it is the only thing we know...[...]... Action is language. Words are special cases of actions.

WORDS THAT OBSTRUCT

We need to use words, but we ought, as best as we can, be open to the most concrete and detailed description possible of the phenomenon we are facing. Ambiguities ought to be brought to the fore; labels ought to be avoided as far as possible. Concrete events are the most fruitful starting point. The struggle for comprehension, the fight for the meaning of the actions and the actors is a very central research topic.

But if the big words work to obstruct comprehension and therefore have to be avoided how does one then manage to say the things one wants to say? My take on this is to employ a more narrative form. If the big labelling words are dangerous because of their power to freeze, then the depictions derived from the more complete sequences of events may offer ways of getting closer to understanding of the phenomenon. In order not to be restricted by the all-encompassing words, I choose the narrative form to present brief stories about life in deprived areas, about life on the balconies one Sunday in June, or about youth who, for no real reason, take money they should not take.

'Psychiatry' is one of the all too big words. For a long time there was not much talk about psychopaths in the Nordic countries. Bo Gerle may be responsible for this. In 1947 he published the book "The bankruptcy of the concept of the psychopath". But now this book has disappeared from the bibliographies and the concept of the psychopath is returning at full speed – returning together with the forensic psychiatrist. Lists of negative qualities are drawn up, and then one studies how many points the person studied scores. If the subjects get more than a certain number they are seen as psychopaths. From the literature, I understand that psychopaths exist in large numbers in our prisons. Using broad definitions, it applies to nearly all prisoners, by more narrow ones at least one out of four prisoners are counted as psychopaths. Rosenqvist and Rasmussen (2001: 214) have this to say about the same theme.

> It is assumed that psychopaths make up approximately one per cent of the general population while 20–25 per cents of the prison population are psychopaths (Hare and Hart, 1993). These are taken to be responsible for more than half of all serious criminality.

I do understand that in a society in which we know each other less and less – as complete human beings – a need arises for someone to tell us who 'the others' are. But at the same time this will be a situation which requires the uttermost vigilance. The story about what 'the others' are like has to be a complete story. If the psychiatrists and the psychologists are to help us, it has to be as narrators of stories about human beings. Otherwise, they will just turn in to salaried employees, the judicial system's assistants by applying simple words to complex lives.

But it will become so ambiguous; it is not standardised, the psychiatrists will say. And I will reply: Yes, as ambiguous as a good poem. Precisely because it is ambiguous it gives us the possibility of moving on. The story is not closed off or 'sticky', as Sartre would have said, but open, due to the possibilities of ambiguousness for further growth. Maybe we should aim at establishing social systems with a maximum of doubt about who we are – and who 'the others' are. Recreate ourselves and others as mysteries. If the psychiatrist were to play any role it has to be as mediators of the complexity of who 'the other' is. They ought to write short stories about the people they meet. Then the lawyers and the rest of us could maybe understand something more about people and about the events.

But this would not benefit the criminal justice systems!

Yes, it would be very beneficial for this system. It would return responsibility to the place where responsibility should be – to the judge. She or he would not get any simple answers, but they would meet complete, ambiguous persons. The judge would not face obstructing words coming between him or herself and the person on whom judgement should fall. Then the judge would have a harder time deciding on the extent of intended pain, but it would also be more challenging. All experience suggests that the closer people get to each other, the harder it is for them to cause suffering to each other. That is good.

1 As a comment to Butler and Mayock's chapter on 'Big fat words' (this volume), Nils Christie suggested we translated a section from his Norwegian book 'Små ord for store spørsmål', Universitetsforlaget, Oslo 2009, pp 21–25; 39–42. The text is translated by Torsten Kolind and Betsy Thom and permission is kindly given by Universitetsforlaget. This brief chapter is also in commemoration and admiration of the great criminologist and humanist Nils Christie.

2 In Norwegian: 'Begrep betyr å gripe om.'

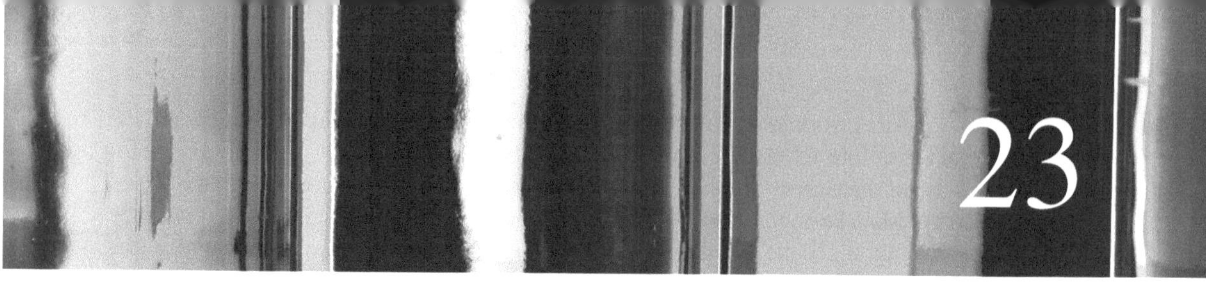

The Increasing Visibility of Gender in the Alcohol and Drug Fields

Geoffrey Hunt, Tamar Antin, Jeanett Bjønness and Elizabeth Ettorre

INTRODUCTION

All too often, reviews of the literature examine past and current research as though the research had been wholly developed in an intellectual environment free of any social, economic, or political influences. We know this is not so: research topics and interests are guided as much by contemporary social and cultural pressures as by theoretical paradigms. To understand developments within any research area, it is essential to consider not only the conceptual heritage (i.e. theoretical developments) that have taken place but also the dominant cultural perspectives of the researchers themselves and the diverse social, political, and cultural contexts in which these researchers have operated (Burawoy, 2004; Leach, 1984). This is particularly true for a discussion of gender in the alcohol and drug research arenas. General and scholarly interest in issues of gender and women's studies ultimately has had an impact on the drugs and alcohol fields. By 1994, McDonald noted that at least in the UK 'gender has become commonplace in book titles. Its popularity has been due in part to a realization that women had been relatively invisible in social science texts prior to the 1970s and to a growth in feminism' (McDonald, 1994:1). However, some more recent feminist scholars (Campbell and Ettorre, 2011) would question how influential this impact has been on the field, noting that merely adding 'gender' or 'women' to the title of a published work is insufficient unless it is developed within a gender perspective.

Nevertheless, the significance of feminist scholarship on contemporary developments in examining the drugs and alcohol fields cannot be understated. The publication of West and Zimmerman's (1987) 'Doing gender' in *Gender and Society*, although outside the field of drugs and alcohol research, had an important impact on recent developments in the drugs and alcohol fields especially in terms of their more nuanced discussion of notions of gender, both in terms of femininity (Ettorre, 1986, 1989, 1992; Measham, 2002; West and Fenstermaker, 1995), and to some extent, masculinity (Collison, 1996; Connell, 1995; Connell and Messerschmidt, 2005). Furthermore, developments occurring outside of the academy have also significantly shaped research in the alcohol and drugs fields. This wider context is particularly significant in understanding research developments and interests on gender and alcohol and drugs. Controls on who can produce alcohol, who can consume it and in what situations or contexts, and the resulting consequences for transgressing these norms have been critical issues in studies of alcohol. Because of their contested and illegal nature, understanding the social and historical contexts has also been important for research on illicit drugs where the consequences for producing, selling, and consuming drugs are different for men and for women (Measham, 2002). The impact of changes in social policy and legislation and in societal attitudes towards the users have had a direct influence on the type of research funded, and consequently, on the type of research conducted.

At different times, different substances have been at the center of public policy. As a result of the War on Drugs, by the late 1980s, illicit drugs were the central focus of much research in the US and issues surrounding alcohol consumption much less important. However, in early 2000, research increasingly centered on alcohol issues, intoxication, and the night time economy (Chatterton and Hollands, 2003; Griffin et al., 2013; Szmigin et al., 2008) due in part to the perceived social problems associated with public intoxication. Consequently, an upsurge in research publications especially began to focus on studies of youthful drunkenness (Bailey et al., 2015; Keane, 2009; Measham and Brain, 2005; Measham et al., 2001; Peralta, 2007). This shifting socio-political context has fostered and influenced research on specific areas that generally are in line with current political thinking.[1]

The evolving social positioning of women and men have also influenced developments in the drugs and alcohol fields. Researchers have suggested that a number of significant changes in the wider society including the erosion of strict gender roles, delaying and limiting childbearing, women's expanded social networks, increases in women's income and disposable income, alcohol marketing and advertising contributing to a shift towards gender convergence, and changes in drinking and drunkenness norms (Chatterton and Hollands, 2003; Fillmore, 1987; Johnson and Gerstein, 2000; Kuntsche et al., 2011; McConville, 1983; Otto, 1981; Szmigin et al., 2008; Wilsnack and Wilsnack, 1991). Hence, changes such as these not only impact issues of alcohol and drug consumption but also influence both the types of research undertaken and the theories utilized to explain these changes.

Although this chapter does not intend to provide an encyclopedic account of all the research that has taken place on gender issues related to alcohol and drugs – an account that would be too extensive for the confines of the Handbook – we will nevertheless inform the reader about the exclusion and inclusion of research on women in the drugs and alcohol fields and the contribution that feminist scholars and the feminist movement have made and are making to these fields. While research done by psychologists and epidemiologists will be referenced in passing, this chapter is influenced by our own disciplines and research interests in sociology, anthropology, cultural studies, feminist research, criminology, social policy, and social history. It is these disciplines that will provide a backcloth to the central discussions within the chapter. Finally, most of the works referred to in this overview are written in English. There are, of course, feminist scholars working in other languages, but much of their work is inaccessible to the wider alcohol and drugs research community as it appears in documents with limited circulation, either by language or region. Also, while much of the work has emphasized research conducted in the US or the UK, we have, where possible, referred to research conducted in other countries.

To explore research on gender in the drugs and alcohol fields, we have divided the paper into three sections: early research on gender and drug and alcohol issues; gendered themes in contemporary research; and emerging gender perspectives.

EARLY RESEARCH ON GENDER AND DRUG AND ALCOHOL ISSUES

The male gaze in studies of alcohol

Until the 1970s, research on women in the drugs and alcohol fields was largely absent, due in part to the preponderance of male researchers, who focused on male drinkers and drug users, and more generally, because of an interest in men by social researchers (see, for example, Bales, 1962; Bemko and Davidson, 1978; McClelland et al. 1972; Kalant, 1980). As Maher (1997) suggests, the theoretical tools to study women's substance use were inadequate and Kalant (1980) even went as far as arguing that research on women and drugs was a 'non-field', as the subjects of research were 'frequently males and sex differences tended to be overlooked' (Ettorre, 2004: 328). Whatever the reasons, most of the research was based on men's lives. As Weibel-Orlando noted 'those theories that do exist about why women drink are offshoots of theories about male drinking... women's drinking looks like a paler version of male drinking behavior' (Weibel-Orlando, 1984: 162). This was the case whether one examined drinking among ethnic minority women in the US (Weibel-Orlando, 1984) or explored drinking practices in Finland, where alcohol culture was seen as synonymous with male culture (Natkin, 1984). Comparable research on gender and drugs was virtually nonexistent.

However, having noted this focus on men, it would be inaccurate to argue that all researchers ignored women, particularly in the domains of drinking and alcohol production. In fact, *The British Journal of Inebriety* featured a number of articles in the early 1900s that focused on women drinkers (inebriates) and/or the effects of women's drinking on their children (Booth, 1911; Reid, 1929; Scharlieb, 1907; Shaw, 1903; Waugh, 1903; Westcott, 1903; Zanetti, 1903) (see also Pescor, 1944). As Heath remarked in discussing the alcohol field:

> There is a presumption that virtually nothing is known about drinking by women prior to the mid-1960s...[however]...The facts are very different from the presumptions. Occasional studies comparing male and female alcohol use appeared in scientific journals early in [the 20th Century]. (Heath, 1991: 176)

For example, Margaret Bacon, following up on Horton's (1943) cross-cultural study of drinking in 32 different cultures, further examined the Human Relations Area Files[2] and discovered that the widespread notion that women tended to drink less in industrialized societies led 'to the erroneous belief that in all societies men drink more than women' (Bacon, 1976: 29). On the basis of her analysis of 113 societies, she concluded that, 'clearly the tendency for men to drink more than women is a frequently observed pattern cross-culturally but it is by no means universal' (1976: 30). Moreover, Keller (1965), in examining 139 societies, where alcohol use was well documented found that only four of them forbade women from drinking and 'only one...accepted drunkenness on the part of men but not women' (Heath, 2000: 73).

While it is nevertheless clear that few researchers considered research on women's drinking as a significant focus in their research, there was one notable exception. In 1934, Elisabeth Hellman, an anthropologist, examined the role of women in beer production in the 'skokiaan' yards of Johannesburg. The role of women in beer production reflected their dominance in agricultural production in many African societies and the brewing of beer allowed women an increased economic and social status. Hellman's work stands out as one of the very few examples of an investigation of the social implications of women's relationship to alcohol.

Social historians also produced some significant research on women and the drinking place in the pre-modern period. Peter Clark's study of the Alehouse (1983) examined the role of women in alcohol production, noting their importance as owners and as brewers. In fact, most of the beer-houses and alehouses in London 'were owned by women and the ale-wife was a noted character in rural England' (Oakley, 1974:12). The importance of women within the trade was even reflected in the accepted use of brewster, the feminine term for a brewer. Historians' interest in women and alcohol was not only confined to research on the Medieval period but also extended to the Victorian era, focusing in particular on women's involvement in the Temperance Movement (Borodin 1981: Gusfield, 1955; Hyslop, 1976; Longmate, 1968; Tyrrell, 1983). Working class women's access to alcohol and the urban pub was an issue of much concern to public commentators, especially to middle class women, who were becoming increasingly involved in the Temperance Movement (Harrison, 1971). Noted in Harrison's book (1971) '*Drink and the Victorians*', the association between female drinking in pubs and sexual encounters was viewed as a significant problem by Victorian reformers, who 'often saw prostitution where none existed' (Harrison, 1971: 50). As a result, greater restrictions were introduced to control women's access to pubs, including restricting women as barmaids.

Although some significant research exists on women and gender in the alcohol field (see, for example, Bemko and Davidson, 1978; Blume, 1985; Cuskey et al., 1972; d'Orban, 1970; Finnegan, 1975, 1978; Finnegan et al., 1973, 1976; Lisansky, 1957, 1958; Litman, 1975, 1978; Litman, and Wilson, 1978; Mondanaro, 1977; Perry, 1979), it is nevertheless the case that prior to the 1980s, little work had been produced on theorizing notions of gender. Epidemiological research on women at this time tended to suggest that drinking by women was an indication of sex role confusion and some sort of psychological malaise (Ettorre, 1997). Given this problem-oriented perspective, socio-cultural researchers largely ignored women's involvement in drinking or even considered how women's access to alcohol, in different historical periods, had been restricted. Instead, much of this early research emphasized the extent to which drinking produced, established, and confirmed masculinity, male solidarity, and male dominance (Dennis et al., 1956; Griffin et al., 2013; Pack, 1982; Sargeant, 1967; Taussig, 1980; Tunstall 1962).

Women's pathologization

During this early stage, the stereotypical image of a drug user was male. When women appeared in the literature, it was traditionally within a 'pathology and powerlessness' perspective (Anderson, 2005, 2008; Maher, 1997) and as a high risk group (Finnegan, 1975, 1978a; 1978b; Finnegan et al., 1973, 1976; Gomberg,1982). Women drug users were portrayed as perpetual victims, their drug use treated as pathological, and notions of women's agency or pleasures were largely absent.[3] In tracing women's drug using experiences, themes of dysfunction, moral depravity, dependence, and exploitation predominated. Although men comprised the norm in drug research, their gender typically remained unanalyzed or invisible (Broom, 1994). Similarly, when sexuality was discussed within drug research, generally, it was reduced to a problem status, such as analyzing the links between drug use and sexual disease transmission (Ostrow and Shelby, 2000; Ross and Williams, 2012). Rarely foregrounded were issues of embodiment, gender, sexualities, sexual identities, or pleasure and agency (Rosenbaum 1981 is an exception).

Due to the stigmatized nature of women's substance use during this early period, it is perhaps no surprise that studies of treatment are among the earliest examples where issues related to women and substance use begin to emerge. The early 1900s marks a period of significant concern about female inebriates. Charles Booth (1969) in '*Life and Labour of the London Poor*', noted that while drunkenness had declined, drinking had increased and this could be laid at the feet of women. In response, the UK Parliament passed the Inebriate Act in 1898, which enabled local authorities to establish State and Certified Reformatories to treat habitual drunkards. Although public drunkenness among both men and women was common during this period,[4] what was significant about these reformatories was that of the 4,590 inebriates who were committed to the reformatories, 81 percent were women (Hunt et al., 1989).

The earliest studies on drug treatment for women were done in the United States (Cuskey et al., 1972; Ellinwood, 1966; Waldorf, 1973). Much of this work was problem-oriented and considered drug using women through the lens of male-oriented psychiatry that defined them as suffering from maladaptation to the female role (Beckman, 1978; Ettorre, 1985; Rosett and Weiner, 1984). This work focused on clinical populations where 'sex differences in treatment outcome' were central and discussions around any social, economic, and/or political issue related to substance use for women (or men) in both non-clinical and clinical populations were absent.[5] Nevertheless, early work in the treatment field has been important in establishing valuable pointers to those working in the field, specifically exposing male bias (Vanicelli and Nash, 1984) and the arguably sexist assumption that women are no different from their male counterparts. Although some early attempts to develop treatment programs specifically for women existed, they were often met with resistance, and of those programs that were started, they tended to be 'set up along masculinist lines with little or no exploration of what drug-using women might need from their own perspective' (Campbell and Ettorre, 2011: 35. See also Du Rose 2015).

Important feminist critiques of these mainstream approaches to alcohol and drug treatment did emerge at this time, arguing that the special treatment needs of women must be considered (MacLennan, 1976) to 'develop services for an under-catered for and stigmatised group' (Waterson and Ettorre, 1989: 124). Stephenson contended that we must not be 'seduced' by theories that present only an 'individual and intrapsychic basis for problems' (Stephenson 1980: 12). Instead, treatment professionals should help women 'substance users to become aware that…their problems mirror the inequalities experienced by all women' (1980: 12). Their problems of living, which were often 'confused with psychiatric disorders', were 'not neurotic'. An exploration of the need for women only services was important in moving towards the creation of services 'visibly' sensitive to women (Jessup and Green, 1987). Connor and Babcock (1980) suggested that until sexism was recognized and worked through from all angles of these women's experiences (including treatment), it would continue to exist as a fuel for their 'pathology'.

The emergence of research on women

In spite of the increasing visibility of women in public domains and influential theoretical contributions from feminist researchers in many of the social sciences well before the 1990s (Ardener 1975; Duelli-Klein, 1983; Stanley, 1990; Stanley and Wise, 1990), significant research on women in the drugs and alcohol fields only began to emerge in the final decades of the twenty-first century. This shift was due in part to the increasing numbers of women involved in drugs and alcohol research who advocated for the development of research on women. For example, Jane Prather and Linda Fidell (1978) published an overview paper in the *International Journal of Addictions* arguing that little research existed on the female drug user, and it was 'imperative that women be included as subjects or respondents' (1978: 880). Such advocacy gradually had an impact on drugs and alcohol research in the contemporary period, as we will discuss below.

GENDERED THEMES IN CONTEMPORARY RESEARCH

Contesting the pathology/ powerlessness paradigm

By the 1990s, research on gender and alcohol and drugs began to situate women in opposition to the marginal realm they had previously occupied. Feminist researchers started to challenge the 'pathology or powerlessness' perspective (Anderson, 2008; Maher, 1997; Moore and Devitt, 1989; Murphy and Rosenbaum, 1999; Taylor, 1993). Research began to shift the lens of inquiry from women as abusers to consumers (Ettorre, 1992, 1997), from women's use as problematic to that of recreational (Henderson, 1993, 1996, 1999), and from abnormal or deviant to normal (Anderson, 1995, 1998; Ettorre, 2004, 2007; Measham, 2002). This paradigm shift highlighted the visibility of women in drugs and alcohol research both by investigating women's engagement with alcohol and drugs in contemporary settings, and specifically in public settings, as well as *making visible* the ways in which women had always been involved in the production and/or consumption of alcohol and drugs (Enefalk, 2015; Hunt et al., 2002; Miller and Carbone-Lopez, 2015; Moloney and Hunt, 2011). Importantly, research at this time begins to emphasize women's agency (Ettorre, 1992; Henderson, 1993, 1997; Maher, 1997; Measham, 2002; Taylor, 1993). Studies began to situate women's alcohol and drug use as active (though not always explicit) symbolic acts of resistance or power (Anderson, 2008; Miller and Carbone-Lopez, 2015; Moloney et al., 2015) or as markers for the construction of identities and lifestyles for young women (Ettorre, 1992; Hutton, 2006; Mullins, 2008; Pini, 2001).

Although epidemiologic research examined gendered comparisons of substance use prevalence, quantities, and frequencies (Bloomfield et al., 2001; Fillmore, 1987; Plant and Plant, 2001; Wilsnack et al., 2000, 2009), what was missing was a focus on the effects of drugs and alcohol on the construction of gendered identities. Yes, gender influences drugs and drinking practices (e.g. men and women have different rates of drug use or prefer different substances), but 'drug use itself can be seen as a way of doing gender' (Measham, 2002: 335). By drawing on Messerschmidt's (1997) ideas of gender as structured action, which are rooted in the sociological analysis of the accomplishment of gender (West and Fenstermaker, 1987, 1995), doing gender considers gender not as a static individual-level trait tightly connected to biological sex but as a process whereby gender is not possessed but rather accomplished in social interactions.

> [P]eople construct their gender identity, their masculinities and femininities... through their experiments with and experiences of drugs, the socio-cultural context of drugs cultures, and the drug-related attitudes and behaviors of women and men within those drug cultures. (Measham, 2002: 351)

Drugs, alcohol, and pleasure

Contemporary research in the drugs and alcohol fields has emphasized the ways in which engagement with drugs and alcohol contributes to how people accomplish their gendered identities in various socio-cultural contexts. For example, at the beginning of the 1990s, research in the drugs field was given a new fillip as a result of the development of the global rave scene and club cultures (Redhead, 1990, 1993, 1997), which was inextricably tied to an increasing consumption of ecstasy and other party or club drugs.[6] Unlike previous developments in illegal drug consumption, the consumption of ecstasy was tied not to any particular drug subculture (see Hunt and Joe-Laidler, 2016), but to mainstream youth cultures, shifting the status of drug users from 'marginal and "other"' to 'mainstream, ordinary and a part of the paramount reality of everyday life' (Measham, 2002: 344). Due to the significant number of young women participating in club cultures (McElrath and McEvoy, 2002; Solowij et al., 1992), this shift in status also applied to women who use drugs.

The rave and club dance scene, which began in the UK, provided an important alternative space where young women were allowed a greater degree of freedom. Dominant stereotypes of drug-using women, in which women were characterized as mad, bad, or sexually available (Hutton, 2006), came to be challenged. In responding to Ettorre's call (1992) to place pleasure at the center of the analysis of women's drug use, Henderson (1996) produced a seminal study of women, drugs, and pleasure. Listening to young women involved in the dance scene, highlighted, according to Henderson, the extent to which these women 'were not being frog-marched into drug use by men and were not leading unhappy lives as a result of their drug use' (1999:41). In fact, the central feature of their participation in the scene was *pleasure*. Moreover, Henderson argued that new analytical tools to understand pleasure were needed because the literature on gender and drug use had remained exactly where Ettorre (1989) had described it.

> Pleasure for most women appears as a subverted or hidden reality [and what was needed was] to look...more closely at the pleasurable effects of substances and in particular to ask ourselves why and how women experience their substance use as pleasurable. (Ettorre, 1989: 598–9).

To create these new tools, Henderson argued that researchers examine the importance of consumption for defining an individual's identity, including performing a gendered identity.[7]

Female drug taking was no longer considered a personal pathology. In fact, Pini (2001), in her work on clubs and raves, describes 'how early rave spaces provided an opportunity for women to experience themselves outside the prescribed structures of normative femininity' (chapter 7, this volume). Exploring how young women seek experiences of adventure, exploration, discovery, and pleasure, she found that women discovered a new freedom in using drugs. The dance floor coupled with the use of drugs allowed women to explore new kinds of femininity and challenge the boundaries of appropriate gendered behavior. This freedom was unusual, especially given the presence of men in the dance scene, because in most other situations young women's ability to become intoxicated had been strictly controlled both by men and by other women (see Hunt et al., 2000, 2002). However, as other writers have noted (McRobbie, 1994; Moloney and Hunt, 2011; Richard and Kruger, 1998), the shift in gender relations was not only for young women, it also influenced young men. As McRobbie notes:

> Laddishness has been replaced by friendliness... working class boys...undergo a conversion to the soft, the malleable and the sociable...Through the addictive pleasure of dance [and ecstasy] they also enter into a different relationship with their own bodies, more tactile, more sensuous, less focused round sexual gratification. (McRobbie, 1994:168)

Although research in the 1990s, especially in the UK, was dominated by work on drugs, raves, and clubs, by the early 2000s, young consumers began to change their 'drug of choice' from ecstasy to alcohol. Moreover, substantial changes occurring in young people's drinking cultures, changes to the drinks industry, and alcohol advertising and marketing all contributed to the development of more 'female-friendly' drinking spaces (Szmigin et al., 2008). Young women were also 'now playing an active part in a new and widespread culture of "extreme drinking" based on the regular normative practice of drinking to intoxication' (Griffin et al., 2013: 187). The apparent increase in public intoxication by women became a hot issue, which was given much attention in the public media. Although, within the public arena, female intoxication was viewed as solely an example of a growing public health and social order problem, a few researchers began to examine the meaning of intoxication for women and explore the extent to which female intoxication was a way of accomplishing femininity. Research on the night-time economy had emphasized the increasing feminization of drinking spaces and argued that the changing social position of women prompted changes to the gendered make up of public drinking venues (Chatterton and Hollands, 2003; Measham, 2005; Measham et al., 2001). With these changes, debates emerged about how women negotiated femininity within these new spaces previously defined by a masculine culture of drinking. Women were now expected to be able to drink heavily *like a man,* while also demonstrating restraint and 'respectability' (Bailey et al., 2015; Gill, 2007; Griffin et al., 2013; Hutton et al., 2013; Lyons and Willott, 2008; McRobbie, 2000; McRobbie, 2009; Measham and Brain, 2005; Montemurro and McClure, 2005; Sheehan and Ridge, 2001).

For example, Waitt and colleagues (2011) argued that becoming intoxicated from alcohol allowed women to perform gender differently by 'assert[ing] an alternative femininity that embraces the risks of drinking and drunkenness' (Waitt, 2011:271). They examined how young women in Australia negotiated their subjectivities through their drinking practices and used intoxication and losing control as a way of breaking everyday boundaries and escaping the demands of living in a neo-liberal society. Their research suggested that in drinking heavily with other women, young women emphasized the pleasures of drunkenness. They used drunkenness as a way of engaging in behaviors deemed to violate normative gendered expressions. However, though supportive of this emancipatory perspective that situates young women's use of intoxication as a form of liberation, others have cautioned against the simplicity of this post-feminist emancipatory framework by also highlighting the other side of this new alcohol order: the competing pressures for women to be able to navigate and manage the risks associated with becoming intoxicated including maintaining notions of feminine respectability. For example, Griffin and colleagues argue that young women today, involved in new cultures of intoxication, are presented with an 'impossible space to occupy' (Griffin et al., 2013: 186).

Gender identity, masculinity, drugs, and alcohol

Significant contributions by contemporary feminist scholars also paved the way for discussions of gender identity and ultimately notions of masculinity as it relates to men's engagement with alcohol and drugs. Interest in studying masculinities within the social sciences more generally came much later than research on women and gender. As Mac an Ghaill notes, 'until recently masculinity has tended to be absent from mainstream academic research' (1996:1). Studies of gender focused on women and a largely unitary notion of masculinity operated. Connell's seminal works (1987, 1995) on masculinity emphasized the importance of examining the multiple forms of masculinities, just as feminist scholars had emphasized the multiple forms of femininity. He argued that not only were masculinities differentiated, they also stood against one another in relations of power. Adopting Gramsci's (1971) notion of hegemony, Connell argued that hegemonic masculinity is 'established by the domination of one masculinity over others' (Mac an Ghaill and Haywood, 2007: 30). Thus, masculinities are 'not fixed character types but configurations of practice generated in particular situations in a changing structure of relationships' (Connell, 1995: 81).[8]

Although limited in number, studies in this vein have tended to focus on the use of alcohol and drugs in the construction of a hegemonic masculine ideal, whereby men are expected to 'act like real men' by being 'wild, tough, popular, youthful, aggressive, competitive, confident, and anti-feminine' (De Visser and McDonnell, 2012; De Visser and Smith, 2007; Peralta, 2007: Schacht, 1996). This has been supported in contemporary epidemiologic studies that have focused on masculine norms and alcohol-related aggression and violence (Graham and Wells 2003; Miller et al., 2014; Wells et al., 2011, 2013). For example, Bourgois' (1996) ethnographic work on urban drug economies in the United States describes marginalized Puerto Rican men's participation in a misogynistic and violent street life and drug culture as a way to reclaim masculine status in a society where women's rights are continually expanding and traditional working class patriarchies are disappearing.[9] Similarly, Peralta's (2007) work on gender and alcohol use among college students in the United States considers the role of alcohol in the construction of hegemonic masculinity. His work suggests that the predominance of heavy drinking by white men marks a hegemonic masculine status, whereby heavy drinking becomes associated with demonstrations of power and light consumption with '"weakness" or otherness' (2007: 750). However, as West (2001) shows, masculinities can also 'be contradictory, challenged, [and] paradoxical…in other words, quite complex…men can express deeply felt emotions when drunk ("crying in your beer") even to their buddies (homosocial love with sexual undertones)' (2001: 373). De Visser and Smith (2007), in their examination of multiple masculinities, argue that it is critical to explore the links between different forms of masculinity and different patterns of alcohol consumption. They note the linkage between hegemonic masculinity and excessive alcohol consumption but also acknowledge that other forms of masculinity can be associated with abstinence or moderate alcohol consumption.

Studying drug economies

Although research on youth cultures contributes significantly to gendered themes in contemporary research (McRobbie, 1995), analogous themes have emerged in studies on drug economies and treatment. Debates about a post-feminist emancipatory framework (McRobbie, 2009) have also been central in research on the changing role of women in drug markets. Although early drug sales research was male-dominated (both in terms of researchers and research subjects), a number of important studies on women drug sellers and their participation in drug markets have contributed important gendered perspectives in contemporary research on drugs (Anderson, 2005; Baskin and Sommers, 2008; Denton and O'Malley, 1999; Fagan, 1994; Maher and Daly, 1996; Maher and Hudson, 2007; Morgan and Joe, 1997; O'Malley and Valverde, 2004). For instance, Maher's work on gendered resistance in the Brooklyn drug market (1997) suggests that street life, although an arena for harassment and victimization (Adler and Adler, 1985; Maher, 1997; Miller, 2001), may offer women opportunities to have a sense of mastery, independence, individual accomplishment, and immediate reward. Several debates have emerged about women's relative levels of empowerment in drug markets versus their continuing exploitation, victimization, or powerlessness; the changing roles of women in the drug economies, from heroin markets to growing opportunities in crack cocaine era to diversified roles in contemporary drug markets (Anderson, 2005; Baskin and Sommers, 2008; Fagan, 1994; Maher and

Daly, 1996; Maher and Johnson, 2007; Miller 2001; Morgan and Joe, 1997). Although women have had an increasing role in the drug economy (Anderson, 2005, 2008; Griffin and Rodriguez, 2011; Hutton, 2005), women's participation largely remains in the lower level roles, and drug markets continue to be highly gender stratified (Maher and Johnson, 2007).

Some researchers (Anderson, 2005; Driscoll, 2000) have argued that while recent studies have highlighted the role of women in the illicit drug economy, they have failed to adequately capture the complexity of power relations within the drug economy and the ways in which power relates to and structures gender. Most studies have only looked at how women *respond* to the male dominated structure of the illicit drug market (Denton and O'Malley, 1999; Dunlap et al., 1994; Johnston et al., 2000; Morgan and Joe, 1996). By focusing solely on the pressures and responses by women in the drug economy, this theoretical perspective overlooks the more active and potentially powerful aspects of their role in it (Anderson, 2005; Driscoll, 2000; Taylor, 1993). As Anderson (2005) contends, while men may hold the structural sources of power in the drug market, this is possible only because of women's relational power. That is, 'women's...relational power assists males' accumulation of structural power and is therefore fundamental to "successful" (i.e. stable and lasting) illicit drug world organization' (Anderson, 2005: 373). Consequently, men and women's power and roles in the world of drug selling are interdependent.

Treatment and gender

Contemporary studies on treatment also began to question the male bias in treatment studies and situate women's drug and alcohol use within a broader structural, or at least social, context (Bjønness, 2012, 2015; Thom, 1986, 1987). The treatment of women involves a complex process in which the needs of women should be recognized as different from men's (Thom, 1984). At the end of the twentieth century, feminist researchers began to challenge the stigmatization of women's drug and alcohol use, arguing for 'a "woman-sensitive perspective" where the "genealogy of women's collective struggle"' (Ettorre, 1997: 165) was made a central feature. For example, in her book, *Women and Alcohol,* Ettorre argues that:

> There is a continual need to examine women's experiences with alcohol and to recognize that these experiences reflect the constant struggle for women to maintain their integrity and self-worth in a substance-using, anxiety-ridden society that does not value women. (Ettorre, 1997: 165)

Undeniably, treatment work carried out within the past two decades accentuates the importance of gender sensitive and/or feminist perspectives for treatment and policy (Du Rose, 2015; Friedman and Alicea, 2001; Kandall, 1996; Klee et al., 2001; Sterk, 1999, Sterk et al., 2002; Stevens and Wexler, 1998; Raine, 2001) and theoretical developments (Boyd, 1999; Campbell, 1999, 2000; Denton and O'Malley, 1999; Evans et al., 2002; Henderson, 1999; Hunt et al., 2002; Irwin, 1995; Murphy and Rosenbaum, 1999; Wright, 2002; Measham, 2002). Rather than grand theories, local narratives of normalization were constructed that focused on consumers or users with specific needs and demands. This perspective also created space for the development of Afrocentric treatment principles (Roberts et al., 2000: 903) or treatments sensitive to indigenous people (Segal, 2001).

NEW DIRECTIONS

Intersectionality

Nuanced considerations of gender have increasingly been incorporated into studies of drugs and alcohol, shedding light on the contextually-dependent performances of multiple masculinities and femininities and the relationships between these multiple identities and the meaning of drugs and alcohol use. Though feminist researchers have been acutely aware of the limitations of gender as a single analytical category, much of the field is still constrained by gender dualism, neglecting a focus on the fluidity of genders and the transformative processes involved. Moreover, the field continues to largely overlook other social identities defined by, for example, ethnicity, social class, and/or sexuality that intensify disadvantage for certain people (Thorne, 1993; Miller and Carbone-Lopez, 2015). Future directions in the drugs and alcohol fields, as Miller and Carbone-Lopez argue, should move beyond simply a 'doing gender' framework and incorporate an investigation of the multiple and intersecting social inequalities that people experience and that shape their gender performances (Miller and Carbone-Lopez, 2015).

Although no widely agreed upon definition exists, the theory of intersectionality or 'multiracial feminism'[10] is a feminist sociological paradigm that focuses on the complicated ways in which overlapping social inequities shape lived experiences and social identities (Crenshaw, 1989, 1991; Hancock, 2007; Hankivsky and Cormier, 2009; McCall, 2005). While the theory emerged both from black feminism and queer and postcolonial theory (Collins, 1990; hooks, 1984; Sedgwick, 1990), the term was officially used by Crenshaw (1989, 1991) who contributed significantly to the field of intersectionality by highlighting the invisibility of black women, as well as arguing that social identity categories were wrongly conceptualized as independent, with one assumed to be dominant. Intersectionality moves beyond the use of single categories of analysis such as class, gender, race, and instead, suggests that the interaction between 'different aspects of social identity (e.g. race, ethnicity, indigeneity, gender, class, sexuality, geography, age, ability, immigration status, religion) as well as the impact of systems and processes of oppression and domination (e.g. racism, classism, sexism, ableism, homophobia)' (Hankivsky and Cormier, 2009: 3) should be central in research. These processes produce what Collins (2000) has called 'the matrix of domination', 'in which people are situated according to their differences from one another' (Burgess-Procter, 2006: 36). A key element to class-race-gender 'is that social relations are viewed in multiple and interactive terms – not as additive' (Daly, 1993: 56).

Although the field has largely neglected an intersectional approach, some important studies exist (Bailey et al., 2015; Dunlap et al., 1997; Maher, 1997; Miller and Carbone-Lopez, 2015; Peralta and Jauk, 2011; Windsor et al., 2010). Maher (1997) was one of the first feminist researchers in the drugs and alcohol fields to grapple with the issue of multiple inequalities in her study of women drug users in New York drug markets. She explored the intersections of race, class, and gender in their lives, explaining how their involvement in the street-level drug economy had shifted from 'primarily class-based explanations towards acknowledgement of a more complex set of cross-cutting influences – race/ethnicity, sex/gender, age, immigrant status, and other social relations' (Maher, 1997:169). She argues that these cross-cutting influences exclude some while privileging others. Maher produces a nuanced understanding of women's agency that 'sees women neither exclusively as victims nor as unfettered actors' (Britton, 2000: 62). She also highlights the ways in which the enforcement of gender and racial divisions within the informal drug economy limited 'women's economic opportunities, placed them at disadvantage to men and channeled them into sex work' (Daly, 2006: 207).

Significant critical studies of US drug policies have also relied on theories of intersectionality to examine the potential consequences of Eurocentric policymaking that arguably further disadvantage communities of color (Benoit, et al., 2003; Windsor and Dunlap, 2010; Windsor et al., 2010, 2012). For example, Windsor and Dunlap (2010) considered the incongruence between the lived experiences of low-income African American drug users and sellers and the assumptions underpinning US drug policies designed to criminalize use and require forced treatment for offenders. They found that participants were not deterred from using because of fears of imprisonment and instead such threats only intensified their distrust of police. Furthermore, coerced treatment was not considered a long-term solution for alleviating use but instead a 'rest period' from drug use in exchange for avoiding criminal charges and lengthy prison sentences. Such investigations have highlighted the multiple disadvantages that confront drug users and sellers who hold overlapping and stigmatized social identities.

More recently, Miller and Carbone-Lopez (2015) critically compared the usefulness of a 'doing gender' framework with theories of intersectionality in examining methamphetamine use among white, working class women in rural Missouri. While acknowledging the debt to the 'doing gender' approach (West and Zimmerman, 1987) in advancing our understanding of gender, they nevertheless raised concerns about the disproportionate emphasis on the normative features of gender. They emphasized the importance of moving beyond this approach to also investigate 'doing race, class and place'. In examining drug use among this population of white methamphetamine users, they were able to explore the 'racialized cultural understandings of white womanhood' (Miller and Carbone-Lopez, 2015:7). Women perceived their drug use in opposition to stereotypes of crack use among black mothers. These notions of white womanhood could be seen in their narratives that emphasized narrative frames of 'supermom', 'superwoman', and 'superthin'. Such narrative frames, while available to these white women, may be less readily available for drug users who are women of color, whose narrative accounts may be more influenced by reacting to dominant media accounts of crack mothers, crime, and prostitution.

To date, multiple debates and developments of intersectionality have dominated the social sciences (Brown, 2012; May, 2014; Phoenix and Pattynama, 2006). However, in spite of the popularity of this approach in feminist sociology, criminology, ethnic studies, and gender studies, it is largely neglected in the drugs and alcohol fields, a surprising oversight given the larger contemporary context of third wave feminism which has highlighted the centrality of diversity and the existence of multiple genders, races, and sexualities (Burgess-Procter, 2006). One possible explanation for this omission may be the under-representation or invisibility of feminist scholars in our fields, who themselves hold other overlapping and stigmatized social identities. Nevertheless, despite the reason for this oversight, the drugs and alcohol fields can be arguably defined by 'epistemologies of ignorance' (Tuana, 2004, 2006: Ettorre 2014), suggesting that knowledge is produced within a social system defined by hegemonic structures and inequalities (Campbell and Ettorre, 2011). Both knowledge and ignorance are imbedded within our field.

Within the context of the need for intersectionality, Campbell and Ettorre (2011) trace the ways in which the production of knowledge in research and treatment have made the drugs and alcohol fields resistant to gendered, classed, and racialized power differentials that structure the lives of drug-using women. By overlooking these power differentials, women's specific needs remain unknown. Indeed, 'epistemologies of ignorance' (Tuana, 2004, 2006) have been an integral component of 'doing gender as well as race, class and place' in an effort to better understand women substance users' experiences and needs.

CONCLUSION

A recent special issue on studies of gender within drugs and alcohol research (Frank and Hunt, 2015) noted that although gender had long been a central feature in research on drug and alcohol users, until recently, much of the research had suffered from two tendencies. First, research had viewed alcohol and drug consumption primarily from a male perspective, and second, the existing research had been slow to incorporate new theoretical developments on gender from the wider social sciences (Hunt et al., 2015). In writing this paper on the study of gender in research on alcohol and drugs, we have sought to explore these two tendencies, noting how the field, until the early 1990s, had focused primarily on men and had viewed women and alcohol and drugs primarily from a pathological perspective. Since then, feminist thinking in gender studies gradually has had an impact on drugs and alcohol research and has had the effect of questioning the pathology perspective and of introducing instead a framework that emphasized women's agency. Feminist thinking not only influenced research on women, it also stimulated research on notions of masculinity, which, in turn, has begun to shape some research on drugs and alcohol.

The impact of recent sociological and feminist critiques has also led to a more vigorous questioning of studies that have focused solely on gender and the extent to which this research is constrained by notions of gender dualism. Theorists have begun to adopt an intersectionality approach that permits not solely an analysis of gender, but also, and equally important, a focus on the intersecting influences of race, ethnicity, social class, and sexuality. Along with this approach has been a developing interest in embodiment theory (see for example Ettorre 2010, 2014) However, while such developments are critically important for feminist and social science research on drugs and alcohol, they are, at the moment, relatively few, and consequently, have had little or no impact on the ever-expanding epidemiological research that dominates the field. This research appears both blissfully ignorant of alternative perspectives and seemingly happy to continue their research on gender as though it were merely a socio-demographic characteristic. To end this overview from a more personal perspective, we would wish to note that for those of us who have conducted research in this field for many years and have sought to introduce a more feminist approach to the study of gender and alcohol and drugs, we are somewhat less than optimistic of the impact of feminist thinking within our fields. While we have been both excited and frequently energized by feminist developments, we have nevertheless found ourselves enmeshed in examining the existing literature on gender and drugs and alcohol and wondering if the field will ever take account of these feminist developments. In charting the history of this research since the early 1900s, we have emphasized new developments that have occurred but we still continue to wonder how long it will be before our fields place gender issues at the center and expose our own 'epistemologies of ignorance'.

NOTES

1 For a further discussion of the impact of social policy on research, see Chauncey (1980) and Mauss (1991).
2 The Human Relations Area Files, based at Yale University, began in 1949 with the aim of developing and distributing files of organized information to enable comparative studies of human societies and cultures.
3 For exceptions, see Ettorre (1989, 1992; 2010).
4 During this period, approximately 250,000 committals to prison annually for drunkenness occurred (Hunt et al., 1989).
5 Women substance users experience a variety of problems of living or what Murphy and Rosenbaum (1987) referred to as 'polyproblems'. These 'polyproblems' do not allow these women to fit comfortably within established treatment systems. Specifically, for women substance users,

fundamental issues such as domestic stress, violence in the family, 'sex role conflict', recreational drug use, the heterogeneity of women as a social group, the need for a gender sensitive perspective, and a broad focus on women's 'polyproblems' remain hidden if not ignored.

6 Although the rave scene gradually developed into a global phenomenon, its early flowering occurred in the UK in the late 1980s and early 1990s. Consequently, much of the seminal literature, which initially examined issues of raves and drugs, was UK based. However, since then, studies of raves, clubs, and drugs have been conducted in number of different countries including the US, Denmark, Hong Kong, Australia, India, and Canada (Hunt et al., 2010; Joe-Laidler et al., 2014; Ravn, 2012; Saldanha, 2007; St. John, 2009).

7 For an extended discussion of identity and consumption, see Campbell (1989), Featherstone (1991), Miles (2000), and Miller (1995).

8 For a critique of the notion of Hegemonic masculinity, see Connell and Messerschmidt (2005).

9 For a critique of Bourgois' use of an emancipation thesis and his failure to elaborate the nature of women's participation in the drug economy and the ways in which their gendered status structures their participation, see Maher (1997).

10 For a fuller explanation of this term, see Baca Zinn and Dill (1996).

REFERENCES

Adler, P. and Adler, P. (1985) 'Women drug users: an ethnography of a female injecting community', *Journal of Contemporary Ethnography*, 24(2):229–232.

Anderson, T. (1995) 'Toward a preliminary macro theory of drug addiction', *Deviant Behavior: An Interdisciplinary Journal*, 16: 353–72.

Anderson, T. (1998) 'A cultural identity theory of drug abuse', *Sociology of Crime, Law and Deviance*, 1: 233–62.

Anderson, T. (2005) 'Dimensions of women's power in the illicit drug economy', *Theoretical Criminology*, 9(4): 371–400.

Anderson, T. (ed.) (2008) *Neither Villain nor Victim: Empowerment and Agency Among Women Substance Abusers*. New Brunswick: Rutgers University Press.

Ardener, E. (1975) 'Belief and the problem of women', In S. Ardener (ed.), *Perceiving Women*. London: Dent and Sons, pp. 1–17.

Baca Zinn, M. and Dill, B. (1996) 'Theorizing difference from multiracial feminism', *Feminist Studies*, 22(2): 321–31.

Bacon, M. (1976) Cross-cultural studies of drinking: integrated drinking and sex differences in the use of alcoholic beverages. In M.W. Everett, J.O. Waddell and D.B. Heath (eds.), *Cross-Cultural Approaches to the Study of Alcohol*. The Hague: Mouton, pp. 23–33.

Bailey, L., Griffin, C. and Shankar, A. (2015) '"Not a good look": impossible dilemmas for young women negotiating the culture of intoxication in the United Kingdom', *Substance Use and Misuse*, 50(6): 747–58.

Bales, R.F. (1962) 'Attitudes towards drinking in the Irish Culture', In D. Pittman and C. Snyder (eds), *Society, Culture and Drinking Patterns*. New York: Wiley and Sons, pp. 157–85.

Baskin, D. and Sommers, I. (2008) 'Demonstrating a female-specific agency and empowerment in drug selling', In T. Anderson (ed.), *Neither Villain nor Victim: Empowerment and Agency among Women Substance Abusers*. New Brunswick: Rutgers University Press, pp. 49–64.

Beckman, L. (1978) 'Self-esteem of women alcoholics', *Journal of Studies on Alcohol*, 39(3): 491–8.

Bemko, J. and Davidson, V. (1978) 'International review of women and drug abuse (1966–1975)', *Journal of the American Women's Medical Association*, 33(12): 507–18.

Benoit, E., Randolph, D., and Dunlap, E. (2003) Code Switching and Inverse Imitation Among Marijuana-Using Crack Sellers. *British Journal of Criminology* 43(3): 506–525

Bjønness, J. (2012) 'Between emotional politics and biased practices – prostitution policies, social work and women selling sexual services in Denmark', *Sexuality Research and Social Policy*, 9(3): 192–202.

Bjønness, J (2015) Narratives about necessity – constructions of motherhood among drug-using prostitutes in Denmark. *Substance Use and Misuse*, 50(6): 783–93.

Bloomfield, K., Gmel, G., Neve, R. and Mustonen, H. (2001) 'Investigating gender convergence in alcohol consumption in Finland, Germany, the Netherlands, and Switzerland: a repeated survey analysis', *Substance Abuse*, 22: 39–53.

Blume, S.B. (1985) 'Women and alcohol: a review', *JAMA*, 256: 1467–70.

Booth, B. (1911) 'The management of the inebriate woman', *The British Journal of Inebriety*, 9(2): 53–108.

Booth, C. (1969) Charles Booth's London: a portrait of the poor at the turn of the century,: Drawn from 'Life and labour of the people in London'. London: Hutchinson.

Borodin, R. (1981) *Women and Temperance: The Quest for Power and Liberty 1873–1990*. Philadelphia: Temple University Press.

Bourgois, P. (1996) *In Search of Respect: Selling Crack in El Barrio*. New York: Cambridge University Press.

Boyd, S. (1999) *Mothers and Illicit Drugs*. Toronto: University of Toronto Press.

Broom, D. (ed.) (1994) *Double Bind: Women Affected by Alcohol and Other Drugs*. St. Leonards: Allen and Unwin PTY Ltd.

Britton, D. (2000) 'The epistemology of the gendered organization', *Gender and Society*, 14(3): 418–34.

Brown, M. (2012) 'Gender and sexuality I: intersectional anxieties', *Progress in Human Geography*, 36(4): 541–50.

Burawoy, M. (2005) '2004 American Sociological Association Presidential address: for public sociology', *American Sociological Review*, 70(1): 4–28.

Burgess-Procter. A. (2006) 'Intersections of race, class, gender, and crime future directions for feminist criminology', *Feminist Criminology*, 1(1): 27–47.

Campbell, C. (1989) *The Romantic Ethic and the Spirit of Modern Consumerism*. Oxford: Basil Blackwell Ltd.

Campbell, N. (1999) 'Regulating "maternal instinct": governing mentalities of late twentieth century US illicit drug policy', *SIGNS: Journal of Women in Culture and Society*, 24(4): 895–923.

Campbell, N. (2000) *Using Women: Gender, Drug Policy and Social Justice*. London: Routledge.

Campbell, N.D. and Ettorre, E. (2011) *Gendering Addiction: The Politics of Drug Treatment in a Neurochemical World*. Houndmills: Palgrave MacMillan.

Chatterton, P. and Hollands, R. (2003) *Urban Nightscapes: Youth Cultures, Pleasure Spaces and Corporate Power*. London: Routledge.

Chauncey, R. (1980) 'New careers for moral entrepreneurs: teenage drinking', *Journal of Drug Issues*, 10(1): 45–70.

Clark, P. (1983) *The English Alehouse: A Social History 1200–1830*. London: Longman.

Collins, P.H. (1990). *Black Feminist Thought: Knowledge, Consciousness, and the Politics of Empowerment*. Boston: Unwin Hyman.

Collins, P. (2000) *Black Feminist Thought: Knowledge, Consciousness, and the Politics of Empowerment*, 2nd edn. New York: Routledge.

Collison, M. (1996) 'In search of the high life: drugs, crime, masculinities and consumption', *British Journal of Criminology*, 36(3): 428–44.

Connell, R.W. (1987) *Gender and Power*. Stanford: Stanford University Press.

Connell, R.W. (1995) *Masculinities*. Berkeley: University of California Press.

Connell, R.W. and Messerschmidt, J. (2005) 'Hegemonic masculinity: rethinking the concept', *Gender and Society*, 19(6): 829–59.

Connor, B. and Babcock, M. (1980) 'The impact of feminist psychotherapy on the treatment of women alcoholics', *Focus on Women: Journal of Addictions and Health*, 1(2): 77–92.

Crenshaw, K. (1989). 'Demarginalizing the intersection of race and sex: a black feminist critique of antidiscrimination doctrine, feminist theory and antiracist politics', *University of Chicago Legal Forum*, 139: 139–67.

Crenshaw, K. (1991) 'Mapping the margins: intersectionality, identity politics, and violence against women of color', *Stanford Law Review*, 43(6): 1241–99.

Cuskey, W. R., Premkumar, T. and Sigel, L. (1972) 'Survey of opiate addiction among females in the United States between 1850 and 1970', *Public Health Reviews*, 1: 7–39.

d'Orban, P. (1970) 'Heroin dependence and delinquency in women – a study of heroin addicts in Holloway prison', *British Journal of Addiction*, 65: 67–78.

Daly, K. (1993) 'Class-race-gender: sloganeering in search of meaning', *Social Justice*, 20: 56–71.

Daly, K. (2006) 'Feminist thinking about crime and justice', In S. Henry and M. Lanier (eds), *The Essential Criminology Reader*. Boulder: Westview Press, pp. 205–13.

Dennis, N., Henriques, F. and Slaughter, C. (1956) *Coal is Our Life*. London: Eyre and Spottiswoode.

Denton, B. and O'Malley, P. (1999) 'Gender, trust and business: women drug dealers in the illicit economy', *British Journal of Criminology*, 39(4): 513–30.

de Visser, R.O. and McDonnell, E. (2012) 'That's OK. He's a guy': a mixed methods study of gender double standards for alcohol use', *Psychology and Health*, 27(5): 618–39.

de Visser, R.O. and Smith, J. (2007) 'Alcohol consumption and masculine identity among young men', *Psychology and Health*, 22(5): 595–614.

Driscoll, L. (2000) *Reconsidering Drugs: Mapping Victorian and Modern Drug Discourses*. New York: Palgrave.

Duelli-Klein, R. (1983) 'How to do what we want to do: thoughts about feminist methodology', In G. Bowles and R. Duelli-Klein (eds), *Theories of Women's Studies*. London: Routledge & Kegan Paul, pp. 88–104.

Dunlap, E., Johnson, B.D. and Maher, L. (1997) 'Female crack dealers in New York City: who they are and what they do', *Women and Criminal Justice*, 8(4): 24–55.

Dunlap, E., Johnson, B.D. and Manwar, A. (1994) 'A successful female crack dealer: case study of a deviant career', *Deviant Behavior,* 15: 1–25.

Du Rose, N. (2015) *The Governance of Female Drug Users: Women's Experiences of Drug Policy*. Bristol: Policy Press.

Ellinwood, E., Smith, W. and Vaillant, G. (1966). 'Narcotic addiction in males and females: a comparison', *International Journal of the Addictions*, 1(2): 33–45.

Enefalk, H. (2015) 'Alcohol and femininity in Sweden c. 1830–1922: an investigation of the emergence of separate drinking standards for men and women', *Substance Use & Misuse*, 50(6): 736–46.

Ettorre, E.M. (1985) 'A study of alcoholism treatment units: some findings on patients', *Alcohol and Alcoholism*, 20(4): 361–9.

Ettorre, E.M. (1986) 'Women and drunken sociology: developing a feminist analysis', *Women's Studies International Forum*, 9(5): 515–20.

Ettorre, E.M. (1989) 'Women and substance use/abuse: towards a feminist perspective or how to make dust fly', *Women's Studies International Forum*, 12(6): 593–602.

Ettorre, E. M. (1992) *Women and Substance Use*. Houndmills: Macmillan.

Ettorre, E. M. (1997) *Women and Alcohol: From a Private Pleasure to a Public Problem?* London: Women's Press.

Ettorre, E.M. (2004) 'Revisioning women and drug use: gender sensitivity, gendered bodies and reducing harm', *International Journal of Drugs Policy*, 15(5–6): 327–35.

Ettorre, E.M. (2007) *Revisioning Women and Drug Use: Gender, Power and the Body*. Basingstoke: Palgrave Macmillan.

Ettorre, E.M. (2010) 'Bodies, drugs and reproductive regimes', In E. Ettorre (ed.), *Culture, Bodies and Sociology of Health*. Aldershot: Ashgate, pp. 155–72.

Ettorre, E. M. (2014) 'Embodied deviance, gender and epistemologies of ignornance: Re-visioning drug use in a neurochemical, unjust world' *Substance Use and Misuse*, 50(6):794–805.

Evans R.D., Forsyth, C.D. and Gauthier, D.K. (2002) 'Gendered pathways into and experiences within crack cultures outside of the inner city', *Deviant Behavior: An Interdisciplinary Journal*, 23(6): 483–510.

Fagan, J. (1994) 'Women and drugs revisited: female participation in the cocaine economy', *Journal of Drug Issues*, 24(2): 179–225.

Featherstone, M. (1991) *Consumer Culture and Postmodernism*. London: Sage.

Fillmore, K.M. (1987) 'Women's drinking across the adult life course as compared to men's', *British Journal of Addiction*, 82: 801–11.

Finnegan, L.P. (1975) 'Narcotic dependence in pregnancy', *Journal of Psychedelic Drugs,* 7: 299.

Finnegan, L.P. (1978) 'Management of pregnant drug dependent women', *Annals of the New-York Academy of Sciences*, 311: 135–46.

Finnegan, L.P., Emich, J.P. Connaughton, J.F., and Wieland, W. (1973) 'Comprehensive care of the pregnant addict and its effect on maternal and infant outcome', *Contemporary Drug Problems,* 1: 795–809.

Finnegan, L.P., Bookhart, P.R., Moten, L., Cohen, C. and Goodman, N. (1976) 'Comprehensive services to drug dependent women and their children', In A. Schecter, H. Alksne and E. Kaufman (eds), *Critical Concerns in the Field of Drug Abuse*. New York: Marcel Dekker, Inc., pp. 745–9.

Frank, V, and Hunt, G. (2015). "Rethinking Gender within Alcohol and Drug Use Research" Special Issue. *Substance Use and Misuse*. 50(6).

Friedman, J. and Alicea, M. (2001). *Surviving Heroin: Interviews with Women in Methadone Clinics*. Gainesville: University Press of Florida.

Gill, R.C. (2007). *Gender and the Media*. Cambridge: Polity Press.

Gomberg, E.S.L. (1982) 'Historical and political overview: women and drug use', *Journal of Social Issues*, 38(2): 9–23.

Graham, K. and Wells, S. (2003). '"Somebody's gonna get their head kicked in tonight!" Aggression among young males in bars—a question of values?' *British Journal of Criminology*, 43(3): 546–66.

Gramsci, A. (1971) *Selections from the Prison Notebooks*. London: Lawrence and Wishart.

Griffin, M. and Rodriguez, N. (2011) 'The gendered nature of drug acquisition behavior within marijuana and crack drug markets', *Crime and Delinquency*, 57(3): 408–31

Griffin, C., Szmigin, I., Bengry-Howell, A., Hackley, C. and Mistral, W. (2013). 'Inhabiting the contradictions: hypersexual femininity and the culture of intoxication among young women in the UK', *Feminism and Psychology*, 23(2): 184–206.

Gusfield, J. (1955) 'Social structure and moral reform: a study of the Woman's Christian Temperance Union', *American Journal of Sociology*, 61(3): 221–32.

Hancock, A. (2007). 'When multiplication doesn't equal quick addition: examining intersectionality as a research paradigm', *Perspectives on Politics*, 5(1): 63–79.

Hankivsky, O. and Cormier, R. (2009). *Intersectionality: Moving Women's Health Research and Policy Forward*. Vancouver: Women's Health Research Network.

Harrison, B. (1971) *Drink and the Victorians: The Temperance Question in England 1815–1872*. London: Faber and Faber.

Heath, D. (1991) Women and alcohol: cross-cultural perspectives. *Journal of Substance Abuse*, 3: 175–85.

Heath, D. (2000) *Drinking Occasions: Comparative Perspectives on Alcohol and Culture*. International Center for Alcohol Policies: Series on Alcohol in Society. London: Taylor and Francis.

Hellman, E. (1934) 'The importance of beer brewing in an urban native yard', *Bantu Studies*, 8: 38–60.

Henderson, S. (1993) 'Fun, frisson and fashion', *International Journal of Drug Policy*, 4(3): 122–9.

Henderson, S. (1996) 'E Types and dance divas: gender research and community prevention', In T. Rhodes and R. Hartnoll (eds), *AIDS, Drugs and Prevention: Perspectives on Individual and Community Action*. London: Routledge. pp. 66–85.

Henderson, S. (1999) 'Drugs and culture: the question of gender', In N. South (ed.), *Drugs: Cultures, Controls and Everyday Life*. London: Sage Publications, pp. 36–48.

hooks, bell. 1984. *Feminist Theory: From Margin to Center*. Cambridge: South End Press.

Horton, D. (1943) 'The functions of alcohol in primitive societies: a cross-cultural study', *Quarterly Journal of Studies on Alcohol*, 4: 199–230.

Hunt, G. and Joe-Laidler, K. (2016) 'The culture and subcultures of illicit drug use and distribution', In H.H. Brownstein (ed.), *The Handbook of Drugs and Society.* Malden: Wiley-Blackwell, pp. 460–81.

Hunt, G., Mellor, J. and Turner, J. (1989). '"Wretched, hatless and miserably clad": women and the inebriate reformatories from 1900–1913', *British Journal of Sociology*, 40(2): 244–70.

Hunt, G., Joe-Laidler, K. and MacKenzie, K. (2000) '"Chillin', being dogged and getting buzzed": alcohol in the lives of female gang members', *Drugs: Education, Prevention and Policy*, 7(4): 331–53.

Hunt, G., Joe-Laidler, K. and Evans, K. (2002) 'The meaning and gendered culture of getting high: gang girls and drug use issues', *Contemporary Drug Problems*, 29(2): 375–411.

Hunt, G., Moloney, M. and Evans, K. (2010) *Youth, Drugs and Nightlife*. London: Routledge.

Hunt, G. Frank, V. and Moloney, M. (Eds.) (2015). Rethinking Gender within Alcohol and Drug Research: Introduction, Substance Use and Misuse. Special Issue. 50(6): 685–692.

Hutton, F. (2005) 'Risky business: gender, drug dealing and risk', *Addiction Research and Theory*, 13(6): 545–54.

Hutton, F. (2006) *Risky pleasures? Club cultures and feminine identities*. Burlington: Ashgate.

Hutton, F. Wright, S. and Saunders, E. (2013) 'Cultures of intoxication: young women, alcohol, and harm reduction', *Contemporary Drug Problems*, 40: 451–80.

Hyslop, A. (1976) Temperance, Christianity and feminism: the Woman's Christian Temperance Union of Victoria, 1887–1997. *Historical Studies*, 17(66): 27–49.

Irwin, K. (1995) 'Ideology, pregnancy and drugs: differences between crack-cocaine, heroin and methamphetamine users', *Contemporary Drug Problems,* 22: 613–37.

Jessup, M. and Green, J. (1987) 'Treatment of the pregnant alcohol-dependent woman', *Journal of Psychoactive Drugs*, 19(2): 193–203.

Joe-Laidler, K., Hunt, G. and Moloney, M. (2014). '"Tuned out or tuned in:" spirituality and youth drug use in global times', In P. Withington and A. McShane (eds), *Cultures of Intoxication, Past and Present Supplement* 9: 61–80.

Johnson, B.D., Dunlap, E., and Tourigny, S.C. (2000) 'Crack distribution and abuse in New York', In M. Natarajan and M. Hough (eds), *Illegal Drug Markets: From Research to Prevention Policy*. Monsey: Criminal Justice Press. pp. 19–77

Johnson, R.A. and Gerstein, D.R. (2000) 'Age, period, and cohort effects in marijuana and alcohol incidence: United States females and males, 1961–1990', *Substance Use and Misuse*, 35: 925–48.

Kalant, O.J. (1980). Introduction. In O.J. Kalant (ed.), *Alcohol and Drug Problems in Women*. New York: Plenum Press. pp. 1–24.

Kandall, S. (1996) *Substance and Shadow: Women and Addiction in the United States,* Cambridge: Harvard University Press.

Keane, H. (2009) 'Intoxication, harm and pleasure: an analysis of the Australian National Alcohol Strategy', *Critical Public Health*, 19(2): 135–42.

Keller, M. (ed.) (1965). A Cross-Cultural Study of Drinking (Supplement 3), New Haven, CT: Quarterly Journal of Studies on Alcohol.

Klee, H., Jackson, M. and Lewis, S. (eds) (2001) *Drug Misuse and Motherhood*. London: Routledge.

Kuntsche, E. Simons-Morton, B. and Bendtsen, P. (2011) 'Cultural and gender convergence in adolescent drunkenness', *Journal of the American Medical Association Pediatrics*, 165: 152–8.

Leach, E. (1984) 'Glimpses of the unmentionable in the history of British social anthropology', *Annual Review of Anthropology*, 13: 1–23.

Lisansky, E.S. (1957) 'Alcoholism in women: social and psychological concomitants', *Quarterly Journal of Studies on Alcohol,* 18: 588–623.

Lisansky, E.S. (1958) 'The woman alcoholic', *Annals of the American Academy of Political and Social Science,* 315: 73–81.

Litman, G. (1975) 'Women and alcohol: facts and myths', *New Behaviour*, 24: 126–9.

Litman, G. (1978) 'Clinical aspects of sex role stereotyping', In J. Chetwynd and C. Hartnett (eds), *The Sex Role System*. London: Routledge & Kegan Paul, pp. 109–26.

Litman, G. and Wilson, C. (1978) *A Review of Services for Women Alcoholics in the UK*. Paper presented at the 24th International Institute on the Prevention and Treatment of Alcoholism, Zurich, Switzerland.

Longmate, N. (1968) *The Waterdrinkers: A History of Temperance*. London: Hamish Hamilton.

Lyons, A. and Willott, S. (2008) 'Alcohol consumption, gender identities and women's changing social positions', *Sex Roles*, 59: 694–712.

Mac an Ghaill, M. (1996) *Understanding Masculinities: Social Relations and Cultural Arenas*. Buckingham: Open University Press.

Mac an Ghaill, M. and Haywood, C. (2007) *Gender, Culture and Society: Contemporary Femininities and Masculinities*. Houndmills: Palgrave.

MacLennan, A. (ed.) (1976) *Women: Their Use of Alcohol and Other Legal Drugs: A Provisional Consultation–1976*. Toronto: Addiction Research Foundation.

Maher, L. (1997) *Sexed Work: Gender, Race, and Resistance in a Brooklyn Drug Market*. Oxford: Clarendon Press.

Maher, L. and Daly, K. (1996) 'Women in the street-level drug economy: continuity or change?' *Criminology*, 34(4): 465–91.

Maher, L. and Hudson, S. (2007) 'Women in the drug economy: a metasynthesis of the qualitative literature', *Journal of Drug Issues*, 37(4): 805–26.

Mauss, A. (1991) Science social movements and cynicism: appreciating the political context of sociological research in alcohol studies. In P.M. Roman (ed.), *Alcohol: The Development of Sociological Perspectives on Use and Abuse*. New Brunswick: Rutgers Center of Alcohol Studies, pp. 187–204.

May, V. (2014) '"Speaking into the void"? Intersectionality critiques and epistemic backlash', *Hypatia*, 29(1): 94–112.

McCall, L. (2005) 'The complexity of intersectionality', *Signs*, 30(3): 1771–800.

McClelland, D., Daviss, W., Wanner, E. and Kalin, R. (1972) *The Drinking Man*. Glencoe: Free Press.

McConville B. (1983) *Women Under the Influence: Alcohol and its Impact*. New York: Shocken Books.

McDonald, M. (ed.) (1994) *Gender, Drink and Drugs*. Oxford: Berg.

McElrath, K. and McEvoy, K. (2002) 'Negative experiences on ecstasy: the role of drug, set and setting', *Journal of Pyschoactive Drugs*, 34(2): 199–208.

McRobbie, A. (1994) *Postmodernism and Popular Culture*. New York: Routledge.

McRobbie, A. (1995) 'Recent rhythms of sex and race in popular music', *Media Culture and Society*, 17: 323–31.

McRobbie, A. (2000) *Feminism and Youth Culture*, 2nd edn. Houndmills: Palgrave Macmillan.

McRobbie, A. (2009) *The Aftermath of Feminism: Gender, Culture and Social Change*. Thousand Oaks: Sage.

Measham, F. (2002) '"Doing gender" – "Doing drugs": conceptualising the gendering of drugs cultures', *Contemporary Drug Problems*, 29(2): 335–74.

Measham, F., Aldridge, J. and Parker, H. (2001). *Dancing on Drugs: Risk, Health and Hedonism in the British Club Scene*. London: Free Association Books.

Measham, F. and Brain, K. (2005) '"Binge" drinking, British alcohol policy and the new culture of intoxication', *Crime Media and Culture*, 1: 262–83.

Messerschimdt, J. (1997) *Crime as Structured Action: Gender, Race, Class, and Crime in the Making*. Thousand Oaks: Sage.

Miles, S. (2000) *Youth Lifestyles in a Changing World*. Philadelphia: Open University Press.

Miller, D. (1995) *Acknowledging Consumption: A Review of New Studies*. New York: Routledge.

Miller, J. (2001) *One of the Guys: Girls, Gangs, and Gender*. New York: Oxford University Press.

Miller, J. and Carbone-Lopez, K. (2015) 'Beyond "doing gender": incorporating race, class, place, and life transitions into feminist drug research', *Substance Use and Misuse*, 50(6): 693-707.

Miller, P., Wells, S., Hobbs, R., Zinkiewicz, L., Curtis, A. and Graham, K. (2014) 'Alcohol, masculinity, honour and male barroom aggression in an Australian sample', *Drug and Alcohol Review*, 33(2): 136–43.

Moloney, M. and Hunt, G. (2011) 'Doing drugs, gender and accountability in the world of raves', In G. Hunt, H. Bergson and M. Milhet (eds), *Drugs and Culture: Knowledge, Consumption and Policy*. Farnham: Ashgate, pp. 171–94.

Moloney, M., Hunt, G., and Laidler, J. (2015) Drug sales, gender and risk: Notions of Risk from the perspective of gang-involved young adults. *Substance Use and Misuse*, 50(6): 721–732.

Mondanaro, J.E. (1977) 'Women: pregnancy, children, and addiction', *Journal of Psychedelic Drugs*, 9(1): 62.

Montemurro, B. and McClure, B. (2005) 'Changing gender norms for alcohol consumption: Social drinking and lowered inhibitions at bachelorette parties', *Sex Roles*, 52(5/6): 279–88.

Moore, J. and Devitt, M. (1989) 'The paradox of deviance in addicted Mexican American mothers', *Gender and Society*, 3(1): 53–70.

Morgan, P. and Joe, K.A. (1996) 'Citizens and outlaws: the private lives and public lifestyles of women in the illicit drug economy', *Journal of Drug Issues*, 26(1): 125–42.

Morgan, P. and Joe, K. (1997) 'Uncharted terrain: contexts of experience among women in the illicit drug economy', *Women and Criminal Justice*, 8(3): 85–109.

Mullins, C. (2008) 'Negotiating the streets: women, power and resistance in street-life social networks', In T. Anderson (ed.), *Neither Villain nor Victim: Empowerment and Agency among Women Substance Abusers*. New Brunswick: Rutgers University Press, pp. 65–83.

Murphy, S. and Rosenbaum, M. (1999) *Pregnant Women on Drugs: Combating Stereotypes and Stigma*. New Brunswick: Rutgers University Press.

Murphy, S. and Rosenbaum, M. (1987). 'Women and substance abuse: Introduction to a special issue.' *Journal of Psychoactive Drugs*. 20(4):125–128.

Natkin, R. (1984) 'The suburban pub in Finland: a woman's viewpoint', In E. Single and T. Storm (eds), *Public Drinking and Public Policy*. Toronto: Addiction Research Foundation, pp. 127–138.

Oakley, A. (1974) *Housewife*. Harmondsworth: Penguin.

O'Malley, P. and Valverde, M. (2004) 'Pleasure, freedom and drugs: the uses of "pleasure" in liberal governance of drug and alcohol consumption', *Sociology*, 38(1): 25–42.

Ostrow, D. and Shelby, R. (2000) 'Psychoanalytic and behavioral approaches to drug-related sexual risk taking: a preliminary conceptual and clinical integration', *Journal of Gay and Lesbian Psychotherapy*, 3(3/4): 123–39.

Otto S. (1981) 'Women, alcohol and social control', In B. Hunter and G. Williams (eds), *Controlling Women: The Normal and the Deviant*. London: Croom Helm, pp. 154–67.

Pack A. (1982) *Nelson's Blood: The Story of Naval Rum*. Annapolis: Naval Institute Press.

Peralta, R. (2007) 'College alcohol use and the embodiment of hegemonic masculinity among European American men', *Sex Roles*, 56(11): 741–56.

Peralta, R. and Jauk, D. (2011) 'A brief feminist review and critique of the sociology of alcohol use and substance abuse treatment approaches', *Sociology Compass*, 5(10): 882–97.

Perry, L. (1979) *Women and Drug Use: An Unfeminine Dependency*. London: Institute for the Study of Drug Dependence.

Pescor, M.J. (1944) 'A comparative study of male and female drug addicts', *American Journal of Psychiatry*, 100: 771–4.

Plant, M. and Plant, M. (2001) 'Heavy drinking by young British women gives cause for concern', *British Medical Journal*, 323: 1183–9.

Phoenix, A. and Pattynama, P. (2006) 'Intersectionality', *European Journal of Women's Studies*, 13(3): 187–92.

Pini, M. (2001) *Club Cultures and Female Subjectivity: The Move from Home to House*. Houndmills: Palgrave Macmillan.

Prather, J. and Fidell, L. (1978) 'Drug use and abuse among women: an overview', *The International Journal of the Addictions*, 13(6): 863–85.

Raine, P. (2001) *Women's Perspectives on Drugs and Alcohol: The Vicious Circle*. Aldershot: Ashgate.

Ravn, S. (2012) *Intoxicated Interactions: Clubbers Talking About Their Drug Use*. PhD Dissertation. Aarhus: Centre for Alcohol and Drug Research, Aarhus University.

Redhead, S. (1990) *The End-of-the-Century Party: Youth and Pop Towards 2000*. New York: St. Martin's Press.

Redhead, S. (ed.) (1993) *Rave Off: Politics and Deviance in Contemporary Youth Culture*. Brookfield: Avebury.

Redhead, S. (1997) *Subcultures to Clubcultures: An Introduction to Popular Cultural Studies*. Malden: Blackwell.

Reid, J. (1929) 'The treatment of female inebriates and drug addicts', *The British Journal of Inebriety*, 24(2): 58–62.

Richard, B. and Kruger, H. (1998). Ravers' paradise? German youth cultures in the 1990s. In Skelton, T. and Valentine, G. (eds.) Cool Places: Geographies of Youth Cultures. London: Routledge. Pp. 161–174.

Roberts, A., Jackson, M. and Carlton-Laney, I. (2000) 'Revisiting the need for feminism and Afrocentric theory when treating African-American female substance abusers', *Journal of Drug Issues*, 30(4): 901–18.

Rosenbaum, M. (1981) *Women on Heroin*. New Brunswick: Rutgers University Press.

Rosett, H.L. and Weiner, L. (1984) *Alcohol and the Fetus: A clinical Perspective*. New York: Oxford University Press.

Ross, M. and Williams, M. (2012) 'Sexual behaviour and illicit drug use', *Annual Review of Sex Research*, 12(1): 290–310.

St. John, G. (2009) *Technomad: Global Raving Countercultures*. Oakville. The David Brown Book Company.

Saldanha, A. (2007) *Psychedelic White: Goa Trance and the Viscosity of Race*. Minneapolis: University of Minnesota Press.

Sargeant, M. (1967) 'Changes in Japanese drinking patterns', *Quarterly Journal of Studies on Alcohol*, 28: 709–22.

Scharlieb, M. (1907) 'Alcohol and the children of the nation', *The British Journal of Inebriety,* 5(2): 59–71.

Schacht. S. (1996) 'Misogyny on and off the pitch: the gendered world of male rugby players', *Gender and Society*, 10(5): 550–65.

Sedgwick, E.K. (1990) *Epistemology of the Closet*. Berkeley: University of California Press.

Shaw, T.C. (1903) 'The psychology of the inebriate mother', *The British Journal of Inebriety*, 1(2): 58–60.

Segal, B. (2001) 'Responding to victimized Alaska Native women in treatment for substance use', *Substance Use and Misuse,* 36(6): 845–65.

Sheehan, M. and Ridge, D. (2001) '"You become really close… You talk about the silly things you did, and we laugh": the role of binge drinking in female secondary students' lives', *Substance Use and Misuse*, 36(3): 347–72.

Solowij, N., Hall, W. and Lee, N. (1992) 'Recreational MDMA use in Sydney: a profile of "ecstasy" users and their experiences with the drug', *British Journal of Addiction*, 87(8): 1161–72.

Stanley, L. (1990) 'Feminist praxis and the academic mode of production', In L. Stanley (ed.), *Feminist Praxis: Research, Theory and Epistemology in Feminist Sociology*. London: Routledge, pp. 3–19.

Stanley, L. and Wise, S. (1990) 'Method, methodology and epistemology in feminist research processes', In L. Stanley (ed.), *Feminist Praxis: Research, Theory and Epistemology in Feminist Sociology*. London: Routledge, pp. 20–60.

Stephenson, S. (1980) 'Special issues of women in therapy', In J. Dowsling and A. MacLennan (eds), *The Chemically Dependent Woman: Recognition, Referral and Rehabilitation*. Toronto: Addiction Research Foundation, pp. 9–17.

Stevens, S.J. and Wexler, H.K. (eds) (1998) *Women and Substance Abuse: Gender Transparency*. Binghamton: Haworth Press.

Sterk, C. (1999) *Fast Lives. Women Who Use Crack Cocaine*. Philadelphia: Temple University Press.

Sterk, C.E., Theall, K.P. and Elifson, K.W. (2002) 'Health care utilization among drug-using and non-drug-using women', *Journal of Urban Health: Bulletin of the New York Academy of Medicine*, 79(4): 586–99.

Szmigin, I., Griffin, C., Mistral, W. and Bengry-Howell, A. (2008) 'Re-framing "binge drinking" as calculated hedonism: empirical evidence from the UK', *International Journal of Drug Policy*, 19(5): 359–66.

Taussig, M. (1980) *The Devil and Commodity Fetishism in South America*. Chapel Hill: University of North Carolina Press.

Taylor, A. (1993) *Women Drug Users: An Ethnography of a Female Injecting Community*. Oxford: Clarendon Press.

Thom B. (1984) 'A process approach to women's use of alcohol services', *British Journal of Addiction*, 79: 377–82.

Thom B. (1986) 'Sex differences in help-seeking for alcohol problems. I The barriers to help-seeking', *British Journal of Addiction*, 81: 777–88.

Thom B. (1987) 'Sex differences in help-seeking for alcohol problem. II Entry into treatment', *British Journal of Addiction*, 82: 989–97.

Thom, B. (1997) 'Women and alcohol: a policy dilemma', *Policy Studies*, 18(1): 49–65.

Thorne, B. (1993) *Gender Play: Girls and Boys in School.* New Brunswick: Rutgers University Press.

Tuana, N. (2004) 'Coming to understand: orgasm and the epistemology of ignorance', *Hypatia,* 19(1): 194–232.

Tuana, N. (2006) 'The speculum of ignorance: the women's health movement and epistemologies of ignorance', *Hypatia,* 21(3): 1–19.

Tunstall, J. (1962) *The Fishermen*. London: MacGibbon and Kee.

Tyrrell, I. (1983) 'International aspects of the Women's Temperance Movement in Australia: the influence of the American WCTU, 1882–1914', *Journal of Religious History*, 12: 292–4.

Vanicelli, M. and Nash, L. (1984) 'Effects of sex bias on women's studies on alcoholism', *Clinical and Experimental Research*, 3: 334–6.

Waitt, G., Jessop, L. and Gorman-Murray, A. (2011) '"The guys in there just expect to be laid": embodied and gendered socio-spatial practices of a "night out" in Wollongong, Australia', *Gender, Place and Culture*, 18: 255–75.

Waldorf, D. (1973) *Careers in Dope*. Englewood Cliffs: Prentice Hall.

Waterson, J. and Ettorre, B. (1989) 'Providing services for women with difficulties with alcohol and other drugs: the current UK situation as seen by women practitioners, researchers and policy makers in the field', *Drugs and Alcohol Dependence*, 24: 119–25.

Waugh, B. (1903) 'The restoration of the female inebriate', *The British Journal of Inebriety*, 1(2): 73–5.

Weibel-Orlando, J.C. (1984) 'Indian alcoholism treatment programs as flawed rites of passage', *Medical Anthropology Quarterly*, 15(3): 62–7.

Wells, S., Graham, K., Tremblay, P.F. and Magyarody, N. (2011) 'Not just the booze talking: trait aggression and hypermasculinity distinguish perpetrators from victims of male barroom aggression', *Alcoholism: Clinical and Experimental Research*, 35(4): 613–20.

Wells, S., Tremblay, P.F. and Graham, K. (2013). Understanding men's aggression in bars: development of the beliefs and attitudes toward male alcohol-related aggression (BAMARA) inventory. *Alcoholism: Clinical and Experimental Research*, 37(Suppl. 1): E260–70.

West, C. and Zimmerman, D. (1987) 'Doing gender', *Gender and Society*, 1(2): 125–51.

West, C. and Fenstermaker, S. (1995) 'Doing difference', *Gender and Society*, 9(1): 8–37.

West, L. (2001) 'Negotiating masculinities in american drinking subcultures', *The Journal of Men's Studies*, 9(3): 371–92.

Westcott, W.W. (1903) 'Inebriety in women and the overlaying of infants', *The British Journal of Inebriety*, 1(2): 65–8.

Wilsnack, S. and Wilsnack, R. (1991) 'Epidemiology of women's drinking', *Journal of Substance Abuse*, 3(2): 133–57.

Wilsnack, R., Vogeltanz, N., Wilsnack, S. and Harris, T. (2000) 'Gender differences in alcohol consumption and adverse drinking consequences: cross cultural patterns', *Addiction*, 95: 251–65.

Wilsnack, R., Wilsnack, S., Kristjanson, A., Vogeltanz-Holm, N. and Gmel, G. (2009) 'Gender and alcohol consumption: patterns from the multinational Genacis project', *Addiction*, 104: 1487–500.

Windsor, L., Benoit, E. and Dunlap, E. (2010) 'Dimensions of oppression in the lives of impoverished black women who use drugs', *Journal of Black Studies*, 41(1): 21–39.

Windsor, L. and Dunlap, E. (2010) 'What is substance use about? Assumptions in New York's drug policies and the perceptions of African Americans who are low-income and using drugs', *Journal of Ethnicity in Substance Use*, 9(1): 64–87.

Windsor, L., Dunlap E. and Armouret, M. (2012) 'Surviving oppression under the rock: the intersection of New York's drug, welfare, and educational polices in the lived experiences of low-income African Americans', *Journal of Ethnicity in Substance Abuse*, 11: 339–61.

Wright, S. (2002) 'Women's use of drugs: gender specific factors', In H. Klee, M. Jackson and S. Lewis (eds), *Drug Misuse and Motherhood*. London: Routledge, pp. 15–31.

Zanetti, F. (1903) 'Inebriety in women and its influence on child-life', *The British Journal of Inebriety*, 1(2): 45–57.

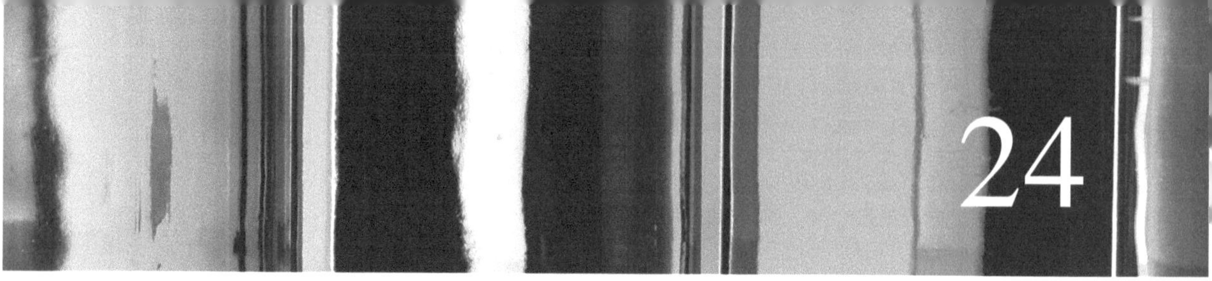

24

Ethnicity and Drug Policy in the USA

Bill Sanders

INTRODUCTION

Stereotypes linking ethnicity to drug use have emerged in the USA. Such allegories have provided support for policies and practices that have marginalized and criminalized minorities. Results have included disproportional rates of arrest and incarceration for drug-related offenses. The ramping up of the war on drugs that began in the 1970s has particularly impacted African Americans and Latinos. Most American prisoners are either black or Latino, and many are incarcerated on drug-related charges.

A longstanding pattern surrounding drug policy is evident in the US. Two dominant themes are found: (i) a specific drug or drug-using practice is linked to the cause of a social ill – promiscuity, corruption, the loss of innocence, child endangerment, crime, terrorism, immigration, the decay of the American way of life; and (ii) such drug or drug-using practice is related to certain groups (cf. Cohen, 1972; White, 1979; Goode and Ben-Yehuda, 1994; Glassner, 2000, 2002; Critcher, 2008). These groups are often ethnic minorities (Hall et al., 1978; cf. Jefferson, 1993). What then emerges is the perception that the minority communities *themselves* are responsible for the social ills – despite the lack of empirical evidence. The end results have negatively impacted them.

This chapter discusses ethnicity and drug policy in the US. It begins by examining contemporary rates of substance use by ethnicity and then comparing these to arrest rates for drug-related offenses. These data indicate that despite the fact that more whites use drugs in general and are more likely to report problematic drug use, blacks and Latinos are arrested and incarcerated for drugs at higher rates. The chapter then provides some examples of the link between ethnicity and the enforcement of substance use prohibition laws: opium smoking among the Chinese; Mexican-Americans and marijuana; and cocaine and African Americans. Various explanations that attempt to explain why these groups have been disproportionality targeted are then offered. The chapter concludes with a discussion on the connection between ethnicity and drug policy, drawing parallels between the US and England. In doing so, it argues that overt and institutionalized racism has explanatory power to explain the cross-national phenomenon of the differential impact of drug laws upon particular ethnic minority communities.

SUBSTANCE USE AND ARREST PATTERNS BY ETHNICITY

The empirical data on differential rates of alcohol and substance use between whites and non-whites often do not line up with popularly perceived notions. Among young people, evidence from *Monitoring the Future* (MTF) – one of the longstanding and reliable sources of data on drug use among youth of the US – suggests that crack cannot be considered a black drug nor can marijuana be considered a Latino drug. Rather, what emerges is that white youths have higher rates of use for most drugs of abuse. Terry-McElrath et al. (2009) reviewed 30 years of data from MTF and found that for all drugs except heroin, past year prevalence rates were significantly higher among whites compared to blacks and Latinos, and regarding the annual prevalence rates of heroin use, only Latinos reported significantly higher rates of use than blacks and whites.

Other sentinel data, such as the *National Survey on Drug Use and Health* (NSDUH), offers a slightly different picture. Between all (juvenile and adult) blacks, whites, and Latinos between 2002 and 2012, rates of past month illicit drug use were highest among blacks and lowest among Latinos with whites in between (SAMHSA, 2013). Between the three ethnic groups, current, binge and heavy alcohol use was highest among whites, followed by Latinos and blacks (SAMHSA, 2013). The rates of problematic substance use as indicated by dependence or abuse were similar for all ethnic groups: 8.7 percent for whites, 8.8 percent for Latinos, and 8.9 percent for blacks (SAMHSA, 2013).

Other researchers have indicated that alcohol and substance use disorders are comparable between, and most prevalent among, whites and Latinos compared to blacks, but that blacks had higher rates of marijuana use disorders compared to whites and Latinos (Pacek et al., 2012). Bernstein et al. (2005) in their review of about 1,000 problematic adult heroin and/or cocaine users reported that whites had higher drug and psychiatric problems compared to blacks, and that Latinos had higher drug severity problems compared to whites. The study of Bourgois et al. (2006) of homeless heroin addicts in San Francisco reported that whites viewed their drug addiction as a form of defeat and needed to use heroin to stave off withdrawal, but blacks viewed their addiction more as a form of defiance and pleasure seeking. Terry-McElrath and colleagues (2009) findings supported this, in that white high school seniors were more likely to report social reasons for using alcohol and substances whereas Latinos and blacks were more likely to report compulsive reasons. However, the authors are keen to point out that these reasons for substance use were not examined by socioeconomic status, which may be more salient than ethnicity regarding different reasons for substance use.

What is important to keep in mind when reading overall rates of substance use, is that they belie actual numbers of substance users. Take problematic substance use as an example. In 2010, the US had a population of about 309 million, of which approximately 12 percent were African American (about 37 million people). Of them, 8.9 percent had drug problems – or about 3.3 million. Latinos were approximately 16 percent of the 2010 census (about 49 million people). Of them, 8.8 percent had drug problems – about 4.3 million people. Whites were about 72 percent of the total US population of the 2010 Census (about 222.5 million). Of them,

8.7 percent had drug problems or about 19.3 million. When looking at the total numbers of Americans with problematic substance abuse issues in 2010, whites constituted more than twice the combined number of blacks and Latinos. Problematic – not recreational and occasional – is what is most linked to crime and violence (Sanders et al., 2009; White and Gorman, 2000).

National alcohol and substance use data do not link up with arrest data. Blacks and Latinos are significantly more likely to be arrested and incarcerated on drug-related charges. Below are some facts [Mauer, 2009; National Association for the Advancement of Colored People (NAACP), n.d.][1]:

- Between 1999 and 2005, blacks constituted about 12 percent of the US population. During this time, they accounted for about 47 percent to about 58 percent of all those in a state prison for a drug offense; for Federal prisoners, the numbers are between about 43 percent to 44 percent.
- Between 1999 and 2005, Latinos constituted about 12 percent of the US population. During this time, they accounted for about 20 percent of all those in state prison on a drug offense; for Federal prisoners, this number climbs to about 33 percent.
- In contrast, during this time, whites were about 70 percent of the US population but averaged about 25 percent of those in a state prison for a drug offense; for Federal prisons, the average is about 23 percent.
- The US has five times as many white compared to black drug users (14 versus 2.6 million), but blacks are 10 times more likely than whites to be sent to prison on drug-related charges.
- About two-thirds of all those incarcerated in state prisons on drug charges are black or Latino.

Even so-called white drugs, such as crystal methamphetamine, disproportionately affect blacks. Whites are significantly more likely to use crystal methamphetamine than non-whites, but blacks are more likely to be arrested for using the drug (Fellner, 2009). The impact that drug laws are having in contemporary African American and Latino communities is an example of a longstanding pattern within the US whereby drug policy unfairly targets and further marginalizes ethnic minorities.

LINKS BETWEEN ETHNICITY AND DRUG POLICY

Three distinct ethnic minority populations in the US have been linked to the use of certain illegal drugs: Chinese and opium smoking; Mexican-American and marijuana; and blacks and cocaine. Policies were enacted that targeted the use of such drugs, which, in effect, targeted these minorities. The mass media fabricated stories about these drugs gave minorities superhuman powers and turned them into crazed lunatics. This spread fear and provided public support for policies. Rather than a concern to curb drug use, though, they served as proxies for broader issues, such as immigration or other forms of control. They also provided a distraction for larger, more pressing social problems. In each of these instances, drug policy clearly assumes an ethnic bias.

Chinese immigrants and opium smoking

An economic crisis occurred in California in the 1870s. Rather than blaming the business class, the focus instead turned to the turpitude of Chinese culture and how this contributed to the economic and moral decay of America (Morgan, 1978; Hardaway, 2003). Part of this culture was opium smoking and the opium dens in the Chinatown district of San Francisco that catered to such use (Morgan, 1978). Within 20 years of the arrival of Chinese in the US, opium smoking began to be recorded within the white 'sporting classes or demi-monde' (Ahmad, 2000: 54). As use spread into the white community, physicians began to take notice, decrying how opium smoking was related to all sorts of ills that faced Americans (Ahmad, 2000). Other forms of opiate use, including morphine and laudanum (aka 'mother's little helper'), continued to enjoy widespread professional recommendation by physicians (Davenport-Hines, 2002). Strangely, doctors knew that all forms of opiates were addictive, but only smoking the drug was believed to cause a lapse in morals; one even likened it to worshiping Satan in a demonic temple (Ahmad, 2000; Hardaway, 2003).

The distinction between smoking opium and using the drug in other ways was replicated in popular fiction. In the late nineteenth century, Conan Doyle's famous celebrated detective, Sherlock Holmes, was an occasional morphine user: he injected the drug. But Holmes deplored the opium dens, which reflected a general viewpoint in Victorian England and America.[2] Music also captured the threat. Ahmad (2000) talks about one in particular, 'Chung Hi Lo and Mary', which is about a white woman who enters the opium den of a Chinese man and quickly becomes addicted to the drug and dies. Other media fueled the humiliation (Hardaway, 2003). Newspapers ran sensationalized and exaggerated stories about the medical impact of Chinese opium smoking dens. One reported how sharing an opium pipe, particularly with a Chinese person, could transmit leprosy (Ahmad, 2000). Another belief circulating at the time was that smoking opium caused 'Orientalness' – a change in customs, attitude and even appearance to that of a Chinese person (Ahmad, 2000). A particular concern expressed by both the media and police was the impact that Chinese opium smoking was having on masculinity, perversity, and the corruption of white women (Ahmad, 2000; Hardaway, 2003). Chinese opium dens were linked to prostitution, which, in some cases, was due to the fact that brothels were located adjacent to the dens (Ahmad, 2000). Fear emerged in relation to the inter-mingling of the sexes given this connection, with the deterioration of US civilization on the brink with the rise in bi-racial children (Ahmad, 2000). Chinese opium smoking, if not curbed, was detrimental to the continued success of an entire way of life.

The federal government viewed smoking opium differently than other administrations. Smoking the drug was banned in the US in 1909 (Hardaway, 2003). Opium use in other forms, though, such as tinctures, was widely available (e.g. laudanum). Tincture overdoses occurred regularly. This gave rise to the 'labeling law' – the Pure Food and Drug Act of 1906. This Act did not outlaw the use of opiates, but rather required that any product that contains opium needed to indicate such (i.e. that they label the contents of the product). At the turn of the twentieth century, opiate use was very common in American culture and such use was hardly censured. Opiates could be ordered via mail order (Ahmed, 2000). Only opium smoking, which was a distinct practice introduced by the Chinese, was illicit. This was despite the fact that only about 6 percent of the Chinese population at the time in America actually used opium (Hardaway, 2003).

The end result of the concern over Chinese opium smoking impacted immigration. Doctors went before the California State Senate on Chinese Immigration in 1876 and warned of the health ills related to opium (Ahmad, 2000). One of the problems with opium they warned was its negative impact on labor: the drug's lethargic effects dimmed workers' drive and determination (Ahmad, 2000). Medical opinion on the threat associated with opium smoking and its relation to the Chinese helped strengthen the Chinese Exclusion Act of 1882, which forbade Chinese immigrant workers from entering US soil (Ahmad, 2000).

MEXICAN-AMERICANS AND MARIJUANA

In the twentieth century in America, the pattern linking ethnicity to substance use is first found among Mexican immigrants. More people began to use marijuana in the late 1920s with the signing of the Eighteenth Amendment (aka the Volstead Act – prohibition of alcohol). Marijuana was used by all kinds of people across the US (Siegel, 1989). The drug was not really considered problematic until the rise of immigrants from Mexico in southern and western states (Hardaway, 2003). Mexican immigrants have a history of using marijuana for medicinal and recreational purposes (Siegel, 1989). Prohibition of marijuana was enacted because the perception was that the drug was used primarily by such immigrants and was the cause of crime, violence, and sexual promiscuity (Hardaway, 2003). In order to strengthen the connection, marijuana was considered as the Mexican herb, Mexican opium, or killer weed (Hardaway, 2003). Hardaway provides an excerpt from a newspaper in Montana in which a physician says the following to a House Health Committee in relation to the state's consideration of a marijuana prohibition bill: 'When some beet field peon takes a few rares of this stuff', explained Dr. Fred Fulsher of Mineral County, 'he thinks he has just been elected president of Mexico so he starts out to execute all his political enemies' (Hardaway 2003: 92).

The problem was not necessarily Mexican immigration, but the high unemployment rate in the 1930s (i.e. the Great Depression; Abel, 1980). As the Chinese before them, Mexican immigrants were scapegoated as the cause of lost jobs, high rates of crime and violence, and the threat that the country would start to become un-American (Musto, 1999; Hardaway, 2003). The press largely fueled this. Newspapers ran stories about Mexicans torturing or killing babies and children because their supply of marijuana had run out, or about Mexicans selling marijuana to schoolchildren (Hardaway, 2003).

The panic surrounding marijuana and the increase in Mexican immigration only impacted southwestern states – where such immigration was heavy – but was not considered problematic in the east – where Mexican immigration was practically non-existent (Hardaway, 2003). This gave further support to the notion that the concern about marijuana was a thinly veined disguise at immigration reform.

The link between Mexican-Americans and marijuana lasted well into the twenty-first century. In major cities in California, Latinos – most of whom are Mexican-American – are two to three times more likely to be arrested for marijuana (Levine et al., 2010). They are significantly overrepresented in marijuana offenses in other states as well (e.g. New York; Geller and Fagan, 2010).

AFRICAN AMERICANS AND COCAINE

Cocaine once enjoyed widespread use throughout American society. Like morphine, many tinctures were made from it, including *Vin Coca Mariani* – coca leaves steeped in wine – that was once used by a former Pope (Hardaway, 2003). All sorts of professionals and artists used cocaine. So, too, did construction laborers and miners in order to work longer hours (Davenport-Hines, 2002; Hardaway, 2003). Cocaine use was widespread among whites, including prostitutes, pimps, and gamblers, but was only considered problematic among blacks (Davenport-Hines, 2002). This concern emerged at a height of lynching (i.e. violent murders), legal segregation, voting restrictions, and other efforts to disempower African Americans (Hardaway, 2003). African Americans using cocaine were thought to be imperious to bullets – they would not stop a coked-up black man – and it caused them to commit violence, especially rape (Musto, 1999; Hardaway, 2003). Even physicians indicated that cocaine turned black men into super humans bent on perversion and lust for white women (Spillane, 2000).

The lopsided connection of cocaine with the African American community continued in the 1980s and 1990s in the form of crack.

The effects of deindustrialization and the removal of the welfare state already set an ominous stage within black inner city communities (see Wilson, 1987; Sampson and Wilson, 1995). A surplus of cocaine and illegal government-sponsored operations led to the introduction of crack – a combination of the drug and baking soda (or ammonia) in a hard form that allowed less affluent people to use it.[3] The crack cocaine trade became a significant part of the illicit economy, which attracted marginalized and disempowered African Americans (see work by Hagedorn, 1988; Taylor, 1990; Jacobs, 1999; Venkatesh, 2008). Drug gangs formed to control the market and both the morgues and the jails began to fill up quickly with young black men. In the late 1980s and early 1990s, large cities such as Los Angeles and Chicago were claiming around 1,000 murders a year, half of them considered gang-related (Klein, 1995; Spergel, 1995).

The media sensationalized the event (Reinarman and Levine, 1997). Gangsta rap emerged and helped to cement in the minds of the public the tight relationship between poor black communities, gangs, and crack cocaine. Crack babies – children born to mothers addicted to the drug – became a national phenomenon, and crack became intrinsically connected to violence, AIDS, and super predators. The government enacted harsh penalties in relation to the perceived threat that crack posed (Reinarman and Levine, 1997; Mauer, 2009). These penalties associated with offenses linked with selling or using cocaine were significantly higher than for powder cocaine – even though both drugs are essentially the same (Fellner, 2009; Mauer, 2009).[4] The Drug Policy Alliance reported that five grams of crack cocaine has the same community penalty as 500 grams of powder cocaine.[5] Whites arrested for powder cocaine use would serve a fraction of the time compared to black crack cocaine users.[6] The focus of crack was in black communities and the police reaction was hard (Fellner, 2009). In cities such as Los Angeles, the police force became militarized, including the use of checkpoints, low flying helicopters, and in one case, a tank (Krisberg, 2005). Approximately 80 percent of those serving time in a Federal prison on crack-cocaine related charges are black (Mauer, 2009).

Drug policy has so negatively impacted black communities so as to be considered the New Jim Crow laws (Alexander, 2010). Whereas the original Jim Crow laws in southern US states were once legalized forms of discrimination that impacted employment and educational opportunities among blacks, modern day drug policy has essentially had the same effects (Alexander, 2010). Criminal records limit the types of jobs that can be obtained and the massive number of African American men with such records have contributed to economic destabilization within their communities (Alexander, 2010). The high incarceration rates have also impacted rates of HIV/AIDS, which disproportionately affects African Americans. This has occurred in at least two ways. Incarceration interrupts primary sexual relations relationships, leading to an increase in sexual risks in the community, such as multiple partners (Blankenship and Smoyer, 2013). The lack of HIV/AIDS prevention and care services inside jails and prisons contributes to exposure among inmates (Sanders et al., 2013).

UNDERSTANDING THE DISPROPORTIONALITY

Several reasons have been offered to explain the disproportional arrest and incarceration rates of Latinos and African Americans compared to whites. These explanations are not necessarily mutually exclusive and may overlap and influence one another (Brownsberger, 2000; Kautt and Spohn, 2002; Fellner, 2009; Mauer, 2009).

One is that Latinos and African Americans have more risk factors or variables at the individual and community level that predispose them to using and selling drugs (Brownsberger, 2000; cf. Huizinga et al., 2007; Fellner, 2009). However, as Huizinga et al. (2007) note in their study of disproportionate minority confinement among juveniles, risk factor backgrounds helped explain some, not all, of the discrepancy between whites, blacks, and Latinos.

Another proposed reason is that Latinos and blacks are more likely to live in poorer areas and as such have less access to indoor, private areas to use and sell drugs (Tonry, 1995; Curtis, 1998; Brownsberger, 2000; Fellner, 2009; Mauer, 2009). Drug sellers in poor communities are also more likely to sell openly to strangers. The combination of these practices makes them more visible to law enforcement (Tonry, 1995; Curtis, 1998; Mauer, 2009). However, as Fellner (2009) points out, poor whites also sell crack in outdoor areas, but have been ignored by the police in favor of targeting poor blacks doing the same thing. Furthermore, as Beckett et al. (2006) have reported, outdoor drug sales occur in relatively affluent areas, and blacks account for disproportional amounts of those arrested for selling drugs indoors. Others have noted that whites sell drugs outside as well, including crack, but the police have largely focused on blacks selling this drug (Beckett et al., 2006; Fellner, 2009). Policing is differential for drug use. In New York City, for instance, evidence suggests that police were more likely to patrol for and make marijuana arrests in black and Latino neighborhoods; they largely ignored whites smoking the drug in public and were less likely to arrest them for open use (Golub et al., 2006, 2007; Geller and Fagan, 2010).

Another dent in the argument that blacks are more likely to smoke marijuana outdoors and more likely to be detected than whites comes from states where marijuana has been decriminalized (e.g. Colorado, Washington). For instance, in Colorado, as expected, the arrest rates for marijuana use plunged when the drug was legalized. However, non-whites were *still* arrested more for marijuana use infractions (e.g. smoking outdoors; Wyatt, 2015). Blacks were twice as likely as whites to be arrested. In Colorado, African Americans are less than 4 percent of the population; nationwide the number is about 13 percent. Given these small numbers, the idea that more blacks than whites smoke marijuana outdoors loses credibility.

Another reason for disproportionate minority arrests and incarceration for drug charges is decision making at the judicial and prosecutorial level (Brownsberger, 2000). Here, the argument is that, out of all those arrested on drug charges, non-whites are much more likely to receive community penalties, such as fines and incarceration (Blumstein, 1993). Krisberg (2005) has reported Latino and black juveniles are significantly more likely to be convicted and placed outside their home for drug-related charges compared to whites. Related reasons are mandatory sentencing laws. These laws have been applied to certain drug offenses, such as crack-cocaine selling and using, which are much harsher compared to the sentences related to other drugs, and most crack sellers and users arrested have been black (Brownsberger, 2000; Fellner, 2009; Mauer, 2009).

Racial profiling is a reason for the disproportionate number of Latinos and African Americans arrested and incarcerated on drug-related offenses.[7] Ample evidence of police officers across the US over many years doing this has emerged (Banks, 2003). Among the most profound findings in relation to racial profiling stems from rulings about New York City's search and seizure practices and marijuana (Geller and Fagan, 2010). The enforcement of the 'stop, question, and frisk' practices and aggressive targeting of low-level offenses by the New York Police Department (NYPD) has dramatically increased arrests for marijuana; those arrested are disproportionately black or Latino (Geller and Fagan, 2010). Geller and Fagan continue by saying 'non-whites bear a racial tax from contemporary policing strategy' (Geller and Fagan 2010: 2). Stop and frisk policy employed by the NYPD were found to be in violation of the Fourth and Fourteenth Amendments, and Fagan's analysis contributed to this decision (Cassidy, 2013). Others have argued that police departments in other large cities in the US (e.g. Philadelphia) employ very similar stop and frisk practices as the NYPD that are also likely unconstitutional (Rudovsky and Rosenthal, 2013).

What is the source of racial profiling? Beckett et al. (2006) note that race matters in relation to the overrepresentation of blacks and Latinos in drug offender statistics, but that it might not necessarily be racist attitudes. Rather, the authors indicate that the true culprit is 'implicit racial bias: the unconscious impact of race on official perceptions of who and what constitutes [a] drug problem' (2006: 130). Beckett et al. (2006) supply evidence that the perception that links blacks to drug use is widely held and not limited to law enforcement. Most Americans, they note, think that the typical drug user is black, despite a substantial amount of empirical evidence to the contrary.

Another contribution is the overall sensitivity of the approach towards America's drug problem. Mauer (2009) notes that substance use in Latino and black communities is viewed as a criminal justice problem, but in white communities, drug use is considered a medical/public health one (see also Sanders et al., 2013). Beckett et al. concur with this when they say that 'members of the public generally prefer "tougher" policy and legal responses when perpetrators are depicted as black' (2006: 107). Fellner also offers a similar comment:

> To the extent that the white majority in the United States identified both crime and drugs with racialized 'others', it has no doubt been easier to endorse or at least acquiesce to punitive penal policies that might have been rejected if applied at equivalent rates to members of their own families and communities. Politicians have been able to reap the electoral rewards of endorsing harsh drug policies because the group that suffered most from those policies – black Americans – lacked the numbers to use the political process to secure a different strategy. (Fellner, 2009: 277)

Fellner (2009) writes about how the impact of the war on drugs upon black communities itself constitutes a form of discrimination and as such should be ruled unconstitutional. She indicates that while discrimination might not exist in the intent of the enforcement of drug laws, the impact has undeniably been cockeyed. According to Fellner (2009), this differential impact of drug enforcement is discriminatory under the International Convention on the Elimination of All forms of Racial Discrimination (ICRDEA), which the US has ratified. She says that the lack of action that the US has taken to redress the imbalance of the War on Drugs upon minority communities is its greatest examples of failure to comply with the ICRDEA. Fellner (2009) continues by arguing that unless the focus of punitive responses in relation to drugs change, the prospects in minority communities will continue to be grim.

Unnever et al. (2009) have found that discrimination is an important consideration in the etiology of crime and delinquency – including substance use – among African Americans, even when controlling for the presence of strong social bonds. They found that one reason blacks committed crime was due to their experiences of discrimination, a form of strain as outlined in general strain theory (Agnew, 1992). Unnever et al. (2009) also indicate that many African Americans across the US feel that racial discrimination is a significant part of their daily, lived realities. Racial bias thus can trap black people in a vicious circle in relation to drug-related offenses: discrimination is related to the reasons they commit crime (including drug use and sales) and why they are more likely to be stopped, arrested, convicted, and incarcerated for drug-related offense.

DISCUSSION

The roots of discrimination linking ethnicity to drug use and policy extend into colonial

America. Alcohol sales were then restricted to free and slave blacks and Native Americans (Lender and Martin, 1982). Native Americans were particularly impacted by alcohol, giving rise to the firewater myth (Lender and Martin, 1982). Traders took advantage of them by selling them sub-standard alcohol and profiting while they were intoxicated (Beauvais, 1998). Hard drinking was routine behavior among all sorts of white colonists (Beauvais, 1998). Native Americans were simply aping such behavior, but myths prevailed that only they were the true drunkards who could not help but to commit violence (Frank et al., 2000). Native Americans in these times did become violent after binge drinking – just as many whites did – but rather than attacking white colonists or other enemies, they largely committed violence against themselves – friends and family (Frank et al., 2000). In this regard, their violence fits a common pattern: alcohol-related violence (and violence more generally) is often committed against people of the same ethnicity who also know one another. Contrary to popular beliefs at the time, little evidence has emerged to suggest Native Americans behaved any more or less violently while intoxicated than those from other ethnicities.

Examples of the link between drug policy and ethnicity unfairly targeting minority communities is found in England. England and the US are aptly compared. Both countries are majority white, with a shared colonial history. Both have similar democracies, economies, and dominant religious institutions. Both have minority populations of non-whites, either brought there as slaves or through immigration opportunities. Both have deep-seated hostilities between the police and certain minority communities. And both have a history of overt and institutional racism that have negatively impacted non-whites for many years. Even their drug policies emerged at similar times, ranking the dangerousness of several drugs the same way (e.g. Controlled Substance Act of 1970; Misuse of Drugs Act 1971). England has a much shallower history of ethnic relations than the US, but Asians and Afro-Caribbean immigrants there have had similar experiences as blacks and Latinos in the US.

In an effort to rebuild after the destruction caused by World War Two, England opened its borders to the Commonwealth nations. Hundreds of thousands of people from the Indian subcontinent (i.e. Asians) and the West Indies (i.e. Afro-Caribbeans) immigrated. For the first time in its history, England contained non-white populations *en masse*. Rather than being welcomed, the newcomers faced housing and employment restrictions due to racial discrimination (Pryce, 1979; Gilroy, 1987). They were relegated to substandard housing conditions, with many families living in homes built for one (Glass, 1960; Patterson, 1963 Pryce, 1979). Only menial, low paying jobs were available to them (Pryce 1979; Harris and James 1993). They were concentrated in specific inner city urban locales. Over time, these areas became synonymous with crime and disorder (Campbell, 1993; Keith, 1993; Back, 1996). Violence and drugs particularly impacted black communities. Fomenting hostilities between black youth and the police over decades culminated in some of the worst riots in the history of the country. In 1981, race riots occurred in Brixton, London, Moss Side, Manchester, and Toxteth, Liverpool; in 2011, the same thing happened in several areas with large populations of black youths: Tottenham, Brixton, Peckham, Croydon, and Lewisham – as well as in a few other English cities. Inquiries into these riots have indicated negative police-community relations were a significant factor (Scarman, 1981; MacPherson, 1999).

The perception of black youth as drug users and offenders has contributed to hostilities between their communities and the police (Spencer and Hough, 2000; Holdaway, 2003). Police stop and search practices have disproportionately targeted black youth and suspicion of drugs is a major reason they are stopped (Spencer and

Hough, 2000; Holdaway, 2003; Eastwood et al., 2013). One report found that blacks were stopped and searched more than six times the rate as whites; Asians were two and a half times more likely (Eastwood et al., 2013; see also Holdaway, 2003). This is despite the fact that drug use among blacks and Asians is *lower* than whites (Eastwood et al., 2013). Blacks were also more likely to receive harsher penalties when compared to whites on drug charges. They are more likely to be charged instead of cautioned, more likely to go to court, and more likely to receive a prison sentence (Eastwood et al., 2013). More than half of the drug possession court cases are for cannabis (Eastwood et al., 2013). The evidence suggests that in England, despite major investigations and recommendations regarding police relations with minority communities, Asian and black youth were more likely to be stopped and searched in the 2010 compared to the 1980s (Eastwood et al., 2013).

The link between ethnicity and drug policy in the US and England has been too strong for such a long period of time to be explained away as pure happenstance. Rather, the overrepresentation of minorities on drug-related arrests and incarcerations is another outcome of overt and institutionalized racism. This racism permeates multiple aspects of white dominant society, including the justice systems. Racism is also the reason blacks and Latinos in the US and Asians and Afro-Caribbeans in England are more likely than whites to live in conditions that give rise to drug use and other problematic behaviors in the first place. US and English drug policies are an extension of a long tradition of officialdom targeting non-whites due to xenophobic, prejudiced beliefs, to scapegoat them for larger social ills not of their making, to demoralize and control them, to limit their influence and movement, or a combination of these reasons. From colonial times to the present day, drug policy has been linked to ethnicity and the principal reason for this is racism.

In the US, the percentage of African Americans and Latinos incarcerated on drug-related charges has decreased, while whites incarcerated for the same offenses have increased (Mauer, 2009). President Obama signed into the law, in 2010, the Fair Sentencing Act, part of which did redress the imbalance between crack cocaine and powder cocaine community penalties. In July 2014, the US Attorney General called for the release of approximately 46,000 non-violent drug offenders, many who are black or Latino, who received relatively harsh sentences. These are hopeful trends and actions towards reducing the disproportionate rates of ethnic minorities on drug-related charges.

NOTES

1 Available from: http://www.naacp.org/pages/criminal-justice-fact-sheet.

2 Compare *The Sign of Four* (1890) when Holmes injects morphine with *The Man with the Twisted Lip* (1891) when he attends an opium den dressed as a vagrant in order to extract information from an addict.

3 The story outlined by Gary Webb in *Dark Alliance* (1999) while at one point controversial, has come to be viewed as history. The US Congress and other key players in his story have verified Webb's reporting. In brief, Webb's account is as follows: the Reagan-era CIA helped coordinate efforts to channel money to pro-democratic forces, the Contras, in Communist-influenced Nicaragua. Cocaine was a chief export of that country; the CIA helped funnel that cocaine to black inner city areas, this occurred through 'Freeway' Rick Ross, who was credited as being one of the few people at the time to know how to make a new form of cocaine – crack. Crack allowed smaller amounts of the drug to be sold, enabling less affluent people to use cocaine; the drug was an instant success, and sales of cocaine skyrocketed. The money generated from such cocaine sales was funneled back to the Contras. The movie *Kill the Messenger* (2014) is about this. Since Rick Ross has been released from prison, he has told his story in the documentary, *How to Make Money Selling Drugs* (2012).

4 Assuming that both drugs are pure, powder cocaine would contain only that drug, whereas

crack cocaine is a mixture of the powder with a legal product (e.g. baking soda, ammonia). Whether or not one form of the drug is more addictive than the other has generated some debate. One argument is that smoking the drug could be more addictive than other administrations (see Samaha and Robinson, 2005). Powder cocaine can be smoked and injected and crack cocaine can be injected, so the form of the drug does not necessarily dictate how it will be administered (e.g. smoked, snorted, injected).

5 Available from: http://www.drugpolicy.org/docUploads/NewJimCrowFactSheet.pdf.

6 These are the Anti-Drug Abuse Acts of 1986 and 1988.

7 Racial profiling refers to when a police officer (or other member of law enforcement) specifically investigate an individual based on the belief that that individual is a member of a particular racial group that are more to engage the behavior under investigation more so than other racial/ethnic groups (see Banks, 2003).

REFERENCES

Abel, E. (1980) *Marijuana: The First 12,000 Years.* New York: Plenum Press.

Agnew, R. (1992) 'Foundation for a general strain theory of crime and delinquency', *Criminology*, 30 (1): 47–88.

Ahmad, D.L. (2000) 'Opium smoking, anti-Chinese attitudes, and the American Medical Community, 1850–1890', *American Nineteenth Century History,* 1(2): 53–68.

Alexander, M. (2010) *The New Jim Crow: Incarceration in the Age of Color Blindness.* New York: The New Press.

Back, L. (1996) *New Ethnicities and Urban Culture: Racism and Multiculturalism in Young Lives.* London: UCL Press.

Banks, R.R. (2003) 'Beyond profiling: race, policing and the drug war', *Stanford Law Review,* 56(3): 571–603.

Beauvais, F. (1998) 'American Indians and alcohol', *Alcohol Health and Research World,* 22(4): 253–9.

Beckett, K., Nyrop, K. and Pfingst, L. (2006) 'Race, drugs, and policing: Understanding disparities in drug delivery arrests', *Criminology,* 44(1): 105–37.

Bernstein, E., Bernstein, J., Tassiopoulos, K., Valentine, A., Heeren, T., Levenson, S. and Hingson, R. (2005) 'Racial and ethnic diversity among a heroin and cocaine using population: Treatment system utilization', *Journal of Addictive Disorders*, 24(4): 43–63.

Blankenship, K.M. and Smoyer, A.B. (2013) 'Between spaces: understanding movement to and from prison as an HIV Risk Factor', In B. Sanders, Y. Thoma, and B. Griffin-Deeds (eds), *Crime, HIV and Health: Intersections of Criminal Justice and Public Health Concerns.* New York: Springer Press, pp. 299–326.

Blumstein, A. (1993) 'Racial disproportionality of U.S. prison populations revisited', *University of Colorado Law Review,* 64 (3): 743–760.

Bourgois, P., Martinez, A., Kral, A., Edlin, B.R., Schonberg, J. and Ciccarone, D. (2006) 'Reinterpreting ethnic patterns among White and African American men who inject heroin: a social science of medicine approach', *PLoS Medicine,* 3(10): 452.

Brownsberger, W.H. (2000) 'Race matters: disproportionality of incarceration for drug dealing in Massachusetts', *Journal of Drug Issues,* 30(2): 345–74.

Campbell, B. (1993) *Goliath: Britain's Dangerous Places.* London: Methuen.

Cassidy, J. (2013) 'The statistical debate behind he stop-and-frisk verdict', *The New Yorker,* 13 August. Retrieved from: http://www.newyorker.com/news/john-cassidy/the-statistical-debate-behind-the-stop-and-frisk-verdict.

Cohen, S. (1972) *Folk Devils and Moral Panics: The Creation of the Mods and Rockers.* London: MacGibbon and Kee.

Critcher, C. (2008) 'Moral panic analysis: past, present and future', *Sociology Compass,* 2(4): 1127–44.

Curtis, R. (1998) 'The improbably transformation on inner-city neighborhoods: crime, violence, drugs and youth in the 1990s', *Journal of Criminal Law and Criminology,* 88(4): 1233–76.

Davenport-Hines, R. (2002). *The pursuit of oblivion.* New York: Norton & Comapny.

Eastwood, N., Shiner, M. and Bear, D. (2013) *The Numbers in Black and White: Ethnic Disparities in the Policing and Prosecution of Drug Offenders in England and Wales.* London: Release.

Fellner, J. (2009) 'Race, drugs and law enforcement in the United States', *Stanford Law and Policy Review,* 20(2): 257–91.

Frank, J.W., Moore, R.S. and Ames, G.M. (2000) 'Historical and cultural roots of drinking problems among American Indians', *American Journal of Public Health*, 90(3): 345–51.

Geller, A. and Fagan, J. (2010) *Pot as Pretext: Marijuana, Race and the New Disorder in New York City Street Policing.* Available from: http://www.econ.brown.edu/fac/Glenn_Loury/louryhomepage/teaching/Ec%20137/Pot%20As%20Pretext_Submitted_JELS.pdf.

Glassner, B. (2000) *The Culture of Fear.* New York: Basic Books.

Glassner, B. (2002) 'Narrative techniques of fear mongering', *Social Research,* 71(4): 819–26.

Gilroy, P. (1987) *Ain't No Black in the Union Jack: The Cultural Politics of Race and Nation.* London: Hutchinson.

Glass, R. (1960) *Newcomers: The West Indians in London*. London: George Allen and Unwin.

Golub, A., Johnson, B.D. and Dunlap, E. (2006) 'Smoking marijuana in public: the spatial and policy shift in New York City arrests, 1992–2003', *Harm Reduction Journal*, 3: 22–45.

Golub, A., Johnson, B.D. and Dunlap, E. (2007) 'The race/ethnicity disparity in misdemeanor marijuana arrests in New York City', *Criminology and Public Policy*, 6: 131–64.

Goode, E. and Ben-Yehuda, N. (1994) 'Moral panics: culture, politics, and social Construction', *Annual Review of Sociology,* 994(20): 49–171.

Hagedorn, J. (with Perry Macon) (1988) *People and Folks: Gangs, Crime and the Underclass in a Rust Belt City.* Chicago: Lake View Press.

Hall, S, Critcher, C., Jefferson, T., Clark, J. and Roberts, R. (1978) *Policing the Crisis: Mugging, the State, and Law and Order*. London: Macmillan.

Hardaway, R.M. (2003) *No Price Too High: Victimless Crimes and the Ninth Amendment.* New York: Praeger.

Harris, C. and James, W. (1993) Introduction. In: James, W. & Harris, C. (eds.) *Inside Babylon: Caribbean diaspora in Britain.* London: Verso, pp. 1–8.

Holdaway, S. (2003) 'Police race relations in England and Wales: theory, policy, and Practice', *Police and Society,* 7: 49–74.

Huizinga, D., Thornberry, T., Knight, K. and Lovegrove, P. (2007) *Disproportionate Minority Contact in the Juvenile Justice System: A Study of Differential Minority Arrest/Referral to Court in Three Cities*. Washington, DC: US Department of Justice.

Kautt, P. and Spohn, C. (2002) '*Crack*-ing down on black drug offenders? Testing for interactions among offenders' race, drug type, and sentencing strategy in Federal drug sentences', *Justice Quarterly,* 19(1): 1–35.

Keith, M. (1993) *Race, Riots and Policing: Lore and Disorder in a Multi-Racist Society.* London: UCL Press.

Klein, M (1995) *The American street gang: Its nature, prevalence and control*. New York: Oxford University Press.

Lender, M.E. and Martin, J.K. (1982) *Drinking in America: A History.* New York: The Free Press.

Levine, H.G., Geltman, J.B. and Siegal, L. (2010) *Arresting Latinos for Marijuana in California: Possession Arrest in 33 Cities, 2006–08.* New York City: Drug Policy Alliance. Retrieved from: http://marijuana-arrests.com/docs/Arresting-Latinos-For-Marijuana-California.pdf.

Jacobs, B.A. (1999) 'Crack to heroin? Drug markets and transition', *British Journal of Criminology,* 39: 555–74.

Jefferson, T. (1993) 'The racism of criminalization: policing and the reproduction of the criminal other', In L. Gelsthorpe (ed.), *Minority Ethnic Groups in the Criminal Justice System*. Cambridge: University of Cambridge, pp. 26–43.

Krisberg, B. (2005) *Juvenile Justice: Redeeming Our Children.* Thousand Oaks: Sage.

Mauer, M. (2009) *The Changing Racial Dynamics of the War on Drugs.* Washington, DC: The Sentencing Project.

MacPherson, W. (1999) *The Stephen Lawrence Inquiry: Report of an Inquiry by Sir William MacPherson of Clung*. London: The Stationary Office.

Morgan, P.A. (1978) 'The legislation of drug law: economic crisis and social control', *Journal of Drug Issues,* 8(1): 53–62.

Musto, D.F. (1999) *The American Disease: Origins of Narcotic Control*, 3rd edn. New York: Oxford University Press.

Pacek, L.R., Malcolm, R.J. and Martins, S.S. (2012) 'Race/ethnicity differences between alcohol, marijuana and co-occurring alcohol and marijuana use disorders and their association with public health and social problems using a national sample', *The American Journal on Addictions,* 21: 435–44.

Patterson, S. (1963) *Dark strangers: A sociological study of the absorption of a recent West Indian migrant group in Brixton, South London*. London: Tavistock.

Pryce, K. (1979) *Endless Pressure: A Study of West Indian Lifestyles in Bristol*. Harmondsworth: Penguin.

Rudovsky, D. and Rosenthal, L. (2013) 'The constitutionality of stop-and-frisk in New York City', *University of Pennsylvania Law Review Online,* 117. Retrieved from: http://www.pennlawreview.com/debates/index.php?id=49.

Reinarman, C. and Levine, H.G. (1997) 'The crack attack, politics and media in the crack scare', In C. Reinarman and H.G. Levine (eds), *Crack in America: Demon Drugs and Social Justice*. Berkeley: University of California Press, pp. 18–51.

Samaha, A.N. and Robinson, T.E. (2005) 'Why does the rapid delivery of drugs to the brain promote addiction?', *TRENDS in Pharmacological Sciences,* 26(2): 82–7.

Sampson, R.J. and Wilson, W.J. (1995) 'Towards a theory of race, class, and urban inequality', In J. Hagan and R.D. Peterson (eds), *Crime and Inequality*. Stanford: Stanford University Press, pp. 37–56.

Sanders, B., Lankenau, S., Jackson Bloom, J. and Hathazi, D. (2009) 'A typology of drug-related offending among homeless young injection drug users', *Journal of Drug Issues,* 39(4): 777–802.

Sanders, B., Thomas, Y. and Griffin-Deeds, D. (2013) 'Intersections of public health and criminal justice', In B. Sanders, Y. Thomas and B. Griffin-Deeds (eds), *Crime, HIV and Health: Intersections of Criminal Justice and Public Health Concerns*. New York: Springer Press, pp. 1–15.

Scarman (1981) *The Scarman Report: The Brixton Disorders 10–12 April 1981: Report of an Inquiry by Lord Scarman*. Harmondsworth: Penguin.

Spencer, A.B. and Hough, M. (2000) *Policing Diversity: Lessons from Lambeth*, London: Home Office.

Spergel, I. (1995) The youth gang problem: A community approach. Oxford: Oxford University Press.

Spillane, J.F. (2000) *Cocaine: From Medical Marvel to Modern Menace in the United States, 1884–1920*. Baltimore: Johns Hopkins University Press.

Siegel, R.K. (1989) *Intoxication: Life in Pursuit of Artificial Paradise*. New York: E.P. Dutton.

Substance Abuse and Mental Health Services Administration (SAMHSA) (2013) *Results from the 2012 National Survey on Drug Use and Health: Summary of National Findings*. Rockville: Substance Abuse and Mental Health Services Administration.

Taylor, C.S. (1990) *Dangerous Society*. East Lansing: Michigan State University Press.

Terry-McElrath, Y.M., O'Malley, P.M. and Johnson, L.D. (2009) 'Reasons for drug use among American youth by consumption level gender, and race/ethnicity: 1976–2005', *Journal of Drug Issues,* 39(3): 677–714.

Tonry, M. (1995) *Malign Neglect: Race, Crime, and Punishment in America*. New York: Oxford University Press.

Unnever, J.D., Cullen, F.T., Mathers, S.A., McClure, T.E. and Allison, M.C. (2009) 'Racial discrimination and Hirschi's criminological classic: a chapter in the sociology of knowledge', *Justice Quarterly,* 26(3): 377–409.

Venkatesh, S.A (2008) *Gang Leader for a Day: A Rogue Sociologist Takes to the Streets*. New York: Penguin.

White, W.L. (1979) *Themes in chemical prohibition*. Washington, DC: National Institute on Drug Abuse.

White, H.R. and Gorman, D.M. (2000) 'Dynamics of the drugs-crime relationship', In G. LaFree., R.J. Bursik, J. Short and R.B. Taylor (eds), *The Nature of Crime: Continuity and Change. Criminal Justice 2000*, Volume 1. Washington, DC: National Institute of Justice, pp. 151–218.

Wilson, W.J. (1987) *The Truly Disadvantaged: The Inner City, the Underclass, and Public Policy*. Chicago: University of Chicago Press.

Wyatt, K. (2015) 'Racial disparities persist with legal pot', *The Denver Post*, 25 March.

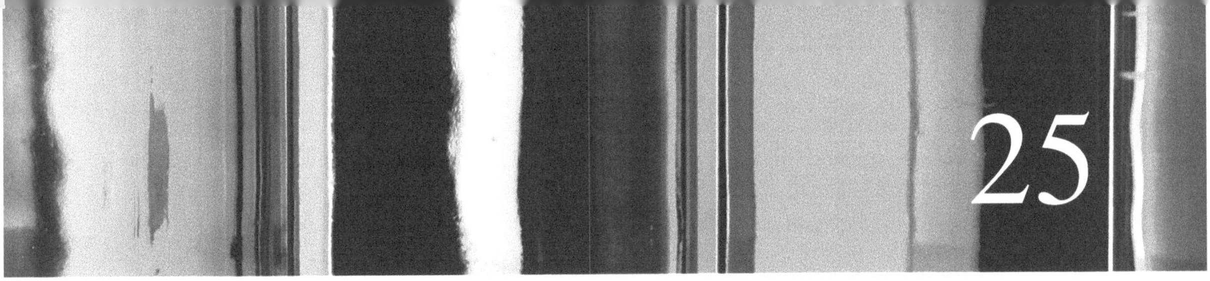

25

Social Class and Deprivation

Angus Bancroft

INTRODUCTION

The subject of this chapter is the material and intangible differences of wealth, occupational position and status that shape the experience and consequences of drug and alcohol use for users, their families and communities. Health behaviours and outcomes are socially patterned. A web of behavioural habits, health beliefs, physical, financial and symbolic resources, life course and intergenerational effects, occupational, neighbourhood and spatial segregations, global and nation-bounded processes and institutions and local environmental conditions determine health and quality of life (Marmot and UCL Institute of Health Equity, 2013). As far as drug and alcohol behaviours are also health behaviours, then the harms caused by them follow the same health gradient where rising affluence means better health. Drug and alcohol use are also culturally symbolic behaviours and that aspect of them is shaped by the same processes. Their meaning and significance for personal identity, social networks, self-actualisation and social status vary by the same measures. For that reason, we cannot approach the topic of drug/alcohol use and social class and deprivation solely as one of the distribution of risk and harm, without also considering it as involving the distribution and operation of power, status and opportunity (Bambra et al., 2005).

In this chapter, I will introduce competing perspectives on the question of what class and deprivation are and what they mean. Very broadly speaking, social class perspectives start by examining how the economic system structures inequality through the labour market. In contrast, deprivation perspectives look at how individuals, families and communities are rendered marginal, which is to some extent external to the labour market system. Drug and alcohol consumption is patterned by class and deprivation, and just as important, the experience of drug and alcohol use is mediated by them. The central claim of this chapter is that material and status privilege positively structures the meaning and outcome of drug and alcohol use, and this is especially noticeable where high affluence and privilege is associated with higher consumption. The framework and patterns presented here are not straightforwardly transferable between societies, however, a constant feature across different societies is the powerful effect that class status has on blunting or sharpening the impact of drug and alcohol problems on users and communities.

DEFINING SOCIAL CLASS AND DEPRIVATION

These two terms are often thrown together. However, they give different theoretical starting points and impart different tones to the discussion of alcohol and drug use. Social class is active, while deprivation is reactive. Studying social class means focusing on status, solidarity and differentiation, workplace organisation and labour process, capital accumulation and state ownership, competing and crosscutting identities, national labour markets and cycles of economic change (Buchmueller and Zuvekas, 1998; Gilman et al., 2011; Home Office, 2013; Sandberg, 2013). Deprivation studies tend to focus on spatial ghettoisation, relative isolation, material disadvantage, ethnicity and gender identities, state intervention, structural violence, surveillance and dependence, occasionally global flows, resource distribution and basic needs (Epele, 2011; MacDonald and Marsh, 2002; Shaw et al., 2007). Both perspectives cross cut each other and frequently make use of the same datasets and concepts. Measures of deprivation often combine a social class element. Both relate in different ways to the distribution of drug and alcohol related risks and harms.

Social class is often taken to mean occupation, however, it involves a network of different qualities linking to stratification and differentiation – education, cultural capital, and group identity. In this way, there is a tendency for measures of social class to become reified, forgetting that it is both a technical classification and also a recognisable 'folk category' (Bourdieu, 1987). The much-used occupation based British Registrar General's social class categories had dominated British social science for a century (Chandola, 2000). There is a natural inertia, in that data is categorised in that way because it has always been so. Consistency allows for comparability but also limits the conceptual grasp of the terms used and sometimes disguises the changing nature of these categories. In the UK and other Western industrialised countries, those changes are recognisable in the historical hollowing out of working class occupations, processes of deskilling and reskilling, the re-entry of women into the labour force and internal and international migration. They are all major changes that have altered the composition and texture of social class categories since 1945 (Jaumotte, 2003; Standing, 2011).

Established concepts of social class related to the capitalist labour market may have little relevance to non-Western countries. Analyses of divisions and changes in the UK and USA labour markets have emphasised market forces and the accumulation of capital. In contrast in China, the role of the state and the Communist Party are far more important, and to some extent, restrain capitalist class formation. The former cadre class has taken advantage of marketisation to reproduce and embed its status while retaining political authority (Bian et al., 2005). In each state, therefore, the relationship between power, opportunity and class position varies depending on history, ideology, overall material wealth, political opportunity, welfare state structure, taxation and redistribution and other factors.

Social class describes an economic or status *relationship*, which may be one of stratification or competing control over key political, social and economic resources. Typically, structured inequalities of resources and power are involved. In contrast, deprivation and associated terms such as poverty and disadvantage describe an *absence*, a comparative or absolute lack and vulnerability. Deprivation models try and capture the many faceted, gradational and constantly shifting nature of the object of study, although they also tend to be less theorised than social class models. The Scottish Index of Multiple Deprivation, for instance, seeks to nail down the combination of material resources, health and wellbeing, labour market stability, educational, cultural and democratic participation and other factors that mark inclusion and exclusion (Office of the Chief Statistician, 2006). Understanding what different aspects of social life the terms social class and deprivation capture is useful as they both shape drug and alcohol use in different ways.

SOCIO-ECONOMIC FACTORS IN POPULATION DISTRIBUTION OF DRUG AND ALCOHOL USE

Health and income tend to correlate. However, risky drug and alcohol use patterns do not straightforwardly match that relationship. This is an area where social class and deprivation perspectives inform the picture, but do so sometimes in unexpected ways – for example, where risk exposure is not positively correlated with social disadvantage (Parker et al., 2002; Wadsworth et al., 2004). Population consumption of drugs and alcohol is patterned by three class related factors: the ability and means to obtain them, the meaning attached to consumption and the risks involved. With alcohol, as a widely legitimated and valorised commodity, it is not surprising to see that consumption is highest among the most privileged groups, while risk is highest among the least privileged.

In some developing countries, such as China, individuals in more affluent categories are more likely to have less healthy lifestyles in general, the opposite relationship to that holding in the USA, for instance (Kim et al., 2004). This relationship is modified again by cross-cutting factors such as life course stage. A study of university students in the USA showed that heavy alcohol use and alcohol related harms were less likely among women, older students, ethnic minority students and students from less privileged class backgrounds (Weitzman and Chen, 2005). A comparison of 15-year old children in China and Finland showed that Chinese individuals from more affluent families were more likely to drink alcohol, whereas in Finland there was no relationship between affluence and alcohol consumption in this group (Liu et al., 2012). Other developing countries demonstrate similar class gradients in consumption to that of China, with privilege correlating with higher consumption (Ritterman et al., 2009). Being wealthy or poor in a wealthy country has a very different meaning than in a less wealthy, developing country. In Brazil, there are higher levels of binge drinking among more affluent male school pupils and among those attending private as opposed to public schools (Sanchez et al., 2013a). Regional data from Brazil also provides some support for the thesis that there is a relationship between income inequality and damaging health behaviours (Pickett and Wilkinson, 2015). In this case, higher inequality is associated with riskier health behaviour among the better off.

Higher income, class and occupational position are often positively correlated with alcohol consumption, but the reverse is the case with alcohol related harms and heavier drinking (Huckle et al., 2010). Members of less privileged social groups are frequently more likely to abstain entirely from alcohol, but these groups also often contain higher proportions of harmful drinkers than in more privileged social groups, who drink more heavily and exhibit less harmful behaviours and outcomes (World Health Organisation, 2014). A Canadian study showed a mildly U-shaped relationship between affluence and alcohol consumption for men, but not women, illustrating how gender modifies class (Matheson et al., 2012). Men living in more affluent neighbourhoods drunk more than those in mid-range neighbourhoods (4.5 to 3.7 drinks per week). Men living in the least affluent areas had 8.5 drinks per week. In the USA, higher education can be used as a very broad proxy for higher social class. Higher education enrolled young adults (18 to 22 years) are more likely to engage in binge drinking than those of the same age not in higher education (44.2 per cent compared to 35.6 per cent). Employed adults are more likely to drink (64.8 per cent) compared to the unemployed (56.1 per cent), but the unemployed have higher levels of extreme consumption (Substance Abuse and Mental Health Services Administration, 2011).

The relationship between consumption and class is heavily mediated by age and sex. In one 15-country study, it was found that the relationship breaks down by gender and country wealth (Bloomfield et al., 2006). Heavy episodic drinking (HED) increases by country wealth. The preponderance of male HEDs over female is greatest in middle income countries and least in low and high income countries, largely due to a much higher proportion of women drinking in high income countries. Many studies have found that the class relationship between risk and alcohol use is really a class plus gender relationship (Almeida-Filho et al., 2004; Barr et al., 1993). Men in less privileged socioeconomic groups are more likely to engage in harmful drinking and have alcohol problems, but this relationship does not hold true for women.

Turning to illicit drug use, we can observe similar influences sometimes resulting in different patterns. For example, the Crime Survey for England and Wales (Home Office, 2013) indicates that the highest levels of powder cocaine use are among those with a household income of either less than £10,000 or of £50,000 or more. However, for any drug overall, the highest use group is that earning less than £10,000. For cannabis, a strong curvilinear relationship was exhibited in the 1998 survey with 14.1 per cent of respondents with a household income of less than £10,000 and 12.3 per cent with one of £50,000 or over using the drug in the past year – the two highest use categories. This relationship had ironed out somewhat by 2013 into a linear relationship with falling levels of use now positively correlated with increasing income. Taking the figures for any drug use, there appears to be a phenomenon wherein for the UK's 'drugwise' generation of the 1990s and early 2000s (Parker et al., 2001) a somewhat curvilinear relationship is common. Middle income groups, those earning over £10,000 and less than £50,000, had lower use for all illicit drugs in 1998. With the fall in drug use among all groups since 2003/4, use among those with a household income of £50,000 or more has fallen faster than other groups. The consequence is an emerging relationship where illicit drug use in general, and specifically more harmful forms of use, is more concentrated in the lowest income category.

The UK Home Office has also classified illicit drug use data from 2001/2 according to the ACORN classification, which combines financial, geographical and lifestyle data (Shelton et al., 2006). It modifies this relationship again and shows a combined income, spatial and cultural relationship, with the 'Urban Prosperity' group having the highest levels of drug use in 2013, followed far behind by the 'Hard Pressed' group. However, again the levels of drug use have fallen more in the Urban Prosperity group from a strikingly high level of 22.4 per cent in 2001/2 to 13 per cent in 2012/13. So what we have is one better off group located by income, area and attitude, that is much more sensitive to changes in consumption trends and is more likely to take up and change its drug use in response to changing trends and leisure activities.

That sensitivity illustrates how the relationship between social class and drug use is one that involves both economic and social position and resources. It could be the case that the Urban Prosperity group is the ablest to defend and justify its consumption choices and deal with possible negative outcomes, so is most likely to temporarily engage in higher risk behaviour. That group is also a highly self-selecting one and likely to be attracted to urban living precisely because it affords opportunities for leisure activities that include drug use. We may also be looking at life stage factors. Families that have children and move into suburban areas will tend to be those on middle incomes and at a stage in their life where consumption patterns change away from riskier patterns of drug and alcohol use. The key finding here is that social class composition affects the form drug and alcohol use takes, and to an extent, the relationship is recursive.

Looking at attitudinal data, in the UK, the middle and less privileged income groups are much more likely to hold disapproving or risk averse attitudes to illicit drug use and drunkenness. Forty-one per cent of those with household income of £50,000 or over agree with the statement that 'it is okay to take cannabis occasionally', which falls to 24 per cent agreement for those with an income of under £10,000. With ecstasy and cocaine there is a similar pattern, and a much lower level of approval overall. So the less privileged income group is more likely to include drug users, harmful drinkers *and* people who exhibit blanket disapproval of these activities. Again there seems to be an 'urban culture effect' in the UK where there are more accepting attitudes to cannabis use among city dwellers, which is somewhat inverted in the case of drunkenness where rural dwellers are rather less likely to think if it as unsafe.

What explains the occasional greater propensity to engage in high-risk drinking and drug use behaviour among some of the more affluent social classes in some locations? The 'edgework' hypothesis (Lyng, 2005) proposes that the class position of individuals disposes them to engage in high risk activity as part of their self-identity. Voluntary risk taking is undertaken to display class position, which relies on class privilege mitigating the consequences of risk. That would certainly fit with the high drug use among the Urban Prosperity group and the attitudes of drug dealers from affluent backgrounds (Mohamed and Fritsvold, 2010). Drug and alcohol use then forms one way in which people perform social class. People in this social class have a more individuated identity stemming from their professional roles, and rely less on communal, solidaristic or institutional resources for self-identity (Turner, 1976). They take on more personal risk as a way of exploring and asserting their individual selves. In contrast, the coping hypothesis proposes that drinking and drug use among the hard-pressed group is a way of self-medicating and dealing with high stress environments (Terry-McElrath et al., 2009). However, it is hard to see either motivation as distributed by social class itself. It works better to see employment and class position as supporting localised drinking cultures around workplaces or positional identity. An example would be the compulsory after work drinking among Japanese white collar workers executives, obligations that increase with the occupational hierarchy (Ben-Ari, 2000; Hagihara et al., 2000). In the UK, individualised workplace cultures, such as white collar and more female dominated workplaces, promote leisure drinking and the 'big weekend' (Measham and Moore, 2009). Nevertheless, claims about high-risk consumption among the more affluent have to be modified by the fact that the connection between risk and harm is heavily mediated by class and deprivation.

THE DISTRIBUTION AND EXPERIENCE OF HARM

Multiple harms are typical of drug and alcohol use in the context of deprivation. They become most powerful in the context of multiple overlapping challenges that might include high incidence of disability and chronic illness, family disruption, employment insecurity and environmental risks such as unsafe substandard housing, service disruption, digital exclusion and high levels of crime and coercion (Shaw et al., 2007). Psychological stressors, exposure to physical risk and the absence of formal and informal safety nets, multiply harm and make it harder to mitigate. Harms have to be understood as being produced and distributed politically. It is a political choice to expose some members of society to greater harm than others.

Rhodes (2009) sets out a very useful typology for understanding the risk environment that generates or ameliorates risk in the context of the users' own situation. It allows us to separate out the distinct ways in which socio-economic risks are distributed and created in each context. It guides us to think more coherently about the patterning of risk and the effective public health responses to it. It also alerts us to how consumption and risk have to be thought of in a global context where people, products and practices transfer and transmit themselves around the world rapidly, contributing to a fast evolving risk environment. He divides risks into those manifesting in the micro environment and the macro environment. The micro environment consists of those elements of the situation that the user and those around them directly interact with, and the macro environment consists of the political, social and economic context structuring the situation that they are in. Class and deprivation operate differently here. For example, an aspect of risk distributed by class would be the power relationship between different groups. Middle and upper class drug users are generally better placed to avoid institutional and workplace drug surveillance (Campbell, 2004). That ability is an extension of the power and agency they enjoy in relation to their workplaces and the institutions they deal with, which is structured by social class – an aspect of the macro environment. Conversely, drug users living in deprived circumstances often lack the resources to avoid exposure and stigma – an aspect of the micro-environment (Stengel, 2014).

Rhodes additionally identifies distinct domains in which risk operates: the spatial and personal, the social, economic and policy. In the spatial and personal domain, micro risks associated with deprivation might consist of poor quality housing conditions that compound health problems and create psychological stressors along with lack of access to safe, controlled spaces for alcohol and drug consumption. Those associated with the macro environment include the concentration of open air drug markets in deprived neighbourhoods, which relates to concentration of users and the greater power of those in the more privileged classes to make demands on policing resources (Martínez et al., 2008). In the social domain, we can see how, in terms of the micro environment, more deprived users are exposed to greater stigmatisation. In the macro environment, middle class users of drugs and alcohol tend to have social and media representations that support their use, that valorise and excuse it. For example, the image of university as a time for hedonism permits extreme intoxication within a largely middle class, time bounded context (Vander Ven, 2011). In economic terms, deprived users are typically in economically precarious positions. Jobs are insecure and low paid, making planning difficult. On the macro level, social security payments are contingent and can be withdrawn. Social security payments accruing to middle class individuals tend to be citizenship rights based. For example, Medicare in the US and pension payments in most countries are not contingent on the behaviour of the recipient. The part of the welfare state that services the poor, in contrast, is increasingly reconfigured to treat poverty as the outcome of individual pathology (Wiggan, 2012). Support is then made increasingly dependent on them modifying their behaviour, such as entering treatment for drug and alcohol use or maintaining a drug free lifestyle. Therefore, the politics of class and deprivation fundamentally texture the relationship of the individual drug or alcohol user and the state.

In the policy domain, punitive drug and alcohol polices tend to fall on deprived users. There is targeting of marginal groups by police and paramilitary agencies, which disrupts the survival strategies they have to employ in highly precarious situations (Parkin and Coomber, 2009; Ribeiro, 2008). In terms of macro-level policy, social segmentation can be supported by housing and welfare policies. Risks also arise from policy decisions about the legal status of each chemical substance. Some of these are essentially arbitrary, such as the distinction between alcohol and illicit drugs. That exposes deprived drug users to much greater risk of arrest and imprisonment. Users can then be exposed to 'secondary punishments' for illicit drug offences and the weight of these falls much more on those who lack other resources. In the USA, this can take the form of withdrawal of social security payments, denial of access to college loans and denial of the right to vote arising from a felony drug use conviction (Blumenson and Nilsen, 2002; Travis, 2002). While in theory these punishments can fall on anyone, in practice, their impact is heaviest upon the most deprived and marginalised (Jürgens et al., 2010). The division is particularly apparent in the terms on which drug and alcohol treatment is accessed. More privileged groups can set the terms on which they access support, they have choice over the form, place and time of it, and they can enter and leave with much greater freedom than those in less privileged positions (Hunt and Stevens, 2004). The overall effect is to diminish the citizenship of more deprived users. They are exposed to greater surveillance, are more likely to received custodial sentences and then find themselves deprived of other rights and entitlements.

To these specific changes, we can add global and historical changes that encompass and work through these different domains. The intensifying relationship between drug and alcohol use and harm is the result of the reconfiguration of labour markets and welfare states around the world, affecting community and personal stability, income, social mobility and disrupting formal and informal supports (McCartney et al., 2012). This can be seen in countries that have endured severe and traumatic de-industrialisation. Leyland et al. (2007) examined the relationship between area deprivation and various causes of mortality in Scotland in three cohorts since 1980. Their data show rising mortality for chronic liver disease among the most deprived group in 2000 to 2002 compared to previous decades, a condition for which alcohol is a major risk factor. There are other vulnerabilities affecting this group, such as the rise in hepatitis infections among intravenous drug users (Hutchinson et al., 2006). Macro and micro environmental risks can be identified in this data. Changes in the labour market, and the availability of drugs and alcohol, are macro risks. Changing habits related to intravenous drug use are micro risks. It was particularly striking in this dataset how harm was multiplied for those suffering multiple kinds of deprivation.

The work of Rhodes and many others points us towards the political economy of health (Bambra et al., 2005). Social economic status inequalities are actively produced and risks distributed. Interest groups lobby and generate constituencies for particular standpoints, known as 'astroturfing' (Edgar, 2013), markets and institutions are shaped by the state (Graeber, 2010) and policies reflect the prejudices and priorities of powerful interest groups and industries more than objective need or harm (Stevens, 2007). Being healthy is part of an achievement of normality, of being an acceptable member of society (Lupton, 1995). Prevailing ideas of what that means are patterned by class, and stigma attaches to ways of using drugs and alcohol that are associated with lower status groups (Blaxter, 1997).

STIGMA, LOSS AND IDENTITY

Stigma can be defined as a pathologised social status, by which structured deprivation connects to personal harm (Hatzenbuehler et al.,

2013). Occupying a stigmatised status – which may be on account of one's sexuality, occupation, caste, religion, ethnicity, mental illness, criminal record, alcoholism or being a user of an illicit drug – frequently reduces the ability to access resources, gain employment, education, credit and have one's needs and demands acknowledged by mainstream services. It creates secondary stressors, isolating and exposing the stigmatised to psychological strain, interpersonal violence and other harms (Richardson et al., 2015). People possessing a stigmatised status often have to expend considerably time and energy dealing with its consequences, putting effort into managing and sometimes concealing it (Lavin, 2014).

Stigma attaches to blameworthy categories, in which people are defined as of lower social worth and authors of their own misfortune. In one ethnographic study in the USA, it was found that medical staff were reluctant to use anaesthetic or analgesics on 'junkies', on the assumption that they would be ineffective, that they should suffer or they could take the pain (Bourgois and Schonberg, 2009). One effect of stigma is on the differential publically acknowledged social loss that occurs in relation to drug related deaths. Drug related deaths are culturally categorised according to the status of the victim. Deaths of young, white, middle class females from illicit drug use represent the epitome of the innocent victim (Forsyth, 2001). Bad, problematic, deaths are of those who are older, poorer and who have been using drugs volitionally for a long time and who are therefore held culpable for their own demise (Guy and Holloway, 2007). Deaths attributed to particularly stigmatised drugs, such as heroin, methamphetamine or crack, render the dead person suspect and make grieving for family members particularly difficult (Valentine et al., 2015). On a personal level the manner of the death calls the moral status of the dead person, and by the process of courtesy stigma (Goffman, 2009), the family itself, into question. A therapeutic part of the grieving process is the creating of a narrative around the dead person, a set of eulogies to their life and those they leave behind (Gillies and Neimeyer, 2006). The public and community response to 'bad' drug related deaths make this difficult.

Stigma is bound up with personal identity and one's agency – the capacity to act autonomously in the world. It has a strong class inflection, for example, with working class, female smokers being heavily stigmatised in societies where smoking levels have fallen rapidly (Berridge, 2007). In South America, chicha – an often illicitly brewed alcoholic drink – was presented in public discourse as the toxic, crime generating, stupefying drink of the indigenous poor (Meléndez, 2003). The drink was prohibited in Colombia, where beer was promoted as a healthy, modern, hygienic drink. Chicha and other locally produced, non-commoditised, alcohols persisted in South America as a focus for local customs, identity, culture and economic reciprocity (Daughters, 2014). Using a stigmatised substance can therefore also become a way of resisting social class or other dominant identities. Stigma can change drug use patterns in very specific ways. For example, the use of blunts – cannabis laced cigars – emerged among Southeast Asian Americans as a way of avoiding what they perceived as stigmatised drug use forms and patterns (Soller and Lee, 2010)

These resistant identities and attitudes developed by stigmatised groups point to the structural injustices that contribute to their situation and seek to push the responsibility for health outcomes back onto institutions (Pilnick and Coleman, 2003). Parkin (2013) identified public injecting among highly marginalised drug use as a meaningful, purposeful activity with the potential to establish and confirm valued social relationships and social capital, in a situation where opportunities for self-actualisation were otherwise highly constrained by welfare and policing institutions. The 'righteous dopefiend' was a more cohesive resistant identity, identified in urban ethnographies of black communities in the USA of the 1960s (Sutter, 1966). The righteous dopefiend was a dealer and a hustler, usually young, black and male, who defined his separation from, and contempt for, the straight white world by his heroin use and his ability to stay one step ahead of the authorities. Once young and an outsider, in the West, users of heroin are now old and marginal even amidst the marginalised (Bourgois and Schonberg, 2009). These examples illustrate how even marginalised, stigmatised drug and alcohol consumption can be a source of valid cultural capital and can reaffirm valued social networks.

SPACE, SOCIAL NETWORKS AND CULTURAL CAPITAL

Non-economic resources have a profound impact on health and patterns of social behaviour (Abel, 2008). Cultural capital is the combination of non-economic resources people can command: educational qualifications, cultural confidence and know-how. Social capital is the relationships that they can leverage, such as community networks, family ties and the more diffuse social recognition that comes with reputation. When these bonds break down, have never existed or do not work as they are meant to, then the problems caused by a lack of economic resources become especially bleak and horizons diminish.

Social capital is key in how communities and individuals are able to respond to economic shocks, such as those of de-industrialisation. In the UK during the 1980s, heroin use took off rapidly and became much more a habit of the poor and excluded (Seddon, 2006). It spread rapidly to urban and rural areas affected by post-industrial blight such as Fife, Edinburgh, Glasgow, Manchester and Liverpool. The collapse of coal and heavy industries, rapid deskilling and high male unemployment combined with longstanding poverty and housing problems to create rapid social disintegration. Looking at how social capital is concentrated – or missing – spatially, there is a distinct spatial stress effect associated with deprived neighbourhoods, with one USA study showing high levels of heavy drinking in low income neighbourhoods related to anxiety and depression (Hill and Angel, 2005). Deprived areas often suffer more problems with public drug use independently of other economic factors (Boardman et al., 2001) and are likely to be the location of public, open air drug markets. As well as generally reducing the amenity of the area, they expose residents to risks of violence (Kadushin et al., 1998). The same phenomenon can be seen in the spread of crack cocaine, and later methamphetamine use, in the USA among urban black and rural white communities (Acker, 2010). There is an intricate relationship between space, class and drug/alcohol consumption. Brazil's social class gradient for binge drinking was modified by region, and there is a stronger relationship in the poorer regions between higher social class and binge drinking (Sanchez et al., 2013a).

In response to these problems, social networks can be mutually advantageous or they can involve a dangerous combination of social fragmentation and mistrust. A study of young drug users in a deindustrialising region of Arctic Russia showed social life to be a constant *dvizhukha* or hustle for them (Pilkington and Sharifullina, 2009). Fencing stolen property, manipulating those in need of cash through predatory lending and drug dealing were ways in which social networks were exploited to personal advantage. However, successes in achieving profitable drug trades, in obtaining money for drugs and in avoiding being ripped off are always contingent and temporary. Hustling in the illicit drug economy can expose men and women to violence, robbery, abuse and arrest while also providing those who can manage in it a temporary step-up in local recognition (Sommers et al., 2000).

Structural factors pattern the HIV risks of injecting drug use practice (Rhodes et al.,

2005). Network effects are strong. HIV and drug injection spread along trafficking routes, creating cross border point to point risk relationships. Social change and development can also disrupt protective neighbourhood networks (McCord and Freeman, 1990). Disintegrating social networks can lead to higher levels of drug use and more dangerous drug use practices and higher levels of drug market violence (Werb et al., 2011). The bodies of deprived heroin users are marked by trauma, scars from untreated wounds, exposure to open air, track marks, collapsed veins and so on. They are both physical memories of the damage of marginalised heroin use and structural marginality.

Resilience is the other side of the coin from risk. It captures the way in which many, often most, people exposed to a particular risk factor mange to achieve better than predicted life outcomes. It is a combination of social capital and personal agency (Backett-Milburn et al., 2008). Children of parents with drug and alcohol problems are exposed to high levels of disruption, crime and poverty. Providing support focused on life transitions and particularly on the transition from adolescence to adulthood is effective in supporting more positive outcomes. Social and network capital are key features of health protective ideas, lay theorising and lay support for health treatment (Cattell, 2001). Drug and alcohol use spreads along social networks, and plays its part in cohering social networks around sociable activities. Chloroform use in Brazil among better off high school students is diffused by their dense social networks, for instance, among pupils at private schools (Sanchez et al., 2013b). Protective knowledge and lay support are also inherent to social networks.

SOCIAL CLASS, POLITICS AND POLICY

Power – meaning the ability and capacity of specific groups to identify and act in their own interests – is crucial in mediating the relationship between health risks and health outcomes (Link and Phelan, 2014; Navarro and Shi, 2001). This perspective highlights that health and social problems resulting from drug and alcohol use are a policy, as well as, or more than, a personal, choice (Navarro, 2007). In the USA, the differential criminal justice focus on crack cocaine, mainly used and traded by socially marginal, urban black populations, in contrast to powder cocaine, typically used by suburban, better off whites is one example where exposure to harm comes together with the power to defend one's group interests (Stuntz, 1998). Power legitimates behaviour. For instance, the ability of alcohol industry organisations to influence licensing, taxation and public discourse to the benefit of some of its consumers can be contrasted with the arbitrary use of force against Afghan opium producers (Bakke and Endal, 2010; Chouvy, 2009). In contrast to the responsibility placed on illicit drug producers, alcohol problems are individualised – blamed on the minority of individual drinkers who were said to be unable to control their intake (Nicholls and Greenaway, 2015).

In the UK, the evening and night-time economy (ENTE) has been licensed to generate revenue and regenerate city and town centres through the provision of easy to drink alcohol and high volume drinking spaces. The ENTE has evolved to provide multiple drinking spaces that are targeted according to social class, gender and related culture, style and taste factors (Hollands and Chatterton, 2003). So when thinking about the class distribution of alcohol use we should consider the meaning of different drink products, drinking styles, spaces and habits and the structuring of these by social class. Commodification of the ENTE has meant greater social segmentation. Corporations have sought to create and define drinking spaces and products to appeal to particular market segments and classes (Hollands and Chatterton, 2003). Products that are advertised as 'reassuringly expensive' are clearly designed and priced to appeal to affluent and aspirational groups. The urban playgrounds that have emerged in globalised cities from Melbourne to Manchester service them (Chatterton and Hollands, 2002). Drinking at home has arisen in many Western countries as a form of withdrawal from the ENTE. Home drinking can be a way of dealing with high prices and also avoiding the violence and exclusion of the public drinking world or preparing to enter it by pre-drinking (Bancroft, 2012). Looking beyond the UK, commercial developments can support changes in consumption practice. In Japan, where female drinking has long been defined as a problem, there is the development of new entertainment services for white collar woman around alcohol consumption and *asobi*, or 'play' (Ho, 2015).

Illicit drug markets operate on different dynamics but are shaped by some of the same forces – globalisation, technological change, product development, aspirational identities and the emergence of niche markets (Ruggiero and South, 1997; see also Chapter 37, this volume). Illicit flows tended to follow licit ones. For example, the diversified Colombian heroin trade with the USA grew with the North American Free Trade Agreement. The image of illicit drug markets in deprived areas is one of open air selling and using, with frequent violence as deals go sour. A study in England and Wales indicated the advent of mobile technology and responses to law enforcement surveillance have migrated much drug selling away from open air settings (Lupton et al., 2002). The growth of online drug markets changes the dynamic of drug purchase. Users of encrypted drug markets are less exposed to violence and the risk of rip off or arrest compared to more marginalised users who have to make cash only on-street trades (Aldridge and Décary-Hétu, 2014). Violence and stigma add to the stress of deprivation for those living in the neighbourhood whether they are directly involved or not. Spatial analysis shows that while violence may cluster around some drug markets, there is no certain relationship, with factors such as law enforcement activity, competition and the type of drug for sale being more influential (Lum, 2011).

CONCLUSION

Unsurprisingly, social class and deprivation shape both the propensity to take up drug and alcohol consumption and the harms that might result. In general, the social consumption gradient varies between societies and at different times, while the social harm gradient runs in one direction. Consumption might be higher in more wealthy groups, as in several developing countries, while harm still clusters at the least well off end of the scale. A very basic division would be that social class changes the meaning and level of drug and alcohol use, while deprivation changes the impact. Factors involved include spatial segregation, inequality, differential access to support services and exposure of some individuals to more punitive consequences and stigma for similar activities. Most worrying is where, as in the UK and USA, harms have become more severe and concentrated over time. The longer poverty and unemployment lasts for individuals, the greater its impact (Mossakowski, 2008). Therefore, declining mobility for the most deprived sections of society has especially grave consequences.

This encourages us to think about how harm reduction might move beyond individual risk behaviour and, following Rhodes (2009), understand how risk is produced and becomes institutionalised and hidden through some of the same mechanisms that perpetuate social class inequality. As I have shown in this chapter, there is a politics of harm. Harm is produced and distributed politically, according to decisions and choices made about the labour market, the welfare state, the prohibition of some substances and the promotion of others, gender relations, neighbourhood and community supports and a myriad of other factors that cluster around class and deprivation. Just as there is a politics of harm, there can be a politics of harm reduction that draws attention to how these harms are produced and distributed.

REFERENCES

Abel, T. (2008) 'Cultural capital and social inequality in health', *Journal of Epidemiology and Community Health* 62(7): e13.

Acker, C.J. (2010) 'How crack found a niche in the American ghetto: the historical epidemiology of drug-related harm', *BioSocieties* 5(1): 70–88.

Aldridge, J. and Décary-Hétu, D. (2014) *Not an 'Ebay for Drugs': The Cryptomarket 'Silk Road' as a Paradigm Shifting Criminal Innovation*. SSRN Scholarly Paper: 2436643. Available from: http://ssrn.com/abstract=2436643 (Accessed 31 March 2016).

Almeida-Filho, N., et al. (2004) 'Alcohol drinking patterns by gender, ethnicity, and social class in Bahia, Brazil', *Revista de Saúde Pública* 38(1): 45–54.

Ben-Ari, E. (2000) '"Not-precisely-work": golf, entertainment and imbibement among Japanese business executives in Singapore', In E. Ben-Ari and J. Clammer (eds), *Japan in Singapore: Cultural Occurrences and Cultural Flows*. Oxford: Routledge, pp. 150–74.

Backett-Milburn, K., et al. (2008) 'Challenging childhoods: young people's accounts of "getting by" in families with substance use problems', *Childhood* 15(4): 461–79.

Bakke, Ø. and Endal, D. (2010) 'Alcohol policies out of context: drinks industry supplanting government role in alcohol policies in Sub-Saharan Africa', *Addiction* 105(1): 22–8.

Bambra, C., et al. (2005) 'Towards a politics of health', *Health Promotion International* 20(2): 187–93.

Bancroft, A. (2012) 'Drinking with and without fun: female students' accounts of pre-drinking and club-drinking', *Sociological Research Online* 17(4): 7. Available from: http://www.socresonline.org.uk/17/4/7.html (Accessed 31 March 2016).

Barr, K.E.M., et al. (1993) 'Race, class, and gender differences in substance abuse: evidence of middle-class/underclass polarization among black males', *Social Problems* 40(3): 314–27.

Berridge, V. (2007) *Smoking and The Sea Change in Public Health, 1945–2007*. London: Institute of Contemporary British History.

Bian, Y., et al. (2005) 'Occupation, class, and social networks in urban China', *Social Forces* 83(4): 1443–68.

Blaxter, M. (1997) 'Whose fault is it? People's own conceptions of the reasons for health inequalities', *Social Science and Medicine* 44(6): 747–56.

Bloomfield, K., et al. (2006) 'Social inequalities in alcohol consumption and alcohol-related problems in the study countries of the EU Concerted Action "Gender, Culture and Alcohol Problems: A Multi-National Study"', *Alcohol and Alcoholism* 41(Suppl. 1): i26–36.

Blumenson, E. and Nilsen, E.S. (2002) 'How to construct an underclass, or how the war on drugs became a war on education', *Journal of Gender, Race and Justice* 6: 61–110.

Boardman, J.D., et al. (2001) 'Neighborhood disadvantage, stress, and drug use among adults', *Journal of Health and Social Behavior* 42(2): 151–65.

Bourdieu, P. (1987) 'What makes a social class? On the theoretical and practical existence of groups', *Berkeley Journal of Sociology* 32: 1–17.

Bourgois, P. and Schonberg, J. (2009) *Righteous Dopefiend*. Berkeley: University of California Press.

Buchmueller, T.C. and Zuvekas, S.H. (1998) 'Drug use, drug abuse, and labour market outcomes', *Health Economics* 7(3): 229–45.

Campbell, N.D. (2004) 'Technologies of suspicion: coercion and compassion in post-disciplinary surveillance regimes', *Surveillance and Society* 2(1): 79–92.

Cattell, V. (2001) 'Poor people, poor places, and poor health: the mediating role of social networks and social capital', *Social Science and Medicine* 52(10): 1501–16.

Chandola, T. (2000) 'Social class differences in mortality using the new UK National

Statistics Socio-Economic Classification', *Social Science and Medicine* 50(5): 641–9.

Chatterton, P. and Hollands, R. (2002) 'Theorising urban playscapes: producing, regulating and consuming youthful nightlife city spaces', *Urban Studies* 39(1): 95–116.

Chouvy, P.A. (2009) *Opium: Uncovering the Politics of the Poppy*. Cambridge: Harvard University Press.

Daughters, A. (2014) 'Of chicha, majas, and mingas: hard apple cider and local solidarity in twenty-first-century rural southern Chile', In G. Pierce and Á. Toxqui (eds), *Alcohol in Latin America: A Social and Cultural History*. Tuscon: The University of Arizona Press, pp. 242–60.

Edgar, A. (2013) 'The dominance of big pharma: power', *Medicine, Health Care and Philosophy* 16(2): 295–304.

Epele, M.E. (2011) 'New toxics, new poverty: a social understanding of the freebase cocaine/paco in Buenos Aires, Argentina', *Substance Use and Misuse* 46(12): 1468–76.

Forsyth, A.J.M. (2001) 'Distorted? A quantitative exploration of drug fatality reports in the popular press', *International Journal of Drug Policy* 12(5–6): 435–53.

Gillies, J. and Neimeyer, R.A. (2006) 'Loss, grief, and the search for significance: toward a model of meaning reconstruction in bereavement', *Journal of Constructivist Psychology* 19(1): 31–65.

Gilman, N., et al. (2011) *Deviant Globalization: Black Market Economy in the 21st Century*. London: Bloomsbury Publishing.

Goffman, E. (2009) *Stigma: Notes on the Management of Spoiled Identity*. New York: Simon and Schuster.

Graeber, D. (2010) *Debt: The First 5,000 Years*. Brooklyn: Melville House.

Guy, P. and Holloway, M. (2007) 'Drug related deaths and the "special deaths" of late modernity', *Sociology* 41(1): 83–96.

Hagihara, A., et al. (2000) 'Work stressors, drinking with colleagues after work, and job satisfaction among white-collar workers in Japan', *Substance Use and Misuse* 35(5): 737–56.

Hatzenbuehler, M.L., et al. (2013) 'Stigma as a fundamental cause of population health inequalities', *American Journal of Public Health* 103(5): 813–21.

Hill, T.D. and Angel, R.J. (2005) 'Neighborhood disorder, psychological distress, and heavy drinking', *Social Science and Medicine* 61(5): 965–75.

Hollands, R. and Chatterton, P. (2003) 'Producing nightlife in the new urban entertainment economy: corporatization, branding and market segmentation', *International Journal of Urban and Regional Research* 27(2): 361–85.

Home Office (2013) *Drug Misuse: Findings from the 2012 to 2013 Crime Survey for England and Wales*. London: National Statistics.

Ho, S.L. (2015) '"License to drink": white-collar female workers and Japan's urban night space', *Ethnography* 16(1): 25–50.

Huckle, T., et al. (2010) 'Socio-economic status predicts drinking patterns but not alcohol-related consequences independently', *Addiction* 105(7): 1192–202.

Hunt, N. and Stevens, A. (2004) 'Whose harm? Harm reduction and the shift to coercion in UK drug policy', *Social Policy and Society* 3(4): 333–42.

Hutchinson, S.J. et al. (2006) 'Hepatitis C virus infection in Scotland: epidemiological review and public health challenges', *Scottish Medical Journal* 51(2): 8–15.

Jaumotte, F. (2003) 'Labour force participation of women: empirical evidence on the role of policy and other determinants in OECD countries', *OECD Economic Studies* 37(2): 51–108.

Jürgens, R., et al. (2010) 'People who use drugs, HIV, and human rights', *The Lancet* 376(9739): 475–85.

Kadushin, C., et al. (1998) 'The substance use system: social and neighborhood environments associated with substance use and misuse', *Substance Use and Misuse* 33(8): 1681–710.

Kim, S., et al. (2004) 'Contrasting socioeconomic profiles related to healthier lifestyles in China and the United States', *American Journal of Epidemiology* 159(2): 184–91.

Lavin, M.F. (2014) 'If you want it, you can get it right here: space and drug use in strip clubs', *Humanity and Society* 38(2): 132–57.

Leyland, A., et al. (2007) 'Cause-specific inequalities in mortality in Scotland: two decades of change. A population-based study', *BMC Public Health* 7(1): 172.

Link, B.G. and Phelan, J. (2014) 'Stigma power', *Social Science and Medicine* 103: 24–32.

Liu, Y., et al. (2012) 'Socioeconomic inequalities in alcohol use of adolescents: the differences between China and Finland', *International Journal of Public Health* 58(2): 177–85.

Lum, C. (2011) 'Violence, drug markets and racial composition challenging stereotypes through spatial analysis', *Urban Studies* 48(13): 2715–32.

Lupton, D. (1995) *The Imperative of Health: Public Health and the Regulated Body*. London: Sage.

Lupton, R., et al. (2002) *A Rock and a Hard Place: Drug Markets in Deprived Neighbourhoods*. London: Home Office.

Lyng, S. (2005) *Edgework: The Sociology of Risk Taking*. London: Routledge.

MacDonald, R. and Marsh, J. (2002) 'Crossing the Rubicon: youth transitions, poverty, drugs and social exclusion', *International Journal of Drug Policy* 13: 27–38.

Marmot, M. and UCL Institute of Health Equity (2013) *Review of Social Determinants and the Health Divide in the WHO European Region: Final Report*. Geneva: World Health Organisation.

Martínez, R., et al. (2008) 'Social disorganization, drug market activity, and neighborhood violent crime', *Urban Affairs Review* 43(6): 846–74.

Matheson, F.I., et al. (2012) 'Drinking in context: the influence of gender and neighbourhood deprivation on alcohol consumption', *Journal of Epidemiology and Community Health* 66(6): e4.

McCartney, G., et al. (2012) 'Has Scotland always been the "sick man" of Europe? An observational study from 1855 to 2006', *European Journal of Public Health* 22(6): 756–60.

McCord, C. and Freeman, H.P. (1990) 'Excess mortality in Harlem', *New England Journal of Medicine* 322(3): 173–7.

Measham, F. and Moore, K. (2009) 'Repertoires of distinction: exploring patterns of weekend polydrug use within local leisure scenes across the English night time economy', *Journal of Criminology and Criminal Justice* 9(4): 437–64.

Meléndez, M. (2003) 'Women and alcohol: cultural essence and social deviance in early twentieth-century South America', *Confluencia* 18(2): 53–66.

Mohamed, A.R. and Fritsvold, E.D. (2010) *Dorm Room Dealers: Drugs and the Privileges of Race and Class*. Boulder: Lynne Rienner Publishers.

Mossakowski, K.N. (2008) 'Is the duration of poverty and unemployment a risk factor for heavy drinking?', *Social Science and Medicine* 67(6): 947–55.

Navarro, V. (ed.) (2007) *Neoliberalism, Globalization, and Inequalities: Consequences for Health and Quality of Life*. Amityville: Baywood Publishing Company.

Navarro, V. and Shi, L. (2001) 'The political context of social inequalities and health', *Social Science and Medicine* 52(3): 481–91.

Nicholls, J. and Greenaway, J. (2015) 'What is the problem? Evidence, politics and alcohol policy in England and Wales, 2010–2014', *Drugs: Education, Prevention, and Policy* 22(2): 135–42.

Office of the Chief Statistician (2006) *Scottish Index of Multiple Deprivation 2006 Technical Report*. Edinburgh: Scottish Executive.

Parker, H., et al. (2001) *UK Drugs Unlimited: New Research and Policy Lessons on Illicit Drug Use*. Houndmills and New York: Palgrave.

Parker, H., et al. (2002) 'The normalization of "sensible" recreational drug use: further evidence from the North West England Longitudinal Study', *Sociology* 36(4): 941–64.

Parkin, S. (2013) *Habitus and Drug Using Environments: Health, Place and Lived-Experience*. Farnham: Ashgate.

Parkin, S. and Coomber, R. (2009) 'Informal "Sorter" Houses: a qualitative insight of the "shooting gallery" phenomenon in a UK setting', *Health and Place* 15(4): 981–9.

Pickett, K.E. and Wilkinson, R.G. (2015) 'Income inequality and health: a causal review', *Social Science and Medicine* 128: 316–26.

Pilkington, H. and Sharifullina, E. (2009) 'The mutual extraction industry: drug use and the normative structure of social capital in the Russian far north', *International Journal of Drug Policy, Risk Environment and Drug Harms* 20(3): 251–60.

Pilnick, A. and Coleman, T. (2003) '"I'll give up smoking when you get me better": patients' resistance to attempts to problematise smoking in general practice (GP) consultations', *Social Science and Medicine* 57(1): 135–45.

Rhodes, T., et al. (2005) 'The social structural production of HIV risk among injecting drug users', *Social Science and Medicine* 61(5): 1026–44.

Rhodes, T. (2009) 'Risk environments and drug harms: a social science for harm reduction approach', *International Journal of Drug Policy* 20(3): 193–201.

Ribeiro, M.O. (2008) 'Street children and their relationship with the police', *International Nursing Review* 55(1): 89–96.

Richardson, L.A., et al. (2015) 'Socioeconomic marginalisation in the structural production of vulnerability to violence among people who use illicit drugs', *Journal of Epidemiology and Community Health* 69: 686–92.

Ritterman, M.L., et al. (2009) 'Objective and subjective social class gradients for substance use among Mexican adolescents', *Social Science and Medicine* 68(10): 1843–51.

Ruggiero, V. and South, N. (1997) 'The late-modern city as a bazaar: drug markets, illegal enterprise and the "barricades"', *British Journal of Sociology* 48(1): 54–70.

Sanchez, Z.M., Locatelli, D.P., et al. (2013a) 'Binge drinking among Brazilian students: a gradient of association with socioeconomic status in five geo-economic regions', *Drug and Alcohol Dependence* 127(1–3): 87–93.

Sanchez, Z.M., Noto, A.R., et al. (2013b) 'Social rank and inhalant drug use: the case of lança perfume use in São Paulo, Brazil', *Drug and Alcohol Dependence* 131(1–2): 92–9.

Sandberg, S. (2013) 'Cannabis culture: a stable subculture in a changing world', *Criminology and Criminal Justice* 13(1): 63–79.

Seddon, T. (2006) 'Drugs, crime and social exclusion', *British Journal of Criminology* 46(4): 680–703.

Shaw, A., et al. (2007) *Drugs and Poverty: A Literature Review*. Edinburgh: Scottish Drugs Forum.

Shelton, N.J., et al. (2006) 'Where not to live: a geo-demographic classification of mortality for England and Wales, 1981–2000', *Health and Place* 12(4): 557–69.

Soller, B. and Lee, J.P. (2010) 'Drug-intake methods and social identity: the use of marijuana in blunts among Southeast Asian adolescents and emerging adults', *Journal of Adolescent Research* 25(6): 783–806.

Sommers, I.B., et al. (2000) *Workin' Hard for the Money: The Social and Economic Lives of Women Drug Sellers*. Huntington: Nova Science.

Standing, G. (2011) *The Precariat: The New Dangerous Class*. London: Bloomsbury.

Stengel, C. (2014) 'The risk of being "too honest": drug use, stigma and pregnancy', *Health, Risk and Society* 16(1): 36–50.

Stevens, A. (2007) 'Survival of the ideas that fit: an evolutionary analogy for the use of evidence in policy', *Social Policy and Society* 6(01): 25–35.

Stuntz, W.J. (1998) 'Race, class, and drugs', *Columbia Law Review* 98(7): 1795–842.

Substance Abuse and Mental Health Services Administration (2011) *Results from the 2010 National Survey on Drug Use and Health: Summary of National Findings*, NSDUH Series H-41. Rockville: Substance Abuse and Mental Health Services Administration.

Sutter, A.G. (1966) 'The world of the righteous dope fiend', *Issues in Criminology* 2(2): 177–222.

Terry-McElrath, Y.M., et al. (2009) 'Reasons for drug use among American youth by consumption level, gender, and race/ethnicity: 1976–2005', *Journal of Drug Issues* 39(3): 677–713.

Travis, J. (2002) 'Invisible punishment: an instrument of social exclusion', In M. Mauer and M. Chesney-Lind (eds), *Invisible Punishment: The Collateral Consequences of Mass Imprisonment*. New York: The New Press, pp. 17–36.

Turner, R. (1976) 'The real self: from institution to impulse', *The American Journal of Sociology* 81(5): 989–1016.

Valentine, C., et al. (2015) 'There are limits on what you can do biographical reconstruction by those bereaved by alcohol-related deaths', In T. Thurnell-Read (ed.), *Drinking Dilemmas:*

Space, Culture and Identity. London: Routledge.

Vander Ven, T. (2011) *Getting Wasted: Why College Students Drink Too Much and Party So Hard*. New York University Press.

Wadsworth, E.J.K., et al. (2004) 'Factors associated with recreational drug use', *Journal of Psychopharmacology* 18(2): 238–48.

Weitzman, E.R. and Chen, Y.Y. (2005) 'Risk modifying effect of social capital on measures of heavy alcohol consumption, alcohol abuse, harms, and secondhand effects: national survey findings', *Journal of Epidemiology and Community Health* 59(4): 303–9.

Werb, D., et al. (2011) 'Effect of drug law enforcement on drug market violence: a systematic review', *International Journal of Drug Policy* 22(2): 87–94.

Wiggan, J. (2012) 'Telling stories of 21st century welfare: the UK Coalition Government and the neo-liberal discourse of worklessness and dependency', *Critical Social Policy* 32(3): 383–405.

World Health Organisation (2014) *Global Status Report on Alcohol and Health 2014*. Geneva: World Health Organisation.

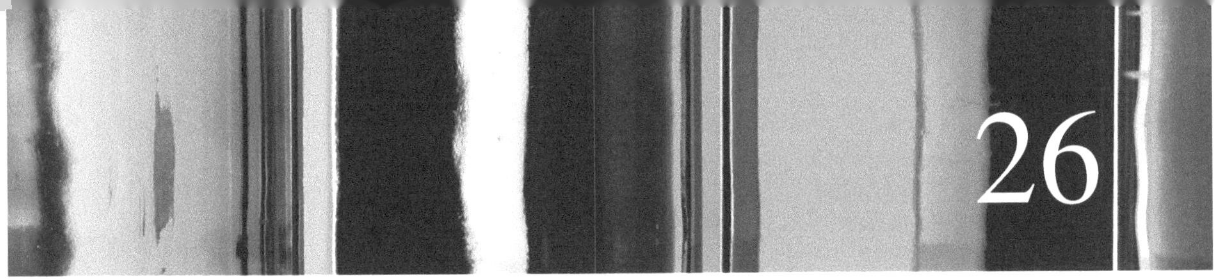

Maturing on a High: An Analysis of Trends, Prevalence and Patterns of Recreational Drug Use in Middle and Older Adulthood

Lisa Williams and Rebecca Askew

INTRODUCTION

Recreational drug use is commonly perceived as a youthful activity that decreases as age increases. The direction of trends in drug taking in many Western countries also shows a general decline over time over the past couple of decades. However, as we outline in this chapter, in spite of these overall reductions in use, in recent decades, drug use is extending further into adulthood at higher rates of prevalence than has traditionally been the case. The Crime Survey for England and Wales (CSEW) (Home Office, 2013) reported recent drug use had increased for all adults aged 35 and over, whilst simultaneously decreasing for all adults aged under 35. Inspired by this emerging trend, what follows is an analysis of prevalence, patterns and trends of recreational drug use from around the end of early adulthood into middle and older adulthood. For our purposes, we define early adulthood as age 18 to 29, middle adulthood as age 30 to 49 and older adulthood as age 50 onwards. We analyse survey data from the United States, Australia and England and Wales. Although we make comparisons between these countries, our aim is to demonstrate the potential extent of adult recreational drug taking and direction of trends, rather than compare each country in a league table fashion. There are lessons to learn for other countries that have similar prevalence rates, patterns and trends in recreational drug use that we describe here, or may in the future. Our analysis does not include alcohol. Whilst we recognize that its consumption may possibly be widespread in adulthood, and it can act as a replacement or substitute for illegal drugs, particularly for former drug takers, here our focus is upon analysing and explaining the current developing trend we identified from the CSEW in respect of illegal drugs.

The chapter begins by outlining the extent, patterns and trends in recreational drug use in adulthood. We then go on to offer some explanations for these. In doing so, we demonstrate how a cohort replacement effect helps us to understand current prevalence and recent trends, we contemplate the utility of the notion of maturing out and the impact of transitions to adulthood to explain why recreational drug use decreases with age, and we also consider the functions and nature of recreational drug taking to explain why it persists into middle and older adulthood. We follow this with a discussion of the research and policy implications of what we have summarized and end the chapter with some concluding thoughts.

DATA SOURCES AND THE LIMITATIONS OF USING QUANTITATIVE DATA TO ANALYSE ADULT RECREATIONAL DRUG USE

We begin with a brief description of the data sources we use to establish the extent and patterns of recreational drug use towards the end of early adulthood into middle and older adulthood and trends. We analyse, at the time of writing, the latest published data from three established household trend studies: the CSEW[1]; the American National Survey on Drug Use and Health (NSDUH); and the Australian National Drug Strategy Household Survey (NDSHS). In addition, we draw on data from the longstanding cohort panel study, the American Monitoring the Future (MTF) study, which has followed a subsample of its panel from adolescence through to leaving college and into older adulthood.[2] All dataset use large representative samples, have collected data on a range of illicit drugs[3] for at least 18 years, and in most cases, much longer, and track drug use from adolescence through to older adulthood.[4] We have chosen these countries because they are relatively similar culturally, they have some of the highest rates of drug prevalence in the Western world (UNODC, 2013) and, in recent times, they have experienced periods that have been described as the 'normalization of recreational drug use' (see Aldridge et al., 2011; Parker et al., 1998) or a 'drug epidemic' (see Johnston et al., 2013).[5]

There are several problems with relying upon ongoing surveys to measure and estimate drug use that we do not have the space to fully detail here; however, it is likely, for various reasons, such as problems with respondent recall and social desirability effects, that these surveys under-estimate drug taking. Furthermore, our piecing together of this jigsaw of prevalence, patterns and trends from these data sources is complicated by differences in published data. For example, the Australian NDSHS and the American MTF study publish recent drug use data measured using both annual and monthly indicators, whereas the CSEW and the American NSDUH only publish results for past year or past month prevalence, respectively. Additionally, there are variations in the detail of data reported for each survey whereby some provide data analysed by distinct small age categories and others use more broad age ranges for specific variables. For these reasons, we do not always systematically report the results from all of the surveys. Finally, in relation to trend data, it is useful to report levels of statistical significance to ascertain whether the results represent real changes over time or arise from changes in methodology. Unfortunately, the different data sources do not always report these, so we include them where they are available.

RECREATIONAL DRUG USE IN MIDDLE AND OLDER ADULTHOOD: PREVALENCE, PATTERNS AND TRENDS

Our analysis, which follows, reveals how recreational drug use extends into middle and older adulthood. How, for some, rates of recent consumption are not decreasing with age, instead they are stabilising in middle and older adulthood and how recreational drug use now extends into middle and older adulthood at prevalence rates that exceed those previously recorded.

The degree of recreational drug experience in adulthood

To illustrate the first finding and to assess the extent of drug experience amongst adults, we will examine lifetime rates of drug use (having 'ever' taken a drug), for the consumption of any illicit drug.[6] The surveys reveal that a significant proportion of adults are drug experienced. Here, we focus on the data from the 2012 American MTF study and the Australian 2010 NDSHS which, unlike the other surveys, provide a detailed breakdown of lifetime prevalence for the consumption of at least one drug by age. Primarily, we note the situation in America is somewhat unique because it currently has the highest lifetime prevalence across all age groups in adulthood, compared to the data from England and Wales and Australia.[7] Examining lifetime prevalence of drug use for at least one drug by age reveals how it differs across age groups. Focusing on the period towards the end of early adulthood, the 2012 MTF study (Johnston et al., 2013) demonstrates that as respondents reach age 30, lifetime prevalence for any drug stands at 65 per cent.[8] It remains around this figure for adults with a modal age of 35 or 40, and then increases to 73 per cent for adults aged 45, and, again, to 79 per cent for those aged 50. The long-term trends in lifetime prevalence indicate that for many adults aged over 30, rates have been in decline. For example, lifetime prevalence for adults with a modal age of 45 was higher 10 years ago (82 per cent), than it is today (73 per cent). These data clearly reveal how current older adults in America are more likely to have tried drugs than younger adults, and older lifetime drug abstainers are in a minority.

Turning to the data from Australia, the pattern of lifetime prevalence for any drug presents a slightly different picture. The age groups with the highest rates of lifetime prevalence are 20 to 29 year olds (51.3 per cent) and 30 to 39 year olds (59.3 per cent). Lifetime prevalence for the 40+ age category is lower at 32.6 per cent. Taking a long view, the NDSHS (Adhikari and Summerill, 2000; AIHW, 2002, 2005, 2008, 2011) data also record a downward trend in lifetime prevalence for any drug across adult age groups. Lifetime rates for adults aged between 20 and 29, and 30 and 39, peaked in 1998 at 67.5 per cent and 61.3 per cent respectively, and they have been in decline ever since. However, lifetime prevalence for adults aged 40 and over is currently at an historical high (32.6 per cent) compared to when it last peaked in 1998 at 30.2 per cent. The evidence presented here indicates that many adults, including middle and older adults, are drug experienced.

Regular recreational drug use in middle and older adulthood: prevalence and changing trends

Lifetime rates of drug use are a useful measure to identify the extent of drug experience, yet they distort the picture of drug taking because they include one-off triers who may briefly experiment with drugs, but never become regular users. It is particularly important, given some of the high lifetime rates of drug use outlined above, that we are able to distinguish the level of and trends in current drug use[9] in these surveys and assess how far regular drug consumption extends from the end of early adulthood into middle and older adulthood. Evidence from all three countries indicates how, in general, the prevalence of recent drug use for the consumption of at least one drug decreases as age increases (see Table 26.1).[10] On the one hand, this common trend confirms that for many, drug use is a youthful activity; however, on the other hand, a

Table 26.1 Prevalence of recent drug use for any drug

CSEW 2012/13		*NDSHS 2010**		*NSDUH 2012*		***MTF 2012*	
Age	%	Age	%	Age	%	Age	%
25–29	12.8	20–29	27.5	26–29	14.6	25–26	30.0
30–34	8.6	30–39	18.8	30–34	13.2	27–28	32.0
35–44	5.9	40–49	12.8	35–39	8.8	29–30	25.0
45–54	3.5	50–59	8.8	40–44	7.3	35	21.0
55–59	2.3	60+	5.2	45–49	7.7	40	18.0
				50–54	7.2	45	19.0
				55–59	6.6	50	19.0
				60–64	3.6		
				65+	1.3		

**Excludes* pharmaceuticals.

***Recent* drug use is measured by past month. For all other sources reported here, past year use is an indicator of recent drug use.

substantial minority are continuing to take drugs into middle and older adulthood. As an illustration of the potential extent of recent drug use in older adulthood, the American NSDUH 2012 estimates that 7 million adults aged 50 and over have taken a drug in the past year (SAMHSA, 2012).

There is also evidence to support our earlier contention that rates of recent drug use are not decreasing with age, instead, for some, they are stabilising in middle and older adulthood. This pattern is discernible in the American data sources (see Table 26.1). The 2012 NSDUH (SAMHSA, 2012) reveals a plateau effect in past month prevalence for at least one drug for adults aged between 40 and 54. Rather than reducing incrementally with each consecutive age group, past month rates of drug taking have stabilized around 7 per cent. Furthermore, they do not drop significantly in the next age band, 55 to 59. Thereafter, past month prevalence almost halves at 3.6 per cent for 60 to 64 year olds and substantially lowers to 1.3 per cent for 65 year olds and over. The greatest percentage reduction in past month prevalence occurs between the age groups 30 to 34 and 35 to 39 when it decreases by 4.4 per cent. The 2012 MTF data also show a similar pattern of recent drug use, for at least one drug, initially decreasing with age and a plateau effect between the ages of 40 and 50 (Johnston et al., 2013). These data clearly demonstrate that recent drug use extends into middle and older adulthood and the evidence presented from the US, illustrates how it does not always decrease in a steady fashion with age.

Whilst it is apparent that many adults are drug experienced and some of these are continuing to take drugs in middle and older adulthood, one of the most striking emerging trends we found in recent drug use in all three countries is that it is rising annually for middle to older adults (see Table 26.2). More and more middle and older adults are continuing to take drugs. In the short-term, the proportions are gradually increasing on a yearly basis and in the long-term prevalence of recent drug use for some adult age groups has escalated substantially. To illustrate, since 2011/12, the CSEW has revealed increases in past year prevalence for any drug for all adults aged 35 and over, whilst in 2012/13, all age groups under 35 reported decreases in past year use (Home Office, 2013). Likewise, a similar trend for middle and older adults is surfacing in the Australian NDSHS data, with increases in past year prevalence for any illicit drug for all adults aged 30 and over in the last two surveys in 2007 and 2010 (AIHW, 2011). These rises

Table 26.2 Recent upward trends in current drug use for at least one drug for adults aged 30 and over

CSEW			*NDSHS**			*MTF*			*NSDUH***		
Age	*2011/12*	*2012/13*	*Age*	*2011*	*2012*	*Age*	*2007*	*2010*	*Age*	*2011*	*2012*
35–44	5.6	5.9	50–54	6.7	7.2	30–39	16.7	18.8	40	16.9	17.6
45–54	3.1	3.5	55–59	6.0	6.6	40–49	11.6	12.8	45	17.8	18.6
55–59	1.8	2.3	60–64	2.7	3.6	50–59	7.0	8.8	50	16.8	18.6
						60+	4.3	5.2			

**Excludes* the non-medical use of pharmaceuticals.
***Recent* drug use is measured by past month. For all other sources reported here, past year use is an indicator of recent drug use.

are statistically significant ($p < 0.05$) for adults aged 30 to 39 and 50 to 59. A consecutive annual increase was also present in the 2012 MTF data for adults aged 40 and over (Johnston et al., 2013). Data from the American NSDUH (SAMHSA, 2012) exhibit this general trend too, with a consecutive annual increase in rates of past month drug use for any illicit drug since 2011 for all age groups 30 and over. This increase is statistically significant ($p < 0.05$) for adults aged 30 to 34.

A longer view displays similar upward trends for some adult age groups, such that rates of recent drug use have climbed considerably. From 2002, the American NSDUH (SAMHSA, 2012) reveals how the rate of recent drug use increased for adults aged between 50 and 59. Past month prevalence for adults aged 50 to 54 more than doubled from 3.4 per cent in 2002 to 7.2 per cent in 2012 and tripled, during the same period, for adults aged 55 to 59, from 1.9 per cent in 2002 to 6.6 per cent in 2012.[11] Analysing data from the CSEW, the prevalence of recent drug use for any illicit drug for adults aged 45 to 54 and 55 to 59 in England and Wales rose by 1.6 per cent and 1.3 per cent respectively since 1996 (Home Office, 2013). These increases are statistically significant ($p < 0.05$). Similarly, the Australian NDSHS data indicates increases in recent drug taking for any illicit drug for all adults aged 40 and over since 1995 (AIHW, 2011). Although younger cohorts may still have higher rates of past year or month prevalence than their older counterparts, this trend data on the whole indicates that recent drug use by older adults is generally increasing yearly, and for some age groups in the countries we examined, it is greater than periods when recent drug use for many adults had reached an historical high. There are three important conclusions we can draw from the data on recent drug use: (i) some adults are taking their drug use with them into middle and older adulthood; (ii) for some their recent drug use is not incrementally decreasing with age, as we might expect, rather, rates are remaining stable for some years in middle and older adulthood; and (iii) for some drug taking is extending further into adulthood at a higher rate than has traditionally been the case.

Patterns of, and trends in, recreational drug use in middle and older adulthood

We now turn to expand our analysis by focusing on the most common drugs consumed in adulthood. Here, in respect of individual drugs, we highlight the levels of recent drug use and how the short and long-term trends we have identified for the consumption of at least one drug play out. We present and analyse data (see Table 26.3) from the CSEW 2012/13 (Home Office, 2013), the Australian NDSHS 2010 (AIHW, 2011) and the American 2012

Table 26.3 Prevalence of past year drug use by age and most common drugs

CSEW 2012/13				*NDSHS 2010*				*MTF 2012**				
										*Pharmaceuticals***		
Age	Cannabis (%)	Cocaine (%)	Ecstasy (%)	Age	Cannabis (%)	Ecstasy (%)	Cocaine (%)	Age	Cannabis (%)	Tranquilizers (%)	Sedatives (%)	Cocaine (%)
25–29	9.4	4.4	2.7	20–29	21.3	9.9	6.5	25–26	25.6	5.1	1.9	3.8
30–34	6.4	2.4	1.3	30–39	13.6	3.9	3.7	27–28	26.5	6.6	2.9	4.2
35–44	4.4	1.6	0.6	40–49	9.4	0.5***	0.4***	29–30	19.8	4.1	2.2	3.3
45–54	2.6	0.5	0.3	50–59	5.5	-	-	35	14.4	3.1	3.1	2.3
55–59	1.7	0.1	0.0	60+	0.5	-	-	40	12.5	3.3	2.8	1.5
								45	12.3	4.6	2.3	1.5
								50	12.2	4.3	2.3	1.8

**Data* in relation to ecstasy is not collected from respondents aged 30 and over.
***For* analysis purposes, pharmaceuticals were combined in the 2012 MTF report and identified as the second most common drug used in the past year. Here, we provide prevalence data for the two main drugs within this category.
****These* figures represent all adults over 40.

MTF study (Johnston et al., 2013).[12] All three surveys observe how the patterns of consumption we describe here emerge, for many adults, during their twenties.[13] They also demonstrate how different drugs comprise adult drug-taking repertoires across the three countries. In addition, further evidence is provided for how drug use generally declines with age and we can again observe how rates of drug use do not always decrease in a regular manner and may plateau in middle and older adulthood.

In all countries, cannabis is the most common drug used in the past year by adults. The next most common drugs consumed in the past year, in England and Wales, and Australia, are stimulant type drugs: cocaine and ecstasy, which have notably lower rates than cannabis. In England and Wales, cocaine is more prevalent than ecstasy as a past year drug, whilst in Australia, this pattern is reversed. So far, the most popular drugs we have identified are those associated with recreational drug taking. However, in America, the non-medical use of pharmaceuticals is, when the frequency for both tranquilizers and sedatives within this category are combined, more prevalent than the past year use of cocaine. This form of consumption does not neatly fit definitions of recreational drug use, especially when it is frequent and involves substantial quantities. In these circumstances, it may be labelled as drug misuse or abuse. The data presented demonstrate how different drugs form part of adult drug-taking repertoires in their twenties, thirties, forties and fifties across the countries. These variations in patterns of drug consumption reflect different usage patterns and consumption preferences in the countries examined.

Earlier we highlighted how, in England and Wales, and Australia, recent drug use is on the increase for adults in their thirties and beyond and in America for adults aged 40 and over. We now outline how these emerging trends appear in relation to the most common drugs consumed in adulthood. Beginning with cannabis, in England and Wales (see Home Office, 2013), there have been recent consecutive annual increases in past year use for all adults aged 35 and over. The largest percentage increase occurred in the 35 to 44 age group, from 3.7 per cent in 2011/12 to 4.4 per cent in 2012/13, followed by the 45 to 54 age group, from 2.0 per cent in 2011/12 to 2.6 per cent in 2012/13. A long-term perspective demonstrates how past year prevalence for cannabis for 35 to 44 year olds is at a similar figure to that recorded in 1996,[14] yet, since then, it has almost doubled for 45 to 54 year olds and more than tripled for 55 to 59 year olds. Both these increases are statistically significant ($p < 0.05$) and current past year prevalence for 55 to 59 year olds has peaked. Similarly, these upward trends in respect of cannabis are evident in Australia (see AIHW, 2011), with a statistically significant ($p < 0.05$) increase in past year consumption for adults aged 50 to 59 from 3.8 per cent in 2007 to 5.5 per cent in 2010. Nevertheless, the largest consecutive annual increase in recent use occurred in the 30 to 39 age group. Long-term trends reveal how recent cannabis consumption peaked for all adult age groups in 1998, however, current prevalence for adults aged 50 to 59 is close to when it peaked at 6.3 per cent. Turning to America (see Johnston et al., 2013), the recent trends in cannabis consumption confirm the upward trends we identified earlier for any drug for adults aged 40 and over. The largest percentage consecutive annual increases occurred amongst adults with a modal age of 40, from 10.6 per cent in 2011 to 12.5 per cent in 2012, and 50, from 10.8 per cent in 2011 to 12.6 per cent in 2012. As data were first collected from adults with a modal age of 50, the recent consumption of cannabis has now reached an historical high.

The short-term trend for cocaine in England and Wales is identical to that for cannabis with the greatest percentage increase in annual prevalence occurring in the 35 to 44 age group, from 1.3 per cent in 2011/12 to 1.6 per cent in 2012/13. In the long-term, since 1996, there have been statistically significant

($p < 0.05$) increases in the recent consumption of cocaine for all adults aged between 30 and 54. The largest increase has occurred in the 35 to 44 age group from 0.2 per cent in 1996 to 1.6 per cent in 2011/12. This represents a substantial rise by a factor of eight with current rates being the highest they have ever been since data was first collected. In Australia, cocaine presents a slightly different situation with increases in past year prevalence from 2007 to 2010 across all adult age groups. Long-term trends reveal how past year prevalence has increased the most, since 1995, by a multiple of four, amongst adults aged 30 to 39. Recent trends in America show consecutive annual increases in cocaine consumption in middle adulthood. In particular, small rises have occurred amongst adults with a modal age of 40 (from 1.3 per cent in 2011 to 1.5 per cent in 2012) and 50 (from 1.6 per cent in 2011 to 1.8 per cent in 2012). However, current past year prevalence has not yet reached previous peaks for these age groups.

In England and Wales, the short-term trends for ecstasy show a mixed pattern across adult age groups, yet when we examine the long-term trends since 1996, overall past year prevalence has either doubled or tripled for adults aged 30 to 54. These increases are statistically significant ($p < 0.05$) for adults aged 35 to 44 and current prevalence is close to when it peaked in 2003/4 at 0.8 per cent. In Australia, short-term trends in respect of ecstasy indicate reductions in past year prevalence across all adult age groups. It peaked in 2007 at 4.7 per cent (now 3.9 per cent) for adults aged 30 to 39 and at 0.6 per cent (now 0.5 per cent) for adults aged 40 and over. Short-term trends for sedatives and tranquilizers, the second most common drugs consumed in the past year by adults in America, have been upward in middle adulthood. There have been annual consecutive increases for adults with a modal age of 40 or 45 for sedatives and 40, 45 and 50 for tranquilizers. Current rates of consumption of sedatives for these adults are lower than when they previously peaked, however, the use of tranquilizers has reached a peak for adults with a modal age of 45 (4.6 per cent) and 50 (4.3 per cent).

These data illustrate how the upward trends in recent drug use outlined earlier in the chapter are present for cannabis, the most common drug used in the countries examined. Recent consumption of cannabis is increasing for adults aged 30 and over in Australia, 35 and over in England and Wales and 40 and over in America. Notably, current prevalence has reached a peak for adults aged 55 to 59 in England and Wales and adults with a modal age of 50 in America. Recent cocaine consumption is also increasing for adults aged 35 and over in England and Wales and current prevalence has peaked for adults aged 35 to 44. Upward trends for cocaine are also present in the Australian and American data. Trends in relation to ecstasy are more mixed across the countries with increases occurring across many adult age groups. However, in England and Wales, the long-term trend reveals how recent ecstasy consumption has increased substantially amongst those in middle and older adulthood and is near to an historical high for adults aged 35 to 44. The data from Australia show a similar trend with current prevalence close to peak levels recorded in 2007. Similarly, the recent trends in the non-medical use of pharmaceuticals in America are mixed with increases across different age groups in adulthood. However, the long-term trend for tranquilizers has now peaked for adults with a modal age of 45 or 50. Again, these different short and long-term trends in all of the countries examined reflect drug consumption practices within each country. Increases and decreases in prevalence for individual drugs are, therefore, dependent upon the usage patterns in each country.

So far, we have outlined how adults in the countries we have examined are drug experienced. Lifetime prevalence data and trends suggest that older cohorts are currently more drug experienced than their younger counterparts. The data on recent drug use indicates that for many adults in middle and older adulthood, rates of recent drug use are rising. Whilst drug taking does generally decline with age, a minority are continuing to take drugs into middle and older adulthood, typically cannabis, followed by stimulant type drugs or the non-medical use of pharmaceuticals. We cannot, therefore, always assume recent drug use will decrease incrementally as age increases and there is evidence for how it can plateau in middle and older adulthood. These findings have implications for how we define recreational drug use as a youthful activity. Consequently, drugs researchers need to develop a detailed understanding of the persistence of drug use in middle and older adulthood. In the following section, we begin this task by offering some explanations for our findings.

EXPLAINING ADULT RECREATIONAL DRUG USE: THE COHORT REPLACEMENT EFFECT, THE JOURNEY TO ADULTHOOD AND THE PERSISTENCE AND NATURE OF RECREATIONAL DRUG USE

In this part of the chapter, we consider how a cohort replacement effect operates to help us understand the prevalence and trends in lifetime and recent drug use summarized above. In this regard, we draw on the concept of the normalization of recreational drug use (see Aldridge et al., 2011; Parker et al., 1998, 2002). In addition, we outline how social or environmental influences experienced during the journey to adulthood impact upon recreational drug journeys over time. Here, we reflect on how and why recreational drug use, for some, decreases with age, and, for others, persists into middle and older adulthood. In addition, to develop our explanations, we contemplate the functions and nature of recreational drug taking. These explanations are by no means exhaustive and individually they can only offer a partial account for what we have observed. However, we assert that collectively, they provide a more comprehensive understanding of prevalence and trends in adult recreational drug use.

The cohort replacement effect

The evidence we presented from the American 2012 MTF study (Johnston et al., 2013) uncovered adults in their forties and fifties with high rates of lifetime prevalence in respect of the trying of at least one drug, such that current lifetime abstainers at this age are in a minority, and lifetime prevalence is greater than amongst younger age groups. In contrast, data from the Australian 2010 NDSHS illustrated how lifetime prevalence rates for at least one drug were highest between 50 and 60 per cent for adults aged 20 to 40 and lowest for adults from age 40 onwards. The long-term trends in lifetime prevalence data from both countries also revealed two further different situations. In America, the trend in lifetime prevalence for most age groups 25 and over is downward, suggesting that many adults today are less drug experienced than their peers were in the past. Whilst this downward trend is also apparent in Australia for adults aged between 20 and 40, it is in ascent for adults aged 40 and over indicating that despite their lower rates of lifetime prevalence than younger adults, they are more drug experienced than adults in this age group were in the past. Furthermore, evidence from all the data sources demonstrates how short-term trends in recent use for any drug, and cannabis in particular, are rising in middle and older adulthood, at least from around age 30 in some of the countries, and, again, the long-term trends reveal how some of these age groups are recording higher prevalence rates now than their peers did in the past.

The concept of a cohort replacement effect is particularly useful for explaining our findings. With data like these, the goal for social researchers is to disentangle the effects of age, cohort and period upon behaviour.[15] The notion of a cohort replacement effect to explain, at least in part, the current prevalence and trends we have described here has been given some weight by researchers (see Aldridge, 2008; Fahmy et al., 2012; Han et al., 2009; Johnston et al., 2013). This concept has been used to understand both increases and decreases in drug prevalence amongst specific age groups. A cohort replacement effect operates through the movement of a comparatively drug experienced age cohort into older age groups and results in two outcomes: (i) an increase in prevalence within older age groups; and (ii) a decrease in prevalence within younger age groups. The former is explained by a drug experienced generation taking their higher levels of drug use with them into older age or recommencing their drug use in later adulthood, and the latter, by a less drug involved cohort moving into younger age groups.

As we have shown in relation to the data we have outlined above, many in middle and older adulthood have greater lifetime rates of drug use compared to their predecessors and, in America, their successors. For some older adults today, their drug experience may have been adolescent experimentation and never led to regular drug taking during the life course. For others, as the data on prevalence of recent drug use has demonstrated, they have brought their drug use with them into middle and older adulthood. Indeed, Johnston et al. (2013) argue that American adolescents of the early 1990s have taken their higher levels of drug use with them into adulthood. As they note: 'This pattern reflects a classic cohort effect, in which different age groups are not all moving in parallel; rather, different age groups show increases when the cohorts (i.e. high school classes) having heavier use at an earlier stage in development reach the relevant age level' (2013: 132). The upward trends in recent drug use for some adults aged 30 and over, as well as the levelling of the prevalence of recent drug use amongst adults around the age of 40 and 50 can, therefore, be explained as a consequence of this type of phenomenon. In their analysis of American NSDUH data for the period 2002 to 2007,[16] Han et al. (2009) offer a similar explanation. They conclude that the upward trend in past year drug use for adults aged 50 to 59 is largely determined by the ageing of the baby boom population who were born during the period from 1946 to 1964, particularly those born after 1950, and who had higher rates of drug use during adolescence and young adulthood than older cohorts.

We argue that some of the current prevalence rates and upward trends we have highlighted in this chapter can be understood as a product of specific drug experienced birth cohorts moving into older age groups. As we have noted, the concept of a cohort replacement effect is premised on the interaction between age and a time period. So what was so unique about the era in which these cohorts grew up and became drug experienced? The normalization thesis (Aldridge et al., 2011; Parker et al., 1998) helps us to appreciate this further. The concept was formulated to explain the unprecedented increases in the prevalence of recreational drug use amongst young people during the 1990s in the UK (Parker et al., 1998). Despite causing some controversy and dispute (see Shiner and Newburn, 1997, 1999), it has since been applied to a range of cultural settings (see, for example, Cheung and Cheung, 2006; Duff, 2003, 2005; Pearson, 2001; Pennay and Moore, 2010; Measham et al., 2001). This pioneering work, published in *Illegal Leisure*,[17] tracked a cohort of adolescents from the early 1990s into young adulthood and concluded that recreational drug use had undergone a process of normalization whereby it had become accommodated and accepted into the everyday lives of young people, an accommodation and acceptance that was even evident to an extent amongst drug abstainers. The adults who form part of this cohort replacement effect that we have described, which has resulted in levels of recreational drug use reaching historical highs for adults in their thirties, forties and fifties, grew up during periods that fit with the notion of drug normalization, and, in the countries we consider here, persisted for many years.[18] Hence, the comparatively high rates of lifetime prevalence of drug use amongst current older adults and lower rates in younger adults who have grown up in times when overall prevalence has generally been in decline in the countries we have examined.

The concept of drug normalization also helps to explain the plateau effect we have identified in relation to older adult drug users in the US: it represents successive age cohorts who grew up during times when drug use was relatively normalized. Furthermore, this idea also explains why prevalence of lifetime and recent drug use is highest in different older age groups across the countries we have examined. These variations in prevalence by age reflect the different periods in which recreational drug use was undergoing a process of normalization in these countries. To illustrate, during the 1990s, the *Illegal Leisure* generation had unparalleled levels of drug use and were the most drug involved cohort of the twentieth century in the UK. Now they are approaching their late thirties, it appears, as the data on recent drug use we have presented from the CSEW 2012/13 indicates, that some of them are taking their high levels of consumption with them into middle adulthood. In America, what has been described as a 'drug epidemic' (see Johnston et al., 2013) occurred earlier, from the late 1970s through to the early 1990s (see Han et al., 2009; Johnston et al., 2013), and in Australia, academics were identifying the process of drug normalization during the mid to late 1990s (see Duff, 2003, 2005). The cohort replacement effect, therefore, provides an explanation for variations in the prevalence and trends of recreational drug use amongst distinct age groups that we outlined earlier in this chapter. However, Han et al. (2009) and Johnston et al. (2013) note it is only a partial explanation. To further develop our analysis of the data in this chapter, we turn to consider social or environmental factors, which can help us to understand some of the changes in adult recreational drug use that occur across the life course.

The effect of the journey to adulthood upon recreational drug use

We have also highlighted how for some adults, the prevalence of recent drug use decreases as age increases. To explain this phenomenon, researchers have emphasized the impact of accomplishing the journey, or making the transition, from adolescence to adulthood (see Bachman et al., 1997, 2002; Hathaway, 2004; Shiner, 2009). This idea develops the notion of 'maturing out'; the process that underpins desistance from drug use (Winick, 1962). From the transitions to adulthood perspective it is argued that adolescence is a period of life characterized by freedom from adult responsibilities, which, in turn, facilitates drug taking. With the adoption of adult roles and responsibilities, for instance, gaining full-time employment, getting married or becoming a parent, and the new identities they endow, values and social relationships they bring, drug desistance becomes more likely (Bachman et al., 1997, 2002; Shiner, 2009; Vervaeke and Korf, 2006). Shiner (2009) argues that recreational drug use begins to decline at precisely the point when adult roles start to bed in during the mid-twenties. In Williams and Parker (2001), the lead author of this chapter observed that the roles and responsibilities associated with adulthood are delayed, the road to adulthood is longer, and consequently, recreational drug use has extended further into adulthood than has traditionally been the case. Marriage and parenthood statistics from the countries we examined are consistent with this idea. The marriage rate is in decline (ABS, 2013a; Cohn et al., 2011; ONS, 2014), for instance, in the UK the overall number of marriages has reduced by 30 per cent since the 1970s (ONS, 2014). Moreover, the age of first marriage has increased. Now, women are more likely to get married in their late, rather than early twenties, and men in their early thirties, rather than their early to mid-twenties (ABS, 2013a; Cohn et al. 2011; ONS, 2014). Likewise, the age of parenthood, at least for women, is also delayed with many first-time mothers now in their mid-twenties (Matthews and Hamilton, 2009), and there has been a substantial increase in the number of first-time mothers in their thirties and forties (ABS, 2013b; Livingston and Cohn, 2010; Matthews and Hamilton, 2009; ONS, 2013). The data we presented in Table 26.1 showed steep reductions in recent drug use around the late twenties and into the early thirties at the age when, for many, transitions to adulthood like these are now accomplished.

Whilst we do not, on the whole, disagree with the analysis of the relationship between transitions to adulthood and desistance from recreational drug use, we believe a more nuanced understanding that reveals how desistance can be a gradual process and, in some cases, it may not always be guaranteed or permanent, is required. We have argued elsewhere (e.g. Aldridge et al., 2011; Williams, 2013) that the relationship between the journey to adulthood and drug journeys has been over-simplified and that the transition to adulthood does not always constrain drug journeys. Drawing on the work of Giordano et al. (2002), who offer an explanation for desistance from crime, adult transitions can be understood as 'hooks for change' that make change possible, but not certain. Collecting further data from the *Illegal Leisure* cohort when they were age 28, Williams (2013) found that many had achieved most of the transitions associated with adulthood *and* continued on their drug journeys, albeit at a slower pace. The nature of transitions is crucial here. For example, gaining full-time employment may not significantly curtail drug journeys and seems to depend on career evolution, in which greater responsibilities at work are associated with moderation in, or desistance from, drug taking. Williams, therefore, contends transitions within transitions occur that affect drug journeys. Furthermore, Williams argues permanent drug desistance may be associated with the simultaneous impact of a number of adult transitions. To illustrate, the drug journeys of female drug takers were: 'often constrained after the accomplishment of several adult transitions and by the full weight of responsibilities which accompany being a mother, maintaining a home and working full-time.' (Williams, 2013: 113; see also Measham et al., 2011). Continuing to take drugs in these circumstances, therefore, becomes more complicated and difficult. These ideas help to explain how recreational drug use may persist or desist, for some, in middle or older adulthood. Adult transitions may not always lead to drug desistance, rather a reduction in the frequency of drug taking may transpire, especially when the responsibilities associated with them are not too demanding. Desistance can, therefore, be understood as a product of accomplishing a transition to adulthood that develops over time or the concurrent effect of multiple adult transitions, such that, in both circumstances, much greater demands are placed on adult lives. Again, it is in the thirties this is likely to occur for many, perhaps accounting for the further reductions in recent drug use during this time.

As we have already noted, some adults do not desist from recreational drug use and, as the data we have analysed in this chapter also demonstrates, it extends, albeit for a relatively few, into the thirties, forties, fifties and beyond. The emphasis placed upon desistance during early adulthood neglects to consider how drug use for some may evolve and persist across the whole life course. In our own work (e.g. Williams, 2013), we have highlighted the zigzagging nature of recreational drug journeys whereby drug use may temporarily cease, prompted, for example, by taking on a new adult role, such as parent, spouse or employee, and then, at another point in the future, continue. Becoming a parent, for instance, does not always lead to permanent desistance from drug use. Female interviewees discussed how they initially stopped taking drugs when they were new to motherhood, but once their children placed less demands on their time, and they had appropriate available social networks to help look after them, they recommenced their drug journeys (Williams, 2013; see also Measham et al., 2011). The literature on recreational drug use and the role of adult transitions is often premised on the journey to adulthood being straightforward and linear. Yet, we know living in contemporary society is fraught with risk (Beck, 1992; Giddens, 1991), such that life is characterized by setbacks and change. By way of illustration, intimate relationships end, which leads to separation, a return to being single and possibly a change in living arrangements. As Williams (2013) has observed, events like these can instigate recommencement of drug journeys. Some of the increasing trends in recent recreational drug use in middle to older adulthood that we have identified may be, in addition to a cohort replacement effect, explained by former drug users resuming their drug journeys after negotiating adult transitions or when their transitions have reversed. In addition, these increasing trends in recent drug use can be partly accounted for by the late onset of drug use in adulthood. Han et al. (2009), in their analysis of upward trends in recent drug use for American adults aged 50 to 59, correctly dismiss this idea providing evidence that only 3 per cent initiated drug use after age 50. However, their data also reveals that just over 10 per cent started taking drugs after age 30. Our own work (e.g. Askew, 2016), with a sample of adult drug users aged 30 to 59, has also found evidence to support this idea, with drug journeys commencing in the twenties and thirties. Findings such as these question assumptions that drug use in adulthood always originates as a result of adolescent experimentation.

The persistence and nature of adult recreational drug use

Explanations for the continuity of recreational drug use in adulthood focus on the absence of adult roles and responsibilities in some drug users lives. In this respect, persistence is associated with unemployment, not being married and not being a parent (Bachman et al., 1997, 2002; Han et al., 2009; Shiner, 2009). Whilst this may account for some adult recreational drug users, others, as we have noted, continue on their drug journeys despite occupying adult roles. We now turn to consider how and why recreational drug use is accommodated in the lives of conventional adults, focusing on the function it plays and how it is controlled.

When explaining how decisions about recreational drugs are made, research (Aldridge et al., 2011; Coffield and Gofton, 1994; Parker et al., 1998; Williams, 2013) has drawn on a cost-benefit assessment in which the perceived costs are weighed up against the perceived benefits. If the benefits offset the costs, then recreational drug use is likely. Whilst decisions about drugs may not always be rational and can be based upon unbridled hedonism (see Aldridge et al., 2011; Measham et al., 2001), in adulthood they become more about making strategic 'reasoned choices' (Williams and Parker, 2001). In this regard, Williams (2013) argues that when some of the benefits of recreational drug use, for example, feeling relaxed, lowering inhibitions or increasing energy, are considered in the context of adults' everyday lives, decisions to take drugs make more sense. The motives for recreational drug use are founded upon the functions drugs can provide, for instance, time-out and stress-relief, to balance against the demands of adult lives (see also Osborne and Fogel,

2008). The survey data we presented earlier demonstrated that cannabis is the most common drug consumed in adulthood, a drug that is perceived to relax users and, therefore, undoubtedly functions in this way for many adults after a challenging day or week at work or home. Similarly, cocaine or ecstasy, which may be consumed less frequently, is often perceived to provide both pleasure and an escape from the responsibilities of everyday life (Hinchliff, 2001; Williams, 2013). In the United States, the non-medical use of pharmaceuticals was the next most common category of drug consumed in adulthood after cannabis. Again, the effects of these drugs either as calming and anxiety reducing, pain relieving or stimulants no doubt operate in the context of stressful adult lives. In this respect, recreational drug use can be viewed as functional, it may help to improve or forget, even if temporarily, current situations or daily life, much like alcohol can. Elsewhere, we have observed how drug takers emphasize the functional nature of recreational drug use (Askew, 2016; Williams, 2013). In her discourse analysis of the ways in which recreational drug use is legitimized in adult lives, Askew (2016) interviewed 26 current drug takers aged between 30 and 59 whose drug repertoires included cannabis, cocaine and/or ecstasy. Participants described their drug use as a leisure activity that functioned to enhance an evening with friends or intimate partners or, cocaine consumption, for example, combatted tiredness and increased stamina during a social event. Exploring the functions associated with recreational drug use, in the context of adult lives, helps to explain why, for some, it persists into middle and older adulthood.

The persistence of recreational drug use in adulthood is also assisted by the ways in which adults exert control over their consumption. During adulthood, choices about which drugs to consume change, drug use becomes less frequent and the quantities per drug taking episode may be reduced (Aldridge et al., 2011; Askew, 2016; Duff et al., 2012; Hathaway, 2004; Parker et al., 2002; Williams, 2013). Drugs that are perceived to have some negative effects, for example the 'come down' after consuming ecstasy, may no longer be taken as frequently in adulthood and instead replaced by cocaine, which is perceived to have less adverse after effects (Williams, 2013). Indeed, this may partly explain why cocaine is more popular than ecstasy amongst many adults in England and Wales. As Pearson (2001) observed in his ethnographic study of adult recreational drug use amongst 30 to 50 year olds, and in particular the consumption of cocaine, it was: 'used occasionally and regulated. This is perhaps what one might expect among people who have other valued life commitments such as family life and work, and who despite regular illicit drug consumption have reached maturity without encountering any major crises with their drug use' (Pearson, 2001: 191). Again, the significance of adult roles is highlighted here: recreational drug use is controlled by reference to other responsibilities at work or home (see also Decorte, 2001; Notley, 2005; Vervaeke and Korf, 2006; Williams, 2013; Zinberg, 1984). Moreover, Williams (2013) emphasized how drug journeys and life journeys intersect and influence decisions about which drugs to consume, how often and how much. It can be argued then, that recreational drug use in middle and older adulthood is controlled and functional. As such, it is interwoven and accommodated within, when appropriate, routine daily activities (see also Notley, 2005; Osborne and Fogel, 2008). This further highlights the ways in which recreational drug use, for many, continues to be normalized in adulthood (see Aldridge et al., 2011; Measham et al., 2011). In this sense, as the data we analysed earlier in the chapter revealed, it may not be normalized with regard to prevalence rates, however, for those who do continue to take drugs in middle and older adulthood, it is normalized by virtue that it is accommodated alongside everyday life, but does not take precedence over it.

In this section of the chapter, we have offered some explanations for the prevalence and trends we outlined earlier. By no means are these exhaustive; however, together they provide insights into the current prevalence, patterns and trends in adult recreational drug use that we sketched out previously. The cohort replacement effect helps us to appreciate why rates of recent drug use have increased and, in some cases plateaued, for middle and older adults in the countries we have examined. They are a result of experienced drug cohorts, who grew up during periods of drug normalization, moving into older age groups. We have also outlined how and why recent drug use decreases with age with reference to the journey to adulthood. In this regard, we argue a more refined understanding of drug desistance is required, which can appreciate the nature of different adult transitions and account for the gradual slowing down and the fluctuating quality of drug journeys across the life course. Although, for many, drug use does eventually permanently cease with age, there are a minority who continue to take drugs in middle and older adulthood. The persistence of recreational drug use in this respect can be understood as a consequence of the nature of it: for many it is functional and controlled and does not take priority over other responsibilities.

INNOVATIONS IN RESEARCH AND DRUG POLICY: BROADENING OUR UNDERSTANDING OF ADULT RECREATIONAL DRUG USE IN THE NEW MILLENNIUM

We now highlight some important research and policy implications arising from what has been discussed so far. In respect of research implications, we identify key issues that should form future research agendas and make some recommendations in relation to accessing adult populations and research design. Our discussion of policy implications focuses on the nature of current policies and what should be developed and focused on in the future.

Research dilemmas: themes, access and research design

A considerable portion of research on recreational drug use focuses on young people and perpetuates the idea of recreational drug use as a young person's activity. Our findings challenge this notion and indicate there is a range of topics that requires further research with participants in middle or older adulthood, using qualitative or mixed methods strategies. They are in relation to the nature, context and motivations for the non-medical use of pharmaceuticals in America, cannabis, cocaine or ecstasy consumption, poly-drug use and drug initiation. Current research on adult recreational drug use tends to access samples, with the exception of large scale nationally representative surveys, from early adulthood or the beginning of middle adulthood, the typical age at which drug use begins to decline. Even though a broad age range may have been selected that includes much older adults, the mean age is typically around 30 (see Duff et al., 2012; Hathaway, 1997, 2004; Notley, 2005; Osborne and Fogel, 2008; Shukla, 2006). The data we have analysed reveals how current age cohorts in their thirties, forties and fifties, who grew up during a time of drug normalization, are taking their drug use with them into middle and older adulthood. Researchers should focus their efforts upon understanding the nature of their recreational drug use and the benefits and problems associated with it.

A lack of research with middle and older adults is connected to difficulties in accessing these samples, who may be unwilling to participate because they are concerned about the ramifications of discussing their drug use, especially when they have positions of responsibility at work, or as parents or even grandparents, in the domestic sphere. Often adult drug users are recruited in relatively accessible venues, for instance, drug services or nightclubs; however, they do not represent most recreational drug users in middle or older adulthood. Typically, snowball sampling is used to recruit participants from hard to reach populations, yet it can create a biased sample. To counter this problem, in our own research (e.g. Askew, 2016), snowball sampling was combined with theoretical sampling to produce a varied sample of drug users aged between 30 and 59. Others have suggested developing snowball sampling through the method of respondent driven sampling (Heckathorn, 1997; Johnston and Sabin, 2010). Although similar to snowball sampling, through peer recruitment and the offer of incentives to participants, it can also access a more varied sample (Johnston and Sabin, 2010). With the advent of virtual technologies and the development of virtual methodologies, social media, such as *Facebook*[19] or drug forums, such as *Blue Light*, can be useful to locate hard to reach populations, especially under-researched groups, although problems with bias may still remain (see Miller and Sonderland, 2010). Clearly, recruiting middle and older adult recreational drug users poses a challenge. Researchers, therefore, need to develop innovative ways, using some of the ideas outlined here, to access adult recreational drug users who fit general population norms and do not appear in easily accessible venues such as drug treatment services or nightclubs. When they do find them, they should be recruited with tact and reassured about confidentiality and anonymity.

Three of the surveys we have analysed are cross-sectional trend studies: the CSEW, the Australian NDSHS and the American NSDUH. This type of research design is effective at identifying changes in overall populations, but cannot tell us about changes at an individual level. As we have noted, some of the increasing trends in recent drug use can be explained by the zigzagging nature of drug journeys, whereby drug users temporarily desist and begin their journey again at a later stage of their life. Appreciating how drug use evolves across the whole life course is essential and longitudinal panel studies, such as the MTF and *Illegal Leisure* projects, are fundamental in this regard. Moreover, a mixed methods approach can provide a more comprehensive account collecting data on both the extent and meaning of recreational drug use. Research funding should be allocated for the continuation of studies like these, as well as for the development of future longitudinal research beginning at various stages of the life course.

Drug policy dilemmas: how to tackle adult recreational drug use

In general, international drug policies are focused upon prevention and enforcement. However, in both cases, these efforts are usually directed at young people. Evidence from the US, for instance, reveals how drug possession/use arrest rates peaked at age 18 in 2010, and middle and older adults were far less likely to be arrested (Snyder, 2012). Furthermore, Reuter and Stevens (2007) argue that only a small proportion of drug users are detected or subject to sanctions. In relation to adult recreational drug users, especially those with many years of experience, Pearson (2001: 195) asserts: 'It is difficult to conceive of an enforcement response to this kind of drug use and this kind of drug user, because they have successfully negotiated their way around enforcement measures for 30 years in some cases'. As we have outlined in this chapter, most recreational drug use in adulthood is functional and controlled, and, therefore, does not cause significant problems for drug takers. Pearson (2001) argues their stake in society, as employees or parents, often keeps their drug use in check. Generally, as the data we have examined demonstrates, recreational drug use in adulthood involves the consumption of low-risk drugs, such as cannabis, and more harmful drugs are taken less frequently (see Nutt, 2009). Moreover, recreational drug takers can be described as 'risk managers' who are mindful of the pleasures associated with their drugs consumption, as well as the risks, which they often perceive as acceptable or manageable (Williams, 2013). This notion of functional, pleasurable, low-risk recreational drug use is absent in many policy debates (Askew, 2016; Williams, 2013).[20] Acknowledging its existence can have numerous benefits, not least in reducing the stigma attached to drug use, and, in turn, making it more likely that adult recreational drug users will seek help and support if they need it in the future (Global Drug Survey, 2014). The policy response to adult recreational drug use does not, therefore, require enforcement nor will prevention methods be effective. To introduce more methods of controlling adult recreational drug use, for example, drug testing in the workplace, is counter-productive. As Perrone et al. (2013) found, drug testing for cannabis can lead users to switch to legal highs, such as synthetic cannabinoids, which are undetectable, but we know little about in terms of harm. We argue that international drug policies need to develop, or continue to develop, responses based upon harm reduction and public health models and respecting the human rights of recreational drug takers.

Although the proportion of recreational drug users in middle and older adulthood is relatively small, the evidence from the countries we have examined, indicate they are growing. It is likely that some of this ageing population of drug users will experience problems in the future and require help or treatment from public health services. Han et al. (2009) predict that there will be an increase in the number of adults aged 50 and over presenting with a past year substance use disorder, such that it is estimated there may be 5.7 million in America by 2020. Health services will need to prepare for this potential increase, and previously unforeseen, demand by developing screening, harm reduction strategies and primary care services for adult recreational drug users. Furthermore, our findings provide fuel for debates about drugs as a human right. We recognize there are competing human rights. However, given recent calls for new drug regulatory systems (see Seddon, 2014; Transform, 2009), the decriminalization of some drugs in many countries across the world, and the legalization of cannabis for recreational purposes in four states of America, the time is ripe to capitalize on these new developments. The surveys we examined revealed a substantial minority who are taking drugs in middle and older adulthood. As we noted earlier, drug use in this respect is likely to be more strategic, functional and a reasoned choice. Moreover, as van Ree (1999) asserts, drugs are often enriching to individual lives. Therefore, it seems unreasonable to us to ignore or violate the following principle: 'people should be entitled to determine what they ingest, even if it does them harm' (Hunt, 2005: 5). Respecting this tenet will require the removal of drug prohibition and incorporating the core principles of human rights into drug policies (see Barrett, 2010). In turn, this is likely to improve the health, well-being and daily lives of adult recreational drug users.

CONCLUDING THOUGHTS

Frequently, when overall prevalence of drug use is in decline, governments claim success in the *War on Drugs*. However, as we have revealed, this masks what is occurring across different age groups. Whilst drug use may be decreasing for younger age cohorts who form the bulk of recreational drug users, recent use is on the increase in middle and older adulthood. It is, therefore, no longer the case, in the countries we have examined, that we can define recreational drug use as a youthful activity. It now extends into adulthood at higher rates than it has done in the past, and in some cases, prevalence of recent drug use for individual drugs is greater than when drug use had previously peaked. Although recent consumption of drugs does, on the whole, decline with age, in America, there is evidence that drug use can plateau in middle and older adulthood and may, for some, become firmly established at this stage of the life course. It is worth noting, that America experienced its 'drug epidemic' earlier than when the process of normalization of recreational drug use began in the UK (see Parker et al., 1998), and Australia (see Duff, 2003, 2005). Therefore, as the adolescents of the 1990s from these countries move towards the end of middle adulthood and into older adulthood, we may also see the plateauing of recent drug use occur. Whilst most recreational drug use is not harmful nor does it take priority over daily life, there may be problems for adults who have extensive, long-term, regular recreational drug careers that began when they were teenagers. Governments must consider appropriate public health responses for their ageing recreational drug using populations. Moreover, international policies need to be developed to respect the rights of drug users.

NOTES

1 Formerly the British Crime Survey.
2 We use this study mainly to supplement the findings of the NSDUH or as an alternative. For example, the NSDUH does not report data on annual prevalence of drug use. When making comparisons in relation to past year prevalence across these countries, we present data from the MTF study.
3 All of the sources collect data about legal, illegal and the non-medical use of some pharmaceuticals.
4 The age range varies for each of the household surveys. The CSEW has an upper age limit of 59, whilst the NSDUH and NDSHS do not have an upper age limit. The MTF is a panel study and so far has followed its cohort through to age 50.
5 The analyses presented here can be extended further to include other countries, particularly those which have implemented decriminalization policies, such as Holland, Portugal and Spain.
6 It should be noted that these data measure recreational and non-recreational drugs, such as crack cocaine and heroin. Surveys like these, however, which sample household or student populations are less likely to capture non-recreational drug use, and therefore, the data discussed here are likely to comprise mainly of recreational drugs. Later in the chapter, we present analyses of the most popular recreational drugs across the three countries.
7 For information, the available published data from the CSEW indicate that 35.9 per cent of 16 to 59 year olds had tried a drug at least once in their lifetime (Home Office, 2013).
8 To address inconsistency in self-reports across the study, Johnston et al. (2013) provide two results for lifetime prevalence of drug use. Here, we use the unadjusted percentages which are lower than the adjusted figures.
9 Current or recent drug use is considered to provide a proxy measure for more regular drug taking. However, it is possible that it may pick up some chaotic drug taking, although this is likely to be minimal.
10 The data presented in Table 26.1 from the 2012 NSDUH report mainly analyses recent drug use data by past month rather than past year. Whilst it is not directly comparable with the other data sources, the aim again is to paint a picture of the trend by age in recent drug use rather than compare prevalence rates across the selected countries.
11 It is not possible to provide a comparable analysis from the 2012 MTF survey because data have only been collected from 50 year olds since 2008, which, so far, indicates a small overall reduction in past year prevalence for any drug by 0.6 per cent.
12 Detailed data in respect of comparable age groups and individual drugs were not available from the American 2012 NSDUH report. Nevertheless, it identifies cannabis, the non-medical use of pharmaceuticals and cocaine as the most common drugs consumed in adulthood, as does the 2012 MTF study.
13 Patterns of drug use often change across the life course. In the UK, for example, we know during adolescence, that the most common drugs consumed may be quite different to those in adulthood. Whilst cannabis predominates across adolescence and adulthood, hallucinogens or amphetamines may also be more common in adolescence and cocaine typically replaces these drugs in adulthood (see Aldridge et al., 2011).
14 Drugs data were first collected as part of the CSEW in 1996.

15 Age effects can be seen as a result of the ageing process, whereas a period effect is the product of living during a certain time or through an event, for example, 9-11, which affects everyone regardless of age. A cohort effect arises through a reciprocal relationship between age and period; the result of being born and/or socialized during a specific time period (see Bell and Jones, 2013; Glenn, 1976).

16 NSDUH data up to 2012, as we have found, indicate the overall trend in recent drug use for adults aged 50 to 59 is rising, which suggests subsequent age cohorts are even more drug experienced.

17 Lisa Williams has been involved in the panel study since 1999. So far, it has followed participants until the age of 28. The results have been published in the following monographs: *Illegal Leisure* (Parker et al., 1998), *Illegal Leisure Revisited* (Aldridge et al., 2011) and *Changing Lives, Changing Drug Journeys* (Williams, 2013), as well as numerous journals.

18 We note, however, it can be argued that drug normalization has prevailed in many Western societies, despite overall drug prevalence reducing in recent years.

19 Although *Facebook* has initially been popular with young people, in 2010, the fastest growing group of users were aged 34 and over (Fletcher, 2010).

20 Even when the growing population of older adult drug users are acknowledged, it is in relation to the dependent use of drugs such as heroin and how treatment services should respond to this problem (see EMCDDA, 2010).

REFERENCES

ABS (2013a) *Marriages and Divorces, Australia, 2012*. Available from: http://www.abs.gov.au/ausstats/abs@.nsf/Products/3310.0 2012 Chapter Marriages?OpenDocument (Accessed 5 August 2014).

ABS (2013b) *Births, Australia 2012*. Available from: http://www.abs.gov.au/AUSSTATS/abs@.nsf/DetailsPage/3301.02012?OpenDocument (Accessed 31 March 2016).

Adhikari P. and Summerill A. (2000) *1998 National Drug Strategy Household Survey: Detailed Findings*. Drug Statistics Series no. 6. Canberra: AIHW

AIHW (2002) *2001 National Drug Strategy Household Survey: Detailed Findings*. Drug statistics series no. 11. Canberra: AIHW.

AIHW (2005) *2004 National Drug Strategy Household Survey: Detailed Findings*. Canberra: AIHW

AIHW (2008) *2007 National Drug Strategy Household Survey: Detailed Findings*. Drug statistics series no. 22. Canberra: AIHW.

AIHW (2011) *2010 National Drug Strategy Household Survey Report*. Drug Statistics Series no. 25. Canberra: AIHW.

Aldridge, J. (2008) 'Decline but no fall? New millennium trends in young people's use of illegal and illicit drugs in Britain', *Health Education*, 108(3): 189–206.

Aldridge, J., Measham, F. and Williams, L. (2011) *Illegal Leisure Revisited: Changing Patterns of Alcohol and Drug Use in Adolescents and Young Adults*. London: Routledge.

Askew, R. (2016) Functional fun: Legitimising adult recreational drug use. *International Journal of Drug Policy*, (published online 5th May 2016), http://dx.doi.org/10.1016/j.drugpo.2016.04.018

Bachman, J. G., Wadsworth, K. N., O'Malley, P. M., Johnston, L. D. and Schulenberg, J. E. (1997) *Smoking, Drinking and Drug Use in Young Adulthood: The Impacts of New Freedoms and Responsibilities*, New Jersey: Lawrence Elbaum Associates.

Bachman, J., O'Malley, P., Schulenberg, J., Johnston, L., Bryant, A. and Merline, A. (2002) *The Decline of Substance Use in Young Adulthood*. London: Lawrence Elbaum Associates Publishers.

Barrett, D. (2010) 'Security, development and human rights: normative, legal and policy challenges for the international drug control system', *International Journal of Drug Policy*, 21(2): 140–4.

Beck, U. (1992) [1986] *Risk Society*. London: Sage.

Bell, A. and Jones, K. (2013) 'The impossibility of separating age, period and cohort effects', *Social Science and Medicine*, 93: 163–5.

Cheung, N. and Cheung, Y. (2006) 'Is Hong Kong experiencing normalization of adolescent drug use: Some reflections on the normalization thesis', *Substance Use and Misuse*, 41(14): 1967–90.

Coffield, F. and Gofton, L. (1994) *Drugs and Young People*. London: Institute for Public Policy Research.

Cohn, D., Passel, J., Wang, W. and Livingston, G. (2011) *Barely Half of U.S. Adults Are Married – A Record Low*. Washington, DC: Pew Research Center.

Decorte, T. (2001) 'Drug users' perceptions of "controlled" and uncontrolled use', *International Journal of Drug Policy,* 12(4): 297–320.

Duff, C. (2003) 'Drugs and youth cultures: is Australia experiencing the normalization' of adolescent drug use?' *Journal of youth Studies*, 6(4): 433–46.

Duff, C. (2005) 'Party drugs and party people: examining the "normalization" of recreational drug use in Melbourne, Australia', *International Journal of Drug Policy*, 16(3): 161–70.

Duff, C., Asbridge, M., Brochu, S., Cousineau, M., Hathaway, A., March, D. and Erickson, P. (2012) 'A Canadian perspective on cannabis normalisation among adults' *Addiction Research and Theory*, 20(4): 271–83.

EMCDDA (2010) *Treatment and Care for Older Drug Users*. Lisbon: European Monitoring Centre for Drugs and Drug Addiction.

Fahmy, V., Hatch, S., Hoftopf, M. and Stewert, R. (2012) 'Prevalence in illicit drug use in people aged 50 years', *Age and Ageing*, 41(4): 553–6.

Fletcher, D. (2010) 'How Facebook is redefining privacy', *Time* (20 May), at http://www.time.com/time/business/article/0,8599,1990582,00.html, accessed 16 March 2016

Giddens, A. (1991) *Modernity and Self-Identity: Self and Society in the Late Modern Age*. Cambridge: Polity Press.

Giordano, P. C., Cernkovich, S. A. and Rudolph, J. L. (2002) 'Gender, crime and desistance: towards a theory of cognitive transformation', *American Journal of Sociology,* 107: 990–1064.

Glenn, N. D. (1976). 'Cohort analysts futile quest – statistical attempts to separate age, period and cohort effects', *American Sociological Review*, 41: 900–4.

Global Drug Survey (2014) *The Global Drug Survey 2014 Findings*. Available from: http://www.globaldrugsurvey.com/facts-figures/the-global-drug-survey-2014-findings/ (Accessed 2 July 2014).

Han, B., Gfroerer, J. and Colliver, J. (2009) *An Examination of Trends in Illicit Drug Use Among Adults Aged 50 to 59 in the United States*. Rockville: OAS Data Review.

Hathaway, A. (2004) 'Cannabis careers reconsidered: transitions and trajectories of committed long-term users', *Contemporary Drug Problems,* 31(3): 401–23.

Hathaway, A. (1997) 'Marijuana and lifestyle: exploring tolerable deviance', *Deviant Behaviour,* 18: 103–24.

Home Office (2013) *Drug Misuse: Findings from the 2012/13 Crime Survey for England and Wales*. London: Home Office. Available from: https://www.gov.uk/government/uploads/system/uploads/attachment_data/file/225122/Drugs_Misuse201213.pdf (Accessed 30 June 2014).

Heckathorn, D. D. (1997) 'Respondent-driven sampling: a new approach to the study of hidden populations', *Sociological Problems*, 44(2): 174–99.

Hinchliff, S. (2001). 'The meaning of ecstasy use to women in the late 1990s', *International Journal of Drug Policy*, 12(5–6): 455–68.

Hunt, N. (2005) 'Public health or human rights?', *International Journal of Drug Policy*, 16: 5–7.

Johnston, L. and Sabin, K. (2010) 'Sampling hard-to-reach populations with respondent driven sampling', *Methodological Innovations Online*, 5(2): 38–48.

Johnston, L. D., O'Malley, P. M., Bachman, J. G. and Schulenberg, J. E. (2013). *Monitoring the Future National Survey Results On Drug Use, 1975-2012. Volume II: College Students and Adults Ages 19–50*. Ann Arbor: Institute for Social Research, The University of Michigan.

Livingston, G. and Cohn, D. (2010) *The New Demography of American Motherhood*. Washington, DC: Pew Research Center.

Matthews, T. and Hamilton, B. (2009) *Delayed Childbearing: More Women Are Having Their First Child Later in Life*. NCHS Date Brief, Number 21. Hyattsville: US Department of Health and Human Service.

Measham, F., Aldridge, J. and Parker, H. (2001) *Dancing on Drugs: Risk, health and Hedonism in the British Club Scene*. London: Free Association Books.

Measham, F., Williams, L. and Aldridge, J. (2011) 'Marriage, mortgage, motherhood: what longitudinal studies can tell us about gender, drug "careers" and the normalisation of adult "recreational" drug use', *International Journal of Drug Policy*, 22(6): 420–7.

Miller, P. G. and Sonderlund, A. L. (2010) 'Using the internet to research hidden populations of illicit drug users: a review', *Addiction*, 105(9): 1557–67.

Notley, C. (2005) 'Four groups of illicit substance users amongst the adult "hidden" non-problematic community', *Drugs: Education, Prevention and Policy,* 12(4): 279–90.

Nutt, D (2009) 'Equasy – an overlooked addiction with implications for the current debate on drug harms', *Journal of Psychopharmacology*, 23(1): 3–5.

Office for National Statistics (ONS) (2013) *Live Births in England and Wales by Characteristics of Mother 1, 2012*, Statistical Bulletin. Available from: http://www.ons.gov.uk/ons/dcp171778_330664.pdf (Accessed 30 June 2014).

Office for National Statistics (ONS) (2014) *Marriages in England and Wales (Provisional), 2012*. Statistical Bulletin. Available from: http://www.ons.gov.uk/ons/dcp171778_366530.pdf (Accessed 30 June 2014).

Osborne, G. and Fogel, C. (2008) 'Understanding the motivations for recreational marijuana use among adult Canadians', *Substance Use and Misuse,* 43: 539–72.

Parker, H., Aldridge, J. and Measham, F. (1998) *Illegal Leisure: The Normalization of Recreational Drug Use*. London: Routledge.

Parker, H., Williams, L. and Aldridge, J. (2002) 'The normalization of "sensible" recreational drug use: further evidence from the North West England Longitudinal Study', *Sociology*, 36(4): 941–64.

Pearson, G. (2001) 'Normal drug use: ethnographic fieldwork among an adult network of recreational drug users in inner London', *Substance Use and Misuse*, 36(1&2): 167–200.

Pennay, A. and Moore, D. (2010) 'Exploring the micro-politics of normalisation: narratives of pleasure, self control and desire in a sample of young Australian "party drug" users', *Addiction Research and Theory*, 18(5): 557–71.

Perrone, D., Helgesen, R. D. and Fischer, R. G. (2013) 'United States drug prohibition and legal highs: how drug testing may lead cannabis users to Spice', *Drugs: Education, Prevention and Policy*, 20(3): 216–24.

Reuter, P. and Stevens, A. (2007) *An Analysis of UK Drug Policy*. London: UKDPC.

SAMHSA (2012) *Results from the 2012 National Survey on Drug Use and Health: Summary of National Findings*. Rockville: SAMHSA.

Seddon, T. (2014) 'Drug policy and global regulatory capitalism: the case of new psychoactive substances (NPS)', *International Journal of Drug Policy*. Available from: http://www.sciencedirect.com/science/article/pii/S095539591400070X (Accessed 30 July 2014).

Shiner, M. (2009) *Drug Use and Social Change: The Distortion of History.* London: Palgrave.

Shiner, M. and Newburn, T. (1997) 'Definitely maybe not? The normalisation of drug use amongst young people', *Sociology*, 31(3): 511–24.

Shiner, M and Newburn, T. (1999) 'Taking tea with Noel: the place and meaning of drug use in everyday life', 139-159, In N. South (ed.), *Drugs: Cultures and Controls in Everyday Life*. London: Sage.

Shukla, R. (2006) 'Using marijuana in adulthood: the experience of a sample of users in Oklahoma City', *Journal of Ethnicity in Substance Abuse*, 4(3–4): 153–81.

Snyder, H. (2012) *Arrest in the United States, 1990–2010*. Washington, DC: Bureau of Justice Statistics.

Transform (2009) *After the War on Drugs: Blueprint for Regulation*. Bristol: Transform.

van Ree, E. (1999) 'Drugs as a human right', *International Journal of Drug Policy*, 10(2): 89–98.

UNODC (2013) *World Drug Report 2013*. Austria: UNODC

Vervaeke, H. K. E. and Korf, D. J. (2006) 'Long-term ecstasy use and the management of work and relationships', *International Journal of Drug Policy*, 17: 484–93.

Winick, C. (1962) 'Maturing out of narcotic addiction', *Bulletin on Narcotics,* 14(1): 1–7.

Williams, L. (2013) *Changing Lives, Changing Drug Journeys: Drug Taking Decisions from Adolescence to Adulthood*. Abingdon: Routledge.

Williams, L. and Parker, H. (2001) 'Alcohol, cannabis, ecstasy and cocaine: drugs of reasoned choice amongst young adult recreational drug users in England', *International Journal of Drug Policy*, 12(5–6): 397–413.

Zinberg, N.E. (1984) *Drug, Set and Setting: The Basis for Controlled Intoxicant Use*. New Haven and London: Yale University Press.

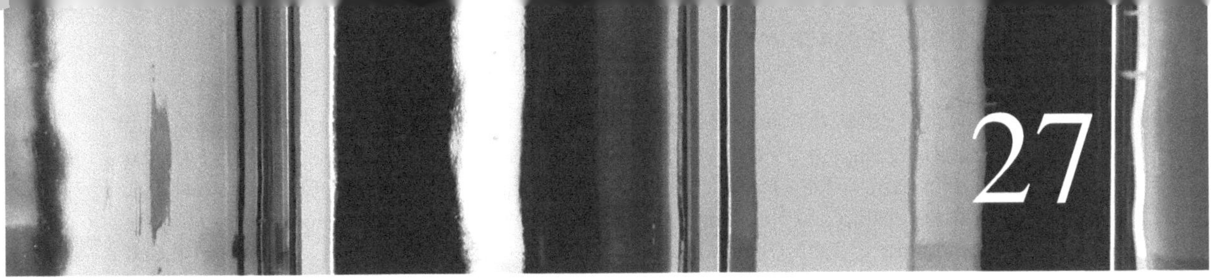

27

Sex Work, Illicit Drug Use and The Risk Environment

Lisa Maher

INTRODUCTION

Increasing evidence supports the role of settings or environments in mediating drug-related harms and, in particular, vulnerability to blood-borne viral infections (Maher, 2002; Rhodes, 2002; Latkin and Knowlton, 2005; Rhodes et al., 2006). Studies have shown how social, spatial and organizational contexts, such as injecting locations (Ouellet et al., 1991; Latkin et al., 1994; Maher et al., 1998; Koester et al., 2003; Rhodes et al., 2006), legislative/policy frameworks and policing practices (Bluthenthal et al., 1999; Maher and Dixon, 2001; Rhodes et al., 2003; Burris et al., 2004; Wood et al., 2004; Cooper et al., 2005; Small et al., 2006; Friedman et al., 2006), social networks and relations (Curtis et al., 1995; Costenbader et al., 2006; Davey et al., 2007) and structural inequalities (Bourgois et al., 1997, 2004; Maher, 2002; Strathdee et al., 2008a) interact to define and organize injecting risk behaviour. Hostile environments may promote harmful drug use and disrupt harm reduction strategies. Homelessness and unstable housing have been associated with elevated rates of drug-related harms, including vulnerability to HIV infection (Bourgois et al., 1997; Bourgois and Bruneau, 2000; Patrick et al., 2001; Miller and Neaigus, 2002; Reyes et al., 2005; Corneil et al., 2006; German et al., 2007). Evidence indicates that intensive policing amplifies drug-related harms, including needle and syringe sharing, rushed injections and the risk of overdose, displaces street-based injectors and deters access to harm reduction services (Bluthenthal et al., 1997, 1999; Maher and Dixon, 1999; Wood et al., 2003; Cooper et al., 2004; Davis et al., 2005; Kerr et al., 2005a; Small et al., 2006; Pollini et al., 2008; Hayashi et al., 2013).

The spatial, social and structural contexts of street-based sex work may similarly encourage risk and facilitate vulnerability, with studies showing how weather conditions, traffic flow, physical locations, legal/policy frameworks and policing can compromise sexual and physical safety (Maher and Curtis, 1992; Vangelder and Kaplan, 1992; Pyett and Warr, 1997; Hubbard, 1998, 1999; Church et al., 2001; Blankenship and Koester, 2002; Hubbard and Sanders, 2003; Shannon and Csete, 2010; Maher et al., 2011a; Shannon et al., 2015). While the literature illustrates a range of strategies and tactics employed by street-based sex workers to avoid violence and manage risk, including working in designated areas and disseminating information about violent or non-paying clients (Barnard, 1993), these are primarily individual-level risk reduction interventions. And while evidence suggests that environmental interventions, including peer-based outreach and mobile resources, sex work cooperatives and managed sex work zones, are effective in promoting safe sex work environments (West, 2000; Gibson et al., 2006; Kerrigan et al., 2006; Bellis et al., 2007; Sanders and Campbell, 2007; Shannon and Csete, 2010; Maher et al., 2011a) much of this research has focused on venue-based sex work.

Unlike most venue-based sex work, street-based sex work is characterized by high rates of injecting drug use (Ward et al., 1993; McKeganey and Barnard, 1996; Cusick, 1998; Shannon et al., 2008a). Increased exposure to a range of harms, including HIV infection, unprotected sex, injecting risk behaviours, violence and assault, poverty, homelessness, stigma and social isolation (Edlin et al., 1994; Maher, 1997; Sterk, 1999; Romero-Daza et al., 2003; Bourgois et al., 2004; Choi et al., 2006; Wood et al., 2007; Shannon et al., 2009) has been reported among street-based sex workers who inject drugs. Many of these harms appear to be linked to environmental conditions, resulting in a concentration of harms among sex workers in low status, street-based sex markets (Maher and Curtis, 1992; Miller, 1993; Maher, 1996; Pyett and Warr, 1997; Kuyper et al., 2005; Wood et al., 2007; Shannon et al., 2008b).

The co-location of street sex and drug markets is increasingly recognized as an important factor shaping patterns of drug use, commercial sex transactions and related risk behaviours (Maher, 1997; Shannon et al., 2008b). This chapter explores the synergies between drug and sexual risks in street-based environments and identifies implications for interventions designed to reduce harm and facilitate safer sex work environments. Utilising a data-driven approach based on observational fieldwork and in-depth interviews (Maher et al., 1998; Maher and Dixon, 1999, 2001; Maher, 2002; Maher and Hudson, 2007; Hudson, 2010; Topp et al., 2010), it attempts to explore general issues related to sex work and drug use in a local context. By focusing on three Sydney neighbourhoods (Cabramatta, Bankstown and Kings Cross) over a 10-year period (1998 to 2008), the chapter illustrates aspects common to sex work in a range of settings such as psychostimulant use, patterns of income generation and violence, as well as issues specific to local settings such as physical environments, availability of harm reduction services, policing and homelessness.

SETTINGS

Exchanging sex for payment is not illegal in any state of Australia. In New South Wales (NSW), sex work was decriminalized in 1979 and in 1995 amendments to the sex industry regulatory framework gave local councils regulatory power over brothels. While there is no general legal prohibition of sex work, this is qualified by laws and regulations that criminalize sex work under certain conditions or in specific settings. Street-based sex work in NSW is restricted by the Summary Offences Act, 1988 (NSW), which prohibits soliciting in a public street, near or within view from a dwelling, school, church or hospital. Breaches of this act may result in move-on orders or arrest (Bligh and Rasaiah, 2001).

Cabramatta

Cabramatta is a suburban ethnic enclave located 32 kilometres from the Sydney central business district. Two-thirds of Cabramatta residents were born in a non-English speaking country and Vietnamese is the most frequently spoken language (Australian Bureau of Statistics, 2001). During the 1990s, Cabramatta developed a reputation as the 'heroin capital' of Australia (Maher et al., 1998; Maher and Dixon, 1999, 2001; Maher, 2002). Since 2001, the street drug market has constricted, likely due to the cumulative impact of successive and sustained police intervention and a nationwide reduction in the availability of heroin (Degenhardt et al., 2005). During the 1990s, sex work in the neighbourhood was initially characterized by informal sex-for-drug trades between women heroin users and local dealers. As the drug market expanded and diversified, particularly following the introduction of cocaine in 1998, growing numbers of women seeking to support their drug use led to an increase in open soliciting and the emergence of a street-based sex market.

Bankstown

Like Cabramatta, Bankstown is both a residential suburb and a busy cultural and commercial hub. Almost half of all Bankstown residents were born overseas in non-English speaking countries and 70 per cent of residents speak a language other than English (Bankstown City Council, 2005). In contrast to Cabramatta, the drug market in Bankstown has always been relatively low key, characterized by a small street market focused on heroin and dominated by user-dealers. Since the 1980s, the street sex market in Bankstown has centred in and around a major arterial road. At the time of the study, sex workers were located along several kilometres of this road and adjacent side-streets and an outreach needle syringe programme (NSP) operated in the area three evenings a week.

Kings Cross

Located approximately 2 kilometres from the Sydney central business district, the 'red light' district of Kings Cross has been associated with injecting drug use since the early 1960s (McCoy, 1980). A densely populated area, Kings Cross is a hub of restaurants, adult entertainment venues and an open drug market with zones that allow for street-based sex soliciting. Despite increasing gentrification and shifting demographics (Salmon et al., 2007), the area maintains a substantial concentration of health and welfare services, including a Medically Supervised Injecting Centre (MSIC) targeting street-based injectors. There are also numerous cheap accommodation venues, such as backpacker hostels and budget motels, as well as several refuges and hostels. Soliciting for sex occurs on and around the main arterial road linking Kings Cross to the Sydney central business district. Gentrification of the adjacent residential areas has resulted in tensions between street-based sex workers and residents. Unique to this area are two local government-sanctioned 'safe houses', which are privately run businesses that provide women with access to safe and clean working spaces. Rooms with shower facilities and condoms are available for a minimum of 20 minutes at a cost of $AUD15. Intended to reduce the need for street-based sex workers to conduct sex jobs in cars, the safe houses also serve as informal drug consumption sites.

PSYCHOSTIMULANT USE AND STREET-BASED SEX WORK

A synergism identified in the literature is the development of street sex markets or prostitution 'strolls' in tandem with the evolution of street-based drug markets (Curtis and Maher, 1993). In a similar way, and despite the fact that Cabramatta hosted a thriving drug market since the mid-1990s, it was not until the advent of cocaine that street-based sex work emerged as a visible enterprise.

The literature suggests that psychostimulant use is associated with higher levels of problematic drug use, risk behaviours and lower levels of health and social functioning (Booth et al., 1993; Cross et al., 2001; Semple et al., 2004; Bogart et al., 2005; Barr et al., 2006; Couture et al., 2012). However, some women suggested that cocaine and methamphetamine or ice was functional for sex workers, helping them to cope with the long working hours and the demands of the job (Maher et al., 2011b).

> The coke is mad at keeping you up, it means that I can work all night and not feel tired and then I can make more money, not fall asleep on the job. (Julia, 19-year-old Anglo-Australian female)

Despite this, almost all of the women who reported intravenous cocaine or ice use had experienced significant health and economic problems related to their use of these drugs.

> I was making $500 to $1,000 dollars every night in the week. Every night of the week and I didn't even have money left over to buy a packet of cigarettes. All my money went to coke. I had to constantly have a shot, have a shot. The purpose of my whole day was to get another shot of coke. (Dani, 24-year-old Latin-Australian female)

In particular, women identified the compulsiveness and paranoia engendered by frequent cocaine and ice use as amplifying the health risks faced by street-based sex workers.

> Ever since I was on the coke – that was when I got raped by those four guys – I was like a stunned mullet all the time. People can just pick you. It eats you away, like termites on a bit of wood. (Dani, 24-year-old Latin-Australian female)

> [Y]ou just lose it [using ice]. Paranoia. Totally terrible, think people are following you umm, think you are being stalked, you know what I mean? Just crazy things, out of normal things, yeah that you are being followed and that you are going to get killed…it's just crazy. (Bunny, 22-year-old Filipino-Australian female)

Sex work conducted under the influence of drugs has been associated with lower rates of condom use (Plant et al., 1989; de Graaf, 1995; Shannon et al., 2011). Our data suggest that the disinhibiting effects of cocaine may facilitate increased sexual risk taking, both by sex workers and their clients.

> I know for a fact that only about two out of all the guys [using cocaine] I was with used a condom. The rest, they never bothered. They pick up any junkie girl off the street and take them to a hotel and just have sex with them without a condom…Cause they don't care, they just wanna do the business like, you know, have the sex. They're just so hot for it they don't really care about getting a disease or anything… They don't give a shit. (Johnny K, 20-year-old Anglo-Australian male)

The effects of cocaine in extending the time it took for men to ejaculate were negatively perceived by women.

> I think for us girls I reckon it's, for me I reckon it's like it's shit man, I reckon for the blokes yeah cause it takes long. Yeah fuckin takes ages man. Um benefit for guys but not for girls man. Oh for me, no, I just like to fuckin hurry up. (Bizzy, 19-year-old Samoan-Australian female)

Some women spoke about not using condoms in this situation in order to encourage clients to complete the sex act.

> If they've been using coke then right there, number one, they are not gonna to come straight off. Number two, if you use a condom then it's gonna take even longer. (Vanessa, 20-year-old Aboriginal-Australian female)

Drug dependent women clearly have less power and fewer incentives to negotiate safe sex than other sex workers. Sex workers may be less likely to use condoms with clients if they are chasing cocaine or ice or withdrawing from heroin. In particular, the synergies between street sex work and psychostimulant use identified here, manifest in both unsafe sex transactions and unsafe injecting (Shannon et al., 2011). Intravenous psychostimulant use further compromises the health and safety of women involved in street-based sex work by affecting rest, nutritional intake and physical safety.

PATTERNS OF INCOME GENERATION

High frequency injection patterns associated with cocaine use among sex workers have been associated with increased vulnerability to HIV infection (Astemborski et al., 1994; Paone et al., 1999). The economic contexts of street-based sex work shape injecting risk by influencing patterns of drug consumption and injection. The structural positioning of many women who inject drugs within the lowest tier of the sex industry means that they often earn less, relative to other sex workers, which may lead to a higher turnover of clients. Strathdee et al. (2008b) found that sex workers who injected drugs had more clients but received significantly less for sex than sex workers who did not inject drugs. In the context of injecting drug use, low price/high volume street-based sex work transactions may encourage risky behaviours such as unprotected sex (Maher and Curtis, 1992; Van Beek et al., 2001; Degenhardt et al., 2006).

> It's not like they pay by the hour. They're paying to get their release so the quicker they come, the less time you spend with them and the more jobs you do, the more money you make, the more drugs you can use. [So sometimes you don't use condoms?] Depends on the job cause it's quicker if you don't. (Dani, 24-year-old Latin-Australian female)

The structural positioning of women in street-level drug markets (Maher, 1997; Maher and Hudson, 2007) is exacerbated by psychostimulant use, and cocaine use in particular, where most women reported an exhaustive pattern of generating income, purchasing drugs and generating more income.

> [Why not buy a whole lot at once?] Because no matter how much money you have, no matter how much you use, you'll still want more. When you get enough money you just go back. It's like a compulsion, you've just got to have another shot. So you make the money, score and start again. (Angel, 22-year-old Filipino-Australian female)

Our data indicate, that unlike sex workers who do not inject drugs, many women injectors barely generated enough income to support their drug use and their basic needs. Sometimes women turned to scamming or ripping off clients/prospective clients in order to generate income (Maher and Curtis, 1992). For many women, the opportunity to 'rort' a client not only afforded income but the opportunity to avoid sex work for a period of time.

> [S]he [friend] says 'Come with me, like this client, I'm gonna fuckin rip him off'. I said 'Na I don't want nothin to do with it mate'. She said 'No you don't have to have anything to do with it. We'll go up the road, I'll drop you off, take him round the corner and fuckin get the money, go and get the fuckin gear'. (Emma, 39-year-old Anglo-Australian female)

Several of the women interviewed in Kings Cross appeared to specialize in rorting, indicating that, where possible, they would rort a client in order to avoid a sexual transaction.

> I will rort people but only if I know that they are just, you know, dumb cunts. I mean some of the guys that approach you are just asking for it, you know, they are dirty bastards and well, yeah there is no way you want to fuck them. I see an opportunity and I take it, that's that. [Can you describe one of those situations?] Guys off the street you see them cruising and like you will get in the car and make a deal, and then you will tell them you need to get on first and that they might like a little something [drugs] too, so you tell them that they have to give you the money and that you will go and get the gear and tell them to meet you somewhere and then if they are stupid enough to give you the money then you just do a runner. (Tiny, 21-year-old Anglo-Australian female)

Further synergies between street sex and drug markets were apparent in women's relationships with sex work clients who also used drugs. Women in Kings Cross reported being approached by clients to purchase drugs on their behalf. These clients often shared the drugs with the women and sometimes provided them with additional income as well.

> I am always scoring for guys. I met one last night and he was on the coke and he wanted me to go score him some heroin and like, he was an older guy and all he wanted was a back massage and someone to score him some heroin so, that was it and so he shouted me some heroin and coke, fuckin, yeah and then he gave me an extra 50 and I got paid for that anyway so it was only like 20 minutes and he gave me like a 145 dollars for that. (Justice, 21-year-old Anglo-Australian female)

Strathdee et al. (2008b) found that nearly half of the 924 female sex workers they studied in Mexico reported that their clients used drugs and one-fifth reported sharing needles and syringes with clients. Some of the women in our studies also reported injecting clients with drugs.

> A lot of people that they just can't do it properly or, yeah, people who have never done it…If it's coke then yeah, I would give them half a cap, because I mean yeah, coke is a different story to heroin you know. And then I just think you poor silly cunt. (Kobie, 29-year-old Aboriginal-Australian female)

For many of the women in our studies, sex work was an ad hoc and opportunistic income generating strategy facilitated by the spatial contiguity of street-based sex and drug markets. In addition to sex work, many of the women we interviewed relied on a range of sources of income including rorting or robbing clients, procuring (and injecting) drugs for clients, as well as property crime and government benefits.

PHYSICAL ENVIRONMENTS

Research has identified the existence of geographic 'hotspots' or risk environments for street sex work, typically characterized by spatial and social isolation and high levels of drug use (Barnard, 1993; Church et al., 2001; Shannon et al., 2008b; Maher et al., 2011a). Street-based sex workers tend to be more likely to engage in unprotected sex with clients than venue-based sex workers (Pyett and Warr, 1997; Larios et al., 2009; Rusch et al., 2010) and transacting sex in cars and public places has been associated with lower levels of condom use due to decreased control over the environment (Shannon et al., 2009). The physical locations that women used to solicit clients varied widely between the three study sites. In Cabramatta, street-based soliciting took place in an area surrounding a public car park and the adjacent residential streets. Some women also sought clients in local hotels. In Bankstown, the focus of street soliciting was a major arterial road and the surrounding side streets, located in and around an industrial estate. The industrial nature of Canterbury Road provided a particularly isolated and desolate environment. Women often worked in side streets, which, during the day, housed a variety of vehicle repair enterprises. At night, these streets were deserted and poorly lit, and although women often worked within sight of each other, there was little sense of a safety network whereby women watched out for each other.

> It's ok if you're on the main road but down here [side street] it's kind of dark and hard to see into the car. The main thing is to make sure he hasn't got his mates in the back. I always try and check the door handles when I get in. If I feel something's not quite right then I'd call out something to one of the other girls just so he knows that someone saw me get into his car. It's not much protection and half the time she's not even going to remember but he doesn't know that. (Cindy, 24-year-old Anglo-Australian female)

In Bankstown, a small number of Asian background women who injected drugs also solicited for clients in local hotels and bars frequented by Vietnamese men – these women provided vaginal and oral sex in parks and cars.

> She was off her face, heroin, pills, whatever and she came up to me and said '*Anh di choi khong*?' I was shocked. I said 'What?' And she said '*Anh di choi khong*?' I told her please don't ever ask me that again. The next thing I see her walk out with Thang. And then about 10 minutes later, not even, she came back with you know, like stains [semen] on her face. (Minh, 29 year-old Vietnamese-Australian male)

The street settings in which women solicit for sex in Bankstown mean that sex work is not illegal. However, their relatively isolated nature and the lack of street traffic in these locations made women drug users and potential clients highly visible to police. By contrast, in Kings Cross, there were designated zones where women were legally able to solicit for sex work. In particular, a small section of a main thoroughfare allowed women to access the safe houses while remaining in close proximity to the drug market. However, women also worked in the residential areas on the south side of William Street, prompting clashes with residents and police as they attempted to solicit clients close to homes, churches and a private school.

The locations of sex acts also varied widely between the study sites. In Bankstown, while women sometimes accompanied clients to private homes or hotel rooms, sex work primarily took place in parked cars. Similarly, in Kings Cross, the majority of sexual transactions took place in clients' cars. As noted by Kurtz et al., getting into a client's car 'gives almost total control to the customer' (2004: 375). Despite being considered hazardous, women reported that sex jobs conducted in cars were perceived as a quicker option and more likely to consist of oral sex transactions.

> I only really want to have to do oral, so going in the car is better for that, you know, it's quicker. Over and done with, and no hanging around. (Lily, 20-year-old Anglo-Australian female)

Street-based sex work in Bankstown and Kings Cross was generally a swift commercial transaction with women spending their evenings jumping in and out of clients' vehicles. However, the risk of violence and injury represents significant personal safety issues in such settings, particularly when women (and sometimes their clients) are intoxicated. In Cabramatta, women reported engaging in commercial sex in parked cars on residential streets or nearby public parks and reserves, discount hotels, private homes and physical spaces such as laundries and garages. In particular, domestic laundries equipped with a mattress or bedrooms in flats were rented out to women for $5 to $10 per 'job', sometimes with the condition that women provide the owner with sex as well.

The main benefits of these informal arrangements were in providing women with a place to work and, sometimes, a place to stay as well. By virtue of their drug use and depleted economic and social resources some women came to rely on successive short-lived associations with older neighbourhood males. These associations meant that women no longer had to solicit on the street, developing an informal network of clients and reducing their public visibility and vulnerability to arrest. However, the shift from public to private sex work may also reduce women's opportunities for contact with, and support from, other workers and health outreach services.

In both Cabramatta and Kings Cross, the street drug and sex markets are socially and spatially contiguous. In particular, the spatial proximity of street drug markets was identified as an important factor influencing patterns of drug consumption for street-based sex workers. In Kings Cross, drug deliveries meant that the cycle of working and using could continue without interruption.

> They [women] get on the phone, and they will come out to you. [A runner or?] Yeah a runner or the guy himself, depends how they have it sorted. They might come out or jump in a car, they jump in the back seat, they grab the drugs, hand over the cash, drive around the corner, drop them off in a different place and then they will continue on. (TJ, 22-year-old Anglo-Australian male)

In contrast, work sites in Bankstown were relatively isolated from the drug market. For some women this enabled better management of their drug use and, in particular, cocaine use, by delaying purchases until they had finished working for the evening. However, women in Bankstown also reported problems in relation to managing opioid use and averting the onset of withdrawal symptoms. Indeed, withdrawal from heroin while working was identified by women as a risk factor for unsafe sex.

> Like in the Cross you can just keep working all night because they will come and do a drop off and you just have a quick shot and keep going. But somewhere like Bankstown is different. You have to get the money and then go get on so you have to pace yourself kind of. Whereas in the Cross you earn a 50 you get a 50 and it just kind goes on like that. (Cathy, 34-year-old Anglo-Australian female)

AVAILABILITY OF HARM REDUCTION SERVICES

A major synergistic influence on the ability of sex workers who inject drugs to negotiate and enact safe sex and safe injection practices is the availability of harm reduction services and, in particular, condom distribution and NSPs. Access to harm reduction services was influenced by both spatial and temporal dimensions and varied significantly across the three field sites. Injectors in Kings Cross were perhaps the best resourced with access to sterile injecting equipment through the Kirketon Road Centre's (KRC) fixed site and outreach NSP, as well as several pharmacies, a 24-hour vending machine and supervised injecting facilities through the Sydney MSIC. Women who worked in Kings Cross often spoke positively about the services they utilized, particularly those provided by KRC, noting that most services operated outside business hours and/or provided outreach services to locations where women worked. However, even with extended hours, most services were unable to keep the same hours as street-based sex workers, leading to the use of budget hotels, sex clubs and safe houses as informal injecting rooms. Unlike hotels and sex clubs, safe houses provided clean injecting equipment for sex workers.

> I'll use here [safe house], if I score...in the lane [Williams Lane] then I use here. But it's better if they [clients] get a room, you know. I don't like red-lighting myself and that when I am on it. They've got fits here and that. (Lily, 25-year-old Anglo-Australian female)

In Cabramatta, sterile injecting equipment was available through a mobile van and pharmacy programmes and an after-hours pedestrian outreach service two nights a week. Access to primary health care was available during business hours in Cabramatta through the Drug Intervention Service Cabramatta (DISC) until 2001 when this service was closed in response to police and community pressure. The lack of access to after-hours NSP and the absence of vending machines in Cabramatta have been repeatedly identified as factors driving high rates of incident HCV infection in the area (Maher et al., 2006).

> What do they think – that we all go to bed at 7 o'clock? Honestly there is nowhere around here [Cabramatta] after about 7 pm at the latest. What do they expect us to do? Quit? (Suzie, 33-year-old Anglo-Australian female)

Canterbury Road is spatially isolated and at least a 15-minute walk to the Community Health Centre that provides NSP during business hours. Like Cabramatta, there is limited after-hours access to sterile injecting equipment. While a mobile outreach van services the area three nights a week, some women relied on male partners and clients to provide them with lifts to access injecting equipment. While women reported obtaining bulk supplies of free condoms, ensuring ready access when working, they were reluctant to carry supplies of needles and syringes while working in case they were used as incriminating evidence in the event of a police search.

While some women were aware that it is not an offence to carry unused syringes in NSW, the intensive police presence in Cabramatta and Bankstown effectively served to deter women from carrying supplies of clean injecting equipment.

Women also identified an inability to predict how much they would earn on a given night as an important factor influencing their relative lack of preparedness. As noted previously (Maher et al., 1998), the demand for heroin displays some elasticity even among severely dependent users and is responsive to variations in income. Within this uncertain environment, 24-hour access to sterile injecting equipment is essential.

> You don't know how much money you will make so you don't know how much you're gonna use. So it's hard to plan ahead. Every day is different. Like tonight I might only need one fit but say tomorrow I make more or I decide to get some coke, I might need five. Or you end up getting on with customers or friends and they don't have any [syringes]. It's hard to plan ahead. (Cindy, 24-year-old Anglo-Australian female)

South western Sydney differs from other areas of Sydney, including Kings Cross, in that approximately 70 per cent of NSP distribution is provided by pharmacies compared to approximately 25 per cent in other areas. Restricted opening hours, the location of NSPs, limited outreach services and having to purchase injecting equipment were identified by women as potential barriers to safe injection practices. The confluence of these factors in Cabramatta and Bankstown created a significant disincentive for sex workers who worked late at night.

Supervised injecting facilities have been associated with reductions in needle and syringe sharing, overdoses, public injecting and numbers of publicly discarded syringes (Hedrich, 2004; Wood et al., 2004; Kerr et al., 2005b, 2006; Thein et al., 2005; Stoltz et al., 2007), increased uptake of drug detoxification and treatment (Wood et al., 2006b) and have not led to increases in drug-related crime or rates of relapse (Kerr et al., 2006; Wood et al., 2006a). In Kings Cross, the MSIC provided a unique service for sex workers who injected drugs.

> [What are some of the good things about the injecting centre?] The best is that you can relax. You're not scared or anything. The cops aren't allowed. You just go in, give 'em your password and that's it. Oh they ask you what you're gonna have and if you had anything before that. They don't need your name or nothing. It's free and clean and they give you a clean fit. If people drop they look after them, bring 'em back to life, not rob 'em. We could use something like that around here [Cabramatta]. (Shannon, 29-year-old Aboriginal-Australian female)

The Sydney MSIC clearly provides sex workers who inject drugs with the opportunity to inject in a safe environment free from the risks of violence and predation that occur on the streets. While approximately 8 per cent of the more than 10,000 registered MSIC clients report sex work in the last month (NCHECR, 2007), restricted opening hours mean that there is a significant gap in the MSIC's ability to provide coverage to this group. Outside the MSIC's opening hours, sex workers who inject drugs in Kings Cross, like their counterparts in Bankstown and Cabramatta, resort to riskier environments such as illegal shooting galleries, hotel rooms, clients' cars, public toilets and street settings.

VIOLENCE

Previous research has identified violence against sex workers as a significant barrier to HIV prevention efforts (Pyett and Warr, 1997; Wojcicki and Malala, 2001; Romero-Daza et al., 2003; Kerrigan et al., 2006; Shannon et al., 2008a; Shannon et al., 2009; Shannon and Csete, 2010). Violence is clearly associated with reduced condom use and HIV and STI transmission and environmental and structural factors – including homelessness, inability to access drug treatment, transacting sex in cars or public spaces and enforcement based policing strategies – have also been independently associated with violence against sex workers (Shannon et al., 2009, 2015). In Kings Cross, many women started working in clubs that provided drugs on 'tic' (like a tab) or 'subbed' (loaned) women cash until such time that their use escalated and they had no way of paying it back. In some cases, women described situations where they would attempt to leave the club in order to make money on the street, only to be found and beaten and brought back to the club.

> She tells me that when she had difficulty working because she was hanging out, the club would 'sub' [advance] her so that she could score. Ella tells me she has been in trouble before with the clubs for being found working on the street rather than working there. 'I am trapped now' she tells me. (Hudson, Field note, 22 June 2006)

Street-based or outdoor sex workers are at higher risk of sexual assault than other sex workers (Sanders and Campbell, 2007). Roxburgh et al. (2006) found that in a Sydney sample of 72 street-based sex workers, 33 per cent reported having been raped. Several women provided accounts of sexual assault, both in the context of intimate relationships and while they were working. Some women drug users appeared to accept the risk of forced sex as an inevitable fact of their working conditions.

> I have been raped by customers. What can you do? It's not like we can go to the cops and say we've been raped. They know we're out there so they're just going to say we deserve it. (Cindy, 24-year-old Anglo-Australian female)

Rape is an immediate danger and one that appears to occur with disturbing regularity among street-based sex workers (Shannon and Csete, 2010).

> I have been raped several times in my life. I have been bashed…I have lost probably eight girlfriends, as in they were working girls that were murdered, raped and murdered, you know. (Cathy, 34-year-old Anglo-Australian female)

Women reported being raped by clients. Some women reported that intoxicated clients were sometimes unable to maintain erections, resulting in anger and embarrassment, which they took out on women. Women also reported being robbed by male drug users, gangsters and police. Women who inject drugs are often vulnerable to abusive and economically parasitically relationships that encourage male control of drug acquisition, preparation and administration (Bourgois et al., 2004). These relationships are embedded in broader cultural scripts around masculinity and male control over women (Maher, 1997). Most of the women in our studies who were in relationships reported supporting their partner's drug use as well as their own.

> I have had like boyfriends like umm, you know Abe and I had a thing once and umm, he would sort of come out and that and wait around for me when I would go off on a job. But that was just so he could get the money to score, he didn't give a shit about me just as long as the money came back. (Tiny, 21-year-old Anglo-Australian female)

Intimate relationships with male partners were often fraught with tension and violence.

> He used to beat the shit out of me. When I didn't make enough or if the coke ran out and he wanted to keep using, he would start on me. It's too hard to be in a relationship with the drugs. (Dani, 24-year-old Latin-Australian female)

The literature also indicates that sexual relationships are valued by some women drug users who live and work on the street, both as a means of protection and avoiding predation by other males (MacRae and Aalto, 2000; Bourgois et al., 2004). However, in practice, most women reported that male partners provided little in the way of material or emotional support.

POLICING

Disruption of health service utilization among people who inject drugs (PWID) as a result of intensive policing of drug markets undermines harm reduction and outreach efforts (Maher and Dixon, 2001; Cooper et al., 2004; Kerr et al., 2005a). Intensive policing and police crackdowns have been associated with harms such as risky injecting practices and reduced access to NSP (Bluthenthal et al., 1997; Maher et al., 1998; Csete and Cohen, 2003; Wood et al., 2003; Small et al., 2006). Policing practices have also been independently associated with prevalent HIV infection with PWID who report being arrested for having track-marks more likely to be infected with the virus (Strathdee et al., 2008a).

Our data suggest that intensive policing or police crackdowns also have the potential to disrupt the street-based sex work environment, creating uncertainty and increasing risk by encouraging women to conduct furtive or hurried transactions. Police crackdowns on street-based sex work reduce the number of potential customers by arresting and charging some and deterring others. When this happens, workers are placed under increased pressure to compete with each other for clients and engage in price cutting and truncated negotiations (Maher, 1997). Within this context, physical locations and their degree of public visibility determine the risk of arrest (Chapkis, 2000). A highly publicized crackdown on kerb crawling that occurred in Bankstown over a six-week period in 2001 resulted in the arrests of 55 men and one woman (*Sydney Morning Herald*, 2001). While sex workers were not the primary targets of this operation, women reported that potential clients had been scared off by the arrests and the accompanying spate of publicity.

> It's bad for business. There's no customers. It's in the papers and everything so they think they're gonna get busted...You've still got the same number of girls as you had before, the same number of habits to support, but no customers...things get a little desperate because everyone is out to take care of themselves and you're more, like competing with each other, trying to get customers. (Angel, 22-year-old Filipino-Australian female)

Within this environment, women were also less likely to discriminate or select their clients or to negotiate in advance the terms and conditions of the transaction.

> You can't be picky. When there's no customers, any job is a good job. (Shannon, 29-year-old Aboriginal-Australian female)

Police crackdowns on drug markets that produce changes in the price and availability of drugs may also have collateral effects on street-based sex work. For example, the crackdown on kerb crawling that occurred in Bankstown in early 2001 coincided with the peak period of a national reduction in the availability of heroin in Australia.

> And now when the gear is dry and the dealers have all put the price up, you know, if you can get it that is, at the same time we need to work more than before. We need to do more jobs just to get the same amount of gear that we got before. (Cathy, 34-year-old Anglo-Australian female)

Faced with a decline in potential clients, women were also less likely to negotiate in relation to the physical locations of jobs, with safety less of a priority than the ability to secure jobs, particularly following the reduction in heroin availability and subsequent increase in price. Within such hostile and uncertain environments, individual police also presented threats to health and safety.

> [T]he police are a different story. They are the law, you know, you don't have much say in anything because they are the law. Basically they can do whatever they want. If they want to search you or drive you to another area, what can you do? (Kelly, 22-year-old Anglo-Australian female)

Police harassment of street-based sex workers is not uncommon. One study found that more than half of the street sex workers interviewed reported being harassed by police and more than a quarter reported that they had been sexually or physically assaulted by police in the last five years (Woodward et al., 2004). In response to police crackdowns, street-based sex workers may shift to isolated, secluded, poorly lit or less visible sites (Alexander, 1998; Shannon et al., 2008b; Maher et al., 2011a). In Cabramatta, this was reflected in the shift to providing services in private settings such as flats, laundries and garages. In Bankstown, women shifted further away from the main arterial road into poorly lit side streets. The displacement of street sex workers to private spaces and isolated industrial settings forces marginalized women further away from harm reduction services, reducing their access to health care and social support. In a study in Mexican border cities, female sex workers with an unstable main place of work had more sexual partners, lower self-efficacy scores for using condoms and fewer gynaecologic visits and were less likely to have ever had an HIV test, suggesting that providing sex workers with stable workplaces facilitates the uptake of HIV/STI and reproductive health interventions (Chen et al., 2012).

HOMELESSNESS

Homelessness disrupts the capacity of street-based sex workers to protect their health and safety and presents serious impediments to safer injecting practices. Many of the women in all three study sites had experienced periods of homelessness and residential instability that served to cement and intensify their involvement in drug use and street life.

Women in all three sites described living in temporary accommodation including refuges, caravan parks and short-stay hotels and motels. Many women, particularly those interviewed in Cabramatta, reported exchanging sex for shelter or a roof over their heads.

> Well just, females like, um, have more opportunity of having a place to stay for the night you know. Some guy might walk up, see you're on the street, feel sorry for you, you know, and whether he's got a good heart or not often 'Yeh you can stay here for the night if you want for nothing or you can do this for that' you know? (Tracey, 27-year-old Anglo-Australian female)

In Cabramatta, the sex market was structured by relationships with local neighbourhood men. Like Kings Cross, many women, particularly Anglo-Australians, ended up in Cabramatta because of the availability of drugs. However, unlike Kings Cross, there is no sex tourism in Cabramatta, and women were dependent on the patronage of local drug dealers and older neighbourhood males.

> Sometime early in the morning girl come at our door, desperate for the drug. An Asian girl, decent girl got addicted and hanging out bad. She will do anything for a cap so the guy let her in. (Star, 29-year-old Vietnamese-Australian female)

While these excerpts indicate that women drug users were vulnerable to predation and exploitation by drug dealers, many women identified benefits to forming relationships with older neighbourhood men. These relationships provided 'gendered solutions' (Maher et al., 1996) to the problems of homelessness and residential instability experienced by many women. Relative to the women, older men possessed significant resources, including jobs or pensions and a place to stay. While women often viewed these arrangements as mutually beneficial, many of the situations described by participants and observed during fieldwork were clearly exploitative.

> Sugar daddies. Yeh pretty much. Just for a place to stay really. Sometimes that involves sex. Sometimes it doesn't. And they give you money all the time and support ya habit just to keep you there. He put me in hotels… but you can't, they don't like you having a boyfriend. (Billie, 24-year-old Anglo-Australian female)

Older males, and 'sugar daddies' in particular, by virtue of their structural positioning vis-a-vis homeless and drug dependent women, provided a source of refuge and respite from the street. Some sugar daddies offered their affections as well as tangible support in the form of shelter, food and small amounts of money. Sometimes these relationships enabled women to reduce the number of paid sex acts by avoiding basic expenditures.

These informal arrangements with older neighbourhood men represent an adaptive response by women to the exigencies of life on the margins. However, these arrangements were often characterized by hidden costs associated with the tenuous and temporary nature of such relationships.

CONCLUSIONS

While ethnographic research possesses the capacity to elucidate the relativity of risk across different environments, the analytic focus of most research to date has been on individual risk behaviour and few efforts have been made to unpack the range of factors that create and maintain these environments or to identify the synergies between them. We currently lack conceptual frameworks for understanding changes in risk environments and for making comparisons between different types of environments. This chapter attempts to provide a starting point for such enquiries by identifying synergies between street sex and drug markets and their role in promoting and sustaining risk environments.

Research on drug-related harms indicates a clear need for safe environment interventions that promote increased access to sterile injecting equipment and are supported by legal and policy reforms (Rhodes et al., 2006). Street-based sex work environments share many of the same characteristics as street-based drug markets, including public injecting, intensive policing and high rates of homelessness and residential instability. The synergistic relationships between street-based sex and drug markets work to exacerbate vulnerability by creating environments that over-determine risk. Within these environments, women exercise agency or choice by prioritizing and choosing between multiple and competing risks including the risk of withdrawal, having little or no income, robbery, assault, rape, arrest and homelessness.

Unpacking the range of market characteristics, social mechanisms and structural features that create these environments, the data presented here show how safe sex and safe injecting are frequently traded off against other priorities. These data illustrate the structural characteristics of street sex markets, including low unit prices that encourage high frequency sex acts, are related to gender-segmented drug markets and the price and availability of drugs. The synergistic relationship between street sex and drug markets illustrated by psychostimulant use indicates how particular patterns of drug use shape income generating practices in ways that promote unsafe sex and unsafe drug use. Our data also illustrate how spatial features of street-based sex and drug markets, including the location and accessibility of harm reduction services, interact to shape risk and protective practices. Violence against sex workers places them at increased risk of blood-borne and sexually transmitted infections (Shannon et al., 2009; Shannon and Csete, 2010). Other structural factors, such as a lack of affordable housing, work to undermine attempts by women to control their occupational environments and their drug use (Shannon et al., 2015). Injecting drug use is an important driver of informalization and the under-development of occupational norms that compounds the exclusion of sex workers from official protection and public health prevention efforts and impedes collaboration and community development.

These results point to a need for interventions designed to address the synergisms that create and shape risk within the context of street sex and drug markets. Negative synergisms between street sex and drug markets increase the harms associated with street-based sex work by encouraging risky patterns of income generation and eroding or preventing the development of occupational norms. Synergisms between the policing of street drug and sex markets create environments characterized by uncertainty and risk and may result in harms such as driving sex workers who use drugs into isolated public or unregulated private spaces. Similarly, drug supply control efforts that reduce availability and drive up the price of drugs may force reductions in the market rates for sexual services and increase risky sexual transactions.

To date, drug harm reduction policies have primarily focused on individual behaviour change. However, environmental interventions designed to provide drug users, including sex workers, with supervised injecting environments have been shown to reduce public injecting and increase public amenity (Maher and Salmon, 2007). The sex industry has also sought to reduce harm by seeking to regulate the occupational environments and conditions of sex work (Sanders and Campbell, 2007) and a recent systematic review identified the need for supportive managerial practices and policies to reduce violence and increase consistent condom use among venue-based sex workers (Shannon et al., 2015). While a structural approach does not necessarily exclude a focus on individual agency, and indeed the literature identifies a range of strategies and tactics employed by street-based sex workers to avoid violence and manage risk (Barnard, 1993), there is a need to go beyond individual-level risk reduction interventions.

This chapter has highlighted the need for structural level interventions, supported by legal and policy reforms, that attempt to reduce the environmental risks of street-based sex work. These include the risks presented by working in deserted settings late at night, being intoxicated or withdrawing from drugs, restricted access to sterile injecting equipment, the risk of arrest or detention and homelessness. In particular, interventions that provide women drug users with stable work sites, access to affordable housing, reduce their exposure to violence and police harassment and facilitate their access to health services, including drug treatment, may provide women with more control over their drug use and promote safer occupational environments for street-based sex workers.

Peer-based interventions such as providing street-based workers with greater access to local knowledge about abusive or violent clients are also important vehicles for environmental risk reduction. Programmes such as the 'Ugly Mugs' programme developed by the Prostitutes' Collective in the Australian state of Victoria circulate information about these clients and their vehicles within the sex worker community. Other sex industry strategies such as working in pairs, writing down number plates, avoiding cars with more than one person in them and checking car door handles to ensure doors can be opened from the inside, are also part of a pro-active community development approach. However, these strategies require time. The data presented here suggest that features of the risk environment, such as police crackdowns and the demands of heavy psychostimulant use, may impede or prevent attempts by sex workers to adopt these strategies.

While regulatory policies and practices are increasingly identified as vehicles for both producing and preventing a range of harms, harm reduction discourses in relation to street-based sex work are dominated by the risk of infectious disease transmission and few studies have explored the potential impact of strategies designed to increase the safety and rights of sex workers to negotiate their working environments and conduct safer transactions. As Sanders and Campbell (2007) note, it will not be enough to simply reduce or 'design out' the risks of sex workers' working environments. There is a need to build respect into these environments by acknowledging sex workers, including street-based sex workers, as members of an occupational community engaged in a form of labour. Women who inject drugs are vulnerable and often marginal members of this community and their needs for safety and security within the occupational settings of street sex work are particularly acute and further compromised by the spatial, social and structural synergies between street sex and drug markets.

ACKNOWLEDGEMENTS

I am grateful to the participants in the ethnographic studies reported here for their stories and their insights, to Dr Heidi Coupland for assistance with data collection in Cabramatta, and to Dr Susan Hudson who collected data in Kings Cross as part of her PhD thesis. Lisa Maher is supported by the award of an Australian National Health and Medical Research Council (NHMRC) Senior Research Fellowship.

REFERENCES

Alexander P (1998) Sex work and health: a question of safety in the workplace. *Journal of the American Medical Women's Association* 53: 77–82.

Astemborski J, Vlahov D, Warren D, Solomon L, Nelson KE. (1994) The trading of sex for drugs or money and HIV seropositivity among female intravenous-drug-users. *American Journal of Public Health* 84: 382–7.

Australian Bureau of Statistics (2001) *Labour Statistics: Concepts, Sources and Methods*. Canberra: Australian Bureau of Statistics.

Bankstown City Council (2005) *Bankstown Community Profile*. Bankstown: Bankstown City Council.

Barnard MA. (1993) Violence and vulnerability: conditions of work for streetworking prostitutes. *Sociology of Health and Illness* 15: 683–705.

Barr AM, Panenka WJ, MacEwan GW, Thornton AE, Lang DJ, Honer WG, Lecomte T. (2006) The need for speed: an update on methamphetamine addiction. *Journal of Psychiatry and Neuroscience* 31: 301–13.

Bellis MA, Watson FL, Hughes S, Cook PA, Downing J, Clark P, Thomson R. (2007) Comparative views of the public, sex workers, businesses and residents on establishing managed zones for prostitution: analysis of a consultation in Liverpool. *Health Place* 13: 603–16.

Blankenship KM and Koester S (2002) Criminal law, policing policy, and HIV risk in female street sex workers and injection drug users. *The Journal of Law, Medicine and Ethics* 30: 548–59.

Bligh A and Rasaiah C (2001) *Street Sex Workers and the Law in Sydney*. Sydney: University of Technology Sydney.

Bluthenthal RN, Kral AH, Erringer EA, Edlin BR. (1999) Drug paraphernalia law and injection-related infectious disease risk among injectors. *Journal of Drug Issues* 29: 16.

Bluthenthal RN, Kral AH, Lorvick J, Watters JK. (1997) Impact of law enforcement on syringe exchange programs: a look at Oakland and San Francisco. *Medical Anthropology* 18: 61–83.

Bogart LM, Kral AH, Scott A, Anderson R, Flynn N, Gilbert ML, Bluthenthal RN. (2005) Sexual risk among injection drug users recruited from syringe exchange programs in California. *Sexually Transmitted Diseases* 32: 27–34.

Booth RE, Watters JK and Chitwood DD (1993) HIV risk-related sex behaviors among injection-drug users, crack smokers, and injection-drug users who smoke crack. *American Journal of Public Health* 83: 1144–8.

Bourgois P and Bruneau J (2000) Needle exchange, HIV infection, and the politics of science: confronting Canada's cocaine injection epidemic with participant observation. *Medical Anthropology* 18: 325–50.

Bourgois P, Lettiere M and Quesada J (1997) Social misery and the sanctions of substance abuse: confronting HIV risk among homeless heroin addicts in San Francisco. *Social Problems* 44: 155–73.

Bourgois P, Prince B and Moss A (2004) The everyday violence of hepatitis C among young women who inject drugs in San Francisco. *Human Organization* 63: 253–64.

Burris S, Blankenship KM, Donoghoe M, Sherman S, Vernick JS, Case P, Lazzarini Z, Koester S. (2004) Addressing the 'risk environment' for injection drug users: the mysterious case of the missing cop. *Milbank Quaterly* 82: 125–56.

Chapkis W (2000) Power and control in the commercial sex trade. In: R Weitzer (ed.), *Sex for Sale: Prostitution, Pornography, and the Sex Industry.* New York: Routledge, pp. 181–201.

Chen NE, Strathdee SA, Rangel G, Patterson TL, Uribe-Salas FJ, Rosen P, Villalobos J, Brouwer KC. (2012) HIV risk behaviours differ by workplace stability among Mexican female sex workers with truck driver clientele. *Journal of Public Health Research* 1: 208–13.

Choi SYP, Cheung YW and Chen KL (2006) Gender and HIV risk behavior among intravenous drug users in Sichuan Province, China. *Social Science and Medicine* 62: 1672–84.

Church S, Henderson M, Barnard M, Hart G (2001) Violence by clients towards female prostitutes in different work settings: questionnaire survey. *British Medical Journal* 322: 524–5.

Cooper H, Moore L, Gruskin S, Krieger N. (2004) Characterizing perceived police violence: Implications for public health. *American Journal of Public Health* 94: 1109–18.

Cooper H, Moore L, Gruskin S, Krieger N. (2005) The impact of a police drug crackdown on drug injectors' ability to practice harm reduction: a qualitative study. *Social Science and Medicine* 61: 673–84.

Corneil TA, Kuyper LM, Shoveller J, Hogg RS, Li K, Spittal PM, Schechter MT, Wood E. (2006) Unstable housing, associated risk behaviour, and increased risk for HIV infection among injection drug users. *Health Place* 12: 79–85.

Costenbader EC, Astone NM and Latkin CA (2006) The dynamics of injection drug users' personal networks and HIV risk behaviors. *Addiction* 101: 1003–13.

Couture MC, Evans JL, Sothy NS, Stein ES, Sichan K, Maher L, Page K. (2012) Correlates of amphetamine-type stimulant use and associations with HIV-related risks among young women engaged in sex work in Phnom Penh, Cambodia. *Drug and Alcohol Dependence* 120: 119–26.

Cross JC, Johnson BD, Davis WR, Liberty HJ. (2001) Supporting the habit: income generation activities of frequent crack users compared with frequent users of other hard drugs. *Drug and Alcohol Dependence* 64: 191–201.

Csete J and Cohen J (2003) *Abusing the user: Police Misconduct, Harm Reduction and HIV/AIDS in Vancouver*. New York: Human Rights Watch.

Curtis R and Maher L (1993) Highly structured crack markets in the southside of Williamsburg, Brooklyn. In: Fagan J (ed.), *The Ecology of Crime and Drug Use in Inner Cities.* New York: Social Science Research Council.

Curtis R, Friedman SR, Neaigus A, Jose B, Goldstein M, Ildefonso G (1995) Street-level drug markets - network structure and HIV risk. *Social Networks* 17: 229–49.

Cusick L (1998) Female prostitution in Glasgow: drug use and occupational sector. *Addiction Research* 6: 115–30.

Davey MA, Latkin CA, Hua W, Tobin KE, Strathdee S. (2007) Individual and social network factors that predict entry to drug treatment. *American Journal on Addictions* 16: 38–45.

Davis CS, Burris S, Kraut-Becher J, Lynch KG, Metzger D. (2005) Effects of an intensive street-level police intervention on syringe exchange program use in Philadelphia, PA. *American Journal of Public Health* 95: 233–236.

de Graaf R (1995) *Prostitutes and Their Clients: Sexual Networks and Determinants of Condom Use*. Amsterdam: Ponsen & Looijen.

Degenhardt L, Day C, Conroy E, Gilmour S. (2006) Examining links between injecting cocaine use and street based sex work in NSW, Australia. *Journal of Sex Research* 43: 107–14.

Degenhardt L, Reuter P, Collins L, Hall W. (2005) Evaluating explanations of the Australian 'heroin shortage'. *Addiction* 100: 459–69.

Edlin BR, Irwin KL, Faruque S, McCoy CB, Word C, Serrano Y, Inciardi JA, Bowser BP, Schilling RF, Holmberg SD. (1994) Intersecting epidemics - crack cocaine use and HIV-infection among inner-city young-adults. *New England Journal of Medicine* 331: 1422–7.

Friedman SR, Cooper HLF, Tempalski B, Keem M, Friedman R, Flom PL, Des Jarlais DC. (2006) Relationships of deterrence and law enforcement to drug-related harms among drug injectors in US metropolitan areas. *AIDS* 20: 93–9.

German D, Davey MA and Latkin CA (2007) Residential transience and HIV risk behaviors among injection drug users. *AIDS and Behavior* 11: S21–30.

Gibson K, Bowen R, Janseen P, Spittal P. (2006) *Evaluation of the Mobile Access Project (MAP)*. Vancouver: Vancouver Agreement Women's Strategy Task Team.

Hayashi K, Small W, Csete J, Hattirat S, Kerr T. (2013) Experiences with policing among people who inject drugs in Bangkok, Thailand: a qualitative study. Plos Medicine 10: e1001570.

Hedrich D (2004) *European Report on Drug Consumption Rooms*. Lisbon: European Monitoring Centre for Drugs and Drug Addiction.

Hubbard P (1998) Community action and the displacement of street prostitution: evidence from British cities. *Geoforum* 29: 269–86.

Hubbard P (1999) Researching female sex work: reflections on geographical exclusion, critical methodologies and 'useful' knowledge. *Area* 31: 229–37.

Hubbard P and Sanders T (2003) Making space for sex work: female street prostitution and the production of urban space. *International Journal of Urban and Regional Research* 27: 75–89.

Hudson SL (2010) *Sex, Drugs and 'Ugly Mugs': An Ethnographic Study of Women Who Inject Psychostimulants and Engage in Street-Based Sex Work in Kings Cross, Sydney*. Sydney: University of New South Wales.

Kerr T, Small W and Wood E (2005a) The public health and social impacts of drug market enforcement: a review of the evidence. *International Journal of Drug Policy* 16: 210–20.

Kerr T, Stoltz JA, Tyndall M, Li K, Zhang R, Montaner J, Wood E. (2006) Impact of a medically supervised safer injection facility on community drug use patterns: a before and after study. *British Medical Journal* 332: 220–2.

Kerr T, Tyndall M, Li K, Montaner J, Wood E. (2005b) Safer injection facility use and syringe sharing in injection drug users. *Lancet* 366: 316–18.

Kerrigan D, Moreno L, Rosario S, Gomez B, Jerez H, Barrington C, Weiss E, Sweat M. (2006) Environmental-structural interventions to reduce HIV/STI risk among female sex workers in the Dominican Republic. *American Journal of Public Health* 96: 120–5.

Koester S, Heimer R, Baron AE, Glanz J, Teng W. (2003) Risk of hepatitis C virus among young adult injection drug users who share injection equipment. *American Journal of Epidemiology* 157: 376.

Kurtz SP, Surratt HL, Inciardi JA, Kiley MC. (2004) Sex work and 'date' violence. *Violence against Women* 10: 357–85.

Kuyper LM, Palepu A, Kerr T, Li K, Miller CL, Spittal PM, Hogg RS, Montaner JSG, Wood E. (2005) Factors associated with sex-trade involvement among female injection drug users in a Canadian setting. *Addiction Research and Theory* 13: 193–9.

Larios SE, Lozada R, Strathdee SA, Semple SJ, Roesch S, Staines H, Orozovich P, Fraga M, Amaro H, de la Torre A, Magis-Rodriguez C, Patterson TL. (2009) An exploration of contextual factors that influence HIV risk in female sex workers in Mexico: The Social Ecological Model applied to HIV risk behaviors. *AIDS Care-Psychological and Socio-Medical Aspects of AIDS/HIV* 21: 1335–42.

Latkin CA and Knowlton AR (2005) Micro-social structural approaches to HIV prevention: a social ecological perspective. *AIDS Care-Psychological and Socio-Medical Aspects of AIDS/HIV* 17: S102–13.

Latkin CA, Mandell W, Oziemkowska M, Vlahov D, Celentano D. (1994) The relationships between sexual behaviour, substance use and personal network characteristics in injecting drug users in Baltimore, Maryland. *Journal of Sexually Transmitted Disease* 21: 161–7.

MacRae R and Aalto E (2000) Gendered power dynamics and HIV risk in drug-using sexual relationships. *AIDS Care-Psychological and Socio-Medical Aspects of AIDS/HIV* 12: 505–15.

Maher L (1996) Hidden in the light: occupational norms among crack-using street-level sex workers. *Journal of Drug Issues* 26: 143–73.

Maher L (1997) *Sexed Work: Gender, Race and Resistance in a Brooklyn Drug Market*, New York: Oxford University Press.

Maher L (2002) Don't leave us this way: ethnography and injecting drug use in the age of AIDS. *International Journal of Drug Policy* 13: 311–25.

Maher L and Curtis R (1992) Women on the edge of crime - crack cocaine and the changing contexts of street-level sex work in New York City. *Crime Law and Social Change* 18: 221–58.

Maher L and Dixon D (1999) Policing and public health: law enforcement and harm minimization in a street-level drug market. *British Journal of Criminology* 39: 488–512.

Maher L and Dixon D (2001) The cost of crackdowns: policing Cabramatta's heroin market. *Current Issues in Criminal Justice* 13: 5–22.

Maher L and Hudson SL (2007) Women in the drug economy: a metasynthesis of the qualitative literature. *Journal of Drug Issues* 37: 805–26.

Maher L and Salmon A (2007) Supervised injecting facilities: how much evidence is enough? *Drug and Alcohol Review* 26: 351–3.

Maher L, Dixon D, Lynskey M, Hall W. (1998) *Running the Risks: Heroin, Health and Harm in South West Sydney*. Sydney: National Drug and Alcohol Research Centre.

Maher L, Dunlap E, Johnson BD, Hamid A. (1996) Gender, power, and alternative living arrangements in the inner-city crack culture. *Journal of Research in Crime and Delinquency* 33: 181–205.

Maher L, Jalaludin B, Chant KG, Jayasuriya R, Sladden T, Kaldor JM, Sargent PL. (2006) Incidence and risk factors for hepatitis C seroconversion in injecting drug users in Australia. *Addiction* 101: 1499–508.

Maher L, Mooney-Somers J, Phlong P, Couture MC, Stein E, Evans J, Cockroft M, Sansothy N, Nemoto T, Page K, for the Young Women's Health Study Collaborative. (2011a) Selling sex in unsafe spaces: sex work risk environments in Phnom Penh, Cambodia. *Harm Reduction Journal* 8: 30.

Maher L, Phlong P, Mooney-Somers J, Keo S, Stein E, Couture MC, Page K. (2011b) Amphetamine-type stimulant use and HIV/STI risk behaviour among young female sex workers in Phnom Penh, Cambodia. *International Journal of Drug Policy* 22: 203–9.

McCoy AW (1980) *Drug Traffic: Narcotics and Organized Crime in Australia*. Sydney: Harper and Row.

McKeganey NP and Barnard M (1996) *Sex Work on the Streets: Prostitutes and Their Clients*. Buckingham: Open University Press.

Miller J (1993) Your life is on the line every night you're on the streets: victimization and resistance among street prostitutes. *Humanity and Society* 17: 422–46.

Miller M and Neaigus A (2002) An economy of risk: resource acquisition strategies of inner city women who use drugs. *International Journal of Drug Policy* 13: 409–18.

NCHECR (2007) *Sydney Medically Supervised Injecting Centre Evaluation Report 4: Evaluation of Service Operation and Overdose-Related Events*. Sydney: National Centre in HIV Epidemiology and Clinical Research, University of New South Wales.

Ouellet LJ, Jimenez AD, Johnson WA, Wiebel WW. (1991) Shooting galleries and HIV disease – variations in places for injecting illicit drugs. *Crime and Delinquency* 37: 64–85.

Paone D, Cooper H, Alperen J, Shi Q, Des Jarlais DC. (1999) HIV risk behaviours of current sex workers attending syringe exchange: the experiences of women in five US cities. *AIDS Care-Psychological and Socio-Medical Aspects of AIDS/HIV* 11: 269–80.

Patrick DM, Tyndall MW, Cornelisse PGA, Li K, Sherlock CH, Rekart ML, Strathdee SA, Currie SL, Schechter MT, O'Shaughnessy MV. (2001) Incidence of hepatitis C virus infection among injection drug users during an outbreak of HIV infection. *Canadian Medical Association Journal* 165: 889–95.

Plant ML, Plant MA, Peck DF, Setters J. (1989) The sex industry, alcohol and illicit drugs - implications for the spread of HIV infection. *British Journal of Addiction* 84: 53–9.

Pollini RA, Brouwer KC, Lozada RM, Ramos R, Cruz MF, Magis-Rodriguez C, Case P, Burris S, Pu M, Frost SDW, Palinkas LA, Miller C, Strathdee SA. (2008) Syringe possession arrests are associated with receptive syringe sharing in two Mexico-US border cities. *Addiction* 103: 101–8.

Pyett PM and Warr DJ (1997) Vulnerability on the streets: female sex workers and HIV risk. *AIDS Care-Psychological and Socio-Medical Aspects of AIDS/HIV* 9: 539–47.

Reyes JC, Robles RR, Colon HM, Matos TD, Finlinson HA, Marrero CA, Shepard EW. (2005) Homelessness and HIV risk behaviors among drug injectors in Puerto Rico. *Journal of Urban Health-Bulletin of the New York Academy of Medicine* 82: 446–55.

Rhodes T (2002) The 'risk environment': a framework for understanding and reducing drug-related harm. *International Journal of Drug Policy* 13: 85–94.

Rhodes T, Kimber J, Small W, Fitzgerald J, Kerr T, Hickman M, Holloway G. (2006) Public injecting and the need for 'safer environment interventions' in the reduction of drug-related harm. *Addiction* 101: 1384–93.

Rhodes T, Mikhailova L, Sarang A, Lowndes CM, Rylkov A, Khutorskoy M, Renton A. (2003) Situational factors influencing drug injecting, risk reduction and syringe exchange in Togliatti City, Russian Federation: a qualitative study of micro risk environment. *Social Science and Medicine* 57: 39–54.

Romero-Daza N, Weeks M and Singer M (2003) 'Nobody gives a damn if I live or die': violence, drugs, and street-level prostitution in inner-city Hartford, Connecticut. *Medical Anthropology* 22: 233–59.

Roxburgh A, Degenhardt L and Copeland J (2006) Posttraumatic stress disorder among female street-based sex workers in the greater Sydney area, Australia. *BMC Psychiatry* 6: 24.

Rusch MLA, Brouwer KC, Lozada R, Strathdee SA, Magis-Rodriguez C, Patterson TL. (2010) Distribution of sexually transmitted diseases and risk factors by work locations among female sex workers in Tijuana, Mexico. *Sexually Transmitted Diseases* 37: 608–14.

Salmon AM, Thein HH, Kimber J, Kaldor JM, Maher L. (2007) Five years on: what are the community perceptions of drug-related public amenity following the establishment of the Sydney Medically Supervised Injecting Centre? *International Journal of Drug Policy* 18: 46–53.

Sanders T and Campbell R (2007) Designing out vulnerability, building in respect: violence, safety and sex work policy. *British Journal of Sociology* 58: 1–19.

Semple SJ, Grant I and Patterson TL (2004) Female methamphetamine users: social characteristics and sexual risk behavior. *Women and Health* 40: 35–50.

Shannon K and Csete J (2010) Violence, condom negotiation, and HIV/STI risk among sex workers. *JAMA-Journal of the American Medical Association* 304: 573–4.

Shannon K, Kerr T, Allinott S, Chettiar J, Shoveller J, Tyndall MW. (2008a) Social and structural violence and power relations in mitigating HIV risk of drug-using women in survival sex work. *Social Science and Medicine* 66: 911–21.

Shannon K, Kerr T, Strathdee SA, Shoveller J, Montaner JS, Tyndall MW. (2009) Prevalence and structural correlates of gender based violence among a prospective cohort of female sex workers. *British Medical Journal* 339: b2939.

Shannon K, Rusch M, Shoveller J, Alexson D, Gibson K, Tyndall MW. (2008b) Mapping violence and policing as an environmental-structural barrier to health service and syringe availability among substance-using women in street-level sex work. *International Journal of Drug Policy* 19: 140–7.

Shannon K, Strathdee SA, Goldenberg SM, Duff P, Mwangi P, Rusakova M, Reza-Paul S, Lau J, Deering K, Pickles MR, Boily MC. (2015) Global epidemiology of HIV among female sex workers: influence of structural determinants. *Lancet* 385: 55–71.

Shannon K, Strathdee S, Shoveller J, Zhang R, Montaner J, Tyndall M. (2011) Crystal methamphetamine use among female street-based sex workers: moving beyond individual-focused interventions. *Drug and Alcohol Dependence* 113: 76–81.

Small W, Kerr T, Charette J, Schechter MT, Spittal PM. (2006) Impacts of intensified police activity on injection drug users: evidence from an ethnographic investigation. *International Journal of Drug Policy* 17: 85–95.

Sterk C (1999) *Fast Lives: Women Who Use Crack Cocaine*. Philadelphia: Temple University Press.

Stoltz JA, Wood E, Small W, Li K, Tyndall M, Montaner J, Kerr T. (2007) Changes in injecting practices associated with the use of a medically supervised safer injection facility. *Journal of Public Health* 29: 35–9.

Strathdee SA, Lozada R, Pollini RA, Brottwer KC, Mantsios A, Abramovitz DA, Rhodes T, Latkin CA, Loza O, Alvelais J, Magis-Rodriguez C, Patterson TL, Proyecto El Cuete. (2008a) Individual, social, and environmental influences associated with HIV infection among injection drug users in Tijuana, Mexico. *JAIDS-Journal of Acquired Immune Deficiency Syndromes* 47: 369–76.

Strathdee SA, Philbin MM, Semple SJ, Pu M, Orozovich P, Martinez G, Lozada R, Fraga M, de la Torre A, Staines H, Magis-Rodriguez C, Patterson TL. (2008b) Correlates of injection drug use among female sex workers in two Mexico-US border cities. *Drug and Alcohol Dependence* 92: 132–40.

Sydney Morning Herald (2001) Kerb crawlers curbed. Sydney: *Sydney Morning Herald.*

Thein HH, Kimber J, Maher L, MacDonald M, Kaldor JM. (2005) Public opinion towards supervised injecting centres and the Sydney Medically Supervised Injecting Centre. *International Journal of Drug Policy* 16: 275–80.

Topp L, Hudson SL and Maher L (2010) Mental health symptoms among street-based psychostimulant injectors in Sydney's Kings Cross. *Substance Use and Misuse* 45: 1180–200.

Van Beek I, Dwyer R and Malcolm A (2001) Cocaine injecting: the sharp end of drug-related harm! *Drug and Alcohol Review* 20: 333–42.

Vangelder PJ and Kaplan CD (1992) The finishing moment - temporal and spatial features of sexual interactions between streetwalkers and car clients. *Human Organization* 51: 253–63.

Ward H, Day S, Mezzone J, Dunlop L, Donegan C, Farrar S, Whitaker L, Harris JRW, Miller DL. (1993) Prostitution and risk of HIV – female prostitutes in London. *British Medical Journal* 307: 356–8.

West J (2000) Prostitution: collectives and the politics of regulation. *Gender, Work and Organization* 7: 106–18.

Wojcicki JM and Malala J (2001) Condom use, power and HIV/AIDS risk: sex-workers bargain for survival in Hillbrow/Joubert Park/ Berea, Johannesburg. *Social Science and Medicine* 53: 99–121.

Wood E, Kerr T, Small W, Li K, Marsh DC, Montaner JSG, Tyndall MW. (2004) Changes in public order after the opening of a medically supervised safer injecting facility for illicit injection drug users. *Canadian Medical Association Journal* 171: 731–4.

Wood E, Kerr T, Small W, Jones J, Schechter MT, Tyndall MW. (2003) The impact of a police presence on access to needle exchange programs. *JAIDS-Journal of Acquired Immune Deficiency Syndromes* 34: 116–18.

Wood E, Schachar J, Li K, Stoltz JA, Shannon K, Miller C, Lloyd-Smith E, Tyndall MW, Kerr T. (2007) Sex trade involvement is associated with elevated HIV incidence among injection drug users in Vancouver. *Addiction Research and Theory* 15: 321–5.

Wood E, Tyndall MW, Lai C, Montaner JSG, Kerr T. (2006a) *Substance Abuse Treatment Prevention and Policy* 1: 13. Updated citation 1: 13 is correct

Wood E, Tyndall MW, Zhang R, Stoltz J, Lai C, Montaner JSG, Kerr T. (2006b) Attendance at supervised injecting facilities and use of detoxification services. *New England Journal of Medicine* 354: 2512–14.

Woodward C, Fischer J, Najam J, Dunne M. (2004) *Selling Sex in Queensland.* Milton: Prostitution Licensing Authority.

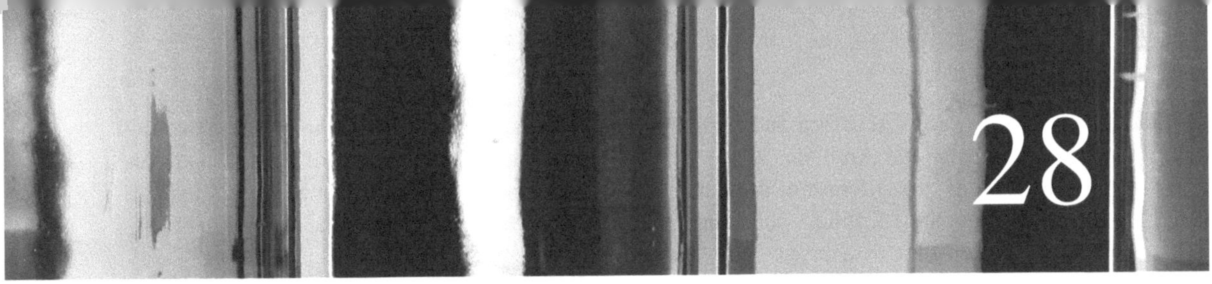

28

Homelessness and Substance Use

Betsy Thom and Carmen Aceijas

INTRODUCTION

There is an extensive literature on problem substance use and related harms and there is a growing research literature on homelessness. However, there is little research that brings these two together. Where homelessness and substance use is addressed, studies are largely country specific, often examining the issues as they affect sub-groups (e.g. Beck et al., 2009; Cottrell-Boyce, 2010; McNaughton, 2008; Neale and Stevenson, 2014; Philippot et al., 2007) and the literature is biased towards developed 'Western' countries where the problems, the responses and the national contexts are very different. The available research does, however, point to enormous variation across countries regarding the experience of homelessness and substance use and regarding approaches to prevention and intervention. There is, too, wide variation in the availability of information and statistics on homelessness and substance use. Even in countries where there are sufficient resources to collect information, it is not possible to give precise figures on numbers of homeless people and we do not know for sure what the causal links are between problem substance use and homelessness. Certainly, all homeless people do not misuse substances and all substance users are not homeless. In part, the uncertainty stems from the difficulty of defining both 'homelessness' and 'problem substance use' and from the variability found in official statistics, research studies and practice responses to these problems. While some research has identified individual characteristics and marginalisation processes as factors associated with homelessness and substance use, other work has emphasised structural factors such as poverty. More recent theories emphasise the complex interaction between structural, institutional, interpersonal and individual factors and highlight the need to consider the mechanisms that generate homelessness and substance use within different systems and contexts (see discussion and references in Benjaminsen and Andrade, 2015). What is clear from the literature is that both homelessness and problem substance use are very often part of a bigger package of social, health and mental health problems that can push individuals and families to the margins of society and keep them there. The individuals and groups affected are highly diverse and ever changing. Responses at policy and practice level reflect not only the level of need in a particular country or region but also specific political and social contexts at any particular time and the moral frameworks that portray homeless people and substance users as worthy or unworthy citizens.

The chapter begins with an examination of the concept of homelessness that highlights substantial differences across the globe in the understanding and measurement of the problem. The following section discusses how, even within a country, it is difficult to assess the number of homeless people at any one time and even more difficult to know how many of these are problem substance users. The chapter then provides a broad overview and illustrative examples of the characteristics and lifestyles of homeless substance users. We then consider individual and structural explanations for homelessness and, finally, comment briefly on responses to homeless substance users.

Throughout the chapter, we aim to illustrate how the category of homeless substance user is socially constructed and located within specific political, social and moral frameworks that impact on the extent and nature of the problem, on official and unofficial responses to the problem and on the lived experiences of those affected by homelessness and problem substance use. We talk about the problems as they manifest in 'Western' or 'developed' countries as compared to 'developing' countries. In doing so, we are aware that grouping countries in this way is a very rough and ready approach to organising information and discussion. Herrick (Chapter 32, this volume) is rightly critical of such broad categorisations, arguing that they can obscure rather than illuminate the situation in different geographical locations with very different social and political systems and different histories and cultures of substance use. With that reservation in mind, the aim was to draw attention to the importance of context as well as individual behaviour in understanding and responding to the issue of homelessness and substance use.

CONCEPTS AND THEIR MEASUREMENT

There are numerous definitions of the concept of 'homelessness'. Together these definitions describe a continuum of homelessness from sleeping rough to living in inadequate or insecure housing and highlight a number of domains of homelessness – physical, legal and social; the issue of social exclusion is often closely interwoven into definitions (Busch-Geertsema, 2010; Edgar, 2012). The European Federation of National Associations Working with the Homeless (FEANTSA, 2013) definition of homelessness reads as 'a person experiences homelessness when he or she does not have somewhere to live in security, peace and dignity'. This definition allows for a broader understanding of the concept to include:

- having no shelter at all necessitating sleeping in the streets or open air (sometimes called rooflessness or primary homelessness);
- having a roof but in temporary conditions where the homeless person moves between private dwellings, hostels or other institutions (sometimes called secondary homelessness); and
- living in sub-standard or insecure housing accommodation such as a caravan on an illegal site, in a tent, in extremely overcrowded conditions or poor and insecure housing, having no legal rights to the accommodation (sometimes called tertiary homelessness).

The importance of taking account of the cultural and social context on our understanding and definition of homelessness is well illustrated by considering what 'homelessness' means in low or middle income countries. Research by Tipple and Speak (2005), based on an examination of homelessness in nine developing countries, found wide variability in official definitions (used in land and housing policies and in censuses) as well as in working definitions used by non-governmental organisations (NGOs) to focus and prioritise their activities. Examples from their research illustrate the variability in understanding and application of the concept. In Zimbabwe, they found that the government definition covered everyone '*without a house to his name*'. In India, pavement dwellers, Hindu Sadhus (wandering ascetics), Bamjardas (gypsies) and Loharas (a nomadic tribe) were not included among the homeless. In Ghana, children living in poor accommodation were not considered homeless, whereas they were included in the broader definition applied by an NGO working in the Ashanti region. In South Africa, NGOs consider shack-dwellers and squatters to be homeless – living conditions that would not be seen as homelessness in some other countries. Tipple and Speak (2005) argue that in developing countries, it is important to differentiate inadequate housing (without land tenure or services) and homelessness. They point out that living in crowded accommodation does not necessarily equate with homelessness (in the sense of sub-standard or inadequate accommodation). They give the example of Kumasi, Ghana, where 73 per cent of all households live in a single room but where no one thinks of such crowding as homelessness.

There have been attempts to promote definitional standardisation. The European Typology on Homelessness and Housing Exclusion (ETHOS) is widely accepted in European countries and referred to in other countries as a useful conceptual framework (Busch-Geertsema, 2010). This four-part classification, which includes rooflessness, houselessness, living in insecure housing and living in inadequate accommodation, was intended to provide a definition applicable to all EU countries (Edgar, 2012). At the same time, the appropriateness of having an elaborated standard definition and what elements it should contain is contested (Amore, 2011, 2013; Edgar, 2012).

Clearly, then, across the world, perspectives differ considerably as to who is included within the homelessness category. The same is true when we look at how people using alcohol and drugs have been categorised for official or research purposes. In some cases, use itself is defined as a problem, whereas in other cases, use is problematic only when it becomes defined as 'misuse' or 'abuse' or 'addiction'. The definition applied in any particular context is influenced by many factors – religion, the age of the user, the amount consumed and the nature of consumption and the behaviour associated with consumption, being only a few examples. Indeed, as is argued in other chapters (e.g. see Chapter 21, this volume), the understanding of addiction and problem substance use can be seen as historically, socially and culturally determined (Fraser et al., 2014; Room et al., 2015).

THE EXTENT OF THE PROBLEM

Definitional differences mean that it is difficult to measure how many people are homeless and how many people have a problem of substance use. It is even more difficult to put the two together and estimate how many homeless people also experience problems of alcohol or drug use. Added to that, homelessness is not a stable condition; people pass in and out of a homeless state and homelessness can endure for any length of time. Definitional variability in official statistics and in research studies make it difficult to know how many people are homeless at any one time, to trace trends in homelessness across time or to compare within and across countries. At the same time, it is important to have measures that allow policy makers to monitor their efforts to reduce homelessness – to know, for instance, the number of people who have become homeless, ceased to be homeless, have experienced homelessness over a given period of time and the type of homelessness experienced. Again, the same can be said about an individual's alcohol and drug use – it is equally fluid, changes over time and is influenced by many factors.

Political, social and practical issues play into the definitions and measurement of both homelessness and substance use/misuse/addiction and have implications for how the issues are defined and measured for policy purposes. The uncertainties created by stakeholders' competing interests are commented on by Busch-Geertsema:

> The quantitative extent of homelessness is often controversial and hotly debated at local, regional and national levels. There is a tendency for those responsible for policies and the funding of services to underestimate the extent in order to minimise public responsibilities and to keep the problem they are expected to deal with manageable. On the other hand, pressure groups tend to overestimate the number of homeless people in order to increase their political relevance and the resources made available to them. (Busch-Geertsema, 2010: 28)

Similar observations could be made about substance use and problem use. For instance, what is defined as problem use, addiction or dependence has implications for the provision of prevention, early intervention and treatment responses; it also determines the number of people who may be categorised as in need of intervention or treatment.

Our knowledge about homelessness and substance use derives from two main bodies of information, studies of people who are homeless and studies of people who experience problems related to their drug and alcohol use. For practical reasons, in many developed countries estimates are often based on people attending treatment services for substance use, using hostels for the homeless or sleeping rough on the streets. For instance, based on a single night count, it was estimated that there were 2,414 rough sleepers in England in 2013; London had 543 rough sleepers. Over a longer time span, 2012 to 2013, outreach workers counted 6,437 rough sleepers across the country (Wilson, 2014). In Australia, in 2011 to 2012, 229,247 people received support from specialist homelessness services with an average of 19,128 people accommodated each night (Homelessness Australia, 2013). A report from the Canadian Homelessness Research Network found that at least 30,000 people were homeless on any given night and at least 50,000 people were part of the 'hidden homeless' – staying with friends or relatives on a temporary basis (Gaetz et al., 2013). The Irish Department of Environment estimated that 5,581 individuals were homeless during one week in March 2002; of those, 4,060 were in Dublin. Rough sleepers accounted for 312 individuals, while the remainder reported staying in emergency or insecure accommodation (Lawless and Carr, 2005). In Denmark, based on numbers in touch with a range of services, 1.0 per 1,000 (5,447) inhabitants were homeless in 2007. Slightly higher figures were recorded in Norway (1.2 in 1,000) and Sweden (1.3 in 1,000) (Benjaminsen and Dyb, 2008). Although approximations, these figures amply demonstrate that even in rich countries there are considerable numbers of people who are homeless at any one time and a far larger number who experience homelessness in their lifetime.

As Doherty and Stuttaford (2007) note in their review of homelessness and drug use in Europe, all homeless people do not suffer from drink or drug problems. However, the links are strong; sources cited by the authors indicated that around 18 million people in Europe (approximately 1 in 20) experienced homelessness in 2000, and 1.5 million (approximately 1 in 300) were problem drug users. Local and national estimates suggested that in most European countries up to and sometimes over 30 per cent of homeless people have associated drug addiction problems. A research briefing published by Crisis, a UK charity for single homeless people, indicated that:

> It is a stark fact that drugs and alcohol are major causes of death amongst homeless people. The links between drug and alcohol abuse and homelessness are well established. (Crisis, 2011: 2)

The point was illustrated by showing that 21.7 per cent of deaths among the homeless were due to drug use compared to 0.3 per cent among the general population and 14.4 per cent were due to alcohol compared to 1.3 per cent among the general population. Evidence, from a review by Lawless and Carr (2005), indicates the extent to which there is an association between homelessness and substance use in UK and Irish populations. They cite studies that found high levels of substance use among different groups of people, including: homeless young people (76 per cent to 88 per cent using drugs/alcohol in different studies) and rough sleepers (up to 83 per cent using drugs/alcohol in different studies), as well as increasing incidence of homelessness among the clients of drug treatment services.

Across studies, it is agreed that the prevalence of drug abuse and alcoholism is significantly higher among homeless people than among the general population. Taking the USA as an example, the prevalence of alcoholism in the homeless population was calculated as 38 per cent compared to 15 per cent in the general population; and the prevalence of drug abuse was calculated as 26 per cent among the homeless compared to 8 per cent in the general population (National Coalition for the Homeless, 2009; Substance Abuse and Mental Health Services Administration, 2006). However, prevalence ranges for alcohol and drug abuse among homeless populations, while consistently higher than among general populations, have shown high levels of variability depending on the study methodology, the specific populations and the measurement tools. Johnson et al. (2005), for instance, found a prevalence interval as wide as 24 per cent to 71 per cent across different studies of homeless and runaway adolescents.

It is even more difficult to arrive at an estimation of problem substance use among homeless groups in developing countries or in countries where there are few sources of official statistics or information. However, a report from United Nations Centre for Human Settlements indicates considerable numbers of homeless people in India, Bangladesh, Korea, China South Africa and Nigeria. Drug and alcohol addiction is frequently mentioned as an associated issue but the general conclusion is that 'poverty is *the* common denominator of homelessness' (United Nations Centre for Human Settlements, 2000: 51).

The links between problem substance use and homelessness are particularly strong for some groups compared to others. Studies indicate that rough sleepers and street homeless populations are especially likely to experience alcohol and drug-related harm, often as part of a much more complex set of mental, physical and social problems (Doherty and Stuttaford, 2007; Lawless and Carr, 2005). However, figures based on these groups may be an underestimate of the extent of the problem as those who are literally 'roofless', in shelters for the homeless or in treatment services, are more visible and easier to count. Less visible groups, such as people in temporary squats or moving between temporary shelters, are less likely to be included in the statistics. The data has other limitations; for instance, studies use different methodologies so that results are not comparable or are incomplete, prevalence counts are undertaken more often in urban than rural areas and research tends to focus on dependent/problematic or chaotic substance use and misses occasional or recreational use – as a result missing populations at risk of developing associated alcohol or drug use problems (e.g. Patel et al., 2004, discuss young refugees and asylum seekers, often living in inadequate housing, as a group at risk of problem substance use). Surveys rely on self-report – and some people may prefer not to be seen as homeless or may be wary of reporting how much they drink. Discussing the methodology used in surveys in France, Beck et al. (2009: 163–4) suggest that, in surveys of homeless people, respondents may minimise the amount they drink 'so as not to give an overly unfavourable image of him/herself, an image close to the stereotype of the "alcoholic tramp"'. For women with children, it is especially important to retain the image of being a 'good mother' and to avoid the stigma that clings to the drinking woman.

For all those reasons, available estimates are at best patchy, and moreover, taken in isolation, they provide only limited snapshots of realities. For estimates of a given issue to be useful, we need to have a measure of the burden they represent in the context of the population in general or of those at risk; and to do this, we need to be able to assess the prevalence of the issue – in this case, homelessness and problem substance use. To illustrate it let us consider the estimation of homelessness in the case of England.

Estimating homelessness in England: an example

Recent estimates for England acknowledge 2,141 people slept rough on any one night during 2013. How important is this figure in numerical terms? To determine the burden of a problem in a given country we need to know how prevalent the issue is among the population at risk. Such determination involves that we are able to quantify: (i) the population at risk and the exposure time. That would be our denominator: (ii) The number of cases. In other words, we have an unequivocal definition of rough sleeper. That would be our numerator

Determining the denominator: Population at risk

Determining the size of population at risk presents the first challenge: is the whole population at risk? Are all individuals considered at risk at the same level of vulnerability? The following example illustrates what would happen if we do not consider different levels or risk.

The population in England in 2013 was estimated at 53.5 million. If we consider the whole population at risk of becoming homeless and that such a risk is constant throughout time and for different population groups, we can calculate the prevalence point (P) of homelessness as:

P = (cases/population at risk) × 100

Translated into the specific homelessness issue:

P = (2,141/53,500,000) × 100 = 0.004% of the population in England was sleeping rough on any one night during 2013.

In London, we have an estimate of 6,508 rough sleepers throughout 2013/14 and a population of 8,416,535 in 2013. Applying the same formula, we obtain:

P = (cases/population at risk) × 100

Translated into the specific homelessness issue:

P = (6,508/8,416,535) × 100 = 0.07% of the population in London were rough sleepers throughout 2013/14.

However, both calculations offered an image of a minor problem and might lead to very wrong conclusions because the differential risk suffered by specific groups and the impact of certain vital events that increase the likelihood of becoming homeless have not been taken into account in the denominator estimate. So, to overcome the risk of offering a biased figure, we need to reconsider and increase precision on the denominator: the real population at risk and exposure time. For instance, excluding privileged and upper middle class people from the population at risk would already significantly decrease the denominator and hence increase the final prevalence.

Determining the number of cases (numerator)

However, we still have the problem of producing an accurate estimate of homeless people (cases) to place in the numerator and this leads us again to the issue of the lack of a unified definition of what conditions must be in place to consider a person as homeless; the broader the definition, the higher the prevalence will be. Let us consider the example of London, with a population of over 8 million people and with a rough sleeper's population of 6,500 individuals which, when applications for homelessness assistance received by Local Authorities (112,070 in 2013) are factored in, we have a numerator (number of cases) much higher: 118,570. In this case, calculating the prevalence of rough sleepers plus homeless people would return a 1.4 per cent prevalence of rough sleepers in London:

> P = (cases/population at risk) × 100 = (118,570/8,416,535) × 100 = 1.4% of the population in London was sleeping rough or homeless last year.

As we can see, the more precise we are in both defining the cases [numerator] and the population at risk [denominator] the higher the figure is.

Additional issues, as already mentioned, are also important. We need to take into account different population groups that are more or less vulnerable to homelessness and the exposure time to social and/or physical risk factors for homelessness. Still, even all this would not allow for cross-country comparisons unless standardised measures are created to facilitate comparisons between countries with different structures in terms of age, gender and social measures relevant to the problem of homelessness.

HOMELESS SUBSTANCE USERS: CHARACTERISTICS AND LIFESTYLES

The costs of homelessness to the individual's physical health, mental health and social well-being – whether problem substance use is a factor or not – have been well documented for both developed and developing countries (for example, see the review of studies in Philippot et al., 2007: Chapter 7). Personal problems can include a wide array of issues such as loss of self-esteem, institutionalisation, increase of substance abuse and reduction of safe measures to consume drugs (such as compromised access to or availability of clean injecting equipment), loss of ability and will to care for oneself, increased exposure to abuse, violence and the risk of HIV infection, risk of sexually transmitted diseases, increased likelihood of entering the criminal justice system and development of behavioural problems, among others. All these can be summarised as amounting to poor physical and mental health, often leading to disempowerment, isolation and poverty. Box 28.1 illustrates the range of problems reported by a sample of 2,500 homeless people in the UK. The links between substance use and other problems are clearly demonstrated.

Box 28.1 Links between substance use and other problems

Problem	*Percentage*
Diagnosed mental health problem	45
Reported mental health issues: diagnosed and undiagnosed	80
Reported physical health problems	73
Reported long-term physical problems	41
Taking drugs or recovering from drug problem	39
Have alcohol problem or recovering from alcohol problem	27
Used drugs and/or alcohol to cope with mental health issues	50
Consume more than recommended amounts alcohol each time they drink	66

Source: Homeless Link (2014).

Homelessness often has devastating effects on individuals that are exacerbated and may become chronic if homelessness becomes a long-term situation. But who are these people and what are their lives like? Much of the research confirms that it is largely men who make up the homeless (i.e. roofless) population, but other groups have also been identified as particularly vulnerable to becoming homeless. From the work of Philippot et al. (2007) and O'Sullivan et al. (2010) we gain an overview of homeless populations in Western Europe. They distinguish:

- Women who have lost their house for family reasons (family breakdown)
- Families (often women and children)
- Socially 'disaffiliated' youth (foster home placement, parental divorce)
- Socially excluded men over 35 years of age (unemployed, without professional qualification, separated, migrants)
- Socially assisted men over 45 years of age (homeless for more than five years, with social welfare or charities as their only financial resources)
- People from ethnic minority and immigrant groups

A key aspect to keep in mind when discussing homelessness and substance use, is that there are major differences between groups and between individuals. This is illustrated by taking a look at three examples – the 'skid row' drinker, women and young people. Even within these groups, there is great variability and the sections below provide merely a glimpse into the issues.

The 'skid row' drinker

Mention homeless substance user and a typical image comes to mind – the ageing skid row drinker, the down-and-out alcoholic or drug addict sleeping in doorways or in the local park. This is the image that dominates the research literature coming from the USA and the UK in the 1950s to 1970s. The moral imputations that underpinned UK post-war policy towards this group are noted in a paper by Wood (1976). Ministry of Health policy to deal with vagrancy outlined different categories of men with different responses to their plight depending on whether they were in work, disabled, incapable of work and unsuitable for training, young men in need of 'mental or moral rehabilitation', or 'hard core' habitual vagrants. The latter were to be offered suitable treatment or 'when necessary dealt with by firmness to "discourage the spread of idle vagabondage"' (Wood, 1976: 390). As Wood found in her study of one London reception centre, drinking was a key issue for this group of men with some severely dependent on alcohol. Furthermore, Wood commented, any attempt to address their situation required an appreciation of their life and their world-view – something that was generally lacking in policy and service provision.

However, we do find a detailed account of the life of homeless alcoholics in a study by Peter Archard (1979). Archard used participant observation methods as one way of understanding life on the streets. His account offers a vivid picture of a sub-culture that includes alcoholics – estimated to be around 25 per cent to 45 per cent of those on skid row – but also includes teetotallers and moderate and heavy drinkers. Through contact with a skid row man, he was able to join a drinking school and participate over a six-month period in the daily activities:

> Drinking cider and cheap wine, making small donations to the school's finances, making 'the run' to the off-license, warning the alcoholics present of the approach of police patrolmen, and helping to remove the more inebriate members in cases of imminent arrest. (Archard, 1979: Appendix: 177)

Archard reveals a complex street life with its own norms, rules and boundaries that define relationships between the men and with the outside world, contains a hierarchy of different types of street drinkers and illustrates strategies of survival to counter chronic poverty. The drinking school becomes a primary group that enables men to act meaningfully within their culture. Classic studies from the USA also illustrate the significance of the *bottle gang* for homeless men as a means of developing and sustaining social links (e.g. Rubington, 1968).

'Invisible' women

Discussing women and homelessness in Europe, Baptista (2010) noted that, despite country differences, four consistent findings were commonly reported: typically, homelessness among women was hidden – especially when homelessness was equated with rough sleeping; all the same, up to a fifth of street homeless were women and around a third of all homeless people were women; women were increasingly presenting at services for the homeless; at the time of writing, there was a noticeable increase in homelessness among younger women and among women from ethnic minority and immigrant backgrounds. Baptista suggested that women may be less visible than men because they try to avoid the risks of sleeping on the streets or in unsuitable shelters or because they are part of a homeless family and under the support of welfare systems. Women with children are often involved with a range of different services (in countries where services are available) and may, therefore, be missed in counts of the homeless and of substance users. Those who are living on the streets develop a range of protective strategies. Sex work, often accompanied by drug use – in both developed and developing countries – can be a survival strategy and a reason for invisibility as women may find temporary shelter with men. (Issues of sex work and substance use are examined in Chapter 27, this volume.)

It may also be that women are more afraid of the stigma that attaches to homelessness – something that has also been recognised as a reason for gender differences in hiding alcohol and drug problems. Indeed, as mentioned already, Beck et al. (2009) draw attention to a universal problem for many marginalised women, including those with problems of substance use. Having a home and being seen to be a 'good mother' – that is, one who does not have a problem of alcohol or drug use – is a prerequisite for retaining custody of children and a probable reason to under-report substance use and related problems. Women who become homeless in Western countries are likely to be poor and single – a finding that is echoed elsewhere. For instance, female-headed households, particularly single mothers living in poverty, were identified as being one of the groups most vulnerable to homelessness in Nicaragua, Argentina, Costa Rica and Australia (Tipple and Speak, 2009). As Tipple and Speak (2009) point out, the visibility and experience of homelessness is influenced greatly by the cultural context. They note the dangers of abuse, kidnapping and trafficking in some countries. In Islamic countries, living on the streets is not an option for women who therefore become reliant on relatives for accommodation. Moreover, as Speak (2005) comments, women in developing countries have the added disadvantage that, even if housing is available, for some the social, cultural and economic context prevents them from accessing it.

It is important, therefore, to recognise the heterogeneity of homelessness among women and, at the same time, to keep in mind 'shared gender experiences' (Neale, 1997), which may be a factor in explaining invisibility.

Children and young people

Europe has its share of young people – generally in their teens – who live on the streets, in short term hostels or squats or in other unstable accommodation. Philippot et al. (2007) found that homelessness among young people in Europe seemed to be most prevalent in the UK. Indeed, in one report from the UK Home Office, youth homelessness and substance use was considered to be a major social problem as levels of substance use in this group (young people age 16 to 24) were much higher than in young people who were 'housed'. Interviews with 160 young people in five major cities showed that 95 per cent had used drugs and that many had become homeless at an early age (Wincup et al., 2003). Indeed, studies have identified an inverse relationship between age at first time homelessness and length of homelessness, the younger the first time, the higher the chances of becoming a long term homeless person (Social Exclusion Unit, 2001).

In developing countries, attention has focussed on street children and it is here we find the richest material on the role of substances and their significance for the lifestyles of young users. To take one example, Cottrell-Boyce (2010) describes the political and economic background to the rise in the number of street children in Kenyan cities and discusses the use of solvents by street children in one of the towns, Ruiru. Observation indicated that around 70 to 100 children were homeless and nearly all were sniffing solvents. The street children adopt a 'base' and join a 'street-family'. This provides friendship, practical support and a measure of safety from the violence of the streets; but it also entails new arrivals accepting glue sniffing 'as a non-negotiable condition of membership of a "base"'. Solvent use is central to the collective identity and the glue bottle is an emblem of belonging and solidarity (Cottrell-Boyce, 2010: 96–7). As with skid row drinkers, studies have shown how subcultures can form around substance use and drug dealing among homeless individuals, especially if we use the wider definition of 'homeless' to include those in inadequate or unstable housing.

However, research on street children illustrates only one aspect of the complexity and diversity of homelessness in developing countries. Tipple and Speak (2009) note that the majority of the homeless population in both industrialised and developing countries fall within the adult age range, between 18 and 59 years old and they highlight the plight of older people as both a cause and effect of inter-generational poverty and homelessness, especially in Africa. (For a detailed discussion of children and homelessness in developing countries see Tipple and Speak, 2009: Chapter 12.)

Examples of the characteristics and lifestyles of homeless substance users given earlier in the chapter, and the literature on homelessness and substance use as a whole, tend to highlight the ways in which vulnerable groups are 'different' from other people: they have complex problems, they require support and services and their problems are perhaps a result of their own behaviour. A distinct barrier is drawn between the affected group and the rest of the population. The reality is rather different. Commenting on the results of a large French survey, Join-Lambert notes that:

> The homeless do not inhabit a world apart from the rest of society. Nearly a third have a job...most are manual workers or unqualified employees. A near majority say that they have family and friends, and nearly three quarters say that they are quite frequently in contact with them... They have contact with social institutions (70% had at least one contact in the previous twelve months), and more frequently with doctors and social workers. (Join-Lambert, 2009: 7)

The homeless, as this study indicated, have much in common with the poorest sectors in society. However, when homelessness is linked with problem substance use and other mental and physical problems, there is a greater risk of stigmatisation and marginalisation that becomes a vicious circle of exclusion. It is this group that features more visibly in research and in publications.

EXPLANATIONS FOR HOMELESSNESS AND PROBLEM SUBSTANCE USE

There is no straightforward answer to the question of why people become homeless, why some people have problems of alcohol or drug misuse or why some homeless people experience problem substance use and others do not. Issues of cause and effect are complex and debated. On the one hand, we find explanations and theories that focus on individual vulnerabilities and characteristics as 'risk factors'. For instance, research consistently finds a majority of males both among homeless people and among people with problem substance use. On the other hand, it is recognised that social, economic and political conditions – structural factors – are also associated with homelessness and problem substance use. Changing labour markets, the nature of the welfare system and the housing system, poverty and living in a deprived or disrupted community are frequently reported as risk factors and causes. Explanations often emphasise 'structure' and 'agency' indicating the interaction between actors and the wider social structures (Neale, 1997). Furthermore, it has been argued that adapting to environmental conditions (as in the case of the street children described above) can explain the behaviour of homeless people, including their substance use (Johnson and Chamberlain, 2008).

A summary of risk factors and triggers for adolescent substance use (Box 28.2) provides an example of this approach to understanding the causes of homelessness. Here, the factors are predominantly individual characteristics – and drug and alcohol misuse is listed as one of the risk factors. These factors emerge also from other European studies [see a review of the literature by Philippot et al. (2007)].

The literature on risk factors for illicit drug use and problem alcohol use is vast. Much of the emphasis is on identifying risk and protective factors among young people. For example, McKeganey et al. (2006) examined use of, and exposure to, illegal drugs among children aged 10 to 12 in the UK. They found that factors associated with use and exposure were gender (boys more than girls), age (more common among 12 year olds), deprivation, use of licit drugs, having a family member who used drugs, having run away from home on more than two occasions, living in a step family, having parents who exercised a low level of supervision, having friends who initiated illegal drug use, having older friends and being involved in a range of problem behaviours. Generally, analyses of risk factors are categorised into sets of factors; the European Monitoring Centre for Drugs and

Box 28.2 Summary of main risk factors and triggers of homelessness in England

Risk factors	*Triggers*
• Sexual or physical abuse in childhood or adolescence • Family disputes and breakdown • A background of local authority care • Offending behaviour and/or experience of prison • Previous service in the armed forces • Lack of a social support network • Debts, especially rent or mortgage arrears • Causing nuisance to neighbours • Drug or alcohol misuse • School exclusion and lack of qualifications • Mental health problems • Poor physical health	• Leaving the parental home after arguments • Marital or relationship breakdown • Widowhood • Discharge from the armed forces • Leaving care • Leaving prison • A sharp deterioration in mental health or an increase in alcohol or drug misuse • A financial crisis of mounting debts • Eviction from a rented or owned home

Source: adapted from Fitzpatrick et al. (2001: 34).

Drug Addiction (EMCDDA), for instance, includes a range of individual and structural factors divided into individual/peers, family, community and school. Box 28.3 shows the factors for each category extracted from a range of research.

Although these are only small examples of the 'risk factor' approach in research on homelessness and on drug use, we can see that there are similarities in the types of characteristics found to increase an individual's risk of becoming homeless or of using alcohol and drugs harmfully. However, it is also important to consider the wider societal factors that may contribute to both problems. Benjaminsen and Andrade (2015), for example, have shown how homelessness is closely linked to welfare policies. In countries such as Denmark, generally considered to be a social-democratic welfare state, the biggest group of homeless people were those with complex health and social needs. In the USA, a liberal welfare state, people who were too poor to afford housing but otherwise had low support needs comprised a substantial proportion of the homeless. The authors concluded that the type of welfare system affected both the scale and nature of homelessness in the two countries: 'the overall macroeconomic and social structures have a deep impact on the level of social marginalisation and exclusion, with severe implications for the people it affects' (Benjaminsen and Andrade, 2015: 16).

The interplay between macro and micro-level factors also emerged in a study of homeless people in the UK experiencing problems of substance use (McNaughton, 2008). The study found that these outcomes should be

Box 28.3 Risk factors for adolescent substance use

Individual/peer

- Association with friends/peers who model problem behaviour, for example, use drugs
- Attitudes favourable to substance use, knowledge about drugs
- Involvement in delinquency (e.g. shoplifting and gang fighting)
- Early and persistent problem behaviours, for example, early age at first drug use
- General sense of hopelessness about life
- Genetic predisposition: behavioural under-control
- Low expectations of success
- Low self-esteem
- Personality: lack of social bonding, alienation, rebelliousness, resistance to authority
- Physiological factors, for example, sensation-seeking, curiosity, boredom, poor impulse control
- Poor social adjustment
- Poor coping skills

Family

- Chaotic home environments
- Family conflict
- Low bonding, lack of mutual attachment and nurturing, and poor family relationships
- Parents and/or other family members use substances or have an attitude that favours substance use
- Poor and inconsistent parenting skills, for example, ineffective parenting and negative communication patterns
- Unrealistically high expectations

Community

- Availability of substances
- Exposure to violence
- Extreme economic deprivation
- Lack of legislation and law enforcement
- Lenient laws and norms about drug and alcohol use
- Neighbourhood disorganisation, including war and refugee camps
- Perceptions of approval of substance-using behaviours in community environments

School

- Academic failure, poor school achievement
- Low degree of commitment to school
- Peer rejection in elementary grades
- Poor academic adjustment and commitment
- Unrealistically high expectations

Source: adapted from EMCDDA. Available from: http://www.emcdda.europa.eu/attachements.cfm/att_93778_EN_Analysis%20Of%20Risk%20And%20Protective%20Factors.pdf (Accessed 7 September 2014).

understood as part of a process of social and material marginality. The interaction between individual characteristics, risk factors and the conditions of modern society – accelerated trends towards individualisation and increased forms of insecurity over the life course – may explain the continuing existence of apparently individual problems such as addiction or homelessness. All but two of McNaughton's sample of 13 women and 15 men gave substance use as a key factor in their homelessness. Their explanations included describing substance use as a strategy to cope with traumatic events such as violence, with mental health issues and with their dwindling material resources that resulted in homelessness. Once caught in the cycle, substance use became a key factor in perpetuating the cycle.

A review of European studies of homelessness supports the trigger effect of problem alcohol and drug use. Philippot et al. (2007) conclude that:

> One of the most striking features of this research is the high prevalence of substance abuse and dependence, especially of alcohol...Every study reports that an overwhelming majority of homeless people suffering from substance abuse or dependency was already facing this problem *before* the onset of homelessness. (Philippot et al., 2007: 492)

While poly-drug use is common among some homeless populations, differences have been found among groups regarding which substance came first. For instance, the National Advisory Committee on Drugs in Ireland (Lawless and Carr, 2005) reported than the majority (87 per cent) of homeless started using drugs before losing their accommodation. The first drug of choice was alcohol (70 per cent), cannabis was the most reported lifetime drug (69 per cent) and the majority of individuals included in that study reported poly-drug use (72 per cent). Generational differences are also possible, as older homeless people tend to report alcohol misuse and younger people report illicit drug use.

However, as we have already said, all homeless people do not have problems of substance use and explanations for homelessness given to researchers and service professionals may reflect the individual's specific circumstances at the time of the survey or research and the specific context in which the account is given. Beck et al. (2009), drawing on a national survey of homelessness in France, emphasise that 'alcohol is not always omnipresent in the lives of homeless people and that excessive consumption most often corresponds to states of great insecurity'. They continue:

> For individuals consuming excessive amounts of alcohol, it would be important to analyse how temporary this consumption is and its context in order to discover in which emergency situations and unfavourable conditions alcohol is systematically consumed, and to what extent consumption reduces as the environment improves. (In Join-Lambert, 2009: 12)

There is, however, a clear *association* between homelessness and problem substance use and a self-perpetuating cycle of related difficulties that push people to the margins of society and keep them there. The issue of which comes first – homelessness or problem substance use – may seem important in trying to understand these problems and in developing policy and practice responses. But the reality is that responses are needed to tackle the dynamics of the whole cycle of marginality.

RESPONSES TO HOMELESS SUBSTANCE USERS

There are numerous different programmes aiming to address the problem, ranging from soup kitchens through to crisis intervention centres, day centres and hostels, residential programmes, various forms of welfare provision and temporary health care clinics aiming to reach vulnerable, unstable populations, harm reduction services such as needle exchange and prevention interventions to reduce the risk of associated infections and diseases such as hepatitis. But, even in the developed countries, where services are more likely to be available, homeless drug and alcohol users face specific challenges that may include:

- Practicalities of being unable to provide a contact address while on waiting lists, in treatment or for treatment follow-up
- Losing contact with services (and continuity of treatment – such as substitution treatment) when they move from one geographical area to another
- Use of exclusion policies that prevent problem drug and alcohol users from gaining entry to some services – for example, homeless services and hostels or housing schemes
- Lack of knowledge among homeless people regarding what support is available
- Being unable to find a place in overcrowded night shelters and hostels
- Feeling unsafe in some forms of hostel or other accommodation (and unwilling to use these services) due to experiences of violence, bullying, substance use and general chaos and poor hygiene
- Returning post drug and alcohol treatment to crisis accommodation or other accommodation with a high risk of exposure to substance use
- Returning post treatment to the circumstances and problems that precipitated their homelessness and substance use
- Finding appropriate accommodation to match high support needs (Beck et al., 2009; Briggs et al., 2009; Brunette et al., 2004; Lawless and Carr, 2005)

Philippot et al. (2007) noted that the main focus of most services targeted at the homeless was primary assistance in emergency situations and that there was insufficient networking and coordination among the different services. Often, homeless people travel from one service to another on a daily basis as well as for the duration of their homelessness:

> For instance, they are forced to leave the night shelter in the morning, they then go to a soup kitchen in another part of town, and then may spend part of the afternoon in a day center that closes in the early evening hours, and have to wait for the opening of the night shelter, hoping they can get in. (Philippot et al., 2007: 495)

Accessing services for their substance use is an added burden and, as mentioned above, while hostels can provide a safe environment (in comparison to sleeping outdoors) they also constitute a 'risk environment'. Briggs et al. (2009) report how respondents in their study described hostels as places where they experienced 'relentless pressure' to use drugs, bullying and intimidation to share drugs, money and paraphernalia, and where they were drawn into new drug-injecting relationships and networks. Moreover, within shelters and hostels, the dominant ideology of 'self-reliance' may require clients to sign a contract, receive counselling, participate in educational groups or in other coercive activities and limit their stay – thus conveying the message that clients should not take advantage of the system (United Nations Centre for Human Settlements, 2000). Some researchers have concluded that residential withdrawal programmes are often the only viable option for the majority of homeless problem substance users, as lack of a home and personal support networks along with the complexity of their needs makes home and community-based programmes unfeasible (Brunette et al., 2004; Lawless and Carr, 2005). Of course, for many homeless substance users throughout the world residential treatment is not an option.

At the strategic level, different intervention models have been identified in the literature (Anderson, 2010; Benjaminsen and Dyb, 2010).

- *The staircase model* (also called the 'staircase of transition') requires the individual to demonstrate the ability to live independently by progressing through a series of steps on a housing ladder, where relevant, with advancement attached to success in substance use treatment. Service providers gradually reduce support and control. This model often requires abstinence as a condition of housing.
- *The tiered model* has two phases with a period in transitional housing between, for instance, a stay in a hostel and independent housing.
- *The normalisation model* is a variant of the housing first approach (see below). Normalisation refers to the individual's housing situation and

there is an emphasis on early stabilisation of the housing situation, preferably in ordinary housing with appropriate services as needed. This approach is supported by research evidence, although most of the evidence is from the USA.

- *The housing first model,* emerging in New York, places homeless people with addictions and other complex needs directly into permanent housing. An analysis of European policy responses found that national strategies to address homelessness have emerged mainly in the advanced welfare regimes of northern and western Europe and in just a few countries in southern and eastern Europe. A clear pattern in almost all of those countries is the spread of the housing first paradigm. This approach emphasises consumer choice and separates housing from any prior requirement for treatment or lifestyle change. Interventions focus on harm reduction. The desired outcome is reducing the use of temporary accommodation, reducing stays in shelters, providing long-term or permanent accommodation and providing individualised services and support. The Danish strategy, for example, explicitly acknowledges a 'housing first' approach (Box 28.4). The statement also highlights the importance of adopting an integrated approach and taking account of economic factors.

Anderson (2010: 52) considers the housing first model as illustrative of a wider policy trend towards 'a "new way of governing" that entails a shift from traditional forms of government to governance structures involving a broad range of stakeholders able to respond to the multiple needs of homeless people'. The Danish strategy, for instance, provides one example of how responsibility is devolved to the municipalities.

However, as Doherty and Stuttaford (2007) warn, we cannot assume that an effective model in one place can be transferred to another place where the social and cultural histories and available resources may be very different. In particular, these models are unlikely to apply in transition or developing countries with very different approaches to housing availability and tenure, and different systems of health care and social welfare provision. In some instances, for example, reform of land and property rights may be the most effective method of preventing homelessness. Strategies based on human rights and empowerment need to be put in place. For street children, a range of interventions going beyond housing and aiming at social integration need to be provided and tailored to their specific circumstances [see United Nations Centre for Human Settlements (2000) for some examples of strategies to combat homelessness across the globe and Tipple and Speak (2009) for discussion of the issues in developing countries, including responses and strategies].

Box 28.4 Homelessness strategy: Denmark

The Homelessness Strategy takes its starting point in a 'housing first' approach. Experience from other countries indicates that an early housing solution for homeless people can help to stabilise their life situations. This requires, however, that housing solutions for homeless people are combined with other forms of social support, depending on the individual problems and needs of the individuals concerned.

The assumption behind the housing first strategy is that by solving the housing issue for the individual, it is possible to achieve a stabilisation of the person's situation, both with regard to housing and other social problems. The goal of the housing first approach is, in other words, to quickly provide a permanent housing solution for the homeless person in combination with the necessary social support.

It should however be emphasised that:

- Housing first cannot stand alone as an initiative in the area, but must be supported by associated initiatives that will contribute to managing the problems of the individual citizen.
- Housing and support must be goal-directed and tailored to the specific needs of the individual.
- It is important that the solution also focuses on the citizen's economic situation.

The Government's Homelessness Strategy – A Strategy to Reduce Homelessness in Denmark 2009 to 2012. Indenrigs-og- Socialministeriet, Denmark.

CONCLUSION

This chapter has aimed to provide an understanding of the complexity of defining, measuring and responding to the needs of homeless people with problem substance use. It has emphasised the heterogeneity of the groups of people who become homeless and indicated the strong association between homelessness and problem substance use. We have tried to illustrate the ways in which structural and cultural contexts as well as individual risk factors have a bearing on experiences of homelessness and substance use and on policy and service responses to these issues. At the same time, we have noted that, despite the particularity of their circumstances, homeless people often have much in common with the poorest sectors in their societies. But, homelessness is often associated with a range of physical and mental health problems and with social care needs in addition to problem substance use, and for those most affected, there is often a cyclical decline into social marginalisation that is difficult to address. Responses to homelessness and problem substance use depend very much on issues discussed earlier – on perceptions of the problems – as having individual or structural roots, on how problems are measured, the adequacy of resources for gathering information, the known extent and nature of the population experiencing or at risk of developing the problems and on the dominant moral frameworks that define homeless substance users as worthy or unworthy. Clearly, across the globe, state responses to homelessness are enormously variable and dependent on political, economic and social contexts and on what is politically palatable at any particular time (see United Nations Centre for Human Settlements, 2000). However, the significant association between homelessness and substance use has implications for policy makers, relevant authorities and practitioners to consider how best to prevent and address the problems of affected population groups in their countries.

REFERENCES

Amore, K., Baker, M. and Howden-Chapman, P. (2011) The ETHOS definition and classification of homelessness: an analysis. *European Journal of Homelessness* 5(2): 19–37.

Amore, K. (2013) Focusing on conceptual validity: a response. *European Journal of Homelessness* 7(2): 223–36.

Anderson, I. (2010) Services for homeless people in Europe: Supporting pathways out of homelessness? In: E. O'Sullivan, V. Busch-Geertsema, D. Quilgars and N. Pleace (eds), *Homelessness Research in Europe. Festschrift for Bill Edgar and Joe Doherty*. Brussels: FEANTSA, pp. 41–63.

Archard, P. (1979) *Vagrancy, Alcoholism, and Social Control*. London: Macmillan Press.

Baptista, I. (2010) Women and homelesness. In: E. O'Sullivan, V. Busch-Geertsema, D. Quilgars and N. Pleace (eds), *Homelessness Research in Europe. Festschrift for Bill Edgar and Joe Doherty*. Brussels: FEANTSA, pp. 163–86.

Beck, F., Legleye, S. and Spilka, S. (2009) Alcohol consumption among homeless adults: challenging a stereotype. *Économie et Statistique. Special issue on The Homeless*. English version. Document de travail F 2009/06. Paris: Institut National de la Statistique et des Études Économiques, pp. 159–81.

Benjaminsen, L. and Andrade, S.B. (2015) Testing a typology of homelessness across welfare regimes: shelter use in Denmark and the USA. *Housing Studies* 30(6): 858–76.

Benjaminsen, L. and Dyb, E. (2008) The effectiveness of homelessness policies – variations among the Scandinavian countries. *European Journal of Homelessness* 2: 45–67.

Benjaminsen, L. and Dyb, E. (2010) Homelessness strategies and innovations. In: E. O'Sullivan, V. Busch-Geertsema, D. Quilgars and N. Pleace (eds), *Homelessness Research in Europe. Festschrift for Bill Edgar and Joe Doherty*. Brussels: FEANTSA, pp. 123–42.

Briggs, D., Rhodes, R., Marks, D., Kimber, J., Holloway, G. and Jones, S. (2009) Injecting drug use and unstable housing: scope for structural interventions in harm reduction *Drugs: Education Prevention and Policy* 16(5): 436–50.

Brunette, M.F., Mueser, K.T. and Drake, R.E. (2004) A review of research on residential programs for people with severe mental illness and co-occurring substance use disorders *Drug and Alcohol Review* 23: 471–81.

Busch-Geertsema, V. (2010) Defining and measuring homelessness. In: E. O'Sullivan, V. Busch-Geertsema, D. Quilgars and N. Pleace (eds), *Homelessness Research in Europe. Festschrift for Bill Edgar and Joe Doherty*. Brussels: FEANTSA, pp. 19–40.

Cottrell-Boyce, J. (2010) The role of solvents in the lives of African street children: an ethnographic perspective. *African Journal of Drug and Alcohol Studies* 19(2): 93–112.

Crisis (2011) *Homelesness: A silent killer. A Research Briefing on Mortality Amongst Homeless People*. London: Crisis. Available from: http://www.crisis.org.uk/data/files/publications/Homelessness%20-%20a%20silent%20killer.pdf (Accessed October 2014).

Doherty, J. and Stuttaford, M. (2007) Preventing homelessness among substance users in Europe. *Journal of Primary Prevention* 28: 245–63.

Edgar, B. (2012) The ETHOS definition and classification of homelessness and housing exclusion. *European Journal of Homelessnes* 6(2): 219–25.

FEANTSA (2013) *Health and Wellbeing for All. Holistic Health Services for People Who are Homelessness*. Brussels: FEANTSA.

Fitzpatrick, S., Kemp, P. and Klinker, S. (2001) *Single Homelessness. An Overview of Research in Britain*. York: Joseph Rowntree Foundation. Available from: http://www.jrf.org.uk/sites/files/jrf/jr073-homelessness-research-britain.pdf (Accessed 12 August 2014).

Fraser, S., Moore, D. and Keane, H. (2014) *Habits: Remaking Addiction*. Hampshire: Palgrave Macmillan.

Gaetz, S., Donaldson, J., Richter, T. and Gulliver, T. (2013) *The State of Homelessness in Canada 2013*. Toronto: Canadian Homelessnes Research Network Press. Available from: http://www.homelesshub.ca/sites/default/files/SOHC2103.pdf (Accessed October 2014).

Homelessness Australia (2013) *Homelessness in Australia*. Factsheet. http://www.homelessnessaustralia.org.au/images/publications/Fact_Sheets/Homelessness_in_Australia_v2.pdf (Accessed October 2014).

Homeless Link (2014). The unhealthy state of homelessness. *Health audit results* 2014: 3. Available from: www.homeless.org.uk/facts/our-research/homelessness-and-health-research (Accessed October 2014).

Join-Lambert, M.T. (2009) A special survey. *Économie et Statistique. Special issue on The Homeless*. English version. Document de travail F 2009/06. Paris: Institut National de la Statistique et des Études Économiques, pp. 3–15.

Johnson, K.D., Whitbeck, L.B. and Hoyt, D.R. (2005) Substance abuse and disorders among homeless and runaway adolescents. *Journal of Drug Issues* 35(4): 799–816.

Johnson, G. and Chamberlain, C. (2008) Homelessness and substance abuse: which comes first? *Australian Social Work* 61(4): 342–56.

Lawless, M. and Carr, C. (2005) *Drug Use Among the Homeless Population in Ireland*. Dublin: The Stationery Office.

McKeganey, N., McIntosh, J., MacDonald F., Gilvarry E., McHardle P., McCarthy S. and Hill M. (2006) Preteens and illegal drugs: use, offers, exposure and prevention. *Drugs: Education, Prevention and Policy* 12(Suppl. 1): 98–104.

McNaughton, C.C. (2008) Transitions through homelessness, substance use, and the effect of material marginalization and psychological trauma. *Drugs: Education, Prevention and Policy* 15(2): 177–88.

National Coalition for the Homeless (2009). *Substance Abuse and Homeleessness*. Washington, DC: National Coalition for the Homeless. Available from: http://www.nationalhomeless.org/factsheets/addiction.pdf (Accessed October 2014).

Neale, J. (1997) Theorising homelessness: contemporary sociological and feminist perspectives. In: R. Burrows, N. Pleace and D. Quilgars (eds), *Homelessness and Social Policy*. London: Routledge, pp. 35–49.

Neale, J. and Stevenson, C. (2014) Social and recovery capital amongst homeless hostel residents who use drugs and alcohol. *International Journal of Drug Policy* 26(5): 475–83.

O'Sullivan, E., Busch-Geertsema, V., Quilgars, D. and Pleace, N. (eds) (2010) *Homelessness Research in Europe. Festschrift for Bill Edgar and Joe Doherty*. Brussels: FEANTSA.

Patel, K., Buffin, J., Underwood, S., Khurana, J., McQuade, C., Brako, M., Keeling, P. and Crawley, H. (2004) *Young Refugees and Asylum Seekers in Greater London: Vulnerability to Problematic Drug Use*. London: Greater London Authority.

Philippot, P, Lecocq, C., Sempoux, F., Nachtergael H. and Galand, B. (2007) Psychological research on homelessness in western Europe: a review from 1970 to 2001. *Journal of Social Issues* 63(3): 483–504.

Room, R., Hellman, M. and Stenius, K. (2015) Addiction: the dance between concept and terms. *International Journal of Alcohol and Drug Research* 4(1): 27–35.

Rubington E. (1968) The bottle gang. *Quarterly Journal of Studies on Alcohol* 29: 943–55.

Social Exclusion Unit (2001) *Preventing Social Exclusion*. London: His Majesty's Stationery Office.

Speak, S. (2005) Relationship between children's homelessness in developing countries and the failure of women's rights legislation. *Housing, Theory and Society* 22(3): 129–46.

Substance Abuse and Mental Health Services Administration (2006) *Results from the 2005 National Survey On Drug Use and Health: national findings. Office of Applied Studies 67–73*. In: K. Philips (ed.), *Homelessness: Causes, Culture and Community. Development as a Solution*. Salve's Dissertations and Thesis. Newport: Salve Regina University, p. 19.

Tipple, A.G. and Speak, S. (2005) Definitions of homelessness in developing countries. *Habitat International* 29(2): 337–52.

Tipple, G. and Speak, S. (2009) *The Hidden Millions. Homelessness in Developing Countries*. London: Routledge.

United Nations Centre for Human Settlements (Habitat) (2000) *Strategies to Combat Homelessness*. Nairobi: UNCHS.

Wilson, W. (2014) *Rough Sleeping (England) Standard note SN/SP/2007 (updated 2014) Social Policy Section*. London: House of Commons Library. http://www.parliament.uk/business/publications/research/briefing-papers/SN02007/rough-sleeping-england (Accessed 22 July 2014).

Wincup, E., Buckland, G. and Bayliss, R. (2003) *Youth Homelessness and Substance Use: Report to the Drugs and Alcohol Research Unit Home Office Research Study 258*. London: Home Office Research, Development and Statistics Directorate.

Wood, S.M. (1976) Camberwell Reception Centre: a consideration of the need for health and social services of homeless, single men. *Journal of Social Policy* 5(4): 389–99.

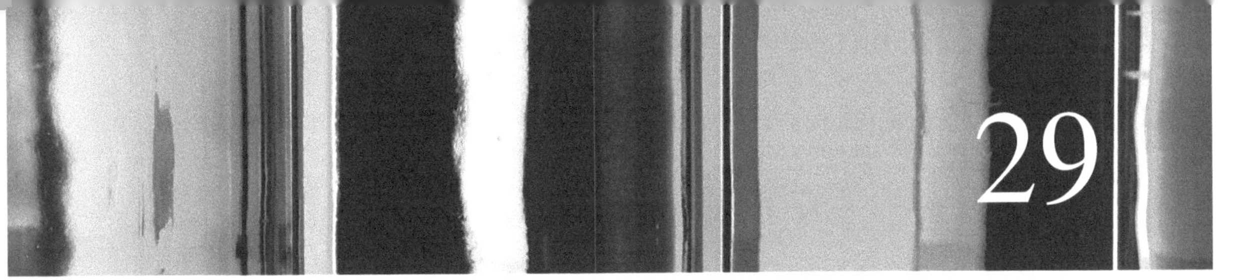

The Prison Population and Illegal Drug Use

Karen Duke and Torsten Kolind

INTRODUCTION

According to the World Prison Population List, more than 10.2 million people are held in penal institutions throughout the world and prison populations are increasing in all five continents. Since 1998, the world prison population rate has risen by about six per cent from 136 per 100,000 of the world population to the rate of 144 in 2013. In 2013, the United States had the highest prison population rate in the world at 716 per 100,000 of the national population. This is significantly higher than other countries and territories, for example, more than half (54 per cent) have rates below 150 per 100,000 (Walmsley, 2013). Based on the World Prison Population List, Table 29.1 provides the rates of a selected number of countries to illustrate some of these variations.

As Drake (2012) argues, the increased reliance on imprisonment and its persistent use over time demonstrates its popularity as a sanction and crime control tool. Prisons are seen as fundamental in producing security and order in society and a key mechanism to deal with drug-related offending. For example, in the United States, drug offenders accounted for 50 per cent of the male federal prison population and 58 per cent of the female prison population in 2012 (US Department of Justice, 2013). Drug offences were the main reason for imprisonment of between 0 per cent and 38.8 per cent of the prison populations in European countries, with a median value of 16.7 per cent (Aebi and Delgrande, 2014). Studies in many countries have also highlighted the over-representation of drug users in prisons and that prison populations have higher rates of lifetime drug use, injecting drug use and problematic drug use compared to the general population (Fazel et al., 2006; EMCDDA, 2012). Prisons are high risk environments for initiation into drug use (Fazel et al., 2006; Stöver and Weilandt, 2007), for more damaging and unsafe forms of drug using behaviour, such as injecting

Table 29.1 Prison population rates (per 100,000 of national population)

Country/territory	*Prison population rate*
United States	716
Russian Federation	475
Lithuania	329
Poland	217
New Zealand	192
Czech Republic	154
England and Wales	148
Spain	147
Portugal	136
Australia	130
Canada	118
Greece	111
Croatia	108
Belgium	108
Italy	106
France	98
Austria	98
Ireland	88
Netherlands	82
Switzerland	82
Germany	79
Denmark	73
Norway	72
Sweden	67
Finland	58

Source: World Prison Population List, 10th edn (Walmsley, 2013).

and needle sharing (Niveau and Ritter, 2008; Jurgens et al., 2009; Carpentier et al., 2012; Kinner et al., 2012) and for transmission of HIV and other blood borne infections (Dolan and Wodak, 1999; Macalino et al., 2004; Small et al., 2005). The rates of HIV and hepatitis C infection, poor health and mental illness are significantly higher among prisoners than the general population (Fazel and Danesh, 2002; Fazel and Baillargeon, 2010). Moreover, in many countries, the majority of prisoners come from minority and marginalized groups (Kerr et al., 2004; Penal Reform International, 2007). Responding to drug-related issues has become an important security and public health priority in prisons throughout the world (WHO, 2005, 2014). For example, in the most recent EU Drug Strategy and Action Plan for 2013 to 2020, a key action is to 'scale up the development, availability and coverage of health care measures for drug users in prison and after release with the aim of achieving a quality of care equivalent to that provided in the community' (European Commission, 2012: C402/4, para 19.6).

This chapter will begin by examining the patterns and levels of drug use among the prison populations in Europe, North America and the Antipodes (Australia and New Zealand), the health profiles of prisoners and their risk behaviours. The chapter will then explore the key theoretical approaches within the social sciences that have been developed to explain prisoners' drug use, their experiences of drugs within prisons and how policies have been developed and implemented. Employing a comparative, cross-national perspective, the ways in which drugs and drug users have been managed and controlled within prison environments will be analysed. Drawing on two case studies (i.e. the Nordic countries and England), the various strategies for treatment and control will be explored and compared. The cases were chosen in order to show how countries with different penal ideologies and traditions in policy and practice nonetheless grapple with the same fundamental dilemma of managing the tensions and contradictions between therapeutic and disciplinary strategies inherent in the prison setting.

PATTERNS AND PROFILES OF DRUG RELATED ISSUES IN PRISON ENVIRONMENTS

The data available on drug issues in prisons have a number of limitations in relation to validity and reliability. This is due to the sensitive nature of the topic (i.e. illicit drugs) and the particular environment of the prison.

Many prisoners will be reluctant to self-report an illegal, stigmatized activity, particularly in the prison setting, where they could be targeted for further punishment and sanctions for their drug use. There are also huge variations in the monitoring of drug-related issues in prisons between different countries and continents. This is due to methodological differences and the absence of standardized instruments in the data collection procedures as well as a lack of agreed international definitions of key terminology such as 'dependence', 'problematic drug use', 'risk behaviour' etc. For example, the European Monitoring Centre on Drugs and Drug Addiction (EMCDDA) is required to collect information on drugs and drug addiction at the European level, including the issue of drugs in prison. Although it is possible to draw a general picture of the situation in European prisons based on the data available (see EMCDDA, 2012), there are significant limitations and wide gaps in the availability of the data (Carpentier et al., 2012). The EMCDDA (2014) recognized the variation in surveys of drug use and drug users in prisons and developed a methodological framework and a standardized European questionnaire on drug use among prisoners. In the future, data collection will focus on several priority areas including information on drug use prevalence (before/inside prison and initiation/continuation); patterns of drug use (frequency, route of administration and risk behaviours); infectious diseases; demographic data; service use; and needs inside prisons.

From the existing statistics, it is possible to draw a rough picture of the drugs 'problem' in prisons across Europe, the United States, Canada, Australia and New Zealand.

Drug use prevalence before prison

It is clear from the available statistics that the use of illicit drugs is more common among prisoners than the general population in a number of countries and regions. For example, the EMCDDA (2012) reports that of the 17 European countries that have reported data on drug use among prisoners, the proportion of prisoners who have ever used any illicit drug before imprisonment ranges from 16 per cent in Romania to 79 per cent in both England and Wales and the Netherlands. In New Zealand, 69 per cent of prisoners reported ever having used drugs prior to entering prison (Ministry of Health, 2006). In 2012, the proportion of Australian prison entrants who reported using illicit drug in the last 12 months was 70 per cent (AIHW, 2013).

Based on the available statistics, prison populations also have high rates of drug dependence, heroin use, injecting and needle sharing. Two-thirds (64.5 per cent) of the American inmate population met the medical criteria for alcohol and/or drug abuse and/or dependence in the year prior to arrest (CASA, 2010). In Canada, the majority (80 per cent) of male offenders in federal custody had a substance abuse problem requiring an intervention response (Weekes et al., 2009). Similar to the general population, the most frequently used drug by prisoners is cannabis. However, prisoners have much higher rates of reported experience of heroin use compared to the general population. For example, the EMCDDA (2012) found that the European countries that were able to provide data on lifetime heroin use reported levels of 15 per cent to 39 per cent compared to less than 1 per cent of the general population. Levels of injecting drug use are also high in prison populations. For example, 44 per cent of Australian prison entrants reported that they had injected drugs (Butler et al., 2011) and 20 per cent reported that they had shared injecting equipment (AIHW, 2013). In the United States, the figures for injecting and needle sharing were lower with 17 per cent of federal and state inmates reporting that they had ever injected drugs and 7 per cent that they had shared needles (CASA, 2010).

Drug use prevalence inside prison

Many prisoners reduce and/or stop their drug taking when imprisoned (Turnbull et al., 1994, 2000; Swann and James, 1998; Dillon, 2001; Bullock, 2003; Stöver et al., 2008). Some prisoners view imprisonment as an opportunity to become drug free, while others are forced to reduce their drug taking due to supply, price and resource issues in the prison setting (Penfold et al., 2005). Crewe (2005: 474) argues that the 'depressing irony' is that some prisoners use drugs as a respite from prison while others find prison a respite from drugs and an opportunity to improve their physical and mental health and repair their personal relationships.

Although it is difficult to obtain valid and reliable data, there is also evidence that some prisoners are 'initiated' into drug use in prison and that existing drug users continue to use drugs in prison, begin to experiment and use different drugs (due to availability issues), start to use drugs again after a period of abstinence or change to more harmful modes of administration (e.g. injecting) (see Strang et al., 2006; Stöver and Weilandt, 2007; Indig et al., 2010). For example, a British survey reported that between 7 per cent and 8 per cent of all prisoners in the sample started using heroin whilst in custody (Ministry of Justice, 2010a). The EMCDDA (2012) collated studies from 15 European countries since 2000, which estimated that between 2 per cent and 56 per cent of prisoners had used an illicit drug while in prison and nine countries reported levels in the range from 20 per cent to 40 per cent. In Australia, 13 per cent of prison dischargees had used illicit drugs while in prison (AIHW, 2013). In Europe, cannabis is the drug most frequently used by prisoners followed by cocaine and heroin. Estimates of heroin use in prison ranged from 1 per cent to 21 per cent. Based on the data available to the EMCDDA, Table 29.2 provides information on lifetime prevalence of drug injecting before and during imprisonment in selected European countries. Estimates of ever injecting drugs in prison ranged from 2 per cent to 31 per cent (see Table 29.2).

Table 29.2 Lifetime prevalence of drug injecting before and during imprisonment in selected European countries

Prevalence of drug injecting (%)			*Year of study*
	Prior to imprisonment	*During imprisonment*	
Belgium	15.2	2.3	2010
Bulgaria (heroin)	7.3 (2009 data)	2.7 (2006 data)	2009/2006
Czech Republic	22.1	8.4	2010
Germany	31.0	22.2	2007
Spain	25.7	3.1	2007
France	7.0	–	2003
Italy	30.4	–	2001 to 2002
Latvia (heroin)	21.1	8.5	2010
Luxembourg	–	31.0	2005
Hungary	10.4	0.7	2008
Poland (adult males)	5.9	3.3	2001
Portugal	12.6	1.9	2007
Romania	6.0	–	2006
United Kingdom (England) (female prisoners)	37.8	6.9	2004 to 2005
United Kingdom (England and Wales)	–	1.0	2001 to 2002
United Kingdom (Scotland)	–	7.5	2009
Croatia	2.5	–	2010

Source: EMCDDA (2012: 12, Table 1). Data provided to EMCDDA by Reitox national focal points.

Prisoners who inject in prison often do so in a higher risk fashion by sharing syringes and constructing syringe substitutes that increases the risk of venous injury, scarring and infection (Kerr et al., 2004). In Australia, 7 per cent of prison discharges reported injecting drugs and 7 per cent used a needle that had been used by someone else while in prison (AIHW, 2013). In Canada, 34 per cent of men and 25 per cent of women in federal prisons admitted to using drugs in the past six months in prison and 17 per cent of men and 14 per cent of women admitted to injecting drugs (Zakaria et al., 2010). Ten per cent of prisoners in New Zealand reported having used a needle to inject, tattoo or pierce themselves while in prison (Ministry of Health, 2006).

In British prisons, the use of novel psychoactive substances (NPS), which are also referred to as 'legal highs' (see Chapter 33, this volume) has been increasing. For example, seizures of NPS in prisons in England and Wales increased from 16 in 2010 to 436 in the first seven months of 2014 with 400 of these for Spice (i.e. synthetic cannabinoid). This increase prompted the Ministry of Justice to introduce new powers to test and punish prisoners using NPS (Ministry of Justice, 2015).

Social, health and demographic profiles of drug users in prisons

There is a paucity of data on the social, health and demographic characteristics of drug users in prisons. However, this information can be gleaned from the data on drug users entering treatment in prison and also from data on the wider prison population. The data on drug users entering treatment in prison indicates that these prisoners have generally experienced deprivation, low educational attainment, unemployment and problems with stable housing (EMCDDA, 2012). In relation to general health issues, prisoners suffer poor physical and mental health when compared to the general population. They also experience high levels of physical and psychiatric problems, including infectious diseases such as HIV/AIDS, hepatitis C and B and psychiatric co-morbidity such as personality and post-traumatic stress disorders and psychosis (WHO, 2014). In the United States, one quarter (24.4 per cent) of inmates have both a substance use disorder and a co-occurring mental health disorder (CASA, 2010). There are also high rates of problem drinking and smoking within prison populations (Ministry of Health, 2006; CASA, 2010; AIHW, 2013). Poor prisoner health can be exacerbated by the overcrowded and unsanitary conditions of some prisons. Risk of suicide in prison may be particularly high for prisoners with drug problems (Fazel et al., 2011). Research studies have also shown that there are high rates of drug related deaths, particularly opioid overdoses, on release from prison (Christensen et al, 2006; Farrell and Marsden, 2008; Merrall et al., 2010).

The prevalence of drug use among prison populations and their corresponding needs in terms of service provision varies between groups depending on age, gender and race and ethnicity. In Europe, for example, the number of women in prison increased by 27 per cent between 2000 and 2010 (EMCDDA, 2012). This rise in the female prison population could partly be explained by the increase in female drug couriers who are often sentenced harshly for their minor roles in the drug supply chain (see Fleetwood, 2014). Women prisoners are more likely to have serious drug related health problems (Fazel et al., 2006) and infectious disease than men (UNODC, 2008). In England and Wales, almost half (49 per cent) of women and one-third (29 per cent) of men reported needing help with a drug problem on entry to prisons (Light et al., 2013). Given their different pathways to drug use and histories of physical violence, sexual abuse and mental health problems, unique drug treatment services need to be developed to meet their specific needs (see Carlen, 1998; WHO, 2009).

THEORETICAL APPROACHES

In this section, we provide a brief overview of some of the different theoretical approaches in the social science literature on drugs and prison. These can be divided into micro-sociological and macro-sociological approaches. The first aims at explaining prisoners' drug use and their experiences in relation to drug taking in a prison setting, while the second focuses on prison drug policies, policy processes and power in the study of drugs and prison.

Micro-sociological approaches

In prison sociology and ethnography, two key theoretical approaches have been applied in order to explain prison life: *indigenous influence theory* and *cultural drift theory* (also termed *deprivation* and *importation* theories, see, for example, Thomas, 1977). The first explains prison life and prisoners' behaviour by reference to intra-institutional processes and influences such as prisonization, the pains of imprisonment, the prisoner culture and identity stripping (Clemmer, 1940; Goffman, 1961; Sykes, 1957). The other approach points to extra-institutional circumstances such as the prisoners' pre-prison lives, personalities, social networks and extra-prison contacts (Irwin, 1970; Cohen and Taylor, 1972; Jacobs, 1983). These two different modes of explanation are also reflected in contemporary social scientific explanations of prisoners' drug use. It should be noted however, that most contemporary studies attempt to merge the two approaches and analyse the interrelatedness of inner and outer institutional circumstances. In this section, therefore, we will discuss examples of how these two modes of explanations are employed.[1]

Explanations of prisoners' drug use in prisons concentrating on intra-institutional circumstances have shown how such drug use can be understood as an answer to the pains of imprisonment encountered by the prisoners, such as boredom, violence, loss of privacy, deprivation of personal autonomy and denial of important social relations. On an individual level, drug use is analysed as a way of coping or as self-medication. Moreover, it has been argued that the prison environment in fact encourages drug use at times and causes prisoners to take up or enlarge their drug taking after being imprisoned (Swann and James, 1998). Along the same lines, Boys et al. (2002) argue that although prisoners' pre-prison drug use influences their drug use in prison and a history of drug dependence is likely to increase the risk of being imprisoned (see also: Liebling, 1999; Stöver and Michels, 2010), prison is to be regarded as a high-risk environment for drug initiation, especially for heroin use. Stated otherwise, inmates' outside vulnerabilities such as problematic drug and alcohol use, psychosocial problems and poor coping skills combined with a detrimental prison environment can promote drug use in prisons (Wheatley, 2007: 403). Seen in this way, prisoners' drug use is explained as an interplay of outer *and* inner prison dynamics. In support of the theory explaining prisoners' drug use as primarily a strategy to reduce the pains of imprisonment however, is the finding that most prisoners, despite their pre-prison drug preferences, prefer drugs such as heroin and cannabis due to their sedative and calming effects (Boys et al. 2002). Similarly, studies also suggest that non-prescribed tranquillizers and opioid substitution drugs, such as methadone and buprenorphine, are increasingly used in prisons in several jurisdictions (Penfold et al., 2005; Plugge et al., 2009; Tompkins et al., 2009; Doyle, 2013; Mjåland, 2015).

In relation to cannabis use, it has been documented that in prisons in Switzerland (Ritter et al., 2013), Denmark (Kolind, 2015) and the UK (Keene, 1997), the estimated level of cannabis use among prisoners is relatively high and is clearly a part of the daily life in prisons. One of the primary reasons for this high level of cannabis use, according to both officers and prisoners, is its perceived effect as an analgesic to relieve stress, to facilitate sleep and ultimately to relieve the experience of imprisonment. Interestingly, the same studies also show that many officers indirectly tolerate or turn a blind eye to prisoners' cannabis use as this tends to help keep prisoners calm and quiet making their work in upholding institutional order easier, but also because officers recognize that cannabis use helps prisoners cope with prison life (see also Carlin, 2005).

Central in many prisoners' experiences with prison life is the feeling that time is void of content and meaning, that time is mainly controlled by external forces, such as judges and prison staff, and that time passes slowly but in retrospect feels empty (Cohen and Taylor, 1972; Toch, 1977). Consequently, boredom is often the dominant feeling related to prison life. In order to cope with this condition, research has shown that prisoners often use drugs to manipulate time and to cope with long sentences. For example, Cope (2003) argues that drugs are used strategically and deliberately by prisoners in order to make time go faster. A key strategy for many prisoners is to use drugs, especially cannabis, to create a 'time vacuum' (i.e. sleeping, relaxing, withdrawing and avoiding interaction) and thereby minimizing the influence of the prison on their pre-prison identity. In this way, prisoners do not deny the fact of their sentence, but deny its impact on their lives. Cope, however, does not only explain prisoners' drug use by reference to the inter-prison life (the indigenous influence theory). In fact, she argues that the context and use patterns of prisoners before their incarceration is important to understand their drug use inside (Cope, 2000). For instance, high levels of cannabis use outside are often related to inside cannabis use and low levels of outside heroin use means that this substance is often not used inside prison. Similarly, gang structures can be imported from the outside and dominate the drug market inside prison. However, as Cope argues, the meanings of drug use change when imported into the prison context. For instance, outside it is not the sedative quality of the drug that is the main motive for using drugs as is the main reason inside. Along the same lines, Keene (1997) argues that although prisoners' drug use may change due to imprisonment, in a broader sense, prison should be seen as solely another context in which they tackle their drug problems (see also Gillespie, 2005: 226).

Another body of research within the micro-sociological approach, which attempts to integrate the intra and extra-institutional processes in order to understand prison life, has argued that prison drug use should not merely be seen as part of individual prisoners' coping strategies – as argued in the theories presented above. It also has to be understood in light of the social contexts and the everyday social lives of prisoners: the prisoner culture, social networks, economics, cultural capital and so on (Wheatley, 2007: 403–6). Based on long-term ethnographic fieldwork, Crewe (2005, 2006) argues that although prisoners use drugs in order to alleviate the pains of imprisonment, such pains are interpreted differently depending on the prisoners' pre-prison biographies. Moreover, at the same time as drugs are used as a coping mechanism, they exacerbate the problems of drug using prisoners. For instance, he shows that drug use and dealing tend to accentuate existing inequalities in prisons between powerful and more vulnerable prisoners, and although drugs do not create a low trust environment, they add to it. Moreover, noting that very few studies have focused on the aspect of drug supply and drug dealing in prisons (however see Munson et al., 1973), Crewe argues that drug dealing in a prison context must be understood as more than simply an economic activity (although drug financial power is important). Drug selling is also strongly related to and bound up with masculinity, self-identity, emotion and internal hierarchies. Drug dealing (and even a culture of drug sharing, see Mjåland, 2014) also plays a role in creating important social and personal interactions in the prison. In this way, drug dealing can enhance the dealers' status and symbolic capital (i.e. by being able to bring drugs into prisons, making connections to outside drug and criminal networks and displaying courage) and the feeling among prisoners that they are part of a larger social group. In addition, drug trafficking can also carry subversive meanings for prisoners in a highly controlled and stigmatized environment (Goffman, 1974; Mjåland, 2015). The importance of the influence of prison culture and social context on prisoners' drug use is also highlighted in the study of Wilson et al. (2007), which traces how the development of a local anti-injecting culture shared among prisoners and staff helps most drug users refrain from injecting and sharing because of the risk involved. Therefore, although drug use should be seen as part of prisoners' individual strategies, it is also strongly determined by the general cultural and social contexts of individual prisons.

In summary, a range of studies has attempted to explain prisoners' drug use by looking at both the specificities of prison life and the extra-institutional lives of the prisoners, although some research, as we have seen, tends to focus more on one of these aspects compared to the other (i.e. the studies tend to focus either on individual coping strategies or the social context and values).

Macro-sociological approaches

In contrast to the micro-sociological attempts at explaining prisoners' drug use and their subjective experiences and strategies in relation to drug taking, another body of research has focused more on prison drug policies, policy processes and power in the study of drugs and prison. Such macro-sociological approaches have investigated both how prison authorities try to counter and manage prisoners' drug use and deal with, and treat, prisoners with drug problems, and how such policies create new forms of subjectivities to which the prisoners must conform.

In a study of English prison drug policy, Duke (2000, 2003; see Case Study 2 below) traces the key shifts in drugs policy approaches from 1980 to 2000 from denial of the existence of prisoner drug use, to partly experimenting with harm reduction during the HIV outbreak in the late 1980s, to a revival of control, punishment and zero tolerance and an increasing focus on managerialism in the late 1990s. Duke concludes that particular 'policy networks' are able to set the agenda in their response to the shifting drug situation in prisons. That is, the drug problem in prisons may change, grow and decline, but the policy reactions toward such changes also have a life of their own and help to determine what in fact constitutes the 'problem' and how the prison system should react. In a similar vein, a study of Nordic prison drug policy has shown that different and even opposing prison drug policy approaches can, in fact, coexist as long as this is considered opportune by the policy actors (Kolind et al. 2013; see Case Study 1 below). On a more general level, changes in prison drug policy reflect and also contribute to the larger societal transformations in governance and ideology. That is, prison drug policy does not only have a life of its own, but is (also) a clear product of its time (Garland, 2001). In their study of the recent 'criminal justice turn' in British drug policy away from former penal-welfare thinking[2] (Garland, 1985), Seddon et al. (2012) argue that this development is related to a more general societal development characterized by a preoccupation with risk and security and influenced by neo-liberal principles of efficient management of welfare services. Increasingly, drug problems, as well as social problems more generally, are understood and tackled as well as produced within this framework of risk and risk assessment. This is apparent at different levels of policy: from national policy frameworks, to the drug interventions delivered on the ground and to the practices of the drug workers and officers (see also Bullock 2011; for officers see Crewe 2011).

However, as suggested by Hardy (2013), it may be more correct to see the prison as being in a state of flux, characterized not by a wholesale rejection of the past penal-welfare ideal, but by a mixture of welfare and risk.

Another set of research studies within the macro-sociological approach has focused on the relationship between power and subjectivity in prison drug policy and practice. This Foucault inspired line of research has investigated how new prison drug related policies and practices create new spaces of identities sketching out new ways to be and experience oneself as an offender. In this way, it is argued, prison policy and practices play a role in constructing (inventing) not only social problems but also 'troubled selves' (Loseke, 2001). For example, in a study of US drug courts, it is argued (Whetstone and Gowan 2011, Gowan and Whetstone 2012) that this court system should be seen as central in identifying low-level drug users, reifying the diagnosis of them as addicts and linking this ultimately biochemical diagnosis (i.e. addiction as a brain disease) to moral culpability. Such classification work is on the face of it class and colour-blind, and thereby, serves as a 'medicalised label disguising a moral crusade to reform the badly behaved poor' (Whetstone and Gowan, 2011: 326). Drug treatment does not only cure, but it also produces new individualized addicted subjects devoid of class, race and urban marginality (for a Canadian study with similar argument see Lyons, 2014). Along the same lines, Mackenzie (2008) argues that the US drug courts are engaged in 'an ethnopolitics of moralized pleasure'. That is, the courts' practice is fundamentally a matter of categorizing. It is a mechanism for categorizing and diverting offenders into treatment programmes and labelling them as criminal, addicted and sick, thereby opposing them from people who seek pleasures from legal and socially proscribed sources (2008: 526). The aim of the programmes therefore, is to normalize the client's sources of pleasure to correspond to responsible neo-liberal citizenship (2008: 527; see also O'Malley and Valverde, 2004). Finally, a study of the penal discourse in Canada (Donohue and Moore, 2009) shows that in drug treatment of prisoners, the institutional identity of the 'offender' increasingly coexists with the 'client': a consumer of welfare services in need of therapeutic attention. It is argued that this shift in subject positions coincides with the growing narratives of consumerism and managerialism in recent Western thought and political practice (see also Moore, 2007).

In summary, there are different analytical approaches in the study of the relationship between drugs and prisons. It is useful to divide these into a micro- and a macro-sociological approach, respectively. We would argue however, that it is important to try to combine both approaches in order to understand the institutional, political and discursive framework within which prisoners' experiences, cultures and strategies are situated and to be open to the fact that prisoners' practices may, at times, have a transformative potential acting back on policy and penal thought.

STRATEGIES FOR DRUGS CONTROL IN PRISONS: THE DILEMMA BETWEEN DISCIPLINARY AND THERAPEUTIC STRATEGIES

Within the prison environment the conflicts and contradictions between security, punishment and control measures and treatment, rehabilitation and harm reduction interventions manifest themselves most acutely (Duke, 2003). Depending on the overall context and conditions, these two forms of regulation (i.e. disciplinary and therapeutic) can co-exist, overlap and reinforce, or sometimes clash with each other. Many prison systems throughout the world have adopted a zero tolerance approach to drug use. The primary focus on policy development and resourcing has been on eradicating the drug problem through increased security, surveillance, testing and punishment, rather than reducing the harms associated with drug use (WHO, 2005). Some prison authorities and governments have refused to contemplate a treatment oriented, harm reduction approach because they believe this would give the appearance of condoning an illegal activity in prison, which would be politically untenable (see, for example, Watson, 2014). Over time, harm reduction has been accepted and mainstreamed in a number of settings, but this has proved difficult to extend to prison environments in some countries (see Duke, 2011). However, other prison systems have viewed prison sentences as 'opportunities' for harm reduction, treatment, rehabilitation and recovery from problematic drug use. Harm reduction techniques, including needle exchanges, have been successfully implemented in a number of prison systems including Moldova, Germany, Kyrgyzstan, Luxembourg, Romania, Spain, Switzerland and Tajikistan (Hoover and Jurgens, 2009; WHO, 2014).

Although a number of countries have introduced harm reduction and treatment initiatives within their prison systems, overall progress in this area remains slow and incongruent to policy and practice in the community (WHO, 2005, 2009, 2014; UNODC, 2008). In some countries, such as the United Kingdom, the disjuncture between the community and prison is a recurring theme within the debates on health care for prisoners (Sim, 2002). Historically, the discourse of less-eligibility has underpinned penal policy whereby prisoners should not be seen to be in receipt of services, or living in conditions, which are superior to those living in the community (Melossi and Pavarini, 1981). When this discourse is translated into penal practice however, it has often meant that prisoners receive a standard of service provision well below that offered in the community, particularly in relation to health care (Sim, 2002). Policy debate at the international level has focused on the *principle of equivalence* and the argument that prisoners have a right to a standard of health care provision in prison equivalent to that available in the community (Lines et al., 2006). Since the late 1980s, there has been increasing pressure for governments to implement equivalent health programmes in prisons, including drug treatment and harm reduction initiatives (WHO, 1987, 1993, 2005, 2014; UNHCR, 1996; UNAIDS, 1997; HRI, 2012). In contrast, it is interesting to examine the Nordic countries where penal policies are based on the ideology of *normalization* (Engbo, 2005), whereby life inside prisons should resemble life outside in the community as far as possible, including the services provided (see Case Study 1 below).

In the following sections, drawing on the Nordic countries (Denmark, Finland, Norway and Sweden) and England as case studies, we will explore how the dilemmas between disciplinary and therapeutic strategies and the different approaches to equivalence are negotiated in the different countries. Despite the UK historically adopting a discourse of 'less-eligibility' and the Nordic countries having one of 'normalization', the dilemma seems impossible to overcome and it dominates and permeates all levels of the prison setting in both cases; from policy to staff culture to prisoners' strategies. Moreover, the dilemma is differently accentuated at different periods of time and within different countries' penal ideologies. In other words, the case studies show that differences exist in penal ideologies and practices, but when it comes to tackling drugs in prisons, the fundamental and endemic dilemma of the prison, trying to both punish and rehabilitate, prevails throughout different regions and countries. The Nordic case is based on a three-year qualitative research project that explored prison based treatment, control and rehabilitation in welfare state institutions in the Nordic countries from 2011 to 2014 (Kolind et al., 2013, 2015, Giertsen et al., 2015). The British case study is based on a qualitative study of the development of prison drugs policy in England and Wales from 1980 to 2000 (Duke, 2000, 2003, 2011), which has been brought up to date to account for recent initiatives.

Case Study 1: Prison drug treatment in the Nordic countries

Over the last two decades, the use of prison drug treatment (PDT) has increased markedly in the Nordic countries. For example, the following services are now offered in prisons: drug treatment wings, cannabis treatment, motivational pre-trial programmes, therapeutic communities, substitution treatment and harm reduction counselling. This development has been rapid and PDT is now uncontested in the Nordic political discourse. This is interesting because only 20 years previously, PDT was perceived as an unsound practice that encountered considerable opposition. This was mainly due to the fall of the rehabilitation ideology or penal welfare thinking (Garland, 1985 in the 1970s (Martinson, 1974; Borch, 2005). A number of factors have played a role in triggering the return of the rehabilitation ideology in the Nordic countries including the rise in the numbers of drug users and the 'drug problem' in prisons, the fear of HIV and hepatitis epidemics (see also: Duke, 2000) and the emerging international scientific studies arguing that treatment in prisons could be effective if methods were carefully designed for defined target groups (see for example, Inciardi et al., 2004). It also should be seen in light of the distinctive penal ideology of the Nordic countries termed *Scandinavian exceptionalism* (Pratt, 2008a, 2008b) characterized by a relatively low prison population, relatively humane prison conditions and an ideology of *normalization*, implying that life inside should resemble life outside as much as possible (see however, Ugelvik and Dullum, 2012).

The 'sudden' popularity also relates to the many ways PDT has been utilized in Nordic public penal discourse. First, PDT has been presented as an important strategy to reduce crime in society. Due to an assumed relationship between drug use and criminality, being proactive and seeking out prison drug users in order to offer them relevant treatment is presented by the authorities as a sensible crime-reducing strategy. Furthermore, providing treatment is seen to help uphold institutional order as drug related disturbances in prisons are believed to be reduced. Second, PDT has been perceived as going hand in hand with the strengthening of the rhetoric and strategy of the US inspired *zero tolerance* approach towards drugs of the Nordic governments in the same period. This simultaneous growth of disciplinary thinking may appear contradictory, but the two approaches have been seen as mutually supportive: they both aim to reduce drug use, drug smuggling and drug selling – thereby helping to fight drugs and support the policy of zero tolerance. It also has been argued that a harsher drug control regime will reduce the availability of drugs, thereby improving the effectiveness of drug treatment programmes. Moreover, it has been claimed that increasing control and disciplinary sanctions will put pressure on and motivate prisoners to start drug treatment, as they will fear the consequences of continued use. Third, the Nordic political discourse on PDT has also been related to a rights perspective. Increasingly, citizens in the Nordic welfare states have been regarded as *users* or *consumers* with legal rights to both health and social services, perceived as free, enterprising individuals not clientized by a powerful state (Frank and Bjerge, 2011; and see Chapter 30, this volume). In the political rhetoric on PDT, this idea of the consumer with rights can be seen in the way drug treatment is presented as a service alongside other services, such as education or work, from which the prisoner can choose. Within this rhetoric, prison does not rehabilitate – instead it *offers* rehabilitation programmes. In Denmark for example, prisoners (as other citizens) have a *Treatment Guarantee*, giving them the right to be offered a drug treatment service within two weeks of request. The political focus on citizens' rights in PDT is also linked to a discussion of prisoners' health with reference to WHO or EU guidelines when discussing substitution treatment and harm reduction (Bruce and Schleifer, 2008; Stöver and Michels, 2010). Basically, it is argued that prisoners are entitled to the same social and health-care services (including drug treatment) as the outside population. Fourth and finally, in the official rhetoric, PDT is linked to the general growth in *managerialism* in the running of present welfare states. According to this rationale, in the Nordic countries, PDT is increasingly judged and not least legitimized on the basis of whether services are delivered on time, reach estimated targets, whether evidence-based drug treatment methods are applied and can be documented and subjected to standardized evaluations. Furthermore, by applying the language of *managerialism* to PDT, the prison services represent themselves publicly as modern, efficient and well-managed welfare institutions.

In summary, PDT has come into existence and been legitimized in the political discourse through a diversity of rationales. It can be argued that this elasticity in public discourse on PDT can explain some of its popularity; it is a practice that can serve different political purposes. At a more general level, PDT may also help to legitimize Nordic prisons per se. By evoking PDT as a rational and humane undertaking, prisons are reinventing themselves as important modern welfare institutions that help to solve a key problem in society: the drug problem.

It should be noted that political rhetoric often differs markedly from actual policy in practice (Shore and Wright, 1997). For instance, placing drug treatment programmes inside prison walls will often change and restrain the content and aims of these programmes, attuning them more to disciplinary practices. In the Nordic prisons we have seen, counsellors adapt the programmes and their individual practices to the control and sanctions of the prison regime. Consequently, the drug treatment programmes inside prison walls come to differ markedly from outside drug services. As an example, some counsellors have integrated the disciplinary sanctions of isolation cells as a response to illegal drug use in their treatment approach, arguing that such sanctions can, in fact, be used as a reflexive process in the work with the prisoners. Conversely, prison officers working in drug treatment wings report how they start changing their own attitudes towards prisoners by being more respectful and understanding. They also interact more with prisoners and use their discretionary power to support prisoners in drug treatment. It is also important to recognize, that seen from the prisoners' perspectives, PDT makes sense primarily in relation to a concrete everyday prison life characterized by disciplinary sanctions, impersonal relations with officers and a tough and inflexible prisoner culture. Thus, prisoners may seek drug treatment primarily in order to mitigate this demanding milieu. The legitimacy of the programmes, therefore, cannot only be judged in relation to declining recidivism and abstinence, but also in the way programmes are able to present an alternative to the detrimental prison culture. The institutional setting and arrangements, therefore, play a major part in shaping the motives, experiences and strategies of the prisoners regarding PDT. For instance, they may stay in treatment primarily to prepare for an early parole, to obtain a transfer to an open prison or to escape drug debts or threats of violence from other prisoners.

In conclusion, the unique Nordic penal tradition focusing on normalizing the life inside the walls making it resemble life outside as much as possible may have facilitated the integration and growth of rights based drug treatment programmes in prisons. However, this growth has also been possible, because of the 'elasticity' of PDT in public discourse. PDT fulfils several dissimilar purposes in official rhetoric. However, when policy is implemented in practice it often changes. Hence, we see how PDT programmes adjust to the disciplinary and control environment inside the walls, as well as how the officers adjust their practices and approaches accordingly. Also, prisoners' motives for engaging in, and experiences with, PDT will often be strongly influenced by the structural setting of the prison. Finally, despite the fact that drug treatment programmes are often viewed positively within a prison setting, this does not necessarily imply that prisons are the best places for conducting drug treatment.

Case Study 2: Prison drugs strategies in England

Previous research has traced the development of prison drugs policy in England from 1980 to 2000 and identified a number of key phases in policy development (Duke, 2000, 2003). The drugs 'problem' in prisons has evolved from being a relatively obscure policy issue to a mainstream one that now occupies prominent places on both the prison and drug policy agendas. The first phase of development from 1980 to 1986 was characterized by a denial and a form of institutionalized collusion around the drugs issue within prisons (Duke, 2003). There was no formal document outlining the Prison Service's policies for dealing with drugs and drug users. In a context of an increasing epidemic of new heroin users in the community (see Pearson, 1987) and an exploding penal crisis characterized by overcrowding, inadequate conditions and unrest (see Fitzgerald and Sim, 1982), drugs, particularly the sedating effects of cannabis, played important control functions in prisons by keeping prisoners contained, quiet and under control (Duke, 2003). With the decline of the rehabilitative ideal in the 1970s (Martinson, 1974), the prison system had been left with a 'crisis of legitimacy' (Fitzgerald and Sim, 1982). The loss of faith in rehabilitation as the primary goal of imprisonment allowed for the rhetoric of 'law and order', 'just deserts' and 'punishment' to emerge as the legitimising rationalities of penal policy (Hall, 1980). However, various sources pointed to a growing problem of drug users in prisons and the inadequacy of the treatment they received compared to community provision (see ACMD, 1980; House of Commons Social Services Committee, 1986). There was increasing pressure for a more explicit prison drugs policy to deal with the growing number of drug users requiring treatment and rehabilitation.

In the period between 1986 and 1993, the HIV crisis was the key factor precipitating the shift towards a more formal, explicit and defined drugs policy in British prisons (Duke, 2003). The denial and collusion around drugs in prisons were no longer sustainable because prisons were seen to be a key site for HIV transmission. The fear of 'contamination' into the 'general population' forced policy makers into responding to the drugs problem in prisons. The liberal, harm reduction response to HIV/AIDS that had been established in community drug services, which included methadone maintenance treatment and needle exchange, proved difficult to implement in the prison setting (Berridge, 1996). Such initiatives were constrained by the institutional context of the prison and the political pressure to adopt a hard-line, abstinence based approach (Duke, 2003). Reflecting increasing crime and imprisonment rates, penal policy became more rational and pragmatic in its approach with growing emphasis on 'just deserts' (i.e. making punishment 'fair' and proportionate to the gravity of the crime) and 'punishment in the community' (i.e. providing alternatives to imprisonment) (Collison, 1993; Hudson, 1993).

From 1993 to 1997, significant shifts occurred in the development of prison drugs policy. This was linked to the dramatic reversal in penal policy characterized by a renewed faith in the deterrent and incapacitative effects of prison and the discourse that 'prison works' put forward by key politicians (Downes, 1997). New 'austerity' measures were introduced and any privileges, such as home leave, temporary release and access to telephones were to be earned by prisoners. Penal policy was thus imbued with a new form of 'populist punitiveness' (Bottoms, 1995) and increasing managerialism with the development of key performance indicators and targets for the Prison Service. Within this context, drugs use in prisons could no longer be ignored or tolerated and became a highly politicized issue. It was framed as a problem of control, order and discipline that threatened the security of the prison system (Duke, 2003). The first prison drugs strategy was introduced in 1995 to tackle and measure the drugs 'problem' in prison and its overarching goal was to eradicate drugs in prisons (HM Prison Service, 1995). It introduced controversial plans to test prisoners for drugs (i.e. mandatory drug testing), increased security measures and emphasized treatment and rehabilitation. The strategy was dominated by a punitive framework of testing, measurement, surveillance and punishment for drugs, while treatment and harm reduction provision lagged behind and remained inadequate (Duke, 2003).

In 1997, the new Labour government placed increasing emphasis on crime reduction through the development of drug treatment initiatives within the criminal justice system. This growth in the drug intervention industry indicated processes of 'criminalization' of drug treatment and rehabilitation, a preoccupation with the drugs-crime link, a growing merger between treatment and punishment and repositioning of treatment to serve crime reduction and public protection goals (see Parker, 2004; Duke, 2006; Seddon et al., 2008; Stevens, 2010). Drugs treatment had thus become a key crime reduction tool for all offenders, including those in prison. In a review of the 1995 prison drugs strategy, the imbalance between disciplinary and treatment initiatives was examined. The revised strategy was to place more emphasis on treatment and throughcare provision and to explore harm reduction initiatives for prisoners who continued to inject. However, at the same time, responses that emphasized security and punishment aspects, such as testing and supply reduction measures, were enhanced and strengthened. The punishment oriented measures converged with the new treatment initiatives. Prisoners involved with drugs were identified through testing and searching procedures and then referred to treatment programmes.

With the establishment of the National Treatment Agency (NTA) in 2001, there was further emphasis and resources made available for prison drugs treatment. The Drugs Intervention Programme (DIP) was set up to provide opportunities for treatment at every point of the criminal justice system including arrest, bail, sentencing, imprisonment and aftercare. In particular, the development of the National Offender Management Service (NOMS) and DIP increased the focus on throughcare, offender management and integrating community services with those in prisons. The emphasis on supply reduction continued with the development of new technologies to detect drugs, including introducing mobile phone blocking technologies and drug detection chairs (i.e. Body Orifice Security Scanners) (see Ministry of Justice, 2008). By 2008, the Integrated Drug Treatment System (IDTS) was established within the prison system to ensure integration between different drug services and provide end-to-end care to prisoners coming in from the community, during imprisonment, on transfers between prisons and post-release. Compared with patchy provision in the 1980s, there is a much wider range of treatment initiatives in British prisons including therapeutic communities, detoxification, opioid substitution treatment, rehabilitation programmes, cognitive behavioural therapy, 12-step abstinence programmes, mandatory and voluntary drug testing and more recently, the development of drug recovery wings. However, these programmes are rarely equivalent to what is offered in the community. For example, methadone treatment is often offered as part of detoxification or for a short period only, rather than on a maintenance basis (Hughes, 2000; Stallwitz and Stöver, 2007). Programmes are also hampered by institutional issues such as overcrowding, staff shortages and a lack of co-ordination (PricewaterhouseCoopers, 2008).

The most recent 2010 national drug strategy places increasing emphasis on abstinence and 'recovery' (HM Government, 2010). Rather than focusing on the harm and crime reduction benefits of treatment, the goal of drugs policy is to offer support to drug users to become 'drug free', choose 'recovery' as a way out of dependency and become active, responsible and contributing members of society. Within this neo-liberal framework, much emphasis is placed on individuals to take responsibility for their drug use, recovery and citizenship (see Duke, 2013; Lancaster et al., 2015). This intersects with initiatives for a 'rehabilitation revolution' in the criminal justice system whereby prisons are to become places of hard work and industry, and 'payment by results' ensures that only those providers that succeed in punishing offenders, protecting the public and reducing offending will be rewarded (Ministry of Justice, 2010b). In relation to prison drugs policy, drug recovery wings are being piloted and will measure key outcome indicators such as recidivism rates and reductions in drug use. These are wing-based, abstinence focused, drug recovery services in adult prisons. Preliminary observations emerging from the first stage rapid assessment of the drug recovery wing pilots highlight a number of positive benefits of the wings for both prisoners and staff in terms of promoting recovery based support and treatment (Lloyd et al., 2014). However, many of the past tensions in prison drugs policy remain unresolved. The policy rhetoric is focused on 'abstinence' and getting prisoners completely free from all drugs, including substitution treatment. However, the expectations regarding full recovery (i.e. complete detoxification/abstinence) versus reduction of methadone prescriptions varied between the different drug recovery wings. Tensions between the recovery agenda and the security/discipline agenda revolving around interactions between staff and prisoners were also highlighted in the preliminary assessment.

In conclusion, the English case study highlights the contradictions and tensions between disciplinary and therapeutic strategies and how these have altered and been managed over time. Treatment and harm reduction strategies have lagged behind the disciplinary strategies such as mandatory drug testing and drug surveillance technologies. Treatment and throughcare provision has been extended and improved in the recent phases of the policy, but has also converged with the security and control aspects of the drugs strategy. Both aspects work in tandem to fulfil the same goals in terms of reducing drugs and crime. The official discourse is focused on 'control', 'order' and 'punishment' and this is the rhetoric that is most often articulated publicly to counter the perceptions of some sectors of the public who believe that prisons are 'soft' on drug users. As Pratt (1999) argues, the doctrine of less eligibility is often kept alive in the official rhetoric by reference to public opinion.

These two case studies have highlighted a number of common themes, including the development of prison drugs treatment as a crime reduction tool, the intersection between treatment and zero tolerance approaches, the emphasis on rights and responsibilities of individual prisoners to take responsibility for their drug use and the opportunities for treatment and the increasing managerialism within the delivery of treatment emphasizing targets, economy and efficiency. However, the Nordic case reflects the ideology of normalization that underpins their penal policy (i.e. that prison services should resemble community provision), while the theme of 'less eligibility' has been a pervasive theme in the English case study where there has been a constant battle to ensure that provision of treatment and harm reduction services in prison are congruent to those in the community. However, this does not mean that community programmes are replicated exactly in the prison setting, rather they are often adapted to fit the institutional context and practices of the prison, as the Nordic case demonstrates. Moreover, the institutional context and arrangements in prisons shape the motives, experiences and strategies of prisoners engaging in such treatment.

CONCLUSION

This chapter has highlighted the nature and the extent of the drug 'problem' in prisons. A number of groups can be identified in relation to drugs with prison populations around the world: the increasing number of offenders who are sentenced to prison for drug offences and who may also be drug users, those who are sentenced for non-drug offences, but who are drug users and those who begin to use drugs in prison. Compared to the general population, prisoners have high rates of drug use, problematic drug use and injecting (Fazel et al., 2006; EMCDDA, 2012). Prisons populations suffer multiple disadvantages in relation to poor health, unemployment, poverty and deprivation, lack of social support and access to health care (Vandevelde et al., 2006; Fazel and Baillargeon, 2010; Stöver and Michels, 2010). Infectious diseases, such as HIV and hepatitis C, are higher in the prison population compared to the general population, particularly for those who are injecting drug users (Fazel and Baillargeon, 2010). The prison setting amplifies and exacerbates the problems experienced by drug users (Boys et al., 2002). When injecting occurs in the prison environment for example, it is often carried out in a more 'high risk' fashion than in the community, which increases the risk of injury and transmission of blood-borne viruses (Shewan et al., 2008).

Explanations for patterns of drug use in the context of the prison can differ to those in the community. Micro-sociological approaches focus on individual prisoners and explain their drug use in prison by reference to intra-institutional processes such as prisonization, the pains of imprisonment, the prisoner culture and identity stripping and by reference to extra-institutional processes such as their pre-prison lives, personalities, social networks and extra prison contacts. Macro-sociological approaches emphasize the response to drugs within prisons and focus on the development of policies and strategies and the administration and distribution of power. Much of the existing research on drugs and prisons has employed either a micro-sociological or a macro-sociological approach. Future research needs to employ a combination of the two approaches in order to better understand the interaction between the individual prisoners' experiences, cultures and strategies and the overall institutional, political and discursive structures.

A variety of rationales has been employed to legitimize the different strategies developed in prisons to deal with drugs including punishment, crime reduction, public health, human rights, rehabilitation and recovery. In recent policy development, both case studies have highlighted the growing convergence of treatment and punishment goals. Historical analyses demonstrate how the tensions between the two have shifted and been managed over time (Foucault, 1991; Mathiesen, 2006). Both treatment and punishment initiatives now coalesce around the overarching, mutual goal of crime reduction (see also: Seddon et al., 2012). It is evident that the discourse around rehabilitation and recovery has been revived, but this has taken on new forms with a distinctively neo-liberal turn where individuals are expected to take responsibility for their drug use and recovery and take up the opportunities on offer for treatment and rehabilitation in prisons. The Nordic case illustrates the elasticity of prison drug treatment with its capacity to fulfil different political purposes by appeasing both the left and the right politically. On the one hand, it can be portrayed as humane and rehabilitative, while on the other hand, it also can be put forward as a zero tolerance approach as a means of taking control of the drug problem and reducing crime.

Various international organizations, including WHO, UNHCR, UNAIDS and HRI, have argued for the principle of equivalence in relation to the provision of policies and services in prison (WHO, 1993, 2005, 2009, 2014; UNHCR, 1996; UNAIDS, 1997; HRI, 2012). This has emerged to counter the doctrine of less eligibility that has been present in the debates around prison policy reform historically. The doctrine of less eligibility can be detected in the types of drugs treatment offered in prisons in some countries, particularly in relation to harm reduction oriented initiatives. However, as the Nordic case demonstrates, even when the principle of normalization underpins prison policy and community programmes are directly transferred into the prison setting, they are often adapted and limited to conform to the institutional framework of the prison. This links to the argument that prisons are not optimal locations for providing drug treatment and rehabilitation services. There is increasing emphasis in many countries on developing alternatives to imprisonment for drug involved offenders, so that they are diverted from custody and can be offered treatment services in the community. For example, in the most recent EU Drugs Action Plan, Member States are encouraged to provide 'alternatives to coercive sanctions (such as education, treatment, rehabilitation, aftercare and social integration) for drug using offenders' (European Commission, 2012: C402/6, para 22.11). Future policy, practice and resources need to be focused on developing these initiatives so that they can become 'real' alternatives to imprisonment.

NOTES

1 It is also possible to discern a third approach in understanding prisoners' drug use: *the treatment perspective* (Gillespie, 2005: 224). Although not clearly a theoretical alternative, this body of research stands out by its empirical focus on public health instead of criminal justice (see Chapter 36, this volume) and examines prevalence of drug use, patterns of use, types of drugs used, drug treatment and harm reduction and the relationship between pre-prison, prison and after prison use.
2 The penal-welfare thinking is characterized by a strong focus on treatment and rehabilitation.

REFERENCES

Advisory Council on the Misuse of Drugs (ACMD) (1980) *Report on Drug Dependants within the Prison System in England and Wales*. London: Home Office.

Aebi, M.F. and Delgrande, N. (2014) *Annual Penal Statistics Space I – 2012*. Strasbourg: Council of Europe.

Australian Institute of Health and Welfare (AIHW) (2013) *The Health of Australia's Prisoners 2012*. Canberra: AIHW.

Berridge, V. (1996) *AIDS in the UK: The Making of Policy 1981–1994*. Oxford: Oxford University Press.

Borch, C. (2005) *Kriminalitet og magt. Kriminalitetsopfattelser i det 20. århundrede*. Copenhagen: Politisk revy.

Bottoms, A.E. (1995) The philosophy and politics of punishment and sentencing. In: C.M.V. Clarkson and R. Morgan (eds), *The Politics of Sentencing Reform*. Oxford: Clarendon Press. pp. 17-49

Boys, A., Farrell, M., Bebbington, P., Brugha, T., Coid, J., Jenkins, R., Lewis, G., Marsden, J., Meltzer, H., Singleton, N. and Taylor, C. (2002) Drug use and initiation in prison: results from a national prison survey in England and Wales. *Addiction*, 97: 1551–60.

Bruce, R.D. and Schleifer, R.A. (2008) Ethical and human rights imperatives to ensure medication-assisted treatment for opioid dependence in prisons and pre-trial detention. *International Journal of Drug Policy*, 19: 17–23.

Bullock, K. (2011) The construction and interpretation of risk management technologies in contemporary probation practice. *British Journal of Criminology*, 51: 120–35.

Bullock, T. (2003) Changing levels of drug use before, during and after imprisonment. In: M. Ramsay (ed.), *Prisoners' Drug Use and Treatment: Seven Research Studies*. Home Research Study No. 267. London: Home Office, pp. 23–48.

Butler, T., Lim, D. and Callendar, D. (2011) *National Prison Entrants' Bloodborne Virus and Risk Behaviour Survey 2004, 2007, and 2010*. Sydney: The Kirby Institute (University of New South Wales) and National Drug Research Institute (Curtin University).

Carlen, P. (1998) *Sledgehammer: Women's Imprisonment at the Millennium*. London: Macmillan.

Carlin, T. (2005) An exploration of prisoners' and prison staff's perception of the methadone maintenance programme in Mountjoy Male Prison, Dublin, Republic of Ireland. *Drugs: Education, Prevention and Policy,* 12: 405–16.

Carpentier, C., Royuela, L., Noor, A. and Hedrich, D. (2012) Ten years of monitoring illicit drug use in prison populations in Europe: issues and challenges. *Howard Journal of Criminal Justice*, 5: 37–66.

CASA (2010) *Behind Bars II: Substance Abuse and America's Prison Population*. New York: The National Center on Addiction and Substance Abuse at Columbia University (CASA).

Christensen, P.B., Hammerby, E. and Bird, S. (2006) Mortality among Danish drug users released from prison. *International Journal of Prisoner Health,* 2: 13–19.

Clemmer, D. (1940) *The Prison Community*. New Braunfels: The Christopher Publishing House.

Cohen, S. and Taylor, L. (1972) *Psychological Survival: The Experience of Long-Term Imprisonment,* Harmondsworth: Penguin Books.

Collison, M. (1993) Punishing drugs: criminal justice and drug use. *British Journal of Criminology*, 33: 382–99.

Cope, N. (2000) Drug use in prison: the experience of young offenders. *Drugs: Education, Prevention and Policy,* 7: 355–66.

Cope, N. (2003) 'It's no time or high time': young offenders' experiences of time and drug use in prison. *The Howard Journal of Criminal Justice,* 42: 158–75.

Crewe, B. (2005) Prisoner society in the era of hard drugs. *Punishment and Society,* 7: 457–81.

Crewe, B. (2006) Prison drug dealing and the ethnographic lens. *The Howard Journal of Criminal Justice,* 45: 347–68.

Crewe, B. (2011) Soft power in prison: implications for staff-prisoner relationships, liberty and legitimacy. *European Journal of Criminology,* 8: 455–68.

Dillon, L. (2001) *Drug Use Among Prisoners: An Exploratory Study*. Dublin: Health Research Board.

Dolan, K. and Wodak, A. (1999) HIV transmission in a prison system in an Australian state. *Medical Journal Australia*, 171 (1): 14–17.

Donohue, E. and Moore, D. (2009) When is an offender not an offender? Power, the client and shifting penal subjectivities. *Punishment and Society,* 11: 319–36.

Downes, D. (1997) What the next government should do about crime. *Howard Journal*, 36: 1–13.

Doyle, P. (2013). *Prevention and Management of Drug Use in Prisons*. Melbourne: Victorian Auditor-General's Office (VAGO).

Duke, K. (2000) Prison drug policy since 1980: shifting agendas and policy networks. *Drugs: Education, Prevention and Policy,* 7: 393–408.

Duke, K. (2003) *Drugs, Prisons and Policy-Making*. New York: Palgrave Macmillan.

Duke, K. (2006) Out of crime and into treatment? The criminalisation of contemporary drugs policy since *Tackling Drugs Together. Drugs: Education, Prevention and Policy*, 13: 409–15.

Duke, K. (2011) Reconceptualising harm reduction in prisons. In: S. Fraser and D. Moore (eds), *The Drug Effect: Health, Crime and Society*. Cambridge: Cambridge University Press. Pp. 209-224.

Duke, K. (2013) From crime to recovery: the reframing of British drugs policy? *Journal of Drug Issues*, 43: 39–55.

Drake, D. (2012) *Prisons, Punishment and the Pursuit of Security*. Basingstoke: Palgrave Macmillan.

Engbo, H. J. (2005) *Straffuldbyrdelsesret*. Copenhagen: Jurist- og Økonomiforbundets Forlag.

European Commission (2012) *EU Drugs Strategy (2013–2020)*. Brussels: European Commission. Available from: http://eur-lex.europa.eu/LexUriServ/LexUriServ.do?uri=OJ:C:2012:402:0001:0010:en:PDF (Accessed 2 April 2016).

EMCDDA (2012) *Prisons and Drugs in Europe: the Problem and Responses*. Lisbon: EMCDDA.

EMCDDA (2014) *Drug Use in Prison: Assessment Report. Reviewing Tools for Monitoring Illicit Drug Use in Prison*. Lisbon: EMCDDA.

Farrell, M. and Marsden, J. (2008) Acute risk of drug-related death among newly released prisoners in England and Wales. *Addiction*, 103(2): 251–5.

Fazel, S. and Baillargeon J. (2010) The health of prisoners. *The Lancet*, 377: 956–65.

Fazel, S. and Danesh, J. (2002) Serious mental disorder in 23,000 prisoners: a systematic review of 62 surveys. *The Lancet*, 359: 545–50.

Fazel, S., Bains, P. and Doll, H. (2006) Substance abuse and dependence in prisoners: a systematic review. *Addiction*, 101: 181–91.

Fazel, S., Grann, M. Kling, B. and Hawton, K. (2011) Prison suicide in 12 countries: an ecological study of 861 suicides during 2003–2007. *Social Psychiatry and Psychiatric Epidemiology*, 46: 191–5.

Fitzgerald, M. and Sim, J. (1982) *British Prisons*, 2nd edn. Oxford: Blackwell.

Fleetwood, J. (2014) *Drug Mules: Women in the International Cocaine Trade*. Basingstoke: Palgrave MacMillan.

Foucault M. (1991) *Discipline and Punish: The Birth of the Prison*. London: Penguin.

Frank, V.A. and Bjerge, B. (2011) Empowerment in drug treatment: dilemmas in implementing policy in welfare institutions. *Social Science and Medicine*, 73: 201–8.

Garland, D. (2001) *The Culture of Control. Crime and Social Order in Contemporary Society*. Oxford: Oxford University Press.

Garland, D. (1985) *Punishment and Welfare*. Aldershot: Gower.

Giertsen, H., Nylander, P.Å., Frank, V.A., Kolind, T. and Tourunen, J. (2015) Prisoners' experiences of drug treatment and punishment in four Nordic countries. *Nordic Studies on Alcohol and Drugs*, 32, 145–164.

Gillespie, W. (2005) A multilevel model of drug abuse inside prison. *The Prison Journal*, 85: 223–46.

Goffman, E. (1961) *Asylums*. Garden City: Doubleday.

Goffman, E. (1974). *Stigma. Notes of the Management of Spoiled Identity*. Harmondsworth: Penguin Books.

Gowan, T. and Whetstone, S. (2012) Making the criminal addict: subjectivity and social control in a strong-arm rehab. *Punishment and Society*, 14: 69–93.

Hall, S. (1980) *Drifting into a Law and Order Society*. London: Cobden Trust.

Hardy, M. (2013) Practitioner perspectives on risk: using governmentality to understand contemporary probation practice. *European Journal of Criminology*, 11: 303–18.

Harm Reduction International (HRI) (2012) *Advocating for Needle and Syringe Exchange Programmes in Prison*. London: HRI.

HM Government (2010) *Drug strategy 2010: Reducing Demand, Restricting Supply, Building Recovery: Supporting People to Live a Drug Free Life*. London: HM Government.

HM Prison Service (1995) *Drug Misuse in Prison: Policy and Strategy*. London: HM Prison Service.

Hoover, J. and Jurgens, R. (2009) *Harm Reduction in Prison: The Moldova Model*. New York: Open Society Institute Public Health Program.

House of Commons Social Services Committee (1986) *Prison Medical Service, Third Report from the Social Services Committee, Session 1985/86*. London: HMSO.

Hudson, B. (1993) *Penal Policy and Social Justice*. London: Macmillan.

Hughes, R. (2000) 'It's like having half a sugar when you were used to three' – drug injectors' views and experiences of substitute drug prescribing inside English prisons. *The International Journal of Drug Policy*, 10: 455–66.

Inciardi, J.A., Martin, S.S. and Butzin, C.A. (2004) Five-year outcomes of therapeutic community treatment of drug-involved offenders after release from prison. *Crime and Delinquency*, 50: 88–107.

Indig, D., Topp, L., Ross, B., Mamoon, H., Border, B., Kumar, S. and McNamara, M.(2010) *2009 NSW Inmate Health Survey: Key Findings Report*. Sydney: Justice Health.

Irwin, J. (1970) *The Felon*. Englewood Cliffs: Prentice-Hall.

Jacobs, J. (1983) *New Perspectives on Prison and Imprisonment*. New York: Cornell University Press.

Jurgens, R., Ball, A. and Verster, A. (2009) Interventions to reduce HIV transmission related to injecting drug use in prison. *The Lancet Infectious Diseases*, 9: 57–66.

Keene, J. (1997) Drug misuse in prison: views from inside: a qualitative study of prison staff and inmates. *The Howard Journal of Criminal Justice*, 36: 28–41.

Kerr, T., Wood, E., Betteridge, G., Lines, R. and Jurgens, R. (2004). Harm reduction in prisons: a 'rights based' analysis. *Critical Public Health*, 14: 345–60.

Kinner, S.A., Jenkinson, R., Gouillou, M. and Milloy, M.J. (2012) High-risk drug-use practices among a large sample of Australian prisoners. *Drug and Alcohol Dependence*, 126: 156–60.

Kolind, T. (2015) Drugs and discretionary power in prisons: the officer's perspective. *International Journal of Drug Policy,* 26: 799–807.

Kolind, T., Frank, V.A., Lindberg, O. and Tourunen, J. (2013) Prison-based drug treatment in Nordic political discourse: an elastic discursive construct. *European Journal of Criminology,* 10: 659–74.

Kolind, T., Frank, V.A., Lindberg, O. and Tourunen, J. (2015) Officers and drug counsellors: new occupational identities in Nordic prisons. *British Journal of Criminology*, 55: 303–20.

Lancaster, K., Duke, K. and Ritter, A. (2015) Producing the 'problem of drugs': a cross national-comparison of 'recovery' discourse of two Australian and British reports. *International Journal of Drug Policy,* 26: 617–25.

Liebling, A. (1999) Prison suicide and prisoner coping. In: M. Tonry and J. Petersilia (eds), *Prison, Crime and Justice Review of Research.* Chicago: University of Chicago Press. pp. 283–360.

Light, M., Grant, E. and Hopkins, K. (2013) Gender differences in substance misuse and mental health amongst prisoners: results from the surveying prisoner crime reduction (SPCR) longitudinal cohort study of prisoners. London: Ministry of Justice.

Lines, R., Jurgens, R., Betteridge, G., Stöver, H., Laticevschi, D. and Nelles, J. (2006). *Prison Needle Exchange: Lessons from a Comprehensive Review of the International Evidence and Experience*, 2nd edn. Toronto: Canadian HIV/AIDS Legal Network.

Lloyd, C., Page, G., Russell, C., McKeganey, N. and Liebling, A. (2014) *Evaluation of the Drug Recovery Wing Pilots: Scoping and Feasibility Report*. York: University of York.

Loseke, D. R. (2001) Lived realities and formula stories of 'battered women'. In: J.F. Gubrium and J.A. Holstein (eds), *Institutional Selves. Troubled Identities in a Postmodern World.* Oxford: Oxford University Press. pp. 107–126.

Lyons, T. (2014) Simultaneously treatable and punishable: implications of the production of addicted subjects in a drug treatment court. *Addiction Research and Theory,* 24: 286–93.

Macalino, G.E., Hou, J.C., Kumar, M.S., Taylor, L.E., Sumantera, I.G. and Rich, J.D. (2004) Hepatitis C infection and incarcerated populations. *International Journal of Drug Policy*, 15: 103–14.

Mackenzie, R. (2008) Feeling good: the ethopolitics of pleasure; psychoactive substance use and public health and criminal justice governance: therapeutic jurisprudence and the drug courts in the USA. *Social and Legal Studies,* 17: 513–33.

Martinson, R. (1974) What works? Questions and answers about prison reform. *Public Interest,* 35: 22–45.

Mathiesen T. (2006) *Prison on Trial*. London: Waterside Press.

Melossi, D. and Pavarini, M. (1981). *The Prison and the Factory: the Origins of the Penitentiary System.* London: Macmillan.

Merrall, E.L., Kariminia, A., Binswanger, I.A., Hobbs, M.S., Farrell, M. (2010). Meta-analysis of drug-related deaths soon after release from prison. *Addiction*. 105 (9): 1545–54.

Ministry of Health (2006) *Results from the Prisoner Health Survey, 2005*. Wellington: Ministry of Health.

Ministry of Justice (2008) *Disrupting the Supply of Illicit Drugs into Prisons. A Report for the Director General of the National Offender Management Service*. (Blakey Report). London: Ministry of Justice.

Ministry of Justice (2010a) *Compendium of Reoffending Statistics and Analysis*. London: Ministry of Justice.

Ministry of Justice (2010b) *Breaking the Cycle: Effective Punishment, Rehabilitation and Sentencing of Offenders.* London: Ministry of Justice.

Ministry of Justice (2015) Press release: new crackdown on dangerous legal highs in prison, 25 January. London: Ministry of Justice. Available from: https://www.gov.uk/government/news/new-crackdown-on-dangerous-legal-highs-in-prison (Accessed 24 June 2015).

Mjåland, K. (2014) 'A culture of shaing': drug exchange in a Norwegian prison. *Punishment and Society*, 16: 336–52.

Mjåland, K. (2015) The paradox of control: an ethnographic analysis of opiate maintenance treatment in a Norwegian prison. *International Journal of Drug Policy*, 26:781–9.

Moore, D. (2007) *Criminal Artefacts: Governing Drugs and Users*. Vancouver: UBC Press.

Munson, N., Rexed, I., Packard, R. and Blum, R. (1973) Prisons. In: R. Blum (ed.), *Drug Dealers: Taking Action*. San Francisco: Jossey-Bass. pp. 171-200

Niveau, G. and Ritter, C. (2008) Route of administration of illicit drugs among remand prison inmates. *European Addiction Research*, 14: 92–8.

O'Malley, P. and Valverde, M. (2004) Pleasure, freedom and drugs: the uses of 'pleasure' in liberal governance of drug and alcohol consumption. *Sociology*, 38: 25–42.

Parker, H. (2004) The new drugs interventions industry: what outcomes can drugs/criminal justice treatment programmes realistically deliver? *Probation Journal*, 51: 379–86.

Pearson, G. (1987) *The New Heroin Users*. Oxford: Blackwell.

Penal Reform International (2007) *Health in Prisons: Realising the Right to Health*. London: Penal Reform International.

Penfold, C., Turnbull, P.J. and Webster, R. (2005). *Tackling Prison Drug Markets: An Exploratory Qualitative Study*. Home Office Online Report 39/05. London: Home Office.

Plugge, E., Yudkin, P. and Douglas, N. (2009). Changes in women's use of illicit drugs following imprisonment. *Addiction*, 104: 215–22.

Pratt, J. (1999) Norbert Elias and the civilised prison. *British Journal of Sociology*, 50: 271–96.

Pratt, J. (2008a) Scandinavian exceptionalism in an era of penal excess. Part I: the nature and roots of Scandinavian exceptionalism. *British Journal of Criminology*, 48: 119–37.

Pratt, J. (2008b) Scandinavian exceptionalism in an era of penal excess. Part II: does Scandinavian exceptionalism have a future? *British Journal of Criminology*, 48: 275–92.

PricewaterhouseCoopers (2008) *Review of Prison-based Drug Treatment Funding. Report to the Department of Health and Ministry of Justice*. London: Ministry of Justice.

Ritter, C., Broers, B. and Elger, B.S. (2013) Cannabis use in a Swiss male prison: qualitative study exploring detainees' and staffs' perspectives. *International Journal of Drug Policy*, 24: 573–8.

Seddon, T., Ralphs, R. and Williams, L. (2008) Risk, security and the 'criminalisation' of British drugs policy. *British Journal of Criminology*, 48: 818–34.

Seddon, T., Williams, L. and Ralphs, R. (2012) *Tough Choices. Risk, Security, and the Criminalization of Drug Policy*. Oxford: Oxford University Press.

Shewan D, Stöver, H. and Dolan, K. (2008) Injecting in prisons. In: R. Pates, A. McBride and K. Arnold (eds), *Injecting Illicit Drugs*. Oxford: Blackwell Publishing Ltd, pp. 69–81.

Shore, C. and Wright, S. (eds) (1997) *Anthropology of Policy. Critical Perspectives on Governance and Power*. New York: Routledge.

Sim, J. (2002) The future of prison health care: a critical analysis. *Critical Social Policy*, 22: 300–23.

Small, W., Kain, S., Laliberte, N., Schechter, M.T., O'Shaunghnessy, M.V. and Spittal, P.M. (2005) Incarceration, addiction and harm reduction: inmates' experiences of injecting drugs in prison. *Substance Use and Misuse*, 40: 831–43.

Stallwitz, A. and Stöver, H. (2007) The impact of substitution treatment in prisons – a literature review. *International Journal of Drug Policy*, 18: 464–74.

Stevens, A. (2010) *Drugs, Crime and Public Health: The Political Economy of Drug Policy*. London: Routledge.

Stöver, H. and Michels, I. (2010) Drug use and opioid substitution treatment for prisoners. *Harm Reduction Journal*, 7: 17.

Stöver, H. and Weilandt, C. (2007) Drug use and drug services in prison. In: L. Moller, H. Stöver, R. Jurgens, A. Gatherer and H. Nikogosian (eds), *Health in Prisons: A WHO Guide to the Essentials in Prison Health*. Copenhagen: WHO Regional Office for Europe, pp. 85–111.

Stöver, H., Weilandt, C., Zurhold, H., Hartwig, C. and Thane, K. (2008). *Final Report on Prevention, Treatment, and Harm Reduction Services in Prison, on Reintegration Services on Release from Prison and Methods to Monitor/Analyse Drug Use Among Prisoners (SANCO/2006/C4/02)*. Brussels: Directorate General for Health and Consumer Affairs.

Strang, J., Gossop, M., Heuston, J., Green, J., Whitely, C. and Maden, A. (2006) Persistence of drug use during imprisonment: relationship of drug type, recency of use, and severity of dependence to heroin, cocaine, and amphetamine in prison. *Addiction*, 10: 1125–32.

Swann, R. and James, P. (1998) The effect of the prison environment upon inmate drug taking behaviour. *The Howard Journal of Criminal Justice*, 37: 252–65.

Sykes, G. (1957) *The Society of Captives.* Princeton: Princeton University Press.

Thomas, C.W. (1977) Theoretical perspectives on prisonization - comparison of importation and deprivation models. *Journal of Criminal Law and Criminology*, 68: 135–45.

Toch, H. (1977) *Living in Prison: The Ecology of Survival.* New York: The Free Press.

Tompkins, C., Wright, N., Waterman, M. and Sheard, L. (2009) Exploring prison buprenorphine misuse in the United Kingdom: a qualitative study of former prisoners. *International Journal of Prisoner Health*, 5: 71–87.

Turnbull, P.J. (2000) The effect of prison on drug use. In: R. Muscat (ed.), *Drug Use in Prison*. Strasbourg: Council of Europe Publishing. pp. 133-144

Turnbull, P.J., Stimson, G.V. and Stillwell, G. (1994) *Drug Use in Prison.* Horsham: AVERT.

Ugelvik, T. and Dullum, J. (eds) (2012) *Penal Exceptionalism? Nordic Prison Policy and Practice.* London: Routledge.

UNAIDS (1997). *Prison and AIDS: UNAIDS Point of View*. Geneva: Joint United Nations Programme on HIV/AIDS.

United Nations Commission on Human Rights (UNHCR) (1996). *HIV/AIDS in Prisons – Statement by the Joint United Nations Programme on HIV/AIDS (UNAIDS)*. Geneva: UNHCR.

UNODC (2008) *Women and HIV in Prison Settings*. Vienna: United Nations Office on Drugs and Crime.

US Department of Justice (2013) *Prisoners in 2012: Trends in Admissions and Releases, 1991–2012.* Washington, DC: Bureau of Justice Statistics.

Vandevelde, S., Palmans, V., Broekaert, E., Rousseau, K. and Vanderstraeten, K. (2006) How do drug-involved incarcerated and recently released offenders and correctional treatment staff perceive treatment? A qualitative study on treatment needs and motivation in Belgian prisons. *Psychology, Crime and Law,* 12: 287–305.

Walmsley, R. (2013) *World Prison Population List*, 10th edn. London: International Centre for Prison Studies.

Watson, T.M. (2014) The politics of harm reduction in federal prisons. *International Journal of Drug Policy*, 25: 916–23.

Weekes, J., Moser, A., Ternes, M. and Kunic, D. (2009) Substance Abuse Among Male Offenders. Ottawa: Correctional Service of Canada.

Wheatley, M. (2007) Drugs in prison. In: Y. Jewkes (ed.), *Handbook on Prisons.* Devon: Willan Publishing. pp. 399–422

Whetstone, S. and Gowan, T. (2011) Diagnosing the criminal addict: biochemistry in the service of the state. In: P. McGann and D.J. Hutsun (eds), *Sociology of Diagnosis (Advances in Medical Sociology).* Bingley: Emerald.

Wilson, G.B., Galloway, J., Shewan, D., Marshall, L., Vojt, G. and Marley, C. (2007) 'Phewww, bingoed!': motivations and variations of methods for using heroin in Scottish prisons. *Addiction Research and Theory* 15: 205–24.

World Health Organization (WHO) (1987). *Statement from the Consultation on Prevention and Control of AIDS in Prisons.* Geneva: WHO Global Programme on AIDS.

World Health Organization (WHO) (1993) *WHO Guidelines on HIV infection and AIDS in Prisons*. Geneva: WHO.

World Health Organization (WHO) (2005) *Status Paper on Prisons, Drugs and Harm Reduction*. Copenhagen: WHO Europe.

World Health Organization (2009) *Women's Health in Prison: Correcting Gender Inequity in Prison Health*. Copenhagen: WHO Regional Office for Europe.

World Health Organization WHO (2014) *Prisons and Health*. Copenhagen: WHO Regional Office for Europe.

Zakaria, D., Thompson, J.M., Jarvis, A. and Borgatta, F. (2010) *Summary of Emerging Findings from the 2007 National Inmate Infectious Diseases and Risk-Behaviours Survey*. Ottawa: Correctional Service of Canada.

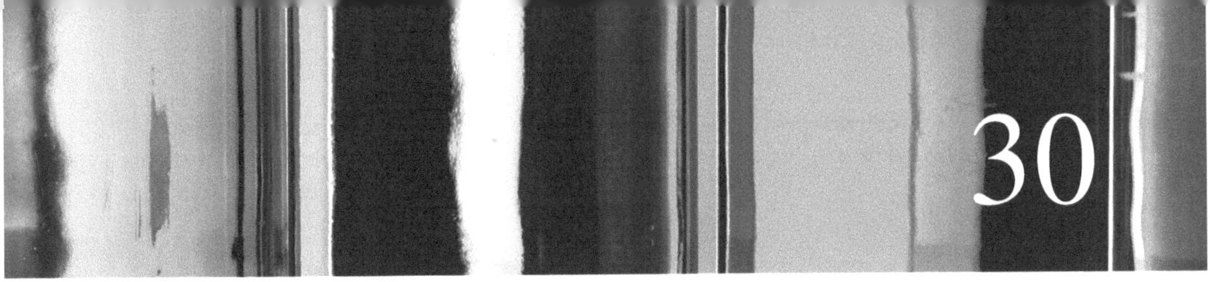

User Perspectives

Bagga Bjerge, Caral Brown and Glenda Daniels

INTRODUCTION

Within the past couple of decades, it has been widely discussed how the perspectives of drug and alcohol users can best be included in public welfare services, service evaluations and policy processes, as well as in non-governmental organizations (NGOs) and private sector organizations. The movement towards an increased focus on the perspectives of users has been debated using different terms such as user involvement, user orientation and user participation, each indicating different levels of participation (Arnstein, 1969; Poulton, 1999). Mostly recognized is perhaps the concept of *empowerment*, generally perceived as a theory of, or a method for, enabling all kinds of users to actively influence, discuss and even take control over important matters regarding their lives (Adams, 1996; Rose, 1996; Andersen et al., 2000). User perspectives, including notions of empowerment are, however, rather fuzzy concepts and are being interpreted and enacted in many different ways (Ward and Mullander, 1991; Sharma, 2008). For instance, the concepts can refer to social movements' fight for participant democracy (Cruikshank, 1999; Rose, 1999; Graham, 2004), user organizations' demands for influence on health and welfare services (Mold and Berridge, 2008; Hunt et al., 2010; Frank et al., 2012) or ways to enable users to gain control over their life via, for example, treatment (Villadsen, 2008; Valenta and Berg, 2010; Bjerge et al., 2014).

In this chapter, we unfold some of the important historical developments and key ideological thoughts, which led to the increased focus on users´ perspectives and empowerment. Further, we address some of the different ways in which user perspectives and empowerment is being enacted amongst service users (SUs) as well as in activist user groups. Subsequently, we provide space for a SU group founder to explain user perspectives from the inside. To conclude the chapter, we critically discuss three types of challenges posed by the interview and literature on the subject.

THE RISE OF USER PERSPECTIVES

Several developments can be identified to have contributed to an increased focus on users´ perspectives. Some developments stem from grass root organizations, new social movements and left-wing aims to decrease 'remote bureaucracies' towards more humanistic perspectives on citizens in need of help (Ward and Mullender, 1991; Adams, 1996; Rose, 1996; Cruikshank, 1999; Graham, 2004). Other developments can be identified as stemming from more economic driven backgrounds and neo-liberal ideas of individual wishes and needs being the driver for society´s development. That is, to enhance individual self-management and freedom as well as to reduce costs of welfare services by tailoring these to the individual person (Rose, 1999; Torfing, 1999; Cruikshank, 2001; Villadsen, 2008; Bjerge, 2012). Common in these different perspectives are attempts to challenge the traditional roles of citizens in need of help as passive welfare recipients. Individuals can then become actively emancipated from the patriarchal (or perhaps rather matriarchal) expertise of welfare professionals. In this regard, the welfare state is criticised for being too rigid and for not including SUs in national or even local problem solving.

Until the mid-1980s and 1990s, the predominant ideas of how to manage citizens in need of help was based on the assumption that 'professionals knew best what would benefit people' (Adams, 1996: 36). Roughly speaking, clients – as these persons were predominantly termed – were not perceived as self-managing, and therefore, needed experts to interpret, define and categorize the nature of their problems as well as the possible solutions to these problems. Clients' needed to adjust to pre-defined services and there was a fairly explicit power relation between client and professional (Bjerge and Nielsen, 2014). Grass roots organizations and civil rights organizations have raised criticism of this prescriptive approach since the 1960s. Right-wing voices have further repeatedly questioned the ideas of the 'Nanny State' and its 'cradle-to-the-grave "coddling"' (Yergin and Stanislaw, 2002: 90). It was not until the 1980s that contours of change in the paradigm could be identified (Adams, 1996; Rose, 1996). In this period the term 'service user', and later 'consumer', began to be used instead of the term 'client', for example, in many social work services. The idea being that when the term 'client' is replaced with 'user', more respect and activity towards the individual is conferred so that they are seen as using a service rather than being a victim in need of help. Morally, the welfare state has to have dialogue with *all* its citizens, no matter how severely marginalized they are (Bjerge, 2009).

The focus on the individual converges with changing ideas of how to manage welfare states more generally. Since the beginning of the 1970s, many Western welfare states – which have expanded widely during the Golden Age after the Second World War – experienced severe economic difficulties due to increasing inflation, unemployment and the decrease of economic resources due to increasing economic globalization (Mann, 1995; Yergin and Stanislaw, 2002). In many countries more and more people became dependent on public services and taxes were raised. That is, the economic costs of the public sector increased and began to challenge the existing ideas of the welfare state. In 1973, the international oil crisis marked a new era. Western economic hegemony decreased due to competition, economic decentralization and strong export of capital towards East Asia (Arrighi, 1997; Robinson and Harris, 2000). Economically and functionally, it became more and more difficult to legitimize public spending. The welfare state became too expensive and inefficient. To accommodate for that, new ideas of how to manage the welfare state emerged, many inspired by concepts from the private sector. Many of the implemented initiatives from the late 1980s and onwards can be understood as part of a new public management (NPM) oriented strategy (Hood, 1991; Pollitt, 2000; Crouch, 2004). The concept of NPM can best be described analytically as a toolbox from which administrators borrow techniques and ideas rather than a well-defined model for public administration. The NPM trend was based on ideas about competition, empowerment, focus on outcome, missions, customers, prevention, decentralization and market mechanisms (du Gay, 2001: 63). The rationale being that if more responsibility and liberty are given to individual users of public services, public spending reduces as less money is needed to ensure the best possible help for the individual. In this perspective, user participation cannot only be seen as a right, but also as an obligation for citizens, including severely marginalized persons, to take responsibility and act more independently from welfare services – and subsequently for the government to decrease support for people in vulnerable living situations.

SERVICE USERS AND ACTIVIST GROUPS

The aim to involve SUs in the development of welfare services has been adopted by many international organizations, for instance, the World Health Organization in Europe, who have recommended the change since 1985 (WHO Europe, 1985). Perspectives of drug and alcohol users have, however, been incorporated less than in fields such as cancer treatment, mental health and older care. Many Western countries have included a stronger focus of SUs in national policies also in the alcohol and drug field (Fischer et al., 2007; Patterson et al., 2009; Thom et al., 2013). For instance, in Danish policies, the Act on Social Services, concerning non-medical issues in drug treatment, states that:

> The aim of help [...] is to improve the individual's possibility to become self-managing [...] or to improve his/her quality of life [...]. Help is based upon the individual's own responsibility for him/herself and his/her family. Help is based upon the individual's need and ability, and help takes place in cooperation with the individual user. (Socialministeret, 2006: 4)[1]

Service users are thus seen as self-managing, and should use their resources to better their life circumstances. Responsibility for change has been increasingly placed on the citizen in need of help and not on the helping profession (for other countries see Fischer et al., 2007; Bryant et al., 2008; Patterson et al., 2009; Van Hout and McElrath, 2012).

Professionals in treatment organizations are encouraged to engage in equal dialogue with users, but are also encouraged or even required to include different kinds of tools to enhance the perspectives of SUs (Fischer et al., 2007; Bryant et al., 2008; Frank and Bjerge, 2011). One such tool can be an individual action plan where goals of a social work intervention are documented, for example, planning in detail how a drug using user becomes stabilized first and then eventually becomes abstinent if that is his or her personal goal. Ideally, the SU will be highly involved in the development of the plan (Bjerge et al., 2014). As a second tool, SUs can be involved in joint meetings and planning daily activities at their treatment centre; for example, planning menus, organizing excursions and discussing ongoing problems. Joint meetings should prepare users to voice opinion and experience how to reach majority decisions, ultimately preparing users toward better forms of self-management (Fischer et al., 2007; Bjerge et al., 2014). A third tool, service evaluations, where individuals are invited to voice opinion and discuss experiences can be used to increase the perspectives of users on quality in local, organizational services as well as in more general, national recommendations or policies (Kolind, 2007; Patterson et al., 2009; Pulford et al., 2011).

There are differences between what has been described above as SU involvement and activist user groups (Mold and Berridge, 2010; Van Hout and McElrath, 2012). The first activist user group was established in the 1970s in Holland (Hunt et al., 2010; Frank et al., 2012). In other countries, such as the UK, activist user groups were established in the 1980s, originally emerging from fears of an HIV/AIDS epidemic among injection users (Mold and Berridge, 2010; Thom et al., 2013). However, a large variety of activist user groups emerged in the 1990s (Anker et al., 2006; Hunt et al., 2010; Mold and Berridge, 2010). Activist user groups do not only address treatment related issues, but have wider political, social and health subjects on their agenda such as rights, de-stigmatization, de-criminalization, increased access to health care facilities and harm reduction. These user groups range from small local or national groups aiming to challenge local conditions to international networks and associations such as the International Harm Reduction Association, International Network of People Who Use Drugs and the European Coalition for Just and Effective Drug Policies.[2] These international organizations have been important players in the emergence of national drug user organizations and many national user groups continue to be affiliated with them (Hunt et al., 2010). Further, these international networks have become more and more prominent with lobbying and participation in policy conferences and organizations. Although, activist user groups are often confronted with challenges in regards to funding, accreditation and visible political influence (Mold and Berridge, 2010; Frank et al., 2013). It is worth mentioning some examples of how user perspectives via activist groups influence decision making processes. For instance, in 1995, the Danish Drug Users Union was invited by the then Narcotics Council under the Ministry of Social Affairs to be represented in the council. The union participated in task groups that discussed a number of drug use(r)-related issues until 2002, when the board was discontinued due to a change in government. This cooperation led to, among other things, a significant report on substitution treatment (Houborg, 2012; Frank et al., 2013). Harsh critique emerged relating to the strict ways substitution policies were managed. It was recommended that substitution treatment should become a medical specialty combined with – not subordinated to – psychosocial treatment or administrative concerns. The legislation regulating drug treatment was subsequently modified, giving drug users the right to complain over the treatment that they received (Houborg, 2012). Internationally, the influence of user groups and networks has been somewhat less direct, yet there still have been important players relating to, for example, the development of harm reduction initiatives (Hunt et al., 2010). For instance, the International Network of People Who Use Drugs are annually invited to speak and participate in the Commission for Narcotic Drugs high level sessions at the United Nations office in Vienna.

GLENDA DANIELS AND THE OXFORD USER TEAM

Having presented a detailed history on the emergence of SU involvement and SU groups, we now give space to Glenda Daniels to present her story. In this narrative, Daniels speaks about how she began a SU group and takes us through her journey of running the Oxford User Team (OUT). Daniels founded OUT, a SU group who promote social inclusion, provide opportunities for people who are overcoming drug and alcohol issues and advocate for local drug/service users to gain evidence based, humane drug and alcohol treatment. The team works with drug service providers, commissioners and related organizations to improve treatment provision and to reduce the impact of drug use on health, safety and social wellbeing of individuals in the wider community. Daniels talks about the difficulties and developments, highs and lows over the years for SU involvement in contemporary society.

Daniels is in ongoing recovery and has personal experience of various treatment modalities including substitution treatment, harm reduction services, residential treatment (Therapeutic Community and 12-step based) and prison drug treatment. She has lived in homeless accommodation and bail hostels and has wide ranging personal experience of being a service user and service user representative. Daniels amongst other things is involved with advocacy, overdose prevention, hepatitis C prevention and care, a school based project where she and her team deliver drug use prevention training in schools, and most recently, a recovery café where other SUs can gain valuable work experience and support at various stages of recovery.

How did you start working in the addictions field?

When I got into early recovery, and was recently released from prison, it seemed like the addictions field may be the only career I would be good at.

I was living in a hostel, by chance I met a drug service worker who had been approached by the local DAAT (Drug and Alcohol Action Team) to do some overdose prevention work and was looking for someone in recovery to help her. I was beginning college, but I was really naïve about (my criminal) offences and how they would impact on getting a job and even a work placement. From my criminal records check, the tutors from the college worryingly said that I wouldn't get a placement so I needed to find myself one if I was to be able to complete this course. Due to my involvement with the OD prevention project, I thought it only natural to do the same with hepatitis C and I began thinking of developing a SU Group. I used this as my work experience and completed the course with flying colours.

If I hadn't started doing this type of work, I may still be using now – I had lost my home, custody of my child and more at this point and this was my last chance to get it right.

How did OUT begin?

There were no SU groups in the south of England except in London. The National Drug Users Development Agency (NDUDA) was the national body and then the Methadone Alliance. The regional manager of the NTA (National Treatment Agency) invited me to spend a day with him, the DAAT commissioner and my mentor. They taught me everything I needed to know about how services were commissioned and monitored. At the time, Models of Care[3] was coming in and it helped me learn what I could argue for and what the evidence base was. They encouraged me and involved me in high level decision making so we felt supported and encouraged that a SU group would benefit SUs in Oxford.

It was going to be a full-time job requiring funding, so we set it up as a charity. Requests started to pour in to share our thoughts on SU involvement and we explained it to commissioners, managers, front line staff and best of all, to SUs themselves. Our regional manager for the NTA commissioned us to create a manual and asked me to work part-time to mentor and assist to set up user involvement mechanisms so that's how OUT began.

Can you give me examples of the types of service user involvement work you do?

Advocacy[4] – Around medication, their script is messed up, or they can't get a script, for instance, waiting times are long. Or their relationship with their key worker has deteriorated or they are generally upset with the services they use. Advocacy relates to the saying 'no good deed goes unpunished'. Services do not like complaints, and feel negatively towards the advocate, so if you, as an advocate receive your treatment at the service, it can suffer because many staff cannot separate you from the job you do.

Commissioning – We aid decisions about which local services would be funded and we help monitor those services. You can have real impact with commissioning – at a tender meeting, you can have seven or eight people and none of them have experienced the treatment that they're reading about and about to fund.

Conferences – I used to be at one conference a month, from the National Drug Treatment or the Royal College of General Practitioners conferences, down to small local conferences. Once we went to Parliament and spoke to a load of MPs. That was probably the most influential one. Now it is one or two conferences a year. SU involvement should be so embedded now that you shouldn't need to have a specialist session but I fear that as the recovery agenda grows, the rights of those users not yet in recovery are being overlooked.

Training – We facilitate overdose and hepatitis C training to current drug users and we train those in recovery who are OUT volunteers if they are interested in becoming advocates. We use standard OUT training and nationally recognized advocacy courses. I most enjoy working with individual SUs, training them to understand their own rights and to get good quality treatment.

How did the recovery café start?

After the Recovery Agenda (HM Government, 2010), we needed to provide real voluntary work if 'full recovery and reintegration' was to be possible. The DAAT funded the set-up. It took about six months to open the café. One big issue in recovery is the ability to gain work and a career – many SUs have lots of transferrable skills, we help them find out what they want to do with their life and with their time every day, it becomes very difficult to maintain recovery without things to do.

Getting a niche in the market is hard. We don't advertise that everybody working there is in recovery. I remember going to the hairdressers and they said, 'Oh, you're not going to have this, that and the other type in there, are you? We won't come in there if that's the case'. So we had to be careful about how we set it up.

How does the recovery café operate on a day-to-day basis?

Some recovery cafés allow SUs to come and talk to other people in recovery. We wouldn't have been able to do it because we're not funded on an on-going basis. We have to have money coming in and we have got to work as a café, otherwise we can't pay the bills. I cover the manager's role as well as my other user involvement work and looking after OUT. We have one part-time paid staff member in the café and every day we have two or three volunteers. Volunteers come from various areas of the community.

When people come, they know that they are going to be working in a café for a couple of weeks just seeing how they feel. Most consider all of the things we do, like the Care Quality Commission work we do, care home inspection, rehabs, hospitals and GP surgeries, etc., the overdose and Hep C training, the advocacy and the school education work. Then volunteers put a plan together that sees them doing a little bit of everything. It's mostly about giving people the opportunity to find out what they can do with their lives. If café work and catering is something that they want to do, great. Others just want to show that they can get up and go out every day and work, get into a routine, function as a normal human being, prove it not just to prospective employers, but to themselves too.

What has your experience of working with local drug services been like?

What people from the NDUDA, the Methadone Alliance, the NTA and our local

DAAT said a SU group was, clashed with what local services thought it should be. They thought SU Involvement was just volunteering for the service you'd used once you'd been off drugs for two years. But SU Involvement is about SUs having a voice in their own treatment, knowing their rights, and services and commissioners consulting and working alongside them to improve provision.

Local services were unhappy about what we were doing and it has not changed since then. For example, if services change what they provide, they don't tell us, the one group they should tell so we can spread the word, you would think they would want us to know. This bad relationship is down to one thing – we raise the issues that SUs are not happy with – we are SUs and should accept what treatment we are given; we are drug addicts after all.

What are relationships between service users and professionals like more generally?

Many SUs have fantastic relationships with their workers and local services, but some do not. For those, more often than not you will be on the back foot. The worker is believed over the SU if any conflict of information or misunderstanding occurs – it would never happen in any other health service.

It doesn't matter what your background is, where you started, where you are now, SUs are always on the back footing. I still have it in my own treatment, after 13 years. My nurse changed again and last week he phoned me and said, 'You've got an appointment' and I said, 'Well I can't come today, I told you this last week, I'm at work and am doing a visit for the DAAT' he replied, 'Oh well, I will trust that you're telling the truth'. He doesn't know me, but automatically I am not being truthful. You would never, ever say that to another patient. The bottom line is you're seen as a drug user so you shouldn't have as many rights. You can pretty much guarantee if you see your GP, once the patient screen comes up, everything you talk about will be put down to methadone or Subutex being the cause. It's very frustrating and very unfair.

What are your links with other local (non-drug) service user organizations?

We don't work with many of them an awful lot because drugs and alcohol are received very differently.

What are your relationships with service commissioners and managers like?

Some are dismissive yet others are inclusive. It is often personality driven. I think it can come down to whether they have a background in drug and alcohol work and how much they get to know you as a person. My experience is great, we've had the same commissioners for a while and they've been very supportive of OUT and of me in general, and of my children and my whole life. But, there are still commissioning decisions to be made and issues to bring up so we have our ups and downs.

Even though everyone says how fantastic SU involvement is, people still think drug users shouldn't really have rights because they are bad people, they should be grateful for getting treatment. Some commissioners are still old fashioned in their approach to SU involvement.

Do you get any support from others?

Not really. The DAAT have been very supportive but now they are in PH (public health) we don't see much of them, their agenda changes when the political landscape changes and that's hard to fit in with at times. You can't get much support from drug and alcohol services because your work conflicts with theirs.

So you have to rely on either trustees or outside support. If you work in drug services, especially in the NHS, they have got clinical supervision, group supervision and others. When you work in small organizations like ours, you don't get that level of supervision and have little support.

What have been the best things for you about running service user-led services?

The best things have been things like our user group being a model of good practice in the country. That was fantastic and it went on for four or five years. During that time, we were going from one place to the next, setting up a SU group in a service or in an area for a DAAT to work with. The overdose and Hep C projects as well, they have been good. It is about being able to have a hand in changing drug treatment in an area for the better – getting things off the ground and letting SUs know that they have rights. In the past it was punitive and non-person centred. People would never have dreamt that they would be able to have a hand in planning their own treatment. Now they wouldn't dream they weren't able to do that.

Having the café has also been good for our advocacy work. People who haven't got a phone, money or who aren't sure where OUT is, still know where the café is. So they will turn up there, they can come in and eat or drink and just wait for me to come. We have finally been able to get the local residential rehab service to send volunteers to us. This is a big achievement because their treatment is abstinence-based and we have people in the café who are on medication. So now the rehab is starting to accept that people in treatment in the community are not going to hurt their residents or be damaging to their recovery.

Another real positive from the café is that we have local people who will come in and say, 'I have got this job. Have you got anybody that would be suitable?' I think we are on our eighth or ninth person that has got a job that way.

Overall, I think our biggest achievement to date must just be that the other local drug services have changed hands many times, but we are still here.

And what has been the hardest thing for you in running service user-led services?

The worst part is how it impacts on relationships with other people in the same field, mostly because of the advocacy. If you challenge people's way of working, they are defensive. I don't think I have met anybody who has worked in SU involvement or advocacy who has said that they are treated fantastically because of the job that they do. You are seen as a drug user and that is never going to change, no matter how much training you do with people.

In terms of the café, the daily business side is probably the hardest part. But that is because I have to deal with everything. People think you go to the suppliers, cook the food and give it out. But there is a lot of behind the scenes stuff and when every staff member working there is in recovery, they come with a lot of issues. Often they just don't turn up. And as soon as somebody gets to a stage where they can come in every day and hold down a voluntary job, then you shouldn't keep them any longer. You should then start pushing them towards getting a paid job. Once you get people who are reliable, you have to encourage them to go, though it would be easier to keep them.

What about funding?

When we first started OUT, we didn't have a contract from the DAAT for three or four years. We would just talk about what was going to happen the following year, and things just happened organically. We were also selling our manual for £200 and people would fund us to train their SU groups. Eventually, we got a small rolling contract. But because of funding changes, our work has now been put out to tender along with everything else. The funding of SU organizations is bad. Once you've been around for a bit, it can become easier but initially, trying to get people to take you seriously and believe in you. As drug users, I think you have to prove yourself more than anybody else.

Do you think all drug users can be involved in service delivery?

I think if somebody is still using heroin and crack daily, it would be difficult for them to take on the running of a SU organization, but they can still 100 per cent be involved in their own treatment and in the services they use. They have the most valuable voice and most important role because they are the people who can get to SUs. But being a user or an ex-user involved in SU Involvement isn't enough to be a support/drug worker. You might be able to deliver some brief interventions, but I don't think anybody should be doing structured one-to-one work unless they have been trained and the next step in recovery isn't really supporting drug users without some time in between.

Has service user involvement changed over the years?

I feel that SU involvement is a lot less now, but I think services are happy with it that way, it gives them less problems. Nowadays hardly anyone ever talks about SU involvement compared with the past. In drug and alcohol services, it's all about recovery involvement. SU involvement isn't as 'sexy' as it once was.

What is the future for service user involvement?

I'm not sure. I think we have come a long way, there are now proper services that are SU-led. But it always seems that drug and alcohol SUs will only ever be allowed to go so far in running organizations solely by themselves. I think that organizations would be a lot more attractive to SUs if they were run by SUs. But nobody is going to give SUs public money. There will always have to be an organization behind it that isn't user led and that defeats the object.

Where would you like to be in five to 10 years?

I would like to have the café standing on its own feet and have OUT in a position where we don't have to run around doing so much work just to keep things going and have funding coming in. That sounds doom and gloom, doesn't it? Actually, it's a day-to-day thing. Some days you enjoy it and other days you think, 'I can't be bothered anymore'. But then I would be lost without it, so I will carry on until I can't do it any longer. Personally, in five to 10 years I'd like to own a home and see my children happy and independent.

DISCUSSION

Glenda Daniels´ experiences with founding and running the OUT is a good example of how user perspectives can be managed. As the OUT deals both with SU experiences and activist activities, it displays how different overall notions can be transformed into local, well-functioning practices. At the same time. Daniels' experiences and opinions point to some of the general challenges that are at play when user perspectives are to be given a more prominent voicc in the drug and alcohol field. One of the main lessons learned, not only from the case of OUT, but from all kinds of user involvement projects is that it can be hard work to implement in practice (Fischer et al., 2007; Van Hout and McElrath, 2012; Bjerge and Nielsen, 2014). Despite good intentions from politicians, NGOs, social workers and users, a variety of different types of challenges can be traced. In this last section, we discuss three of these challenges.

1 One type of challenge is that though user perspectives and empowerment are concepts that have been discussed within the past decades, traditions, experiences and values from the treatment paradigm are still present in the treatment field (Adams, 1996; Bjerge and Nielsen, 2014). As Daniels points out, users often have a sense of being on the 'back foot' in relation to, for example, social workers or nurses. In practice, there are still unequal power relations (Bryant et al., 2008). This is institutionalized by traditions and prior experiences of drug users not being fully trustworthy such as Daniels describes. Being a drug user is still associated with ideas of unreliability in the field. Furthermore, in line with Daniels' experiences, research by Bryant et al. (2008) focusing on user participation in Australian drug treatment suggests that many users do not have knowledge about participation activities available to them revealing a lack of communication between providers and users and lacks higher levels of activities such as, for example, decision-making (2008: 132).
2 Inequality between users and service providers is also institutionalized by policies and rules on, for example, substitution medication and control (Dahl, 2007). Exercising control to avoid overdose fatalities, errors in medication or to prevent substitution drugs from being diverted into the black market are strong elements in these rules (Frank and Bjerge, 2011). However, professionals are often ambiguous about the control aspect of drug treatment, because many of them believe that trustfulness and equality should be the cornerstones of 'real' treatment (Lilly et al., 2000; Frank and Bjerge, 2011). In that sense, inequality between user and professional is deeply embedded in the structural set up of welfare services, whilst user perspectives are promoted as the way forward. Therefore, the promise of user involvement often receives the status as a political 'fetish', as Cowden and Singh (2007: 15) discuss. Politically, user involvement is represented as state of the art in drug and alcohol treatment, but in practice, it has limited impact due to prior traditions and experiences.
3 It is often challenging and demanding for users to act in accordance with the ideas of a more self-managing citizen. As Daniels points out, for example, running the OUT café is hard work, because users '*come with a lot of issues*'. That is, users' lives are often highly unstable, affecting the possible outcome of user driven activities. Similarly, a Danish methadone treatment project shows that giving users more responsibility in forms of participating in joint meeting, taking a more active role in treatment was perceived as being too demanding for many SUs. Some actively chose to 'dis-empower' themselves for periods of time, pushing responsibility back to professionals to lead more stable lives (Bjerge and Nielsen 2014). Grand schemes of user involvement are often scaled down from, for example, ideas of collective decision making and responsibility to more individually based initiatives such as trying to formulate individual aims on a day-to-day basis. Further, as the OUT café shows, active user involvement often relies on a few active and reliable users such as Daniels herself. In that sense, the demands of being active and empowered can be highly difficult to enact when issues such as addiction, physical and mental illness, homelessness etc. are also on the personal agenda of many users (Patterson et al., 2009; Van Hout and McElrath, 2012). As Daniels points out, when users are in fact stable and reliable, it is time to '*encourage them to go*', though the OUT café would benefit from their stable manpower.
4 This leads to the last, more theoretically driven challenge in the turn towards more inclusion of user perspectives. For whose sake are we doing it? Could it be that behind the positive buzzwords and the managerial incorporation of criticism of the treatment paradigm, there

is also still an underlying, societal demand for drug and alcohol users to correct themselves and eventually, through the right kind of empowerment and guidance, become productive citizens (Cruikshank, 1999; Rose, 1999). Being perceived as free and self-managing in contemporary welfare states is strongly linked to discourses of user responsibility; a 'capacity and will to make self-conscious choices' (Villadsen, 2008: 100). The aim of a responsible, self-managing user mirrors the idea that choices are meant to liberate users from the bonds restraining them, including a liberation from the expertise of social workers (Gomart, 2002; Bjerge et al., 2014). Users are subsequently articulated as autonomous, free and self-managing subjects responsible for their own health and wellbeing (Moore, 2009). Freedom to act and rational choice are thus imagined as embodied qualities in individual subjects, all of whom are imagined as sovereign subjects that goes hand in hand with the trends of NPM and a more market oriented welfare state (Hood, 1991; du Gay, 2005; Villadsen, 2008; Bjerge, 2012). This perception of freedom, however, is a negative perception; the individual is only free when he or she acts on his or her own, they are not subject to any external forces upon them (Gomart, 2002: 519–20). That is, the criticism of the treatment paradigm has been incorporated into welfare policies and services based in managerial and market oriented rationales rather than democratizing, grass root driven demands (Cruikshank, 1999; Rose, 1999; Cowden and Singh, 2007; Villadsen, 2008). Therefore, it is worth discussing if the strive to include user perspectives and emancipate users from former ways of hegemonies, can also be regarded as new ways to govern these citizens in the 'right' direction. In the extreme, this would imply that rather than liberating users from the strings of notions of 'normal' citizens in more anarchistic perspectives – for example, via a societal acceptance that not all citizens have to be equally productive in a market oriented sense and live their lives according to majority norms (cf. Rose, 1999) – new sets of tools, strategies, methods and ideas of how to guide marginalized citizens in the 'right' direction are being implemented by the use of empowerment and user involvement.

Despite some negative undertones we can see that there is scope to improve the culture for SU involvement. As should be clear from the article, it is an important but an equally difficult endeavour. Therefore, it needs special attention from politicians, administrators, frontline workers and not least users to be transformed from idealistic notions into meaningful practice. Changing the official vocabulary from 'client' to 'user' and setting up user-oriented initiatives does not do it alone. If the inclusion of user perspectives and empowerment is something that we as society want to emphasize, there is a need for specialist support (based on users and service providers' experiences) to set-up treatment facilities and cafés that recognize users' participation – self-management and freedom are phenomena that come in many different colours and shapes. Perhaps this may help to break down the culture of SUs being on the back foot when working in recovery. Although we recognize that welfare services are constituted by a variety of (often conflicting) policies and services of care, support and control, more political and bureaucratic willingness to experiment and delegate responsibility to SUs seems to be needed if we are being serious about the subject. That is, to make sure that user involvement and empowerment continue to develop and become more than a political fetish or new ways to govern citizens, but something that has an impact on an increasing number of users, such as it has had for Glenda Daniels and her team.

NOTES

1 All empirical examples of user involvement in the drug field stem from research in Western countries, as user involvement in this particular field has mainly been set up in the West. Further, as one of the authors has worked extensively with the subject in Denmark, examples from these studies will used to put our findings into perspective (Bjerge, 2007; Frank and Bjerge, 2011; Frank et al., 2013; Bjerge and Nielsen, 2014; Bjerge et al., 2014).

2 For a detailed description of user organizations, see Hunt et al. (2010).

3 A national framework for commissioning the treatment of adult drug misusers in England, describing best practice in drug treatment provision. Established in 2002.
4 The four mentioned topics have been identified by the authors after the interview.

REFERENCES

Adams, R. (1996). *Social Work and Empowerment*. New York: Macmillan Press Ltd.

Andersen, M. L., Brok, P. N. and Mathiassen, H. (2000). *Empowerment - Teori Og Praksis - Empowerment På Dansk*. Frederikshavn: Dalofo forlag.

Anker, J., Asmussen, V., Kouvonen, P. and Tops, D. (2006). Introduction. In J. Anker, V. Asmussen, P. Kouvonen and D. Tops (eds), *Drug Users and Spaces for Legitimate Action*. Helsinki: Nordic Council for Alcohol and Drug Research (NAD), pp. 5–22.

Arnstein, S. (1969). A ladder of citizen participation. *Journal of the American Institute of Planners* 35(4): 216–24.

Arrighi, G. (1997). *Globalisation, State Sovereignty and the 'Endless' Accumulation of Capital*. Irvine: Conference on States and Sovereignty in the World Economy, University of California.

Bjerge, B. (2007). *Empowerment, selvforvaltning og metadonbrugere*. In B. Bjerge and B. Selmer (eds), *Det Sociale Arbejdes Daglige Praksis. Perspektiver På Brugerinddragelse Og Retssikkerhed*. Aarhus: Aarhus Universitetsforlag, pp. 115–130.

Bjerge, B. (2009). *Mellem Vision Og Praksis: Strukturreformen, Rusmiddelbureaukrati Og New Public Management*. PhD thesis. Copenhagen: Sociologisk Institut, Copenhagen University.

Bjerge, B. (2012). Structural reform as New Public Management policy. Three dilemmas in Danish substance misuse treatment. In M. Hellman, G. Roos and J. V. Wright (eds), *A Welfare Policy Patchwork – Negotiating the Public Good in Times of Transition*. Stockholm: NVC, pp. 181–201.

Bjerge, B. and Nielsen, B. (2014). Empowered and self-managing users in methadone treatment? *European Journal of Social Work* 17(1): 74–87.

Bjerge, B., Nielsen, B. and Frank, V. A. (2014). Rationalities of choice and practicalities of care. *Contemporary Drug Problems* 41: 57–90.

Bryant, J., Saxton, M., Madden, A., Bath, N. and Robinson, S. (2008). Consumer participation in the planning and delivery of drug treatment services: the current arrangements. *Drug and Alcohol Review* 27(2): 130–7.

Cowden, S. and Singh, G. (2007). The 'user': friend, foe or fetish? A critical exploration of user involvement in health and social care. *Critical Social Policy* 27: 5–23.

Crouch, C. (2004). Post-democracy and the commercialization of citizenship. In C. Crouch (ed.), *Post-Democracy*. Oxford: Polity Press, pp. 8–103.

Cruikshank, B. (1999). *The Will to Empower*. New York: Cornell University Press.

Cruikshank, B. (2001). Revolutions within: self-government and self-esteem. In A. Barry, T. Osbourne and N. Rose (eds), *Foucault and Political Reason. Liberalism, Neo-Liberalism and Rationalities of Government*. London: Routledge, pp. 231–53.

Dahl, H. V. (2007). The methadone game: control strategies and user responses. In J. Fountain and D. J. Korf (eds), *Drugs in Society: European Perspectives*. Oxford and New York: Radcliffe Publishing Ltd, pp. 102–15.

du Gay, P. (2001). Entrepreneurial governance and public management: the anti-bureaucrats. In J. Clarke, S. Gewirtz and E. McLaughlin (eds), *New Managerialism, New Welfare?* London: The Open University in association with Sage Publications, pp. 62–81.

du Gay, P. (2005). Bureaucracy and liberty: state, authority, and freedom. In P. du Gay (ed.), *The Values of Bureaucracy*. Oxford: Oxford University Press, pp. 1–16.

Fischer, J., Jenkins, N., Bloor, M., Neale, J. and Berney, L. (2007). *Drug User Involvement in Treatment Decisions*. York: Joseph Rowntree Foundation.

Frank, V. A., Anker, J. and Tammi, T. (2012). Drug user organizations in the nordic countries - local, national, and international dimensions. *Substance Use and Misuse* 47(5): 462–73.

Frank, V. A. and Bjerge, B. (2011). Empowerment in drug treatment: dilemmas in implementing policy in welfare institutions. *Social Sciences and Medicine* 73: 201–8.

Frank, V. A., Bjerge, B. and Houborg, E. (2013). Shifts in opioid substitution treatment policy in Denmark from 2000–2011. *Substance Use and Misuse* 48(11): 997–1009.

Gomart, E. (2002). Towards generous constraint: freedom and coercion in a French addiction treatment. *Sociology of Health and Illness* 24(5): 517–49.

Graham, M. (2004). Empowerment revisited – social work, resistance and agency in black communities. *European Journal of Social Work* 7(1): 43–56.

HM Government (2010) Drug Strategy 2010: Reducing Demand, Restricting Supply, Building Recovery: Supporting People to Live a Drug Free Life. HM Government. ISBN Number: 978-1-84987-388-8

Hood, C. (1991). A public management for all seasons? *Public Administration* 69: 3–19.

Houborg, E. (2012). The political pharmacology of methadone and heroin in Danish drug policy. *Contemporary Drug Problems* 39: 155–92.

Hunt, N., Albert, E. and Sanchez, V. M. (2010). User involvement and user organizing in harm reduction. In T. Rhodes and D. Hedrich (eds), *Harm reduction: Evidence, Impacts and Challenges*. Luxembourg: European Monitoring Centre for Drugs and Drug Addiction, pp. 333–54.

Kolind, T. (2007). Form or content: the application of user perspectives in treatment research. *Drugs: Education, Prevention and Policy* 14(3): 261–75.

Lilly, R., Quirk, A., Rhodes, T. and Stimson, G. (2000). Sociality in methadone treatment: understanding methadone treatment and services delivery as a social process. *Drugs: Education, Prevention and Policy* 7: 163–78.

Mann, M. (1995). As the twentieth century ages. *New Left Review* (I/214): 104–24.

Mold, A. and Berridge, V. (2008). 'The rise of the user'? Voluntary organizations, the state and illegal drugs in England since the 1960s. *Drugs: Education, Prevention and Policy* 15(5): 451–61.

Mold, A. and Berridge, V. (2010). *Voluntary Action and Illegal Drugs: Health and Society in Britain Since the 1960s.* Basingstoke: Palgrave Macmillan.

Moore, D. (2009). 'Workers', 'clients' and the struggle over needs: understanding encounters between service providers and injecting drug users in an Australian city. *Social Science and Medicine* 68(8): 1161–8.

Patterson, S., Weaver, T., Agath, K., Rutter, D., Albert, E. and Crawford, M. J. (2009). User involvement in efforts to improve the quality of drug misuse services in England: a national survey. *Drugs: Education, Prevention and Policy* (16): 364–77.

Pollitt, C. (2000). Is the emperor in his underwear? The impacts of public management reform. *Public Management* 2(2): 181–99.

Poulton, B. C. (1999). User involvement in identifying health needs and shaping and evaluating services: is it being realised? *Journal of Advanced Nursing* 30(6): 1289–96.

Pulford, J., Adams P. and Sheridan, J. (2011). What do clients want from alcohol and other drug treatment services? A mixed methods examination. *Addiction Research and Theory* 19(3): 224–34.

Robinson, W. I. and Harris, J. (2000). Towards a global ruling class? Globalization and the transnational capitalist class. *Science and Society* 64(1): 11–54.

Rose, N. (1996). The death of the social? - Refiguring the territory of government. *Economy and Society* 25: 327–56.

Rose, N. (1999). *Powers of Freedom - Reforming Political Thought*. Cambridge: Cambridge University Press.

Sharma, A. (2008). *Logics of Empowerment: Development, Gender, and Governance in Neoliberal India*. Minneapolis: University of Minnesota Press.

Socialministeret (2006). *Vejledning Om Formål Og Andre Generelle Bestemmelser I Serviceloven. Vejledning nr. 1 til serviceloven af 5 December 2006.*

Thom, B., Duke K., Frank, V. A. and Bjerge, B. (2013). Stakeholders in opioid substitution drug user treatment policy: similarities and differences in six European countries. *Substance use and Misuse* (48): 933–42.

Torfing, J. (1999). Workfare with welfare: recent reforms of the Danish welfare state. *Journal of European Social Policy* 9(5): 5–28.

Valenta, M. and Berg, B. (2010). User involvement and empowerment among asylum seekers in Norwegian reception centres. *European Journal of Social Work* 13(4): 483–501.

Van Hout, M. C. and McElrath, K. (2012). Service user involvement in drug treatment programmes: barriers to implementation and potential benefits for client recovery. *Drugs: Education, Prevention and Policy* 19(6): 474–83.

Villadsen, K. (2008). Freedom as self-transgression: transformations in the 'governmentality' of social work. *European Journal of Social Work* 11(2): 93–104.

Ward, D. and Mullender, A. (1991). Empowerment and oppression: an indissoluble pairing for contemporary social work. *Critical Social Policy* 11: 21–30.

WHO Europe (1985). *Targets For All.* Copenhagen: World Health Organization.

Yergin, D. and Stanislaw, J. (2002). *The Commanding Heights. The Battle for the World Economy*. New York: Touchstone Book.

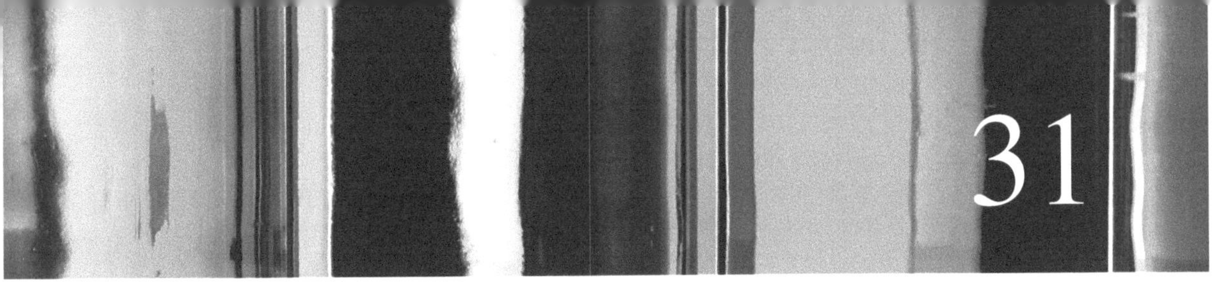

The Relevance of Western Research to Developing Countries: Narrowing the North-South Divide in Drug Policy and Practice

Isidore Silas Obot

INTRODUCTION

Globalization has been a feature of human existence for a very long time. Our forebears had for centuries sought to reach out to people in far flung places for reasons of trade, exploitation of raw materials and cultural exchange. What has changed in recent years is the speed at which this need for socio-economic integration and exchange of ideas and world views has accelerated. There are clear signs of rapid growth across the world in some aspects of modern globalization, namely trade, capital and investment, movement of people and knowledge dissemination (The World Bank, 2000). Today, we live in a world where developments in electronic communications are closing the gap in access to knowledge and, in spite of forces that are uncomfortable with the way the world is shaping up, the march of globalization – the interchange of world views, consumer products, ideas and culture – seems unstoppable.

This chapter focuses on disparities between the global North and South in the availability of knowledge on illicit drug production and psychoactive substance use, and in responses to drug problems. It argues that in spite of globalization, a large gap exists between North and South in access to, and utilization of, knowledge on drugs. Central to the North-South differences and one of the defining qualities of the gap between the two regions of the world is the general lack of evidence-based practices in responding to various drug problems in southern countries. The gaps that exist in knowledge and practice seem not to be affected by globalization and progress in addiction science, calling attention to the need for appropriate and timely interventions at the global level, specifically in the southern hemisphere (Babor, al., 2010; WACD, 2014). Of growing concern is a situation in which a region with the largest population, an increasing use of licit and illicit drugs and a mounting burden of addiction-related health problems is contributing very little to the understanding of these problems. The chapter further discusses the implication of this on policy development, the implementation of interventions and the need for addiction research that takes into consideration the cultural underpinnings and political climate in developing countries.

THE NORTH-SOUTH DIVIDE

The world is divided in many different ways with the most obvious being into continents and countries, but the broadest possible division is into two hemispheres – North and South. In this categorization, the North is made up mostly of industrialized (also known as developed) countries in Europe and North America, while the South consists of a large group of countries in Africa, Asia and Latin America. Population figures show that a highly disproportionate number of people in the world live in southern countries and most of these countries are located in the southern hemisphere. Though this distinction is not totally precise, the 'North' differs from the 'South' not only in population and per capita income but on many other development dimensions. That the great majority of southern countries are usually described as 'developing' or 'less developed' and share the characteristic of being low- or middle-income (LAMI) economies is a reflection of this non-flattering status. This labelling has been described as 'inherently slippery, inchoate, unfixed' (Comaroff and Comaroff, 2012), but it seems to have become an acceptable substitute in many circles for the term 'Third World'.

The North-South dichotomy is no doubt a crude one, but nonetheless, one that has historically defined relationships between the two parts of the world on several economic fronts. For centuries, agricultural products from the southern hemisphere, for example, cocoa, spices and sugar, have fed the appetites of the North, and a certain dependence on southern raw materials by rich northern countries has been a defining feature of the relationship between the two geographic regions. In this age-old economic relationship between poor countries and established economies, both sides have often benefited from each other in ways that are not always easy to quantify but sometimes the relationship has been self-serving, unequal and tumultuous, as best illustrated by the colonial experiences of many countries in the Global South.

Out of a total population of 7.2 billion people in the world today, more than 5.7 billion live in LAMI countries and a little over 1 billion in high income countries, that is, a much larger number of people in the world, up to 80 per cent, live in LAMI (or developing) countries in the three continents (The World Bank, 2014). The differences between the inhabitants of these worlds are stark and disconcerting: LAMI countries are mostly of low to medium human development; they account for only 20 per cent of the global gross domestic product (GDP) and, as shown in Table 31.1, major disparities exist in life expectancy at birth, infant and child mortality rates and level of education. In economic and social terms, it is indeed an unequal world, a world in which

Table 31.1 Selected indicators by human development status

Indicator	*Very high human development*	*High human development*	*Medium human development*	*Low human development*
Life expectancy at birth	80.1	73.4	69.9	59.1
Mean years of schooling	11.5	8.8	6.3	4.2
Gross national income per capita (current USD)	33,391	11,501	5,428	1,633

Source: UNDP (2013).

many people continue to live on less than a dollar day, and where the gap between North and South shows little sign of closing.

While a wide economic gap exists, the picture is not totally bleak. There have been positive signs of economic growth in some developing countries in recent years suggesting that the South is indeed rising. A good number of the countries with fast changing living conditions in the world today are in the South, represented more visibly by membership in the BRICS countries (Brazil, Russia, India, China and South Africa), and including rapidly developing economies in Africa and Latin America. Though the speed of growth seems to have slowed in some of these countries, the existence of these pockets of economic progress shows that indeed there is 'a "South" in the North and a "North" in the South' (UNDP, 2013). This situation, together with the presence of a host of other factors that accompany and sustain economic development, has major implications for problems associated with the availability and use of licit and illicit psychoactive substances.

PRODUCTION AND TRAFFICKING OF ILLICIT DRUGS

The economic and overall developmental disparities between countries in different regions and between countries within regions have been part of the human experience for a long time. It is in this unequal world that a global regime of illicit drug control is situated and has operated with little success, in part, because the circumstances in poor southern economies are at variance with northern perceptions and expectations, and also because an age-old supply and demand relationship between the two hemispheres has helped to sustain trade in illicit psychoactive substances. This is the reality that will continue to confront drug policy makers or those entrusted to implement policy. It is a reality that an international control regime that seeks to foist near uniform and inflexible policy on every country and group of people cannot ignore.

In general terms, developing countries have served as providers of raw materials for the production of drugs while the North has provided the bulk of the consumers of finished products, but this relationship, which implies a clear division of labour, is not that simple. On the one hand, consumption of an expanding list of psychoactive substances has increased in many southern countries, and on the other, the North contributes to supply in various ways. For example, in the production of heroin, cocaine and amphetamines, northern countries play a significant role in the provision of precursor chemicals, and the worldwide distribution of ecstasy, initially from the Netherlands, has helped to modify the view that illicit drugs only originate from the South. Therefore, where drugs are concerned, there is no fine line separating producing from consuming countries. This is increasingly the case in several African countries (e.g. Nigeria, Kenya, Senegal) where for years the concern was about trafficking but where substances such as heroin and amphetamine-type stimulants (ATS) are now known to be consumed by a growing number of young people (UNODC, 2012, 2014). It is also noteworthy that in some West African countries (especially Nigeria) there is now local production of ATS based on reports of discovery and destruction of clandestine laboratories by drug law enforcement agencies (UNODC, 2015).

Yet a broad categorization of countries can still be made in terms of roles in the chain of activities leading from production of raw materials to consumption of finished products. Table 31.2 shows the global distribution of producing, manufacturing, transit and consuming countries based on figures published by the United Nations Office on Drugs and Crime (UNODC) and the certification determination of the US Government. Production refers to the cultivation of raw materials such as the opium poppy, cannabis or the coca plant; while manufacturing is the conversion

Table 31.2 Major illicit producing/manufacturing, trafficking and consuming countries or regions for opium/heroin, coca/cocaine, cannabis and amphetamine-type stimulants (ATS)

Drug category	*Producing/manufacturing countries*	*Transit/trafficking countries/ regions*	*Consuming countries*
Opium/heroin	Afghanistan, Myanmar, Lao PDR, Colombia	Iran, Pakistan, Central America, Mexico	Iran, USA
Coca/cocaine	Colombia, Peru, Bolivia	Mexico, the Caribbean, Nigeria, Spain, the Netherlands	USA, Latin America, Europe
Cannabis herbs and resin	Herbal production widely dispersed; resin in Morocco, Pakistan, Afghanistan	Trafficking is widely dispersed in Europe and Africa.	Use is widely dispersed globally
ATS	Europe (amphetamine), China, Myanmar, the Philippines, North America (methamphetamine), Netherlands, Belgium (ecstasy)	Thailand, China, USA, Philippines, UK, Netherlands, Australia, West and Central Europe	East and South-East Asia, Oceania, West and Central Europe, US

Source: Based on figures from UNODC and US certification decisions (various years).

of these raw materials into consumable end-products, for example, heroin, morphine or cocaine. Transit or trafficking countries serve to connect producers and manufacturers to drug markets in major consuming countries.

The primary contribution of developing or 'southern' countries to the availability of drugs globally is in the production of opium and its products, coca and cocaine, and cannabis. Producing countries also participate in drug trafficking but the central role of delivering these drugs to users is often under the control of citizens of other countries who have developed networks to move the drugs through national borders to distant markets. The reality today in many developing countries, as stated above, is that markets are not that distant anymore. Demand for drugs has become a common feature of life in these countries and there are clear concerns about the consequences of illicit drug use leading to global and regional calls for appropriate policies in different regions. For example, the Global Commission on Drug Policy (2011) and the West Africa Commission on Drugs (WACD, 2014) have both advocated for a shift from the prevailing criminal justice orientation to a public health perspective on drug use in addressing the global drug problem.

DRUG USE AND ITS CONSEQUENCES

Globally, between 3.5 per cent and 7 per cent of people aged 15 to 64 years (or 162 million to 324 million) have used an illicit drug at least once in the past year (UNODC, 2014). The great majority of them have consumed cannabis and as the data presented in Table 31.3 shows, cannabis is the illicit substance most often used in the developing countries of Africa, Asia and South America, with the prevalence of use in West Africa (12.4 per cent) more than in other regions and double the global average of 3.8 per cent.

The pattern of illicit drug use globally shows that no part of the world is spared. It seems that in spite of spirited efforts at the global and national levels, the availability of drugs has not decreased in any significant way. Analysts of the UN drug control system and policy makers in countries with drug production and trafficking activities attribute this to a variety of factors, some related to weaknesses in the control regime itself (Bewley-Taylor, 2005) and others to the relationship between demand and supply. What seems clear and occasionally voiced by policy makers and politicians in southern countries is that successful supply reduction

Table 31.3 Estimated annual prevalence of illicit drug use in different regions of the world, 2012 (best estimates as per cent of population of 15 to 64 year olds)

Region	*Opiates*	*Cocaine*	*Cannabis*	*Amphetamine-type stimulants*
Africa	0.3	0.4	7.5 (West Africa 12.4)	0.9
Asia	0.3	0.05	1.9	0.7
Americas	0.3	1.5	8.1 (North America 11.2)	1.0
Europe	0.5	0.7	4.3	0.5
Global	0.4	0.4	3.8	0.7

Source: UNODC (2014).

has to be a shared responsibility between 'supply nations' and 'consuming nations'. From Nigerian drug czars in the 1990s to Latin American leaders, the voices warn that where there is demand supply will follow, hence more work is needed in northern countries to reduce demand. In 2006, a former Executive Director of the UNODC added his voice to this concern by warning that 'while Colombia, Laos and other countries have made significant progress in curbing supply, their efforts are still not reciprocated on the demand side' (Costa, 2006: 6). This call to the West to 'get serious about tackling demand for illegal drugs' also serves as a warning to southern countries that because what gets in does not always go out – they should expect increasing consumption of new substances on their shores. As already stated above and highlighted with the information presented in Table 31.2, this is already happening in many southern countries where illicit drug use has expanded to include imported and local substances with addictive properties (e.g. khat) and new patterns of high-risk use of other drugs (e.g. injection drug use).

DRUGS AND UNDER-DEVELOPMENT IN PRODUCING AND TRANSIT COUNTRIES

The availability of large pools of unemployed youth in developing countries provides ideal recruiting environments for drug production, trafficking and retail distribution. In spite of extreme measures used to prosecute the 'war on drugs' (including long jail sentences and the death penalty in some countries), many young people from poor backgrounds continue to be used in various drug-related criminal enterprises. An example of this is Nigeria where, in spite of heightened enforcement activities over the years, drug trafficking within and through the country has not been affected significantly and, indeed, where new developments, such as local production of ATS, have complicated the situation on the ground (NDLEA, 2011, 2012). Nigeria is certainly not alone in what, according to new data, seems like a failing effort to significantly affect the supply of drugs to markets in major consuming countries (UNODC, 2014).

The involvement of poor countries in the global drug trade has serious economic, health and social implications for affected countries beyond the personal tragic consequences experienced by their young citizens. These negative consequences include corruption (which has a direct effect on economic and political development), weakening of state institutions and loss of social capital or the networks that help to sustain productivity in the population. Worse still, is the fact that the bulk of the profit made from drugs does not accrue to the farmer or the low level trafficker in the South but to dealers in the North, a situation with historical antecedents in the legal supply of raw materials such as cocoa and coffee beans, where farmers are known to earn relatively little for their labour.

Because sooner or later drug abuse emerges in a producing or trafficking country, the impact on health, education, productivity, crime, social cohesion and other adverse consequences is not far behind. While all countries with rampant drug use are witnessing increases in these problems today, the effect is greater in poor countries where there is lack of resources to counter the impact and where there are often no policies implemented to address the problem of abuse and its consequences (WHO, 2010).

NORTH-SOUTH DISPARITIES IN RESPONSES TO DRUG SUPPLY AND DEMAND

Drug trafficking, psychoactive substance use and drug use disorders have become a major issue in many countries across the world and increasingly so in developing countries. It is not surprising, therefore, that there are attempts to address the problem using various approaches. Unfortunately, some of the popular approaches applied in these countries have not proven effective (Babor et al., 2010). In many developing countries, drug control efforts are primarily focused on the enforcement of stringent laws with punishment for various use and possession offences. Overall, there is an over-dependence on ineffective strategies, which have not been shown to be effective either in curbing supply or reducing demand for drugs.

CURBING SUPPLY WITH ALTERNATIVE DEVELOPMENT

There are many strategies that the global community uses to reduce the supply of drugs other than enforcing laws against drug production and trafficking. One of these is alternative development. Alternative development is 'a process to prevent and eliminate the illicit cultivation of plants containing narcotic drugs and psychotropic substances through specifically designed rural development measures' (UN, 1998: 34). It is the responsibility of affected nations but with support from the international community, to use this strategy to achieve two objectives: elimination of illicit crops and the eradication of poverty in communities that depend on illicit drug cultivation.

Alternative development through crop substitution has been known for a long time to have only limited impact in the control of drug supply (Farrell, 1998). This may be due to a variety of reasons: profits from alternative crops tend not to match profits derived from illicit crops and access to international markets for licit crops is limited because of trade restrictions in some countries and regional groupings. Hence, local growers of crops (e.g. coca in Bolivia or opium poppy in Afghanistan) that are used to produce illicit drugs are faced with the dilemma of abandoning a lucrative activity for an uncertain venture, one with the potential of jeopardizing the economic fortunes of their families (Mansfield, 2001).

Crop eradication and substitution might also be seen as an attempt to eradicate the cultural practices of a people and, therefore, for this reason alone is likely to receive little support. For example, plants such as cannabis sativa, coca, opium and khat play social roles in different societies around the world. Resistance to crop eradication in countries where it has been tried is, therefore, not just an economic concern but might be perceived as an attack by the West on the culture of indigenous people. This is the sentiment expressed in the quip about the difference between coca and cocaine: 'yes to coca, no to cocaine'. The fear in rich industrialized countries is, of course, that a Yes to coca is a Yes to cocaine, not only in traditional consuming countries but in producing countries. Here lies another source of rift between North and South in global drug control with implications for curbing supply and reducing demand.

REDUCING DEMAND WITH EFFECTIVE PREVENTION AND TREATMENT

Addressing the global drug situation involves efforts on all fronts and in recent years there has been a widely expressed fondness for an 'integrated and balanced strategy' proposed by the United Nations (ECOSOC, 2009), a strategy in which the gap between supply and demand interventions would be bridged. As stated earlier, demand reduction – which comprises efforts aimed at preventing drug use or treating addiction – has historically received little attention when compared to supply reduction either in terms of national budgets allocated or in the involvement of bilateral partners.

Hence, there are continued deficits in developing countries in the availability and coverage of effective prevention and treatment programmes. From Asia to South America and the African continent, people with drug problems are invisible at best or persecuted at worst. As noted earlier, drug policy in these countries often means drug control through law enforcement and rarely the provision of treatment and rehabilitation services to people in need, even if these people are now becoming more visible by their numbers. And what often passes for prevention activities are awareness/sensitization campaigns using posters, other media or law enforcement officers to deliver messages that aim to frighten young people and keep them from experimenting or increasing their involvement with drugs but often have little impact (Babor et al., 2010; Hawks et al., 2002). For example, several evaluations of Drug Abuse Resistance Education (DARE), one of the most well-known fear-based prevention campaigns, which has been implemented in schools in many developed and developing countries, have shown the programme to be ineffective in preventing drug use (West and O'Neal, 2004).

Lack of adequate attention to drug demand reduction has been a troubling aspect of international drug control for many years. While signatories to the three UN conventions try to observe the stipulations of these conventions in their declared or undeclared war on drugs, they have showed less interest in investing in policies and strategies to reduce demand at home. One reason for this is probably that in many of the developing countries illicit drug use was not a problem of significant proportion until recently. Another reason is that the conventions generally sought not to address demand reduction but to control supply of 'narcotics' and 'psychotropic substances' (UN, 1961, 1971). Hence, local investment, and bilateral and multilateral efforts between producing and trafficking countries and the West, have tended to focus more on controlling supply of illicit substances and less on the local demand side of the drug issue. This lopsided nature of drug control was one of the central themes of the 'Special Session of the [UN] General Assembly Devoted to Countering the World Drug Problem' held in New York in 1998. Although 'measures to enhance international cooperation' in controlling supply occupied the attention of participants at the Assembly, declarations were made that had policy implications for drug demand reduction.

The 'political declaration' that came out of this meeting recognized demand reduction as 'an indispensable pillar in the global approach to countering the world drug problem' (UN, 1998: 5). In the accompanying declaration on the 'Guiding principles of drug demand reduction', principle (a) stated that: 'There shall be a balanced approach between demand reduction and supply reduction, each reinforcing the other, in an integrated approach to solving the drug problem' and principle (b) (i) that policies should 'aim at preventing the use of drugs and at reducing the adverse consequences of drug use' (1998: 9).

In spite of these declarations and action plans the fact remains that while treatment and care are lacking or inadequate in most countries across the world, it is in developing countries that the gap between demand

and availability is widest. This is supported by various global and regional surveys of the availability of resources for treatment and prevention of alcohol and drug problems. For example, in an assessment by the World Health Organization conducted in 2010, 100 per cent of high-income countries reported that they had a national substance abuse policy, 93.2 per cent in the European region and only 32.6 per cent in the African region (WHO, 2010). In Africa, legal and policy frameworks to address drug demand reduction are generally lacking, and when specific components of demand reduction are considered, the regions present a much more diverse picture (Harm Reduction International, 2012), further highlighting the gap between North and South in responding to drug issues, including the knowledge dimension.

KNOWLEDGE AND INFORMATION GAP

The knowledge and information gap between North and South, rich and poor countries, has been an important subject of discussion and action in development circles in the past few decades. Because scientists in poor countries generally lack the capacity and financial support to address the health problems in their countries, a 10/90 gap has developed, according to the Global Forum for Health Research. This gap means that 10 per cent of expenditure on health research and development is devoted to problems that affect 90 per cent of the world's population. Twenty years ago, the World Health Organization noted that 'the regions where the burden is greatest, and changing most rapidly, are severely disadvantaged by the small numbers of their scientists, the invisibility of the work of their scientists, and the lack of incentives for excellence and productivity' (WHO, 1996). Therefore, research capacity building in less developed countries and access to research information for development have become a double plank for a number of global efforts to close the gap. The lack of 'voice' of scientists in poor countries compared to their counterparts in rich countries cuts across all disciplines. For example, out of nearly 90 academic journals that publish addiction science, less than a handful are domiciled in developing countries (Stenius et al., 2008).

In the substance abuse field, systems of regular data collection exist in many European and North American countries and comprehensive regional mechanisms for the evaluation of progress in drug policy and programmes have also been implemented in these two regions. But few of these drug monitoring systems exist in the less developed countries and regions of North Africa and the Middle East, Sub-Saharan Africa and East and South Asia. This is probably not a surprising situation considering that most of these countries also have less developed mechanisms for data collection and reporting in other areas of knowledge. It should be pointed out that there are indeed projects aimed at setting up epidemiologic networks for secondary data and drug observatories, for example, the West Africa Epidemiology Network on Drug Use (WENDU), which is sponsored by the Economic Community of West African States (ECOWAS), but this is still in its infancy.

The chronic lack of data on illicit drugs in poor countries is a major hindrance to how these countries respond to drug problems in their midst. Hence, this divide between North and South in the production and utilization of knowledge from research is an issue requiring attention by both national and international drug control experts. Such knowledge is needed to guide prevention activities, treatment and care efforts that are context specific and sustainable.

PREVENTING DRUG USE

One of the most popular areas of drug abuse intervention is the prevention of use with programmes that typically target young people (especially those at high risk of initiating drug use). For these interventions to be effective, they should take place in a range of settings, focus on a broad range of life-skills and be sustained over a long period (Babor et al., 2010). Unfortunately, what often passes for prevention in many developing countries is actually information dissemination, school education and awareness campaigns, which are usually sporadic and restricted in scope. In many of these countries, prevention is carried out by civil society organizations (CSOs) with funds from external agencies and little support from individual governments (Obot, 2004b) they tend not to be sustainable. In terms of specific strategies, the most popular ones are the use of electronic mass media and posters and the least used strategy is targeting people in the workplace. The statement by the UNODC that 'the consistency, professionalism and measurability of impact of these efforts may provide some cause for concern in some regions' is unfortunately as true today as it was about 10 years ago (UNODC, 2005: 19).

TREATING SUBSTANCE USE DISORDERS

While the issue with preventive interventions is not availability but scope and sustainability, the problem with treatment is lack of it even in the face of increased demand in recent years, a reflection of rising trends in the use of psychoactive substances. Again, surveys of resources for the management of drug use disorders show a clear disparity in the availability of, and access to, evidence-based treatment. This disparity can be seen not only in the number and spread of facilities offering treatment services but also in the number of beds available per population, the lack of trained manpower and the non-adoption of substitution therapy (WHO, 2010) in developing countries.

Surveys have shown that what exists in most countries is some form of medical detoxification, not as a step towards therapeutic intervention but as end in itself. As stated in the 2005 UNODC report: 'Some regions such as Central and South-West Asia and Sub-Saharan Africa seem to rely excessively on detoxification, placing less emphasis on the subsequent stages of treatment and rehabilitation, thereby failing to offer a continuum of care and diversification of services' (UNODC, 2005: 13). More than 10 years hence not much has changed in the treatment situation in these parts of the world – ineffective interventions continue to dominate while effective strategies are neglected and just often ignored by policy makers, for example, harm reduction.

NEGLECT OF SUBSTITUTION THERAPY AND HARM REDUCTION

The term harm reduction refers to the following:

> Policies, programmes and practices that aim to reduce the harms associated with the use of psychoactive drugs in people unable or unwilling to stop. The defining features are the focus on the prevention of harm, rather than on the prevention of drug use itself, and the focus on people who continue to use drugs. (Harm Reduction International, 2015)

The focus of harm reduction is on preventing death, disease, injury and other negative consequences often associated with some forms of drug use (e.g. injecting heroin or cocaine) and not on eliminating use of a substance. It is a pragmatic approach that recognizes that a substantial part of the risk involved in drug use has little to do with the substance itself but with the method and context of use. In spite of evidence showing that harm reduction strategies prevent death and improve the quality of life of persons in the programme, resistance to the approach has remained in many developing countries.

Among the strategies that qualify as harm reduction are methadone maintenance and other substitution therapies, needle exchange programmes, medical prescription of heroin and the provision of safe injection sites. The most well-known and probably least controversial strategy among these is substitution therapy, especially methadone maintenance (MM). Though MM has been practiced for decades in some countries, it is a rare initiative in LAMI countries and illegal in some. Indeed, there are clear differences between North and South and within countries in terms of its availability.

Substitution therapy is perceived negatively by health care workers, policy makers and the public in most countries in the global South because it is regarded as encouraging continued use of drugs. Also, the need for this form of treatment has not always been there because opioid use is a relatively new phenomenon in some of these countries. However, in some cities in countries with growing opioid dependence, such as Iran, China and Tanzania, there are signs of spirited acceptance of harm reduction through drug substitution as an intervention strategy (Harm Reduction International, 2012; WHO, 2004).

DISPARITY IN THE AVAILABILITY OF OPIOID ANALGESICS

On a related matter, there is wide disparity in the average consumption of narcotic drugs for legitimate medical purposes between countries with high levels of development (mostly northern countries) and those with low to middle levels of development. For example, while the defined daily doses per million inhabitants are nearly 11,000 in Germany, 12,545 in Denmark and more than double that (29,5009) in the USA, they are 83 in Mexico, 41 in China, eight in India and three in Senegal. Other than codeine, Fentanyl and Pethidine, narcotic analgesics are not available at all in some of the poorer countries, but in developed countries, there is a rising trend in use of synthetic and semi-synthetic substances for pain and palliative care. In 2000, the 10 countries with the highest rates of use consumed up to 80 per cent of morphine as analgesic; in 1998, the average per capita use in the 10 countries with the highest levels of use reached 31 grams per 1,000 inhabitants. In the next 10 highest consuming countries, the rate was 16 grams per 1,000 inhabitants, in the next 60 countries, it was only 2 grams per 1,000 inhabitants and in the remaining 120 countries, use was almost non-existent (INCB, 2000). In 2007, only six countries (all developed) accounted for 79 per cent of morphine consumption (INCB, 2009; Milani and Scholten, 2011).

According the World Health Organization, about 83 per cent of the world's population live in countries where access to controlled medicines is low or non-existent (WHO, 2009). Of all the people who live in Africa and South-East Asia, for example, none lives in a country with low to adequate consumption of controlled substances; almost all live in countries with very low to virtually no consumption (Seya et al., 2011). And in spite of the increasing number of people suffering and dying from non-communicable diseases in developing countries, the situation has not shifted much, and even with current interest in the popular media (e.g. Guru-Murthy, 2014), the situation may remain so for a long time.

Why does this disparity in the consumption of pain medications continue to exist in a globalized world? There are several reasons. The first has to do with national regulatory and drug control systems that create obstacles in the process of drug acquisition and dispensation. The second reason is the attitude and knowledge of health care workers and policy makers who are often worried about the potential for addiction to a potent medication such as morphine or ketamine, as in the case of China that is currently lobbying for the global restriction of this drug because of growing prevalence of abuse by young people

(Convention on Narcotic Drugs, 2015). A third reason is the extra work involved in administering these controlled drugs. Finally, economic and procurement impediments get in the way of supply even though some of the drugs are now rather affordable (Scholten, 2013). Countries report difficulties in estimating their needs and put up barriers in strong legislations aimed at preventing diversion without adequate mechanisms to ensure utilization for medical and scientific purposes. Because the right to health should mean freedom from pain, the challenge for developing countries is to ensure adequate availability of the drugs and at the same time prevent diversion from legal markets to private illicit use. This can be achieved with a review of guidelines for rational use of analgesics, education of health care professionals (pharmacists and physicians) and training in rational prescribing.

DEVELOPING COUNTRIES AND THE POLITICS OF DRUG CONTROL

Beginning from the earliest days of international drug control efforts, developing countries have experienced serious negative effects of what has become a long-standing 'war on drugs'. Major producing countries in the southern hemisphere have borne the consequences of limitless attempts to rid the world of illicit substances in several ways. The march to a 'drug-free' world has sometimes been seen as a burden on poor countries struggling to develop and this has been a source of conflict between the two sides of the divide for several decades. The most often cited example of how one northern country can influence drug policy in other (southern) countries is the US certification/designation programme, a programme that is known to have played a critical role in bilateral relations between the US and many countries of the South over the years (Obot, 2004a).

As an instrument of US drug control strategy, the certification programme originated from the Foreign Assistance Act (FAA) of 1961, which requires the President to submit to Congress a list of countries engaged in drug production and/or transit with impact in the US and fail to cooperate with the US on the war against drugs. Each year, this list includes mostly producing countries of the southern hemisphere, although being listed may not always affect relations with the US. The President has three options: full certification, denial certification or certification due to 'vital national interest'. A country with significant drug production or trafficking can receive full certification if the country 'during the previous year...cooperated fully with the United States, or has taken adequate steps on its own, to achieve full compliance with the goals and objectives of the 1988 UN Drug Convention' (Bureau of International Narcotics and Law Enforcement Affairs, 2000: 1–2). The certification programme has been widely criticized because it is not always easy to determine cooperation in an objective manner, but also because it often seems to serve as an instrument of foreign policy as well as a drug control mechanism (Ayling, 2005; Nadelman, 1993; Obot, 2004a).

The process of certifying countries was modified in 2002 in such a way that it now requires the President to identify countries that have 'failed demonstrably...to make substantial efforts [as opposed to the more difficult task of "fully" cooperating with the US] to adhere to counter-narcotics agreements and take counter-narcotics measures set forth in U.S. law' (US Department of State, 2002: 1–5). According to the Office of the National Drug Control Policy (ONDCP):

> If a country is not certified, most foreign assistance is cut off and the United States is required to vote against funding by six multilateral development banks to that country. However, assistance may be provided if the President determines at any time after his initial determination that the provision of assistance during the fiscal year is a vital national interest or that the country has made substantial efforts to comply with the standard. (ONDCP, 2006).

The penalty can be stiff and one country that has experienced the intended and unintended consequences of decertification is Nigeria, especially in the 1990s, when the country's drug control officials engaged in extreme measures to achieve certification benchmarks (Obot, 2004a).

Reports of the involvement of Nigerians in international drug trade date back to the 1960s when the popular media carried stories of arrests and prosecution of Nigerians for cannabis trafficking in the UK (Lambo, 1965). What followed in the 1980s was the expansion of trade in illicit drugs to include cocaine and heroin and the image was created that Nigeria had become a significant transit point for drugs heading to Europe and the US (Obot, 1990, 1992, 2004a). Indeed, available data from law enforcement bodies showed large increases in the number of arrests for trafficking in cocaine and heroin through the country, and in 1994, the US government reacted by decertifying the country. For many years after, Nigeria experienced a variety of negative consequences for not cooperating enough with the US in its war on drugs as Nigerian citizens continued in what seemed like their high-level involvement in the global drug trade. The effects were clearly felt as 'decertification resulted in significant economic, social, and psychological consequences for Nigeria and Nigerians', including 'missed economic opportunities, diminished international support for civil society initiatives, the experiences of humiliation at airports' in different parts of the world (Obot, 2004a: 25). A more important consequence in the long-term was that:

> [B]ecause drug control in Nigeria... was focused solely on the achievement of certification benchmarks, a domestic perspective on the solution of drug problems has failed to evolve. Decertification contributed to an existing neglect of demand reduction, abuse of human rights... and solidified a war mentality in dealing with the problem [of drug use] in the country. (Obot, 2004a: 25)

Today, Nigeria is fully certified, but while the overall picture of drug trafficking through the country might have improved (NDLEA, 2012), few would argue that victory has been achieved.

The certification/designation programme is one of many ways of curbing the movement of illicit drugs from the global South to the North but it is not clear how effective it has been in achieving this goal. This programme and other instruments of international drug control and drug diplomacy have been widely criticized by experts from both sides of the divide. McAllister, for example, asserts that efforts to control drug supply 'reflect...attempts by western industrialized states to impose their standards and values upon the rest of the world' (2000: 254). In addition, some critics of the certification exercise argue that political considerations seem to influence decertification decisions; that the exercise is unfair, ineffective and a source of conflict instead of cooperation with developing countries; that it distorts priorities in affected countries seeking to be certified; and that it encourages a war mentality in dealing with drug problems (Ayling, 2005).

The certification/designation programme is but one example of how a policy initiative focusing solely on the control of supply can influence action on drugs in southern countries in a way that does not respond to the needs of these countries. Although there has been much talk about a balanced approach to the global drug problems dating back to the 1972 Convention and emphasized in the Political declaration and Guiding principles of drug demand reduction (UN, 1998), attention has been fixed on the control of supply in most countries. The main strategy to achieve this and, indeed, to reduce demand has been law enforcement. In countries of the southern hemisphere, control policies that focus on repressive measures for curbing production and trafficking do not help these countries domesticate the drug problem even as serious use problems begin to emerge in many of them. What it does is reinforce the impression among policy makers and citizens of these countries that the drug war is a foreign war, fought to protect the interests of northern countries and that ultimately they are the victims of an unjust war. A situation like this does little to limit the problems associated with drugs either in rich industrialized countries with high demand or in the global South currently experiencing increasing problems associated with the use of drugs.

NARROWING THE NORTH-SOUTH RESPONSE TO DRUGS

The United Nations General Assembly Session (UNGASS) on illicit drugs held in New York in 1998 reached several conclusions on the future of drug policy and control. Two of the conclusions with direct relevance to this chapter are the need for an 'integrated and balanced approach' to addressing drug problems and the emphasis on 'shared responsibility'. It is not unusual that disagreements have existed between North and South on how to tackle the global drug problem. Representatives of producing/transit countries have accused their northern counterparts of neglecting demand reduction in their countries while focusing on supply in foreign lands. They point to the fact that the drug question often features prominently in bilateral and multilateral discourse between northern and southern countries. In their dealings with Latin American, Asian and African countries, some Western nations have spoken too loudly in the language of drugs, often to the surprise and consternation of leaders and citizens of the rest of the world, where the major concern is economic development. Not only is the perception that this concern is secondary to the West's preoccupation with drugs, the rest of the world feels that they are being blamed for drug problems in Western countries and wonder why greater attention is not paid to the demand for drugs at home that may be the driver of supply.

In addition, people in both South and North are also confused about an international drug control regime that has criminalized or seeks to criminalize the use of substances that have been part of their culture for centuries. However, because certain types of drug use come at a price to society some kind of social control of availability and use will also continue to be needed. The problem to be solved is how to do this in ways that are less disruptive of individual lives and international relations than we are experiencing today. A successful international drug control regime calls for efforts at different levels and in many spheres of experience to bridge the divide – in perception and human development – between North and South, rich and poor countries.

As earlier noted, one persistent aspect of the drug question in developing countries is the lack of valid and reliable data. The capacity to conduct research and sustain a research infrastructure is sorely lacking in all but a few countries. Support from bilateral partners and international organizations have tended to focus on supply reduction (mostly law enforcement) activities to the neglect of demand reduction and research. Assuming that this focus was driven by the perceived role of southern countries in the availability of drugs and the self-interest of funders, there is reason now for a revision in how drug control bodies formulate and execute country programmes and the kind of support Western donors provide to developing countries. The recent examples of European Union development funding for programmes in Nigeria (EU, 2013) and the ECOWAS region, in which data collection and demand reduction projects feature prominently, is a good example of what future relationships might look like. Also worthy of support are North-South collaborative efforts that aim to build capacity in public health and policy research in southern universities and research institutes, for example, the consortium for advanced research training in Africa (CARTA) (Ezeh et al., 2010).

CONCLUSION

Psychoactive substance use is a global phenomenon and effective responses to the problem (both supply and risky use) require a concerted action by all nations in every part of the world. It is possible to bridge the North-South gap in understanding and dealing with the problem because the differences that currently exist serve no useful purpose in implementing effective and integrated global and national responses. There are countries that are easily identifiable with drug supply because of geography and history but risky drug use has become a problem for all. In 2016, the world will be presented with a golden opportunity to reassess our responses to drugs at the United Nations General Assembly Special Session on the World Drug Problem. With recent well publicized reports by two groups from the South – the Organization of American States (OAS, 2013) and the West Africa Commission on Drugs (WACD, 2014) – the stage seems set for what is expected to be robust and far-reaching debates on current responses to a problem that indeed affects us all, one that requires that we work towards closing the gaps in knowledge and actions that hinder progress towards finding and sustaining effective solutions.

REFERENCES

Ayling, J. (2005). Conscription in the war on drugs: recent reforms to the U.S. drug certification process. *International Journal of Drug Policy*, 16: 376–83.

Babor, T., Caulkins, J., Edwards, G., Fischer, B., Foxcroft, D., Obot, I., Rehm, J., Reuter, P., Room, R., Rossow, I. and Strang, J. (2010). *Drug Policy and the Public Good*. Oxford: Oxford University Press.

Bewley-Taylor, D.R. (2005). Emerging policy contradictions between the United Nations drug control system and the core values of the United Nations. *International Journal of Drug Policy*, 16: 423–31.

Bureau of International Narcotics and Law Enforcement Affairs. (2000). *Majors list and the certification process*. Fact Sheet released by the Bureau of International Narcotics and Law Enforcement Affairs. Washington, DC: U.S. Department of State.

Comaroff, J. and Comaroff, J. (2012). Theory from the South: a rejoinder. *Cultural Anthropology Online*, 25 February 2012. Available from: http://www.culanth.org/fieldsights/273-theory-from-the-south-a-rejoinder (Accessed 30 August 2015).

Convention on Narcotic Drugs (2015). Further information provided by the People's Republic of China on the proposed scheduling of ketamine. Available from: https://www.unodc.org/documents/commissions/CND/CND_Sessions/CND_58/ECN72015_CRP5e_V1501482.pdf (Accessed 31 August 2015).

Costa, A. M. (2006). Drug trade thrives on the West's denial. *International Herald Tribune*, 3 February 2006: 6.

Economic and Social Council (ECOSOC) (2009). *2009 Political Declaration and Plan of Action on International Cooperation towards an Integrated and Balanced Strategy to Counter the World Drug Problem*. New York: ECOSOC.

European Union (2013). Response to Drugs and Related Organized Crime in Nigeria. Abuja: EU.

Ezeh, A. C., Izugbara, C. O., Kabiru, C.W., Fonn, S., Kahn, K., Manderson, L., Undieh, A. S., Omigbodun, A. and Thorogood, M. (2010). Building capacity for public health research in Africa: the consortium for advanced research training in Africa (CARTA) model. *Global Health Action*, 3: 5693.

Farrell, G. (1998). A global empirical review of drug crop eradication and United Nations' crop substitution and alternative development strategies. *Journal of Drug Issues*, 28(2): 395–436.

Global Commission on Drug Policy (2011). *War on Drugs: Report of the Global Commission on Drug Policy*. Available from: http://www.globalcommissionondrugs.org/reports/ (Accessed 20 June 2014).

Guru-Murthy, K. (2014). The African cancer patients dying in unnecessary pain.

The Guardian, 29 May 2014. Available from: http://www.theguardian.com/world/2014/may/29/african-cancer-patients-dying-unnecessary-pain. (Accessed 1 June 2014)

Harm Reduction International (2012). The Global State of Harm Reduction: Towards an Integrated Response. London: HRI.

Harm Reduction International (2015). *What is Harm Reduction? A Position Statement from Harm Reduction International*. Available from: http://www.ihra.net/what-is-harm-reduction (Accessed 31 August 2015).

Hawks, D., Scott, K. and McBride, M. (2002). Prevention of Psychoactive Substance Use: A Selected Review of What Works in the Area of Prevention. Geneva: World Health Organization.

International Narcotics Control Board (INCB) (2000). *Report of the International Narcotics Control Board for 2000*. Vienna: INCB.

International Narcotics Control Board (INCB) (2009). *Report of the International Narcotics Control Board for 2009*. Vienna: INCB.

Lambo, T.A. (1965). Medical and social consequences of drug addiction in West Africa. *Bulletin on Narcotics*, 27(1): 3–13.

Mansfield, D. (2001). Alternative development in Afghanistan: the failure of quid pro quo. Available from: http://www.scottshelmand-valleyarchives.org/docs/nar-01-03.pdf (Accessed 30 August 2015).

McAllister, W. B. (2000). *Drug Diplomacy in the Twentieth Century: An International History*. London: Routledge.

Milani, B. and Scholten, W. (2011). *The World Medicines Situation 2011: Access to Controlled Medicines*. Geneva: WHO.

Nadelman, E. (1993). *Cops Across Borders: The Internationalization of U.S. Criminal Law Enforcement*. University Park: Penn State University Press.

National Drug Law Enforcement Agency (NDLEA) (2011). *2011 Annual Report*. Lagos: NDLEA.

National Drug Law Enforcement Agency (NDLEA) (2012). *2012 Annual Report*. Lagos: NDLEA.

Obot, I. S. (2004a). Assessing Nigeria's drug control policy, 1994–2000. *International Journal of Drug Control Policy*, 15: 17–26.

Obot, I. S. (1992). Ethical and legal issues in the control of drug abuse and drug trafficking: the Nigerian case. *Social Science and Medicine, 35*(4), 481-493.

Obot, I. S. (2004b). Responding to drug problems in Nigeria: the role of civil society organizations. *Substance Use and Misuse*, 39(8): 1289–301.

Obot, I. S. (1990). Substance abuse, health and social welfare in contemporary Africa: An analysis of the Nigerian experience. *Social Science and Medicine, 31*(6), 699-704.

Office of National Drug Control Policy (ONDCP) (2006). *Certification for Major Illicit Drug Producing and Transit Countries:* ONDCP Fact Sheet: Available from: http://www.whitehousedrugpolicy.gov/publications/international/factsht/certification.html (Accessed 15 May 2006).

Organization of American States (2013). The Drug Problem in the Americas. Washington: OAS.

Seya, M.J., Gelders, S.F.A.M., Achara, U.A., Milani, B. and Scholten, W.K. (2011). A first comparison between the consumption of and the need for opioid analgesics at country, regional and global level. *Journal of Pain and Palliative Care Pharmacotherapy*, 25: 6–18. Available from: http://apps.who.int/medicinedocs/documents/s17976en/s17976en.pdf (Accessed 20 June 2014).

Scholten, W. (2013). *Access to Opioid Analgesics: Essential for Quality Cancer Care*. Geneva: WHO.

Stenius, K., Obot, I., Kerr-Correa, F., Furtado, E. and Babor, T. (2008). Beyond the Anglo-American world: advice for researchers from developing and non-English-speaking countries. In T. Babor, K. Stenius, S. Savva and J. O'Reilly (eds), *Publishing Addiction Science: A Guide for the Perplexed*, 2nd edn. ISAJE: London, pp. 37–49.

United Nations (UN) (1961). *Single Convention on Narcotic Drugs of 1961 as Amended by the 1972 Protocol*. Available from: http://www.unodc.org/documents/commissions/CND/Int_Drug_Control_Conventions/Ebook/The_International_Drug_Control_Conventions_E.pdf (Accessed 30 August 2015).

United Nations (UN) (1971). *Convention on Psychotropic Substances of 1971*. Available from: http://www.unodc.org/documents/commissions/CND/Int_Drug_Control_

Conventions/Ebook/The_International_Drug_Control_Conventions_E.pdf (Accessed 30 August 2015).

United Nations (UN) (1998). *Political Declaration, Guiding Principles of Drug Demand Reduction, and Measures to Enhance International Cooperation to Counter the World Drug Problem*. Vienna: United Nations.

United Nations Development Program (UNDP) (2013). *Human Development Report 2013. The Rise of the South: Human Progress in a Diverse World*. New York: UNDP.

United Nations Office on Drugs and Crime (UNODC) (2005). *2005 World drug report*. Vienna: UNODC

United Nations Office on Drugs and Crime (UNODC) (2012). *West Africa – 2012 ATS Situation Report*. Vienna: UNODC.

United Nations Office on Drugs and Crime (UNODC) (2014). *World Drug Report*. Vienna: UNODC.

United Nations Office on Drugs and Crime (UNODC) (2015). *World Drug Report*. Vienna: UNODC.

US Department of State (2002). *International Narcotics Control Strategy Report, 2001*. Washington, DC: Bureau of International Narcotics and Law Enforcement Affairs.

West Africa Commission on Drugs (WACD) (2014). *Not Just in Transit: Drugs, the State and Society in West Africa*. Geneva: WACD.

The World Bank (2000). *The World Development Report*. Washington, DC: The World Bank.

The World Bank (2014). *Country and Lending Groups*. Available from: http://data.worldbank.org/about/country-and-lending-groups (Accessed 27 June 2014).

West, S. L. and O'Neal, K. K. (2004). Project D.A.R.E. outcome effectiveness revisited. *American Journal of Public Health*, 94: 1027–9.

World Health Organization (WHO) (2009). *Access to Controlled Medications Programme: Improving Access to Medications Under International Drug Conventions: Briefing Note*. Geneva: WHO. Available from: http://www.who.int/medicines/areas/quality_safety/ACMP_BrNoteGenrl_EN_Feb09.pdf (Accessed 20 June 2014)

World Health Organization (WHO) (2010). *ATLAS on Substance Use 2010: Resources for the Treatment and Prevention of Substance Use in the World, 2010*. Geneva: WHO.World

World Health Organization (1996). *Investing in Health Research and Development*. Report of the Ad Hoc Committee on Health Research Relating to Future Intervention Options, Geneva: WHO.

World Health Organization (2004). Neuroscience of psychoactive substance use and dependence. Geneva: WHO.

32

The Relevance of 'Western' Alcohol Research and Policy to Developing Countries

Clare Herrick

INTRODUCTION

In their recent work on 'ecological public health', Rayner and Lang put forward the contention that 'there is a battle for the soul of public health as a project' (2012: 58). In large part, and as I will explore in this chapter, this is a battle being waged over evidence: what it is; how it is produced and by whom; its validity; generalisability; and relevance. With the rise and rise of evidence-based policy and evidence-based medicine (Dobrow et al., 2004; Smith and Joyce, 2012), evidence itself has become an important object of inquiry and critique. Yet, despite the swathe of writings that use the terms 'evidence', 'evidence based' and 'hierarchies of evidence', Petticrew and Roberts argue that there is still relatively little reflexivity concerning 'the types of evidence' that such work advocates or rejects (2003: 528). In this chapter therefore, my primary concern will be to dissect the 'evidence' that emerges from, and, in turn, shapes alcohol research and policy. In the process, I will critically reflect on the degree to which this is relevant to developing countries of the Global South. At present, the geographic coverage of alcohol research and its findings is restricted largely to Anglophone and Scandinavian countries. This inevitably raises the question of whether the assertion of Room et al. that 'the *general principles* based on these findings are also applicable in other countries, but the *implementation* needs to be adapted to the specific culture' (2005: 525) has any degree of traction from an interdisciplinary social science perspective. The idea that policies can be universally applied with only the processes of implementation tweaked to account for local culture and context does, however, seem somewhat optimistic. The possibility of evidence being applicable to multiple contexts is constrained by many factors, not least countries' vastly different drinking cultures, political economic structures, regulatory and judicial systems, healthcare provision, public health architectures, income inequality, education and civil society involvement. In this chapter, I therefore explore the argument long made by health geographers and medical anthropologists that *context matters* (Adams et al., 2014; Dunn and Cummins, 2007). Within this school of thought, the possibility of 'general principles' or 'best buys' (World Health Organisation 2011a) for alcohol control policies seems deeply counterintuitive. This is perhaps even more so in the multiple contexts of the Global South where alcohol control policies are only just starting to be developed.

The 2010 endorsement of the World Health Organisation's (WHO) *Global Strategy to Reduce the Harmful use of Alcohol* has provoked concerted efforts to act on and enhance the 'knowledge base' on the 'magnitude and determinants of alcohol-related harm and on effective interventions to reduce and prevent such harm' (2010a: 41). There is no doubt that alcohol control policies are urgently needed in low and middle-income countries where alcohol harms are felt along a host of interlinked domains: health, economic, social and cultural (Herrick, 2014; Parry, 2000). However, the vital question that motivates this chapter is whether the whole population 'evidence-based policies' that currently constitute the global gold standard – controlling access through restricted opening hours and days, increased taxation/minimum unit pricing, government monopolies at the retail tier and limits on advertising, product placement and promotion (Room et al., 2002) – are relevant to those countries that are currently least likely to have the capacity (or, indeed, will) to either implement or enforce them. In turn, this raises far broader points about the constitution of alcohol as an embedded 'wicked problem' (Pennay, 2012; Weber and Khademian, 2008). It is not that alcohol is necessarily any more 'wicked' a problem within developing countries, but rather that the historical, cultural, economic, structural and political genesis of its wickedness often undermines the very capacity of the state and individuals to manage their vulnerabilities to alcohol-related harms. There is also the crucial question of what alcohol policy is supposed to achieve. Should it reduce rates of alcohol-attributable disease? Should it reduce the incidence of injuries, violence and crime? Should it target the infectious or non-communicable disease (NCD) burden or rather be used as a vehicle to reduce health or socio-economic inequities? Countries will all have different priorities in relation to alcohol-related harms depending on how such harms are manifested, yet the overriding public health paradigm dictates that policy should reduce population-scale *total consumption* in order to reduce the prevalence of individual harms (Babor et al., 2010). However, in many developing countries where informal and formal liquor markets coexist, alcohol control policies may be in fundamental tension with the pursuit of household livelihoods (Herrick, 2013). In seeking evidence to support policy development, we can ask what works and for whom, but we also need to inculcate the local contextual factors that might generate unintended consequences from even the most well-intentioned, evidence-based policy.

To explore these ideas, this chapter is structured in three sections. In the first, I explore the nature and use of evidence in alcohol research. To do so, I consider the types of knowledge said to constitute evidence and how this evidence base is collated and (selectively) deployed. In so doing, I critically reflect on the use and possible flaws of a 'hierarchy of evidence', which places systemic reviews and randomised controlled trials (RCTs) at its apex. In arguing the case for the context-specific limitations of relevance, I draw upon recent anthropological work arguing for the importance of 'people-centred evidence' (Biehl and Petryna, 2013: 19). While public health perspectives have long been antagonistic towards the 'problem deflation' tendencies of ethnographic research (Room, 1984), more recent work has conceded that ethnographic approaches may feasibly form 'their own coherent body of scientific evidence' (Schmidt and Room, 2013: 53). This is a significant admission and an important moment for alcohol's inclusion within a rapidly developing 'critical global health' research field (Brown and Moon, 2012). The second section will dwell in more detail on the question of whether this body of evidence is relevant to the multiple contexts of developing countries. It does so through three 'interjections'. The first reflects on the geographical fallacies of the alcohol public health evidence base and the implications of this for the kind of evidence-based policies that become public health lore. The second explores the frequent disjuncture between the intended and actual outcomes of policy recommendations in Southern contexts. To do so, it draws on specific examples from Botswana and South Africa and explores the potential for harms inherent when well-meaning policies have unintended consequences. The third considers how alcohol has become enfolded within debates over globalisation and the 'threats' posed by the rising and uncontrolled consumption of 'unhealthy commodities' (Moodie et al., 2013; Stuckler et al., 2012). The drive to implement alcohol policies in the Global South then becomes an intervention to avoid the same 'diseases of comfort' (Choi et al., 2005) that have befallen the Global North. This raises important and valid questions about the consequences of erasing pleasure, choice and the right to consume from public health framings of alcohol as a problem of, and for, the South. This paper thus makes a case for the importance of different kinds of evidence: non-systematic, anecdotal, individual, local and people-centric in the context of alcohol harms in the South. People, after all, are the ones who drink. It thus only makes sense for people to be placed foremost if research, policy and the genesis of evidence are to be relevant to their everyday lives.

EVIDENCE AND THE 'UNAVOIDABLE SOCIAL' IN ALCOHOL RESEARCH

In January 2014, news stories in the UK reported on collusion between the government and the alcohol industry in killing off plans to introduce minimum unit pricing (MUP), based on a feature piece published in the *British Medical Journal* (Gornall, 2014). The article had a media teaser that offers a good starting point for this exploration of the nature of evidence and its complex relationship with alcohol research and policy. The short description of Gornall's paper states that 'politicians ignored the strong public health evidence in favour of protecting the interests of industry', despite pledging its commitment to evidence-based policy in general and MUP in particular in its 2010 general election campaign. This media teaser is significant to this chapter for two reasons. First, it begs an exploration of not just the 'strength' of the public health evidence, but also the nature of the evidence itself. And, second, given the mantra of evidence-based policy, it raises the question of how, if the evidence was so 'strong', it could plausibly have been ignored. These two points are worth considering in turn. In 2012, the government further confirmed its commitment to MUP in its *Alcohol Strategy* (Home Office, 2012). To do so, it cited evidence of the policy's potential impact on crime and alcohol-related mortality modelled by the same Sheffield Study (SS) that had been commissioned by the Labour government in 2008 (Meier et al., 2009). In the SS, the authors undertook a series of systematic reviews and 'reviews of reviews' of the evidence base in three areas: the effect of pricing and taxation on alcohol consumption, the effect of promotion on alcohol consumption and the effect of alcohol consumption on alcohol-related harms. The inclusion criteria for studies was fourfold: systematic review, research study, data analysis (quantitative) and economic study. In their report, the authors note a number of limitations to the methodology, notably proving causality, the consistency of effects, the difficulties of establishing the existence of a dose-response relationship (and therefore causality) and, finally, the difficulty of developing true experimental conditions when exploring policy and health/behavioural factors. From these reviews, the authors then developed a series of policy statements that were used to steer political commitment to MUP until its unexpected demise.

With respect to the relationship between pricing/tax and consumption/harms, the SS included 284 studies running from 1945 to 2003 from the UK, Australia, Switzerland and the USA. While the evidence base was significant in its magnitude, the authors were cautious about its significance. By way of summary, they tacitly stated:

> When other factors remain unchanged, an increase in price has *generally* led to a decrease in alcohol consumption, and a decrease in price has *usually* led to an increase in alcohol consumption, with the size of the elasticities *sometimes* dependent on the relative presence or absence of other alcohol policy measures. (Meier et al., 2009: 31; emphasis added)

To this, they then added the further caveat that changes in consumption may be reflective of broader societal and socio-economic shifts – such as changes in anti-alcohol sentiment – and not just pricing mechanisms. In light of these uncertainties, the report still makes the very certain evidence statement that 'there is *strong and consistent* evidence to suggest that price increases (including through taxation) have a *significant effect* in reducing demand for alcohol' (Meier et al., 2009: 33). I flag up these two statements to highlight how 'generally', 'usually' and 'sometimes' can seamlessly transmogrify into 'strong and consistent' and 'significant effect' over the space of a few pages. This is not a prelude to a dissection of the methodologies of the study, which have been roundly and unsurprisingly critiqued by right-wing think tanks including the Adam Smith Research Group (2012) and the Centre for Economics and Business Research in a report commissioned by SAB Miller (2012). Instead, I highlight the rapid segue from uncertainty to certainty in order to demonstrate that policy is not always reflective of the state of knowledge or the certainty of the evidence base, but rather appeasing the conflicting social, economic and political needs of a host of actors (Smith, 2014).

It was perhaps inevitable that the Coalition government would announce a U-turn on its commitment to MUP and, in July 2013, they stated their concern that it would 'penalise responsible drinkers'. Instead of MUP, they announced a plan to ban 'below-cost sales' as a result of the findings of its consultation process. In the report outlining the findings of the consultation process, The Home Secretary Teresa May's foreword said:

> That consultation has…not provided evidence that conclusively demonstrates that Minimum Unit Pricing (MUP) will actually do what it is meant to: reduce problem drinking without penalising all those who drink responsibly. In the absence of that empirical evidence, we have decided that it would be a mistake to implement MUP at this stage. We are not rejecting MUP – merely delaying it until we have conclusive evidence that it will be effective. (Home Office, 2013: 3)

From an evidence-based policy perspective, the decision seems somewhat counterintuitive. At the time of the U-turn, the SS authors issued a press release defending the integrity of their research and stating that banning below-cost sales would be 40 to 50 times less effective than a MUP of 45p in terms of hospital admissions, crimes and deaths per year (The University of Sheffield, 2013). The press release was embargoed by the government until two days after the announcement of the U-turn. At this point, the few remaining public health groups on the government's alcohol 'Responsibility Deal' pulled out in protest. Gornall's comprehensive exposé of this messy process clearly highlights the influence the liquor industry had in derailing the MUP plans and ensuring continued partnership and self-regulation. This will no doubt confirm fears of those arguing that the WHO needs to be free from industry influence (Babor et al., 2013), especially as industry is starting to play a policy advisory role in many countries (Bakke and Endal, 2010; Holden et al., 2012). The fall of MUP also demonstrates the industry's tactic of casting doubt on the evidence – a tried and tested method long used by the tobacco trade. It is not my intention to dwell on the lobbying role and tactics of the liquor industry, which have been ably discussed elsewhere (Casswell, 2013), but rather to highlight how the perpetual limitations of evidence can be used in the service of dismantling potentially unpopular policy choices. For, as Marmot has asserted, sometimes 'the policy implications of the science may well [influence] their view of the evidence' (Marmot, 2004: 907). David Cameron's assertion in a March 2012 speech that 'the responsibility of being in government isn't about doing the popular thing, it's about doing the right thing' (Prime Minister's Office, 2012), thus rings hollow in this case. Yet, what is the 'right thing'? Acting on evidence, however imperfect? Acting in advance of perfect evidence (accepting that such a thing is impossible) along the lines suggested by the precautionary principle? Or, discounting the evidence to appease voters in advance of a re-election campaign? Gornall's piece overwhelmingly confirms the latter.

The MUP case also, importantly, highlights the very weaknesses of what we might call the 'evidence system'. In this system, evidence is ordered into a hierarchy in which systematic reviews and meta-analyses sit at the top, followed by RCTs, cohort studies, case-control studies, cross-sectional studies and case reports (Petticrew and Roberts, 2003). Essentially, this hierarchy 'relies on study design as a marker for the credibility of evidence' (2003: 527) without due thought for the notion that different types of research problem are rarely or meaningfully amenable to a universal set of methodologies. Systematic reviews, for example, are roundly critiqued by Petticrew for often concluding 'that little evidence exists to allow the question to be answered' (2003: 756), a problem that is even more common in relation to public health interventions where there are often very few intervention evaluations to actually review. While systematic reviews are only as strong as the studies that comprise them, Petticrew argues that they 'do not replace judgment or compassionate reasoning, and absence of clear evidence from systematic reviews does not mean that inertia is the recommended course of action' (2003: 758). Rather, actions should be guided by the best *available* evidence. This is also important with respect to RCTs, which have come under particular scrutiny from critical medical anthropologists. In their 2013 edited volume, *When People Come First,* Biehl and Petryna take on the hegemony of RCTs within the public health and biomedical landscape and draw attention to the implications of their dominance for theory, practice and the ethics of research. They argue that the current landscape of global health research and funding priorities (which have largely been shaped by Millennium Development Goals) prioritises RCTs as a 'theoretical and technical fix' (2013: 8). As a consequence, they suggest that 'biosocial approaches to disease and health that could help to specify dynamic causal connections and local politics are relegated to the low-authority category of "soft science"' (2013: 8). Indeed, and as they continue, 'the fine-grained excesses of lives and stories are often smoothed over or averaged out by course-grained statistics and plans. Ethnographic granularity impedes generalizable knowledge' (2013: 17). For anthropologists of global health as well as geographers and sociologists, the discounting of qualitative research as evidence is inherently problematic. More than this, from a social science perspective, it is nonsensical when public health problems are, at root, those of the choices people make and the consequences of those choices made by others.

People are, ironically therefore, often an impediment to the progress of public health. By this I mean that if policy requires evidence and evidence requires adherence to the strict principles of systematic reviews or RCTs, then as Adams et al. argue, 'some health problems will never be addressed simply because they cannot generate good numbers' (2014: 190). One of the chief impediments to the production of the kind of numbers required is the complex reality of human 'experience and its contextual contingencies' (2014: 191) that condition the efficacy and effect of any health intervention. As Biehl and Petryna argue, health outcomes are 'multi-layered and multiply determined' (2013: 13) and, as a result, the interplay of local conditions, individual knowledge and experience - or what they aptly term 'the unpredictable social' (2013: 18) – represent the inconvenient truth that will always limit the evidence base as currently conceived. Anthropologists have long argued for the importance of ethnographic research in drawing attention to the local-scale granularity, contingency and detail that helps narrate the everyday lives in which decisions are made (or constrained), risks taken and harms generated. More recently, however, a number of medical anthropologists have drawn critical attention to the global health research field and the limitations posed by its own prerequisites for what constitutes evidence (Farmer, 2004; Nguyen and Peschard, 2003). Biehl and Petryna speak well for this school of thought when they argue that 'in an atmosphere that gives its first allegiance to quantifiable, volume-based audits or replicable scientific knowledge, ethnographic evidence is readily seen as anecdotal and exceptional, unreliable on account of its granularity or the wiliness of its subjects' (2013: 16). This hierarchy of knowledge and evidence thus has consequences. It potentially stops important research questions, for which experimental methods are unsuitable, from being asked. It effectively silences the voices of those who suffer, to whom Paul Farmer and others have long argued that public anthropologists have a moral duty (Farmer, 2004; Janes and Corbett, 2009; Quesada et al., 2011). It contains no capacity or will to register and make sense of individual opinion, experience, explanation, contingency and choice – all the potential mechanisms by which interventions get translated into outcomes. Thus, the evidence base neither expands nor deepens, but rather the 'gaps' in evidence are perpetually highlighted, the need for more research constantly reiterated and remaining knowledge gaps invoked in support of policy caution or inaction. There is very little 'truth' or absolute 'reliability' in evidence relating to complex human behaviours, only a best guess as to which policies might plausibly generate favourable outcomes for the greatest number (without widening inequalities) given the prevailing social and economic conditions.

At present, there is a glaring gap in the evidence base in relation to alcohol consumption, policy and alcohol-related harms from countries of the Global South. This is clearly intensely problematic when the WHO is pushing forward its *Global Strategy* on alcohol and the post-2015 development goals may well catalase the reorientation of global health research and funding. One of the reasons the evidence base in developing countries is so limited is that alcohol research currently falls outside the global health remit by virtue of its categorisation as a risk factor for the global chronic disease burden (Parry et al., 2011). However, should NCDs be incorporated within the revised post-2015 sustainable development goals, this may well lift alcohol from the global health hinterland and into the core of a vastly reworked vision of the key developmental and public health challenges facing the South. At present, tuberculosis, HIV/AIDS and malaria together comprise 80 per cent of all global health funding (Moran et al., 2009). Maternal and child health and vaccinations have more recently been added to this triumvirate by the Gates Foundation, but this has done little to stem the growing concern that the prioritising of technological fixes to complex 'bio-social' health problems is diverting attention from the upstream social determinants of health (McCoy et al., 2009). This, in turn, further disconnects the reality of people's lives and the conditions that structure wellbeing from the concerns of the global health world (Horton, 2013: 509). This is at least the case insofar as global health research structures favour 'outcome investing', 'actionable measurement' and 'generating quality evidence' (Bill and Melinda Gates Foundation, 2014). This commitment to measurement and evaluation is nothing less than laudable. However, it leaves little space to research people and the intersections between their frequently illogical and unpredictable behaviours and their lived realities. At a time of concern with inequality and health justice (Khoo, 2013), the search for the general may well impede the discovery of the particular, the different and divergent. Indeed, as Biehl and Petryna argue:

> The human populations that constitute the subjects of health and development plans are not just the source of problems or so-called cultural obstacles. Their experiential and practical knowledge, all too readily dismissed by champions of quick technical fixes and measurable, generalizable results, can transform paradigms and may well provide the keys to effective solutions. (Biehl and Petryna 2013: 14)

Their work echoes that of Abdu-Maliq Simone's (2010) writings on the city in which he argues that individuals perpetually and inevitably evade the capacity to govern them. This is both a problem, but also a vivacious source of 'cityness' that is one of the defining characteristics of human inhabitation. Turning people from a problem into a solution is thus one element of the global health repertoire that is currently lacking. Alcohol may well be a good starting point in this endeavour.

TRANSLATING EVIDENCE TO EVIDENCE-BASED POLICY IN THE GLOBAL SOUTH

In this final section, I will explore how alcohol has been conceptualised as a particular problem of, and for, countries of the Global South, and how evidence has been implicated within this. I do this through three interjections. First, I consider the geographical fallacies inherent within the alcohol public health evidence base and the ways in which crucial contextual differences may be subsumed within ways of thinking that prioritise the regional over the local. Second, I explore the frequent disjuncture between the evidence base and the reality of its application in fundamentally different contexts. To do so, I draw on specific examples from Botswana and South Africa to examine the unintended consequences of policies. Third, I examine how alcohol has become embroiled in debates over globalisation and the threats posed by development. The evidence base from the Global North suggests that, as incomes rise, so too do levels of consumption. If we subscribe to the population-level model of harms, then rising overall consumption will result in greater harms. As such, the drive to implement alcohol policies in the Global South becomes as much about reducing harms as it does intervening to evade the fate of 'high consumption' countries in western and eastern Europe. This then raises essential questions concerning the importance of demand and pleasure in consumption choices, even amid conditions of poverty and underdevelopment. Alcohol consumption and its harms are often cast as a fundamentally *different* problem when considered in developing countries. While this is correct to a degree, overplaying the differences misses the important synergies between drinkers in both hemispheres. Questions of pleasure are all too often erased in the context of development, where meeting basic needs is seen as more immediate than attending to desires.

Alcohol-related harms emerge as much from choice as circumstance and alcohol control policies have long skirted the need to reconcile the demands of both to achieve positive outcomes for human health and wellbeing.

The geographical fallacies in public health thought

One component of the evidence problem that has been largely ignored by the public health community is the classificatory mechanisms of surveillance data. Our geographical imaginations are corralled by these ways of knowing, such that the world is reduced to WHO regions, World Bank regions, World Bank income bands or even Millennium Development Goal regions. Data is sliced along these constructed lines, creating a vision of the world in which the 47 countries of the African region might be meaningfully compared to the 35 countries of the Americas region. While national data on alcohol consumption and harms allows for cross-country comparisons, there is a broader point to be made here about the ways in which public health data contributes to geographical imaginations of the Global South. The term 'Global South' is, itself, a 'polythetic category' with its members sharing 'one or more – but not all, or even most – of a diverse set of features' (Comaroff and Comaroff, 2012: 126). Often, these countries have only a history of colonisation or protectorate status in common. Thus, the Global South is really only meaningful in relation and opposition to the Global North. Yet, as Comaroff and Comaroff further argue, this is an 'opposition that carries a great deal of imaginative baggage congealed around the contrast between centrality and marginality, free-market modernity and its absence…it obscures as much as it describes' (2012: 126). The label thus reflects a *relationality,* rather than a meaningful category in and of itself. This point is important because the mechanisms and language by which the public health field constructs and presents the objects of its actions can have profound implications for the types of policy and implementation activities that are undertaken and the complex consequences that can result.

At a most basic of levels, engaging with these ideas suggests that even the title of this chapter needs scrutiny. Thus, instead of asking whether Western research and policy is relevant to developing countries, we might rightly ask about the relevance of developing countries to Western alcohol research and policy. Or, put another way, what can the experiences of liquor in the South reveal about the gaps and limits to our current knowledge or evidence base on alcohol and preventing its harms? In the first place, this would mean breaking apart the regionalist fallacy that says we can think of developing countries or the Global South as a geographic, economic, cultural and political entity that exists in contradistinction to a developed Global North. It would also mean reconsidering the extent to which countries of the South have similar cultural relationships to alcohol, drinking occasions and harms, as well as shared constraints with respect to enacting alcohol policies. All too often when reading of 'alcohol in developing societies', there is a marked tendency to generalise and extrapolate across whole regions and continents. For example, writing about Uganda's standing as the country with the world's highest prevalence of alcohol-related harms according to cross-national comparative studies (Graham et al., 2011), Swahn and Tumwesigye suggest that 'the prevalence and urgency of these problems underscore the need for a more targeted vision for alcohol research, also for the need for evidence-based policies and prevention efforts across sub-Saharan Africa' (2013: 14).

Two thoughts spring to mind in relation to their statement. First, there are only seven African countries that are *not* categorised as being in its Sub-Saharan region and, second, while it would be valuable to know more about the nature and harms associated with alcohol in the majority of African countries, what data would we need and how would it have to be collected in order to be considered bona fide evidence? In reality, there are a number of 'evidence-based policies and prevention efforts' already in place in Sub-Saharan Africa: high taxation in Botswana, controls on liquor access in Zimbabwe, reformed licensing regulations in South Africa and advertising restrictions in the Gambia. However, there are only nine countries in the region with written national alcohol policies, although 41 out of 45 countries have licensing systems. Action on alcohol is happening in Africa, however a recent inaugural meeting of the East African Alcohol Policy Network points to a far bigger problem. A press release of the meeting laments that 'from the presentations made at the conference, it is clear that there is lack of alcohol-related research to support policy formulation' (Hyde, 2012). This statement directly contradicts the WHO claim that the evidence base is sufficient to implement its best buy policies. The question remains the degree to which the evidence marshalled by the WHO is relevant to East Africa and why this is important.

When evidence does not work

Room et al. (2002) argue that it would be helpful to develop 'evidence of how people actually use alcohol in their daily lives'. This is the kind of 'people-centred evidence' (Biehl and Petryna, 2013) that is the *sine qua non* of anthropological research but, until recently, was anathema to public health. This type of qualitative evidence is often best derived from ethnographic work, the kind of 'slow research' recently advocated by Adams et al. (2014) for moral as well as intellectual reasons. Indeed, to take an example, although alcohol taxation is advocated as a win-win within alcohol policy 'best buys' as it generates government revenue (which ideally should be ploughed into health promotion activities), but it should also reduce alcohol consumption among those that drink the strongest and potentially most harmful drinks. However, while studies of alcohol's price elasticity often emerge from 'natural experiments' in countries such as Russia where significant climbs in mortality rates in the early 1990s have been ascribed to the relaxation of strict alcohol control regulations as part of wider economic reforms, there have been no studies in countries of the South. It is important to note here that there is some residual uncertainty about whether declines in alcohol control were a *causal* factor for rising Russian mortality rates or a mediating factor linking 'mass psychological stress' (Shkolnikov et al., 1998) with the socio-economic, political, labour-market and cultural shifts that happened after the breakup of the Soviet Union. For many developing countries however, raising tax on liquor may not reduce consumption. Instead, it may prove regressive as well as having a series of unintended, negative consequences. In countries where the illicit or informal trade is well developed, the point of taxation is blurred as the retail sector is often outside the purview of the treasury and local authorities. Moreover, when prices increase, people tend to move to cheaper and stronger forms of alcohol (Meier et al., 2009). Where the illicit or counterfeit trade flourishes, this will not necessarily be to weaker forms of alcohol (i.e. strong cider or spirits to beer), but rather strong, unregulated and potentially harmful products.

This has been a particular problem in South Africa, where a legislative gap enabled the production of unregulated 'ales' of unknown strength and provenance. These products started to be retailed through formal channels and took a significant market share among poorer drinkers before authorities introduced a legal definition of 'ale'. In countries where very high rates of tax have been imposed, such as Botswana – which now has a 50 per cent levy on alcohol – there has been anecdotal reports of people crossing the border to drink as well as shifting to cheaper, strong brands of beer (Burgis, 2009). Indeed, this was repeatedly confirmed by interviewees in my own research in the capital, Gaborone, in 2014. In both these cases, however, we know very little about the decision-making processes and trade-offs that people make in choosing what and how much to drink. Put a different way, we know little about how rates of tax on discretionary (but socially normalised and desirable) products affect everyday practices and experiences. Higher tax and stretched household resources might mean that women have to go without food more often when men drink. It might also mean that children's school fees are paid in arrears (if at all) and parents might not be able to afford text books and uniforms. There is rarely a linear and logical relationship between price shifts and consumption habits as people make exceptions, compromises and trade-offs to ensure access to necessities or rare pleasures. To assume that rational economic man is at play is to thoroughly obscure the effects of people's inherent irrationality, a point that Thaler and Sunstein (2008) have made in their attempts to secure the global dominance of 'nudge' theory.

Another 'best buy' in alcohol policy concerns restricting access to liquor through controls on supply. This means limiting the opening hours and days of sale for off and on-trade premises and regulating outlet density through controls on licenses. The argument is that when liquor is harder to obtain, consumption among the whole population will fall and, as a result, harms. This intervention is seen as 'highly cost-effective, but also feasible and appropriate to implement with local LMIC health systems' (World Health Organisation, 2011a: 7). Obviously for this policy to be feasible, countries need not only to have licensing systems, but these systems need to effectively implemented and, most crucially, enforced. A licensing system in name only is ineffectual without fair and transparent enforcement. However, the ways in which these policies are enforced is also crucial to their success. As an example, together with colleagues, I have explored the unintended consequences of South Africa's Western Cape Liquor Act of 2012. The Act was imposed with the intention of regularising South Africa's huge informal liquor sector and the harms that are said to emanate from it. South Africa has extremely high rates of alcohol-related injury and violence, as well as road traffic fatalities (Matzopoulos et al., 2008a, 2008b; Seedat et al., 2009). These problems are often attributed to a culture of drinking in which weekend-long binges are commonplace (Parry, 2005; Parry et al., 2005) and violence is already a significant and endemic problem.

With respect to the 'evidence' needed to support restrictions on opening hours, reference is often made to the effect of prohibiting the sale of liquor after 11pm in Diadema, Brazil, in 2002, where rates of homicide are comparable to many urban centres in South Africa. The paper by Duailibi et al. (2007) shows that monthly assault rates fell substantially after the imposition of the law and murders fell by 44 per cent. However, closer inspection of the study's findings begs the question of whether these trends were particular to Diadema or reflective of wider falls in crime rates over the same period, especially after the 2004 enactment of tougher gun laws. This is pertinent as the major fall in assault rates only happened two years after the change in closing time. The authors also concede that it is possible that violent individuals may have started to drink elsewhere once restrictions were imposed, thus relocating crime. They also note uncertainty over the link between the opening hours and the fall in assaults against women, stating that 'although the data were consistent with a sizeable reduction in assaults against women, we are less certain that this effect was a result of the new law' (2007: 2279). For the purposes of this chapter, it is important to note that these limitations and uncertainties as to the conclusiveness of the evidence are skimmed over in efforts to set out simplified global policy recommendations in which is stated that 'a reduction of the hours or days of sale of alcoholic beverages leads to fewer alcohol-related problems, including homicides and assaults' (Anderson et al., 2009: 2238).

The findings of Duailibi et al. are the single source supporting this assertion. Given this, it should be noted that Duailibi and colleagues conclude their paper by saying that 'given Diadema's poor socioeconomic conditions and high baseline rate of violence, we would not expect such a dramatic effect of a closing-time law to generalize to all cultures or countries' (2007: 2279), despite then asserting that their findings 'strongly support restrictions on drinking hours as a public health measure' (2007: 2280). The Diadema case study is a clear example of a situation where 'some ideas become accepted as fact though they may not be true. They become "factoids": assumptions or speculations reported and repeated so often that they are popularly considered true' (Cummins and Macintyre, 2002: 436). These are problems of interpretation or *overinterpretation* in which factoids 'can easily and uncritically become part of the apparatus of government health policy when they fit in with broader policy objectives' (2002, 438). In the case of alcohol evidence then, the facts should probably never 'speak for themselves'.

With these major caveats duly noted and caution sounded, I return to the Western Cape Liquor Act. This legislation granted the South African Police Service and a lamentably small number of liquor inspectors (30 for the entire Western Cape Province of 129,500 km^2 and almost 6 million inhabitants) power to raid and close illegal, unlicensed bars or 'shebeens' that operate largely in poor, residential areas. In implementing the Act, shebeeners report being routinely fined, asked for bribes by police and their supplies confiscated. In the South African case, the enforcement of liquor legislation is inextricable from historical antagonisms between non-whites and the police, as well as present concerns about endemic corruption in policing (Herrick and Charman, 2013). However, this example also demonstrates that even the best intentioned policies can have unwanted and unintended consequences. In this case, increased police attention has led to a mushrooming of smaller, survivalist shebeens across many neighbourhoods (Charman et al., 2013). These premises pose threats to human wellbeing in terms of precipitating injury and violence, but their size and access issues make them far harder to police. Indeed, the downsizing of shebeens is a logical survival strategy amid the threat of harassment, theft and robbery as cash-only businesses and the possibility of a criminal record for operating without a licence. It is also a way of mitigating the threat posed by competitors who would be likely to alert the police and, in so doing, ensure a temporary competitive advantage in a saturated marketplace. Given this, it is notable that the City of Cape Town recently rescinded on its restricted opening hours – after survey research suggested the laws were having an adverse effect on businesses (personal communication, 2013) – and has now granted licensed premises the opportunity to re-apply for extended opening hours. This goes against the evidence-based advice of the WHO. While the approach to shebeens has not similarly softened, thought is now turning to how best to lure shebeeners away from selling liquor. The Framework Convention on Tobacco Control makes note of the need to ensure alternative livelihoods for those engaged in the tobacco growing industry, however, the alcohol *Global Strategy* makes little mention of this. If the harms associated with the illicit trade (at production, distribution and retail tiers) are to be managed, then people will need viable economic alternatives. On the other side, if demand for liquor is to be reduced, then consumers will also need attractive and plausible alternatives to drinking as a leisure and coping activity. I shall dwell on the implications of this in the final interjection.

Modernisation as human fate and public health threat

There is a spurious logic at play in the public health framing of alcohol consumption and its harms in countries of the South. It has been commonly argued that higher income countries, in general, have greater rates of per capita alcohol consumption than low income countries. However, middle income countries have the highest burden of alcohol-related harms, despite often having lower overall rates of consumption (WHO, 2010a, 2011b). From a public health perspective therefore, low and middle-income countries are facing a 'perfect storm' of market liberalisation, increased availability of commercially-produced liquor and rising affluence (Caetano and Laranjeira, 2005; Parry, 2000). These attributes of globalisation are further seen as undermining the more traditional pattern of high abstention rates and low incidence of hazardous and harmful drinking. The factors contributing to the 'perfect storm' are, by themselves, arguably desirable from a human and economic development perspective. Who, after all, could argue against the importance of rising affluence to countries of the South (notwithstanding the effect that rising wealth among the few has had on rates of socio-economic inequality in countries such as South Africa, Brazil and Angola)? Yet, a public health approach to alcohol seems unhelpfully ambiguous about the benefits of development.

For example, as Schmidt et al. argue, 'as alcohol is a commodity that requires disposable income to obtain, the poorest segments of the population are usually the least likely to drink. This opens up the possibility that otherwise beneficial decreases in socioeconomic inequity can lead to an increased burden of alcohol-attributable health problems in low-income populations' (2010: 12). They go on further to suggest that 'if the laudable goal of ending extreme poverty throughout the world were attained there is the potential, in the absence of countermeasures, for a substantial increase not only in rates of people who drink but also in rates of heavy drinking' (2010: 15). Under the epidemiological transition model, progression from developing to developed country brings with it, hypothetically and if countries follow the path of the Global North, a diminished threat from infectious disease. By contrast, as countries move towards the consumption and behavioural patterns of the Global North, they face mounting rates of NCDs (Yach and Beaglehole, 2004; Yach et al., 2005a, 2005b). Alcohol is a risk factor for both infectious and NCDs, but from a global heath governance standpoint, sits more squarely within the emergent post-2015 frameworks of the latter. As such, as countries 'globalise' or 'modernise' in the sense of following 'a strong, normative teleology, a uni-linear trajectory toward a particular vision of the future…to which all humanity should aspire, to which all history ought to lead and all peoples should evolve, if at different rates' (Comaroff and Comaroff, 2012: 118), they also face new, emergent risks from political economic forces beyond their immediate control. Development may consequently be undesirable from a risk behaviour standpoint. However, globalised lifestyles – of which alcohol is a clear part – are deeply aspirational and, moreover, a basic right. The internal conflict between health and development, in which progress in the latter provokes new and often more pernicious risks to the former is a debate that has churned for a number of years (Beaglehole and Bonita, 1998), but takes on a renewed salience in relation to the 'industrial epidemics' of alcohol, tobacco and food (Jahiel and Babor, 2007). Here, questions of individual rights and choice must be reconciled with the protective role of public health.

In their publication, *Alcohol in Developing Societies: A Public Health Approach*, Room et al. contend that 'while [alcohol] carries *connotations* of pleasure and sociability in the minds of many, harmful consequences of its use are diverse and widespread' (2002: 26; emphasis added). This sentence is particularly telling. There is little doubt that the consequences of alcohol use can be significant to both drinkers and non-drinkers. However, the suggestion that drinking only carries 'connotations' of pleasure and sociability dramatically underplays the importance and *reality* of both to the genesis of harms. To this, we might also add that the demand for pleasure and socialisation also fuels the possibility of alcohol as a viable and attractive means for many to make a living. In conditions where unemployment may be extremely high, female incorporation into the workplace is low and educational opportunities unevenly distributed, subsistence alcohol production and retailing can be an important livelihood choice. This is particularly and historically the case in southern African countries (Herrick, 2013). While concern has been expressed that the rise of commercially produced liquor in the Global South has actually displaced locally-brewed, traditional products in favour of far stronger and more expensive drinks (Caetano and Laranjeira, 2005), the degree to which this has had an impact on countries is contingent on their varied political economic histories of liquor. It is thus important to acknowledge the persistence of selling liquor as a viable and attractive livelihood choice and its consumption as a source of pleasure, particularly as the two are mutually reinforcing. Accepting the importance of pleasure – even in the Global South – is a crucial step in generating evidence that matters (Coveney and Bunton, 2003). Moreover, without an acceptance of the 'persistence of pleasure' (Measham, 2004) as well as the manifold motivations for drinking – coping, stress, unemployment, boredom, a lack of leisure alternatives – interventions will often fail in the face of human ingenuity. Under conditions of poverty, the motivations for drinking are only more pronounced in their effects and consequences. Thus, it is important for public health to concede that people drink because they have free will and, ultimately, the right to do so. When lives are hard and people are vulnerable, this may be even more so. Working *with* pleasure and embedding it within the research process means asking different kinds of questions about how harms can be reduced, engaging with qualitative research methods and, therefore, generating new kinds of evidence. Such an evidence base may not be universal or generalisable, but it will certainly be people-centred and, moreover, relevant.

CONCLUSION

In this chapter, I have reflected on the 'incalculable mosaic of evidence' (Adams et al., 2014: 3) generated by alcohol research as well as its application within policy. In so doing, I have drawn attention to the ways in which the global public health agenda has reinforced adherence to a hierarchy of evidence that favours RCTs and systematic reviews over what Biehl and Petryna (2013) have termed 'people-centred evidence'. In contrast to the universal, nomothetic and generalising tendencies of public health sanctioned evidence, people-centred evidence asks questions about the 'entanglements between systems and human experiences' (2013: 13). It does so because a 'bio-social' approach to health acknowledges that outcomes are multi-dimensional in their genesis and unfolding. And, moreover, the efficacy of interventions is thoroughly contingent on what Adams (2013: 63) calls the 'unforgiving realities of life'. These realities are important regardless of geographical context, yet it could be argued that some realities and geographies are more unforgiving than others. This may, in turn, undermine the efficacy of interventions that have otherwise shown positive effects elsewhere. This is not to say that the intervention is ineffective per se, but rather that the context renders it unsuitable and irrelevant. In the race to ensure the implementation of the *Global Strategy* amid an international policy climate that finally seems to be waking up to the need to inculcate NCDs within global development goals, it is important public health does not lose sight of the people whose health it seeks to improve. The conditions for evidence preclude experimentation in the very literal sense of the word. In the social and infrastructural maelstrom of many Southern urban contexts, life is changing quickly. Experiments and risks are needed if research is to capture these shape-shifting realities. Controlling for the inconvenient parameters of life is meaningless when life itself is deeply and inherently uncertain. Let us therefore hope that the search for relevance inspires greater freedom to research those questions and problems that matter most to people in ways that are meaningful when set against the complexity of multiple lived realities.

REFERENCES

Adam Smith Research Group (2012) *The Minimal Evidence for Minimum Pricing: The Fatal Flaws in the Sheffield Alcohol Policy Model*. London: Adam Smith Research Group.

Adams, V. (2013) 'Evidence-based global public health: subjects, profits, erasures', In J. Biehl and A. Petryna (eds), *When People Come First: Critical Studies in Global Public Health*. Princeton: Princeton University Press, pp. 54–90.

Adams, V., Burke, N. J. and Whitmarsh, I. (2014) 'Slow research: thoughts for a movement in global health', *Medical Anthropology* 33: 179–97.

Anderson, P., Chisholm, D. and Fuhr, D. C. (2009) 'Effectiveness and cost-effectiveness of policies and programmes to reduce the harm caused by alcohol', *The Lancet* 373: 2234–46.

Babor, T., Caetano, R., Casswell, S., Edwards, G., Giesbrecht, N., Graham, K., Grube, J., Gruenewald, P., Hill, L., Holder, H., Homel, R., Osterberg, E., Rehm, J., Room, R. and Rossow, I. (2010) *Alcohol: No Ordinary Commodity. Research and Public Policy*. Oxford: Oxford University Press.

Babor, T., Hall, W., Humphreys, K., Miller, P., Petry, N. and West, R. (2013) 'Who is responsible for the public's health? The role of the alcohol industry in the WHO global strategy to reduce the harmful use of alcohol', *Addiction* 108: 2045–7.

Bakke, Ø. and Endal, D. (2010) 'Alcohol policies out of context: drinks industry supplanting government role in alcohol policies in sub-Saharan Africa', *Addiction* 105: 22–8.

Beaglehole, R. and Bonita, R. (1998) 'Public health at the crossroads: which way forward?', *The Lancet* 351: 590–2.

Biehl, J. and Petryna, A. (2013) *When People Come First: Critical Studies in Global Health*. Princeton: Princeton University Press.

Bill and Melinda Gates Foundation (2014) *Our Approach to Measurement and Evaluation*. Available from: http://www.gatesfoundation.org/How-We-Work/General-Information/Our-Approach-to-Measurement-and-Evaluation (Accessed 29 January 2014).

Brown, T. and Moon, G. (2012) 'Geography and global health', *The Geographical Journal* 178: 13–17.

Burgis, T. (2009) Botswana sobers up. *Financial Times*, 15 May. Available from: http://www.ft.com/cms/s/0/dc6381e4-3e90-11de-9a6c-00144feabdc0.html#slide0 (Accessed 2 April 2016).

Caetano, R. and Laranjeira, R. (2005) 'A "perfect storm" in developing countries: economic growth and the alcohol industry', *Addiction* 101: 149–51.

Casswell, S. (2013) 'Vested interests in addiction research and policy. Why do we not see the corporate interests of the alcohol industry as clearly as we see those of the tobacco industry?', *Addiction* 108: 680–5.

Centre for Economics and Business Research (2012) Minimum Unit Pricing: Impacts on Consumer Spending and Distributional Consequences. London: CEBR.

Charman, A., Petersen, L. and Piper, L. (2013) 'Enforced informalisation: the case of illegal liquor retailers in South Africa', *Development Southern Africa* 30: 580–95.

Choi, B. C. K., Hunter, D. J., Tsou, W. and Sainsbury, P. (2005) 'Diseases of comfort: primary cause of death in the 22nd century', *Journal of Epidemiology and Community Health* 59: 1030–4.

Comaroff, J. and Comaroff, J. L. (2012) 'Theory from the south: or, how Euro-America is evolving toward Africa', *Anthropological Forum* 22: 113–31.

Coveney, J. and Bunton, R. (2003) 'In pursuit of the study of pleasure: implications for health research and practice', *Health (London)* 7: 161–79.

Cummins, A. and Macintyre, S. (2002) '"Food deserts" – evidence and assumption in health policy making', *British Medical Journal* 325: 436–8.

Dobrow, M. J., Goel, V. and Upshur, R. (2004) 'Evidence-based health policy: context and utilisation', *Social Science and Medicine* 58: 207–17.

Duailibi, S., Ponicki, W., Grube, J., Pinsky, I., Laranjeira, R. and Raw, M. (2007) 'The effect of restricting opening hours on alcohol-related violence', *American Journal of Public Health* 97: 2276–80.

Dunn, J. R. and Cummins, S. (2007) 'Placing health in context', *Social Science and Medicine* 65: 1821–4.

Farmer, P. (2004) 'An anthropology of structural violence', *Current Anthropology* 45: 305–25.

Gornall, J. (2014) 'Under the influence: 1. False dawn for minimum unit pricing', *British Medical Journal* 348: f7435.

Graham, K., Bernards, S., Knibbe, R., Kairouz, S., Kuntsche, S., Wilsnack, S. C., Greenfield, T. K., Dietze, P., Obot, I. and Gmel, G. (2011) 'Alcohol-related negative consequences among drinkers around the world', *Addiction* 106: 1391–405.

Herrick, C. (2013) 'Alcohol control and livelihoods: can public health aspirations and development goals be reconciled?', *Critical Public Health* 24: 361–71.

Herrick, C. (2014) 'Healthy cities from/of the South', In S. Parnell and S. Oldfield (eds), *The Routledge Handbook of Cities of the South*. Routledge: London, pp. 556–69.

Herrick, C. and Charman, A. (2013) 'Shebeens and crime: the multiple criminalities of South African liquor and its regulation', *South African Crime Quarterly* 45: 25–33.

Holden, C., Hawkins, B. and McCambridge, J. (2012) 'Cleavages and co-operation in the UK alcohol industry: a qualitative study', *BMC Public Health,* 12: 483.

Home Office (2012) *The Government's Alcohol Strategy*. London: Home Office.

Home Office (2013) *Next Steps Following the Consultation on Delivering the Government's Alcohol Strategy*. London: Home Office.

Horton, R. (2013) 'Non-communicable diseases: 2015 to 2025', *The Lancet* 381: 509–10.

Hyde, A. (2012) *East Africa Alcohol Policy Alliance Agrees: More Research Required*. London: STRIVE, London School of Hygiene and Tropical Medicine.

Jahiel, R. and Babor, T. (2007) 'Industrial epidemics, public health advocacy and the alcohol industry: lessons from other fields', *Addiction* 102: 1335–9.

Janes, C. and Corbett, K. (2009) 'Anthropology and global health', *Annual Review of Anthropology* 38: 167–83.

Khoo, S. (2013) 'Health justice and capabilities: a turning point for global health?', *International Sociology* 28: 155–67.

Marmot, M. G. (2004) 'Evidence based policy or policy based evidence?', *British Medical Journal* 328: 906–7.

Matzopoulos, R., Myers, J., Butchart, A., Corrigall, J., Peden, M. and Naledi, T. (2008a) 'Reducing the burden of injury: an intersectoral preventive approach is needed', *South African Medical Journal* 98: 703–5.

Matzopoulos, R., Myers, J. and Jobanputra, R. (2008b) 'Road traffic injury: prioritising interventions', *South African Medical Journal* 98: 692–6.

McCoy, D., Kembhavi, G., Patel, J. and Luintel, A. (2009) 'The Bill and Melinda Gates Foundation's grant-making programme for global health', *The Lancet* 373: 1645–53.

Measham, F. (2004) 'The decline of ecstasy, the rise of "binge" drinking and the persistence of pleasure', *Probation Journal* 51: 309–26.

Meier, P. S., Brennen, A. and Putrshouse, R. (2009) *Independent Review of the Effects of Alcohol Pricing and Promotion*. London: Report commissioned by the Department of Health.

Moodie, R., Stuckler, D., Monteiro, C., Sheron, N., Neal, B., Thamarangsi, T., Lincoln, P. and Casswell, S. (2013) 'Profits and pandemics: prevention of harmful effects of tobacco, alcohol, and ultra-processed food and drink industries', *The Lancet* 381: 670–9.

Moran, M., Guzman, J., Ropars, A.-L., McDonald, A., Jameson, N., Omune, B., Ryan, S. and Wu, L. (2009) 'Neglected disease research and development: how much are we really spending?', *PLoS Medicine* 6: e1000030.

Nguyen, V. K. and Peschard, K. (2003) 'Anthropology, inequality, and disease: a review', *Annual Review of Anthropology* 32: 447–74.

Parry, C. (2000) 'Alcohol problems in developing countries: challenges for the new millennium', *Suchtmed* 2: 216–20.

Parry, C., Plüddemann, A., Steyn, K., Bradshaw, D., Norman, R. and Laubscher, R. (2005) 'Alcohol use in South Africa: findings from the first Demographic and Health Survey 1998', *Journal of Studies on Alcohol and Drugs* 66: 91–7.

Parry, C. D., Patra, J. and Rehm, J. (2011) 'Alcohol consumption and non-communicable diseases: epidemiology and policy implications', *Addiction* 106: 1718–24.

Parry, C. D. H. (2005) 'South Africa: alcohol today', *Addiction* 100: 426–9.

Pennay, A. (2012) '"Wicked problems": the social conundrum presented by public drinking laws', *Drug and Alcohol Dependence* 19: 185–91.

Petticrew, M. (2003) 'Why certain systematic reviews reach uncertain conclusions', *British Medical Journal* 326: 756–8.

Petticrew, M. and Roberts, H. (2003) 'Evidence, hierarchies, and typologies: horses for courses', *Journal of Epidemiology and Community Health* 57: 527–9.

Prime Minister's Office (2012) Prime Minister: 'We have to tackle the scourge of violence caused by binge drinking. And we have to do it now'. London: Prime Minister's Office.

Quesada, J., Hart, L. and Bourgois, P. (2011) 'Structural vulnerability and health: Latino migrant laborers in the United States', *Medical Anthropology* 30: 339–62.

Rayner, G. and Lang, T. (2012) *Ecological Public Health: Reshaping the Conditions for Good Health*. London: Routledge.

Room, R. (1984) 'Alcohol and ethnography: a case of problem deflation?', *Current Anthropology* 25: 169.

Room, R., Babor, T. and Rehm, J. (2005) 'Alcohol and public health', *The Lancet* 365: 519–30.

Room, R., Jernigan, D., Carlini-Marlatt, B., Gureje, O., Mäkelä, K., Marshall, M., Medina-Mora, M., Monteiro, M., Parry, C., Partanen, J., Riley, L. and Saxena, S. (2002) *Alcohol in Developing Societies: A Public Health Approach*. Helsinki: Finnish Foundation for Alcohol Studies.

Schmidt, L. A. and Room, R. (2013) 'Alcohol and inequity in the process of development: contributions from ethnographic research', *The International Journal of Alcohol and Drug Research* 1: 41–55.

Schmidt, L., Mäkelä, P., Rehm, J. and Room, R. (2010) 'Alcohol: equity and social determinants', In E. Blas and A. Sivasankara Kurup (eds), *Equity, Social Determinants and Public Health Programmes*. Geneva: WHO, pp. 11–31.

Seedat, M., Van Niekerk, A., Jewkes, R., Suffla, S. and Ratele, K. (2009) 'Violence and injuries in South Africa: prioritising an agenda for prevention', *The Lancet* 374: 1011–22.

Shkolnikov, V. M., Cornia, G. A., Leon, D. A. and Meslé, F. (1998) 'Causes of the Russian mortality crisis: evidence and interpretations', *World Development* 26: 1995–2011.

Simone, A. (2010) *City Life from Jakarta to Dakar: Movements at the Crossroads*. London: Routledge.

Smith, K. E. (2014) 'The politics of ideas: the complex interplay of health inequalities research and policy', *Science and Public Policy* 41: 561–74.

Smith, K. E. and Joyce, K. E. (2012) 'Capturing complex realities: understanding efforts to achieve evidence-based policy and practice in public health', *Evidence and Policy: A Journal of Research, Debate and Practice* 8: 57–78.

Stuckler, D., McKee, M., Ebrahim, S. and Basu, S. (2012) 'Manufacturing epidemics: the role of global producers in increased consumption of unhealthy commodities including processed foods, alcohol, and tobacco', *PLoS Med* 9: e1001235.

Swahn, M. H. and Tumwesigye, S. (2013) 'Global perspective on alcohol research: facilitating interdisciplinary and international collaborations to address prevailing challenges', *The International Journal of Alcohol and Drug Research,* 1: 13–15.

Thaler, R. and Sunstein, C. R. (2008) *Nudge: Improving Decisions About Health, Wealth and Happiness*. New Haven: Yale University Press.

The University of Sheffield (2013) *News Release: Ban on Below-Cost Selling for Alcohol Would Have Smaller Impact Than A 45p Minimum Price*. Sheffield: University of Sheffield.

Weber, E. P. and Khademian, A. M. (2008) 'Wicked problems, knowledge challenges, and collaborative capacity builders in network settings', *Public Administration Review* 68: 334–49.

World Health Organisation (2010a) *Global Strategy to Reduce the Harmful Use of Alcohol*. Geneva: WHO.

World Health Organisation (2010b) *Global Status Report on Non-Communicable Disease*. Geneva: WHO.

World Health Organisation (2011a) *From Burden to 'Best Buys': Reducing the Economic Impact of NCDs in Low- and Middle-Income Countries*. Geneva: WHO.

World Health Organisation (2011b) *Global Status Report on Alcohol and Health*. Geneva: WHO.

Yach, D. and Beaglehole, R. (2004) 'Globalization of risks for chronic diseases demands global solutions', *Perspectives on Global Development and Technology* 3: 213–33.

Yach, D., Kellogg, M. and Voute, J. (2005a) 'Chronic diseases: an increasing challenge in developing countries', *Transactions of the Royal Society of Tropical Medicine and Hygiene* 99: 321–4.

Yach, D., Leeder, S., Bell, J. and Kistnasamy, B. (2005b) 'Global chronic diseases', *Science* 307: 317.

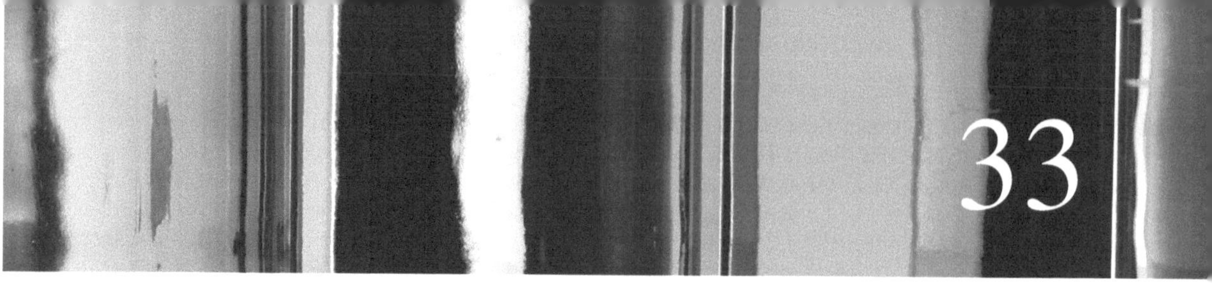

What's So 'New' About New Psychoactive Substances? Definitions, Prevalence, Motivations, User Groups and A Proposed New Taxonomy

Fiona Measham and Russell Newcombe

INTRODUCTION

One of the most interesting developments in the field of drug and alcohol studies in recent years has been the emergence of new psychoactive substances (NPS). This phenomenon is something of a (rapidly) moving target however, in terms of what we know about NPS, how different countries have reacted to their emergence and indeed, what we even mean by the term. This chapter will explore definitions, prevalence and user motivations in order to tease out the broader picture of what characterises NPS use, such that it should warrant a chapter in and of itself in this collection. A new typology of NPS is also proposed here, which combines pharmacological effects with chemical classifications to provide an underlying framework for this review.

Although prevalence of use of NPS remains low by comparison with both established illegal drugs such as cannabis and cocaine and established legal drugs such as alcohol and tobacco, this chapter suggests that the significance of the interest generated by NPS relates to the rapidity of innovation in manufacturing and retail practices; the speed and scale of policy responses; and the relationship between the two, which was initially characterised by commentators as 'cat and mouse'.[1] The authors conclude here that the dynamic interaction between the NPS market and policy change can be better characterised as 'hare and hounds', in that legislative control has been a significant driving force in manufacturing and retail innovations.

DEFINITIONS

The emergence and evolution of the NPS issue parallels the emergence and evolution of the terminology used to describe the appearance of a cluster of psychoactive substances in recent years which, unusually for the drugs field, were identified as a potential global threat *before* a significant physical or social problem emerged. The roots of the NPS debate can be traced back to the 1970s and the development of the term 'designer drug', itself a somewhat imprecise term, used to characterise psychoactive substances that were derivatives of controlled drugs and had been created to circumvent existing legal restrictions specifically for recreational purposes. Buchanan and Brown (1988), who ascribe the coining of the term to a California pharmacologist called Henderson, identify four main categories of 'designer drugs': phenylethylamines (e.g. MDMA), synthetic opioids, methaqualone derivatives and arylhexylamines (e.g. phencyclidine or PCP also known as 'Angel Dust', perhaps the most highly publicised of the 1970s designer drugs in the United States). However, contrary to the implication that these substances were created by street chemists, in fact, many of these 'designer drugs' were the offshoots or rejects of commercial pharmaceutical research and development, and hence, the details of their synthesis had already been published in professional and academic papers [see Brandt et al. (2014) for an overview of the development of NPS nomenclature and definitions]. Whilst the term 'designer drugs' continued to be used throughout the 1980s and 90s, another term started to emerge – 'legal highs' – which was an indication of the broadening array of herbal as well as synthetic substances available as pills, powders, liquids and vegetable matter that were being manufactured and sold to emulate the appearance and effects of existing recreational drugs and to evade legislative control. The shift in emphasis here was towards herbal, and therefore by implication, 'natural' products ('herbal highs'), in contrast to the 'synthetic' associations of 'designer drugs' (also known as 'research chemicals').

In terms of NPS specifically, the watershed moment came in 2008 when the manufacture of synthetic cannabinoids and substituted cathinones became an international concern. Such were the numbers of new psychoactive substances identified by forensic scientists around the world from 2008 onwards that the term novel psychoactive substances (Dargan et al., 2010) or new psychoactive substances was coined (EMCDDA, 2007). For example, the term was widely enough accepted in scientific circles that by 2009 the UK Advisory Council on the Misuse of Drugs (ACMD) established a 'New Psychoactive Substances Working Group' to address concerns.[2] The definition utilised by the ACMD working group was: 'Psychoactive drugs which are not prohibited by the United Nations Single Convention on Narcotic Drugs or by the Misuse of Drugs Act 1971, and which people in the UK are seeking for intoxicant use' (ACMD, 2011: 10.)

Similarly, the definition utilised by the UK Association of Chief Police Officers (ACPO) at this time also emphasised legal status – specifically the lack of legislative control within the UK – as the defining feature in its definition:

> New Psychoactive Substances or so called 'legal highs' are substances which produce the same, or similar effects, to illegal stimulant drugs such as cocaine and ecstasy, but are not controlled under legislation [the Misuse of Drugs Act 1971 in the UK]. They are however, considered illegal under current medicines legislation to sell, supply or advertise for 'human consumption'.(ACPO, 2011: 19)

This emphasis on circumventing legislative control led Newcombe to suggest that 'legal highs', the term still favoured by the media and in everyday conversation, could more accurately be considered 'legal loophole' drugs (Newcombe, 2012a). Most recently, the acronym NPS has increasingly emphasised *New* Psychoactive Substances (e.g. NPS Review Expert Panel, 2014) rather than *Novel* Psychoactive Substances (e.g. ACMD, 2011; Dargan et al., 2010), in recognition that whilst their *recreational* use might be a relatively recent concern, the drugs themselves were not necessarily novel in that at least some of them had an established, if not unproblematic, history of pharmaceutical development. The United Nations Office on Drugs and Crime (UNODC) has clarified the meaning of 'new' in their definition of NPS:

> Substances of abuse, either in a pure form or a preparation, that are not controlled by the 1961 Convention on Narcotic Drugs or the 1971 Convention on Psychotropic Substances, but which may pose a public health threat. The term 'new' does not necessarily refer to new inventions – several NPS were first synthesized 40 years ago – but to substances that have recently emerged on the market and which have not been scheduled under the above Conventions. (UNODC, 2013: 2)

Other variations in the NPS literature include 'emerging' in place of 'novel' or 'new' and 'compounds' or 'drugs' instead of the more general term 'substances'.

The definition and scope of NPS continues to evolve and expand to include both controlled and uncontrolled psychoactive drugs, synthetic and natural substances, as well as substances that are inadvertently consumed as adulterants or substitutes to the drug of choice.[3] With so much emphasis placed on defining, identifying and cataloguing new NPS through national and international warning systems (EMCDDA, 2014a), as well as monitoring the websites that sell them (Schifano et al., 2010), this has resulted in a somewhat 'trainspotter' approach to charting the field. Indeed, the European Monitoring Centre for Drugs and Drug Addiction (EMCDDA) annual report graph that charts the new additions to the NPS cornucopia each year has become an essential element of NPS conference presentations in this field.

Unsurprisingly, given the wide variations in definitions of NPS, the consequent identification and publication of NPS-related problems and mortality rates themselves have been contentious, highly publicised and highly politicised (Goodair et al., 2014; King and Nutt, 2014). Whilst Cope from the UK Office for National Statistics argued that 'there is no official definition of a new psychoactive substance' (Cope, 2014: 1715), perhaps the closest to a consensus is the EMCDDA definition. Article 3 of EMCDDA Council Decision 2005 defines NPSs as

> [A] new narcotic or psychotropic drug, in pure form or in preparation, that is not controlled by the 1961 United Nations Single Convention on Narcotic Drugs or the 1971 United Nations Convention on Psychotropic Substances, but which may pose a public health threat comparable to that posed by substances listed in these conventions. (UK New Psychoactive Substances Ministerial Review Expert Panel, 2014: 4)

A definition that was adapted for use by the UK New Psychoactive Substances Ministerial Review Expert Panel (2014: 4). However, this definition of NPS is weakened by the ambiguity of 'new' and the redundancy of 'may pose a public health threat' given that all drugs carry some degree of risk.

THE LEGAL CONUNDRUM

A notable feature in the evolution of the term has been the reduced emphasis on legal status that leads to the central unanswered question: exactly what is *new* or *novel* about new psychoactive substances? A definition that focuses on legal status (e.g. ACMD, 2011) is no longer relevant for many contemporary legislative jurisdictions as we have a situation where NPS are rapidly and broadly controlled through 'blanket bans', analogue legislation, generic legislation, temporary controls and amendments to existing drug controls.[4] In the UK for example, many NPS are already controlled through generic legislation shortly after, or even considerably before, they make an appearance and without recourse to established risk assessment processes for individual substances that were previously central to many policy structures but which are now considered too cumbersome in the face of the speed and scale of NPS development. This has led to a cycle of rapid and wide ranging legislative change that is illustrated in the UK's use of generic legislation that prohibits the possession and supply of whole families of drugs without individual risk assessments. The government's NPS Review Expert Panel reported that 'over 550 NPS have been controlled since 2009, with 350 controlled since July 2010... The UK has banned the majority of NPS seen in the EU since 2005. Of the 410 NPS identified in Europe up to 2014... over 85% of the main groups are already controlled' (2014: 17).

Whilst most of the changes to NPS terminology have resulted in a net widening effect, it is interesting to note that some definitions have resulted in a reduction in the number or scale of drugs covered. As NPS have been controlled, illegal markets have developed and some NPS use has bedded in and become established into the repertoires of drug users and suppliers. Consequently, some NPS, most notably mephedrone, are now documented separately to other/all NPS in official reports (e.g. Public Health England, 2014).

A definition that centres on the *novel* element overlooks the continuities between pharmaceutical and recreational drug developments in recent years and also the appearance of 'new' drugs and their use by recreational users before, as well as after, 2008. However, as the NPS definition has evolved to include both legal and illegal drugs, so it has come to include 'substances that are not necessarily new but which have recently been increasingly abused' (International Narcotics Control Board, 2013: 36). This net-widening has meant that some of the broadest NPS definitions now include: not particularly 'new' illicit drugs (e.g. ketamine, GHB/GBL) and in some cases more traditional illicit drugs (e.g. psilocybe, khat) whose recreational use has been increasingly noted in some dance club scenes from the 1990s onwards (Measham et al., 2001), and including psilocybe and khat products that were sold from 'headshops' prior to their prohibition (2005 and 2014, respectively) in the UK);a merging of NPS with 'club drugs' or 'dance drugs' (notably ecstasy, cocaine and amphetamines); long standing uncontrolled psychoactive drugs (e.g. nitrous oxide, 'poppers'); medicines that are legally manufactured and prescribed and which again only recently were recognised as having any recreational appeal. Although 'indirectly' psychoactive (intoxication effects are typically described as 'side effects'), these various medications and pharmaceuticals can also be obtained without prescription from online pharmacy websites, some of which also sell the more popular NPS. These include psychiatric drugs (e.g. anti-depressants, anti-psychotics); sleeping pills (e.g. chlorals, Z-drugs); analgesics with recently recognised abuse potential (e.g. tramadol, pregabalin); and wholly or predominantly physiological drugs, including sexual potency drugs (e.g. sildenafil), performance enhancing drugs (notably steroids), cognitive enhancing drugs (e.g. modafinil) and image enhancing drugs (such as melanotan and botox).

Significantly, most definitions of NPS exclude the 'new' forms and uses of the three main legally regulated drugs around the world, namely caffeine (e.g. caffeine tablets, powder and even shampoos; high strength 'energy' drinks); alcohol (e.g. alcohol powder or 'palcohol', inhalable alcohol vapour); and nicotine (e.g. e-cigarettes, shisha and medicinal nicotine products).

As we can see, the ongoing evolution of terms in the field of NPS studies has blurred what were once considered fairly clear distinctions. In particular – and despite 'legal highs' still being the most commonly used term for NPS in the media and everyday conversation – the legal/illegal distinction causes increasing problems given the national and temporal differences in drug laws, along with the variations implicit in the term 'legal' (notably regarding production, supply and use). Consequently, attempts at precise definition often lead to semantic dances about what NPS are *not*, such as any psychoactive drugs that are not legally controlled, more particularly meaning *not* legally controlled for medical use, *not* legally prohibited and *not* licensed for recreational use. Unsurprisingly, a series of alternative terms has emerged, with NPS – which potentially sidesteps the legal/illegal distinction – coming to dominate. The broadest and most flexible definition of the 'new' prefix of NPS would be: legal or illegal drugs that have been recently discovered, marketed and/or notably consumed. An operational definition of 'new' could also specify a cut-off year relating to the rise of these 'new drugs' markets, such as the 2008/9 mephedrone 'watershed' in the UK discussed further below, with NPS relating as much to a new *cultural* phenomenon as to specific psychoactive drugs. In this way, NPS could be characterised as a flexible collective noun more akin to terms such as 'dance drugs' or 'club drugs' (Coomber et al., 2013).

Some colloquial terms for groups of NPS have also been coined by researchers across the globe. The main examples include 'research chemicals' for synthetic NPS (notably hallucinogens); 'herbal highs' for plant-based NPS; 'spice', 'mamba', or 'herbal incense' for synthetic cannabinoids; 'bath salts' for stimulants (particularly for cathinones in North America); and 'smart drugs' or 'nootropics' for eugeroic stimulants (see Table 33.1 below).

To conclude, our assessment of the evolution of the terms and concepts that describe and demarcate NPS includes consideration of the role of historical and socio-cultural context to this definition. Thus, given the semantic ambiguities and cultural variations of this still developing term, this chapter adopts the following operational definition of NPS: those drugs emerging or rising significantly in use after the 2008 mephedrone 'watershed', starting with first generation synthetic cannabinoids and cathinones, followed by a widening array of substances that are typically uncontrolled to begin with. Drugs controlled and/or whose recreational use was established before 2009 and those in the four categories outlined above are largely absent from the later sections of this chapter unless included in our summaries of other studies that include them.

CLASSIFICATIONS OF NPS: TOWARDS A NEW TAXONOMY

In order to review the evidence on NPS – and to design research studies – it is necessary to go beyond the sculpting of clear and precise definitions such as those discussed above, to a principled classification of NPS. Therefore, in this section, we briefly examine the available conceptual frameworks for categorising NPS – that is, models developed to organise and classify specific NPS into broader categories according to rules of inclusion and exclusion. Whilst a variety of classification systems exist in the literature, few are widely accepted across all disciplines and professional groups involved with NPS and the constantly evolving nature of NPS means that they can rapidly become outdated. The most common four dimensions of extant classifications are: by source, by legal/medical status, by psychoactive effect (on the brain and mind) and by chemical group. We discuss these four dimensions below before presenting a new multi-level classification of NPS based on two of the most important dimensions.

Source classification

The source classification is relatively straightforward: NPS can be broadly divided into natural and synthetic drugs. Natural NPS can be sub-divided into plant-based drugs (e.g. salvia, peyote, amanita muscaria) and animal-derived drugs (e.g. cane-toad skin excretions). Plant-based drugs (or plant extracts) are an NPS category frequently used by researchers. Synthetic NPS can be sub-divided into semi-synthetic drugs (production of which starts with a natural drug)

Table 33.1 Drugs controlled in the UK in the twenty-first century by amendments to the 1971 Misuse of Drugs Act

Year	*Drugs*	*Class and schedule*
2001	• 35 phenethylamines	A1
2003	• GHB (gammahydroxybutyrate)	C4i (C2 from 1/15)
2005	• Psilocin-based mushrooms (live/fresh) • Ketamine	A1C4i (B3 from 6/14)
2009	• First generation synthetic cannabinoids • GBL (gammabutyrolactone), 14BD (butanediol) • BZP (benzylpiperazine) and other piperazines	B1CC1
2010	• Mephedrone and substituted cathinones	B1
2012	• 2DPMP (desoxypipradol/Ivory Wave) • Phenazepam • Pipradol esters and ethers (piperidines)	B1C2C3
2013	• Second generation synthetic cannabinoids • Methoxetamine • Desmethyltramadol • Lisdexamphetamine • Zopiclone and zaleplon	B1B1B1B2C4i
2014	• NBOMe compounds • Benzofuran compounds (5-APB, 6-APB) • Khat • Tramadol	A1B1C1C3
2015	• Dimethylaminorex (4,4'-DMAR) • Cyclohexyldiphenylethylpiperazine (MT-45) • Tryptamine compounds (AMT, 5-meo-DALT) • Lysergamides: ALD-52, ETH-LAD, PRO-LAD, AL-LAD, LSZ • AH-7921 (opioid)	A1A1A1A1A1A1
	Planned	
	• Third generation synthetic cannabinoids • Psychoactive Substances Bill proposing 'blanket ban' on sale of all psychoactive substances with some exemptions • Possible ban on all drugs affecting CB1 brain receptor	
	Reclassification and rescheduling	
	2004 Cannabis	C1 (from B1)
	2007 Methamphetamine	A2 (from B2)
	2009 Cannabis	B1 (from C1) – except Sativex (b4i)
	2014 Ketamine	B2 (from C4i)
	2015 GHB	C2 (from C4i)

and fully synthetic drugs (made without recourse to natural drugs). A third classification by source is 'electronic highs', though these are outside the scope of this chapter (Newcombe, 2012b). Also, as noted above, some NPS products contain a mixture of natural and synthetic drugs: notably 'synthetic cannabis' products, which may contain minor plant-based drugs mixed with synthetic cannabinoids (Uchiyama et al., 2010).

Legal classification

Another common way of classifying NPS is by their legal status, which derives from national legislation assigning controlled drugs to classes/schedules, with criminal penalties for possession and trafficking offences reflecting the level of legal categorisation. This system is not fixed but constantly evolves as new legislation to control emerging NPS is introduced, and as laws in different countries are amended to allow new or revised categorisations. National legislation on drugs, typically enacted in Medicine Acts, also covers medical and non-medical aspects of NPS use and supply (notably regulations on prescribing and dispensing). International legislation derives from the United Nations (notably the three drugs conventions) and in Europe from the European Union (EU) Parliament.

Focusing on the UK, NPS are categorised by the Misuse of Drugs Act 1971 (MoDA) in two ways: by three classes (A to C), which determine the penalties for possession and trafficking offences (up to life imprisonment for trafficking class A drugs); and by five schedules (1 to 5), which regulate prescribing and dispensing (the strictest being schedule 1, which means the drug has no recognised medical use). Over the twenty-first century, a growing number of NPS and new/problematic medical drugs have been legally controlled in the UK by successive amendments to the MoDA (see Table 33.1).[5]

Psychopharmacological classification

Perhaps the most common ways of classifying NPS are by their psychoactive effects and chemical groups, including their impact on neurotransmission. The taxonomy of NPS presented here was influenced by several sources including drug definition and classification schemes used on such websites as Wikipedia and Erowid, along with models implicitly or explicitly identified by researchers, trainers and organisations (Dargan and Wood, 2013; EMCDDA, 2014a; Mentor-Adepis, 2014; Zohara et al., 2014).[6] Adley's Drug Wheel is particularly useful, combining seven categories of broad psychoactive effect – depressants, opioids, stimulants, cannabinoids, empathogens, psychedelics and dissociatives – with a two-way classification by legal status in the UK (http://thedrugswheel.com/). By April 2015, it covered 100 drugs/drug groups, including 69 controlled substances and 31 non-controlled substances. Its main limitations are the relevance of its legal classification to the UK only and its basis in just one psychochemical classification level.

In our proposed classification of NPS, psychoactive drugs can be organised according to a conceptual framework founded on two primary orthogonal dimensions of altered brain activity: stimulant-depressant and hallucinogenic-antipsychotic. However, with the notable exception of cannabidiol, there are very few psychoactive substances with predominantly anti-psychotic effects in common use. Accordingly, our scheme bases the first categorisation level (general effect on the CNS) on the tripartite distinction between depressants, stimulants and hallucinogens. The second level categorises NPS into nine families of psychoactive effect, namely: inebriant, sedative and analgesic families of depressants; euphoriant, eugeroic and entactogen families of stimulants; and psychedelic, dissociative and deliriant families of hallucinogens. The third level categorises NPS into 37 chemical groups and the fourth category itemises the hundreds of drugs that come under these headings[7] – these can be further divided into legal and illegal drugs according to national laws. It should be noted that there are many types and levels of chemical classification and the categories used in Table 33.2 are open to further refinement.[8]

Table 33.2 presents the taxonomy of drugs considered to be NPS according to at least some of the many definitions discussed above, which cover both 'new' drugs and 'legal' drugs, as well as drugs available from High Street 'headshops', online websites and other sources in the case of drugs such as laughing gas, poppers, khat and magic mushrooms. The scheme can also be modified and tightened to focus on NPS by our earlier operational definition (at the levels of chemical group and specific drugs). Clearly, given that the effects of drugs vary widely by sub-types

Table 33.2 A new taxonomy of new psychoactive substances

Psychoactive effect			*Chemical classification*
Class	*Family*	*Group*	*Specific NPS*
Depressant	Sedative	• Benzodiazepine • Anti-histamine • GHB-type • Kavalactones • Z-drugs	*phenazepam, etizolam, brotizolamdiphenhydramine, promethazine, cyclizineGHB, GBL, GBK, 14BDmethysticin, yangonin, kavain [kava: 15]zopiclone, zaleplon*
	Analgesic	• Opioid • Kratom compound	*MT-45, AH-7921, doxylam, carfentanil, ocfentanilmitragynine, hydroxymitragynine*
Stimulant	Euphoriant	• Amphetamine • Cocaine analogue • Cathinone - natural • Pyrrolidine • Piperazine • Piperidine • Oxazoline • Aliphatic amine	*fluoroamphetamine, 4-methylamphetaminedimethocaine, fluorotropacocainecathinone, cathine [khat]naphyrone, pyrovalerone, MDPVBZP, TFMPP, mCPP, MeOPPpipradol, 2DPMP, DPMP, ethylphenidatemethylaminorex, dimethylaminorex (DMAR)dimethylamylamine (geranamine)*
	Eugeroic	• Pyridine • Xanthine • Benzhydril-sulfinyl • Ephedrine	*nicotine, arecoline, cotinine, cytisinecaffeine, theobromine/theophyllinemodafinil, armodafinil, adrafinilephedrine, pseudo-ephedrine, cathine*
	Entactogen	• Phenethylamine • Cathinone - synthetic • Aminoindane • Benzofuran	*25B-NBOMe, 25I-NBOMe, bk-2CB, mescalinemephedrone (m-cat), methylone, methedroneMDAI, MMAI, 5-IAI, 2-AI, TAI, ETAI5/6-APB, bromo-dragon FLY, 2C-B-FLY*
Hallucinogen	Psychedelic	• Lysergamide • Tryptamine • Cannabinoid (SCRA) • Harmala alkaloid	*LSA, LSH [ipomea]AMT, AET, 5-MeO-DALT, 4-HO-METJWH-018, AM-2201, CP-47, 5F-AKB-48, XLR-11harmaline, harmine (beta-carbolines)*
	Dissociative	• Arylcyclohexylamine • Other NMDA-RA • Diterpenoid • Isoxazole	*methoxetamine, dephenidine, tiletaminenitrous oxide, dextromethorphansalvinorin-A [salvia]muscimol, ibotenic acid [amanita]*
	Deliriant	• Alkyl nitrite • Anti-cholinergic • Hydrocarbon • Haloalkane	*amyl nitrite, butyl nitrite, isopropyl nitriteatropine, scopolamine, hyoscyaminetoluene, butane, petroleumchloroform, chlorofluorocarbons (CFCs)*

NMDARA, N-methyl-D-aspartic acid receptor antagonist; SCRA, synthetic cannabinoid receptor agonist; [ ], plant source.

and consumption patterns (e.g. route of use, dose, setting), some drugs or drug categories could arguably be classified under alternative headings. For instance, the entactogen family could be included under the class of hallucinogens or stimulants, because entactogens vary widely in their effects and when consumed in different ways. Similar considerations apply to cannabinoids. Even so, our taxonomy provides a useful framework for understanding and discussing NPS and will be used to organise the evidence that follows.

TRENDS IN NPS PRODUCTION, SUPPLY AND USE

This section provides a brief overview of the main evidence concerning the development of NPS markets, including trends in production, distribution, availability, prevalence of use and consumption.

The challenges of defining and measuring drug use in general have been widely discussed elsewhere in this collection and in relation specifically to NPS here. These ongoing challenges make estimating the prevalence of use – across drugs and population groups – even more complex. Moreover, allowing for the usual caveats for drug prevalence research (Newcombe, 2007), NPS research is even more challenging because of the large numbers of substances, their rapid development and changing legal status and the complexities of identifying and matching chemical compounds with branded retail products and the street or slang names adopted by different user groups. The lists of actual and potential drugs cast an increasingly gloomy shadow across research on patterns and prevalence of NPS use. This has led some researchers (including one of the authors) to embrace greater cross disciplinary collaboration and triangulation in order to explore what users have bought and believe they are consuming by comparison with what retailers have bought from manufacturers and believe they are selling – resulting in fertile collaborations between criminologists, chemists and toxicologists (e.g. Archer et al., 2014a, 2014b). Whilst urine testing as a validation tool for self-reported drug use is nothing new (e.g. Measham et al., 2001), the scale of mass pooled urine analysis in recent years across Europe (EMCDDA, 2014b) in large part has been fuelled by the rapid expansion in the number of NPS and the need to ascertain their prevalence of use whilst challenging the constraints of traditional self-report data collection.

Global NPS use

The World Drug Report (UNODC, 2014: 51) has reported that NPS use is now 'a truly global phenomenon'. Of 103 countries on which relevant information was available in December 2013, 94 reported the emergence of NPS markets, up from 70 out of 80 in mid-2012. The total global number of NPS has more than doubled from 166 in 2009 to 348 at the end of 2013 (including 97 NPS identified for the first time in 2013). This has led to the unprecedented situation of 'the number of NPS clearly exceed[ing] the number of psychoactive substances controlled at the international level' (UNODC, 2014: 52): that is, 348 NPS compared with 234 controlled drugs. The main drug groups comprising the 348 NPS included cannabinoids (29 per cent), phenethlyamines (21 per cent), cathinones (15 per cent), tryptamines (8 per cent), plant-based drugs (6 per cent), piperazines (4 per cent), arylcyclohexylamines (3 per cent), aminoindanes (1 per cent) and other NPS groups (11 per cent).

The Global Drug Survey (GDS) accesses predominantly young adults through a range of general and specialist media websites such as The Guardian, Fox News and Mixmag. The 2013 GDS was based on a self-selecting convenience sample of 78,800 people (Winstock, 2014a). Across the 18 countries with sample sizes of over 600 (average sample size: 4,000), 12 per cent reported having used NPS/'legal highs' in the last year (using a broad definition of NPS that includes longstanding and non-synthetic psychoactive substances including nitrous oxide and salvia) and 22 per cent reported having bought drugs online. Of the 10 types of NPS use reported, last year use of nitrous oxide was the most common (6 per cent), reported by 14 countries and ranging from 1 per cent in Portugal to 27 per cent in the Netherlands. The other two most popular NPS were salvia and synthetic cannabinoids, with national rates of use ranging from 1 per cent to 10 per cent. The report on the December 2014 GDS noted that there was a substantial drop in last year NPS use to 7 per cent (Winstock, 2014b). Among the 11 countries with over 1,500 respondents, last year use of NPS varied from below 10 per cent in nine countries to 12 per cent in the UK. Overall, the most commonly reported 'research chemicals and legal highs' were synthetic cannabinoids: 2 per cent reporting having used them in the last year.

A review of the literature on the epidemiology of NPS use by Sumnall and colleagues concluded that aside from mephedrone, *Salvia divinorum* and SCRAs 'most other NPS appear not to have made a significant impact on the drug market with respect to user preference…[and] remain infrequent choices' (Sumnall et al., 2013: 99). They note that 'most data on NPS epidemiology comes from (small) convenience samples', which produce findings with limitations given that 'such data can only reveal drug use behaviours in the respondents surveyed, and cannot easily be generalized beyond the study' (2013: 99). Although the authors did not mention that nitrous oxide use is second only to cannabis in the UK and is the most popular NPS in the UK general population survey (Home Office, 2014), this may be because nitrous oxide only recently was included in (some) definitions of NPS.

USA

The US Office of National Drug Control Policy (2014) reported that the number of new synthetic drugs identified in 2012 reached a record 158, including 51 cannabinoids (compared with two in 2009), 31 cathinones (compared with four in 2009) and 76 other new drugs. The number of hospital emergency department visits involving synthetic cannabinoids more than doubled from 11,406 in 2010 to 28,531 in 2011 (Substance Abuse and Mental Health Services Administration, 2013).

Indeed, research consistently indicates that synthetic cannabinoids are the most popular type of NPS in the USA, although it should be noted that this depends on how NPS are (or are not) defined and classified, including which NPS are itemised in survey questionnaires and which NPS are included under standard drug group headings in surveys. For instance, the Monitoring the Future (MtF) self-report annual surveys of US college students and young adults, based on repeated cross sectional surveys of high school graduates, have been reported from 1976 to 2013 (Johnston et al., 2014). The MtF surveys of over 40,000 secondary school students and several thousand college students and young adults aged 19 to 28 years has reported the prevalence of last year use of three itemised NPS in recent years (see Table 33.3) (Johnston et al., 2014). However, it is likely that drugs classified as NPS in some other studies or reporting systems are incorporated under general drug group headings in the MtF study – including hallucinogens (e.g. NBOMe), inhalants (e.g. nitrous oxide), tranquillisers (e.g. phenazepam) and opioids (e.g. MT-45).

Table 33.3 New psychoactive substances use among eighth to tenth graders in US secondary schools, college students and young adults, 2009 to 2014

	Synthetic cannabis	*Synthetic stimulants*	*Salvia divinorum*												
	8th	*10th*	*12th*	*CS*	*YA*	*8th*	*10th*	*12th*	*CS*	*YA*	*8th*	10th	12th	CS	YA
2009													5.7	5.8	3.5
2010											1.7	3.7	5.5	3.5	3.6
2011			11.4	8.5	7.4						1.6	3.9	5.9	3.1	2.2
2012	4.4	8.8	11.3	5.3	5.3	0.8	0.6	1.3	0.3	0.5	1.4	2.5	4.4	1.5	1.5
2013	4.0	7.4	7.9	2.3	3.2	1.0	0.9	0.9	0.1	0.4	1.2	2.3	3.4	1.0	0.9
2014	3.3	5.4	5.8			0.5	0.9	0.9			0.6	1.8	1.8		

CS, college students; YA, young adults (19 to 28 years).

In 2014, levels of last year use of synthetic cannabinoids (also referred to as 'K2/Spice') ranged from over 3 per cent among eighth graders to almost 6 per cent among twelfth graders. These represent significant drops from the previous year and levels for all three grades have dropped steadily since 2012. Levels of last year use of salvia also dropped two- to three-fold from 2010 to 2014 to below 2 per cent, and last year use of synthetic stimulants ('bath salts') was reported by fewer than 1 per cent of students in all grades in 2014. Levels of last year use of all three NPS have fallen fairly steadily across recent years for both groups, and to lower levels than those for school students by 2013 – 3 per cent or lower for cannabinoid use and 1 per cent or lower for use of salvia and stimulants.

Prevalence of NPS use across Europe

The Early Warning System run by EMCDDA (2015) reported that more than 450 NPS were currently being monitored across the EU. Overall, 299 different NPS were detected in 2013: 101 newly identified and 198 previously identified NPS. The most commonly identified types since 2008 were synthetic cannabinoids (134) and cathinones (77). NPS identified for the first time reached a record 101 in 2014, compared with 81 in 2013, 74 in 2012, 49 in 2011, 41 in 2010, 24 in 2009 and 13 in 2008. The most common new types identified over the last two years were: cathinones (from seven in 2013 to 31 in 2014), cannabinoids (from 29 to 30), phenethlyamines (from 14 to nine), arylalkylamines (from seven to four), opioids (from five to five), tryptamines (from one to five), benzodiazepines (from two to four) and other synthetic substances (from 16 to 13).

Seizure figures for 2013 show that there were a record 46,370 seizures of over 3.1 tonnes of NPS, with the two main types including 21,495 seizures of almost 1.6 tonnes of synthetic cannabinoids and 10,657 seizures of more than 1.1 tonnes of synthetic cathinones. There was a seven-fold increase in reported NPS seizures between 2008 and 2013.

The EMCDDA (2013) identified 651 shops that sold NPS as 'legal high' products or 'research chemicals', a slight decrease on 693 in January 2012, but higher than the 631 in July 2011, 314 in January 2011 and 170 in 2010. The July 2011 snapshot exercise found that the three NPS most commonly sold by the online shops at that time were all plant products: kratom (128), salvia (110) and hallucinogenic mushrooms (72). The next three most commonly sold NPS were synthetic drugs: MDAI (61), methoxetamine (58) and 6-APB (49) (EMCDDA, 2011a, 2011b). The UK was home to 121 of the shops.

The European Commission 'Flash Eurobarometer' survey of 'young people and drugs' was based on telephone interviews with over 13,000 15 to 24 year olds in all 28 EU Member States in June 2013. The average EU figure for reported lifetime use of NPS increased from 5 per cent in the 2011 survey to 8 per cent in the 2014 survey (European Commission, 2014). The top six countries for NPS use all exhibited increases in lifetime use of NPS from 2011 to 2014: Ireland (from 16 per cent to 22 per cent), Slovenia (from 7 per cent to 13 per cent), Slovakia (from 7 per cent to 13 per cent), Spain (from 5 per cent to 13 per cent), France (from 5 per cent to 12 per cent) and the UK (from 2 per cent to 10 per cent). The biggest increase was in the UK, where the proportion of NPS users increased five-fold between the two surveys.

NPS availability and use in the UK

Official statistics

Although national NPS seizure figures are not available, the number of seizures of NPS in prisons in England and Wales has been reported to have increased significantly, from 16 in 2010, 90 in 2011, 138 in 2012, 267 in

2013 and 436 in the first 7 months of 2014 (Parliamentary Question, September 2014). Each year, the vast majority of these seizures involved synthetic cannabinoids (from 15 in 2010 to 430 in the first half of 2014) and the prison authorities have reported that use of these NPS leads to increased violence and disorder among inmates. A qualitative study of NPS that included interviews with prisoners and ex-prisoners also reported that synthetic cannabinoids are the most popular drug in UK prisons (Linnell et al., 2015).

The 2013/14 annual report of the UK Forensic Early Warning System (FEWS) noted that 'so far the Coalition Government has controlled over 350 NPS, by group or generic definitions, including some not seen in the UK, under the 1971 Act' (FEWS, 2014: 4).[9] The total number identified since 2011 was 31, including 10 cannabinoids, four tryptamines, three phenethlyamines and three cathinones. Analysis of NPS samples collected by FEWS found that around nine out of 10 were mixtures of either two (61 per cent) or three (30 per cent) active drug ingredients. In 2013/14, 3 per cent of internet and 4 per cent of headshop samples contained controlled NPS, compared to 16 per cent and 64 per cent in 2012/13. However, 88 per cent of festival samples contained controlled drugs in 2013/14, a similar amount to 2012/13 (84 per cent) (FEWS, 2014).

An NPS was the primary drug[10] of concern for 144 people in drug treatment in England in 2013/14 – just under 0.1 per cent of all drug treatment clients (Public Health England, 2014). However, separate statistics for mephedrone and GHB/GBL indicated that the number of NPS users in treatment had almost tripled over the last three years.

General household surveys

Annual general household surveys of drug use are conducted in all countries of the UK but due to space constraints, we focus here on prevalence surveys in England and Wales only (see UK Drug Focal Point, 2014, for a summary of NPS use across the UK).

The annual Crime Survey for England and Wales (CSEW) includes a general household survey of drug use among over 20,000 adults (Home Office, 2014) and is the most robust national data set on drug prevalence in the UK. Over the six years ending 2014/15, the CSEW has reported on the prevalence of use of seven types of NPS: mephedrone, spice, khat, BZP, GHB/GBL, nitrous oxide and salvia. Overall lifetime and last year use of mephedrone has declined steadily for both adults and young adults since it was controlled and national data was first collected in 2010, although it rose slightly in 2013/14 (see Table 33.4).[11]

Nitrous oxide and Salvia divinorum

Both nitrous oxide and salvia remained uncontrolled drugs in the UK at the end of 2014, although not included in many post-2008 definitions of NPS given their long-standing, if low level recreational usage, they are considered to be 'legal highs' by some commentators based on their legal status, effects and availability (to date) from online retailers and headshops. Between 2012/13 and 2013/14, there were increases in the last year use of both of these drugs, for both adults and young adults, with the change in last year use of salvia among all adults being statistically significant (Table 33.5). Nitrous oxide was the second most commonly used drug by young adults in the UK after cannabis and the third most commonly used drug

Table 33.4 Prevalence of use of mephedrone in England and Wales, 2010/11 to 2014/15 (CSEW)

	Adults 16 to 59		*Young adults 16 to 24*	
	Lifetime	Last year	Lifetime	Last year
2010/11	–	1.3	–	4.4
2011/12	–	1.0	–	3.3
2012/13	1.9	0.5	4.5	1.6
2013/14	2.3	0.6	6.3	1.9
2014/15	2.2	0.5	5.3	1.9

Table 33.5 Prevalence of last year use of salvia and nitrous oxide in England and Wales, 2012/13 to 2013/14 (CSEW; Home Office, 2014)

	Adults 16 to 59		*Young adults 16 to 24*	
	Salvia	Nitrous oxide	Salvia	Nitrous oxide
2012/13	0.3	2.0	1.1	6.1
2013/14	0.5	2.3	1.8	7.6

by all adults after cannabis and cocaine.[12] The figures on last year use also show that mephedrone and salvia are the fifth and sixth most popular drugs among young adults (ecstasy is fourth).

The CSEW also reported on last year use of four other drugs between 2009/10 and 2011/12, which are included in some definitions of NPS. Last year use of 'spice' and BZP both fell from around half a per cent to 0.1 per cent, while last year use of khat and GHB/GBL remained level at about 0.2 per cent and 0.1 per cent respectively. Between 2009/10 and 2010/11, notable drops in last year use of all four of these NPS were evident among 16 to 24 year olds, with 25 to 59 year olds exhibiting stable and lower levels of use. In short, of seven types of NPS assessed by the CSEW, three were fairly popular compared with controlled drugs, while four were used by fewer than 0.2 per cent according to the latest figures available.

MOTIVATIONS AND USER GROUPS

In this final section we draw together some of the evidence discussed above to piece together why the NPS phenomenon shot into the spotlight from 2008 onwards and what might be the motivations of users, which then sheds light on who are the key user groups. Whilst many of the reasons for taking NPS are similar to the motivations for consuming a whole host of other psychoactive substances – legal, illegal or prescription; prohibited, controlled or licensed – it is only through an understanding of the inter relationship between established and 'new' psychoactive substances that we can more fully understand their appearance and appeal.

Purity

A key reason for the emergence of NPS relates to their *relative* purity, by comparison with established drugs across Europe in that particular historical period (Measham, 2013). Forensic analyses of ecstasy and cocaine seizures and submissions to drug checking organisations (such as the Dutch Drug Information and Monitoring System or DIMS) in 2008/10 concur that purity was at its lowest level across Europe just before mephedrone became a concern. In the UK for example, purity levels fell to an all-time low for most established controlled drugs in around 2009. Cocaine purity reached a low point of 20 per cent in 2008 (Table 33.6) and the MDMA content of ecstasy pills fell to a low point of 20 mg in 2009 (UK Focal Point on Drugs, 2014), after the emergence of MDMA crystal (MD, Molly) as a higher priced, higher purity 'premium' product in the mid-2000s in the UK (Smith et al., 2009). Conversely, forensic analyses of mephedrone showed that it was being sold at approximately 95 per cent purity before legislative control in 2008 to 2010 (Miserez et al., 2014). Whilst it could be argued that it was merely coincidence that the purity levels of the most popular established illegal stimulants were at their lowest point in decades at the very same time that mephedrone (a legal stimulant with not dissimilar effects to cocaine and ecstasy) first became a concern, studies with users endorse this connection. Interviews with mephedrone users before legislative control in the UK (Measham et al., 2010) articulate a clear narrative of disillusionment with Class A drugs by both

Table 33.6 Domestic resale mean percentage purity of certain drugs seized by police in England and Wales, 2003 to 2013

	2003	*2004*	*2005*	*2006*	*2007*	*2008*	*2009*	*2010*	*2011*	*2012*	*2013*
Amphetamines	11	9	10	11	11	8	8	8	10	5	7
Cocaine powder	51	42	43	35	33	29	20	24	26	37	38
Crack cocaine	70	64	65	50	52	43	27	31	26	30	36
Heroin (brown)	33	40	47	44	50	43	44	35	18	20	33
Ecstasy*	65	67	66	48	52	33	44	49	71	102	n/a

Source: UK Focal Point on Drugs (2014); *mg of MDMA base per tablet.

recreational drug users and problem drug users:

> I guess it has kind of replaced my desire for ecstasy... because I don't really feel like I can get hold of proper ecstasy. Whereas mephedrone I feel much more comfortable taking because I kind of know what I am getting. So in that way it has probably replaced my, yes I would say it probably has – until I can find, if I find a good source of MDMA – it has replaced my use of that drug. (Professional male, 34, 2009, in Measham et al., 2010)

From 2011 onwards, both DIMS and UK forensic analyses suggest that the purity of cocaine and ecstasy increased again across Europe, with the MDMA content of seized ecstasy pills increasing five-fold from 20 mg to 100 mg in the six-year period from 2008 to 2014 (ACMD, 2015). Conversely, after legislative control of substituted cathinones in 2010, forensic analyses of second generation NPS show that unlike the first generation NPS of high purity, these second generation NPS were of variable content and sometimes even illegal (Brandt et al., 2010). The variable content, effects and legal status of these NPS were widely publicised, capitalised on by politicians and drugs prevention campaigns. This may have dampened some of the initial demand for NPS and resulted in a fall in NPS prevalence rates in annual surveys, including both the general household survey and convenience sample surveys of festival-goers (Measham, 2013) and club-goers (Wood et al., 2012a). The rise and fall in self-reported mephedrone use contrasts with the disillusionment and then reinforcement of ecstasy's appeal as the MDMA content of tablets rose to and surpassed their previous levels (Pidd, 2014). So a key point here is that the appeal of NPS products when they first appeared related to the purity and reliability of their contents *relative* to the purity and reliability of established illegal drugs and the relationship between the two.[13]

It should not be assumed that there was simple displacement from low purity Class A drugs to high purity legal NPS in 2008/9, however. Annual surveys conducted with club-goers at South London gay-friendly dance clubs from 2010 onwards have shown consistently high levels of self-reported mephedrone use each year, with mephedrone becoming the drug most likely to be consumed on a night out and also these club-goers' favourite drug (Measham et al., 2011b; Wood et al., 2012b). However, these surveys found no evidence of wholesale displacement from Class A drugs such as cocaine and ecstasy to NPS, but rather mephedrone appeared to have been added to existing drug-using repertoires and was being used as a supplement, a secondary drug, to 'top up' low purity Class As (Moore et al., 2013). This is supported by the general population survey (Smith and Flatley, 2011), which reports that nine in 10 mephedrone users reported having used other illegal drugs in the last year. These various studies suggest, therefore, that purity was a particular appeal for users who were already experienced Class A drug users, such as club-goers. A further indicator of the elasticity of demand for mephedrone and its possible status as a 'topping up' drug relates to the fact that the price only rose to £20/25/gram after legislative control in 2010 and has stayed at that price since then.[14]

Availability

This has been a significant driver to NPS use: for the first time, psychoactive drugs were widely, cheaply and legally available online, in specialist headshops, market stalls, festivals and (of increasing concern) at small independent convenience stores and petrol garages with variable retail practices (NPS Review Expert Panel, 2014). However, as with purity, availability of NPS is also *relative* and usually gauged in comparison with the access and availability of illegal drugs. So for users who either could not access or did not want access to established drugs through street 'dealers', legal NPS hold an obvious appeal.

The DrugScope 2013 street drug trends survey, based on information from drugs workers at 25 agencies in mainland Britain, revealed that the main source of NPS was not internet websites but specialist 'headshops' and also non-specialist shops such as petrol stations, pet shops, takeaway food shops, newsagents, tobacconists, sex shops and market stalls. While few young people were coming forward to treatment services, outreach workers reported that some young people were at risk of serious health consequences, a finding confirmed in the qualitative study by Linnell and colleagues (2015). Daly (2013) also reported that a snapshot survey carried out in Newcastle of 116 people (mainly teenagers aged 16 to 17) found that, of those who had recently bought 'legal highs', 45 had purchased them from headshops, while 20 had bought them from a petrol station or takeaway food shop.

Availability of NPS appeals particularly to teenagers and novice users without established contact with illicit subcultures and illegal economies (evidenced in the disproportionate numbers of patients in their mid-teens hospitalised for SC-related problems in the UK). Others who may not be able to access illegal drugs through street dealers may be residents in rural areas without easy access to urban street markets and middle class professionals who were suddenly able to order NPS products online with a credit card and without the risks associated with purchasing illegal drugs such as being exploited by street dealers or caught by the police. The converse of this is that once mephedrone was banned, self-reported use fell (e.g. Lader, 2015; Measham, 2013, Winstock, 2014a), suggesting that at least, in part, once availability plummeted, so did use. Furthermore, for those who continued to use controlled NPS, their use was likely to be riskier in terms of both physical and social harms due to greater variations in content and purity in unregulated markets combined with accessing criminal supply networks.

Legality

If prevalence of NPS use falls in the years after legislative control, as indicated with falling mephedrone use in the UK general household survey discussed above (Lader, 2015), then perhaps this can be seen as evidence of a deterrent effect of banning drugs, as distinct from the impact of reduced availability resulting from the ban on legal sales? In general, there is a weak evidence base on the deterrent value of criminal law. What we know from international comparative drug policy analyses (e.g. EMCDDA, 2011c; Stevens, 2011) and regional times-series data (e.g. Wood et al., 2012b) is that there appears to be little impact of drug policy change on drug use in a range of different jurisdictions.

Furthermore, in surveys and interviews, users themselves rarely prioritise legal status when discussing why, or indeed why not, to take illegal drugs (e.g. Parker et al., 1998). Research with users has found that more important reasons for taking or avoiding drugs include price, purity, availability, perceived pleasurable/unpleasant effects, curiosity and the wider social context to use (Norman et al., 2014; O'Brien et al., 2015). Moreover, if, as discussed above, NPS users are more likely to be experienced drug users and take NPS along with illegal drugs in weekend polydrug repertoires, then the legal status of NPS in particular is of little relevance.

Where legal status has been found to result in a significant appeal for uncontrolled NPS has been for those who come into contact with drug testing, through employers, treatment services, the operation of motor vehicles and the criminal justice system more generally. For example, SCRAs have been found to hold a particular appeal amongst US professionals (Perrone et al., 2013), UK professionals (Sumnall et al., 2016), UK prisoners (Brown, 2014), UK ex-offenders (Linnell et al., 2015) and clients in treatment who are drug tested.

Media

A fourth key driver to NPS use has been the media. Intense media scrutiny of NPS drug-related deaths and NPS policy have led to a symbiotic relationship between press coverage, policy makers and user demand for drugs (Forsyth, 2012; Measham et al., 2011a). For NPS at least as much as for any other drug problem, there is a sharp contrast between the lack of information regarding short and long term effects of use, the spiralling numbers of psychoactive substances available and the burgeoning easy access both to information and to retailers themselves through the internet. Although not unique to NPS – the early internet was utilised when ecstasy gained popularity with 1990s dance club cultures[15] – it has been widely noted how pivotal the internet has been to the development of NPS (Forsyth, 2012; Schifano et al., 2010), with NPS being considered the first group of drugs to be born out of the internet age. Indeed, the internet has played a multi-faceted role in relation to the development of NPS, from the facilitation of multimedia news, research data collection and dissemination, dark and clear net retail outlets, to online user forums and virtual communities (Barratt et al. 2014; O'Brien et al., 2015).

CONCLUSION: FROM 'CAT AND MOUSE' TO 'HARE AND HOUNDS'

In answer to the question what is new about new psychoactive substances, it is the speed of innovation combined with the globalisation and virtualisation of drug markets and user groups that have together led to the essential 'newness' of the NPS phenomenon. However, within this innovation also lies another key feature of the NPS debate. The rapidity of NPS manufacturing and marketing innovations move in conjunction with the rapidity of policy developments. This relationship between pharmacological and policy developments was widely characterised in the early years as a 'cat and mouse' relationship (including by the authors elsewhere: Measham et al., 2010), with NPS chemists and entrepreneurs ready to respond to each new piece of legislation. Having seen several generations of NPS and NPS-related legislation now develop, one of the authors[16] has suggested that it is perhaps more accurate to characterise this relationship between NPS development and policy change as 'hare and hounds' rather than 'cat and mouse' because it is the speed of policy change itself that is the driving force behind the faster and faster pace of NPS innovations. Without each set of generic controls of SCRA in the UK, for example, it is highly unlikely that there would have been a further generation of SCRA development within such rapid succession of the previous one.

In conclusion, we see pockets of popularity and differentiated demand for NPS around the world, with legislative control impacting on purity, availability, price and appeal for some drugs in some areas, but persistent use by some others. Although prevalence of use of NPS remains low by comparison with established illegal drugs in most countries, the significance of the rise of 'legal highs' relates to the rapidity of innovation in this area and also the speed and scale of policy responses. In contrast to established illegal drugs, control regimes have been quick to respond to the perceived threat, the level of which has led to innovation and expansion of control regimes. Therefore, rather than a 'consensus fracture' as we have seen in relation to established illegal drugs and the 'war on drugs' (Bewley-Taylor, 2012), global drug prohibition regimes have indicated their capacity for innovation, adaptation and co-operation, with a tightening of the drug policy ratchet and the blanket of prohibition being thrown wider (Stevens and Measham, 2014). Indeed, it is in the response to criticism of prohibition as a creaky structure ill fitted to tackling the emergent NPS problem, that we have seen a reinvigoration, expansion and U-turn away from more liberal regimes with the introduction of the current regime of analogue, generic and 'blanket ban' control measures from 2009 onwards, resulting in a new era for both pharmacological and policy developments.

NOTES

1 Another metaphor applied to the relationship between pharmacological entrepreneurship and NPS legislative control compares this dynamic with 'cutting off the hydra's head' where several more grow back in its place. For example, 'Drugs have been a problem for centuries but legal highs have turned them into a narcotics version of Lernaean Hydra'. Available from: http://www.telegraph.co.uk/men/active/mens-health/11310863/Why-the-problem-of-legal-highs-wont-go-away.html.

2 Measham in attendance, 8 October 2009.

3 Two examples of these: first, BZP which was mis-sold as ecstasy in the UK in 2009/10 and appeared widely in forensic analyses of police seizures but had negligible reported use in general population surveys (Hoare and Moon, 2010) and self-reported surveys (Measham et al., 2011a, 2011b) at that time. PMA/PMMA was banned under UK generic legislation in 1977 and has been mis-sold as ecstasy, particularly from 2012 onwards. Four high profile deaths over the Christmas 2014 holiday period were attributed to pink 'Superman' tablets sold as ecstasy but which contained a high dose of PMMA (http://www.bbc.co.uk-england-suffolk-30709953). Blue 'Batman' tablets sold in the UK in 2014 were reported to contain a large amount of NBOMe, while other tablets sold as ecstasy were reported to contain methylone or 4-MTA (http://www.independent.co.uk/life-style/health-and-families/features/the-evolution-of-ecstasy-from-mandy-to-superman-the-effects-of-the-drug-mdma-9959732.html).

4 Space constraints preclude a detailed discussion of NPS policy options and implications, which can be found elsewhere (e.g. NPS Review Expert Panel, 2014).

5 In 2011, the UK MoDA was amended to allow for the passing of a 'temporary class drug order' (TCDO) that bans the sale (but not possession) of a potentially harmful new drug for a period of approximately 12 months to allow an assessment to be made of the need for permanent restrictions on sale and possession. In the first two years, three drugs were placed under a TCDO – methoxetamine, 5/6-APB and NBOMe compounds – all of which were subsequently banned (see Table 33.1).

6 Recent reviews of the evidence about particular categories of NPS include: amphetamines (Lapoint et al., 2013); cannabinoids (Auwarter et al., 2013; ACMD, 2014; Kickman and King 2014; Linnell, 2014); piperazines (Gee and Schep, 2013); cathinones (ACMD, 2010; Wood and Dargan, 2013); pipradols (White and Archer, 2013); aminoindanes (Brandt et al., 2013); arylcyclohexylamines (Chan et al., 2013; Greene, 2013); phenethlyamines (King, 2013); benzofurans (Greene, 2013); dimethoxyphenethylamines/NBOMe (ACMD, 2013); and tryptamines (ACMD, 2014; Greene, 2013).

7 Specific chemicals sold as NPS branded products are also given trade names by manufacturers and retailers but these are not used here.

8 Space constraints preclude a more detailed discussion here. More detailed definitions of these classes of drugs, covering their chemistry and psychopharmacology, can be found on such websites as Erowid and Wikipedia.

9 Examples of NPS seen in the UK market in the past year are AKB-48 (a synthetic cannabinoid), 25-B-NBOMe (a phenethylamine) and 4-MeO-PCP (a dissociative anaesthetic) as well as substances sold under branded names such as CRITICAL HAZE (containing 5F-AKB-48), SPARKLEE (containing MPA, 5-MeO-DALT and 2-aminoindane) and Black Mamba (containing AM-2201, 5-MeO-DALT and JWH-081) (FEWS 2014: 4).

10 Primary use of NPS is defined by the National Drug Treatment Monitoring System (NDTMS) for England as drug use that meets these two conditions: (i) no use of opiates or crack in the treatment journey; and (ii) report of primary drug in the earliest episode of the latest treatment journey to cross the reporting year in any of the following NPS categories: predominantly stimulant, hallucinogenic, dissociative, sedative/opioid or cannabis or not otherwise specified (Public Health England, 2014).

11 Based on these figures, the total number of lifetime users of mephedrone was estimated to have climbed from 584,000 in 2012/13 to 764,000 in 2013/14, while the total number of last year users climbed from 161,000 to 205,000. By 2013/14, these numbers included 394,000 young adults who had ever used mephedrone and 117,000 young adults who had used mephedrone in the last year (Lader, 2015).

12 It can be extrapolated from these figures that the number of last year users of nitrous oxide in the UK climbed from over half a million in 2012/13 to nearly three quarters of a million in 2013/14.

13 There is some evidence that purity levels and accurate labelling is increasing again amongst third generation NPS products (ACMD, 2015; FEWS, 2014).

14 Whilst it doubled in price compared with its legal price of £10/gram, it remains at about half the price per gram of MDMA and cocaine in the UK.

15 With ecstasy came the advent of ecstasy information and analysis forums and pill report sites, for example, www.ecstasy.org.

16 Measham, F. (2014) The unfathomable foggyiness of being: user motivations, market practises and policy implications. Presentation to NPS conference, Queen Mary College, London, May 2014.

REFERENCES

Advisory Council on the Misuse of Drugs (ACMD) (2011) *Consideration of the Novel Psychoactive Substances ('Legal Highs')*. London: Home Office. Available from: https://www.gov.uk/government/uploads/system/uploads/attachment_data/file/119139/acmdnps2011.pdf.

Advisory Council on the Misuse of Drugs (ACMD) (2015) *Mephedrone: Five Years of Control*. London: Home Office.

Archer, J., Dargan, P., Hudson, S., Davies, S., Puchnarewicz, M., Kicman, A., Ramsey, J., Measham, F., Wood, M., Johnston, A. and Wood D. (2014a) Taking the Pissoir: a novel and reliable way of knowing what drugs are being used in nightclubs. *Journal of Substance Use*, 19(1–2): 103–7.

Archer, J., Dargan, P., Lee, H., Hudson, S. and Wood, D. (2014b) Trend analysis of anonymised pooled urine from portable street urinals in central London identifies variation in the use of novel psychoactive substances. *Clinical Toxicology*, 52: 160–5.

Barratt, M., Ferris, J. and Winstock, A. (2014) Use of Silk Road, the online drug marketplace, in the United Kingdom, Australia and the United States. *Addiction*, 109(5): 774–83.

Bewley-Taylor, D. (2012), *International Drug Control: Consensus Fractured*. Cambridge: Cambridge University Press.

Brandt, S., Sumnall, H., Measham, F. and Cole, J. (2010) Analyses of second-generation 'legal highs' in the UK: Initial findings. *Drug Testing and Analysis*, 2(8): 377–82.

Brandt, S., King, L. and Evans-Brown, M. (2014) The new drug phenomenon. *Drug Testing and Analysis*, 6: 587–97.

Brown, S. (2014) Synthetic cannabis causing serious health problems in English prisons. *The Guardian*, 15 May. Available from: http://www.theguardian.com/society/2014/may/15/synthetic-cannabis-serious-health-problems-english-prisons.

Buchanan, J. and Brown, C. (1988) 'Designer drugs': a problem in clinical toxicology. *Medical Toxicology and Adverse Drug Experience*, 3(1): 1–17.

Coomber, R., McElrath, K., Measham, F. and Moore, K. (2013) *Dictionary of Key Concepts in Drugs and Society*. London: Sage.

Cope, I. (2014) Legal highs: a problem of definitions? *The Lancet*, 383: 1715.

Dargan, P., Albert, S. and Wood, D. (2010) Mephedrone use and associated adverse effects in school and college/university students before the UK legislation change. *QJM: An International Journal of Medicine*, 103: 875–9.

Dargan, P. and Wood, D. (eds) (2013) *Novel Psychoactive Substances: Classification, Pharmacology and Toxicology*. London: Academic Press.

Drugscope (2014) Business as usual? A status report on new psychoactive substances (NPS) and 'club drugs' in the UK. Available from: http://www.drugscope.org.uk/Resources/Drugscope/Documents/PDF/Policy/BusinessAsUsual.pdf.

European Commission (2014) *Flash Eurobarometer 401: Young People and Drugs*. Conducted by TNS Political and Social. Available from: http://ec.europa.eu/public_opinion/flash/fl_401_en.pdf.

EMCDDA (2007) *Early-Warning System on New Psychoactive Substances: Operating Guidelines*. Lisbon: EMCDDA.

EMCDDA (2011a) *Online Sales of New Psychoactive Substances/'Legal Highs': Summary of Results from the 2011 Multilingual Snapshots*. Lisbon: EMCDDA. Available from: http://www.emcdda.europa.eu/publications/scientific-studies/2011/snapshot.

EMCDDA (2011b) *Responding to New Psychoactive Substances*, Drugs in Focus EMCDDA Briefing 22. Lisbon: EMCDDA.

EMCDDA (2011c) *Annual Report 2011: The State of the Drugs Problem in Europe*. Lisbon: EMCDDA.

EMCDDA (2013) *European Drug Report*. Luxembourg: Publications Office of the European Union.

EMCDDA (2014a) *EMCDDA–Europol 2013 Annual Report on the implementation of Council Decision 2005/387/JHA*. Lisbon: EMCDDA. Available from: http://www.emcdda.europa.eu/attachements.cfm/att_229598_EN_TDAN14001ENN.pdf.

EMCDDA (2014b) *Wastewater Analysis and Drugs: A European Multi-City Study*, Perspectives on Drugs. Lisbon: EMCDDA.

EMCDDA (2015) *New Psychoactive Substances in Europe: An update from the EU Early Warning System*. Luxembourg: Publications Office of the European Union.

FEWS (2014) *Annual Report on the Home Office Forensic Early Warning System (FEWS), A system to identify New Psychoactive Substances in the UK*. London: Home Office. Available from: https://www.gov.uk/government/uploads/system/uploads/attachment_data/file/344551/2014-08-12_-_FEWS_Annual_Report_Aug_2014_-_Final__2_.pdf.

Forsyth, A. (2012) Virtually a drug scare: mephedrone and the impact of the internet on drug news transmission. *International Journal of Drug Policy*, 23(3): 198–209.

Goodair, C., Corkery, J. and Claridge, H. (2014) Legal highs: a problem of definitions? *The Lancet*, 383: 1715.

Home Office (2010) Drug *Strategy 2010 Reducing Demand, Restricting Supply, Building Recovery: Supporting People to Live a Drug-Free Life*. London: Home Office. Available from: https://www.gov.uk/government/publications/drug-strategy-2010—2

Home Office (2014) *Drug Misuse: Findings from the 2013 to 2014 Crime Survey for England and Wales*. London: Home Office. Available from: https://www.gov.uk/government/statistics/drug-misuse-findings-from-the-2013-to-2014-csew.

International Narcotics Control Board (2013) *Annual Report 2012*. Vienna: United Nations.

King, L. and Nutt, D. (2014) Deaths from 'legal highs': a problem of definitions. *The Lancet*, 383: 952.

Johnston, D. et al. (2014) *Monitoring the Future National Survey Results on Drug Use, 1975–2013, Volumes 1 and 2: Secondary School Students*. Ann Arbor: University of Michigan: Institute for Social Research.

Lader, D. (2015) *Drug Misuse: Findings from the 2014/15 Crime Survey for England and Wales*, Statistical Bulletin 03/15. London: Home Office.

Linnell, M., Measham, F. and Newcombe, R. (2015), *New Psychoactive Substances: The Local Picture, A Research Study and Needs Assessment for Blackburn with Darwen Borough Council*. Manchester: Linnell Publications.

Measham, F. (2013) Social issues in the use of novel psychoactive substances: differentiated demand and ideological supply. In P. Dargan and D. Wood (eds), *Novel Psychoactive Substances: Classification, Pharmacology and Toxicology*. London: Elsevier, pp. 105–27.

Measham, F., Aldridge J. and Parker, H. (2001) *Dancing On Drugs: Risk, Health and Hedonism in the British Club Scene*. London: Free Association Books.

Measham, F., Moore, K. and Østergaard, J. (2011a) Mephedrone, 'bubble' and unidentified white powders: the contested identities of synthetic 'legal highs'. *Drugs and Alcohol Today*, 11(3): 137–47.

Measham F., Moore, K., Newcombe, R. and Welch, Z. (2010) Tweaking, bombing, dabbing and stockpiling: the emergence of mephedrone and the perversity of prohibition. *Drugs and Alcohol Today*, 10(1): 14–21.

Measham, F., Wood, D., Dargan, P. and Moore, K. (2011b) The rise in legal highs: prevalence and patterns in the use of illegal drugs and first and second generation 'legal highs' in south London gay dance clubs. *Journal of Substance Use*, 16(4): 263–72.

Mentor-Adepis (2014). *The Drugs Wheel*. London: Mentor-Adepis. Available from: http://mentor-adepis.org/drugs-wheel/.

Miserez, B. et al. (2014) Analysis of purity and cutting agents in street mephedrone samples from South Wales, *Forensic Toxicology*, 32: 305–10.

Newcombe, R. (2007) Trends in the prevalence of illicit drug use in Britain. In M. Simpson et al. (eds), *Drugs in Britain: Supply, Consumption and Control*. Basingstoke: Palgrave-MacMillan, pp. 13–38.

Newcombe, R. (2012a) Legal highs in the UK: nature and extent of use. Warrington: *HIT Hot Topics Conference*. Available from: https://www.youtube.com/watch?v=YOOBRRmXLzk.

Newcombe, R. (2012b) Un-drug highs: electronic intoxication. Liverpool: *HIT Hot Topics Conference*, FACT.

NPS Review Expert Panel (2014) *New Psychoactive Substances Review: Report of the Expert Panel*. Available from: https://www.gov.uk/government/uploads/system/uploads/attachment_data/file/368583/NPSexpertReviewPanelReport.pdf.

O'Brien, K., Chatwin, C., Jenkins, C. and Measham, F. (2015) New psychoactive substances and british drug policy: a view from the new domestic cyber-psychonauts. *Drugs: Education, Prevention and Policy*, 22: 217–23.

Parker, H., Aldridge J. and Measham, F. (1998) *Illegal Leisure: The Normalization of Adolescent Recreational Drug Use*. London: Routledge.

Parliamentary Question (2014) Parliamentary question on seizures of NPS in prisons in England and Wales, 2010 to 2013. Available from: http://www.theyworkforyou.com/wrans/?id=2014-09-26.209374.h&s=nps#g209374.r0.

Perrone, D. et al. (2013) United States drug prohibition and legal highs: how drug testing may lead cannabis users to Spice. *Drugs: Education, Prevention and Policy*, 20(3): 216–24.

Pidd, H. (2014) Clubbers warned of overdose risk from super-strength ecstasy, *The Guardian*, 28 November. Available from: http://www.theguardian.com/society/2014/nov/28/clubbers-warn-overdose-risk-from-superstrength-ecstasy-mdma.

Public Health England (2014) *Adult Drug Statistics from the National Drug Treatment Monitoring System (NDTMS) - 1 April 2013 to 31 March 2014*. Available from: http://www.nta.nhs.uk/uploads/adult-drug-statistics-from-the-national-drug-treatment-monitoring-system-2013-14.pdf.

Schifano, F. et al. (2010) Psychonaut web mapping; ReDNet research groups, mephedrone: chemical, pharmacological and clinical issues. *Psychopharmacology*, 214(3): 593–602.

Smith, Z., Moore, K. and Measham, F. (2009) MDMA powder, pills and crystal: the persistence of ecstasy and the poverty of policy. *Drugs and Alcohol Today*, 9(1): 13–19.

Stevens, A. (2011) *Drugs, Crime and Public Health: The Political Economy of Drug Policy*. London: Routledge-Cavendish.

Stevens, A. and Measham, F. (2014) The 'drug policy ratchet': why do sanctions for new psychoactive drugs typically only go up? *Addiction*, 109(8): 1226–32.

Substance Abuse and Mental Health Services Administration (2013) *Results from the 2012*

National Survey on Drug Use and Health: Summary of National Findings, NSDUH Series H-46, HHS Publication No. (SMA) 13-4795. Rockville, MD: Substance Abuse and Mental Health Services Administration.

Uchiyama, N. et al. (2010) Chemical analysis of synthetic cannabinoids as designer drugs in herbal products. *Forensic Science International,* 198: 31–8.

UNODC (2013) *NPS: New Psychoactive Substances*. Vienna: World Drug Campaign, UNODC. Available from: www.unodc.org/drugs.

UK Focal Point on Drugs (2014) *United Kingdom Drug Situation: Annual report to the European Monitoring Centre for Drugs and Drug Addiction (EMCDDA) 2014 Edition*. London: Public Health England.

UNODC (2014) *World Drug Report 2014*. Vienna: United Nations. Available from: http://www.unodc.org/wdr2014/.

US Office of National Drug Control Policy (2014) *Synthetic Drugs (a.k.a. K2, Spice, Bath Salts, etc.)*. Washington, DC: Office of National Drug Control Policy. Available from: http://www.whitehouse.gov/ondcp/ondcp-fact-sheets/synthetic-drugs-k2-spice-bath-salts.

Winstock, A. (2014a) *Global Drug Survey 2013: Last 12-Month Prevalence of Top 20 Drugs*. Available from: http://www.globaldrugsurvey.com/wp-content/uploads/2014/04/last-12-months-drug-prevalence.pdf.

Winstock, A. (2014b). *The Global Drug Survey 2014 Findings*. Available from: http://www.globaldrugsurvey.com/facts-figures/the-global-drug-survey-2014-findings/.

Wood, D., Hunter, L., Measham, F. and Dargan, P. (2012a) Limited use of novel psychoactive substances in South London nightclubs. *QJM: An International Journal of Medicine*, 105(10): 959–64.

Wood, D., Measham, F. and Dargan, P. (2012b) 'Our favourite drug': prevalence of use and preference for mephedrone in the London night time economy one year after control. *Journal of Substance Use*, 17(2): 91–7.

Zohara, J., Nutt, D., Kupfer, D., Mollerd, H., Yamawakie, S., Spedding, M. and Stahlg, S. (2014) A proposal for an updated neuropsychopharmacological nomenclature. *European Neuropsychopharmacology*, 24: 1005–14.

34

The Decriminalization of Drugs

Henry H. Brownstein

The use and sharing of the substances we collectively call drugs has been, and always will be, a part of our experience as human beings. Throughout history, through trial and error, and more recently, through scientific study, humans have discovered some substances that are harmful to themselves or to their relations with others and other substances that contribute in a positive way to their personal or social health and wellbeing. Naturally then at times, some people under some circumstances have gotten themselves into trouble with drugs or have caused trouble for others by their involvement with drugs, and at other times, some people under other circumstances have benefited from their involvement with drugs. Either way, drugs, inevitably, are part of our social world. As Andrew Weil wrote, 'Like the fantasy that drugs can be made to go away, the idea that people who want drugs can be discouraged from using them is an impossible dream that gets us nowhere except in worse trouble' (1972: 189).

In that drugs are an inevitable part of social experience, arguably, it is illogical even to consider that the consumption or distribution of those substances called drugs by people living in society could, or should always and in all circumstances and for all people, be prohibited by either formal or informal standards for personal and social behavior. Further, if the use of some drugs has been found to be harmful and the use of others has been found to be beneficial for some or all people in one way or another in some or all circumstances then an absolute prohibition on any and all drug use or drug involvement would be unreasonable if not irresponsible. Scholars and policymakers have found that given how different drugs in different circumstances used by different people have different outcomes any effective drug policy needs to be nuanced and pragmatic and not limited to a single solution, such as absolute prohibition, to minimize the problems and maximize the benefits of drug involvement (cf. Babor et al. 2010; MacCoun and Reuter

2001; Reuter 2013; Room 2012). This would suggest that public policy including drug policy should be based on scientific evidence, but historically values and assumptions have mattered as much as science (Brownstein 2013; Lancaster 2014; Strang et al. 2012). It is not surprising then that the governing authorities of contemporary societies around the world are deep into their second century of constructing and deconstructing norms and laws, and therefore, programs and policies designed to inhibit and control, or at least manage, the use, production, and distribution of drugs among their citizens. So while this is not to say that other approaches have not been tried or are not now being tried, prohibition has an established and enduring history.

Rightfully so or not, and recognizing that reforms are taking place around the world during the early years of the twenty-first century (Pacula et al. 2014; Pardo 2014; Reuter 2013), in different nations at different times, prohibition has been the focus of drug policy and varying forms of involvement of some or all citizens with different drugs has been criminalized. The first problem with this approach is that it is not now and may never be known with certainty which drugs are harmful under what circumstances to what people in what way, or even what values should be used to identify and select what drugs should be the subject of criminal law. The second problem is that once involvement with a particular drug by particular people under particular circumstances has been criminalized, it is at best very difficult to decriminalize it when new knowledge or changing values indicate that it is no longer advantageous or desirable for involvement with that drug to be treated as a crime.

This chapter addresses the definitions of norms and law and then the meaning of criminalization and decriminalization as they relate to drug involvement. Then it offers a brief overview of the history of drug criminalization and decriminalization efforts in contemporary societies and demonstrates through two examples the problems faced in such efforts involving two very different drugs that have been criminalized: marijuana and methamphetamine. While the focus of this chapter is specifically on decriminalization and not broadly on drug policy, it concludes with a discussion of criminalization and decriminalization of drugs as public policy.

NORMS AND LAW

An ordained minister and professor of political economy and social science, William Graham Sumner, early in the twentieth century explored the contradictory forces of personal freedom and social order (1907). He considered how people living among others would recognize their own needs and be able to both satisfy those needs and to distinguish ways of satisfying them that were pleasurable from those that were painful, and how, over time, in harmony with others around them, they would settle on ways of meeting their needs that would satisfy them and become normal (Sumner 1907: 2–3). These folkways would not be established in any formal code but rather by habit and custom. Adherence would be reasonable given the ability of particular folkways to meet the needs of individuals and collectives of individuals. But by serving as a standard they nonetheless in their way would guide and constrain behavior and action. And people being human would naturally go on to make judgments and seek truths and to impose values on things around them. So it would be with folkways. For Sumner, this informed his notion of mores. Whereas folkways are the product of habit and custom, mores are concerned with the social good or social welfare as defined by the people in the collective who live by them (1907: 30). Nonetheless, they are not formally codified as are laws, which once codified by a governing authority are considered by Sumner to be more utilitarian and practical (1907: 56).

The point here is that to understand criminalization and decriminalization of anything, including involvement with drugs, it is important first to understand law as a form of norms. Social scientists who study drugs and drug policy have considered how both formal and informal standards apply in the way, or ways, governments respond to drug use and drug involvement (MacCoun and Reuter 2001). Sumner's work on folkways, mores, and law provides a foundation for understanding the modern concept of norms, and hence, laws. Therefore, how and why their influence varies on how people act and behave, including how they act and behave in terms of drug involvement.

Mainstream social scientists during the twentieth century defined norms as customary and routine standards guiding social action and individual behavior and in that sense as being central to an understanding of social experience whether it be orderly (e.g. Morris 1956; Parsons and Shils 1951; Zetterberg 1958) or disorderly (e.g. Cloward and Ohlin 1960; Cohen 1955; Merton 1938). By this thinking, for norms to be successful in serving the function of maintaining social order, there would need to be widespread compliance. Ideally, a broad spectrum of people would need to share in the values that underlie any norm and share in the belief that adherence to the norm would be beneficial to them both as an individual and as a member of the society. However, as Hans Zetterberg pointed out, 'Modern society is far from homogeneous in terms of social beliefs, values, and norms' (1958: 183). That is, norms can only serve order and conformity for a social collectivity of people if there is adherence to those norms by members of the collectivity, and just because a norm is believed by some, or even by many, to serve a particular need or function for members of the collectivity as individuals or as a group does not necessarily mean that there will be widespread compliance with or even acceptance of that norm. Sometimes, norms that do serve a function end up being discarded, and at other times, norms that are not effective or efficient at meeting a social need remain in place.

In recognition of this problem, particularly in large and complex contemporary nations, conflict and critical social scientists have questioned the functionalist interpretation of social norms. Rather they focus on how differences in values or beliefs or different circumstances and situations can sometimes make compliance with particular norms undesirable or even can place adherence to one norm in direct conflict with adherence to another. In his analysis of conflicting norms, Samuel Stouffer argued that in any society for some people and under some circumstances there would be a 'strain for conformity' to particular norms so that individuals might conform or not or seek a compromise adhering, for example, in part to one norm and in part to another (1949: 707). Using particular examples, Stouffer acknowledged the importance of this social status or role conflict and highlighted other places where such strain or conflict would be found, such as a foreman in an industry or a non-commissioned officer in the military (1949: 707–8). He went on to observe that the extent of strain or conflict with regard to adherence to norms is closely related to the measure of variation in the values of those with authority to establish sanctioned norms and those who lack that authority but are nonetheless expected to adhere to the norms (Stouffer 1949).

In contemporary complex societies with lots of people from different backgrounds with varying personal characteristics and social experience, there is bound to be a wide range of values and beliefs that are not only not all shared but may easily be in conflict. The selection of whose values and beliefs that will serve as the basis for the formation of both informal and formal norms naturally will be based on who has the power to impose their will on the mass of all people. Power, however, is the probability that one individual or group in relation to others can carry out his or her will even in the face of resistance

(Weber 1947: 152). Therefore, the likelihood that an individual or group of individuals would be able to assert power over others is dependent on whether or not, and to what extent, they grant them authority, defined as the enforceable right to exercise power.

For Weber authority may be legitimated in three different ways (1947: 328). On charismatic grounds, authority would come from the devotion of the others 'to the specific and exceptional sanctity, heroism, or exemplary character of an individual person, and of the normative patterns or order revealed or ordained by him'. One example might be the authority of a religious leader. On traditional grounds authority would come from 'an established belief in the sanctity of immemorial traditions and the legitimacy of the status of those exercising authority under them'. Folkways would be an example of norms with traditional authority. The third type of legitimate authority, rational or legal, is grounded in 'the belief in the "legality" of patterns of normative rules and the right of those elevated to authority under such rules to issue commands'.

A religious leader with charismatic authority may encourage the use of one particular drug for spiritual purposes and might prohibit followers from using another drug for any purpose. But under such authority, the use of the prohibited drug would not be a crime. As crime by definition is a violation of law, the use or production or distribution of drugs can only be criminalized in relation to norms established by a governing agency with the duly granted legitimate authority to propose, ratify, and impose law. In that sense, the question of the criminalization or decriminalization of drugs is fundamentally a legal question.

CRIMINALIZATION AND DECRIMINALIZATION

A crime is an act that by its commission or omission is in violation of a public law that is enforceable by virtue of the recognition and consent of some body of people who have granted authority to a particular governing body to make such law on their behalf and to impose punishment for violations of that law (see http://thelawdictionary.org/crime/ and http://www.justicebc.ca/en/cjis/reporting/crime/). Consequently, to criminalize something such as the use, production, or distribution of one or another drug by all or some people would require placing some or all relevant personal behaviors or social acts in the realm of law and the violation of law. That is, by definition it would be necessary for a legitimate governing authority to enact and enforce laws that would make those behaviors or acts by all, or some people, crimes.

In the middle of the twentieth century, Peter Berger and Thomas Luckmann argued that reality is a social construction in the sense that individuals construct objective facticities from the subjective meanings that they attach to their own actions and interactions and those of others around them (1966). Building on that understanding of social reality, social problems theorists since the late twentieth century have explained social problems as the constructions of individuals with competing claims about the meaning and nature of particular social beliefs, values, and norms (cf. Best 1989, 1990; Brownstein 2000; Miller and Holstein 1993; Spector and Kitsuse 1987; Woolgar and Pawluch 1985). Given the Weberian definition of power as the probability that some people will be able to impose their will on others who may resist, not only the decision about what problems rise to the level of social problems but also under what circumstances, with what people, and how to respond to those problems is inevitably placed in the hands of those who are able to attain power (cf. Brownstein 1996; Quinney 1970). This is relevant to understanding how and why behaviors or actions related to drug involvement could, and would, be criminalized.

Erich Goode described what he calls the process of criminalization in the United States in terms of the construction of social problems specifically as it has been used to address the use of certain drugs by certain people as it is defined by at least some segment of society to be a social problem. He wrote, 'To most Americans, the use of most psychoactive drugs represents both a social problem and a crime. As a result, we should expect that, like social problems, what *makes* drug use a form of crime is the consequence of a process of social construction' (2012: 78).

In terms of the relevance of power for social decisions about the criminalization of drug involvement, he concluded, 'Much of the drug legislation passed during this century has been motivated by political, moral, and economic reasons rather than a genuine concern for the health and welfare of vulnerable members of the society' (2012: 79).

Looking across the last 100 years or more at not only the United States but other nations as well, the competition taking place in the 'marketplace of claims' (Best 1990) about the virtue of the claim for criminalizing the use, production, or distribution of all or some drugs by all or some people is largely being won by those who favor some level of criminalization under some or all circumstances (cf. Currie 1993; Walker 2011). And representatives of those legally established governments favoring criminalization have been exercising their power to authorize and enforce laws that make such drug involvement criminal. In describing competing claims during the time when crack cocaine was the target of much of the criminalization effort in the United States, for example, Currie wrote:

> Even many who support the thrust of our present drug policies would acknowledge that the drug crisis among 'hard-core' users in the more marginal populations is understated by conventional statistics, and that is has proven remarkably resistant to the conventional tools of the drug war. But they would argue that the declines in *middle*-class drug use prove that the drug war is 'on the right track', and that if we only redoubled our efforts we could make it work against the admittedly tougher situation in the inner cities as well. (Currie 1993: 30)

Considering how powerful the process of criminalization of drug involvement by the type of drug and type of user and market participant, he continued, 'the conventional drug war had virtually nothing to do with the declines in drug use among the better-off, for it was never *fought* against their drug use' (Currie 1993: 30). Rather, as he suggests, the construction of drugs as a social problem and the criminalization of that problem by those with the power to make and enforce laws has focused on drugs not manufactured by approved manufacturers and the drug involvement of people distinguished by selected characteristics, such as race, class, and gender (cf. Duster 1970; Inciardi 2007; McWilliams 1990; Sloman 1979).

On a conceptual level, in the same way that criminalization means using legitimate legal authority to define some behaviors or actions by some or all people in some or all circumstances as unlawful, decriminalization means using such authority to define them as lawful after they had earlier been defined as unlawful. On an operational level, decriminalization has been enacted in terms of things such as not enforcing drug laws, responding to drug law offenders with civil rather than criminal sanctions, or eliminating all drug laws (Room 2012). From either perspective, decriminalizing something that had previously been criminalized is not easy (Reuter 2013). If something has never been defined as unlawful, members of society can argue about whether or not it should be, but until such time as those with authority to do so declare it unlawful, it is not. But once something is determined to be unlawful and is recognized and treated as such over time, the process of having the same authority convincing people that what at one time was defined as unlawful is once again okay to do is a more difficult problem. In the case of drugs, the problem is complicated by the fact that some drugs are legal but others are not, some drugs are legal on some occasions or under some circumstances, but not on other occasions or under other circumstances, and some drugs are legal for some people to use but not others. And there is the complication that there are drugs that are known or merely believed to be harmful all or some of the time and others known or merely believed to be helpful all or some of the time. On the helpful side, there are drugs that are commonly used for purposes of health and wellbeing, but there are also drugs that are commonly used just because of the way they make people feel. As Aldous Huxley wrote, 'Most men and women lead lives so painful, at the best so monotonous, poor and limited that the urge to escape, the longing to transcend themselves if only for a few moments, is and always has been one of the principal appetites of the soul' (1954: 62). So sorting out what drugs, when, how, and by whom should be lawful or unlawful has been, and remains, a policy challenge for governing authorities in all nations trying to do the right thing.

CRIMINALIZING DRUGS THROUGH LAW AND POLICY

The twentieth century was a very active time for drug policy makers around the world. Until that time, national and local governments that were granted varying degrees, spheres and types of authority gave limited attention to using that authority in relation to the use, production, and distribution of the substances we call drugs. Then by the early years of the twentieth century, governments of different nations and at different organizational levels within nations, worked independently, collaboratively, and even competitively, to identify areas of authority that could be used to gain control over what was increasingly being defined as a major social problem, although even in the twentieth century, there was some variability in terms of how the problem was defined and the extent to which it was viewed as a criminal problem. By the end of the twentieth century, there was considerable debate about whether drug policy should focus on prohibition and criminalization or the management and reduction of harms related to drug involvement (Brownstein 2013; Room and Reuter 2012). By the early twenty-first century in many nations, including those such as the United States where the war was being fought, efforts to reform drug policy in a less prohibitive or punitive direction were underway, particularly in the case of marijuana (Pacula et al. 2014; Pardo 2014; Room 2012).

David Musto described drug policy in the United States in the late nineteenth century as 'an era of wide availability and unrestrained advertising' (1991: 42). People seeking relief from pain or illness had easy and open access to a number of different home remedies, pharmacological substances with unnamed ingredients that sometimes included opium or cocaine. The retailer, Sears Roebuck, sold hypodermic needles for morphine users, a soft drink company introduced a new energizing drink called Coca Cola with extracts of coca, and a new product for coughs and congestion called Heroin was introduced by the Bayer Company (Inciardi 2007; Musto 1991). During this period, each state independently had authority to regulate medical practice and the use, production, and distribution of pharmaceutical substances so policy was neither centralized nor coordinated. By the early twentieth century in the United States, the federal government pursued areas of legal authority that would allow for greater centralized control and a more consistent and coordinated national drug policy. In the marketplace of claims, the debate over the extent and nature of the problem with drugs pitted the medical community with its concern for what it considered a public health and addiction problem against the criminal justice community with its concern for drugs as public safety and crime problem (Inciardi 2007; Musto 1991, 1999).

Similarly, according to a report by the British Medical Association, 'Opium eating and laudanum (an alcoholic solution of opiates) consumption were widespread in mid-19th century Britain. Opium, and its derivative morphine, were available as patent medicines, in tinctures and other commercial products that were readily accessible through chemists and herbalists' (BMA Board of Science 2013: 87). In the UK, the government began to pay attention to drugs as a serious social problem starting with the 1868 Pharmacy Act requiring that pharmacists maintain records of purchases. Then, at the start of the twentieth century, with the 1908 Pharmacy Act, introducing legislation to more actively control use by placing certain pharmaceuticals containing small amounts of morphine, cocaine, and opium derivatives in the schedule of poisons (BMA Board of Science 2013: 87). And as in the US, in the UK there was tension between those claiming drugs to be a public health concern calling for programs and policies to manage the problem and those claiming drugs to be a concern of public safety calling for programs and policies to control the problem.

During the early years of the twentieth century, nations around the world began in earnest to define drug involvement as a social problem (see Brownstein 2013). Although not all placed the greatest emphasis on the problem as one of public safety (some instead placing greater emphasis on the problem as one of public health), ultimately political activity during this period hastened the criminalization of drug involvement, particularly for some drugs and people under some circumstances. Criminalization of drug involvement became a prominent legislative and policy making theme. Nations around the world independently, and in collaboration, introduced laws and policies that made criminal the personal behavior and social activity of individuals involving the use, production, or distribution of selected drugs, behaviors, and activity that until that time had been commonplace, if not widespread or even encouraged. The late twentieth century and early twenty-first century concern for decriminalization would not have been possible had there never been the period of criminalization a hundred years earlier.

In the US, where crime is the responsibility of individual states, the Federal government sought to find a way to establish its authority to pass legislation that would allow it to address the problem of drugs. In 1906, it used its authority over public health across state lines and passed the Pure Food and Drug Act, giving it the right to set standards for the quality, packaging, and labeling of patent medicines sold through interstate commerce (Musto 1991: 43). Then it found a way to use the tax code to participate in the criminalization of drugs by passing the Harrison Act in 1914 and the Marijuana Tax Act in 1937, thereby giving it some level of authority over the production, importation, sale, purchase, and distribution of narcotic drugs and marijuana (Kaplan 1971; Musto 1999; Smith 1988). By the later years of the twentieth century, the Federal government formally declared war on drugs making some people involved with drugs not only criminals but also enemies of the nation (Inciardi 2007; Weisheit 1990; Wisotsky 1986).

While criminalization of drugs was a common theme across nations, not all nations emphasized it to the extent of the US. Some favored a more balanced approach. In the UK, drug policy in the early twentieth century focused more on the problem as one of public health. In 1920, the Dangerous Drugs Act was passed giving authority to the medical community to prescribe morphine, cocaine, and heroin (BMA Board of Science 2013; also, Bennett 1988). According to the BMA Board of Science report:

> At the suggestion of the Home Office, the Ministry of Health convened an expert committee (Departmental Committee on Morphine and Heroin Addiction) chaired by Sir Humphrey Rolleston, then President of the Royal College of Physicians, to consider and advise on the circumstances in which it was medically advisable to prescribe heroin or morphine to addicts. The report produced by the committee (usually known as the Rolleston Report), reaffirmed the doctor's freedom to prescribe regular supplies of opioid drugs to certain addicted patients in defined circumstances that the committee regarded as 'treatment' rather

than the 'gratification of addiction'. (BMA Board of Science 2013: 89)

But earlier, when soldiers reportedly had been using cocaine during World War I, the Army Council issued an order, in 1916, to limit their access to the drug by prescription only and when that was not successful, they introduced that same year the Defence of the Realm Act, making it law and thereby making violation criminal (BMA Board of Science 2013: 88). That is, in the UK, the establishment of law and policy was more balanced, viewing the social problem of drugs as both a public health and a public safety problem.

In terms of the cooperation and collaboration of nations to address their mutual and growing concern with the social problem of drugs, there were a number of efforts starting in 1909 when 13 nations gathered in Shanghai for the International Opium Commission. The focus was limited to opium and opiates and there were no binding resolutions or treaties but it did open communication. It was followed, in 1911, in The Hague, with a meeting of 12 nations at which they each agreed to enact domestic legislation to control drug trafficking and educate their citizens (Musto 1991: 43). Then later during the middle of the twentieth century, nations continued to meet to reach agreements on drug policy, and ultimately, through the United Nations, three Conventions were negotiated (Bewley-Taylor 2003; Sinha 2001; United Nations 1961, 1971, 1988). Each Convention had its own focus, but broadly, they were focused on the supply of drugs, and in particular, prohibition and criminalization of drug trafficking (Bewley-Taylor 2003; Room and Reuter 2011).

THE CHALLENGE OF CRIMINALIZATION AND DECRIMINALIZATION: CASE STUDIES

By the end of the twentieth century, the criminalization of drug involvement was widespread. In varying degrees, nations across the world had laws and policies directed at criminalizing the behavior and action of people involved in some drugs in some circumstances and much of the dialogue about drug policy reform in the late twentieth century focused on the legalization or decriminalization of drug involvement to one degree or another (compare Brownstein 2013; Goode 1997; Inciardi 1999; Reuter 1991, 1992; Trebach and Zeese 1990). Particularly in nations other than the US, there was also considerable attention to policies of harm reduction that focused on public health rather than public safety (e.g. DuPont and Voth 1995; Erickson and Hathaway 2010; Herring et al. 2010; Inciardi and Harrison 2000; Riley et al. 1999). Just as criminalization was a popular policy theme around the turn of the twentieth century, decriminalization became a popular policy theme for the efforts of advocates of drug policy reform toward the turn of the twenty-first century.

The shift toward decriminalization would have been unnecessary had there not been an earlier period of expansion of laws and policies to criminalize drugs. In that sense, decriminalization is a false issue. The problem is that trying to undo what has already been done is a very complicated and an often confounding process. In the case of drug policy, trying to decriminalize after 100 years of criminalizing may not be possible. Over the years, the laws and policies involving drug involvement have built upon themselves in so many different ways on so many levels that disentangling one piece of the overall policy by changing one or a few laws or modifying a particular policy initiative inevitably has unintended consequences that may make things worse rather than better. Below are two examples from the US, a nation with a strong tradition of criminalization of drugs and drug involvement, of how efforts to change or modify laws and policies for two different drugs that had been criminalized, marijuana and methamphetamine, have had unintended consequences that created new crime problems rather than reducing crime.

Marijuana

The early twentieth century in the US was an era when there was a poor economy and high levels of crime and violence. At least partly in response to those conditions in 1930, the Federal Bureau of Narcotics (FBN) was created and Harry Anslinger was named its first Commissioner. Anslinger served for more than 30 years, and over that time, he devoted much of his attention to the criminalization of marijuana use and trade (Inciardi 2007; Kaplan 1971; McWilliams 1990). He used not only the authority of his position as a senior official in the US government, but also the platform it gave him to advocate for the demonization of all drug involvement, in particular marijuana, and to encourage laws and policies that would criminalize personal behavior and social activity associated with the use, production, and distribution of selected drugs. He also wrote articles for magazines about what he believed to be the dangers of marijuana including 'Marijuana, Assassin of Youth', 'Youth Gone Loco', and 'One More Peril for Youth' (see Inciardi 2007; McWilliams 1990; Sloman 1979).

During the 1930s, there was not much scientific evidence about what different drugs, including marijuana, did and what impact they had on people in terms of their own health and wellbeing or their relationships with others. So, in his advocacy for the criminalization of marijuana, Anslinger depended on stories he had heard or read but could not document or substantiate. He kept a dossier of such stories (see Anslinger and Cooper 1937) in what has come to be known as his gore file (Sloman 1979: 57). Given his position with the FBN his stories were granted a level of credibility they would not otherwise have had. At a conference of the US Treasury Department, which housed the FBN, on January 14, 1937, in the absence of real evidence, he used these stories to ask and answer his own question, although at the end of his presentation he did have a disclaimer stating that he could not provide more details or documentation to support the stories. The question he asked was: 'What are the proofs that the use of marijuana, in any of its forms, is habit-forming or addictive, and what are the indications and positive proofs that such addiction develops socially undesirable characteristics in the user?' (Sloman 1979: 57).

In 1937, the US Congress was considering a bill known as the Marijuana Tax Act. Naturally the Tax Act was a revenue bill, the direct purpose of which was to give the Federal government the authority to collect taxes on marijuana transactions while indirectly establishing Federal authority over marijuana users, producers, and distributors (Inciardi 2007; Musto 1999; Smith 1988). Anslinger, as head of the FBN, was the first to testify at the hearings before the Committee on Ways and Means of the House of Representatives during the First Session of the Seventy-Fifth Congress on April 27, 28, 29, 30, and May 4, 1937, on bill number H.R. 6385, *Taxation of Marihuana*. As he had been doing all along, Anslinger did not have any solid evidence to support his claims, but nonetheless, used the opportunity to advocate for the criminalization of marijuana involvement by telling stories from his gore file. Decades later, just before Anslinger passed away in 1975, John Kaplan wrote:

> In weighing the evidence on the connection between marijuana and aggression, one is struck by two things: one is the relatively large number of statements made by policy-making committees, medical societies, and public officials as compared with the relatively small number of studies that actually bear on this issue; the other is the even more striking fact that the studies and evidence relied on in these statements are of extremely weak probative value. (Kaplan 1971: 92)

By the twenty-first century, much more research had been conducted and the evidence did not support the claims that Anslinger was making when he began his crusade about marijuana as a public safety problem, invariably resulting in higher incidence and rates of crime and violence (e.g. Golub et al. 2007; Harcourt and Ludwig 2006; Pacula and Kilmer 2003; Spunt et al. 1994). This does not necessarily diminish the argument that there may be a negative relationship between marijuana use and health, but the at the same time, there is growing evidence that marijuana or its components may have therapeutic value for the health of individuals (Watson et al. 2000). Therefore, the marijuana debate in the US shifted from criminalization to medicalization and even decriminalization.

On the Federal level in the US, marijuana remains on the list of controlled substances with no medical value, but in recent years, states have increasingly introduced their own legislation decriminalizing the medical use of marijuana for people with particular medical needs such as symptoms of cancer, AIDS, glaucoma, epilepsy, or for persistent pain. According to the National Conference of State Legislatures (NCSL), by 2015, marijuana had been decriminalized for comprehensive public medical use in 23 states plus the District of Columbia and Guam, in 14 states, the use of 'low THC' or 'high cannabidiol' products for limited medical purposes was an acceptable legal defense, and in two states (Colorado and Washington), even marijuana use for recreational purposes was no longer criminalized (see http://www.ncsl.org/research/health/state-medical-marijuana-laws.aspx; Accessed 28 May 2015).

What would seem to be a national movement in the US toward decriminalization is complicated for two reasons. First, there is not common agreement among researchers about what is the medical value if any of marijuana, how the benefits balance against the risks, or even if enough research has been done to have confidence in a particular conclusion (Pacula et al. 2014; Watson et al. 2000). Perhaps a greater barrier in the way of progress toward decriminalization in the US is the fact that while almost half the states favor decriminalization, at least for medical purposes, the Federal government does not (Pardo 2014). As a result, a person who uses, produces, or distributes marijuana according to the laws of his or her own state is still subject to criminal penalty for the violation of Federal law. And Article 6 of the Constitution states:

> This Constitution, and the laws of the United States which shall be made in pursuance thereof; and all treaties made, or which shall be made, under the authority of the United States, shall be the supreme law of the land; and the judges in every state shall be bound thereby, anything in the Constitution or laws of any State to the contrary notwithstanding.

As a result, states that decriminalize marijuana cannot guarantee that they can defend their citizens from Federal prosecution. Further, because the Federal government has authority or at least influence over various aspects of social and economic life, for example, banking, state approved marijuana businesses face restrictions not shared by other legitimate businesses, such as having a bank account or accepting credit card purchases.

The situation in the Netherlands poses an interesting contrast, yet similarly, is not simple. Historically, in the Netherlands, there has been balance in drug policy with a focus on protecting health and minimizing health risks but also on combatting the extent to which the behavior or activity of drug users, producers, and traffickers was a public nuisance (van Laar et al. 2011). Over time, drug policies have emphasized public health concerns and small amounts of marijuana have been accessible to locals and visitors through coffee shops (see Cohen 1996). Then, in 2012, a new law went into effect that continues to permit the sale of marijuana to residents but bans sales to tourists. While in the Netherlands, like any other nation that has signed the international drug treaties making the sale and possession of marijuana technically unlawful, under the practice known as *gedoogbeleid*, the Dutch have practiced discretion and have emphasized enforcement against large scale suppliers, while tolerating the use of smaller amounts (MacCoun and Reuter 1997: 48). Just as in the US during the early decades of the twenty-first century, there will be a challenge to those trying to decriminalize the involvement of people with marijuana, in the Netherlands, there is likely to be a challenge to those trying to criminalize involvement with marijuana.

Methamphetamine

Methamphetamine is a central nervous system stimulant first synthesized in Japan early in the twentieth century and not accessible in the US until the middle of the century. In the 1930s, it was made available to soldiers to keep them alert, in the 1950s, it became popular among people concerned with weight loss and attentiveness, and in the 1960s, it gained attention as a recreational drug until reports of health and safety concerns started to make people wary of its use (Hunt et al. 2005; Weisheit and White 2009). Then, as time passed, concerns about any dangers of using methamphetamine faded, new methods for making it with easily obtainable precursor drugs were developed, and by the 1990s, methamphetamine use increased, particularly in western states and rural parts of the country (National Drug Intelligence Center 2005; National Institute of Justice 2003). Around that time, there was not large scale production with international or even interstate distribution networks, but rather methamphetamine was being produced by individual cooks using chemicals and supplies purchased from legitimate pharmacies and hardware and farm supply stores to make small amounts of meth for local distribution (National Drug Intelligence Center 2005, 2011).

By the early twenty-first century in the US, methamphetamine was considered a serious health and safety problem (Office of National Drug Control Policy 2005). The Federal government passed the Combat Methamphetamine Epidemic Act of 2005 (Title VII of the USA PATRIOT Improvement and Reauthorization Act of 2005, P.L. 109–77) and states followed with similar legislation (McBride et al. 2011). These new laws did not directly make the production of methamphetamine unlawful but cleverly did criminalize easy access to precursor chemicals otherwise available for lawful purposes. The intent was to regulate the sale of these chemicals that were routinely sold in common household products for legitimate purposes, notably the pseudoephedrine contained in common cold medicines, to control their use by meth cooks for making methamphetamine. Unfortunately, there was an unintended consequence that was not what the legislators had planned.

By focusing on the chemicals needed for production, the legislation was aimed at the supply of methamphetamine and not the demand for its use. So the demand for the drug was not diminished. In fact, the effort to regulate the availability of the precursor chemicals, while it did disrupt production by local cooks, it also stimulated the entrepreneurial spirit of methamphetamine producers and suppliers and moved the industry in two inventive and profitable directions (Brownstein et al. 2014). That is, the effort to reduce criminal involvement with methamphetamine by controlling access to the precursor chemicals needed to make methamphetamine inadvertently resulted in new, improved, yet still criminal, ways to produce and distribute the drug.

On the local level, meth cooks found new ways to obtain the precursor chemicals they needed and developed new cooking methods that simplified the process for making small quantities and made it more efficient. With the legislation, local meth cooks could no longer walk into their local pharmacy and walk out with bags full of cold medicine containing the pseudoephedrine they needed. In response, 'smurfing' was invented (National

Drug Intelligence Center 2009). A small group of users would be recruited by the local cook from among his friends and acquaintances and each would go to one or more local pharmacies and purchase as much cold medicine as was allowable under the law. Then they would get together with the cook who would mix up a batch of meth that they would all would share. These collectives of meth users also benefited from the invention of a new technique for making meth known as one-pot or shake-and-bake (Nemes 2011). With this technique, a lesser amount of pseudoephedrine is mixed with ammonium nitrate (found in farm fertilizer or in cold-pack compresses found in any number of stores), and with a few other ingredients, are mixed in a two-liter bottle and shaken, something that can be done anywhere (Blostein et al. 2009). While this technique is simpler, requires fewer chemicals, and does not give off that distinctive odor well known to law enforcement, it is still dangerous and explosions can occur. Nonetheless, in the early twenty-first century after the passage of the legislation to control their use of the drug, in various parts of the US, meth cooks and users continued to gather almost like social clubs in a home or even a car to spend some time together getting high on methamphetamine (Brownstein et al. 2014).

On a national level, the drug conglomerates or cartels that had been operating out of Mexico to produce and distribute other drugs, such as heroin and cocaine, to the vast US drug consumer markets, responded to the legislation to control meth use by adding a high quality and easily transportable form of methamphetamine to their product line (Beith 2010; Keefe 2012; Langton 2012). These organizations operate what are called 'super labs' in Mexico and in parts of the US, producing larger quantities of methamphetamine for wholesale distribution in a crystal form popular among many users (National Drug Intelligence Center 2011: 23). As meth sales historically and culturally have been personal in the US, the Mexican distributors operate on the retail level through local sellers they recruit from among the local meth community making them not only meth users but also participants in the criminal activity of the illicit methamphetamine business (Brownstein et al. 2014).

On an international level, there are also unintended consequences of nations with higher numbers of methamphetamine users introducing laws to criminalize involvement with methamphetamine by introducing laws that control access to precursor chemicals. In spite of efforts by the United Nations to gain control over the accessibility of precursor chemicals needed to make methamphetamine, the United Nations Office on Drugs and Crime estimated during the first decade of the twenty-first century that worldwide there are between 15 and 16 million people using methamphetamine (2007: 17). Based on several studies of methamphetamine markets in Australia (McKetin et al. 2005, 2006), Rebecca McKetin wrote an editorial in which she said, 'As regulation of precursor chemicals in wealthy destination markets become more stringent, responsibility for policing chemical diversion and synthetic drug manufacture and managing harms from synthetic drug use are likely to shift increasingly to developing countries – many of which have limited capacity to manage such problems' (207: 521).

DECRIMINALIZATION AS PUBLIC POLICY

By definition, something is criminal because it is against the law of some governing body with the authority to impose formalized norms known as law over the behaviors and actions of the participants of some organized community of people. Decriminalization then means to remove something, including things such as personal behaviors or social activities from the authority of laws under which it has previously been placed. In the case of drugs in general, in one form or another for one reason or another, they are widely available and easily obtainable in most if not all contemporary communities of people. So, in the case of drugs, to the extent it is reasonable or even possible to criminalize personal behavior or social activity related to drug production, distribution, or use necessarily involves making choices about which drugs used by which people under what circumstances should be declared lawful and which should be declared unlawful. In that sense, both decriminalization and criminalization are essentially the same thing, the process of making political decisions about drugs and the people who are involved with them.

From a social problem perspective, the notion of drugs as a problem is a social construction, as are the public policy responses to drugs, drug use, and drug involvement. There are both negative and positive consequences for individual health and well-being from using or being involved with drugs. Those consequences can be related to the drugs individuals use and also to some extent the decisions they make about how they use them, how often they use them, who they use them with, and even the settings in which they use them. There are also both negative and positive consequences for social relationships, particularly in terms of the social institutions of family and economy, and those by definition are the product of decisions, behaviors and actions of the individuals engaged in the production and distribution of drugs. But at the same time, the decisions and related actions that result in laws to criminalize or decriminalize involvement with drugs in one way or another, for one drug or another, or for some set of people or others, are also social. Therefore, the involvement of any people with any drugs, in any way, is only criminal to the extent that people with authority make it criminal.

Public policy is the product of the decisions and actions of individuals in a society granted the authority to define the problems and challenges of the society and to set priorities and allocate resources to address the problems and challenges they identify as worthy of attention. Throughout the twentieth century in modern societies, those people with the authority to make public policy on drug production, distribution, and use, often favored decisions and actions that criminalized involvement with drugs. This was not true for all drugs, for all people, in all nations, or for all circumstances, but it was the overriding theme of drug policy in the twentieth century. At the start of the twenty-first century in some societies, there is a noticeable shift for at least some drugs, for some people, in some circumstances, to decriminalize drug involvement broadly and to introduce policies that regulate or manage drug involvement to minimize harm without making outlaws of everyone involved with drugs.

Given the inevitability of drug involvement in society, and the different impact of different drugs on different people in different circumstances, any drug policy needs to be nuanced enough to manage and regulate drug involvement in a pragmatic way. Decriminalization itself can be operationalized in many ways – for example, not enforcing drug laws, responding to drug law offenders with civil rather than criminal sanctions, or eliminating all drug laws – but in itself, it is not a policy. Decriminalization is rather the modification of a policy of criminalization. And whatever happens in the end, involvement in one way or another, with some drugs but not all, will remain criminal for some, but not all people under some but not all circumstances. When it comes to something such as drugs that covers such a wide range of substances, many of which are clearly beneficial and desirable to a great number of people, then it is not possible to criminalize or decriminalize, but only to keep shifting the line between legal and illegal.

REFERENCES

Anslinger, H.J. with Cooper, C.R. (1937). Marijuana, assassin of youth. *The American Magazine*, 124, No. 1. Available from: http://www.redhousebooks.com/galleries/assassin.htm (Accessed 26 May 2012). Reprinted in Kaplan, J. (1971). *Marijuana – The New Prohibition*. New York: Pocket Books.

Babor, T., Caulkins, J., Edwards, G., Fischer, B., Foxcroft, D., Humphreys, K., Obot, I, Rehm, J., Reuter, P., Room, R., Rossow, I. and Strang, J. (2010). *Drug Policy and the Public Good*. Oxford: Oxford University Press.

Beith, M. (2010). *The Last Narco – Inside the Hunt for El Chapo, the World's Most Wanted Drug Lord*. New York: Grove Press.

Bennett, T. (1988). The British experience with heroin regulation. *Law and Contemporary Problems* 51: 299–314.

Berger, P.L. and Luckmann, T. (1966). *The Social Construction of Reality – A Treatise in the Sociology of Knowledge*. Garden City: Doubleday & Company.

Best, J. (1989). *Images of Issues: Typifying Contemporary Social Problems*. New York: Aldine de Gruyter.

Best, J. (1990). *Threatened Children – Rhetoric and Concern About Child Victims*. Chicago: The University of Chicago Press.

Bewley-Taylor, D.R. (2003). Challenging the UN Drug conventions: problems and possibilities. *The International Journal of Drug Policy* 14: 171–9.

Blostein, P.A., Plaisier, B.R., Maltz, S.B., Davidson, S.B., Wideman, E.W., Feucht, E.C. and VandenBerg, S.L. (2009). Methamphetamine production is hazardous to your health. *The Journal of Trauma* 66: 1712–17.

BMA Board of Science (2013). *Drugs of Dependence – The Role of Medical Professionals*. London: British Medical Association.

Brownstein, H.H. (1996). *The Rise and Fall of a Violent Crime Wave – Crack Cocaine and the Social Construction of a Crime Problem*. Guilderland: Harrow & Heston.

Brownstein, H.H. (2000). *The Social Reality of Violence and Violent Crime*. Boston: Allyn and Bacon.

Brownstein, H.H. (2013). *Contemporary Drug Policy*. London and New York: Routledge.

Brownstein, H.H., Mulcahy, T.M. and Huessy, J. (2014). *The Methamphetamine Industry in America: Transnational Cartels and Local Entrepreneurs*. New Brunswick: Rutgers University Press.

Cohen, A. (1955). *Delinquent Boys – The Culture of the Gang*. New York: The Free Press.

Cohen, P. (1996). *The Case of Two Dutch Drug Policy Commissions – An Exercise in Harm Reduction 1968–1976*. Paper presented at the 5th Annual International Conference on the Reduction of Drug related Harm., 7–11 March, 1994. Toronto: Addiction Research Foundation. Revised in 1996. Available from: http://dare.uva.nl/document/12561 (Accessed 28 May 2012).

Cloward, R.A. and Ohlin, L.E. (1960). *Deliquency and Opportunity – A Theory of Delinquent Gangs*. New York: The Free Press.

Currie, E. (1993). *Reckoning – Drugs, the Cities, and the American Future*. New York: Hill and Wang.

DuPont, R.L. and Voth, E.A. (1995). Drug legalization, harm reduction, and drug policy. *Annual Internal Medicine* I23: 46I–5.

Duster, T. (1970). *The Legislation of Morality – Law, Drugs, and Moral Judgment*. New York: Free Press.

Erickson, P.G. and Hathaway, A.D. (2010). Normalization and harm reduction: research avenues and policy agendas. *International Journal of Drug Policy* 21: 137–9.

Golub, A., Johnson, B.D. and Dunlap, E. (2007). The race/ethnicity disparity in misdemeanor marijuana arrests in New York City. *Criminology and Public Policy* 6: 131–64.

Goode, E. (1997). *Between Politics and Reason: The Drug Legalization Debate*. New York: St. Martin's Press.

Goode, E. (2012). *Drugs in American Society*. Boston: McGraw Hill.

Harcourt, B.E. and Ludwig, J. (2006). *Reefer Madness: Broken Windows Policing and Misdemeanor Marijuana Arrests in New York City, 1989–2000*. John M. Olin Law and Economics Working Paper No. 317 (2nd Series). Chicago: The Law School the University of Chicago.

Herring, R., Thom, B., Beccaria, F., Kolind, T. and Moskalewicz, J. (2010). Alcohol harm reduction in Europe. In T. Rhodes and D. Hedrich (eds), *Harm Reduction: Evidence,*

Impacts and Challenges. EMCDDA Monograph (10). Lisbon: European Monitoring Centre for Drugs and Drug Addiction, pp. 275–301.

Hunt, D.E., Kuck, S. and Truitt, L. (2005). *Methamphetamine Use: Lessons Learned*. Cambridge: Abt Associates. Report submitted to the National Institute of Justice.

Huxley, A. (1954). *Doors of Perception*. New York: Harper and Row.

Inciardi, J.A. (ed.) (1999). *The Drug Legalization Debate*, 2nd edn. Thousand Oaks: Sage Publications.

Inciardi, J.A. (2007). *War on Drugs IV: The Continuing Saga of the Mysteries and Miseries of Intoxication, Addiction, Crime and Public Policy*, 4th edn. Boston: Allyn & Bacon.

Inciardi, J.A. and Harrison, L.D. (eds) (2000). *Harm Reduction – National and International Perspectives*. Thousand Oaks: Sage.

Kaplan, J. (1971). *Marijuana – The New Prohibition*. New York: Pocket Books.

Keefe, P.R. (2012). Cocaine incorporated. *New York Times Magazine*, 15 June: 36–43, 62–3.

Lancaster, K. (2014). Social construction and the evidence-based drug policy endeavor. *International Journal of Drug Policy*, 25: 948–51.

Langton, J. (2012). *Gangland – The Rise of the Mexican Drug Cartels from El Paso to Vancouver*. Mississauga: Wiley & Sons Canada.

MacCoun, R. and Reuter, P. (1997). Interpreting Dutch cannabis policy: reasoning by analogy in the legalization debate. *Science* 278: 47–52.

MacCoun, R. and Reuter, P. (2001). *Drug War Heresies: Learning from Other Vices, Times, and Places*. Cambridge: Cambridge University Press.

McBride, D.C., Terry-McElrath, Y.M., Chriqui, J.F., O'Connor, J.C., VanderWaal, C.J. and Mattson, K.L. (2011). State methamphetamine precursor policies and changes in small toxic lab methamphetamine. *Journal of Drug Issues* Fall: 253–82.

McKetin, R. (2007). Methamphetamine precursor regulation: are we controlling or diverting the drug problem? *Addiction* 103: 521–3.

McKetin, R., McLaren, J. and Kelly, E. (2005). *The Sydney Methamphetamine Market: Patterns of Supply, Use, Personal Harms and Social Consequences*. Mongraph Series No. 13. National Drug Law Enforcement Research Fund. Sydney: National Alcohol and Drug Research Centre.

McKetin, R., McLaren, J., Riddell, S. and Robins, L. (2006). *The Relationship Between Methamphetamine Use and Violent Behavior. Crime and Justice Bulletin*. Sydney: NSW Bureau of Crime Statistics and Research.

McWilliams, J.C. (1990) *The Protectors: Harry J. Anslinger and the Federal Bureau of Narcotics*. Newark: University of Delaware.

Merton, R.K. (1938). Social structure and anomie. *American Sociological Review* 3: 672–82.

Miller, G. and Holstein, J.A. (1993). Constructing social problems: context and legacy. In G. Miller and J.A. Holstein (eds), *Constructionist Controversies – Issues in Social Problems Theory*. New York: Aldine de Gruyter, pp. 3–18.

Morris, R.T. (1956). A typology of norms. *American Sociological Review* 21: 610–13.

Musto, D. (1991). Opium, Cocaine, and Marijuana in American History. *Scientific American* 265: 40–7.

Musto, D. (1999). *The American Disease*, 3rd edn. New York: Oxford University Press.

National Drug Intelligence Center (2005). *Methamphetamine Drug Threat Assessment*. No. 2005-Q0317-009. Washington, DC: USDOJ.

National Drug Intelligence Center (2009). *Pseudoephedrine Smurfing Fuels Surge in Large-Scale Methamphetamine Production in California*. Situation Report. Product No. 2009-S0787-007. Washington, DC: USDOJ.

National Drug Intelligence Center (2011). *National Drug Threat Assessment 2010*. No. 2011-Q0317-001. Washington, DC: USDOJ.

National Institute of Justice (2003). *2000 Arrestee Drug Abuse Monitoring: Annual Report*. NCJ 193013. Washington, DC: USDOJ.

Nemes, R. S. (2011). Shake and Bake: The Meth Threat and the Need to Rethink 21 USC § 841 (c)(2). *Wash. UL Rev.* 88(4): 993–1020.

Office of National Drug Control Policy (2005). *National Drug Control Strategy*. Washington, DC: The White House.

Pacula, R.L. and Kilmer, B. (2003). *Marijuana and Crime: Is There a Connection Beyond Prohibition?* NBER Working Paper Series. Working Paper Number 10046. Cambridge: National Bureau of Economic Research.

Pacula, R.L., Kilmer, B., Wagenaar, A.C., Chaloupka, F.J. and Caulkins, J.P. (2014). Developing public health regulations for marijuana: Lessons from alcohol and tobacco. *American Journal of Public Health* 104(6): 1021–8.

Pardo, B. (2014). Cannabis policy reforms in the Americas: a comparative analysis of Colorado, Washington, and Uruguay. *International Journal of Drug Policy*, 25(4): 727–35.

Parsons, T. and Shils, E.A. (1951). *Towards a General Theory of Action*, Cambridge: Harvard University Press.

Quinney, R. (1970). *The Social Reality of Crime*. New Brunswick, NJ: Transaction Publishers.

Reuter, P.H. (1991). On the consequences of toughness. *A RAND Note* N-3447-DPRC: 138–164.

Reuter, P.H. (1992). Hawks ascendant: the punitive trend of American drug policy. *Daedalus* 121: 15–52.

Reuter, P.H. (2013). Why has US Drug policy changed so little over 30 years? *Crime and Justice* 42: 1–66.

Riley, D., Sawka, E., Conley, P., Hewitt, D., Mitic, W., Poulin, C., Room, R., Single, E. and Topp, J. (1999). Harm reduction: concepts and practice. a policy discussion paper. *Substance Use and Misuse* 34: 9–24.

Room, R. (2012). *Roadmaps to Reforming the UN Drug Conventions*. Oxford: The Beckley Foundation.

Room, R. and Reuter, P. (2012). How well do international drug conventions protect public health? *The Lancet* 279: 84–91.

Sinha, J. (2001). *The History and Development of the Leading International Drug Control Conventions*. Ottawa: Parliamentary Research Branch, Library of Parliament.

Sloman, L. (1979). *Reefer Madness – Marijuana in America*. New York: Grove.

Smith, M.A. (1988). The drug problem – is there an answer? *Federal Probation* 52: 3–6.

Spector, M. and Kitsuse, J.I. (1987). *Constructing Social Problems*. New York: Aldine de Gruyter.

Spunt, B.J, Goldstein, P.J., Brownstein, H.H. and Fendrich, M. (1994). The role of marijuana in homicide. *Substance Use and Misuse* 29: 195–213.

Stouffer, S.A. (1949). An analysis of conflicting social norms. *American Sociological Review* 14: 707–17.

Strang, J., Babor, T., Caulkins, J., Fischer, B., Foxcroft, D. and Humphreys, K. (2012). Drug policy and the public good: evidence for effective interventions. *The Lancet* 379: 71–83.

Sumner, W.G. (1907). *Folkways—A Study of the Sociological Importance of Usages, Manners, Customs, Mores, and Morals*. Boston: Ginn and Company, the Athenaeum Press.

Trebach, A.S. and Zeese, K.B. (eds) (1990). *The Great Issues of Drug Policy*. Washington, DC: The Drug Policy Foundation.

United Nations (UN) (1961). *Single Convention on Narcotic Drugs, 1961*. Available from: www.unodc.org/pdf/convention_1961_en.pdf (Accessed 5 June 2012).

United Nations (UN) (1971). *The Convention on Psychotropic Substances, 1971*. Available from: www.unodc.org/pdf/convention_1971_en.pdf. online (Accessed 5 June 2012).

United Nations (UN) (1988). *United Nations Conference for the Adoption of a Convention Against Illicit Traffic in Narcotic Drugs and Psychotropic Substances*. Available from: www.unodc.org/pdf/convention_1988_en.pdf (Accessed 5 June 2012).

United Nations Office on Drugs and Crime (UNODC) (2007). *World Drug Report 2007*. Vienna: United Nations.

van Laar, M., Cruts, G., van Gageldonk, A., van Ooyen-Houben, M., Croes, E., Meijer, R. and Ketelaars, T. (2011). *Report to the EMCDDA by the Reitox National Focal Point*. Final Version as approved by the Scientific Committee of the Netherlands National Drug Monitor (NDM) on the 22nd of December 2010. Lisbon: European Monitoring Centre for Drugs and Drug Addiction.

Walker, S. (2011). *Sense and Nonsense about Crime, Drugs, and Communities*, 7th edn. Belmont: Wadsworth.

Watson, S.J., Benson, J.A. and Joy, J.E. (2000). Marijuana and medicine: assessing the science base: a summary of the 1999 Institute of Medicine Report. *Archives of General Psychiatry* 57: 547–52.

Weber, M. (1947). *The Theory of Social and Economic Organization* (translated by A.M. Henderson and T.A. Parsons and edited with an Introduction by T.A. Parsons). New York: Free Press.

Weil, A. (1972). *The Natural Mind – An Investigation of Drugs and Higher Consciousness*. Boston: Houghton Mifflin.

Weisheit, R.A. (1990). Civil war on drugs. In R.A. Weisheit (ed.), *Drugs, Crime and the Criminal Justice System*. Cincinnati: Anderson, pp. 1–10.

Weisheit, R. and White, W.L. (2009). *Methamphetamine: Its History, Pharmacology, and Treatment*. Center City: Hazelden.

Wisotsky, S. (1986). *Breaking the Impasse in the War on Drugs*. New York: Greenwood.

Woolgar, S. and Pawluch, D. (1985). Ontological gerrymandering: the anatomy of social problems explanations. *Social Problems* 33: 159–62.

Zetterberg, H.L. (1958). Compliant actions. *Acta Sociologica* 2: 179–201.

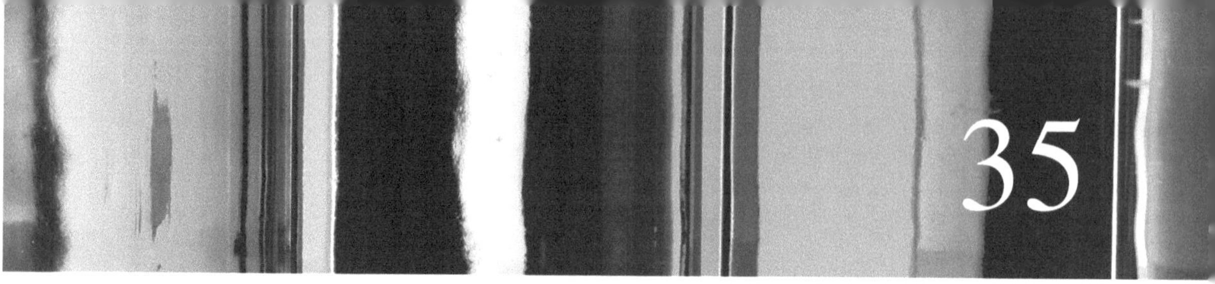

35

The Limits of Evidence-Based Practice in the Pursuit of Specific Treatment Efficacy

Anders Bergmark and Lena Hübner

INTRODUCTION

For almost two decades, the necessity of establishing practices that are based on scientifically secured knowledge, also known as evidence-based practice (EBP), has constituted an important and growing international tendency in many different professional fields. The drive for a scientific underpinning for professional practice is most clearly developed within the medical field, but is also apparent in psychosocial, non-medical interventions.

As, on the whole, the actual establishment of EBP has not been realized – that it still has the character of a project, 'a normative projection of the hopes invested in the future; a legitimacy of potential rather than of what actually has been achieved' (Bergmark and Lundström, 2006: 110, our translation) – the door remains open to a substantial amount of definitional freedom as to what constitutes the content and limits of EBP. In consequence, several interpretations of EBP are simultaneously present in most national contexts (Bergmark and Lundström, 2006).

That different – and sometimes openly contradictory – notions exist as to what EBP is and how it should be practiced does not in itself represent an insurmountable problem. More important is the lack of awareness of this fact. On the whole, serious discussion of the content and forms of EBP is limited to a rather small group of scholars, whereas politicians, administrators and practitioners generally seem to be unaware of any definitional problems. As a result, many of the activities that in practice are recognized as EBP (e.g. the use of standardized assessment of client characteristics) take place under a legitimacy that is based on something much more elaborated. Shlonsky and Gibbs (2004: 137) claim that 'EBP is in danger of becoming a catchphrase for anything that is done with clients that can somehow be linked to an empirical study, regardless of the study's quality, competing evidence, or consideration of clients' needs'.

In the following, we will outline the historical context of the evidence movement and its roots in evidence-based medicine (EBM) including a mapping of the critical appraisal perspective (Sackett et al., 2000) and its rival alternative, EBPs (i.e. the list that identifies effective interventions). We will also provide a condensed description and analysis of the methodological pillars of evidence-based practice; that is, the randomized controlled trial (RCT) and the systematic review, and in connection with this discuss, some of the most important methodological problems that can cause flaws in the many attempts to establish unbiased evidence. We will present actual results from efficacy treatment studies in the alcohol and drug abuse field while also providing examples of different strategies among the organizations (national and international) that produce this type of evidence. Finally, we will discuss the difficulties of implementing EBP, which partly is connected to the fact that there is a shortage of research or reviews that identify interventions that are clearly better than others, and at the same time, elaborate some of the alternatives to the present medical model of treatment effects. Taken together, we intend to illuminate a number of problems that can be considered as internally important for the EBP project, or differently expressed, we intend to discuss the limits of EBP from an empirical and insider perspective rather than dismissing the entire project with a more general and external criticism of its epistemological assumptions (see e.g. Hjørland, 2011).

DIFFERENT FORMS AND CHARACTERISTICS OF EBP

By and large, the growth of the EBP movement has resulted in two completely different methodological tracks; on the one hand, we see that the organizations primarily active in the international arena (the Cochrane Collaboration, Campbell Collaboration, AGREE Collaboration, CONSORT Group and GRADE working group) are constantly standardizing and improving their methodological requirements and demands for general systematic rigour, along with other measures intended to secure the production of unbiased evidence. On the other hand, it is apparent that some national and regional organizations aiming at establishing EBP by and large have developed their regimes in the opposite direction – towards an apparent weakening of the criteria used to identify and delimit evidence.

In the field of EBM, where the demand for a more substantial input of scientific evidence into actual practice has been insistent for a longer time than in any other professional field, Timmermans and Mauk observed the following:

> So many parties have jumped on the EBM bandwagon and so many clinical practice guidelines are churned out by individuals, professional organisations, insurers and others that the benefits of uniformity may disappear in the cacophony of overlapping, conflicting and poorly constructed guidelines. With more than 1,000 guidelines created annually, calls for guidelines for clinical guidelines have been issued. (Timmermans and Mauk, 2005: 19)

EBP is often described as an application or a movement that has taken hold in medicine and spread into other professions, such as nursing, teaching, social work and psychology (see Bohlin, 2011). In the late 1990s, EBP also reached non-medical professionals working with substance abuse treatment; in the same way as doctors, they were expected to base their practice on scientific knowledge. EBP can also be said to stand in opposition to the traditional bureaucratic/judicial approach, where in the handling of alcohol and drug problems interventions and assessments are motivated by legislative and regulatory frameworks, while EBP is directed by the intention to identify and use the best available scientific knowledge. In this way, EBP can also be said to challenge politically controlled treatment practices.

In order to understand the present state of affairs concerning EBP outside of the medical field it is necessary to highlight one specific tradition within that field. One of the leading advocates of what came to be known as evidence-based medicine and that eventually spread further as EBP was David Sackett of McMasters Hospital in Canada, whose name is still strongly associated with the genesis of the evidence movement. The problem that he and his colleagues were trying to solve was that research showed that doctors did not routinely apply the best possible scientific knowledge at their disposal, but were bound by the context they worked in and dependence on authority figures in their environment.

What came to be given priority in the education at McMasters, therefore, was the aspiring doctors' ability to seek out and critically review research results relevant to their clinical questions. Through teaching methods, such as group work and problem-based learning, the intention was to educate physicians who were not authoritarian, but able instead to orient themselves sufficiently in current knowledge and arrive at independent decisions both in research and in clinical practice. The term used to describe the ability to find research and critically review it, and then see how it could be applied in clinical practice, came to be known as critical appraisal and the scientific methods that came to be valued most were the experimental studies of medical interventions and compilations of experimental studies in systematic reviews (Sackett et al., 2000).

One of the most quoted passages in Sackett's and colleagues' texts is the definition of evidence-based medicine: 'The conscientious, explicit, and judicious use of current best evidence in making decisions about the care of individual patients' (Sackett et al., 1996: 71).

Critical appraisal outlines a procedure where we carefully, clearly and with good judgment use the best possible current evidence when deciding on treatment for each individual patient. The actual implementation of EBP, if we start from the Sackett model, can be described in five different steps (Sackett et al., 2000; Gambrill, 2006):

1 Formulation of research questions on the basis of information about the client and/or other relevant factors.
2 Location of the best possible knowledge bases (evidence) with relevance to these issues.
3 Critical reviewing of the knowledge base (the evidence) with respect to validity, importance (in terms of evidence strength) and usability in practice.
4 Application of the evidence-based knowledge in practice, taking into account the client's individual characteristics and preferences.
5 Evaluation of the impact of the intervention and assessment of how to improve the application of steps 1 to 4 in the future.

The critical appraisal perspective has been criticized on one vital point: it is very difficult to implement in practice. Despite many well-organized attempts to train doctors in the critical appraisal version of EBP, it has been shown that they still did not apply the critical appraisal perspective, tending instead to rely on the work of others who had produced guidelines or a list of EBPs. Although there is a substantial difference between critical appraisal and following guidelines, this distinction is often blurred in policy documents and rhetoric concerning the 'true nature' of EBP.

RANDOMIZED, CONTROLLED EXPERIMENTS AND SYSTEMATIC REVIEWS – THE CORNERSTONES OF THE EVIDENCE MOVEMENT'S METHODOLOGICAL PROGRAMME

A relatively large number of methodological considerations can be regarded as related to the idea and implementation of EBP, but it is clear that two methodological components come across as far more central than others;

namely RCTs and systematic reviews. In general, the methodological weight of these components is similar in the two basic perspectives on EBP; both critical appraisal and the guideline model emphasize the necessity of RCTs and systematic reviews, seen as necessary in order to produce unbiased and reliable evidence. When it comes to the RCTs, it is relatively clear that the aspect of this procedure that is attributed the greatest weight is the randomization (random distribution) of individuals into experiment and control groups. The emphasis on systematic reviews as a fundamental basis for the establishment of EBP, on the other hand, is largely associated with the development of information technology, which has led to a whole new availability of scientific publications and a general expansion of the number of published scientific studies. This growth of scientific knowledge has led to the need for large amounts of information to be compiled and synthesized. It is no longer enough to underpin a given position with reference to a single scientific study, as results may vary between studies. An evidence-based judgment must include all relevant knowledge, which can lead to a situation where hundreds of scientific studies must form the basis of choices made. The sheer scale of the number of studies also requires the procedure to be conducted systematically. Over time this also has come to mean that the systematic review in many cases is synonymous with a synthesizing process based on quantitative methodology, mostly including a so-called meta-analysis.

We will now describe in a little more detail the meaning, demarcations and problems associated with the implementation of systematic reviews as well as of RCTs, and as an experimental design of the RCT type can be regarded as a more fundamental methodological component than the systematic review, it seems reasonable that we first tackle description and analysis of the RCT.

The internationally accepted concept of the RCT can be applied in a number of different ways. The basic variant is the version we have presented, the randomized controlled trial, an experimental design characterized by the random breakdown of subjects into experiment and control groups, where other conditions that might affect the outcome variable are kept under control. Both intervention and control conditions must be standardized (controlled) as regards content and scope. The intervention must be directed at individuals with a clear problem profile (i.e. exclude individuals with more complex problems), and an RCT study should also be 'double-blind', with patients as well as staff unaware of what constitutes intervention or control input. This is very hard to accomplish in the psychosocial area, but it is difficult to underestimate the importance of this problem, which should lead to a critical examination of effects obtained under conditions that do not fulfil the double-blind condition. There is an obvious risk that effects identified as related to specific elements de facto are derived from how the implementation of an intervention has been staged (e.g. a placebo effect generated by the fact that the staff delivering the intervention is confident that the intervention is effective).

Sometimes, the acronym RCT is used to refer to a randomized *clinical* trial (see e.g. Bohlin, 2011) and at times the term simply randomized trial is also used as a synonym of RCT. For those who want to orient themselves in the most advanced description and delimitation of the concept we refer to the CONSORT Group (Consolidated Standards of reporting Trials), whose activities aim at the establishment of standardized rules for how RCT should be reported in scientific studies.

The control options that form the basis of the comparison with an experimental intervention can be roughly divided into three different types: (i) where the control group receive no intervention at all (or an intervention that is delayed in time, with the individuals put on a waiting list to be compared, during the time they are not receiving any intervention, with the individuals in the intervention group); (ii) where the control group receive the 'usual' intervention (treatment as usual, abbreviated TAU) sometimes also referred to as the standard treatment; in practice, however, this does not mean that the individuals in the control group de facto receive a standard intervention, the opposite is rather the case, as both the usual and the standard intervention will vary with time and place; and (iii) where the control group receives an alternative intervention that ideally is meant to be effective (*bona fide*, in good faith) and has the same scope and intensity as the experimental intervention, but includes clear differences with regard to the mechanisms that are supposed to influence the individuals included in the experiment. The type of control group used, therefore, is of fundamental importance to the results of an RCT and how it is interpreted (Karlsson and Bergmark, 2015).

The question of whether 'evidence' can be based on RCTs alone or if other types of designs can be accepted as a basis is a controversial issue and in many respects represents a clear watershed in the scientific debate as to how evidence should be produced. Methodologically, there are several alternative approaches, particularly within the framework of quasi-experimental or comparative projects that use so-called matched control (with control groups designed so that on a number of relevant points they have the same composition as the experiment group) or statistical control (where the observable relevant differences that exist between the control group and the intervention group are kept constant by using different statistical techniques). The basic idea is the same as in the RCTs: to create in different ways a counterfactual measurement point in order to compare the ones who get the treatment with those receiving another treatment or no treatment at all. With a quasi-experimental design it becomes possible to study the effects of different treatment interventions under 'natural' conditions, for example, to the extent that a given treatment unit offering both cognitive behavioural therapy and 12-step treatment it can choose – instead of allocating clients randomly between these treatment options – to use a quasi-experimental design that seeks to compensate for differences between the two client groups by using statistical techniques. An arrangement of this kind has the advantage of having the potential to improve external validity, but nevertheless, it is generally considered to be a weaker design than the randomized study (which emphasizes internal validity). In a comparative investigation of RCT studies and non-randomized designs, Kunz and Oxman (1998) conclude that the latter tend to overestimate the effect of a given intervention. Conversely, McKee et al. (1999) found no difference between RCTs and non-randomized studies.

Overall, despite the undeniably prevalent criticism of RCTs, it would probably still be hard to argue that they should take anything other than first place as a basis for evaluation of a given intervention effect. This situation is also reflected in the so-called evidence hierarchies. Let us now move from the methodological considerations that are central to EBP to discuss the results of some of the more important studies in the alcohol field.

MAJOR MULTICENTRE STUDIES ON THE TREATMENT OF ALCOHOL PROBLEMS

Although meta-analysis has come to appear – in a time characterized by a never-ending stream of scientific information – as the only reasonable method of establishing valid knowledge surveys, scientific developments with regard to the treatment of alcohol misuse is primarily influenced by the large multicentre studies rather than by meta-analysis. The unprecedentedly largest and most important multicentre study in the substance abuse field, Project MATCH (matching alcohol treatments to client heterogeneity; Babor and

Del Boca, 2003) is a randomized controlled trial that took over 10 years to complete. Involving 1,726 clients, 159 researchers and assistants, and 95 therapists in 32 different research institutions, it is often described – with reference to its scope as well as its final outcome – as the Titanic of alcohol research. The driving force behind the project was the lack of scientific support for stable effects of the treatment interventions that had been studied in controlled experiments. It was hypothesized that the absence of positive outcomes was to be explained by a lack of matching between different types of client characteristics and specific treatment interventions, also identified as a possible source of a 'dilution effect' in the sense that positive results from the 'proper' matching were counteracted by those cases where the matching between treatment and client did not fit.

Project MATCH was designed to shed light on whether a match could improve outcomes for different types of treatment interventions. This was staged in two parallel 'arms', one open care study and one aftercare study. Three different types of treatment interventions, cognitive behavioural therapy (CBT), motivational enhancement therapy (MET) and 12-step facilitation therapy (TSF) were studied in both these arms.

The project's purpose and design required the treatment options to clearly differ in terms of both theoretical foundations and implementation. For this reason, great emphasis was put on selecting treatment options characterized by distinct differences between them and on the implementation of these interventions via detailed manuals. Despite the extensive theoretical basis and the fact that both the design and the implementation were characterized by excellent methodological quality, Project MATCH could not identify any robust and interpretable matching effects (Babor and del Boca, 2003). In addition to the lack of the hypothesized matching effects was also the rather disappointing outcome of the three different treatment interventions. Regardless of the treatment provided to the individuals in each treatment group, the success rate was about the same. Project MATCH can be regarded, therefore, as a study that provides strong empirical support for the findings within general psychotherapy research on treatment efficacy, that is, the tendency for bona fide treatments to provide the same type of result overall (see Wampold, 2001; Bergmark, 2008a).

Essentially, it was not possible to identify the specific mechanisms that were theoretically postulated. Project MATCH could not, for example, show any support for the hypothesis that MET affects the individual's level of aggression or that CBT affects an individual's coping ability. The main findings from Project MATCH have been labelled as 'unintended' (Babor and Del Boca, 2003) and constitute a substantial empirical argument for a reorientation of research efforts concerning psychosocial interventions (Babor 2008, Bergmark 2008b).

The results from Project MATCH are to a substantial extent also reflected in the UK Alcohol Treatment Trial (UKATT) initiated at the beginning of the twenty-first century, which represents the most comprehensive study of psychosocial treatment interventions ever conducted in the United Kingdom. UKATT is a RCT conducted at five different treatment centres. The study included 742 individuals who either received social behaviour and network therapy (SBNT, the experimental intervention) or motivational enhancement therapy (MET, intended to serve as a control intervention). At the follow-up, 12 months after therapy cessation, no differences could be identified in outcomes between the two treatment groups (UKATT research team, 2005). In retrospect, it was examined whether an analysis of five targeted matching hypotheses could identify some differences in outcomes for individuals who had received a match as any of the five hypotheses. None of the five matching hypotheses was confirmed by analysis of the results after 12 months (UKATT research team 2007). Results from the UKATT study thus show more or less complete accordance with the results of Project MATCH.

As we shall see in the next section, the lack of a reasonable solid scientific base that could support the identification of 'best practice' interventions is not only associated with the high quality multicentre studies, it is also a basic characteristic of the majority of systematic reviews concerning psychosocial interventions.

SYSTEMATIC REVIEWS

By the end of 2006, the National Treatment Agency for Substance Misuse (NTA) in England published a comprehensive narrative overview of the effects of treatment for alcohol problems (Raistrick et al., 2006). On the basis of previous surveys, and some of the results of Project MATCH and UKATT (results from UKATT regarding matching were not available at that time), the authors concluded that 'there is a range of effective treatments with little research evidence of clear differences in effectiveness between them. At the present state of our research knowledge, therefore, there is no 'best' treatment for alcohol problems or treatment of choice' (Raistrick et al., 2006: 41).

The meta-analysis by Imel et al. (2008) was the first proper study in the addiction field, including only studies that compare treatment interventions which are active treatments intended to have effect. After the usual literature searches in relevant databases, the authors identified 30 original studies involving 3,500 individuals that compared psychosocial treatment interventions of a bona fide nature for alcohol problems. The inclusion criteria required individuals participating in the study to be randomly assigned to the various treatment options. The meta-analysis of these 30 studies essentially showed the same type of results obtained from more extensive analyses of general psychotherapy and thus offered no support for the existence of differences in impact between different types of treatment interventions for alcohol problems. In the meta-analysis in Imel et al. (2008), Bruce Wampold acted as co-author. Wampold, who has performed a variety of meta-analyses concerning efficacy in the general psychotherapy field and played a crucial role in the problematizing of the possibilities of identifying psychotherapeutic treatment options that are more efficient than others, has vigorously argued (2001) that it is necessary to distinguish between the concepts of absolute and relative effect (efficacy). Absolute efficacy is determined by comparing the results from a given treatment with results from a non-treated control group (or a control condition not intended to have effect), while relative efficacy implies a comparison between two (or more) different treatment interventions intended to be effective. Wampold uses the bona fide concept in order to specify that the control treatment must be designed in such a way that it can be said to constitute a real treatment intervention. As noted by Karlsson and Bergmark (2015), a variety of control conditions between different original studies within the same review constitute a major problem as this undermines the possibility of drawing conclusions based on the review. It is worth noting, however, that the large multicentre studies discussed in the foregoing section meet the requirements for delivering relative effects, although no relative effects were identified.

GUIDELINES FOR INTERVENTIONS OF ALCOHOL PROBLEMS

In a recent study on the methodological congruence between three different guidelines for psychosocial interventions for alcohol problems, Bergmark et al. (2014) show that not only are the methodological procedures underpinning the guidelines different in many important respects; several of the conclusions concerning specific interventions also deviate from each other. Although the guidelines at hand [Practice Guideline for the Treatment of Patients with Substance Use Disorders, American Psychiatric Association (APA 2006); Alcohol-Use Disorders; the NICE Guideline on Diagnosis, Assessment and Management of Harmful Drinking and Alcohol Dependence, British National Institute for Health and Clinical Excellence (NICE), National Collaborating Centre for Mental Health published by The British Psychological Society and The Royal College of Psychiatrists (2011); Guidelines for the Treatment of Alcohol Problems, Australian Government, Department of Health and Ageing (2009)] are all produced by prestigious organizations, there can be no real doubt that the NICE guidelines are of higher quality, being both more transparent and more elaborated than the other two. The development methods are carefully described and search protocols are clearly identified for each section; the PICO2 frame was used for review questions about interventions and as search protocol, and meta-analyses were initiated when the conditions at hand allowed it. The search protocols for psychological and psychosocial interventions show that only RCT designs were considered to be reliable enough to substantiate the evidence base at NICE. The guideline is also more demanding than the others in its inclusion criteria, as only studies on treatment-seeking populations were included (NICE, 2011: 230). Studies on treatments addressing problems other than an actual alcohol problem were also excluded.

An important difference between the guidelines is how systematic reviews are used in the process of evidence identification. The NICE guidelines do not use external systematic reviews at all (i.e. reviews produced by other organizational bodies than themselves), only making use of the systematic reviews produced by NICE. The Australian guideline producers did not present any new meta-analyses of their own origin, but included earlier meta-analyses from other sources in their review and rated them at the highest level in their evidence hierarchy. In the APA guidelines, systematic reviews are rated very low, number six in their evidence hierarchy.

Differences of this kind contribute to the fact that the guidelines reach different conclusions considering the efficacy of some of the best-known treatment interventions for alcohol problems. In the NICE guidelines, the quality of the evidence regarding motivational interviewing (MI) and MET is evaluated as moderate (here it is important to understand that this assessment does not concern the efficacy of MI/MET, but rather is a statement concerning with what certainty NICE draws its conclusion concerning this intervention). MI/MET is described as suitable to use as part of the initial assessment for all individuals with an alcohol problem, but it is also clearly stated that the present state of evidence is not sufficient for a recommendation of MI/MET as a stand-alone intervention. According to the NICE guidelines there is no evidence for MI/MET being more effective than other interventions. In contrast to this rather restrictive perspective on MI/MET, the APA guideline refers to Project MATCH as providing support for MI/MET as a stand-alone treatment. The Australian guideline identifies MI/MET as a 'first line' or 'stand-alone' intervention, their recommendation graded at the A level, which signifies that it is directly based on category [I] evidence, that is, evidence obtained from a systematic review or meta-analysis of randomized controlled trials.

These types of methodological problems have increased the institutionalized efforts of some actors to implement even more far-reaching standardizations intended to counteract the presence of competing and non-congruent positions concerning which interventions constitute best practice in a given field. An organization such as the Cochrane Collaboration can, to a considerable extent, be seen as built upon a foundation laid down by its protocols, handbooks and databases, which can all be seen as explicit expressions of an aspiration to reduce and control irrelevant influences and to increase transparency concerning the reviews that it publishes. However, the ambition to establish objective and thoroughly scientifically gathered evidence will inevitably be undermined by the exponential growth of published studies in almost any given scientific field, which means that scientific knowledge will consistently be subjected to revisions and thereby also can always to a certain extent be said to be uncertain.

An identified difference between two or more 'evidence' statements from producers concerning the available evidence for a given intervention, as shown in the previous section, is not necessarily always related to a lack of methodological stringency or divergent perspectives on what constitutes a sound methodological procedure. In some cases, the differences seem to be the result of plain omissions. In their analysis of the reviews produced by the Cochrane and the Campbell collaborations on psychosocial interventions for alcohol problems, Karlsson and Bergmark (2015) noted what control group designs were considered suitable for inclusion in the different reviews and analysed the extent to which the reviews argued for chosen comparison conditions. The authors also analysed whether type of control group in the primary studies influenced how the reviews framed the effects discussed and whether this was related to conclusions drawn. The Cochrane Collaboration has explicitly addressed this type of question. Following the Cochrane handbook (7, section 5.3), a main distinction should be drawn between inactive and active control group designs. The first type of comparison provides absolute effects and the latter relative effects. The handbook underlines that reviews should specify the interventions of interest along with the interventions with which these will be compared, in particular whether with an inactive control intervention (i.e. no treatment, standard care or a waiting list) or with an active control intervention (e.g. a different variant of the same intervention, a different drug, a different kind of intervention). Karlsson and Bergmark (2015) provide a straightforward conclusion: little attention is paid to the difference between designs using active and inactive control groups and the differential effect estimates that can be obtained from these. Although there were some exceptions, the majority of the reviews largely ignored this distinction. This conclusion illuminates the fact that the presence of explicit and institutionalized methodological procedures, such as can be found in the Cochrane handbook, are by no means a guarantee for practices among reviewers.

THE EVIDENCE BASE FOR THE TREATMENT OF DRUG PROBLEMS

If the evidence base for alcohol problems can be said to be broad but somewhat shallow, in the sense that 'there is a range of effective treatments with little research evidence of clear differences in effectiveness between them, at the present state of our research knowledge, therefore, there is no 'best' treatment for alcohol problems or treatment of choice' (see above; Raistrick et al., 2006: 41), the situation is quite different for treatment interventions for drug problems. Here the evidence base is narrow and, by and large, only pharmacological substitution treatment for opioid dependence has been able to provide stable and reliable results concerning its efficacy. Over the years, it is mainly methadone maintenance treatment that has dominated both clinical practice as well as research concerning treatment for drug problems.

The main exception is buprenorphine, which became popular during the first years of the new century and also is used for maintenance treatment for opioid dependence. In a recent Cochrane review, Mattick et al. (2014) compared the results for methadone and buprenorphine and noted that the main difference between the two treatment alternatives was that methadone seemed to be better at keeping patients in treatment. On average, the chances of a patient leaving treatment during study periods were 17 per cent lower for methadone.

It is noteworthy that the same type of evidence is interpreted differently by the Cochrane reviewers and the NICE organization expert group. While the Cochrane group, based on the fact that methadone brought about lower health care costs and provided better retention, identified methadone as the default choice, the experts at NICE (technology appraisal TA114) claimed:

> The decision about which drug to use should be made on a case by case basis, taking into account a number of factors, including the person's history of opioid dependence, their commitment to a particular long-term management strategy, and an estimate of the risks and benefits of each treatment made by the responsible clinician in consultation with the person.

The reason for this discrepancy between the Cochrane reviewers and NICE recommendation is not articulated in the Cochrane report.

Among studies concerning treatment effects for problems related to the use of cannabis the most important and well-designed is the Cannabis Youth Treatment (CYT) study (Dennis et al., 2004). This is a multi-site investigation with a design that sets out to identify the effects of treatment intensity as well as of different treatment modalities by comparing a 12-session combination of MET and CBT in different dosages with family support network therapy, parent education group meetings, the adolescent community reinforcement approach (CRA), and multidimensional family therapy. Although all the interventions led to improvements, the authors concluded that 'overall the clinical outcomes were very similar across sites and conditions at 12-month follow-up' (Dennis et al., 2004: 209). Accordingly, the study did not provide any support for the idea that a larger dosage of a given treatment is more effective than a smaller one and neither did it identify any of the interventions as more effective than the others.

While clinical guidelines based on systematic reviews that cover other types of treatment interventions than substitution treatment for opioid dependence are quite rare, there are exceptions: NICE and the National Collaborating Centre for Mental Health (NCCMH) have published a comprehensive review of psychosocial treatment intervention of drug problems (NICE, 2008).

This guideline constitutes an impressive work that covers many aspects of drug misuse: identification, brief interventions, treatment settings, cost effectiveness, and treatment interventions such as contingency management (CM), CBT and the community reinforcement approach. The methodological quality of the different analyses is characterized by a high standard; the aggregation of original studies is essentially completed with a significant precision with respect to such factors as the type of drug, the treatment model, outcome measures and control group. The reader is provided with full transparency through detailed information of included and excluded studies as well as forest plots for the different meta-analyses of the evidence underpinning the recommendations. However, as generally appears to be the case with guidelines and many systematic reviews, the ambition to enhance the objective character of the recommendations seems to restrain a more analytical contextualization. One gets the impression that the manuals and protocols used to produce the guidelines constitute an empirical apparatus that cannot deal with issues that fall outside the predefined work process. For a reader with an interest in some elaboration of the empirical analyses presented, it would have been interesting to see a broader perspective or a critical evaluation.

Robust support for efficacy is by and large only identified for CM, which basically constitutes a rather clear-cut behavioural system of reward and punishment (more rarely the latter). Although the guidelines provide substantial evidence of relatively wide support to suggest that the intervention in question is effective during treatment, by contrast the basis for sustained efficacy after stopping treatment is significantly weaker (Prendergast et al., 2006). For this reason, the strong recommendation for the implementation of CM might have benefitted from an elaboration of the difference between 'during treatment' and 'follow-up' efficacy. Is it reasonable to consider CM a psychosocial intervention, or is it simply a question of getting what you pay for, but only as long as you pay for it?

One of the more surprising results in the guidelines is the relative lack of support for CBT, which generally tends to be described as the evidence-based intervention par excellence, not only for addiction treatment but also among psychotherapies in general. The recommendation that CBT 'should not be offered routinely to people presenting for treatment of cannabis or stimulant misuse or those receiving opioid maintenance treatment' stands out as a clear break with earlier recommendations concerning the usefulness of CBT in addiction treatment and might, in this respect, be considered an important step forward. Conversely, it could also be said to contribute to some confusion, not least among those practitioners who have adopted CBT in their work on the basis of its presentation as effective and evidence-based. Although the project to produce clinical practice guidelines is based on the intention to gain more control over the variability and effectiveness of practice, we can also expect – partly as a result of the ever-growing number of guidelines and systematic reviews and their relative incompatibility – that we will also have to deal with more confusion and refutations among some practitioners.

CONCLUDING REMARKS

In 2005, one of the world's most influential scientists, John Ioannidis, published an article with the provocative title, 'Why Most Published Research Findings Are False', in which it is contended:

> The probability that a research claim is true may depend on study power and bias, the number of other studies on the same question, and, importantly, the ratio of true to no relationships among the relationships probed in each scientific field. In this framework, a research finding is less likely to be true when the studies conducted in a field are smaller; when effect sizes are smaller; when there is a greater number and lesser preselection of tested relationships; where there is greater flexibility in designs, definitions, outcomes, and analytical modes. (Ioannidis, 2005: 697)

Unfortunately, the circumstances that Ioannidis identifies as associated with false research results are quite common among the original treatment efficacy studies in the substance misuse field, and accordingly, also undermine the quality of systematic reviews and meta-analyses. Furthermore, many studies that are concerned with the efficacy of psychosocial interventions are not suitable to interpret within a medical conceptualization.

For more than three decades, the lion's share of the research on psychosocial intervention efficacy has been organized along the lines of the medical model. That is, studies are arranged in accordance with a conceptual scheme where specifically selected interventions are directed towards pathological processes or other biological shortcomings that have been identified through reliable diagnoses. Such a model appears to be absolutely sensible in relation to known and well-described physical problems treated with pharmacological substances or operations, but the overall results of psychotherapy research (Wampold, 2001) and studies of the outcome of psychosocial interventions in the substance misuse field indicate that the medical model should not be the first choice when it comes to the design of studies on psychosocial interventions.

The basic observation that there generally are no differences in outcome between different bona fide psychotherapeutic interventions also includes a direct challenge vis-à-vis the theoretical frameworks that claim that there are specific elements/mechanisms underlying the effects of a given intervention. This challenge also involves a substantial critique directed against the use of the medical model in the psychosocial area. In the same spirit, Morgenstern and Longabaugh (2000) noted that research has not yet been able to identify why CBT is given to be an effective intervention. An even more far-reaching conclusion expressed in a systematic review focused on answering what scientific support there is for MI, CBT, family therapy and 12-step treatment includes specific mechanisms of action. Morgenstern and McKay write, 'the findings of the review suggest that there is minimal support for the propositions that (a) theory-based active ingredients are the primary curative agents and (b) specific therapeutic factors suggested by these models are more important than general factors such as therapist skill and the therapeutic alliance' (Morgenstern and McKay, 2007: 1383). Arguably, the most frequently studied treatment mechanism is the placebo intervention, which precludes the presence of specific mechanisms and must instead be described as contextual, that is, related to the context in which it is included. For many decades, the randomized, double-blind, placebo-controlled study has constituted the preferred experimental design in the medical field. Generally, a placebo intervention is defined with reference to a specific therapeutic theory; a given treatment intervention is regarded as a placebo control to the extent that its contents be regarded as peripheral as opposed to central in relation to the theory being studied. As the mechanism of action of a placebo intervention generally is attributed to psychological categories such as expectation, hope and credibility, it represents a particular problem in the context of the study of psychosocial interventions. While a psychosocial intervention cannot be hidden from the individual who is conducting it (be done blind in the same way that a doctor may be unaware of whether or not he or she is distributing a pharmacological or a sugar pill), an alternative approach may be used. The closest alternative to a pure placebo intervention is reasonably to use a comparison of two interventions that are both bona fide, but clearly different when it comes to central theoretical assumptions. Interventions should also be performed by individuals who can be regarded as clearly allied with the intervention they implement. A design of this type is thus essentially what must be used in order to establish whether a given intervention has a relative effect.

The medical model's emphasis on specific mechanisms entails a corresponding underestimation of the importance of performer effects. A performer effect is the contribution to an overall effect that can be attributed to characteristics of an individual. This is true not only in interventions that involve treatment, such as psychotherapy and other types of psychosocial interventions, even if it is just for this type of activity that it executes the most important effects. Given the indications that performer effects are often much larger than the effects of the technology or the method applied (Wampold, 2001, Bergmark 2008b), there are obvious reasons to remain open to the possibility of new priorities in terms of what kind of targeting future research should have. Our basic alternative direction is essentially a retreat to a more fundamental and traditional scientific paradigm, because the current developments concerning the establishment of EBP in many ways has reduced the notion of what 'science' means in the question of study designs and systematic assessment instruments. Scientific activities must necessarily avoid being reduced to ideology production, a position that also includes a critical review of all types of knowledge pretentions, including those produced by organizations with institutionalized legitimacy (Karlsson et al., 2014).

The objections or criticisms launched against EBP as a global or national project should be balanced against its basic idea, that people in vulnerable positions are entitled to as good and as effective action as possible and that treatment providers should not devote time and resources on interventions that have no effect or may even be harmful. This may be stating the obvious, but what makes the argument stronger in this context is that it actually is formulated as operational and headline targets. Furthermore, based on the fact that EBP is intended to determine how clients are affected by interventions, to systematize this knowledge and use it as the basis for future decisions is above the authority of experience, intuition, anecdotal knowledge or adaptation to local traditions. The anti-authoritarian feature is also strongly emphasized by the influential representatives of the EBP as a means for both practitioners and clients to strengthen their influence over the development of practice (Gambrill, 2006).

The conviction that EBP can represent a host of good values must, however, be balanced against estimates of just how feasible it is in its individual parts and as an overall project. We must try to create a professional environment that is comfortable with uncertainty. We should therefore encourage authors to discuss problems and biases and possible confounding factors, and should acknowledge that most studies should be viewed as hypothesis-generating, rather than as conclusive.

REFERENCES

Babor, T. (2008) When prophecy fails: flying saucers, the second coming, and the treatment matching hypothesis. *Nordic Studies on Alcohol and Drugs*, 25: 294–6.

Babor, T. and Del Boca, F. (2003) *Treatment Matching in Alcoholism*. Cambridge: Cambridge University Press.

Bergmark, A. and Lundström, T. (2006) Mot en evidensbaserad praktik? Om färdriktningen i socialt arbete. [Towards an evidence-based practice? On the future direction of social work.] *Socialvetenskaplig Tidskrift*, 13: 99–113.

Bergmark, A. (2008a) Specific and contextual treatment mechanisms. *Nordic Studies on Alcohol and Drugs*, 25: 285–93.

Bergmark, A. (2008b) On treatment mechanisms – what can we learn from the COMBINE study? *Addiction*, 103: 703–5.

Bergmark, A., von Greiff, N. and Skogens L. (2014) The pursuit of evidence-based practice – comparisons of three guidelines on psychosocial interventions for alcohol problems, *Nordic Studies on Alcohol and Drugs*, 31: 271–88.

Bohlin, I. (2011) Evidensbaserat beslutsfattande i ett vetenskapsbaserat samhälle. Om evidensrörelsens ursprung, utbredning och gränser. In I. Bohlin and M. Sager (eds), *Evidensens Många Ansikten. Evidensbaserad Praktik i Praktiken*. Lund: Arkiv. Pp 31–68.

Dennis, M., Godley, S., Diamond, G., Tims, F., Babor, T., Donaldson, J., Liddle, H., Titus, J., Kaminer, Y., Webb, C., Hamilton, N. and Funk, R. (2004) The Cannabis Youth Treatment (CYT) study: main findings from two randomized trials. *Journal of Substance Abuse Treatment*, 27: 197–213.

Gambrill, E. (2006) Evidence-based practice and policy: choices ahead. *Research on Social Work Practice*, 16: 338–57.

Hjørland, B. (2011) Evidence-based practice: an analysis based on the philosophy of science. *Journal of the American Society for Information Science and Technology*, 62: 1301–10.

Imel, Z., Wampold, B., Miller, S. and Fleming, R. (2008) Distinctions without a difference: direct comparisons of psychotherapies for alcohol use disorders. *Psychology of Addictive Behaviours*, 22: 533–43.

Ioannidis, J. (2005) Why most published research findings are false. *PloS Medicine*, 2; 697–701.

Karlsson, P. and Bergmark, A. (2015) Compared to what? An analysis of control group types in Cochrane and Campbell reviews of psychosocial treatment efficacy with substance use disorders. *Addiction*, 110: 420–8.

Karlsson, P., Bergmark, A. and Lundström, T. (2014) Procedures and claims among US evidence-producing organizations: the case of the Incredible Years programme. *Evidence and Policy*, 10: 61–76.

Kunz, R. and Oxman, A. (1998) The unpredictability paradox: review of empirical comparisons of randomised and non-randomised clinical trials. *British Medical Journal,* 317: 1185e.

Mattick, R.P., Breen, C., Kimber, J. and Davoli, M. (2014) Buprenorphine maintenance versus placebo or methadone maintenance for opioid dependence. *The Cochrane Database of Systematic Reviews*, (2): CD002207.

McKee, M., Britton, A., Black, N., McPherson, K., Sanderson, C. and Bain, C. (1999) Methods in health services research. Interpreting the evidence: choosing between randomised and non-randomised studies. *British Medical Journal,* 319: 312–5.

Morgenstern, J. and Longabaugh, R. (2000): Cognitive and behavioral treatment for alcohol dependence: a review of evidence for its hypothesized mechanisms of action. *Addiction*, 95: 1475–90.

Morgenstern, J. and McKay, J. (2007) Rethinking the paradigms that inform behavioral treatment research for substance abuse disorders. *Addiction*, 102: 1377–1389.

NICE (2008) *Drug Misuse: Psychosocial Interventions*. London: Alden Press.

Prendergast, M., Podus, D., Finney, J., Greenwell, L. and Roll, J. (2006) Contingency management for treatment of substance use disorders: A meta-analysis. Addiction, 101: 1546–60.

Raistrick, D., Heather, N. and Godfrey, C. (2006) *Review of the Effectiveness of Treatment for Alcohol Problems*. London: National Treatment Agency for Substance Misuse.

Sackett, D.L., Rosenberg, W.M., Gray, J.A., Haynes, R.B. and Richardson, W.S. (1996) Evidence-based medicine: what it is and what it isn't. *British Medical Journal*, 312: 71–2.

Sackett, D.L., Straus, S.E., Richardson, W.S., Rosenberg, W. and Haynes, R.B. (2000) *Evidence-Based Medicine: How to Practice and Teach EBM*. Edinburgh: Churchill Livingstone.

Shlonsky, A. and Gibbs, L. (2004) Will the real evidence-based practice please stand up? Teaching the process of evidence-based practice to the helping professions. *Brief Treatment and Crisis Intervention,* 4: 137–53.

Timmermans, S. and Mauk, A. (2005) The promises and pitfalls of evidence-based medicine. *Health Affairs*, 24: 18–28.

UKATT Research Team (2005) Effectiveness of treatment for alcohol problems: findings of the randomised United Kingdom Alcohol Treatment Trial (UKATT). *British Medical Journal,* 331(7516): 541–4.

UKATT Research Team (2007) UK Alcohol Treatment Trial: client-treatment matching effects. *Addiction*, 103: 228–38.

Wampold, B. (2001) *The Great Psychotherapy Debate – Models, Methods and Findings.* Mahwah: Lawrence Erlbaum Associates.

36

Public Health Approaches to Substance Use: A Critique

Susanne MacGregor

INTRODUCTION

At Christmas 2014, representatives of leading doctors, public health campaigners and health charities wrote to a British national newspaper calling for a ban on alcohol firms sponsoring football clubs and other sports events. Signatories to the letter included the Alcohol Health Alliance UK, the Royal Colleges of Physicians, Anaesthetists, Nursing and Psychiatrists and the College of Emergency Medicine, along with 30 others. Their letter said 'It would be considered outrageous if high profile clubs like Everton or Celtic were to become brand ambassadors for tobacco and so why is it acceptable for alcohol?' (*The Guardian*, 26 December 2014). Reports noted that France has banned alcohol sponsorship of sport since 1991 as do Russia, Ukraine and Norway, while Australia, New Zealand, South Africa and the Republic of Ireland are considering similar actions. The Portman Group, which speaks for the alcohol industry in Britain, said a ban was unnecessary as rates of binge drinking among 16 to 24 year olds are in significant decline and emphasised that alcohol sponsorship contributes to the UK's vibrant and diverse economy.

At about the same time, some of the controversies behind a recently published Home Office Report on Drug Policy (Home Office 2014) were revealed by a Minister who had resigned on the issue. The Liberal Democrats, as part of their involvement in the UK 2010 to 2015 Coalition Government, had been pressing for changes in drug policy. The report had concluded that there was little relationship between tough drug laws and patterns of drug use but it had made no policy recommendations. The Minister revealed that three key recommendations proposed in the original draft had been vetoed by the Conservative members of the government. These were: to promote the use of cannabis-based medicines; to pilot a system of decriminalisation similar to that adopted in Portugal; and to encourage more long-term heroin users to seek treatment involving supervised diamorphine injections.

Drug and alcohol issues are high on British policy agendas and continue to be matters of dispute, as they are in other countries. Public health campaigners are often involved in these controversies in alliance with others, arguing for more attention to 'health' matters when policy is being decided: in the case of drugs, 'health' is opposed to 'criminalisation', while with alcohol, it is opposed to 'business interests'. To argue for a 'health' approach to drugs is to oppose prohibition and control through law, police, courts and prisons and replace it with control through treatment and harm reduction measures, such as needle and syringe exchange schemes: this is characterised by its opponents as a move towards 'liberalisation'. To argue for a 'health' approach to alcohol is to oppose the liberalisation that has accompanied the growth of the night-time economy and removal of restrictions on the sale of alcohol, that is, to prefer stricter controls, modelling policy on the perceived success of changes in controls on tobacco. The influence of tobacco in contemporary public health is considerable and looms over debates on alcohol, and to a lesser extent, drugs also.

Where alcohol is concerned, one image of the public health approach is as puritanical, advocating more restrictions and controls, less concern with pleasure, and vocal hostility to 'the industry'. In the drugs field internationally, 'public health' has a more benign image, involving compassion towards drug users, less victimisation, a non-judgemental approach and hostility to punitive law enforcement, especially incarceration and use of the death penalty for traffickers. The self-image of those centrally involved in public health however, emphasises reducing harm and promoting wellbeing, acting pragmatically and ideas of equality, equity, social justice and social solidarity.

The above illustrations show some of the difficulties in attempting to give an overview of 'public health' approaches to drugs and alcohol and offer a critique of these within the space of one short chapter. The situation is extremely complicated. Public health is a multi-faceted phenomenon. Philosophical and ethical issues are involved. Public health is not only a detached scientific and social scientific enterprise but also a living set of social practices. Its central goals are improving health and wellbeing and protecting populations from disease, while at one and the same time, it involves theoretical approaches, day to day practices and policy debates and actions, including campaigning. Campaigning, by its nature, involves selection and promotion of key issues, some exaggeration and use of rhetoric and sensationalism to claim attention in the noisy world of politics. In addition, public health is itself constantly changing, partly in response to developments in scientific and social scientific knowledge and partly because, as a practice, it reflects the historical and cultural contexts in which it is located. There are differences over time and between countries and, to add to the complexity, there are disputes within the field.

Public health approaches specific to drugs and alcohol have also varied in different places at different times. Prohibition has, at times, been the approach to both alcohol and drugs, yet elsewhere, liberalisation has developed. Rarely has either extreme prohibition or full liberalisation existed: today there is strict prohibition of alcohol in Saudi Arabia and strict prohibition of drugs in Russia but use of both substances is still found in each country. What is more common, when comparing across time and place, is to observe *varieties of control*, with public health restrictions and practices forming one possible component of these regulatory frameworks.

Given all these qualifications, this chapter will attempt to outline and critique the main approaches of public health to drugs and alcohol in contemporary societies, considering theories, practices and policies and comparing across drugs and alcohol. It will attempt to show that there is not one but several versions of a public health approach to drugs and alcohol. Variations have reflected changes in the balance between collectivism and individualism as the traditional, collectivist public health approach altered into the individualism of the 'new public health'. There are now signs of the balance moving back with calls for a '*new*, new public health' to return to its original principles of collective social responsibility, ambitions of social reform and challenge to powerful vested interests – identified as multinational corporations in the cases of alcohol and tobacco and the penal-institutional establishment in the case of illicit drugs and the international 'war on drugs'. Key issues within this are questions around the role of the state (punitive or welfare) and the legitimacy of state intervention, around the roles of expert knowledge, science, technology and professionals and their links to actions geared to social reform as well as ideas of individual and/or social rights and responsibilities.

WHAT IS PUBLIC HEALTH?

The shape of public health research, policy and practice has reflected the wider paradigm of social politics within which it has operated: whether within a night watchman state, welfare state (from liberal to social democratic) or current neo-liberal – and each generates supporters and critics (Hellman et al. 2012). As a discourse and set of practices, it has changed in response to internal changes, such as changes in theories, methodologies and techniques of practice, and to external changes in context, especially through the long waves of change towards industrial-urban societies and post-industrial, globalised consumer capitalism. With regard to psychoactive substances, there have been changes in their real nature and in associated pleasures and problems, and changes in perceptions of problems. Variations occur across societies and over time but there are some common features in a paradigm of public health that has developed primarily via Western scientific discourse and is now dominant at the international level and spreading around the world.

Key concepts

The 'public health community' has changed over time, being originally mainly composed of middle class, white men in suits but now involving a much wider range of people from different backgrounds and interests. Accordingly, the lens of public health has changed over time. In most schools of public health today, a broad definition of public health is found. This is one in which a number of academic disciplines take part, with medical framing as just one segment – which may be more or less dominant depending on country or institution. There are battles within the field of public health – crudely between disease prevention and health promotion perspectives – and, especially regarding research, many of the disciplines do not co-operate very closely but operate in silos: practitioners, however, generally have to work together in teams. This diversity is united by three shared assumptions: that the main field of interest is about populations rather than individuals; that it is about action in a social framework; and that it is concerned with interventions and their effects.

There are a number of key concepts that frame its perspective, including especially *populations, environment* and *prevention*. Many are contained, for example, in this definition of public health as 'the *arts* and *science* which advisors to and agents of the *State* employ in exercising their (public) *authority* to identify and address *threats* that derive from sources in the *environment* for the health of *populations'* (Brown 2010: 156–7; my emphasis).

A fundamental concept is that of the *prevention paradox*. Geoffrey Rose pointed out that 'it is a common irony of preventive medicine that many people must take precautions in order to prevent illness in only a few' (Rose 1992: 12). The prevention paradox is that a preventive measure that brings large benefits to the community offers little to each participating individual (Rose 1981). The underlying concept is of some kind of herd immunity being built up in a population through specific preventive measures. This works for 'communicable diseases' tackled through vaccinations. Does it work also for what are termed 'non-communicable diseases', such as lung cancer, obesity, type 2 diabetes or cirrhosis, which are associated with certain behaviours and styles of life such as smoking, over eating and lack of exercise and heavy drinking? What exactly are the modes of communication that influence behaviours at a population level? The line between communicable and non-communicable diseases is hard to draw and the very terms may be misleading.

Understandings of the 'environment' have changed over time from an original focus on the material environment to environment defined as the social, for example, as 'community', a move that paralleled the phenomenon of de-institutionalisation. In some contexts, public health became defined as community medicine.

Key characteristics of public health

The original medical approach to public health developed around specific diseases, especially occurring in epidemics or concentrations, and built on scientific (objective observational) studies and focused on particular populations in towns or institutions or sub-groups such as mothers, soldiers or the poor. With movements for social reform, some solutions proposed were technical, focusing on the material world, improving housing and workplaces and on ways to alter patterns of transmission, especially through various forms of hygiene – hand washing, sewage disposal, quarantine – or population level treatments such as vaccination programmes. This perspective is still important in public health, especially in low and middle income countries and it is emerging again in Western high income countries as the material and social infrastructures – from sewers to social welfare programmes – built during the nineteenth and twentieth centuries – begin to decay – or are deliberately demolished in the name of slimming the state.

Public health is an applied field. Researchers and practitioners come from various disciplinary backgrounds – for example, medicine, psychology, sociology – and have different specialisms – viruses such as HIV or Ebola, specific groups such as mothers, children or injecting drug users – and they tend to focus variably on high, middle or low income countries. These influences shape them into sub-groups within public health. Currently, in general, in the dominant rational scientific discourse of public health, whatever the problem or the setting, a key orientation is to be 'systematic', applying 'targeted, timely, appropriate and effective interventions' based on scientific evidence.

Public health disciplines may use different sets of research methods. There remains a preference for quantitative analysis of large data-sets using either administrative data or survey responses rather than mixed methods or qualitative approaches, although these can play their part in multi-disciplinary teams and there are strong advocates for the qualitative approach, especially within critical public health (Green and Thorogood 2013). However, ideas of 'robust data' and 'gold standards of evidence' give preference to results from randomised controlled trials (RCTs) following a biomedical model. Within public health, there are critics of this trend, arguing it can be wasteful in encouraging expensive, large-scale studies, which produce only trivial results, delaying action until 'robust' results have been delivered and neglecting the role of argumentation in policy deliberations. All approaches, however, aim ultimately to reduce avoidable mortality and morbidity. Health and wellbeing are measured largely by outcomes relating to mortality and morbidity – assumed to be proxy measures of a good and happy life: this is because these can serve as consistent and relatively reliable indicators at population level over time and cross nationally. Attempts have been made to include reference to the quality of life through the development of QUALYS, which measures quality adjusted life years based on assessments by health economists (Weinstein and Stason 1977).

Because of its involvement in the real world, public health is not just an interesting intellectual exercise but also requires engagement in politics and policy. This has often involved working together in alliances or partnerships. Not all those who argue for a 'public health approach' in policy debates are themselves public health specialists. For many of the groups who grow up around a special interest – such as drugs, alcohol, tobacco or AIDS – calls for a 'public health approach' is a flag of convenience, helping to bring together a motley alliance of people who may not be sure or even agree on what they mean by the term.

Throughout its history, the central issues for public health have been about how a disease is defined, identified and understood and who are involved in making these definitions. Such understandings are not solely a matter of science but also are shaped by social, economic and political considerations. The way an issue is framed has consequences for policy responses, and contests about such framing are constantly going on – sometimes becoming more pronounced but always involving a process of negotiation between different interested parties. These debates occur within public health and between public health and other groups involved in the political process. Experts – public health researchers, professionals and practitioners – are key actors in these negotiations but they work in a landscape crowded with other players – industry, lobbyists, the media, politicians and pressure groups among them. As Elisabeth Pisani put it in her ground-breaking book on the politics of AIDS, 'Science does not exist in a vacuum. It exists in a world of money and votes, a world of media enquiry and lobbyists, of pharmaceutical, manufacturing and environmental activism and religions and political ideologies and all the other complexities of human life' (2008: 5)

Social determinants of health

Other key concepts in the public health approach are those of *upstream* and *downstream* interventions. Public health tends to argue against spending time 'fishing bodies out of the river once they have fallen in'. Most argue the need to look upstream at the factors leading people to fall into the river in the first place and try to prevent this happening. To answer this question, public health talks about *social determinants,* the data referred to usually being statistical correlations. These social determinants (influential factors) may be *immediate, proximal* or *underlying*, acting at different *levels* of influence and carrying various *degrees of power*.

This conception is illustrated in Figure 36.1. However, although social and environmental factors are included in this paradigm, the central focus of attention is still 'the individual', who is made up of a number of social characteristics such as age, gender, class, occupation, place of residence and so on. The aim is to alter the behaviour of this 'individual' through various 'interventions'. A common assumption is that by providing information to rational actors, healthier behaviours should follow. Sociologists criticise this viewpoint and argue that, instead of focusing on the 'individual', the object of study and the focus of interventions should be on 'social practices'. Human beings are not desiccated calculating machines but are human beings living in a social world. Public health should instead pay attention to the 'patterned, routine and habitual ways

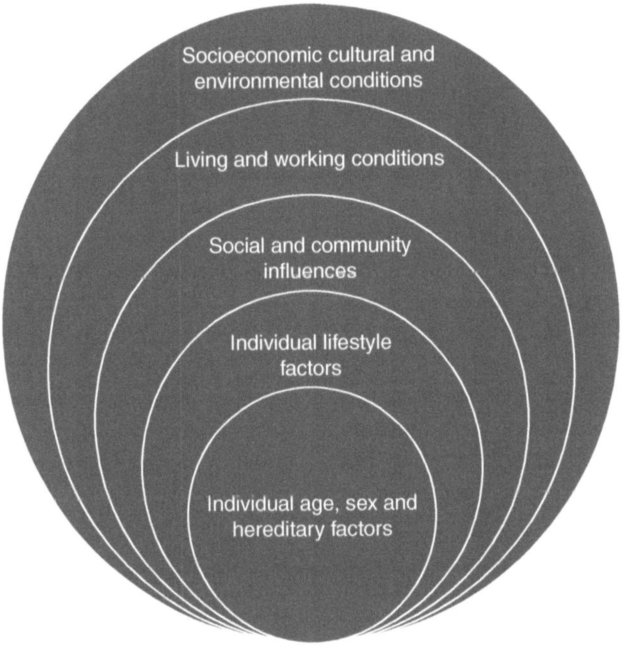

Figure 36.1 Paradigm of social determinants of health status

people live their lives' (Blue et al. 2014). An example of a public health measure aiming to impact on social practices would be the ban on smoking in public places.

The new public health

In the second half of the twentieth century, traditional medicine, centring on the cure of disease, was critically assessed, old administrative and disciplinary barriers were broken, and the active participation of individuals and social groups in improving their health was promoted (Petersen and Lupton, 1996). In turning attention towards the social, economic and physical environment, a new public health sought to avoid the trap of 'blaming the victim' (Ryan, 1976; Ashton and Seymour, 1988).

The essence of this new approach was to stress individual responsibility for health and the internalisation of norms and values conducive to good health among the majority of self-governing citizens: the state's role was to provide information and education for these and reserve more direct interventions for the recalcitrant poor, dangerous and deviant (Rose 1999).

A landmark document published by the then Canadian Minister of Health, Marc Lalonde, in 1974, directed attention to the lifestyle, genetic, and environmental causes of disease, including social factors in health, as well as in medical care itself. This work was a forerunner to the agenda-setting *Ottawa Charter on Health Promotion* (WHO 1986). This conception of public health stressed the value of: a comprehensive approach; coordination of health and social services; community participation and empowerment; cooperation between health and other services; primary care; self-care; monitoring and adoption of scientific knowledge; screening programmes; stimulation of behavioural changes; creation of positive environments; a shared philosophical position; concern with action; advocacy and education; and a focus on vulnerable or at risk groups.

Over time, the community and social aspects of this approach declined and interventions focused increasingly on individual behaviour change, including the roll out of cognitive behavioural therapy delivered by psychologists. The most recent micro-management approach to individual behaviour change is use of contingency management (applied also in some drug and alcohol treatment settings), providing incentives in the form of payments to nudge people towards appropriate behaviour. These techniques, increasingly applied in wider social policy, for example, as conditional cash transfers, have been borrowed from the marketing field and are an example of the libertarian paternalist strategy of health promotion (Thaler and Sunstein 2008).

These approaches have been criticised from within public health itself by those who argue that the focus on individual risk factors has diverted attention from underlying determinants, such as the dominance of the market in healthcare (Stuckler et al. 2010) and this view calls for a *new*, new public health. These critics point out that the public health approach is finding it difficult to manage many of the main conditions now seen as responsible for much ill-health in developed (and increasingly in emerging) economies – especially obesity, alcohol consumption and depression, as well as continuing use of tobacco. To some people, behaviours such as over-eating, heavy drinking and lack of exercise are seen as perverse, self-destructive choices made by irresponsible people who put intolerable costs and pressures on health systems. The fact that many of these seem to be more prevalent in disadvantaged groups is used to justify attitudes of blaming and stigmatising the poor. The alternative view is to see them as victims of environmental pollutants, suffering from 'industrial diseases' (Jahiel and Babor 2007) caused by irresponsible vested interests encouraging hazards such as consumption of processed food and sugary drinks, urban economies based around the car or leisure activities associated with heavy drinking. Such critics argue that the difficulty of getting alternative views across – those which pay attention to social practices and differing power relations – is a reflection of the continuing dominance of the neoliberal paradigm and its notions of individual rights and responsibilities and of individualism and self- management.

Some of these critiques have coalesced under the banner of 'critical public health'. This is an approach that challenges the status quo in public health and questions what have come to be defined as problems: the journal *Critical Public Health* is 'committed to exploring and debating issues of equity, power, social justice and oppression in health' (see also Center for Critical Public Health San Francisco: http://criticalpublichealth.org/about/; accessed 29 December 2014). In general, its adherents hold more respect for sociological and social anthropological approaches to public health and less for medical or scientific disciplines alone. They emphasise the value of qualitative social research methods and place less reliance on solely quantitative methods such as RCTs or surveys. There is also a tendency to side with those blamed for diseases, the cast out and excluded, marginalised and deviant groups. Research and practice here pays more attention to women and minority groups and is generally more understanding of their behaviours.

WHERE DO ALCOHOL AND DRUGS FIT WITHIN PUBLIC HEALTH?

In general, public health has not prioritised drugs and alcohol, leaving these to the field of 'addiction studies'. It has, however, become very concerned about tobacco since the second half of the twentieth century. And with the arrival of HIV and its link to injecting drug use, public health responses grew in importance. Alcohol has recently risen up the agenda as its contribution to the 'global burden of disease' has been calculated (Room et al. 2005; Degenhardt et al. 2008). This is to consider the question in terms of specific public health institutions, policies and practices. However, public health has also played a part in the story of approaches to substance use by providing a lens of ideas and values for various political actors through which they could view drugs and alcohol and justify actions and interventions in the name of the health of society as a whole. As Deborah Stone has explained:

> Problem definition is a process of image-making, where the images have to do fundamentally with attributing cause, blame, and responsibility. Conditions, difficulties, or issues thus do not have inherent properties that make them more or less likely to be seen as problems or to be expanded. Rather, political actors deliberately portray them in ways calculated to gain support for their side... political actors use narrative story lines and symbolic devices to manipulate so-called issue characteristics, all the while making it seem as though they are simply describing facts. (Stone 1989: 282)

So certain concepts have been highlighted in discussions on policies towards drugs and alcohol to support or oppose existing forms of control and these will now be reviewed.

Total consumption theory and total population policies

Total population policies were initially seen as progressive. They focused on the general population in order to avoid the stigmatisation and victimisation of certain categories of drinkers, characteristic of traditional forms of control (Tigerstedt 1999). Segregation within institutions had been a major aspect of general social policy. Similarly, in some countries, asylums were established to which alcoholic and narcotic inebriates could be compulsorily committed. In the United States, institutional approaches to treatment included the famous Lexington centre, first named as the US Narcotic Farm but which changed its name shortly afterwards to the US Public Health Service Hospital. It was in equal parts federal prison, treatment centre, farm and research laboratory. The Farm was shut down 40 years after it opened amid scandal over its drug-testing programme, which involved experiments where inmates were being used as human guinea pigs and rewarded with heroin and cocaine for their efforts (Campbell et al. 2008). Similarly, compulsory institutional care of alcohol abusers was provided in Sweden from 1916. Edman has described how alcohol abusers were eligible for compulsory institutional care only if they *also* displayed one or more of the so-called special indicators: being a danger to other people or themselves (which was understood to mean at risk of suicide rather than cirrhosis of the liver), failing to fulfil their maintenance obligations to their relatives or being an economic burden on their family or society, living a troublesome or wandering life or bringing down a number of drinking arrests on themselves (Edman 2005: 48). The Swedish law led mainly to the compulsory institutional care of socially excluded males.

Social policies of segregation and confinement were challenged by the wave of deinstitutionalisation that occurred after the Second World War. However, observers have noted a parallel rise in the numbers of mentally ill and substance users who were confined in prisons, most notably in the USA. Criminal justice systems, thus, remain important in the control of drug and alcohol users.

As a contrast to segregation and stigmatisation, it was seen as progressive for alcohol controls to be detached from directly governing concrete individuals and replaced by the regulation of abstract risks defined on an aggregate level (Tigerstedt 1999). An influential WHO report, *Alcohol Control Policies in Public Health Perspective* (Bruun et al. 1975), outlined a comprehensive alcohol policy based on governmental measures and primarily directed at controlling the availability of alcohol. The view was that interventions into the consumption level of whole populations is a more efficient way of influencing certain kinds of alcohol-related harm when compared to care of serious individual cases. It was also argued that serious alcoholics are inclined to react to measures directed at the population as a whole, though quite how this process works remains somewhat mysterious. One idea was that, given the social and often reciprocating nature of drinking, lighter and heavier drinkers across the whole population tend to move up and down in concert in terms of changes in levels of alcohol consumption. Rates of alcohol-related problems are said to rise and fall as the population's per capita consumption rises and falls. In this conception, the objectives of public health are to delineate for the drinking population as a whole, the risks of disease and premature death associated with different levels of alcohol consumption and to seek means to minimise the number of drinkers in the hazardous range (Bruun et al. 1975: 29).

So rather than focus on treatment of people labelled alcoholics, the total populations approach argues in favour of tax and price policies, reductions in availability and restrictions on advertising. While some criticise this set of policies as illiberal, initially their aim was to protect individuals (offenders and alcoholics) against arbitrary and unreasonable treatment. At the time, Bruun made this case (1967) in Finland, as many as one-third of all incarcerations were alcohol-related cases.

These policies derive from the total consumption approach that was later further elaborated by Skog (1985). It established a scientific rationale for restrictive 'Nordic' regimes focusing on the general availability of alcoholic beverages and high prices, including the elimination of private profit from parts of the alcohol market and restrictions on the hours of sale and number of sales outlets.

Currently, an influential body of experts criticising relatively liberal policies on alcohol (which focus on providing information and education to encourage individuals to adopt moderate habits) argue instead for what they have labelled a public health approach. They point out that the use of alcohol is associated with some common harms, a mix of acute and chronic health and social problems (Babor et al. 2003; Rehm et al. 2009). These harms are thought to be preventable by introducing population level policies. For example, the AMPHORA manifesto on alcohol states that 'We do not regard that we live in a *reasonable or just* society that allows 1 in 8 of the deaths that occur in our economically productive years (15–64 year olds) to be due to alcohol' and 'We also do not regard that we live in a *fair society*, when the *harm* done by alcohol disproportionally affects *disadvantaged people*' (my emphasis). They cite supporting evidence for the benefit of legally required warning labels on all beverage containers and that alcohol should be less easy to get. Here we see that total population public health approaches refer not only to science and evidence but also to sets of values (Patussi et al 2012).

The coordinated and comprehensive policies suggested by these advocates include education and awareness campaigns, the introduction of warning labels, product disclosure regulations, advertising and sponsorship bans, taxation to raise the price of products, restrictions on consumption in public and work places and cessation support programmes. A current issue is that of the value and acceptability of minimum unit pricing policies for alcohol (Stockwell et al. 2014). Stricter controls and regulations are said to be particularly relevant in those countries, such as in Europe or Australia, where a high proportion of the population are consumers and high proportions drink above recommended levels.

Where relatively small proportions of the total population are consumers, as is the case with some illicit psychoactive drugs, population level policies would logically appear less relevant. However, paradoxically, it is here that strict controls are applied at population level. Policies of prohibition as set out in the international drug control conventions affect whole populations and are justified as a public health measure. The argument of supporters of this regime is that controls on supply of these toxic substances have been effective in preventing widespread use and containing harm. Here the criminal justice system – law and policing and prisons – operates to further public health objectives, it is argued.

The paradigm of drinking patterns or cultures

Stockwell and colleagues questioned the applicability of total population policies in the field of alcohol (Stockwell et al. 1996). The prevention paradox with regard to alcohol use has been said to be that most people who have experienced some adverse consequence relating to their recent drinking typically consume only small or moderate amounts of alcohol *per week*. This argument has been used to justify a shift in prevention efforts away from heavy or excessive drinkers to the more numerous moderate drinkers. Stockwell and colleagues comment that paradoxical findings provide a shaky platform for prevention policies. They do not dispute Kreitman's observation that the largest number of people in the community who experience some form of alcohol-related harm can be found among the majority moderate drinkers (Kreitman 1986). Their criticism is not so much of the fact of this form of prevention paradox but of the feasibility of policies derived from it. They think encouraging everyone to drink less alcohol is hard to defend. They favour devoting more attention to policies designed to limit the violence, accident and injury related to alcohol *intoxication*.

Other critics of the total population approach argue that such 'Nordic' policies may be suitable for their culture but are inappropriate elsewhere and should not be reified at the international level (Beccaria and Sande 2003). They argue that drinking practices are deeply anchored in culture (Rehm et al. 1996). Changes in alcohol policy will not substitute new drinking patterns – as seen in the notorious failed attempt in England to introduce a style of 'continental European' drinking through a liberalisation of licensing regimes (Nicholls 2009). The view here is that there are only limited possibilities for alcohol policy to influence drinking practices. A similar argument can be made regarding drugs policies (Reinarman et al. 2004; Home Office 2014).

The paradigm of drinking patterns specifies a relationship between particular ways of drinking and particular forms of alcohol-related harm and considers the implications of these relationships for policy options and strategies. In terms of regulation, it involves a shift in the main focus of policy from aggregate levels of consumption to *harm and high-risk* drinking in communities. It stresses the need to distinguish between low risk, hazardous and harmful consumption whenever possible with the firm intention to advance and improve harm reduction strategies (Stockwell et al. 1997: 3).

Harm reduction

A particular understanding of a public health approach, which grew out of the focus on risks, equates it with harm reduction. This movement developed alongside the HIV/AIDS epidemic from the 1980s onwards, drawing on the perception that AIDS presents more of a threat to society than drug use itself. *Harmful use* of drugs should be the object of concern not *use per se* and the main harms to be avoided are the risk of communicable disease transmission. Strategies focus on high-risk subsets of the population.

Harm reduction approaches challenge strict control policies, arguing that in order to attract users to services, deliberate attempts have to be made to overcome stigmatisation and exclusion. Harm reduction interventions regarding drugs and alcohol may involve any of a multitude of activities such as: immunisation against hepatitis; NSPs; activities to prevent drinking or drug taking while driving; or use of plastic rather than glass containers. One aim is to provide a safe environment in which to drink or take drugs, reducing the harm to self or others. The focus may also be on the substance, involving, for example, labelling or testing. It may be on the method of consumption (as with e-cigarettes; encouraging oral rather than injecting opioid use; provision of clean needles; or encouraging combining drinking with eating and sitting rather than standing). Those involved in delivering interventions need not be public health professionals themselves but more immediate contacts in the relevant setting, as where naloxone is made available to police, transport workers, family and friends or where bar staff are trained to protect drinkers from intoxication.

Tim Rhodes has refined the analysis of the *environment* by distinguishing between micro and macro level features and physical, social, economic and policy environments (Rhodes 2002). This has practical applications, for example, epidemiological evidence associates elevated blood-borne viral risk with injecting in 'public' and 'semi-public' environments. This leads to awareness of the need for 'safer injecting environment interventions' (Rhodes et al. 2006), such as drug consumption rooms. This contribution also stresses the value of mixed methods, especially including a strong role for qualitative research. In the case of problems linked to homelessness and public injecting, for example, ethnographic research can help to illuminate the 'social relations' of how drug users and risk practices interact with injecting environments. Observation of specific settings and the behaviour of small groups helps to improve effectiveness and prevents prior assumptions and moral judgements influencing the design of programmes. Similar arguments have been made for wet rooms for homeless street drinkers (Archard 1979).

The step-by-step approach of public health practice is also used in developing interventions relevant to local conditions, for example regarding the location of off licences. A more radical approach involving community action (e.g. Holder 2000) proposes a systems approach to the reduction of alcohol problems by changing the community structures that provide the context in which alcohol consumption occurs.

Some look at harm reduction as a distinct approach rather than a sub-set of public health. Gerry Stimson, considering the issue through the case of e-cigarettes, defines the harm reduction approach as one focused on producing a safer product rather than banning it outright (Stimson et al. 2014). The harm reduction approach encourages users to switch their pattern of use – to safer substances, to use safer ways of consuming or use in safer settings. The focus is not on eradicating *use* but on eradicating *harm*. This approach is generally more liberal, both socially liberal and also economically liberal, accepting the role of the market in supply and being sceptical about claims for benign intervention by the state or doctors. There tends to be a greater acceptance of the role of the suppliers – the industry – in the harm reduction approach, whereas more fundamentalist tobacco and alcohol campaigners are hostile to the companies involved in producing and distributing the product (Editorial 2013; McCambridge et al. 2013).

The example of e-cigarettes highlights the contemporary influence of debates on tobacco in public health in general with implications for controversies regarding drugs and alcohol.

Tobacco control

The tobacco control narrative is extremely influential within international public health today (WHO 2013). This narrative sees all tobacco use as bad or risky and argues for an end to the tobacco industry. Banning involvement of the tobacco industry in the policy arena is emphasised and ethical policies restrict some organisations from investing in them (e.g. the Wellcome Trust). All these principles are taken up by some alcohol campaigners today (McCambridge et al. 2014). The success of the notion of harm to others from passive smoking has encouraged attention to the harms caused to others through use/misuse of alcohol with attention to foetal alcohol syndrome, spikes in domestic violence after football matches, road traffic accidents, costs to public services such as in accident and emergency departments and in policing.

The FCTC is seen as the first global health treaty (WHO 2003) (although supporters of the UN Conventions on drugs claim that the underlying goal of these is the protection of health). Portrayed as a model public health approach, its key elements are use of controls on price and taxes to deter consumption; introduction of smoke free areas at work and in public places; restrictions on packaging and labelling to limit positive associations; and restrictions on advertising.

In this international campaign, the goal of a 'tobacco free world' has been identified, reminiscent of the aim of a 'drug free world' promoted at the 1998 UN General Assembly. The problem with such ambitions is that, even if they were socially desirable (and those who enjoy use of nicotine, alcohol or some drugs would dispute this), they may be neither technically feasible nor politically practicable. With regard to policy, the main issue is whether to focus on the demand or supply side. Implementing population level regulations is easier to theorise than implement. Suppliers can be agile in outmanoeuvring controls, as where illicit alcohol is produced and sold locally or smuggled into the country or where a smart tweaking of the chemistry can produce new synthetic drugs. Public health bureaucracies can be slow and cumbersome and their heavy-footed approach beaten by more entrepreneurial smart suppliers. Especially in contemporary globalised societies, controls at national level are less effective because of the increase in online shopping, in conjunction with the rise of underground markets, inadequate inspections, appearance of alternative products and new social media – all these act to counteract controls on advertising, price, labelling and access (Nicholls 2012; McCreanor et al. 2013).

Some have argued that the FCTC should be used as a model for international controls on alcohol (Room et al. 2005). Some drug reformers also see this as a desirable mode of regulation to replace the current 'War on Drugs' approach, critics of which note a range of unintended consequences: displacement from one substance to another; increased involvement of organised crime; geographical displacement of production or markets; violence as competition for control erupts when stable supply chains are disrupted; ecological damage; diversion of resources from health to enforcement; and stigma and marginalisation of users (Rolles et al. 2012).

Critics of the public health approach as it has developed in the case of tobacco, and calls for its extension to alcohol, see it as imbalanced, as inflating the problem and exaggerating the impact of use of tobacco or alcohol on others. For example, the common references to 'binge drinking' in public debate are producing an exaggerated and unbalanced image of the problem, focusing on out of control use by young women and disturbances in city centres and accident and emergency departments, while the real problem and costs to health services come from long-term, quiet tippling at home. Others have warned tobacco campaigners against making the mistakes of the war on drugs (Reuter 2013).

The criticism here is of certain public health activists and the argument is for a more refined and careful analysis and use of qualitative as well as quantitative material. But it could also be seen as an argument for distancing from public life and encouragement to remain within the quiet sophisticated world of experts who view evidence more dispassionately. This would be to challenge the essence of public health, as one of its core characteristics is its active involvement in public life and willingness to challenge power detrimental to the public good wherever it is found. Public health scientists and social scientists have a right (and some say duty) to be stakeholders – along with others, that is, not to be the sole authority but to play a part and engage in discussions.

Such debates about the 'right' public health approach open up the question: what is the 'public' that is being protected from disease and whose wellbeing is being promoted even at the cost of some liberties? And in our increasingly complex and diverse societies – and in a borderless world – is this focus on the public and on defined populations at all feasible? It was such observations that led to the rise of the new public health, which gave a greater role to individuals and self-discipline through following guidance, advice and information rather than leaving it to experts and leaders to decide and enforce what is best for each citizen.

The larger question is about how much state intervention is acceptable. Critics argue that psychoactive substances are not at all in the same category of threat as Ebola or polio. Indeed, they have their place and use in society, for example, use of heroin and morphine for pain relief and the use of alcohol or drugs for pleasure or in rituals (Measham 2004).

CONCLUSION

The public health approach can thus be seen to rest on some shared goals and is identified by its core concepts and key characteristics. There are, however, competing priorities within public health. Change has developed over time as one view has contested another, with challengers to orthodoxies often claiming to be more 'progressive'. Mainstream public health has had many other priorities than drugs, alcohol and tobacco but the importance of these has risen up the agenda as their contribution to ill health has been recognised. There are differences in approaches to drugs and alcohol reflecting their different legal statuses in different societies but the tobacco narrative has become increasingly influential overall at the international level. An interesting contrast currently is that where drug reformers want a move to a more liberal approach, advocates for alcohol and tobacco reform often argue for stricter controls. The issue is where – along a continuum from liberal to prohibitive – appropriate and legitimate frameworks of control would sit. Some have discerned a possible move to a shared common regulatory framework sitting somewhere in the middle.

Underlying these debates are issues surrounding the role of the state, respect for science and the authority of professionals. While all claim to be 'evidence based' most of those involved in these controversies can be seen to be influenced also by their core values regarding especially individualism versus collectivism and freedom versus solidarity. Free market, right-wing think tanks support the libertarian views and criticise the total consumption model that tends to favour restrictions on consumption of alcohol or illicit drugs across the board. They stress that per capita alcohol consumption is very much dependent on the amount of *heavy drinking* in a population (noting that in Britain currently, for example, about 45 per cent of alcohol is drunk by about 10 per cent of the population). Total consumption policies place the burden of costs on moderate drinkers while being ignored by at risk drinkers, it is argued (Duffy and Snowden 2014). Instead, alcohol policy should target excessive drinkers, alcoholics and those who require help rather than the total population. Such ideas are strongly opposed by social groups driven by different values, such as those based on religious beliefs or other moral certainties. Muslims oppose alcohol use. Prohibition of use of heroin or cocaine is strongly supported by the Russian and Chinese governments. Supporters of prohibition of either alcohol or opium see certain substances as uniquely toxic and addictive, destroying lives and undermining families and communities. With the decline of socialist ideas in recent decades, economic liberalism has come to dominate the policy agenda internationally and within many countries. Critics of this tendency argue that now a rebalancing is needed: 'we also need more assertive promotion of the idea that protecting and promoting population health and the interests of society are core duties of government, if effective alcohol policies are to be introduced' (McCambridge et al. 2013: 203).

Some see these as self-indulgent debates within rich countries, ignoring the growing problems relating to drug and alcohol use in developing countries. Singer has described the contribution that the legal and illegal drug trade makes to a set of barriers to development, including: interpersonal crime and community violence; the corruption of public servants and the disintegration of social institutions; the emergence of new or enhanced health problems; the lowering of worker productivity; the ensnarement of youth in drug distribution and away from productive education or employment; and the skewing of economies to drug production and money laundering (Singer 2008). He says:

> It can reasonably be argued that legal drugs like tobacco and alcohol (which, as noted, is not legal in all development contexts) have at least as great if not a considerably greater impact on development internationally than do illegal drugs and that development policy would benefit from a focus on what might be called 'nico-ethanol-terrorism' (e.g. corporate promotion of nicotine and ethanol addiction and disease). Both legal and illegal drugs contribute to the maintenance of social inequality internationally because of their effect in hindering development. (Singer 2008: 476)

Support for such arguments is found in examples from Mexico and West Africa and is encouraging a revival of a broad social reform movement internationally. 'All of these issues are of concern to a growing body of increasingly linked grassroots non-government organizations' (Singer 2008: 476).

Controversy and dispute have marked the history of public health and of policy debates on drugs and alcohol, testifying to the relevance and importance of the issues of drugs and alcohol within public health and more widely in national and international politics and society.

REFERENCES

Anderson P, Braddick F, Reynolds J and Gual A (eds) (2012) *Alcohol Policy in Europe: Evidence from AMPHORA*. The AMPHORA Project. Available from: http://amphoraproject.net/view.php?id_cont=45. [accessed 08/04/2016]

Archard P (1979) *Vagrancy, Alcoholism and Social Control*. London: Macmillan.

Ashton J and Seymour H (1988) *The New Public Health*. Milton Keynes: Open University Press.

Babor T et al. (2003). *Alcohol: No Ordinary Commodity – Research and Public Policy*. Oxford: Oxford University Press.

Beccaria F and Sande A (2003) 'Drinking games and rite of life projects', *Young: Nordic Journal of Youth Research* 11: 99–119.

Blue S and Shore E with Carmona C and Kelly M (2014) *Smoking, Drinking and Eating: Public Health Should Not Be All About The Individual*. Available from: theconversation.com (Accessed 25 November 2014).

Brown L D (2010) 'The political face of public health', *Public Health Reviews* 32(1): 155–73.

Bruun K, Edwards G, Lumio M, Mäkelä K, Pan L, Popham R F, Room R, Schmidt W, Skog O J, Sulkunen P and Österberg E (1975) *Alcohol Control Policies in Public Health Perspective*. Helsinki: Finnish Foundation for Alcohol Studies.

Campbell, N D, Olsen, J P and Walden L (2008) *The Narcotic Farm: The Rise and Fall of America's First Prison for Drug Addicts*. New York: Harry N. Abrams, Inc.

Degenhardt L et al. (2008) 'Toward a global view of alcohol, tobacco, cannabis and cocaine use: findings from the WHO World Mental Health Surveys', *PLOS Medicine* 5(7): 1053–66.

Duffy J C and Snowden C (2014) *Punishing the Majority: The Problems with Alcohol Policy in the UK*. London: Institute of Economic Affairs.

Editorial (2013) 'Who is responsible for the public's health? The role of the alcohol industry in the WHO global strategy to reduce the harmful use of alcohol', *Addiction* 108: 2045–7.

Edman J (2005) 'Treatment of what? Class, gender and work ethics within the compulsory institutional care of alcohol abusers in Sweden during the 20th century', *Nordik Alkohil and Narkotikatidskrift* 22: 45–61.

Green J and Thorogood N (2013) *Qualitative Methods for Health Research*. London: Sage.

Guardian (2014) http://www.theguardian.com/society/2014/dec/25/protect-children-stop-alcohol-sponsorship

Hellman M, Roos G and von Wright J (2012) *A Welfare Policy Patchwork: Negotiating the Public Good in Times of Transition*. Helsinki: Nordic Centre for Welfare and Social Issues.

Holder H D (2000) 'Community prevention of alcohol problems', *Addictive Behaviors* 25(6): 843–59.

Home Office (2014) *Drugs: International Comparators*. London: Home Office.

Jahiel R I and Babor T (2007) 'Industrial epidemics, public health advocacy and the alcohol industry: lessons from other Fields', *Addiction* 102(9): 1335–9.

Kreitman N (1986) 'Alcohol consumption and the prevention paradox', *British Journal of Addiction* 81: 353–64.

Lalonde M (1974) *A New Perspective on the Health of Canadians: A Working Document*. Ottawa: Government of Canada. Available from: http://www.phac-aspc.gc.ca/ph-sp/pdf/perspect-eng.pdf (Accessed 3 April 2016).

McCambridge J, Hawkins B and Holden C (2013) 'Vested interests in addiction research and policy. The challenge corporate lobbying poses to reducing society's alcohol problems: insights from UK evidence on minimum unit pricing' *Addiction* 109: 199–205.

McCambridge J, Kypri K, Drummond C and Strang J (2014) 'Alcohol harm reduction: corporate capture of a key concept', *PLoS Med* 11(12): e1001767.

McCreanor T, Lyons A, Griffin C, Goodwin I, Moewaka Barnes H and Hutton F (2013) 'Youth drinking cultures, social networking and alcohol marketing: implications for public health', *Critical Public Health* 23(1): 110–20.

Measham F. (2004). 'The decline of ecstasy, the rise of "binge" drinking and the persistence of pleasure', *Probation Journal* 5(4): 309–26.

Nicholls J (2009) *The Politics of Alcohol*. Manchester: Manchester University Press.

Nicholls J (2012). 'Everyday, everywhere: alcohol marketing and social media – current trends', *Alcohol and Alcoholism* 47(4): 486–93.

Patussi V, Scafato E, Alunni F, Di Rosa G, Fanucchi T, Gandin C, Londi I, Magri G, Paganelli J. Alcol: manifesto europeo AMPHORA. (In English: Alcohol: The AMPHORA European manifesto) Alcologia. 2012 Nov; 15:8-10. [accessed 08/04/2016]

Petersen A and Lupton D (1996) *The New Public Health: Health and Self in the Age of Risk*. London: Sage.

Pisani E (2008) *The Wisdom of Whores: Bureaucrats, Brothels and the Business of AIDS*. London: Granta Books.

Rehm J, Ashley M J, Room R, Single E, Bondy S, Ferrence R and Giesbrecht N (1996): 'On the emerging paradigm of drinking patterns and their social and health consequences', *Addiction* 91(11): 1615–21.

Rehm J, Mathers C, Popova S et al. (2009) 'Global burden of disease and injury and economic cost attributable to alcohol use and alcohol use disorders', *The Lancet* 373: 2223–33.

Reinarman C, Cohen P D A and Kaal H L (2004) 'The limited relevance of drug policy: cannabis in Amsterdam and in San Francisco', *American Journal of Public Health* 94(5): 836–42.

Reuter P (2013) 'Can tobacco control endgame analysis learn anything from US experience with illegal drugs?', *BMJ Open access* 22: i49–51.

Rhodes T (2002) 'The "risk environment": a framework for understanding and reducing drug related harm', *International Journal of Drug Policy* 13(2): 85–94.

Rhodes T, Kimber J, Small W, Fitzgerald J, Kerr T, Hickman M and Holloway G (2006) 'Public injecting and the need for "safer environment interventions" in the reduction of drug-related harm', *Addiction* 101: 1384–93.

Rolles S, Murkin G, Powell M, Kushlick D and Slater J (2012) *The Alternative World Drug Report: Counting the Costs of the War on Drugs*. Bristol: Transform Drug Policy Foundation.

Room R, Babor T and Rehm J (2005) 'Alcohol and public health', *The Lancet* 365: 519–30.

Rose G (1981) 'Strategy of prevention: lessons from cardiovascular disease', *BMJ* 282: 1847–51.

Rose G (1992) *The Strategy of Preventive Medicine*. Oxford: Oxford Medical Publications, Oxford University Press.

Rose N (1999) *Powers of Freedom*. Cambridge: Cambridge University Press.

Ryan W (1976) *Blaming the Victim*. London: Random House.

Skog O J (1985) 'The collectivity of drinking cultures: a theory of the distribution of alcohol consumption', *British Journal of Addiction* 80(1): 83–99.

Singer M (2008) 'Drugs and development: the global impact of drug use and trafficking on social and economic development', *International Journal of Drug Policy* 19: 467–78.

Stimson G, Thom B and Costall P (2014) 'Disruptive innovations: the rise of the electronic cigarette', *International Journal of Drug Policy* 25: 653–5.

Stockwell T, Hawks D, Lang E and Rydon P (1996) 'Unravelling the preventive paradox for acute alcohol problems', *Drug and Alcohol Review* 15(1): 7–15.

Stockwell, T, et al. (1997) 'Opinion piece: sharpening the focus of alcohol policy from aggregate consumption to harm and risk reduction', *Addiction Research and Theory* 5(1): 1–9.

Stockwell T, Auld M C, Zhao J and Martin G (2014) 'Does minimum pricing reduce alcohol consumption? The experience of a Canadian province', *Health Promotion Practice* 15(1): 100–8.

Stone D (1989). 'Causal stories and the formation of policy agendas', *Political Science Quarterly* 104(2): 281–300.

Stuckler D, Basu S and McKee M (2010) 'Public health in Europe: power, politics, and where next?', *Public Health Reviews* 32(1): 213–42.

Thaler R H and Sunstein C R (2008) *Nudge: Improving Decisions About Health, Wealth and Happiness*. New Haven: Yale University Press.

Tigerstedt C (1999) 'Alcohol policy, public health and Kettil Bruun', *Contemporary Drug Problems* 26(2): 209–35.

Weinstein M and Stason W (1977) 'Foundations of cost effectiveness analysis for health and medical practices', *New England Journal of Medicine* 296(13): 716–21.

World Health Organization (WHO) (1986) *Ottawa Charter for Health Promotion*. Geneva: WHO. Available from: http://www.who.int/healthpromotion/conferences/previous/ottawa/en/.[accessed 08/04/2016]

World Health Organization (WHO) (2003) *WHO Framework Convention on Tobacco Control*. Geneva: WHO. Available from: http://whqlibdoc.who.int/publications/2003/9241591013.pdf. [accessed 08/04/2016]

World Health Organization (WHO) (2013) *WHO Report on the Global Tobacco Epidemic: Enforcing Bans on Tobacco Advertising, Promotion and Sponsorship*. Geneva: WHO.

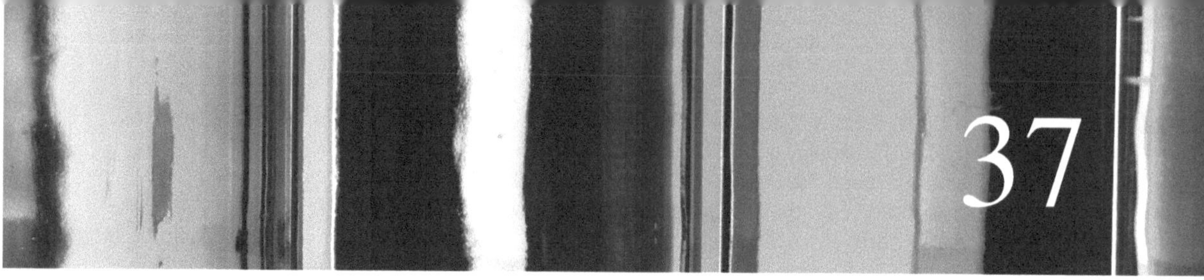

37

Illegal Street Economies and Drugs: Getting Involved, Skilled and Trying to Quit

Philip Lalander

INTRODUCTION

In the influential article 'Taking Care of Business' (1969), Preble and Casey describe the sophisticated division of labour used by American drug dealers in order to minimize detection. Individuals are needed to import, distribute, dilute and portion the product, just as they are needed to sell to resellers, sell on the street, provide connections to dealers for compensation, take care of quality control or look out for the police. In today's urban environments, these roles are still being performed (Parker et al., 1988; Neale, 2002). Looking more specifically at the sale of drugs, one can also see how it is characterized by diversification with different actors working at different levels. For example, Pearson and Hobbs (2001) who have investigated the British drug market, identify a general division into four levels. These are importation (assuming production takes place overseas), wholesale distribution, the middle market and retail-level dealing. There is a considerable distance between the dealer on the street and the person organizing the smuggling of hundreds of kilos. Often a street dealer knows only the person at the next level while other actors remain unknown.

This chapter focuses primarily on those actors who operate on what can be referred to as a street- or retail-level. Thus, it focuses on dealers and drug-users who operate on the lowest level, on the street and at private residences. These individuals receive, distribute and use the drugs that people higher up in the hierarchy administer and deliver. As street level actors, they are resellers and sometimes users of drugs, engaged in selling in order to finance their personal use (Murphy et al., 1990; Bretteville-Jensen, 2002; Lalander, 2003).

A process perspective is applied and addressed through subtitles such as 'learning the game', 'being in the game' and 'leaving the game'. As the aim is to approach drug related economies from an actor's perspective, the chapter is based primarily on ethnographic studies (see, for example, Adler, 1985; Bourgois, 1995/2003; Maher, 1997; Jacobs, 1999; Lalander, 2003, 2008, 2009; Svensson, 2007). In such studies, researchers attempt to understand ideas and actions among participants in local drug economies by spending extended periods of time with them.

The arguments presented in the chapter are strongly influenced by the symbolic interactionist assumption that people 'act towards things on the basis of the meanings that things have for them' (Blumer, 1969: 2). By using this perspective, actions that often are considered insane, unsafe or evil can come to be seen as relatively reasonable from the actors' perspectives, their life situations and life histories. The ambition is to present the reader with perspectives and concepts from research that provide a comprehensive understanding for outsiders of the hidden worlds that illegal street economies represent. However, the chapter does not just focus on perspectives from symbolic interactionism. The studies mentioned above (see e.g. Adler, 1985; Bourgois, 1995/2003; Maher, 1997; Jacobs, 1999; Lalander, 2003, 2008, 2009; Svensson, 2007) also include aspects of class, gender and ethnicity/race, as these are important dimensions of illegal street economies. Therefore, the last sections of the chapter explicitly discuss these structuring aspects that have an obvious impact on the lives of the actors in the illicit economy.

LEARNING THE GAME

The drug market is informally organized with secret purchasing and sales channels. All handling of illicit drugs is done discreetly, as penalties for drug dealing are severe everywhere. These severe penalties for drug crimes lead to strategies and norms within the illicit networks in order to minimize the risk of detection. Strategies can, for example, relate to how drugs are delivered and how to communicate with each other with little risk of detection. These safety measures are important components in maintaining the networks. They are taught to novices and contribute to creating a sense of exclusivity and belonging.

Getting involved in illegal street economies implies a procedure of learning together with other actors (Murphy et al., 1990). In Bourdieu's terms, this learning is incorporated in *habitus*, an ordering structure through which an individual interprets and experiences the world. This term has been used by several researchers studying illicit drug economies from an actor's perspective, such as Fleetwood's (2014) study of women in the international cocaine trade, Lalander's (2003, 2008) study of young heroin dealers and addicts in a Swedish town, Sandberg and Pedersen's (2006, 2009) study of hash dealers of immigrant background in Oslo, Norway, and Lisa Maher's study (1997) on female participation in the crack market in New York City. The term addresses the ways people's economic and social positions leave traces in their behaviour and affects the ways they perceive themselves and their possibilities to act in various situations.

Crossley (2001) stresses that our life experiences are incorporated into our everyday being and are expressed in daily routines and that they, therefore, cannot be seen as cognitive surface awareness that can be quickly unlearned. The actions of individuals are intimately connected to their habitus. Through habitus, we can act smoothly in environments to which a certain habitus is adapted, but this is difficult in environments that require other knowledge and actions than what an acquired habitus entails. Experienced wine tasters feel at home in a wine tasting room while they might feel alienated in a mechanical workshop. An experienced drug dealer can quickly read a situation on the street while having difficulty interpreting situations in other social contexts to which she or he is not accustomed. This feel for the game makes up what Anderson (1990) calls 'being streetwise', but with a Bourdieu-inspired term from Sandberg and Pedersen (2006, 2009) and Lalander (2008), we can talk about *street capital*. This term entails a person's ability to master situations that can arise on the streets coupled with the reputation gained by street actors. For example, individuals might increase their street capital by showing an ability to handle a police interrogation without snitching or needlessly talking about things. Street capital can also be gained by the successful use of violence or by belonging to the 'proper' social networks.

What, then, might the road into the illicit street economy look like? Even though there are many routes into an existence in which the sale and use of illicit drugs are central, it is possible to distinguish a 'typical path'. The typical path is an expression of the way involvement in illicit economies can provide a course of action through which individuals can obtain respect in life situations that are otherwise dismal and hopeless (cf. Sutherland, 1947: Grapendaal et al., 1995; Bourgois, 1995/2003; Jacobs, 1999). This path can be illustrated by Hugo, one of the participants in my own study (Lalander, 2008, 2009) of young men of Latin American backgrounds who became involved in selling heroin in a Swedish town. Hugo became involved in the illicit economy as a child. He grew up in a marginalized and stigmatized section of a Swedish town. Hugo tells of scoring a batch of hash and taking it to the older people that he admired:

> 'You want some smoke, guys?' I said and tossed up smoke, and they were like 'What the fuck?!' [*surprised and high pitched voice*]. 'This fucking kid!' [*still a surprised voice, followed by laughter*] you know, and we smoked and that's how I got in. Then they started to notice [*snaps his fingers, goes quiet*]. I got into fights, and all that and the police got me and I remained silent and stuff like that. It was like 'That fucking kid, we can trust him'. They noticed that they could trust me. I kept quiet about stuff, I did, and then I was there with them, everywhere, and it was then that they started taking care of me and calling me Pequeño [*Spanish for 'the little guy'*]. Not a fuck would touch me, you know. I was the baby that everyone took care of. They all looked after me. (Lalander, 2009: 78, author's translation)

In this quote, it is evident that Hugo comes to be trusted and respected when he first brings the hash and then remains silent when caught by the police. When he tells this story, he does so in a proud tone of voice, as if he was relating the early steps in a career, which later, at only 14 years of age, would have him assisting a major dealer in selling heroin. Early on, others with more experience could tell that he was a potential prospect, a guy who signalled that he did not belong to the crowd of more well-behaved and law-abiding pupils. He describes that when he was given the task of selling heroin it made him feel as if he had been offered a job and given the honour to work with a major dealer. He recalls that he was also easily impressed with this dealer, a man around 45 years old, who was also a master at telling exciting stories in addition to organizing heroin sales. For Hugo, dealing drugs was also, in part, a matter of being seen by others as a competent actor. He was happy neither at home nor school. He often cut classes to hang out with other kids and young adults in those spaces and street corners that were central meeting points for marginalized youth in the area. He was drawn to environments where he felt pride and made social connections with people already there. In the same fashion, he would avoid people and environments that made him feel ashamed (see also Scheff, 1994).

Gradually, Hugo becomes a drug dealer in the sense that the skills and strategies that are valued within the illicit economy become incorporated into his habitus, through which he deciphers and experiences the world. To live in the world of an illicit economy becomes as natural to him as going to work is for other people. He learns the safety precautions, such as reading various signs in the environment indicating that the police are doing surveillance, almost like a mechanic who learns to read the sounds of the engine to diagnose a problem. Incorporation of skills is a question of specialization, of learning from encounters with others who possess the right cultural competence and of handling the risks that can arise from various situations in the environment (see also Murphy et al., 1990).

Thus, as also indicated by Sutherland (1947), Becker (1953), Jacobs (1999) and Fleetwood (2014), becoming skilled is a matter of a gradual involvement, or what Murphy et al. (1990) call 'drifting into dealing', that occurs in a social context and through encounters with other actors. These actors are often individuals who the person is close to, looks up to and trusts, such as friends, partners, relatives or individuals from the same ethnic network (see also Lalander, 2003; Fleetwood, 2014). To get into the illicit networks, no school transcripts or proof of previous employment are needed. All that is necessary is an engagement with, and an ability to live by, the rules that govern the illicit economy. Often the street dealer position is an extension and professionalization of a former role as provider of drugs to friends (Murphy et al., 1990; Taylor and Potter, 2013).

For many who act within illicit drug environments, this gradual involvement also entails what Adler (1985) describes in *Wheeling and Dealing*, an ethnographic study of major cocaine dealers as a separation process. She writes, '[j]oining these social networks required a commitment to the drug world's norms, values and lifestyle, and limited the degree of involvement individuals subsequently had with nondeviant groups' (1985: 122). In the study, *Hooked on Heroin* (2003), Lalander calls this a gradual process of separation in which individuals are socialized into the game and the rules that the game provides. Friends with other interests and a more law-abiding habitus are no longer seen as interesting and are perceived as a risk for detection. In such a way, the socialization taking place in the networks becomes manifested and crystallized.

The illicit networks can be seen as social arenas for learning what differs from what characterizes regular school, for example, theoretical, teacher-led lessons and pre-made rigid schedules. The socialization that takes place on the street is characterized by unpredictability and personal involvement in what is about to happen. The education is administered by more experienced peers, who function as mentors (Murphy et al.,1990; Lalander, 2003).

By committing crimes together, there is a heightened sense of clandestine community and social ties are strengthened (Scheff, 1994; Lalander, 2003). Such actions 'on the edge', give rise to stronger emotional sensations than do more mundane actions, such as eating lunch or riding the bus. Adler (1985) points to something similar when she uses expressions such as 'the fast life', 'hedonism', 'euphoria' and 'living in the present, not worrying about the future'. To be involved in illicit drug economies can be seen in contrast to living like 'the middle class'. 'Drug dealers lived for the present, surrounding themselves with the maximum pleasure they could grab. They did not, as the middle-class ethos suggested, live in reduced comfort so that they could enjoy the fruits of their labour at a later date' (Adler, 1985: 85). Thus, to live in a now-oriented existence, without bureaucratic rules and schedules, outside the institutions of modern society, is an attraction for those who enter these informal and secret systems. Nevertheless, an existence that may feel rewarding and pleasurable can gradually develop into something else, into a struggle for survival, into frustration, suffering, prison life and death (Neale, 2002).

BEING IN THE GAME

Being situated in an environment, in which money circulates quickly and illegally, in addition to handling money and a steady supply of drugs that can generate addiction, involve considerable risk (Svensson, 2007; Moloney et al., 2015). If individuals start using the substances personally and to a large extent, there is a risk that they become less competent and cautious as dealers. Their personal consumption may also increase to the point where the entire profit is needed to finance the personal use. Some may end up owing money to other actors, which can also lead to acquiring a bad reputation (Waldorf, 1993). It is also possible that conspicuous consumption, such as buying various luxury items, attracts the attention of the police, especially if the person lacks the legal income that could make such purchases possible (Lalander, 2003; Moloney et al., 2015).

Drug dealers need to have some personal authority in order to handle price negotiations and setting boundaries with customers. As there is often a considerable risk of being robbed by other actors in the business, some means to gain power needs to be available, either in the form of weapons or physical power (one's own or that of an accomplice) (Jacobs, 2000; Topalli et al., 2002). Besides this, using Goffman's words, there is a need for a strong character, which involves high degrees of self-control.

> These capacities (or lack of them) for standing correct and steady in the face of sudden pressure are crucial (…) I will refer to these maintenance properties as an aspect of the individual's character. Evidence of incapacity to behave effectively and correctly under the stress of fatefulness is a sign of *weak* character (…) Evidence of marked capacity to maintain full self-control (…) is a sign of strong character. (Goffman, 1967: 217)

In relation to local drug economies, having a strong character can entail the ability to limit one's own drug use, resist customers' pleas for discounts or gifts and remain composed in situations involving violence or threat of violence. It also entails the ability to remain silent during police interrogations, even if suffering from withdrawal or being placed in isolation for long periods of time (Lalander 2003, Svensson 2007). Showing strong character and an ability to act properly in a variety of situations contribute to increased street capital.

Possessing this character is especially important when illegality means that participants do not enjoy the same protection against various threats as do others from, for instance, official societal institutions, such as the police and the judicial system (Topalli et al., 2002; Rosenfeld et al., 2003). To a greater degree than in other societal contexts, participants in the illegal economies have to trust their personal abilities or place their trust in the social networks to which they belong. If they have a debt to collect, they cannot take advantage of the usual regulated societal institutions such as courts, credit counsellors, collection agencies or banks (Taylor, 1993). Instead, in line with the code of the street, they have to collect their money, either by negotiations or by threatening or using violence (Brookman et al., 2011).

In such an informal economy, the individual's personal *reputation* is an important resource (Brookman et al., 2011). It determines whether the buyer can be trusted with a credit or whether the seller's wares can be assumed to be of good quality. Reputation also determines personal reliability – is it even possible to get involved in illicit dealings with this person? Finally, reputation encompasses an assessment of the person's power or authority. Is the person capable of collecting a debt? Can he or she defend possessions? (Svensson, 2007). To act forcefully and with strong character – with or without the use of violence – in the face of disrespectful encounters is, therefore, an important part of the display of mastery of prevailing codes. Mastering the codes is necessary to demanding respect (Bourgois, 1995/2003; Brookman et al., 2011).

Many street dealers develop a competent personal performance, an embodied competence for acting smoothly in various situations that might occur in the illicit drug economy, parallel to learning what Bourdieu (1990) calls *a feel for the game*. This competence makes up a part of what was earlier called habitus. A correct habitus means that an individual can quickly interpret situations and also see what potential courses of action are appropriate. Experienced drug dealers will be able to read a drug dealing situation in a different way than the average person would. They can perceive those *signs of alarm* (Goffman, 1967) that may indicate, for instance, that the police are in pursuit. This competence is not an innate or natural quality, but a consequence of learning together with others.

One aspect of having practical skills and a feel for the game, at least if a person is to be successful in the street economy, is the ability to self-present as tough or cool in various encounters. Strongly inspired by Goffman, Katz argues that toughness is created by 'using symbols and practical devices that suggest an impenetrable self' (1988: 81). These can be tattoos that indicate sympathies with dark forces or criminal groups, or other symbols that signal a message of proud outsider status and a rejection of established society. Using a Goffman perspective (1959/1990), symbolic self-presentation relates to what individuals send out to people they encounter, for example, through the way they talk, the tone they use, the words they choose or the ways they move – such as the choice of gait or a bodily display like leaning against the wall while holding a cigarette or a firearm. It is of great importance to be perceived as authentic in one's behaviour and not as someone who is performing a part that does not fit with the image the audience has of the person in question. The relationship between performance and 'reality' determines the audience's perspective of whether or not the actor is judged as being authentic or inauthentic (1959/1990; see also: Katz, 1988; Messerschmidt, 1993).

Katz (1988) argues that a certain sort of violence is done solely to show that the violent actors are 'badasses', that they are capable of using violence without hesitation, such as beating somebody in front of other people in their social networks. Messerschmidt writes about that kind of violence that 'such violence, neither out-of-control nor ungovernable, is situationally determined and regulated' (Messerschmidt, 1993: 123). In Goffman's (1959/1990) words, such violence is an expression of projecting a desirable definition of the situation and of establishing who has the upper hand. It is a form of self-presentation in the illicit economy. However, toughness is also often expressed through silence (Katz, 1988), through making oneself invulnerable to others. In Goffman's (1959/1990) words, individuals 'mystify' themselves by not talking too much or about the wrong things, in order to create an impression of being cool and untouchable.

As explained above, successful self-presentation is a matter of creating an impression of authenticity. However, this authenticity is created not only in present social situations, but also follows from previous situations in which the actor was involved. If a person tries to act tough, it is important that, in reality, he or she has shown to be tough at an earlier stage. In Lalander's study *Respekt* (2009; see also 2008), a completely inexperienced dealer came to a low-income area in the Swedish town of Norrköping. In this area, much of the heroin trade, which was extensive in the town in the late 1990s to early 2000s, was controlled by a group of young men of Latin American background. They used to meet behind the community centre. The inexperienced dealer showed up in a Mercedes as if he wanted to show off his status to the young men. One of the guys, Hugo (see also above), relates how they reacted:

> He came here, to Hageby with his nice car like this and stopped people, Chileans out in the street and said: 'Yeah, do you know anything about ecstasy?' You just: 'What's it to you?' 'Well, I have, like, some to sell', just to brag, just to make himself known or something. You just told him: 'Eeeh, shit, fuck off!' A big guy doesn't do it like that, come to a township and say: 'Yeah, you want ecstasy?' in a Mercedes or something. (Lalander, 2009: 191, author's translation)

It is evident in Hugo's statement that the man was not seen as sufficiently experienced and that he did not have enough street capital to be considered trustworthy. He was seen as a 'freshie' and someone with whom you should not to do business. The inexperienced person was also seen as a safety risk who surely would not be able to show strong character in police interrogations. The only reason they did not beat him up was that he worked closely with 'the man', the big delivery person. Thus, in addition to having the ability to present themselves as strong, tough, cool and authentic, actors worthy of respect also need to be able to account for their history, their accumulation of street capital and their social contacts. If their social contacts are highly respected, they can compensate for a lacking reputation or insufficient street capital.

LEAVING THE GAME

At the age of 25, Hugo wanted to leave his life as a dealer. He had grown tired of constantly worrying about the police and felt a sense of responsibility towards his children. At the beginning of his dealing career, he had found it exciting, like being in a gangster movie where the top guy was like a cinematic Godfather, but that feeling had faded. Now he wanted a steady job and a 'normal' life. He expressed it thus:

> Now I don't live a safe life, I don't feel I do. All the time I have to be worried that the money won't last. I want a job to go to in the morning, my child goes to childcare, my wife goes to school. I go to my job and then return home. Eat supper, have a family life, a proper family life, and not worrying: 'What the hell are we gonna do towards the end of this month, how are we going to pay the bills?' I know that I go to work every day, and I know that I get my money on the twenty-fifth. You see? That's what you strive for. Not like now, now you have nothing to do and just wait for the money from social welfare. It's tough. You see? (Lalander, 2009: 220, author's translation)

He finds himself in a sort of vacuum and a state of ambivalence. If a person has lived for a long time with drugs and drug dealing, it is not easy to just stop and leave that life behind. For Hugo, and others who strive to be drug free, it is crucial to keep away from those friends who are still in the game, those who live for the day, hustle on the stret, and barter hash for pills, stuff or money. Some describe an ambivalence – they like the life of an outsider at the same time as they want to leave such a demanding lifestyle. As discussed above, the style of living has embedded itself in their bodies, in habitus, through the socialization they have undergone. The knowledge they have acquired has no value in established society and the years they have invested in the street culture becomes a gaping hole in their CV that has to be explained to potential employers (cf. Grapendaal et al., 1995; Svensson, 2007). Their acquired street capital cannot be translated into what Bourdieu (1984) calls cultural capital. This type of resource is needed in order to obtain a position in society and is normally manifested through educational transcripts or lists of previous employments.

Ernesto and Primo, also participants in *Respekt* (Lalander 2009), say that they are sometimes completely convinced that they want to quit drugs and dealing, but that it feels like they are 'pulled back', after some days or weeks. They are unable to resist this magnetic force just by way of reason. This force is a consequence both of what they have learned on the street and of the fact that they do not feel accepted by the Joneses. Evidently, this is related to the habitus that they have acquired during their journeys through life, which affects the ways they think about and assess their life chances and options for action. These circumstances are similar to the findings in Maher's (1997) study of drug addicted women involved in the drug economy in three New York neighbourhoods. She argues that their habitus is strongly tied to their marginalized position in society, meant that they found it difficult, for example, to move away from their neighbourhood where they had their livelihood and their networks and where they enjoyed some sort of acceptance and dignity despite their daily crack and heroin use.

The difficulty in leaving the game is also often related to a lack of competence. Bourgois (1995/2003) describes a major dealer called Ray, who also wants to start living a legal lifestyle. Nonetheless, he encounters great practical difficulties in connection with his attempt at establishing himself in legitimate society and he gives up in the face of the bureaucracy and paperwork required to live a legal life. Instead, he goes back to the business to which he is accustomed. Through drug dealing and participating in the local drug economy, he can double or triple the invested cash.

Another financial aspect of trying to leave is that the individuals may be used to having cash in their pockets. Quitting dealing brings considerable loss of income and they are no longer able to enjoy the relative freedom of consumption that was previously available. This loss of income becomes particularly problematic in an extremely consumption-oriented society where products quickly lose their value and must be constantly replaced by new and improved products. Some former dealers experience frustration when they can no longer buy nice Christmas or birthday presents for their children or girlfriend because of poor financial prospects (Adler, 1985; Bourgois, 1995/2003; Lalander, 2008). A drug delivery can bring a rapid and significant improvement to the financial situation. Difficulties in quitting can also be related to having amassed debts within the illicit economy and to the fact that debtors are not interested in whether a person is trying to go legal or not. Thus, in order to pay off the debt, some may start doing business again, with the thought of eventually living a legal life further down the line.

Finally, it is particularly challenging to leave the illicit economy behind for individuals who have developed a strong addiction. One of the greatest risks of being involved is that they start using from their supply of drugs for sale, even if they have told themselves that they are not going to do that. Thus, it is not good for self-discipline and self-esteem, nor for health or finances.

As long as individuals continue to use drugs, there is a strong incentive to maintain those social contacts that previously were needed for participation in the illicit economy. Furthermore, with the gradual process of separation from 'normal' people while learning the game, mentioned earlier, they rarely have many friends left from outside of the drug environment (Skårner, 2001; Neale, 2002). Of major importance to being able to leave the illicit economy is to have or to develop contacts that are involved in the legal economy who can provide access to a legal job (Bourgois, 1995/2003; Skårner, 2001; Neale, 2002; Lalander, 2009).

SOCIAL INEQUALITY AND ILLEGAL STREET ECONOMIES

> Substance abuse in the inner city is merely a symptom – and a vivid symbol – of deeper dynamics of social marginalization and alienation. (Bourgois 1995/2003: 2)

In the previous sections, the illicit street economy has been described primarily from a symbolic interactionist perspective. However, to only use this perspective means that societal structures are rendered invisible and that individuals' positions within the hierarchies of society are not revealed. For that reason, this section and the two following will examine drug dealing as a consequence of social inequality and illegal economies as structured by class, gender and ethnicity/race. Those dimensions can be viewed as intersecting with each other, implying that it is impossible to understand one dimension alone, but rather they need to be understood as interdependent and intertwined. The three dimensions also relate to aspects of power and dominance, on local, national and global levels.

Our opportunities to create stable and harmonious lives are not equally distributed. In his book, *Collateral Damage* (2011), Bauman writes about so-called problem neighbourhoods with high rates of juvenile delinquency, exemplified by drug dealing, vandalism, violence and robbery. Discussing the British city of Bradford, he argues that a one-sided focus on and blaming of youth criminals means ignoring the local, national, and global processes that create the situation. Bauman writes:

> The links to the Bradford phenomenon extend far beyond the confines of the city. The situation of youth in Bradford is a collateral casualty of profit-driven, uncoordinated and uncontrolled globalization. (Bauman 2011: 10)

Forty per cent of teenagers in Bradford live in households where not a single person has steady work. Future prospects for work are not bright for those youth who begin to engage in criminal activities and involve themselves in the illicit economy. A global neoliberal economy with the goal of generating profit has not considered the lives and futures of young people. As Bauman writes, it is hard for those who live under uncertain economic constraints to pull themselves out of poverty in legitimate and socially acceptable ways. Relating to his study of the crack trade in St Louis, Jacobs writes that 'St Louis is developing a population of truly disadvantaged – people with scarce resources and abundant social service needs that cannot be met and are getting worse. Such conditions provide an ideal context for drug use, drug selling, and other serious criminality' (Jacobs, 1999: 8). In the research of both Parker et al. (1998) and Pearson (1987) on the growing influence of heroin in English working-class environments, during the 1980s and 1990s, it is clear that the heroin economies benefit from young people's exposedness. This correlation is strengthened as society is deindustrialized, and a shifting economy creates domestic problems, undermining young people's faith in their future.

Along these lines, exposedness can be magnified when people are indeed trying to manage and lessen the feeling of meaninglessness and lack of hope. The fact that exposedness can increase when people attempt to escape it is also evident in Bourgois' multi-year ethnographic study, *In Search of Respect* (1995/2003). In this work, the local crack market in East Harlem, New York, is seen as an expression of poverty in the world's richest country, the United States, where *the American dream* nurtures the idea of equal opportunities to create a good life for everyone. The life situation for those studied by Bourgois makes participation in the drug market a plausible alternative. At the same time, this leads to an escalation of their problems, in the form of drug addiction, repeated incarcerations, insecure conditions for families and frustration over being unable to get out of problematic life situations by legal means. In Bourgois' study, Primo and Ceasar grow up in a Puerto Rican section of East Harlem. Here people live in poverty and marginalization. Bourgois lived there for five years and got to know the actors on the streets. It is evident that social inequality contributes to the illicit and alternative economy that develops. If Primo and Ceasar had grown up under different and more supportive circumstances, it is likely that they would have chosen different careers, different ways of managing their lives.

In a similar way, in the study *Street Capital* (2006, 2009), Sandberg and Pedersen analyse hash dealing in Oslo, a city that has become one of the richest in Europe as a result of the oil economy. Through extensive fieldwork, the researchers sought to understand how the young dealers see themselves, how they act as dealers and what drives them to become actors in the illicit economy. In most cases, the young dealers were of non-Nordic backgrounds and held a weak social and economic position within Norwegian society. Some were living illegally in Norway and for that reason could not participate in the legitimate labour market. On the other hand, their customers were often of Norwegian background. In Sandberg/Pedersen's (2006, 2009), Bourgois' (1995/2003) and Lalander's (2008) research, it is obvious that illicit means of making a living within a street culture context becomes a solution for managing poverty and challenging life situations, in addition to providing ways of escaping feelings of marginalization and hopelessness. The street people who feel neglected by society can develop knowledge and respect in relation to other actors, earlier referred to as street capital (see Sandberg and Pedersen, 2006, 2009; Lalander, 2008; Fleetwood, 2014).

GENDER IN ILLEGAL STREET ECONOMIES

Possibilities to act and to be seen as a person with credibility and high amounts of street capital in the illegal economy is often strongly gendered. Generally, men have a dominant position in the street economies even if there are exceptions to this dominance (cf. Steffensmeier, 1983; Taylor, 1993; Moore and Hagedorn, 1999; Lalander, 2003; Grundetjern and Sandberg, 2012; Moloney et al., 2015). Acting within the illegal street economy has been a way to stage and perform masculinity, as argued by Messerschmidt (1993) and Katz (1988). In previous research, being tough and cool have often been associated with men who act out certain forms of masculinity and hyper-masculinity in a street setting (Messerschmidt, 1993; Connell, 1995; Frosh et al., 2002), where the actors overcompensate their manliness by presenting a tough front (cf. Dance, 2002).

Women are often seen as victims of various circumstances they are not capable of directing or controlling, as objects (cf. Bourgois, 1995/2003; Maher, 1997) and victims of evil drug dealers and pimps. Maher's ethnographic study *Sexed Work: Gender, Race and Resistance in a Brooklyn Drug Market* (1997) focusing on female crack dealers, criticizes the official image of women as passive victims. It reveals the strategies women use in order to make it on the street and to not be exploited and used in a sexualized economy in which women are seen as inferior to men.

The fact that women are capable of developing strong, independent positions and carving out spaces for agency is confirmed by many studies in, for example, the US (Sterk, 1999; Miller, 2001; Miller and Decker, 2001; Moloney et al., 2015), Australia (Denton and O´Malley, 1999), Norway (Grundetjern and Sandberg, 2012) and Sweden (Lalander, 2003; Richert, 2009). However, these studies also confirm that the illegal street economy is dominated mainly by men, and a gendered logic of thinking, in addition to gendered status hierarchies, make it harder for women to succeed and be seen as competent actors (Moore and Hagedorn, 1999; Moloney et al., 2015). Thus, women often have to work harder than men to succeed in the hierarchy on the street and also to compensate for the fact that they were born women.

The attitude that women are less capable of managing situations and operating in the illegal economy is also present in the Swedish ethnographic study, *Hooked on Heroin* (Lalander 2003), in which some female dealers are interviewed. One of them is Hannah. She handles the heroin sales she and her boyfriend have to carry out every day in order to both make enough money for their personal dose and to save some money for the future. While Hannah heads out on the town to meet people and to deliver 0.2 gram units of heroin to customers, her boyfriend, Steve, is at home sleeping. In their business relations, Steve is the passive one, while Hannah takes care of business and also, to a significant degree, plans her actions by calculating various risks. She has developed a set of useful skills as addressed by Taylor in the book *Women Drug Users* (1993), an ethnographic study conducted in Glasgow. Taylor writes: 'They developed sets of skills which afforded them satisfaction…Shoplifting, fraud, dealing with drugs, all require a variety of skills if they are to be carried out successfully' (1993: 152). In the example above, Hannah does not, however, gain street capital in the same way as her sleeping boyfriend, Steve. According to reputations about their relationship, she has sex with him in order to get drugs while he is the active and resourceful one. Thus, within the network, there are prejudices that ascribe stronger character to men than to women. These prejudices may have the consequence that women see themselves as others do and that they too believe they lack the capacity to be resourceful and commit certain crimes (Steffensmeier and Allan, 1996; Grundetjern and Sandberg, 2012).

Women need to compensate both for being physically weaker and seen as less competent than male actors on the street, with a lower amount of street capital. Grundetjern and Sandberg (2012) analyse how women drug dealers develop strategies in order to prove that they 'belong in the game' despite their gender. These strategies are: desexualization by 'downplaying all signs of femininity to avoid sexual attention' (2012: 627). Violent posture by presenting oneself as even more aggressive and dangerous than men and to be a real 'badass' (Katz 1988) when others are watching. Emotional detachment by hiding the feelings they have for others in order to create emotional distance, and service-mindedness by conducting sales flawlessly so that a relationship of trust is created between seller and customer.

Another strategy for gaining self-respect in a highly gendered street economy is to speak about men as less competent, as some female dealers do in a study by Moloney et al. (2015). The study deals with perceptions of different types of risks in the illegal economy among young gang-involved men and women. Both the men and the women believed that the women did not face the same risks of being arrested or searched as did the men. Many of the women believed that this is a consequence of the fact that men are vain and that they care too much about flashing, looking masculine and presenting themselves as gangsters. One woman says that the men appeared with: 'all kinda big-ass chains, gold teeth, Rolexes, big this and they got no kinda job, nothing' (Moloney et al., 2015). Many of the women describe themselves as more discrete in how they dress and behave. These types of attitudes among women involved in the street economy can probably give them a higher value in their own eyes, in that the male dealers appear a bit stupid in comparison with themselves. It is thus a matter of imaginarily turning the power positions upside down. However, this does not change the overall structural male dominance.

ETHNICITY/RACE AND INTERSECTIONS IN ILLEGAL STREET ECONOMY

> I might be racist, but hell! It's the niggers that are making me this way. They're power tripping (...) Trying to take over the entire show. They didn't used to be like that to me, but once a nigger, always a nigger. That Carter is the fuckin' ringleader. He's the biggest nigger of them all. The big, black nigger. I'm gonna move down with Frank and the whites. I gotta get away from the niggers. (Bourgois and Schonberg, 2009: 41)

Class and gender are two important dimensions on the street: ethnicity/race is the third as the quote above suggests. It is expressed by Felix, a man of Latino American heritage, as a comment about African-American dealers taking over the area. The place is a poor area in San Francisco with high rates of unemployment, crime and social suffering. The everyday life language of the people in Bourgois and Schonberg's study is full of racial and racist expressions. The way the actors on the street reflect about themselves and other people in the surrounding area is, according to Bourgois and Schonberg, a consequence of their life histories that can be traced back to colonialism, racism, and ideas of white supremacy. These phenomena often create unequal opportunities and severe tensions between different groups of people on racial grounds (Hall, 1990, 1996). The quote also relates to segregation, a situation where groups with similar backgrounds move to areas where they can feel that they are with people of their own kind.

Talking about other races as inferior, as difficult to trust and as bad in one way or another, is also a way to subordinate groups and thus create feelings of self-respect and dignity. Using race and ethnicity can, therefore, represent a way for people who are on the margins of society to symbolically and imaginarily create a higher position for themselves. This symbolic subordination can be further reinforced by, for example, refer ring to African-Americans as 'crack monster motherfuckers' (Bourgois and Schonberg, 2009: 41). In addition, the racialization of illegal economies may have the consequence that people cooperate more with actors of the same ethnic origin than with others, as they believe that they can trust these people in the highly risky business in which they are involved (Paoli and Reuter, 2008).

An example of ascribing a certain ethnic heritage to one's self is provided in my own (Lalander, 2008) ethnographic study of young heroin dealers of Chilean descent in a Swedish low-status residential area as also referred to above. Hugo's parents migrated from Chile in the mid-80s, leaving a poor economic situation coupled with limited education opportunities in Chile for a relatively poor and socially vulnerable situation in Sweden. The parents did not have any education that could provide them with steady jobs. The situation was similar to that of most of Hugo's friends whose parents also arrived in Sweden during the mid-80s and who soon began to long for Chile. In order to handle this tough and socially vulnerable situation, the children started to orient themselves towards each other. They also began to create a kind of Chilean ethnicity by using symbols from Chilean street culture, such as tattoos and graffiti. When they talked about other people they would use words such as 'Arab', 'African', 'Swede' etc., indicating that race and ethnicity are important markers in life. This construction of ethnicity was conducted due to experiences of being on the margins of society, in a situation with little hope for the future. The construction was also a response to the identification of themselves and their parents as migrants and to feelings of not being seen as either 'real' Chileans when they went back to Chile on vacations or 'real' Swedes while they were in Sweden. In this situation of suffering, they 'over-communicated' (Barth, 1969; Hylland-Eriksen, 1993) their ethnic origin by symbolising themselves, through talk and other signs and signals, as 'real' Chilean men. Thus, construction of ethnicity can be related to processes of globalization and of 'strengthening of traditional identities' (Hagedorn, 2007: 3; see also Paoli and Reuter, 2008).

The construction of a Chilean identity was clearly a process with intersectional qualities for the young men in the Swedish low-status residential area. Possibilities and limitations based on class, ethnicity and gender intersected with each other in their attempts to create self-respect within a marginal and socially vulnerable position characterized by increased inequality between people and a growing segregation, separating 'Swedes' from people from non-European countries. This moulding of ethnic identity is in line with Hylland-Eriksen's (1993) thoughts that ethnicity does not represent something permanent, but rather something dynamic and under construction, closely related to factors such as class and gender. In relation to this unstable character of ethnicity, researchers (Hall, 1990, 1996; Back, 1996; Alexander, 2000) differentiate between an 'old' and a 'new' perspective on ethnicity. These researchers are using a post-colonial perspective, indicating that colonial inequality between different groups of races prevails.

The old perspective refers to ethnicity as something relatively static, with an essentialist 'cultural' centre, something people are socialized into, quite unproblematically and with distinct boundaries separating one ethnic group from another. The new perspective on ethnicity, conversely, sees it as a socially constructed position (Hall, 1990, 1996) that includes factors such as racism, discrimination and segregation, in which people grow up and carry on with their lives. Thus, ethnicity is created to deal with social positions. The application of ethnic identities is not necessarily related to beliefs about some historical origin. It can also be related to images of popular culture expressed, for instance, through movies and music thematizing life on the street, such as rap and reggae music and the images of tough masculinity which sometimes exist there. Thus, the new perspective on ethnicity involves much more fluidity than the old perspective. For instance, in the study referred to above, young men of Chilean descent pick style elements lifted from Jamaican reggae, American gangster rap and symbols from the streets in their original home town in Chile (Lalander, 2008). Thus, technology creates possibilities for creating hybrid street cultures that are not, as the old ethnicity concept proposes, about one's cultural centre. Thus, the term 'new ethnicity' is tightly linked to social class and the possibilities that late modern society provides through increased mobility and media technology.

The last three sections have dealt with three important dimensions of illegal street economies – class, gender and ethnicity. As stated before, these should be understood together. Understanding how they merge with each other is of critical importance to obtain a comprehensive appreciation of street culture dynamics, the forces that motivate people to enter it and the difficulties involved in leaving it and of the ways these structures operate within the illegal street economy. An overarching condition is that the global neo-liberal economy creates social inequalities (Bauman, 2011). While some groups of people in the world get increasingly wealthy, other groups are marginalized and forced into 'chronic social suffering' (Bourgois, 1995/2003: xxiii). Sassen (2007) argues that the global economy has allowed for the creation of 'marginalised spaces', where illegal economies and networks have become arenas for people who live in severe marginalization (see also Wacquant, 2007).

CONCLUSION

This chapter has shown that the choice to enter into, and become established in, a local drug economy is a gradual social process, in which one 'drifts' (Murphy et al., 1990) into being a dealer. The process occurs in interaction with others. In the same way, individuals' ways of decoding their environment are influenced by the people they encounter, the social and economic contexts in which they live and the surrounding social structures that influence society.

People's experiences in life are internalized in their habitus, the embodied structure they refer to when interpreting various situations and in reflecting on what is desirable and possible for themselves. Several researchers (Maher, 1997; Sandberg and Pedersen, 2006, 2009; Lalander, 2008) have used this concept to analyse how actors begin to think about and experience the world in specific ways when they get involved in illicit economies. To enter into, and become an actor in, such social systems entails an adaptation and learning of those codes that dominate and which, to a great extent, serve to protect the illicit drug economy from the representatives of established society, such as the police and prosecutors. This adaptation includes learning to master the risks involved in the illicit drug economy. The codes are taught in the street environment but also in societal institutions such as juvenile detention and prisons. To act in a way seen as desirable from the perspective of the illicit economies means to be able to act with what Goffman (1967) describes as strong character, and to follow the existing rules. This way of acting improves the dealer's reputation.

With the Bourdieu-inspired concept 'street capital', several researchers (Sandberg and Pedersen, 2006; 2009; Lalander, 2008; Grundetjern and Sandberg, 2009; Fleetwood, 2014) have focused on the fact that local drug economies have their intrinsic system, a symbolic economy for determining what type of actions and experiences are to be seen as valuable and as providing reputation and status, but also as forbidden and worthy of punishment. Partly, street capital relates to the actors' ability to master challenging situations on the street, partly to the reputation they have managed to build by acting in certain situations. Here, the capacity for violence often plays a significant role. In this struggle for status, it is also important for the actors to be able to present themselves as tough, cool and authentic (cf. Goffman, 1959/1990; Katz, 1988). Their status is also dependent on what social capital they can access, in other words what other social connections they can engage in various situations.

People's life conditions, their room to act and motivations to participate in the illegal economy are also grounded in and influenced by structural factors such as class, gender and race and the various ways these influence each other (Bourgois, 1995/2003; Maher, 1997; Jacobs, 1999; Sandberg and Pedersen, 2006; 2009; Lalander, 2008). Local drug economies create opportunities for people who grow up in socially exposed areas to gain respect and make money, to become significant within the illicit economies and to obtain street capital and a sense of self-respect. However, the choice to participate in illicit economies is connected to risks, both internal risks associated with operating in a violent environment with its intrinsic laws and external risks such as long prison sentences. If actors also choose to use the drugs they sell, various potential health risks are added. Thus, even if participating in illegal drug economies may be seen as a way to improve life, at least in the short run, it may have the consequence of further social degradation (Bourgois, 1995/2003; Bourgois and Schonberg, 2009).

As for gender, men are often positioned in a more favourable position than women concerning the possibilities of accessing and gaining street capital. Nevertheless, women may carve out spaces of agency using different forms of everyday life strategies (Grundetjern and Sandberg, 2012; Moloney et al., 2015), thereby compensating for the fact that they are facing various aggravating factors because they are born women. In addition, ethnicity/race is involved in the everyday life of illegal street economies, creating boundaries between different groups of people (Bourgois 1995/2003; Maher, 1997; Bourgois and Schonberg, 2009). Ethnicity/race also intersects with class. Some groups, such as African Americans, Latinos and Asian-Americans in the US (Faupel et al., 2010) or groups of non-European immigrants in the Nordic countries (Dahlstedt and Neergaard, 2013), face more obstacles than others in forming a stable economic and social life. Addressing ethnicity the old way – as something relatively stable – is difficult in contemporary global society. These days, symbols from different forms of popular culture travel worldwide, creating possibilities for hybrid new ethnicities that are merged with aspects of class and gender and comprised of sources from different parts of the world.

In order to understand illegal street economies, it is of major importance not to see them solely as comprising of individual actors and networks that commit crimes and organize themselves on the street. A more comprehensive understanding requires a perspective on how agency on the street is created and limited by structural factors and dimensions such as class, gender and ethnicity/race. Further, understanding the significance of these dimensions, requires an awareness of the restrictions and opportunities provided by overarching economical structures that operate on global, national and local levels.

ACKNOWLEDGEMENTS

I would like to express my gratitude to my colleague, Bengt Svensson, at Malmö University, who has helped me to improve the text by providing valuable comments. I also express my gratitude to Torun Elsrud, also a colleague at Malmö University, who helped in improving the language.

REFERENCES

Adler, P. A. (1985) *Wheeling and Dealing*. New York: Columbia University Press.

Alexander, C. (2000) *The Asian Gang: Ethnicity, Identity, Masculinity*. London: Berg Publishers.

Anderson, E. (1990) *Street Wise: Race, Class and Change in an Urban Community*. Chicago and London: The University of Chicago Press.

Back, L. (1996) *New Ethnicities and Urban Culture: Racism and Multiculture in Young Lives*. London: Routledge.

Barth, F. (1969) *Ethnic Groups and Boundaries: The Social Organisation of Cultural Difference*. London: Routledge.

Bauman, Z. (2011) *Collateral Damage: Social Inequalities in a Global Age*. Malden: Polity Press.

Becker, H. (1953) 'Becoming a marihuana user', *American Journal of Sociology*, 59(3): 235–42.

Blumer, H. (1969) *Symbolic Interactionism*. Englewood Cliffs: Prentice-Hall.

Bourdieu, P. (1984) *Distinction: A Social Critique of the Judgement of Taste*. Cambridge: Harvard University Press.

Bourdieu, P. (1990) *The Logic of Practice*. Stanford: Stanford University Press.

Bourgois, P. (1995/2003) *In Search of Respect: Selling Crack in El Barrio*. Cambridge: Cambridge University Press.

Bourgois, P. and Schonberg, J. (2009) *Righteous Dope Fiends*. Berkeley: University of California Press.

Bretteville-Jensen, A-L. (2002) *Understanding the Demand for Illicit Drugs*. Bergen: Department of Economics.

Brookman, F., Bennett, T., Hochstetler, A. and Copes, H. (2011) 'The "code of the street" and the generation of street violence in the UK', *European Journal of Criminology*, 8(1): 17–31.

Connell, R. W. (1995) *Masculinities*. Berkeley: University of California Press.

Crossley, N. (2001) *The Social Body: Habit, Identity and Desire*. London: Sage.

Dahlstedt, M. and Neergaard, A. (eds) (2013) *Migrationens och etnicitetens epok: Kritiska perspektiv i etnicitets- och migrationsstudier.* Stockholm: Liber.

Dance, L. J. (2002) *Tough Fronts: The Impact of Street Culture on Schooling*. New York and London: Routledge Falmer.

Denton, B. and O'Malley, T. (1999) 'Gender, Trust and Business', *British Journal of Criminology*, 4: 513–30.

Faupel, C., Horowitz, A. M. and Weaver, G. S. (eds) (2010) *The Sociology of American Drug Use*. Oxford: Oxford University Press.

Fleetwood, J. (2014) *Drug Mules: Women in the International Cocaine Trade*. London and New York: Palgrave Macmillan.

Frosh, S., Phoenix, R. and Pattman, R. (2002) *Young Masculinities: Understanding Boys in Contemporary Society*. Basingstoke: Palgrave.

Goffman, E. (1959/1990) *The Presentation of Self in Everyday Life*. London: Penguin.

Goffman, E. (1967) *Interaction Rituals: Essays of Face-to-Face Behaviour*. New York: Anchor Books.

Grapendaal, M., Leuw, E. and Nelen, H. (1995) *A World of Opportunities*. Albany: State University of New York Press.

Grundetjern, H. and Sandberg, S. (2012) 'Dealing with gendered economy: female drug dealers and street economy', *European Journal of Criminology*, 9(6): 621–35.

Hagedorn, J. M. (ed.) (2007) *Gangs in the Global City: Alternatives to Traditional Criminology*. Urbana and Chicago: University of Illinois Press.

Hall, S. (1990) 'Cultural identity and diaspora', In J. Rutherford (ed.), *Identity: Community, Culture, Difference*. London: Lawrence & Wishhart, pp. 222–237.

Hall, S. (1996) 'New ethnicities', In D. Morley and K. H. Chen (eds), *Critical Dialogues in Cultural Studies*. London and New York: Routledge, pp. 441–449.

Hylland-Eriksen, T. (1993) *Ethnicity and Nationalism: Anthropological Perspectives*. London: Pluto Press Limited.
Jacobs, B. (1999) *Dealing Crack: The Social World of Streetcorner Selling*. New York: Northeastern University Press.
Jacobs, B. (2000) *Robbing Drug Dealers. Violence Beyond the Law*. New York: Aldine de Gruyter.
Katz, J. (1988) *Seductions of Crime*. New York: Basic Books.
Lalander, P. (2003) *Hooked on Heroin: Drugs and Drifters in a Globalized World*. Oxford and New York: Berg Publishers.
Lalander, P. (2008) 'The role of ethnicity in a local drug dealer network', *Journal of Scandinavian Studies in Criminology and Crime Prevention*, 9: 65–84.
Lalander, P. (2009) *Respekt: Gatukultur, ny etnicitet och droger*. Malmö: Liber.
Maher, L. (1997) *Sexed Work: Gender, Race and Resistance in a Brooklyn Drug Market*. Oxford: Oxford University Press.
Messerschmidt, J. (1993) *Masculinities and Crime: Critique and Reconceptualization of Theory*. Lanham: Rowman & Littlefield.
Miller, J. (2001) *One of the Guys: Girls, Gangs, and Gender*. New York: Oxford University Press.
Miller, J. and Decker, S. H. (2001) 'Young women and gang violence: gender, street offending, and violent victimization in gangs', *Justice Quarterly*, 18(1): 115–40.
Moloney, M., Hunt, G. and Joe-Laider, K. (2015) 'Drug sales: gender and risk: notions of risk from the perspective of gang-involved youth', *Journal of Substance Use and Misuse*, 50(6): 721–32.
Moore, J. D. and Hagedorn, J. M. (1999) 'What happens to girls in the gang?', In M. Chesney-Lind and J. M. Hagedorn (eds.), *Female Gangs in America*. Chicago: Lake View Press, pp. 177–86.
Murphy, S., Waldorf, D. and Reinarman, C. (1990) 'Drifting into dealing', *Qualitative Sociology*, 13(4): 321–43.
Neale, J. (2002) *Drug Users in Society*. Basingstoke: Palgrave.
Parker, H., Bakx. K. and Newcombe. R. (1988) *Living with Heroin*. Milton Keynes: Routledge.
Parker. H., Bury. C. and Egginton. R. (1998) *New Heroin Outbreaks Amongst Young People in England and Wales*. London: Police Research Group. Home Office.
Paoli, L. and Reuter, P. (2008) 'Drug trafficking and ethnic minorities in western Europe', *European Journal of Criminology*, 5(1): 13–37.
Pearson, G. (1987) *The New Heroin Users*. Oxford: Basil Blackwell.
Pearson, G. and Hobbs, D. (2001). *Middle Market Drug Distribution* (Home Office Research Study 224). London: Home Office.
Preble, W. and Casey, J. J. (1969) 'Taking care of business: the heroin user's life on the street', *International Journal of the Addictions*, 4: 1–24.
Richert, T. (2009) 'Injektionsmissbrukande kvinnors inkomstkällor och anskaffning av droger', *Nordisk Alkohol-och Narkotikatidskrift*, 5: 365–83.
Rosenfeld, R., Jacobs, B.A. and Wright, R. (2003) 'Snitching and the code of the street', *British Journal of Criminology*, 43: 291–309.
Sandberg, S. and Pedersen, W. (2006) *Gatekapital*. Oslo: Universitetsforlaget.
Sandberg, S. and Pedersen, W. (2009) *Street Capital: Black Cannabis Dealers in a White Welfare State*. Bristol: Policy Press.
Sassen, S. (2007) 'The global city: one setting for new types of gang work and political culture?', In J. M. Hagedorn (ed.) *Gangs in the Global City: Alternatives to Traditional Criminology*. Urbana and Chicago: University of Illinois Press, pp. 97–119.
Scheff, T. (1994) *Microsociology*. Chicago: University of Chicago Press.
Skårner, A. (2001) *Skilda världar? En studie av narkotikamissbrukares sociala relationer och sociala nätverk*. Gothenburg: Institutionen för socialt arbete.
Steffensmeier, D. (1983) 'Organization properties and sex-segregation in the underworld', *Social Forces*, 61(5): 1010–32.
Steffensmeier, D. and Allan, E. (1996) 'Gender and crime: toward a gendered theory of female offending', *Annual Review of Sociology*, 22: 459–87.
Sterk, C. (1999) *Fast Lives: Women Who Use Crack Cocaine*. Philadelphia: Temple University Press.
Svensson, B. (2007) *Pundare, Jonkare Och Andra: Med Narkotikan Som Följeslagare*. Stockholm: Carlssons.

Sutherland, E. H. (1947) *Principles of Criminology,* 4th edn. Chicago: J. B. Lippincott.

Taylor, A. (1993) *Women Drug Users*. Oxford: Clarendon Press.

Taylor, M. and Potter, G. R. (2013) 'From "social supply" to "real dealing": drift, friendship, and trust in drug-dealing careers', *Journal of Drug Issues,* 43(4): 392–406.

Topalli, V., Wright, R. and Fornango, R. (2002) 'Drug dealers, robbery and retaliation', *British Journal of Criminology*, 42: 337–51.

Wacquant, L. (2007) 'Three pernicious premises in the study of the American ghetto', In J. M. Hagedorn (ed.), *Gangs in the Global City: Alternatives to Traditional Criminology*. Urbana and Chicago: University of Illinois Press, pp. 34–53.

Waldorf, D. (1993) 'Don't be your own best customer: drug use of San Francisco gang drug sellers', *Crime, Law and Social Change,* 19(1): 1–15.

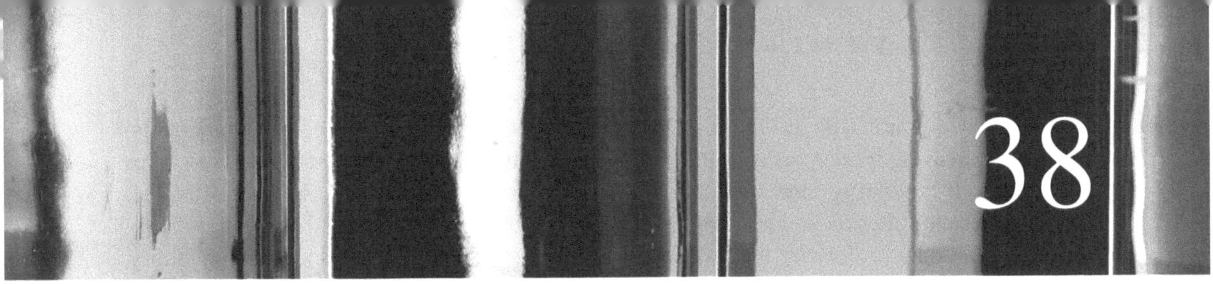

38

Legal Economies: The Role of the Alcohol Industry

Jacek Moskalewicz and Łukasz Wieczorek

INTRODUCTION

The expansion of a neo-liberal economic order at the turn of the twentieth and twenty-first centuries and progressing economic globalisation have been associated with the disappearance of alcohol monopolies, increasing competition and a growing capacity of the alcohol industry and its sophisticated marketing, as well as a diminishing level of state control over the alcohol industry. Legal alcohol industries in search of new profits expand their activities into emerging and developing markets with even lower level of regulations.

The aim of this chapter is to review the crucial impact of the legal alcohol industry on alcohol supply and its consequences for public health and public order in different historical and economic environments, with special focus on the prevailing neo-liberal economic order. We aim to collect and present evidence that regulation of supply and marketing of risky goods, such as alcohol, must not be left to the market, as its regulatory power tends to absorb profits for market forces without any consideration given to economic and social costs that have to be paid by the state and society.

To highlight the role of the alcohol industry, a semi-historical, narrative approach will be used. Lessons from the socio-economic history of alcohol since the industrial revolution will be drawn and then contemporary developments will be discussed focussing on regions mostly affected by a neoliberal economic order, namely countries of central and Eastern Europe and developing countries, against a background of economic globalisation.

HISTORICAL OVERVIEW

Since the early days of the industrial revolution, the alcohol industry tended to maximise its production, minimise cost and increase consumption of its products by means of increasing individual consumption as well as by winning new consumers. Despite acute exploitation and low job security, the new urban proletariat that emerged from industrialisation acquired more or less regular, though low, wages, and therefore, represented substantial purchasing power that could be absorbed by goods whose per unit price was not high and whose provision did not require high investments. Alcoholic beverages, in particular spirits, met these criteria and a history of legal economies may serve as a good example of the destructive potential of legal industries with regard to public health and order. In the following pages, we will give a couple of historical examples as a background to the contemporary story of the alcohol industry's victorious march over public health interests in globalised markets.

The gin craze

The first example reaches back to the beginning of the industrial revolution when gin replaced beers and ales as the drink of choice in England among the urban proletariat. The art of distilling was known already in Europe in medieval ages. Nevertheless, due to imperfect technologies of distilling from grain, its taste was awful and spirits served mainly as medicines. Gin, invented in the Netherlands in the mid seventeenth century, had a much better taste thanks to re-distillation of the malt spirits with juniper berries, giving it a special flavour that appealed to both men and women (Warner 2003). Against a background of enthronisation in Britain of a Dutch prince, *William of Orange*, in 1689, and the war with France that followed, gin found its way to England to generate funds for military campaigns on the continent. Imposition of high taxes on imported spirits stimulated gin production in England. At the turn of the seventeenth century, the British Parliament broke the Distillers Company's monopoly, reduced taxes on spirits and increased taxes on beer by 100 per cent. As a result of that de-regulation, by the 1720s, over 1,000 distilleries operated in London and its vicinity, as well as over 6,000 retail outlets. Gin production increased from 2 million litres in the 1680s to 10 million in the 1720s and 25 million litres in the 1730s. Gin became very cheap indeed. It was estimated that the consumption of gin per adult drinker could be as high as 40 litres annually. Despite the lack of systematic health and crime statistics, there is a lot of anecdotal evidence and media reports that document an acute increase of health and social problems associated with high alcohol consumption whose level appeared to have increased by up to 10 times over about 50 years. Daily newspapers of those times reported a number of deaths due to alcohol poisoning, fire and criminal activities related to alcohol supply or caused by drinking. Eventually, after several decades, attempts were initiated to bring back a degree of regulation to control the unrestricted flow of alcohol. Around the mid eighteenth century, in a series of Parliamentary decisions, high taxes were introduced on distilling and distributing alcohol to control the flow of alcohol in a more effective way and producers were no longer allowed to the retail sale of gin. Moreover, several years of poor harvest increased prices of grain and made its producers less dependent on the demand of the alcohol industry – prices of food went up, while wages diminished. As a result of administrative measures and economic factors, both the demand for, and the supply of, spirits went down and in the late 1750s, the gin craze was over (Warner 2003).

Industrialisation can be blamed for the gin craze not only because it introduced new production technologies that increased the quantity and quality of alcohol supply, but more importantly, because it produced a class of poor consumers, namely the urban proletariat.

The Eastern European vodka epidemic

The industrial revolution moved slowly southward from the United Kingdom to Western Europe and then to its more eastern parts, eventually to Russia, including its Polish partition at the turn of the eighteenth century. Nevertheless, a feudal model of agriculture based on serf labour dominated there throughout the first half of the nineteenth century. Grain – its major export commodity could not compete any longer on international markets. Its surplus production had increasingly been converted to vodka (Bielewicz and Moskalewicz 1986a). Feudal landlords produced alcohol and then forced their serfs to drink in the landlords' inns, paying their wages in alcohol coupons and penalising those who did not obey. Profits from alcohol became a major source of income for large agricultural estates. The production of alcohol increased when potatoes, giving 10 times more starch per hectare, replaced grain as a major raw material. Eventually, a new technological invention called the Pistorius apparatus, which allowed the production of 85 per cent alcohol during single distillation, accelerated the production of spirits even further and brought vodka prices to a very low level. By the 1830s, drunkenness became acutely widespread in Eastern Europe among the rural and urban proletariat affecting men, women and children alike. In some counties, vodka per capita consumption was estimated to be as high as 40 litres annually (Święcicki 1968). Such an extraordinary high alcohol intake had resulted in deteriorating health of generations coming of age. In the 1840s, the governor of the so-called Polish Kingdom reported to the Russian Emperor that the majority of recruits drafted to the army were actually unfit for military service. In response, a decree was issued that imposed a number of restrictions; these included control over the number of distilleries, reducing alcohol content to 46 per cent, imposing high excise taxes, requiring licences for alcohol sales, limiting opening hours and, placing a ban on selling alcohol to drunk individuals (Frieske and Sobiech 1984). Parallel to this, social movements emerged, including so-called sobriety fraternities initiated by the Catholic church, which associated the fight against drunkenness not only with moral revival but also with the fight for national independence as well as with the appearance of working class movements, recognising that the fight against alcohol capital may reinforce the struggle for social emancipation. These concerted actions of the state and the emerging civic society had a long-lasting effect on consumption levels, which dropped from more than 10 litres of 100 per cent alcohol per capita in the 1840s to less than four litres by the end of the nineteenth century (Moskalewicz and Sierosławski 1985).

As in the case of the gin craze a hundred years earlier, the combination of technological innovations and a legal unregulated market led to extremely high consumption levels with all the negative consequences that followed. The introduction of alcohol control reinforced by civic society improved public health and order remarkably.

Sobering up period

Concern about alcohol as a source of social and health problems prevailed over the second half of the nineteenth century and into the beginning of the twentieth century. Numerous lessons from the past were well taken. Most Western countries applied some forms of control over the alcohol economy with a focus on supply reduction measures, including state monopolies which were intended to limit the influence of vested private interests (Room 1985); some countries such as the USA, Canada, Norway, Finland or Russia chose to prohibit alcohol altogether. In addition to having an instrumental purpose, alcohol policies carried strong symbolic meanings. As argued by Joseph

Gusfield (1986), in the USA, prohibition reflected a power struggle, attempts by the traditional American rural middle class to impose its morals on subsequent waves of immigrants often from cultures known for heavy drinking, such as Italians, Irish or Poles (Pennock and Kerr 2005). In fact, prohibition emphasised the moral superiority of old American values and justified the superior political position of those representing them (Gusfield 1986), whereas its repeal implied the moral victory of new urban classes that worshipped the new god of *laissez-faire* economy. Despite a defeat of prohibitive sentiments in the industrialised world, alcohol consumption prior to World War Two was relatively low due to the Great Recession, which drastically lowered the purchasing power of the populations, not only in the USA, but also in other prohibitive countries such as Canada and Finland.

Alcohol and welfare states

After a few years of austerity and poverty following World War Two, the global economy started to grow, in particular, in increasingly affluent Western societies with market economies. However, the countries that adopted a centrally planned model of economic development also enjoyed dynamic economic growth over a few post-war decades. On both sides of the Iron Curtain, economic, as much as socio-cultural developments, encouraged drinking. Incomes tended to grow, the alcohol industry was consolidated, technological innovations increased productivity and reduced costs, a variety of new drinks appeared on the market in addition to traditional alcoholic beverages. In many countries, industrialisation accelerated the flow of young rural people to the cities or to large industrial plants offering them regular wages and the temptations of drink or of entertainment industries strongly associated with the drink industry. Cultural exchange, in particular cinema and to some extent tourism facilitated the transmission of cultural patterns, including drinking patterns (Bielewicz and Moskalewicz 1986b). Temperance sentiments faded away in a new consumerism culture (Pennock and Kerr 2005). Alcohol control measures were thought of as old fashioned, especially against a background of growing popularity of the disease concept of alcoholism. Adoption of the disease concept re-located the focus of control from alcohol to alcoholism, from populations to individuals particularly vulnerable to the disease of alcoholism (Moskalewicz 2001). And again, the disease concept was welcomed on both sides of the Iron Curtain as it diverted attention from structural determinants of social problems related to drinking to individual causes that needed medical treatment. Medicine was to replace social reforms (Wald et al. 1990).

From the 1950s on, the supply of alcohol increased; alcohol became more affordable and available and consumption tended to grow with special impetus in spirit drinking countries where initially there had been low consumption levels, such as the Netherlands, Finland and Poland. Three post-war decades in Poland saw a high rate of annual consumption growth during which consumption increased three- to four-fold between 1950 and 1980 (Sulkunen 1978; Litmanowicz and Moskalewicz 1986). Changes in alcohol consumption reflected progressing cultural homogenisation of the industrialised world (Mäkelä et al. 1981). Parallel to these trends, the homogenisation process affected alcohol control policies as well. Countries with a high level of alcohol control, such as the Nordic countries and Poland, liberalised their control systems facilitating access to alcohol, in particular through its affordability, while countries with very little or no control policies introduced some restrictions (Österberg and Karlsson 2002).

The 1980s saw alcohol consumption levelling off or even declining in Western Europe, as well as in North America, as a result of the combination of administrative measures and the saturation effect, which meant that alcohol consumption was not very likely to increase above certain relatively high levels and the growing position of health in the value systems of affluent societies (WDT 1993).

Alcohol and real socialism: interplay between economic considerations and symbolic meanings

Health arguments happened to be of lesser concern in the countries whose economies were centrally planned. Following a few decades of impressive post-war growth, most of them, in particular the Soviet Union and Poland, suffered from market imbalance and poor productivity. Alcohol emerged as an important economic factor not only because of the budget revenues but also due to its potential to absorb a substantial share of purchasing power, thus reducing the risk of deep economic in-equilibrium. On the other hand, heavy drinking among people in economically productive age groups became seen as an important obstacle to further economic development. This perspective, adopted first in Poland but then in the Soviet Union, had a pragmatic dimension as drinking in the work place could contribute to many problems, including mismanagement, poor productivity, theft, absenteeism and presenteeism, as well as deterioration of the health of the work force. Its symbolic dimension cannot be overlooked as blaming alcohol shifted attention from other, structural sources of economic failure. In the late 1970s, Poland carefully planned its alcohol policy to be built on the Nordic model of comprehensive control that balances public health and economic interests (Wald et al. 1981). The reform was accelerated in the beginning of the 1980s when Solidarity, in its fight for moral superiority, blamed the regime for pushing alcohol in order to increase budget revenues and to manipulate 'drunken society'. To reject this accusation, the state sacrificed direct economic interests for political and symbolic gains (Moskalewicz 1981). The supply of alcohol was cut down almost overnight in the beginning of 1981 'to save grain for bread' and by mid-1981, a rationing system was introduced. In one-year consumption diminished by 25 per cent from eight litres of 100 per cent alcohol per capita to six litres. Health statistics saw an even steeper decline, including a 60 per cent drop in first hospital admissions due to alcoholic psychoses, 30 per cent in hospital admissions due to alcohol disorders and a two-fold decrease in deaths due to liver diseases among men aged 20 to 44 years (Morawski 1983). For almost a decade to come, both consumption and problem statistics showed stabilisation at the relatively low level by international standards (Wald et al. 1990).

A few years later, in 1985, an even more radical alcohol crusade was initiated in the Soviet Union as a benchmark of political reform called *perestroika* that was launched to break a long period of stagnation and to give new impetus for social and economic development. Alcohol reform, which was to destroy deeply rooted traditions and interfere with individual habits, conveyed a message that real change was intended. It could also be read as a symbol of superiority of a new leader – Gorbachev – over drunken society and previous dignitaries who were (in)famous for their heavy drinking. The campaign included the extreme reduction of vodka supplies, uprooting of vine plantations in wine producing republics and shortening hours of operation of alcohol outlets. Over one year, recorded alcohol consumption decreased by half from about 10 litres of 100 per cent alcohol to less than five litres. Initially, the campaign brought significant health benefits having an impact not only on alcohol specific diseases but also on overall mortality figures. Male life expectancy increased by 2 to 3 years, while suicide rates decreased by 50 per cent (Tarschys 1993). Despite these positive outcomes, that top-down campaign, just like *perestroika* itself, did not enjoy popular support (Kollom 2010, 2012). Moonshining slowly replaced recorded licit supply. Sales of alcohol went down while sales of sugar which was the main raw material for moonshine *(samogon)* production rose. Consumption of non-beverage alcohol, such as technical spirits or cosmetics, was on the rise too. Nevertheless, in the beginning of the 1990s, major health indicators still showed positive effects of the anti-alcohol campaign. The situation suddenly reversed as soon as Russia and the countries that emerged after the disintegration of the Soviet Union decided to launch a rapid transition towards a market economy.

GLOBALISATION AND ALCOHOL

Attempts to facilitate international trade in order to prevent global economic crises date back to the late 1940s when a General Agreement on Tariffs and Trade (GATT) was adopted in the course of the so called Bretton Woods negotiations. In general, decisions arrived at Bretton Woods promoted free movement of goods, services, capital and people between countries (Grieshaber-Otto et al. 2000). Even though alcoholic beverages had been treated as an ordinary commodity in all economic treaties that followed (Alavaikko and Österberg 2000; Österberg and Karlsson 2002; Ugland 2002; Babor et al. 2010), until the 1990s, international trade agreements did not directly affect the alcohol policies of individual countries. Although the globalisation process had advanced considerably, nevertheless, the ultimate goal of international agreements was to regulate international economic exchange rather than to make way for unregulated economic relations. This approach was suddenly reversed in the early 1990s, just after the disintegration of the Soviet bloc with its highly regulatory model of economic development. In 1994, a North American Free Trade Agreement was adopted to remove systematically most tariff and non-tariff barriers to trade and investment in Canada, the USA and Mexico. Parallel to this, the European Economic Area emerged, assuring free movement of goods and services not only within the European Union but also within other affluent European countries, namely Iceland, Lichtenstein and Norway. The following year saw the creation of the World Trade Organization (WTO) and the adoption of the General Agreement on Trade and Services (GATS) (Grieshaber-Otto et al. 2000; Ugland 2002; Zeigler 2009). The role of WTO is to supervise and liberalise international trade globally and it is open to all states that meet the criteria of liberal economic order as defined by WTO. As almost 160 countries are members of WTO (all European Union countries), it has a significant impact on national government and national alcohol policy (www.wto.org). WTO also has significant indirect impact on alcohol policy even in countries that did not sign the treaty, as it is important for nonmembers to participate in the global trade system (Hellebø 2003). Countries that want to join the WTO must accept the agreement as a whole and comply with the general obligations including treating products and service suppliers from all WTO countries equally without favouring domestic suppliers. These obligations are convergent with the interests of the alcohol industry, which are 'reduction of the general role of government; restrict governments' ability to regulate; privatize ownership and production of services and goods; reduce public funding generally and, particularly, subsidies to domestic private corporations; and to decentralize administrative and financial procedures' (Zeigler 2009: 14).

The idea of reducing trade barriers (for example, custom duties), import bans and quotas and non-tariff barriers forced by EU and WTO is enthusiastically supported by the alcohol industry, but comes into conflict with strict alcohol policies, placing countries under pressure to abandon their policies and to deregulate the alcohol market (Chenet and McKee 1998; Hellebø 2003; Zeigler 2009). The obligations of WTO members regarding abolishing restrictive regulations, facilitate the entry of alcohol industries into developing markets with relatively low alcohol consumption and an underdeveloped alcohol policy. Those markets lack power and resources in the negotiation stage of economic treaties (Saxena 1997; Casswell and Hill 2006). But the strong pressure exercised by the WTO is also visible in developed economies. Under the pressure of WTO, Japan opened its market in 1996 to spirits such as vodka, gin, rum, brandy, whisky and other beverages and decreased alcohol taxes on imported beverages. Chile and South Korea had similar experiences. Their taxation systems were perceived as discriminatory regarding spirits from other countries and favoured domestic liquor (Zeigler 2009). The process of accession of Finland and Sweden to the European Union and the pressure of the European Free Trade Association (EFTA) in the mid-1990s meant that strict Nordic alcohol policy was broken (Chenet and McKee 1998; Nordlund and Osterberg 2000; Ugland 2002).

GLOBAL ALCOHOL MARKET, GLOBAL ECONOMIC PLAYERS

Production and distribution of alcoholic beverages is closely connected with many other areas of the economy – agriculture, trucking, capital goods manufacturing, packaging industries and the hospitality sector. Alcohol marketing gets involved in advertising, sport and the entertainment industry (including films, television and music) (Jernigan 2009). By the end of the first decade of the twenty-first century, the global alcohol market was worth about $980 billion, of which, the global beer trade was worth almost $500 billion and the spirits market $216 billion (Jernigan 2012) – which represents a 100-fold increase compared to the mid-1970s (Walsh 1997). Jernigan (2009, 2012) observed a growing consolidation across the alcoholic beverage industry. There are only a few global economic players in this globalised sector. In 2005, the 26 largest companies had a total net revenue/turnover from trade of more than $150 billion and a total operating profit of $26 billion. Almost half of sales by volume of globalised brands belonged to the 10 largest alcoholic beverages marketers; these were beer companies responsible for the sale of more than 60 per cent of production of globalised beer. In 2005, total global sales of beer were at the level of 160 billion litres (ICAP 2006a; Jernigan 2009).

Data from alcohol industries shows that the largest beer market is in the Asia-Pacific region, including China (with 62 billion litres of beer sold in 2008), followed by Western Europe and North America (respectively 29 and 28 billion litres of beer sold in 2008) (Ulstein 2009).

North America witnesses progressing concentration of alcohol capital and production. In the USA, the six largest brewers, Anheuser-Busch Inc., MillerCoors, Pabst Brewing Co., D. G. Yuengling and Son Inc., Boston Beer Co. and North American Breweries, control more than 90 per cent of the beer market. In Canada, 90 per cent of beer is produced either by Labatt (which is owned by Anheuser-Busch InBev) or Molson (Giesbrecht 2000). The consolidation of the beer market resulted in Anheuser-Bush InBev, SABMiller and Heineken being present in every region of the world as top producers (Ulstein 2009).

Global marketing of spirits is also consolidated. Since 1991, more than half the volume of spirits sold in the global market is derived from the 10 largest marketers (Jernigan 2009, 2012). A few of the biggest producers are getting even bigger but alongside this trend, there exist about 900 local spirits marketers providing less than a third of the total volume of global production (ICAP 2006a). The fall in demand for legal vodkas in Eastern Europe resulted in slowing down the expansion of the global spirit market.

As regards the wine industry, the level of concentration is lower. Less than 20 per cent of the global wine market is in the hands of the top 10 global economic players. It is worth underlining that the top three global wine marketers are from the USA (Jernigan 2009). Recently, wine sellers are being bought up by players from other alcohol sectors and wine is beginning to catch up in the development of global brand identities and distribution systems. Among the 10 largest producers of wine, at least three are part of global holdings with beer or spirits. The world's largest wine producer, Constellation Brands, also markets beer and spirits (Jernigan 2009).

SOCIAL ASPECT ORGANISATIONS

Parallel to global dynamic developments in the legal alcohol economy, the alcohol industry gave birth to so-called social aspect organisations (SAO), which operate on national and/or international levels. They promote the parent company or the industry itself (Jernigan 2009, 2012) but also attempt to influence alcohol research and alcohol policy. The main SAO in the global arena is the International Centre on Alcohol Policies (ICAP),[1] headquartered in Washington (Room 2006). ICAP was founded in 1995 by global producers[2] and succeeded in involving a former prominent WHO expert as its director. ICAP claims that alcohol policies must focus on patterns of drinking and on teaching responsible drinking; should build public-private partnerships that contribute to the development of alcohol policy; national legislation should be a framework within which self-regulation mechanisms implemented by the alcohol industry could operate; and alcohol, despite its harmful effects, brings a net benefit for society (Jernigan 2009).

ICAP's publications focused on responsible drinking (safe alcohol consumption), cultural aspects (drinking patterns, binge drinking), biological determinants of drinking and some elements of alcohol policy such as warning labels, age limits, alcohol and pregnancy, blood alcohol concentration in drivers, violence and licensed premises, alcohol education and advertisement and alcohol taxes (Bujalski et al. 2007). The ICAP Report 'Alcohol taxation' (2006) is a review of excise taxes on alcohol beverages from the perspective of governments, industry and consumers. The conclusion is that:

> In establishing alcohol policies, governments must weight commercial freedoms and consumers' rights of access to a product against protecting their citizens. This includes determining levels of taxation that do not impose an undue burden on consumers and restrict their choices or penalize producers by restricting fair trade practices. Like any policy measure that addresses the general population, taxation is a blunt tool and does not differentiate between problematic and unproblematic drinking patterns. (ICAP 2006b: 11)

SAOs act in many areas of public life. They finance prevention programmes, are involved in national and international policy trying to influence changes in legislation, become members of organisations and committees, recruit scientists, prepare codes of good practice on alcohol sale and drinking, arrange conferences and produce publications on alcohol issues. In underdeveloped countries and emerging markets, they create other social aspect organisations (Grant and O'Connor 2005; ICAP 2006a; Jernigan 2009, 2012).

In the opinion of the alcohol industry, often echoed by SAO, the globalisation of alcohol sales has many advantages. Alcohol beverages as a product are standardised in all the regions of the world which leads to improving their quality. Globalisation of the alcohol industry also offers an opportunity for the global economy by increasing employment, generating revenues for governments, supporting the hospitality and retail industries as well as the media sector and diffusing technological advantages from more- to less-developed regions. Alcohol marketers also cooperate with other sectors of industry such as transport and distribution networks and plastic, glass or paper packaging. Multinational corporations allow for technology and skills transfers, the introduction of modern business management and production methods (Room and Jernigan 2000; Jernigan 2009). The industry claims that the increased quality of alcoholic beverages represents an advantage for public health, especially in developing countries where many deaths associated with illicitly produced alcohol are recorded. From the perspective of the industry, quality ingredients and technologies ensure product freshness and safety of use (Room and Jernigan 2000).

Employment in the alcohol sector differs from country to country and from beverage to beverage. In France, alcohol related employment amounts to more than 10 per cent of the total work force. ICAP estimated that by 2010, the European Union spirits sector employed about 50,000 people directly in the production of alcohol and about 250,000 were involved indirectly. In the brewery sector, there were 164,000 employees and almost 15 times more (2.6 million) were involved indirectly. In the USA, the beer industry alone employed almost 2 million Americans (ICAP 2006a). Most of these jobs are in the retail sector and services (hotels, restaurants, cafes) and only a quarter are directly involved in production (Lehto 1997). In EU countries, each job in the brewing sector generates one job in retail, two in the supply sectors and almost 12 in the hospitality sector (ICAP 2006a).

Taxes from alcoholic beverages are often an important source of government revenue. In the European Union, average revenue from alcohol taxes generates about 24 billion euros per year, which is about 3 per cent of its total budget. In developing countries, revenues from alcohol beverages are an even more important source for budgets than in developed countries (ICAP 2006a; O'Sullivan et al. 2013).

Provision of all these direct economic benefits constitutes an important asset of the alcohol industry that has significant impact on alcohol policies worldwide. Counter arguments stressing the high cost of alcohol harm are not entirely convincing as revenues from alcohol are immediate and fuel national budgets every day, while loses are long-term and are routinely covered from regular budgets that do not change immediately with the changes in alcohol consumption and harm. Moreover, the increased costs of alcohol treatment or prevention are welcomed by numerous stakeholders having vested interests in the absorption of public funds. Only recently, economic counter arguments have become more sophisticated, noting that employment in alcohol production is very low and a shift of consumer demand to other products and services could generate much higher employment and similar revenues (Anderson and Baumberg 2006).

LEGAL ALCOHOL ECONOMIES IN CENTRAL AND EASTERN EUROPE

Disintegration of the Soviet bloc ended an era of centrally planned economy in Europe. Within a few years, all former members of that bloc, as well as countries that emerged or re-appeared on the ruins of the Soviet Union in the beginning of the 1990s, enthusiastically adopted a path towards a market economy. Building a market economy, however, required substantial capital that was not readily available in economies dominated by state ownership of major economic entities. As large capital flows from abroad were unlikely due to an unstable and changing legal framework and because there was a lack of domestic capital, the first wave of privatisation covered the retail sector; privatising small shops or catering establishments could be done almost overnight without substantial investments (Lehto and Moskalewicz 1994). Alcohol, and in particular, spirits, played an important role in this process as it offered high profit per unit sold and did not demand high storage or staff costs. The profitability of trading in alcohol was largely increased through illegal supplies that were notoriously distributed without any taxes paid. The number of alcohol outlets quickly increased as more and more people wanted to participate in these profits. For example, in Poland, the number of outlets licensed to sell spirits and wines increased three-fold over the course of several years from 30,000 in the late 1980s to about 100,000 in the 1990s (Wald et al. 1990; Moskalewicz and Wieczorek 2009). In Estonia, the number of alcohol shops increased by 80 per cent in only two years, between 1993 and 1995 (WHO 1999; Reitan 2000). Due to a high density of alcohol outlets, which were estimated to be as high as one per 100 to 500 inhabitants, unrecorded sales could not be effectively controlled either by the fiscal apparatus or by law enforcement (Moskalewicz and Simpura 2000). The more so because both the state administration and the police were undergoing internal purges. To increase their profits and to make any controls more difficult, shop owners demanded prolonged opening hours and that all restrictions regarding density be lifted. Alcohol became widely available – round the clock at every street corner (Moskalewicz 1992; Ahven 2000; Waters and Thom 2007). Its price went down due to increased competition at the retail level but also due to the high share of illegal alcohol of which no taxes were paid and all profits were taken over by the private sector (Moskalewicz 1992; Waters and Thom 2007).

As a result of the sudden privatisation that led to increased availability and affordability, alcohol consumption increased remarkably, in particular, in countries affected by Gorbachev's anti-alcohol crusade in the second half of the 1980s, such as the Baltic countries, Belarus, Kazakhstan, Moldova, Russia and Ukraine where consumption doubled from five to six litres of 100 per cent alcohol per capita in the late 1980s to a dozen or so litres in the beginning of the 1990s (Moskalewicz and Simpura 2000; Waters and Thom 2007; Kollom 2010; Nemtsov 2011). The high level of unrestricted alcohol supply had dramatic health consequences and affected general mortality, in particular among males in their productive (and drinking) ages. Male life expectancy decreased in about five years in Lithuania from 68 to 63 and in Ukraine from 67 to 61, while in Russia, it decreased from 65 to 57. Also, Kazakhstan suffered from decreased life expectancy, which dropped by 4 years for men and almost 3 years for women between 1990 and 1997 (Waters and Thom 2007). This unprecedented mortality crisis can be attributed in large part to alcohol consumption, but it was also related to transitional stress (Cornia and Paniccia 2000) affecting mental health and suicide rates (Kollom 2010) and to increased rates of violent crime including homicide. Despite substantial improvement in mortality figures in all countries affected in recent years, male life expectancy is still no higher than 25 years ago and the gap in male life expectancy between Russia and 'old' EU members is about 20 years. In 2006, the life expectancy of Estonian men was still one of the shortest in the European Union (67.4) (Kollom 2010). The gender gap in life expectancy was very large in Central and Eastern European countries, being as high as a dozen or so years, which indicated that men in those countries drink at much higher levels than women.

It seems that legal alcohol producers from the developed countries offered a crucial share of those supplies that not only badly affected the health of societies in transition but also affected their economies by contributing to the grey or black markets and reducing budget revenues. As claimed by Nusupov and Nusupov (1999) the lion's share of what they called 'un-included alcohol' came from licensed companies. Millions of litres of unrecorded spirits were poured every year, seriously affecting public health and order and depriving the state of a significant part of its alcohol revenues. In that period, in the mid-1990s, exports of spirits from Western European countries increased three- to four-fold, substantially contributing to the mortality crisis in Russia and elsewhere.

The absence of any alcohol control measures to counteract the dramatic mortality crisis can also be understood against a background of the failure of the top-down Soviet anti-alcohol campaign that was associated with the previous authoritarian regime. Reinvigoration of active control policies had been delayed as it could be seen as an attempt to awake remnants of communism, the regime whose time was definitely seen as over (Simpura and Moskalewicz 2000; Kollom 2010). Finally, the alcohol question could not have become a central concern compared to the dramatic political and social problems that broke out during transformations towards a market economy (Waters and Thom 2007; Kollom 2010).

LEGAL ALCOHOL ECONOMIES IN DEVELOPING COUNTRIES

In general, consumption of alcohol in developing countries is lower than in developed countries. Nevertheless, unlike developed countries where consumption tends to level off or decline, consumption in developing countries fluctuates with periods of relative economic prosperity or downfalls (Parry 2000; Saxena et al. 2007). Over the long term, a clear upward trend can be observed since the 1960s, as in Thailand, where consumption increased 30 times from 0.26 litre per capita in 1961 to 8.47 litres 40 years later (Thamarangsi 2006), as well as in Brazil, where the annual rate of consumption growth had been 10 per cent leading to doubling consumption in less than 10 years (Pinsky and Laranjeira 2007). In developing countries, per capita consumption figures are less informative than in Europe or North America, as a large proportion of developing societies abstain from alcohol, most prominently, women and adolescents who are not expected to drink under traditional social norms. Abstention rates among men are also much higher compared to the developed world (e.g. Benegal 2005). In a number of developing cultures, traditional, homemade brews represent a substantial share of overall consumption without being recorded by official sale statistics, which means that the disparity between developing and developed countries is not as great as official statistics suggest. Despite the large share of unrecorded consumption, even the recorded consumption alone calculated per drinker has already achieved or surpassed average levels recorded in developed countries. Moreover, some African countries, such as Uganda or Nigeria, have recently become world leaders in alcohol consumption, showing potential for an increase in other developing countries (Obot 2013).

Having been faced with declining trends in Europe and in more affluent parts of the world, the alcohol industry sees developing countries as a crucial area for further expansion (Obot 2013), as they combine a number of factors that make them very promising markets:

- Prospects of economic growth as many developing countries compete successfully on global markets
- Prospects for growing consumption among male drinkers due to urbanisation and attainment of more regular incomes in urban setting
- Prospects for growing consumption among women associated with their attempts at gender emancipation
- Prospects for growing consumption among adolescents who try to avoid traditional social controls
- Replacement of traditional homemade beverages by Western-type beverages provided by the alcohol industry
- Symbolic meaning of Western-type drinks as an expression of Westernisation (Obot 2013)

The alcohol industries do their best to use these opportunities for further growth. They make huge investments in alcohol production, promotion and marketing, including sophisticated advertisement techniques, sponsoring sport and cultural activities, getting involved in charity initiatives but also by influencing alcohol policies directly or indirectly so as to create and sustain an optimal environment for their economic gain (e.g. Benegal 2005).

Also in developing countries, globalisation brought about a high concentration of capital. The alcohol industry actively supports further globalisation and benefits from this process. For example, the Central American Free Trade Agreement was strongly supported by the Distilled Spirits Council of the USA because under the provision of that treaty, Central American countries would immediately remove all duties on USA gin and whiskey (Caetano and Laranjeira 2006). Strong recommendations coming from international agencies such as the WTO or the International Monetary Fund to reduce import restrictions and from local alcohol and entertainment/tourist industries to liberalise developing economies (Assunta 2001; Pyne et al. 2002; Benegal 2005; Thamarangsi 2006), including alcohol control, brought more problems than real benefits (Jernigan 2000).

By the early 1990s, the largest global breweries divided the world into their spheres of influence: Anheuser-Busch conquered North America and some Latin American countries, Carlsberg and Heineken – Asia, while SAB-Miller dominates in Sub-Saharan Africa. As a result, some alcohol producers achieved an almost monopolistic position in local markets as well as incredible economic power that was soon translated into political influence.

The marketing strategies invented for developing countries clearly aim at increasing consumption of current drinkers, in particular, young urban males but also to promote alcohol among women and adolescents. Messages that are spread by alcohol advertising were summarised by Obot (2013). Those contain normative claims such as that drinking is a normal activity as well as building aspirational associations suggesting that drinking and success go together, including success in private, economic and social life. The content of advertising messages and exposure to them, which are regulated in most of the developing countries by codes that are voluntarily adopted by the industry, go far beyond what would be recognised as ethical in the developed world (Assunta 2001; Odejide 2006; de Bruijn 2011). Attempts at the introduction of further restrictions by the state are vigorously resisted by the industry on the basis of freedom of speech (Parry 2010). In those countries where some external restrictions exist, such as in Brazil, India or Thailand, the industry finds ways to evade them (Benegal 2005; Thamarangsi 2006; Pinsky and Laranjeira 2007).

To meet the tastes and aspirations of potential new consumers, new products have been invented and promoted such as wine coolers, alcopops and pre-mixed cocktails. Their taste, generally sweet and fruity, appeals to the tastes of youngsters and women and facilitates transition from non-alcoholic drinks to alcohol-containing beverages (Benegal 2005; Odejide 2006; Thamarangsi 2006). As there is no taste of alcohol, consumers do not control their level of alcohol drinking.

To increase affordability of alcohol, in particular to young people, spirits are sold in small containers, which means that youngsters can enjoy intoxication from their pocket money without investing more in purchasing regular sized bottles or paying a large catering margin just for a drink (Obot 2013).

Apart from modern advertising and products targeting low drinking populations, the industry promotes its products in a more indirect way, sponsoring different events and programmes, which may attract the attention of young people and women, such as fashion shows, beauty contests, sports events, concerts and seasonal carnivals (Obot 2006, 2013). Drinking competitions and free drinks also encourage drinking in excess (Odejide 2005). For example, in Nigeria, Easter parties are organised where alcohol is offered free of charge (Jernigan 2000; Obot 2006). Finally, the industry carries what Parry and Bennetts (1998) call 'below-the-line' advertising, sponsoring cultural events, charity and community level initiatives to improve its image. As early as the beginning of the 1990s, two-thirds of Black South Africans in metropolitan areas believed that liquor companies care for the community by supporting community projects (Parry and Bennetts 1998: 141).

Having achieved enormous economic power in developing countries, as much as globally, the alcohol industry not only interferes with national alcohol policies but also intentionally aims to have a paramount impact on their formulation and implementation (Thamarangsi 2006). In addition to lobbying at the national level, the industry, and namely the International Centre for Alcohol Policy, worked out a national alcohol policy template that is offered to developing countries either directly or from experts whose links with ICAP are blurred. Bakke and Endal (2010) analysed alcohol policy documents sponsored by SABMiller and ICAP in four African countries, namely Lesotho, Malawi, Uganda and Botswana. All four drafts of policy documents were almost identical, disregarding national specificities and strengthening industry vested interests including stressing moderate use of alcohol, which 'has a positive role to play in socialisation and the industry is a major contributor to the economy of Leshoto' (Bakke and Endal 2010: 24). Although negative aspects of drinking are recognised, the document emphasises legitimate 'expectations of adult citizens to purchase and consume alcohol in a well-regulated manner' (Bakke and Endal 2010: 24). The partnership between the industry and the government is also stressed as the industry 'has vested interests in reducing alcohol misuse'. Individually directed interventions and self-regulation in alcohol advertisement are recommended.

Under continuous pressure from the alcohol industry, but also from alcohol exporting developed countries, alcohol control policies do not exist in the majority of developing countries, and if they do exist, they are not properly enforced (Saxena 1997; Pinsky and Laranjeira 2007). Prices of alcohol do not match inflation and tend to decline in relative terms. Density of alcohol outlets seems to be at a high saturation level, for example, South Africa has one liquor outlet per 190 people, taking into consideration formal and informal places (Parry and Bennetts 1998); a similar ratio has been achieved in Brazil (Pinsky and Laranjeira 2007) while in Thailand there is one alcohol dealer per 110 people (Thamarangsi 2006). With some exceptions, such as Islamic countries, exposure to alcohol advertising is overwhelming (de Bruijn 2011). In developing countries, international companies apply marketing strategies and advertising approaches that might not be used in developed countries due to external restrictions and/or self-imposed codes; as formulated by Saxena, it 'would be un-ethical by European standards' (1997: 45).

CONCLUDING REMARKS

Legal alcohol stakeholders are well integrated within the legal economy in developed as well as in developing societies. As with any economic stakeholder, they always look for expansion opportunities disregarding the health and social implications of their activities. However, due to the great potential of harm intrinsic to alcohol – the commodity they provide – it should not be controlled solely by free market forces (Babor et al. 2010). Alcohol is very likely to produce numerous unintended side effects, whose cost, as a rule, overweighs economic benefits. In fact, uncontrolled economic activities by large economic players may lead to what Jahiel called 'corporation induced diseases' (Jahiel 2008: 517–31, quoted in Obot 2013) with catastrophic impact on public health and order. History has recorded a number of such plagues induced by economic interests starting with the eighteenth century gin craze, which affected England at the turn of the seventeenth century, followed by a high tide of alcohol consumption and problems in the first half of the nineteenth century in Eastern Europe and significant consumption growth in the years following the World War II in most developed countries. In all these historical examples, technological or organisational innovations outpaced existing control systems that were helpless to prevent, or even manage, problems related to alcohol consumption.

The most recent high tide of alcohol consumption started as soon as the economic regimes of centrally planned economies disappeared suddenly from Eastern Europe and elsewhere, and when economic freedom and deregulation were prescribed as proper remedies for all economic problems, not only in economies in transition towards a market economy, but also in all other countries, first of all in the developing world. The alcohol industry keenly joined in the wave of economic deregulation achieving substantial economic gains. Decent, law obeying producers from the developed world actively supported semi-legal economic operators who profited from a high level of deregulation adopted in some countries undergoing transition towards a market economy. Under the wings of a new economic order, the alcohol industry invented and implemented new marketing strategies, which included not only traditional advertisement of a product, but also promoting itself as an important economic and social stakeholder boosting the national economy, competing with traditional, unhealthy beverages, supporting modernity, taking care of gender equality, offering new products that appeal to the expectations of young people and building their identity on national sentiments. Out of concern about its image, the industry established what is called 'social aspect organisations', which claim to offer balanced, apparently scientific perspectives in the alcohol debate, including policy advice to developing countries. With growing economic power, the alcohol industry has become an important partner in international and national debates on alcohol policy. Its influence is seen in World Health Organisation which, as noted by Caetano and Laranjeira (2006), in its resolution from the 58th World Assembly, encourages Member States 'to organise open consultations with representatives of industry and agriculture and trade sectors of alcoholic beverages in order to limit the health impact of harmful alcohol consumption'. Current international treaties approach alcohol as an ordinary commodity that has resulted in a significant decline in relative prices and stimulated consumption growth. Domestic economic policies also treat alcohol as an ordinary commodity. As a result, alcohol became widely available, which includes its availability around-the-clock from an abundance of alcohol outlets. This not only increases legal consumption but also opens wide avenues for illegal supply with all its harmful consequences for health and economic order. Economic drawbacks include not only reduced budget revenues but also disastrous effects of the illegal alcohol market on the legal economy, which affects fair competition and corrupts state administration.

All the historical and contemporary evidence clearly documents that market forces alone do not balance overall profits and losses of alcohol supply for society. Without external controls, the industry always tends to maximise consumption, paying no, or very little, attention to the negative consequences its product brings about. Therefore, the state alongside civic society has a legitimate right, as well as evidence-based measures, to intervene to reduce the social and economic costs of alcohol consumption.

ACKNOWLEDGEMENTS

The chapter was prepared within Work Package 2 of the ALICE RAP project funded by the European Commission.

NOTES

1 The name changed in 2014 when the International Center for Alcohol Policies (ICAP) merged with the Global Alcohol Producers Group (GAPG) to form a new organisation, the International Alliance for Responsible Drinking (IARD).

2 Allied Domecq Spirits and Wine (in 2006, split up between Pernod Ricard, Diageo and Beam Global Spirits and Wineon), Bacardi-Martini, Brown-Forman, Coors Brewing Company, Guinness PLC (now part of Diageo), Heineken NV, International Distillers and Vintners (now part of Diageo), Miller Brewing Company (now controlled by SABMiller, which was formed by joining Miller with South African Breweries, with the Philip Morris successor company Altria retaining a 20 per cent share), Joseph E. Seagram and Sons (whose spirits brands were acquired primarily by Pernod Ricard and Diageo in 2000) and South African Breweries (now SABMiller).

REFERENCES

Ahven A. (2000) Social problems in official statistics in Estonia in the 1980s and 1990s. In: H. Leifman and N. Edgren Henrichson (eds), *Statistics on Alcohol, Drugs and Crime in the Baltic Sea Region*. Helsinki: NAD Publications, 37: 17–58.

Alavaikko M. and Österberg E. (2000) The influence of economic interests on alcohol control policy: a case study from Finland. *Addiction*, 95(Suppl. 4): S565–79.

Anderson P. and Baumberg B. (2006) *Alcohol in Europe. A Public Health Perspective. A report for the European Commission*. Saint Ives: Institute of Alcohol Studies.

Assunta M. (2001) Impact of alcohol consumption on Asia. *The Globe*, 4: 4–8.

Babor T.F., Caetano R., Casswell S., Griffith E., Giesbrecht N., Graham K., Grube J., Hill L., Holder H., Homel R., Livingston M., Österberg E., Rehm J., Room R. and Rossow I. (2010) *Alcohol: No Ordinary Commodity: Research and Public Policy*, 2nd edn. Oxford: Oxford University Press

Bakke Ø. and Endal D. (2010) Alcohol policies out of context: drinks industry supplanting government role in alcohol policies in sub-Saharan Africa. *Addiction*, 105: 22–8.

Benegal V. (2005) India: alcohol and public health. *Addiction*, 100: 1051–6.

Bielewicz A. and Moskalewicz J. (1986a) Historia społeczno – kulturowa alkoholu. In: I. Wald (ed.), *Alkohol i związane z nim problemy zdrowotne i społeczne*. Warsaw: Państwowe Wydawnictwo Naukowe.: 11-34.

Bielewicz A. and Moskalewicz J. (1986b) Alkohol a współczesne procesy makrospołeczne. In: I. Wald (ed.), *Alkohol i związane z nim problemy zdrowotne i społeczne*. Warsaw: Państwowe Wydawnictwo Naukowe.: 35-44.

Bujalski M., Dąbrowska K. and Moskalewicz J. (2007) *Alcohol Research and Industry. Potential for Conflict of Interests*. Paper presented at the 33rd Annual Alcohol Epidemiology Symposium of the Kettil Bruun Society, Budapest, Hungary, 4–8 June 2007.

Caetano R. and Laranjeira R. (2006) A 'perfect storm' in developing countries: economic growth and the alcohol industry. *Addiction*, 101(2): 149–52.

Casswell S. and Hill L. (2006) *Economic Treaties and Alcohol in the Western Pacific Region*. Palmerston North: Massey University. Centre for Social Health Outcomes Research and Evaluation; World Health Organization. Regional Office for the Western Pacific.

Chenet L. and McKee M. (1998) Down the road to deregulation. *Alcohol and Alcoholism*, 33(4): 337–40.

Cornia G. and Paniccia R. (eds) (2000) *The Mortality Crisis in Transitional Economies*. Oxford: Oxford University Press.

de Bruijn A. (2011) *Alcohol Marketing Practices in Africa: Findings from the Gambia, Ghana, Nigeria and Uganda*. Brazzaville: World Health Organization. Regional Office for Africa.

Frieske K. and Sobiech R. (1984) *Pijaństwo - Interpretacje Problemu Społecznego*, Warsaw: Instytut Wydawniczy Związków Zawodowych.

Giesbrecht N. (2000) Roles of commercial interests in alcohol policies: recent developments in North America. *Addiction*, 95(Suppl. 4): S581–95.

Grant M. and O'Connor J. (eds) (2005) *Corporate Social Responsibility and Alcohol. The Need and Potential for Partnership*. Abingdon: Routledge.

Grieshaber-Otto J., Sinclair S., Schacter N. (2000) Impacts of international trade, services and investment treaties on alcohol regulation. *Addiction*, 95(Suppl. 4): S491–504.

Gusfield J. R. (1986) *Symbolic Crusade. Status Politics and the American Temperance Movement*. Urban and Chicago: University of Illinois Press.

Hellebø, L. (2003) *Nordic Alcohol Policy and Globalization as a Changing Force*. Bergen: Rokkansenteret, Stein Rokkan senter for flerfaglige samfunnsstudier.

International Center for Alcohol Policies (ICAP) (2006a) *The Structure of the Beverage Alcohol Industry*. ICAP Reports 17. Washington, DC: International Center for Alcohol Policies.

International Center for Alcohol Policies (ICAP) (2006b) *Alcohol Taxation*. ICAP Reports 18. Washington, DC: International Center for Alcohol Policies.

Jahiel R.J. (2008) Corporation induced diseases, upstream epidemiologic surveillance, and urban health. *Journal of Urban Health: Bulletin of the New York Academy of Medicine*, 85(4): 517–31.

Jernigan D. (2000) The alcohol industry in developing countries. *Journal of Substance Use*, 5(1): 14–20.

Jernigan, D. (2009) The global alcohol industry: an overview. *Addiction*, 104: 6–12.

Jernigan D. (2012) Global alcohol producers, science and policy: the case of the International Center for Alcohol Policy. *American Journal of Public Health*, 102: 80–9.

Kollom K. (2010) Estonian non-governmental organisations in alcohol policy planning. *Nordic Studies on Alcohol and Drugs*, 27(2): 165–82.

Kollom K. (2012) How liberal is Estonian alcohol policy? A review of policy development, 1991–2008. *Nordic Studies On Alcohol and Drugs*, 29: 283–302.

Lehto J. (1997) The economics of alcohol. *Addiction*, 92(Suppl. 1): S55–9.

Lehto J. and Moskalewicz J. (1994) Alcohol policy during extensive socioeconomic change. Copenhagen: WHO Regional office for Europe.

Litmanowicz M. and Moskalewicz J. (1986) Wielkość i struktura spożycia alkoholu w różnych krajach. In: I. Wald (ed.), *Alkohol i związane z nim problemy zdrowotne i społeczne*. Warsaw: Państwowe Wydawnictwo Naukowe: 63–78.

Mäkelä K., Room R., Single E., Sulkunen P. and Walsh B. with: Bunce R., Cahannes M., Cameron T., Giesbrecht N., Lint J., Makinen H., Morgan P., Mosher J., Moskalewicz J., Muller R., Osterberg E., Wald I. and Walsh D. (1981) *Alcohol, Society, and the State 1: A Comparative Study of Alcohol Control*. Toronto: Addiction Research Foundation.

Morawski J. (1983) Alcohol related problems in Poland, 1950–1981. In: N. Gisbrecht, M. Cahannes, J. Moskalewicz, E. Österberg and R. Room (eds), *Consequences of drinking. Trends in alcohol problem statistics in seven countries*. Toronto: Addiction Research Foundation:. 1–23.

Moskalewicz J. (1981) Alcohol: commodity and symbol in polish society. In: E. Single, P. Morgan and J. Lint (eds), *Alcohol, Society and the State 2: The Social History of Control Policy in Seven Countries*. Toronto: Addiction Research Foundation: 9–31.

Moskalewicz J. (1992) Privatization of alcohol arena in Poland. In: J. Ferris, R. Dunning, N. Giesbrecht and P. West (eds), *Proceedings of a Symposium Held in Toronto, Canada, October 27–30, 1992*. Toronto: Addiction Research Foundation: 79–91.

Moskalewicz J. (2001) Alcohol policy as a public issue. Reconsidering an old concept and its relevance for mental health. *Epidemiologia e Psychiatria Sociale*, 10(2): 71–6.

Moskalewicz J. and Sierosławski J. (1985) Alkohol i robotnicy. Spojrzenie z perspektywy struktury społecznej. In: P. Wójcik (ed.), *Problemy patologii i przestępczości*. Warsaw: Akademia Nauk Społecznych: 257–343.

Moskalewicz J. and Simpura J. (2000) The supply of alcoholic beverages in transitional conditions: the case of Central and Eastern Europe. *Addiction*, 95(Suppl. 4): S505–22.

Moskalewicz J. and Wieczorek Ł. (2009) Dostępność, konsumpcja alkoholu i konsekwencje picia – trzy dekady doświadczeń. *Alkoholizm i Narkomania*, 22(4): 305–37.

Nemtsov A. (2011) *A Contemporary History of Alcohol in Russia*. Huddinge: Södertörns högskola.

Nordlund S. and Österberg E. (2000) Unrecorded alcohol consumption: its economics

and its effects on alcohol control in the Nordic countries. *Addiction*, 95(Suppl. 4): 551–64.
Nusupov A. and Nusupov A. (1999) 'Bor'ba s ten'yu', *Delovaya nedelya*, 23 July.
O'Sullivan S., Lumibao L., Pustejovsky R., Hill T. and Willhide J. (2013) *State Government Tax Collections. Summary Report: 2012*. Released April 11. Maryland: US Census Bureau. Available from: http://www2.census.gov/govs/statetax/2012stcreport.pdf (Accessed 3 April 2016).
Obot I. (2006) Alcohol use and related problems in Sub-Saharan Africa. *African Journal of Drug and Alcohol Studies*, 5(1): 17–26.
Obot I. (2013) Alcohol marketing in Africa: not an ordinary business. *African Journal of Drug and Alcohol Studies*, 12(1): 63–73.
Odejide O. (2005) *Extreme Drinking Among Young People in Ibadan, Nigeria: A Focus Group Study*. ICAP commissioned study, unpublished report.
Odejide O. (2006) Alcohol policies in Africa. *African Journal of Drug and Alcohol Studies*, 5(1): 27–39.
Österberg E. and Karlsson T. (2002) Alcohol policies at the European Union level. In: E. Österberg and T. Karlsson (ed.), *Alcohol Policies in EU Member States and Norway: A Collection of Country Reports*. Helsinki: STAKES: 43–75.
Parry C. and Bennetts A. (1998) *Alcohol Policy and Public Health in South Africa*. Oxford. Oxford University Press.
Parry C. (2000) Alcohol problems in developing countries: challenges for the new millennium. *Suchtmed*, 2(4): 216–20.
Parry C. (2010) Alcohol policy in South Africa: a review of policy development processes between 1994 and 2009. *Addiction*, 105(8): 1340–5.
Pennock P.E. and Kerr K.A. (2005) In the shadow of prohibition: domestic American alcohol policy since 1933. *Business History*, 47(3): 383–400.
Pinsky L. and Laranjeira R. (2007) Ethics of an unregulated alcohol market. *Addiction*, 102(7): 1038–9.
Pyne H., Claeson M. and Correia M. (2002) *Gender Dimensions of Alcohol Consumption and Alcohol-Related Problems in Latin America and The Caribbean*. Washington, DC: The World Bank.
Reitan T. (2000) Does alcohol matter? Public health in Russia and the Baltic countries before, during, and after. *Contemporary Drug Problems*, 27(3): 511.
Room R. (1985): Alcohol monopoly as an idea and as a reality: some perspectives from history. *Alkoholpolitik: Tidskrift för nordisk alkoholforskning*, 2:,1–6. Available from: http://www.robinroom.net/alcomono.htm (Accessed 3 April 2016).
Room R. (2006) Advancing industry interests in alcohol policy: the double game. *Nordic Studies On Alcohol and Drugs*, 23: 389–92.
Room R. and Jernigan D. (2000) The ambiguous role of alcohol in economic and social development. *Addiction*, 95(Suppl. 4): 523–35.
Saxena S. (1997) Alcohol, Europe and the developing countries. *Addiction*, 92(Suppl. 1): S43–8.
Saxena S., Thornicroft G., Knapp M. and Whiteford H. (2007). Resources for mental health: scarcity, inequity and inefficiency. *Lancet*, 370: 878–89.
Simpura J. and Moskalewicz J. (2000) Alcohol policy in transitional Russia. *Journal of Substance Use*, 5(1): 39–46.
Sulkunen P. (1978) *Developments in the Availability of Alcoholic Beverages in the EEC Countries. Report No. 121, (November)*. Helsinki: Social Research Institute of Alcohol Studies.
Święcicki A. (1968) *Alkohol: Zagadnienia Polityki Społecznej*. Warsaw: Społeczny Komitet Alkoholowy.
Tarschys D. (1993) The success of a failure: Gorbachev's alcohol policy, 1985–88. *Europe-Asia Studies*, 45: 7–25.
Thamarangsi T. (2006) Thailand: alcohol today. *Addiction*, 101: 783–7.
Ugland T. (2002) *Policy Re-Categorization and Integration: Europeanization of Nordic Alcohol Control Policies*. Oslo: ARENA Report No. 3 and SIRUS Report No. 1.
Ulstein A. (2009) *Alcohol Trends – Markets and Innovations. Analyses and Forecasts, Compiled from Business Insights 2008/9 Reports*. Brussels: EUROCARE.
Wald I., Kulisiewicz T., Morawski J. and Bogusławski A. (1981) *Raport O Problemach Polityki W Zakresie Alkoholu*. Warsaw: Instytut Wydawniczy Związków Zawodowych.

Wald I., Morawski J., Moskalewicz J. and Szydłowska T. (1990) II *Raport o polityce wobec alkoholu, Zespół Ekspertów Komisji do Spraw Przeciwdziałania Alkoholizmowi przy Ministrze Zdrowia i Opieki Społecznej*, Warsaw; also published in the series: *Alkohol a Zdrowie*. Dokumenty, raporty, materiały szkoleniowe, nr 2, Biuro Pełnomocnika Ministra Zdrowia i Opieki Społecznej d/s Profilaktyki i Rozwiązywania Problemów Alkoholowych, Warsaw, 1992.

Walsh B. (1997) Trends in alcohol production, trade and consumption. *Addiction*, 92(Suppl. 1): S61–6.

Warner J. (2003) *Craze. Gin and Debauchery in an Age of Reason*. New York: Random House Trade Paperbacks.

Waters E. and Thom B. (2007) Alcohol, policy and politics in Kazakhstan. *Europe Asia Studies*, 59(6): 999–1023.

World Drinking Trends (WDT) (1993) *World Drinking Trends 1993*. Henley-on-Thames: NTC Publications Ltd.

World Health Organization (WHO) (1999) Alcohol and Public Health in 8 Developing Countries. Geneva: WHO.

Zeigler D. (2009) The alcohol industry and trade agreements: a preliminary assessment. *Addiction* 104: 13–26.

39

Natures, Cultures and Bodies of Cannabis

Cameron Duff

INTRODUCTION

It is customary to regard cannabis as a particular kind of object or thing: *a* drug. With its familiar organic materiality, cannabis is treated as a singular substance, routinely manipulated in its preparations for consumption, although maintaining a consistent identity throughout these preparations. Regardless of how it may be consumed, whether smoked in a pipe, rolled into a joint, cooked and eaten, or taken in a tincture, cannabis is understood to describe a stable, knowable entity. Something, indeed, in the ontology of the drug is understood to remain constant throughout its varied iterations. Drawing from the Actor-Network-Theory (ANT) of John Law and Bruno Latour, this chapter departs from 'common-sense' accounts of the ontological character of drugs such as cannabis to explore the myriad relations in which cannabis is enacted. Alert to the ontological contingency of cannabis, the chapter exposes the heterogeneity of the drug, its divergent natures, cultures and materialities. I argue that cannabis should not be regarded as a stable, singular entity, given the diversity of relations, practices, semiotic registers and political squabbles in which the drug is produced as an object of knowledge and practice. It is further the case that efforts to contain the ontological identity of cannabis partially explain the profusion of legal, social, political and medical controversies regarding its use (Room et al., 2010). Presupposing a stable object of analysis, these controversies, in fact, engender different enactments of the drug, including, but not limited to, medical marijuana, recreational pot, synthetic cannabis, a boon to civic finances, personal freedom and a threat to the health of consumers (Hall, 2008; Kilmer, 2014; Lucas, 2008; Pardo, 2014). Within these discourses, cannabis is enacted as a drug, a medicine, a food, a means of restoring municipal finances, a health risk and a signal instance of personal liberty, reflecting some of the ways cannabis may be said to act within the varied contexts of its consumption (see also Duff, 2014: 137–9). Whereas it is common to regard the principal referent in each of these discourses and contexts as the self-same identical substance, this chapter proposes to explore the multiple ontologies characteristic of cannabis.

ANT insists that all objects, whether 'natural' or 'cultural', are produced as 'an effect of stable arrays or networks of relations [which] hold together so long as those relations also hold together and do not change their shape' (Law, 2002: 91). I argue in this chapter that the relations by which cannabis is ostensibly construed as a singular object no longer 'hold together', having splintered and recombined in novel arrays that in each instance produce cannabis anew. Consider, as an example, the differences between cannabis products purchased in an illegal drug market in Melbourne and the products purchased from a legal dispensary in Seattle. Despite a superficial homology, these objects cannot be regarded as identical given the significant legal, social, cultural and political differences that obtain between them. The cannabis consumed in a tincture prescribed by a health care professional is not the same ontological object as the cannabis smoked outside a bar on a Friday night. This chapter examines why it may be useful to maintain a distinction between these objects, how this distinction may help reframe legal, medical and social responses to cannabis and its implications for debates regarding other kinds of drug use. Throughout the chapter, I argue that the 'object materialities' (Law and Singleton, 2005) at work in the production of cannabis distribute this object across the three ontological registers commonly used in the English language to differentiate psychoactive substances: drug, non-drug and medicine (Tupper, 2012: 469). As the discussion below will elaborate, cannabis is no longer (if it ever was) one ontologically discrete object, but several, as it is enacted within discourse and practice as a drug (cannabis), a non-drug ('weed') and as a medicine ('medical marijuana'). Doubtless, the English language struggles to avail a grammar equal to the analytical challenges opened up by ANT, restricted, as one is, to the lexeme cannabis. This chapter responds to these challenges by attempting to pluralize cannabis' referents. Henceforth, I will remind readers of this concern by placing 'cannabis' in scare quotes to indicate the drug's contested ontology. I will return to this issue in the conclusion where I discuss some of the conceptual, analytical and terminological effects of ANT for drug studies.

THE OBJECTS AND FORMS OF 'CANNABIS'

The principal advantage of any attempt to elaborate the ontological fecundity of 'cannabis' lies in the attention this move calls to the diversity of 'cannabis' objects. Health, legal, social and political responses to 'cannabis' insist on maintaining the drug's ontological identity so that, for example, 'cannabis' may be scheduled for the purposes of maintaining and enforcing legal prohibitions, for advancing health promotion and harm reduction messages regarding its consumption, or in order to differentiate 'cannabis' from other kinds of psychoactive substances. Rarely do policy makers, clinicians, researchers or consumers pause to consider the growing diversity of 'cannabis' products (or objects) and the extent to which this diversity troubles existing ontological assumptions regarding the drug's cultural, pharmacological and/or legal identity. Even the emergence of 'synthetic cannabis' (Bright et al., 2013) has done little to shake ontological and epistemological assumptions regarding the drug's identity, with most analyses emphasizing, instead, the pharmacological coherence between synthetic cannabinoid 'analogues' and delta-9-tetrahydrocannabinol (cannabis' 'natural' psychoactive compound). While this coherence has mainly been asserted as a point of law to facilitate the formal prohibition of 'synthetic cannabis' in line with existing legal schedules, the bourgeoning proliferation of 'cannabis' products, both 'natural' and 'synthetic', suggests the value of scrutinizing the object(s) of 'cannabis' more carefully. I would add that such scrutiny is an essential prerequisite for the development of more sophisticated responses to 'cannabis'. Far from treating the drug as one coherent object, the proliferation of 'cannabis' products indicates the need for renewed attention to the manner in which 'cannabis' objects are produced as a function of their own particular agencies (see Gomart, 2002) and by way of their enactments within discourse and practice (Law and Singleton, 2005). The legal and social differentiation of therapeutic from recreational applications of the drug provides just one example of why diverse 'cannabis' objects needs to be articulated so that more refined accounts of 'cannabis' use, its benefits and harms, may be advanced. My argument here proceeds from ANT's account of objects and the means of their 'articulation'.

The first point to make about ANT's approach to the analysis of objects is to observe Law's (2002: 92) insight that if objects may be construed as 'relational contingencies' then it follows that how these contingencies 'stabilize themselves is primarily an empirical matter'. If all objects are produced, maintained, made use of or discarded in material practices, social relations and political discourses, then these same practices, relations and discourses ought to be available for empirical enquiry such that that 'making' and 'unmaking' of objects may be described. Even so, while the role of objects is often highlighted in social science reports of cultural and political affairs, the *agency* of these objects is rarely acknowledged. The result is pervasive exaggeration of the role (human) subjects play in the organization of social affairs, and a corresponding indifference to the work objects perform in 'stabilizing' these states (Latour, 2005: 73–5). By way of correcting this oversight, Law's advice is to focus on the practices and relations in which objects are produced. Importantly, ANT maintains an explicit symmetry between 'cultural' and 'natural' objects by insisting upon the material relationality of each (Latour, 2005). With respect to the former, asserting that 'cultural' objects are produced in an assemblage of relations highlights the socio-technical relationships that underpin the design, production, distribution, adoption, utilization and/or modification of objects such as mobile phones, a tennis racquet, an edited volume of essays or a painting. Various social and material relations are enacted or performed in the production of these 'cultural' objects, yet 'natural' objects, such as organic material, chemical compounds or bacteria, are equally caught up in material and social relations as they are 'objectified' in knowledge and practice (see Latour, 1999: 145–50).

Hence, both 'natural' and 'cultural' objects obtain a use-value in the practices and relations that bodies (mainly human) establish with them. It is for this reason that all versions of ANT emphasize the role of objects in the distribution of action or agency. In a significant move, ANT radically opens the category of the actor to include not only humans but also objects, tools, instruments, plans, logics and so on (Latour, 2005: 64–70). These 'actants' mobilize and extend the array of actions permissible within a network. The greater the array of objects, bodies and signs an actor is associated with, the greater that actor's capacity for action (Latour, 2005: 43–6). If these relations are disrupted or suspended, if relationships break down or actants fail, then an actor's individual capacities will also decline. Object relations may, for these reasons, be described as conduits or mechanisms for the production, distribution and utilization of agency (Latour, 2005: 64–70).

Applying the logic of actor-networks to the study of 'cannabis' suggests, from the very outset, the need to differentiate particular kinds of 'cannabis' objects because such objects are inevitably produced in disparate arrays, just as they generate or sustain disparate agencies (see also Gomart, 2002: 99–105). The 'cannabis' that is grown according to strict organic farming techniques and then sold at a premium in legal retail outlets in Colorado or Washington (see UNODC, 2014), should not be regarded as the same kind of object as the 'cannabis' circulating in illegal drug markets in Australia. It is not just the *context of consumption* that differs in each case. The material relations necessary for the production of each object differ in substantive ways too. Moreover, the 'cannabis' referred to in each case cannot be regarded as 'natural' substances, given the varied actants involved in their production, such as the manipulation of soil, irrigation and lighting conditions; the presence or absence of pesticides and fertilizers; differing modes of formal and informal distribution, marketing and promotion; along with the material technologies active in the consumption of the drug, such as lighters, pipes or vaporizers (see Holland, 2010; Walsh et al., 2013). Unique social and material relations obtain in the case of the legal 'cannabis' consumed in Denver, and the illegal 'cannabis' consumed in Melbourne, such that each object must be regarded as ontologically distinct. Certainly, these substances share some properties, just as similar kinds of social and material relations may be discerned in their production, yet they do not share an identity any more than their effects may be said to remain constant across each context of consumption. One may be tempted to call these substances different drugs, though it will suffice, for now, to describe them as different kinds of objects.

It must be acknowledged, of course, that policy makers, advocates, scholars and clinicians are already in the habit of discriminating between different 'cannabis' objects in distinguishing, for example, therapeutic from recreational contexts of consumption (Holland, 2010). Hence, the 'medical marijuana' prescribed for the elderly cancer patient is normally regarded as a different kind of substance from the 'cannabis' joint passed around among adolescents truanting from school (Walsh et al., 2013). Yet the object-logic proposed in ANT, and briefly introduced above, would suggest that the ontological differentiation of 'cannabis' objects ought to be extended far beyond these therapeutic and recreational contexts. While Law (2002) insists that any such reckoning of the ontological complexity of 'cannabis' should involve empirical verification, I would like to develop Tupper's (2012) insights regarding the polysemic fecundity of the term 'drug' as a way of indicating how this empirical inquiry might proceed. Reflecting on the range of lexical contexts in which the word 'drug' may be said to make sense in English, Tupper (2012: 465–9) identifies three relatively discrete meanings of the term corresponding with the description of drugs as 'medicine', as legal 'non-drugs' and as illegal 'drugs'.

Briefly, the term 'drug' construed as medicine captures the near universal differentiation of pharmaceutical and/or traditional preparations, which are typically indicated for their therapeutic potential from substances consumed primarily for their psychoactive effects. Paracetamol may, for example, be distinguished from cocaine according to this simple binary. Yet Tupper (2012) also notes an important lexical discrepancy between illegal and legal substances such that 'drugs' may be distinguished from 'non-drugs'. The former include substances such as cocaine, ecstasy and heroin that are subject to stringent legal, moral and social prohibitions in most countries, while the latter includes substances such as alcohol, tobacco and caffeine that are legal in most jurisdictions and traded in complex global commodity markets. While strictly speaking, cocaine, ecstasy, heroin, alcohol, tobacco and caffeine are all psychoactive (and thus all 'drugs' at one level of analysis), everyday parlance establishes a distinction between legal and illegal substances that in Tupper's (2012) analysis calls for a distinction between 'drugs' and 'non-drugs'. So endemic is the use of alcohol and caffeine, for example, that these substances are not typically understood as drugs at all, requiring the term 'non-drugs' in Tupper's schema. Bearing this analysis in mind, and reflecting on the variety of networks in which 'cannabis' objects may be said to act, Tupper's medicine/non-drugs/drugs schema offers a means of mapping the ontological divergence of 'cannabis' in contemporary social, legal, medical and political practices. Within the various networks in which 'cannabis' objects are enacted, one may indeed observe the distribution of 'cannabis' across Tupper's three registers. 'Cannabis' is constituted as a *medicine* in debates regarding 'medical marijuana', as a *non-drug* in cultures, practices and discourses redolent of the normalization of 'cannabis' (Parker, 2005), and finally, as a *drug* in statutes maintaining the prohibition of 'cannabis' and the biomedical research that legitimizes this prohibition. I will briefly explore each of these domains before offering some conclusions.

'CANNABIS' OBJECTS (MEDICINES)

The historical record indicates that 'cannabis' has been consumed as a medicine for many thousands of years (Holland, 2010: 17–20), although the drug's therapeutic benefits are explicitly disavowed in contemporary drug laws in most countries (Lee, 2012: 4–5). For example, in the United States, Federal law treats 'cannabis' as a 'Schedule 1' substance, stipulating that the drug has significant potential for misuse with no therapeutic indications (Kilmer, 2014). Existing statutes in the United Kingdom, Canada, Australia and New Zealand contain similar clauses, even in instances where limited trials of the supply of 'cannabis' for medical indications have been initiated (see Room et al., 2010). Despite legal repudiations of the therapeutic benefits of 'cannabis', the resurgence in the last two decades of organized 'medical marijuana' movements in Canada, the United States, Israel, New Zealand, the United Kingdom and in many parts of Europe (Lee, 2012) has done much to transform the object-materialities of 'cannabis'. Principal among these changes has been the rapid proliferation of 'cannabis' products, transforming both the drug itself, along with the ways it may be ingested (Russo, 2013). Notably, a pharmaceutical formulation of tetrahydrocannabinol (THC), with the generic name of dronabinol, has been available under prescription throughout North America and Europe for some time (Holland, 2010). Prescribed to treat a range of conditions, including epilepsy, multiple sclerosis, HIV/AIDS, some cancers, glaucoma and fibromyalgia, dronabinol is available as a tablet or in a liquid preparation and is produced and distributed by global pharmaceutical conglomerates (Vandrey et al., 2013). The drug is subject to stringent regulations with respect to its preparation, marketing, distribution, access and availability, consistent with all legal pharmaceutical medications. Dronabinol has, in these respects, given material form to the therapeutic potential of 'cannabis', reflecting widespread interest in the medical efficacy of THC.

A very different set of object-materialities may be observed in community led efforts to promote the therapeutic benefits of 'cannabis', such as the various 'compassion clubs' or dispensaries that have emerged throughout North America in last two decades (Lucas, 2008; Penn, 2014). These clubs promote 'safe and reliable access' (Penn, 2014: 373) to 'cannabis' products, with many also playing an active role in agitating for the further liberalization of 'cannabis' laws in relation to both medical and recreational uses of the drug. In the United States, dispensaries have opened in each of the states and districts that have passed 'medical marijuana' laws, whereby individuals may legally purchase 'cannabis' products with an appropriate referral from an accredited health care provider. At the time of writing, 23 states have passed legislation enabling access to 'medical marijuana', which consumers may source through licensed dispensaries. Another four states (Colorado, Washington, Alaska and Oregon) have gone further in making the sale, distribution and possession of 'cannabis' legal for both medical and recreational purposes (UNODC, 2014). Licensed dispensaries provide access to a range of 'cannabis' plant materials, based on the known therapeutic and recreational effects of sativa, indica and hybrid strains and consumer demand in relation to these effects. Yet in what is undoubtedly a more significant development given the interests of this chapter, dispensaries in the United States also supply commercially produced therapeutic preparations 'infused' with 'cannabis' 'plant essences'. Examples include massage oils, analgesic ointments and balms, transdermal patches and gels, bath soaks, tinctures and drinks (see www.grassstationco.com for further examples). These products are available with varying concentrations of THC to enable 'exact THC dosing and no resulting cannabis taste' (see http://www.grassstationco.com/#!edibles-in-denver/c141q). Also available are edible 'cannabis' products in a rapidly expanding range. This includes cakes, cookies and bars, which have long been popular among consumers, along with commercially produced confectionary, energy drinks and teas.

All of this suggests that 'cannabis' ought to be regarded as a 'fluid object', to adopt Law's (2002) terminology, an object whose relations have broken apart as they have recombined in the production of novel 'cannabis' objects with differing materialities, effects, identities and cultural meanings. As examples, chocolate bars, candies, salsa sauces, herbal teas and massage oils – each infused with THC in varying dosages and legally available across many parts of the United States – are held together in relational networks that draw together research chemists, entrepreneurs, 'cannabis' activists, bemused journalists, policy makers, municipal authorities, curious consumers and experienced 'cannabis' aficionados (Dowd, 2014). Each such 'cannabis' object has a unique ontology according to the specific spatial, discursive and performative combination of these relations. As a result, the analgesic 'cannabis' cream purchased as a present for a relative must be interrogated in relation to a discrete set of object-materialities that differ in significant ways from the relations constitutive of the 'pot' shared among friends at a party.

The analgesic cream in this example has broken with the networks that constitute the drug 'cannabis'. In its formulation as a medicine, the cream (among any number of analogous therapeutic preparations) dismantles the relations constitutive of 'cannabis' (the *drug*), creating a new 'cannabis' object that has few, if any, of the associations significant of a psychoactive drug. Just as the entrepreneurs who are driving a booming 'cannabis' industry across North America have become the subject of approving profiles in *Forbes* and the *New York Times* (see Vardi, 2014), transforming the status and cultural valence of 'cannabis' in the United States, the growing demand for 'medical marijuana' does away with any simple objectification of the drug 'cannabis'. What the reification of 'cannabis' as medicine means for established scientific tropes regarding the harmfulness of the drug is the subject of renewed controversies (Lee, 2012; Pardo, 2014; Penn, 2014). Mainly, these debates are characterized by an attempt to maintain the same singular object of scientific, social and political analysis. Later in this chapter, I will reflect on how radically expanding the objects of 'cannabis' may transform analysis of the health and social aspects of the drug and its benefits and harms. This analysis is further complicated by studies describing the *normalization* of 'cannabis' (Parker, 2005), which suggest that the drug may be in the process of migrating to the category of 'non-drug' in Tupper's (2012) lexical typology.

'CANNABIS' OBJECTS (NON-DRUGS)

What has come to be known as the 'normalization thesis' was initially proposed by Howard Parker, Judith Aldridge and Fiona Measham on the basis of longitudinal research undertaken during the mid to late 1990s among adolescents and young adults living in the north-west of the United Kingdom (Measham et al., 1994; Parker et al., 1998, 2002). Parker and his colleagues were interested in the nature of young people's transitions from adolescence to adulthood and the place of alcohol and other drug use in these transitions (Parker, 2005). They discovered that this period of 'emerging adulthood' (Arnett, 2005) often involves extended phases of intermittent, recreational drug use, which is regarded by a significant (and growing) number of young people to be an unremarkable, routine and *normal* activity (Aldridge et al., 2011). This process is especially striking in the case of 'cannabis', with studies in the United Kingdom (Parker, 2005), Canada (Duff et al., 2012), Hong Kong (Cheung and Cheung, 2006), Australia (Duff, 2005), Denmark (Frank et al., 2013), Finland (Hakkarainen et al., 2007), the Netherlands (Reinarman and Cohen, 2007), Israel (Harel-Fisch et al., 2012), Sweden and Switzerland (Sznitman, 2007), furnishing strong evidence of the normalization of 'cannabis'. Each of these studies indicates that the normalization of 'cannabis' involves 'reasoned choice' (Parker, 2005: 212), whereby individuals assess a range of factors, including risks to health, getting caught and impairment of school or work performance, in making decisions about the drug. As a result, the normalization of 'cannabis' does not extend to excessive or dependent use of the drug, but rather describes 'recreational' use understood as 'the occasional use [of "cannabis"] in certain settings and in a controlled way' (Parker, 2005: 206). With important implications for the study of 'cannabis' and its characteristic object-materialities, Parker (2005: 205) concludes that normalization proceeds as 'stigmatized individuals become included in many features of everyday life as their identities or behaviour become increasingly accommodated and perhaps eventually valued'.

More broadly, Parker and his colleagues have identified six indicators of drug normalization: increasing access and availability of illicit drugs in the community; increasing prevalence of this drug use; increasingly tolerant attitudes about drug use among both users and non-users; expectations among current abstainers regarding future initiation of illicit drug use; the 'cultural accommodation' of drug cultures in mainstream film, TV and music; and, finally, more liberal policy shifts (Parker, 2005: 206–7). As I have noted, there is now considerable evidence from a range of countries indicating the normalization of 'cannabis' in each of these six domains [see Sznitman et al. (2013) for a review]. The literature points to a number of congruent trends. First, and most significantly, prevalence rates for 'cannabis' use have risen in many countries since the late 1970s, with minor fluctuations from nation to nation that do little to counter the broader trend of increasing consumption (see EMCDDA, 2012; UNODC, 2014). Concurrently, community attitudes towards 'cannabis' use have become more lenient in many countries, with national studies consistently pointing to growing support for the relaxation of existing laws prohibiting personal use of the drug (Angus Reid Strategies, 2010; Holland, 2010; Lee, 2012). 'Cannabis' is also perceived to be readily available in most developed nations with research indicating that availability has either remained the same or become easier over the last 20 years (UNODC, 2014). Meanwhile, representations of 'cannabis' and 'cannabis' use have become more common in popular culture, particularly film, television and music (Gruber et al., 2005; Haines-Saah et al., 2014; Primack et al., 2008). Significantly, these representations are not only more widespread, they are also generally more positive and/or supportive of 'cannabis' use. Finally, there have been tremendous changes in legislative responses to 'cannabis' with nations such as Portugal and Uruguay, along with a number of US jurisdictions, decriminalizing the recreational use of 'cannabis', while many other nations have proceeded with trials of the therapeutic supply of 'cannabis', just as others have maintained formal prohibition (UNODC, 2014).

Taken all together, I would argue that these broad trends indicate significant changes in the object-materialities that constitute 'cannabis' as a particular kind of drug. In keeping with Tupper's (2012) schema, 'cannabis' may be said to be changing its object-relations as it is transformed in diverse contexts from a 'drug' to a 'non-drug', more akin to alcohol than cocaine. The normalization of 'cannabis' documented in Australia, Canada, Israel, the United Kingdom, the United States, Hong Kong, New Zealand and across Europe suggests that 'cannabis' is mutating as an object of knowledge and practice as it settles into the daily lives of ordinary consumers. Studies in each country indicate that many individuals are maintaining 'cannabis' use careers well into middle age, adopting active work and family commitments while integrating 'cannabis' use into their leisure time in much the same way as many other people manage the use of alcohol (Järvinen and Ravn, 2014; Duff et al., 2012). Indeed, it is arguable that 'cannabis' now more closely resembles alcohol in terms of community attitudes and behaviours than drugs such as cocaine and heroin, with which it is still grouped in most nation's extant drug laws (see Room et al., 2010; also Duff and Erickson, 2014; Frank et al., 2013).

Another way of making this argument is to observe that 'cannabis' is breaking free of the networks and relations that constitute the substance as an illegal, stigmatized drug. For much the same reason, Parker and his colleagues stress that drugs such as 'cannabis' should be assessed in terms of lifestyle, leisure and consumption preferences, rather than stigma and deviance. As such, 'cannabis' has become the object of consumption and identity formation in ways that mirror the consumption of other cultural artefacts such as fashion, music, media or technology (Aldridge et al., 2011). What is more, as the drug has become entangled in contrasting object and consumer relations – as it has partially transcended its stigmatized history by way of its 'accommodation' within popular culture – 'cannabis' has ceased to describe a singular, stable object of analysis or practice. The 'weed' that is produced at a party and shared among friends in much the same way as beer or wine shares few of the object-relations that constitute 'cannabis' as a harmful substance, illegal to possess, sell or consume. The 'weed' described in this scenario is not the same object as the 'cannabis' prohibited in statute. The normalization of cannabis, by which the substance has come to resemble 'non-drugs' such as alcohol and tobacco, provides a further indication of the need to dispense with conventional ontological and epistemological assumptions regarding drug 'objects'. And yet, just as 'cannabis' objects have been remade in the form of medicines and 'non-drugs', countervailing trends may be observed as 'cannabis' evolves as an object of biomedical research.

'CANNABIS' OBJECTS (DRUGS)

Despite the normalization of 'cannabis' in various cultural contexts, and renewed interest in the drug's therapeutic benefits, it must be acknowledged, of course, that 'cannabis' is still prohibited almost everywhere, with many jurisdictions continuing to impose heavy criminal sanctions for the possession, distribution and/or consumption of the drug (Room et al., 2010). In other words, for all its ontological proliferations, 'cannabis' remains a prohibited 'drug', even as it is acts elsewhere according to different object-materialities as either a 'medicine' or a 'non-drug' (Tupper, 2012: 372). Much of the rationale for the enduring prohibition of 'cannabis' may be traced to biomedical studies enumerating the harms associated with 'cannabis' use. The health and social costs of consumption have been especially salient topics of inquiry (Thake and Davis, 2011). Consistent with the object-logic presented in ANT, biomedical inquiry may be regarded as another of the major relational networks in which 'cannabis' objects are produced. It differs from the two modes already surveyed to the extent that biomedical research primarily seeks to problematize 'cannabis'. Starting with the epidemiology of 'cannabis' use, biomedical research routinely describes links between regular 'cannabis' use and a range of health and social problems, such as accidents and injuries, road trauma and unemployment, along with mental health problems such as psychosis, cognitive impairment, anxiety and depression (Calabria et al., 2010; Hall and Degenhardt, 2009). While these problems are commonly articulated in relation to vulnerable individuals, other studies identify structural, economic and social processes and their role in the distribution of 'cannabis' related problems (Temple et al., 2011).

A key feature of biomedical analysis of the effects of 'cannabis' use has been the attempt to identify causal relations between consumption and select mental health problems including psychosis, depression, anxiety and cognitive impairment (Hall and Degenhardt, 2009). Over the last 10 to 15 years, a number of important studies have described the effects of 'cannabis' use on various aspects of neurological functioning, with almost all reporting positive correlations between consumption and discrete neurotoxic effects. In particular, a consensus has emerged regarding the link between the persistent use of 'cannabis' and subtle but enduring impairment in memory, attention and the organization and integration of complex information (Hall and Degenhardt, 2009). Much of this research employs sophisticated psychometric tests to assess the effects of 'cannabis' use across a range of indices. Such studies typically report 'subtle cognitive deficits' among participants who regularly consume 'cannabis' (Solowij, 1998: 102–3). The most significant reported deficits include problems with short-term memory retention and higher order cognitive functioning, particularly among long-term users (Lynskey et. al., 2003). Despite enduring controversies regarding the definition and measurement of units of 'cannabis' use, including how to assess the frequency and quantity of consumption and how to distinguish between discrete patterns of long-term use (Asbridge et al., 2014), causal links between 'cannabis' use and significant cognitive impairments are now so well established in the biomedical literature as to be virtually unassailable therein.

A slightly more complicated picture has emerged in research exploring the role of 'cannabis' use in the aetiology of severe and persistent mental illnesses such as schizophrenia, bipolar disorder and depression [see Large et al. (2011) for a review]. Although studies routinely indicate elevated rates of 'cannabis' use among individuals diagnosed with a mental illness (Power et al., 2014), complicating efforts to tease out the causal effects of consumption, there is now strong evidence that 'cannabis' use is a 'component cause' of psychotic disorders such as schizophrenia, insofar as lifetime exposure to the drug accounts for a portion of the global burden of mental illness (Large et al., 2011). Whereas scholars for a long time debated whether 'cannabis' use caused psychotic disorders in otherwise healthy subjects, or was simply correlated with these conditions, research in the last decade has partially confirmed a causal link between consumption of 'cannabis' and the incidence of mental illness (McGrath et al., 2010). Interestingly however, while it is generally accepted among researchers and clinicians that 'cannabis' use accounts for only a 'small amount of the variance' (Power et al., 2014: 1) in the incidence and prevalence of mental illness, such nuances have been lost in popular reporting of the aetiology of 'cannabis' related problems such as depression and psychosis (Ferdinand et al., 2005). Indeed, evidence of a causal link between 'cannabis' use and the incidence of mental illness is commonly cited in efforts to resist the liberalization of drug policies in many countries (Large et al., 2011). Studies describing a high degree of vulnerability among adolescents and young adults to the neuro-cognitive effects of 'cannabis' have been especially salient in this regard (Patton et al., 2002).

In these respects, biomedical analysis of the incidence, prevalence and effects of 'cannabis' use has become a key site of the material and discursive enactment of 'cannabis' objects. Within these research disciplines, in psychology, cognitive neuroscience, addiction studies, psychiatric medicine and related fields, 'cannabis' is constituted as a discrete, uniform substance with measureable, mainly toxic, effects on neurocognitive functioning and development. In its adoption within drug education, prevention and harm reduction initiatives, this research further contributes to the constitution of 'cannabis' as a harmful drug with deleterious effects on health, cognitive functioning, social inclusion, employment, academic achievement and 'positive' development (Catalano et al., 2004). The tangle of material, social and discursive relations wherein 'cannabis' is constituted as a discrete object of knowledge and practice – as a 'drug' in Tupper's (2012) analysis – must be contrasted with the object-materialities reviewed earlier in this chapter whereby 'cannabis' may be said to act either as a 'medicine' or a normalized 'non-drug'. The divergent means by which these contrasting materialities are held together should be understood as the most significant explanation for the proliferation of 'cannabis' objects. Within biomedical research, the object-materialities constitutive of the 'drug' 'cannabis' are held together by networks linking scientists, funding bodies, academic publishers, editors and reviewers and neuroimaging technologies such as positron emission tomography and functional magnetic resonance imaging (Parvaz et al., 2011), as well as the policy communities that take up this research in the design of 'cannabis' education, prevention and treatment initiatives (Copeland et al., 2001).

This network of relations, and the work that is undertaken to stabilize and extend it, contrasts in important ways with the networks constitutive of 'medical marijuana' and 'recreational pot'. These networks occasionally converge, although mainly they function in isolation of one another in the production of discrete, discordant 'cannabis' objects. While researchers, clinicians, consumers and policy makers persist with the illusion of its ontological stability, 'cannabis' continues to break apart and recombine in the organization of novel 'cannabis' objects, each with their own morphology, consumption patterns, effects and identities. I should like to close this chapter by assessing some of the policy and research implications of this divergence.

THE OBJECT-MATERIALITIES OF DRUGS: IMPLICATIONS FOR POLICY AND PRACTICE

Paying closer attention to the social and material networks in which 'cannabis' objects are produced provides unique insights into the legal, social and political controversies that attend the cultivation, distribution and consumption of the drug. Just as 'cannabis' products proliferate in their social and material articulations, so too do controversies regarding these products and their identities, meanings and effects. The problem, as I have characterized it throughout this chapter, is that these controversies rarely attach to the same object, despite efforts to stabilize the referent 'cannabis'. It follows, for example, that debates regarding access to medical marijuana should not automatically be assumed to reference the same object as debates regarding the role of 'cannabis' in the aetiology of mental illness. The object of these debates is ontological distinct in each case, just as the effects these debates typically identify between health and consumption refer to different objects too. Hence, the 'medical marijuana' purchased in Seattle cannot be regarded as the same kind of object as the 'cannabis' obtained illegally in Melbourne, given fundamental differences between the object-materialities constitutive of the 'medicine' in Seattle and the 'drug' in Melbourne. Attempts to reconcile, on the one hand, contrasting perspectives regarding the therapeutic benefits of 'marijuana', and the harms ascribed to 'cannabis' in biomedical research on the other, necessarily falter because these debates refer to different objects. The notion that it is possible to devise a coherent set of health and social policies to regulate the use of 'cannabis' founders for much the same reason.

'Cannabis' has, in these respects, become a 'wicked problem' (Head, 2008) for policy makers, clinicians, scholars and law reform advocates, mainly because 'cannabis' no longer refers to a single, coherent object. While policy makers, jurists and legislators, in particular, struggle to devise responses to the drug capable of accommodating its therapeutic, recreational and deleterious manifestations, the substance itself continues to fragment in diverse object-materialities. 'Cannabis' has become too 'fluid' (Law, 2002) an object to permit the attribution of coherent qualities, materialities, practices or effects necessary for the stabilization of the drug's identity in law, politics, practice or medicine. Of course, international law persists with the attempt to fix the status of 'cannabis' as a harmful illicit drug, while individual nation-states are encouraged to ratify these conventions in their own sovereign arrangements (Pardo, 2014). Contemporary biomedical research evinces similar efforts to articulate a set of stable relations between 'cannabis' use and the onset of discrete harms, deficits or problems (Hall and Degenhardt, 2009). Without ignoring the significance of efforts in either international law or biomedical inquiry to assert the material stability of 'cannabis', the proliferation of 'cannabis' products, the diversity of ways and means of consuming the drug and the ongoing polysemic fragmentation of the drug's cultural identity all betray the folly of persisting with the idea of 'cannabis' as a singular object.

Drawing from Tupper's (2012) analysis, I have argued throughout this chapter that 'cannabis' may now be characterized in relation to at least three distinctive object-materialities, consistent with the notion of 'cannabis' as 'medicine' ('medical marijuana' in all its diverse manifestations); 'cannabis' as 'non-drug' ('weed' as a normalized substance of common prevalence) and 'cannabis' as an illegal 'drug' associated with significant neurocognitive harms. While, notionally, these objects share some common properties, the analysis presented above would suggest that despite these properties, the distinctive object-materialities in which 'cannabis' is variously enacted as a medicine, a non-drug and a drug, hinder (if not prevent) the articulation of coherent social, legal, political and medical responses to 'cannabis'. As a result, public policy, medicine and the law continue to struggle to accommodate a substance that has become so heterogeneous as to permit identifications as both medicine and poison. Working at cross-purposes, the promotion of medical marijuana in scholarly, legal and political discourses inevitably advances the normalization of 'cannabis' by undermining in these same discourses the claim that this substance is too dangerous to use. Attempting to sustain the coherence of 'cannabis' while at the same time admitting of its therapeutic, recreational and injurious qualities has broken the integrity of the 'cannabis' object as it has dissolved into fluidity (Law, 2002).

All of which is to argue for a more sensitive, variegated approach to the analysis of 'cannabis' objects, more alert to the social and material articulations in which 'cannabis' may be said to act in the event of its ontological stabilization (see also Gomart, 2002). If it is true, as I have concluded, that 'cannabis' now describes at least three objects, a medicine, a commodity and a poison, then legal, social, political and medical responses to the drug arguably need to adopt more tailored responses to each of these different entities. The 'reality' as Latour (2005) might have it, is that 'cannabis' acts in certain networks as a medicine, just as it acts in others as a relatively harmless intoxicant enjoyed by millions of individuals worldwide (UNODC, 2014), while in other networks, the drug produces significant psychiatric harms. Instead of attempting to reconcile these divergent realities, to parse available legal, social, medical and political discourses in an effort to uncover the truth of 'cannabis', I would argue instead for a more sophisticated response to 'cannabis' that gives each of these realities their due. Based on the analysis offered in this chapter, one avenue for policy reform may be to promote access to 'medical marijuana' in instances where therapeutic benefits have been demonstrated, while modifying legal arrangements to permit the 'reasonable' and 'controlled' (Parker, 2005: 206) use of 'cannabis' redolent of its normalization, just as policies are devised to combat the heavy, frequent consumption of 'cannabis' that has been most clearly implicated in the onset of health and social problems associated with the drug (Power et al., 2014).

To a greater or lesser extent, the course proposed here mirrors the political compromises observable in responses to the emergence of 'medical marijuana' in countries such as Canada, Denmark and Israel, where attempts have been made to accommodate the drug's therapeutic qualities while maintaining the prohibition of recreational 'cannabis' use (Pardo, 2014; Penn, 2014). My argument is that such responses would be less contradictory and more supportive of public health, individual liberty and civic order were they to give up the illusion of ontological integrity, and instead, address the actual social, material and political circumstances in which 'cannabis' is variously enacted. My feeling is that the push to recognize the legitimacy of 'medical marijuana' has doomed the project of 'cannabis' prohibition because it fundamentally undermines this prohibition's primary rationale: the claim that 'cannabis' use is harmful to health at any volume of consumption (see Mather et al., 2013). Some reconfiguration of existing legal, social and medical responses to 'cannabis' would seem inevitable in this light, the first stirrings of which one might observe in recent developments in the United States, Canada, Australia and across Europe. In each of these countries, moves to promote access to medical marijuana have been accompanied by efforts to repeal the prohibition of recreational 'cannabis' use (see Pardo, 2014).

A better course, in my view, is, first, to acknowledge the heterogeneity of 'cannabis' objects such that policies may be formulated to promote access to medical marijuana in instances where health benefits can be demonstrated; second, to permit controlled, recreational use of the drug in order to protect individual liberty and uphold respect for the rule of law (see Stokes et al., 2000); and finally, to support evidence based interventions to reduce the prevalence of patterns of 'cannabis' use that have been consistently linked to harm (see Hall and Degenhardt, 2009). Such a course is only contradictory and may only be regarded as serving discordant ends, so long as one continues to invest in the illusion of ontological integrity on which all existing health and social policy responses to 'cannabis' rest. The faltering legitimacy, not to mention inconsistent efficacy, of these responses would surely indicate the value of adopting more innovative approaches to the social and legal regulation of 'cannabis' use. The dividend can only be a better fit between the design of public policy and the divergent socio-material realities of 'cannabis' in all its contradictory manifestations.

REFERENCES

Aldridge, J., Measham, F. and Williams, L. (2011). *Illegal Leisure Revisited: Changing Patterns of Alcohol and Drug Use in Adolescents and Young Adults*. London: Routledge.

Angus Reid Strategies (2010). *Majority of Canadians Would Legalize Marijuana, But Not Other Drugs*. Available from: http://angusreidglobal.com/wp-content/uploads/2010/04/2010.04.15_Drugs_CAN.pdf (Accessed 24 July 2014).

Arnett, J. (2005). The developmental context of substance use in emerging adulthood. *The Journal of Drug Issues*, 35: 235–54.

Asbridge, M., Duff, C., Marsh, D. and Erickson, P. (2014). Problems with the identification of 'problematic' cannabis use: examining the issues of frequency, quantity, and drug use environment. *European Addiction Research*, 20(5): 254–67.

Bright, S., Bishop, B., Kane, R., Marsh, A. and Barratt, M. (2013). Kronic hysteria: exploring the intersection between Australian synthetic cannabis legislation, the media, and drug-related harm. *International Journal of Drug Policy*, 24(3): 231–7.

Calabria, B., Degenhardt, L., Hall, W. and Lynskey, M. (2010). Does cannabis use increase the risk of death? Systematic review of epidemiological evidence on adverse effects of cannabis use. *Drug and Alcohol Review*, 29(1): 1–13.

Catalano, R., Berglund, M., Ryan, J., Lonczak, H. and Hawkins, J. (2004). Positive youth development in the United States: research findings on evaluations of positive youth development programs. *Annals of the American Academy of Political and Social Science*, 98: 98–124.

Cheung, N. W. and Cheung, Y. W. (2006). Is Hong Kong experiencing normalization of adolescent drug use? Some reflections on the normalization thesis. *Substance Use and Misuse*, 41(14): 1967–90.

Copeland, J., Swift, W., Roffman, R. and Stephens, R. (2001). A randomized controlled trial of brief cognitive–behavioral interventions for cannabis use disorder. *Journal of Substance Abuse Treatment*, 21(2): 55–64.

Dowd, M. (2014). Don't harsh our mellow, dude. *The New York Times*, 4 June. Available from: http://www.nytimes.com/2014/06/04/opinion/dowd-dont-harsh-our-mellow-dude.html (Accessed 22 July 2014).

Duff, C. (2005). Party drugs and party people: examining the 'normalization' of recreational drug use in Melbourne, Australia. *International Journal of Drug Policy*, 16(3): 161–70.

Duff, C. (2014). *Assemblages of Health: Deleuze's Empiricism and the Ethology of Life*. Rotterdam: Springer.

Duff, C. and Erickson, P. (2014). Cannabis, risk and normalisation: evidence from a study of socially integrated, adult cannabis users in four Canadian provinces. *Health, Risk and Society*, 16(3): 210–26.

Duff, C., Asbridge, M., Brochu, S., Hathaway, A., Marsh, D. and Erickson, P. (2012). A Canadian perspective on cannabis normalization among adults: has all the stigma gone? *Addiction Research and Theory*, 20(4): 271–83.

EMCDDA (2012). *The State of the Drug Problem in Europe*. Annual Report. Lisbon: European Monitoring Centre for Drugs and Drug Addiction.

Ferdinand, R., Sondeijker, F., Van Der Ende, J., Selten, J., Huizink, A. and Verhulst, F. (2005). Cannabis use predicts future psychotic symptoms, and vice versa. *Addiction*, 100(5): 612–18.

Frank, V. A., Christensen, A. S. and Dahl, H. V. (2013). Cannabis use during a life course–integrating cannabis use into everyday life. *Drugs and Alcohol Today*, 13(1): 44–50.

Gomart, E. (2002). Methadone: six effects in search of substance. *Social Studies of Science*, 32(1): 93–135.

Gruber, E., Thau, H., Hill, D., Fisher, D. and Gruber, J. (2005). Alcohol, tobacco and illicit substances in music videos: a content analysis of prevalence and genre. *Journal of Adolescent Health*, 37: 81–3.

Haines-Saah, R., Johnson, J., Repta, R., Ostry, A., Young, M., Shoveller, J., Sawartzky, R., Greaves, L. and Ratner, P. (2014). The privileged normalisation of marijuana use – an analysis of Canadian newspaper reporting, 1997–2007. *Critical Public Health*, 24(1): 47–61.

Hakkarainen, P., Tigerstedt, C. and Tammi, T. (2007). Dual-track drug policy: normalization of the drug problem in Finland. *Drugs: Education, Prevention, and Policy*, 14(6): 543–58.

Hall, W. (2008). The contribution of research to the development of a national cannabis policy in Australia. *Addiction*, 103(5): 712–20.

Hall, W. and Degenhardt, L. (2009) Adverse health effects of non-medical cannabis use. *The Lancet*, 374: 1383–91.

Harel-Fisch, Y., Abdeen, Z., Walsh, S. D., Radwan, Q. and Fogel-Grinvald, H. (2012). Multiple risk behaviors and suicidal ideation and behavior among Israeli and Palestinian adolescents. *Social Science and Medicine*, 75(1): 98–108.

Head, B. (2008). Wicked problems in public policy. *Public Policy*, 3(2): 101–18.

Holland, J. (ed.) (2010). *The Pot Book: A Complete Guide to Cannabis: Its Role in Medicine, Politics, Science, and Culture*. Toronto: Park Street Press.

Järvinen, M. and Ravn, S. (2014). Cannabis careers revisited: applying Howard S. Becker's theory to present-day cannabis use. *Social Science and Medicine*, 100: 133–40.

Kilmer, B. (2014). Policy designs for cannabis legalization: starting with the eight Ps. *The American Journal of Drug and Alcohol Abuse*, 40(4): 259–61.

Large, M., Sharma, S., Compton, M. T., Slade, T. and Nielssen, O. (2011). Cannabis use and earlier onset of psychosis: a systematic meta-analysis. *Archives of General Psychiatry*, 68(6): 555–61.

Latour, B. (1999). *Pandora's Hope: Essays on the Reality of Science Studies*. Harvard: Harvard University Press.

Latour, B. (2005). *Reassembling the Social: An Introduction to Actor Network Theory*. Oxford: Oxford University Press.

Law, J. (2002). Objects and Spaces. *Theory, Culture and Society*, 19(5/6): 91–105.

Law, J. and Singleton, V. (2005). Object lessons. *Organization*, 12(3): 331–55.

Lee, M. (2012). *Smoke Signals: A Social History of Marijuana – Medical, Recreational and Scientific*. New York: Scribner.

Lucas, P. (2008). Regulating compassion: an overview of Canada's federal medical cannabis policy and practice. *Harm Reduction Journal*, 5(5): 1–13.

Lynskey, M., Heath, A., Bucholz, K., Slutske, W., Madden, P., Nelson, E., Satham, D. and Martin, N. (2003). Escalation of drug use in early onset cannabis users vs co-twin controls. *Journal of the American Medical Association*, 289(4): 427–33.

Mather, L., Rauwendaal, E., Moxham-Hall, V. and Wodak, A. (2013). (Re)Introducing medicinal cannabis. *The Medical Journal of Australia*, 199(11): 759–61.

McGrath, J., Welham, J., Scott, J., Varghese, D., Degenhardt, L., Hayatbakhsh, M.R., Alati, R., Williams, G.M., Bor, W. and Najman, J.M. (2010) Association between cannabis use and psychosis-related outcomes using sibling pair analysis in a cohort of young adults. *Archives of General Psychiatry*, 67(5): 440–7.

Measham, F., Newcombe, R. and Parker, H. (1994). The normalization of recreational drug use amongst young people in north-west England. *The British Journal of Sociology*, 45: 287–312.

Pardo, B. (2014). Cannabis policy reforms in the Americas: a comparative analysis of Colorado, Washington, and Uruguay. *International Journal of Drug Policy*, 25(4): 727–35.

Parker, H. (2005). Normalization as a barometer: recreational drug use and the consumption of leisure by younger Britons. *Addiction Research and Theory*, 13(3): 205–15.

Parker, H., Aldridge, J. and Measham, F. (1998). *Illegal Leisure: The Normalization of Adolescent Drug Use*. London: Routledge.

Parker, H., Williams, L. and Aldridge, J. (2002). The normalization of 'sensible' recreational drug use: further evidence from the north west England longitudinal study. *Sociology*, 36(4): 941–64.

Parvaz, M., Alia-Klein, N., Woicik, P., Volkow, N. and Goldstein, R. (2011). Neuroimaging for drug addiction and related behaviors. *Review of Neuroscience*, 22(6): 609–24.

Patton, G., Coffey, C., Carlin, J., Degenhardt, L., Lynskey, M. and Hall, W. (2002). Cannabis use and mental health in young people: cohort study. *British Medical Journal*, 325(7374): 1195–8.

Penn, R. (2014). Establishing expertise: Canadian community-based medical cannabis dispensaries as embodied health movement organisations. *International Journal of Drug Policy*, 25(3): 372–7.

Power, R., Verweij, K., Zuhair, M., Montgomery, G., Henders, A., Heath, A., Madden, P., Medland, S., Wray, N. and Martin, N. (2014). Genetic predisposition to schizophrenia associated with increased use of cannabis. *Molecular Psychiatry*, 19(11): 1201–4.

Primack, B., Dalton, M., Carroll, M., Agarwal, A. and Fine, M. (2008). Content analysis of tobacco, alcohol, and other drugs in popular music. *Archives of Pediatrics and Adolescent Medicine*, 162(2): 169–75.

Reinarman, C. and Cohen, P. (2007). Lineaments of cannabis culture: rules regulating use in Amsterdam and San Francisco. *Contemporary Justice Review*, 10(4): 393–410.

Room, R., Fischer, B., Hall, W., Lenton, S. and Reuter, P. (2010). *Cannabis Policy: Moving Beyond Stalemate*. Oxford: Oxford University Press.

Russo, E. (ed.) (2013). *Cannabis: From Pariah to Prescription*. New York: Routledge.

Solowij. N. (1998). *Cannabis and Cognitive Functioning*. Cambridge: Cambridge University Press.

Stokes, G., Chalk, P. and Gillen, K. (eds) (2000). *Drugs and Democracy: In Search of New Directions*. Melbourne: Melbourne University Press.

Sznitman, S. (2007). An examination of the normalisation of cannabis use among 9th grade school students in Sweden and Switzerland. *Addiction Research and Theory*, 15(6): 601–16.

Sznitman, S. R., Kolobov, T., Bogt, T. T., Kuntsche, E., Walsh, S. D., Boniel-Nissim, M., and Harel-Fisch, Y. (2013). Exploring substance use normalization among adolescents: a multilevel study in 35 countries. *Social Science and Medicine*, 97: 143–51.

Temple, E., Brown, R. and Hine, D. (2011). The 'grass ceiling': limitations in the literature hinder our understanding of cannabis use and its consequences. *Addiction*, 106: 238–44.

Thake, J. and Davis, C. (2011). Assessing problematic cannabis use. *Addiction Research and Theory*, 19(4): 448–58.

Tupper, K. (2012). Psychoactive substances and the English language: 'Drugs', discourses, and public policy. *Contemporary Drug Problems*, 39(3): 461–92.

Vandrey, R., Stitzer, M. L., Mintzer, M. Z., Huestis, M. A., Murray, J. A. and Lee, D. (2013). The dose effects of short-term dronabinol (oral THC) maintenance in daily cannabis users. *Drug and Alcohol Dependence*, 128(1): 64–70.

Vardi, N. (2014) Inside the pot stock bubble. *Forbes*, 26 March. Available from: http://www.forbes.com/sites/nathanvardi/2014/03/26/high-times-inside-the-pot-stock-bubble/ (Accessed 22 July 2014).

Walsh, Z., Callaway, R., Belle-Isle, L., Capler, R., Kay, R., Lucas, P. and Holtzman, S. (2013). Cannabis for therapeutic purposes: patient characteristics, access, and reasons for use. *International Journal of Drug Policy*, 24(6): 511–16.

United Nations Office on Drugs and Crime (UNODC) (2014). *World Drug Report 2014*. New York: United Nations Publication, Sales No. E.14.XI.7.

Index

Page numbers in **bold** indicate tables or boxes and in *italic* indicate figures. End of chapter notes are denoted by a letter n between page number and note number.

FSC
www.fsc.org
MIX
Papier | Fördert gute Waldnutzung
FSC® C083411

Kolibri 360 GmbH
Ferdinand-Jühlke-Straße 7
99095 Erfurt, Deutschland
produktsicherheit@kolibri360.de